Surgical Technology for the Surgical Technologist

A Positive Care Approach

2nd Edition

Surgical Technology for the Surgical Technologist

A Positive Care Approach

2nd Edition

Association of Surgical Technologists, Inc.

Executive Editor
Paul Price, CST, MBA
Executive Director, Accreditation Review Committee on Education in Surgical Technology
Director of Education, Association of Surgical Technologists

Senior Editors
Kevin Frey, CST, MA
Manager, AST Education Department

Teri L. Junge, CST/CFA
Surgical Technology Program Director
San Joaquin Valley College, Fresno, California

THOMSON
DELMAR LEARNING™

Australia Canada Mexico Singapore Spain United Kingdom United States

THOMSON
DELMAR LEARNING

Surgical Technology for the Surgical Technologist, Second Edition

Association of Surgical Technologists, Inc.

Vice President, Health Care Business Unit:
William Brottmiller

Editorial Director:
Cathy L. Esperti

Acquisitions Editor:
Rhonda Dearborn

Developmental Editor:
Marjorie A. Bruce

Marketing Director:
Jennifer McAvey

Channel Manager:
Tamara Caruso

Editorial Assistant:
Debra Gorgos

Marketing Coordinator:
Chris Manion

Production Director:
Karen Leet

Project Editor:
Jennifer Luck

Art/Design Coordinator:
Connie Lundberg-Watkins

Production Coordinator:
Bridget Lulay

Cover photos courtesy of Intuitive Surgical, Inc., Santa Barbara, California

Printed in China
6 7 8 XXX 09 08 07

For more information, contact Delmar Learning, 5 Maxwell Drive, Clifton Park, NY 12065 or find us on the World Wide Web at http://www.delmarlearning.com

Library of Congress Cataloging-in-Publication Data
Surgical technology for the surgical technologist : a positive care approach / Association of Surgical Technologists, Inc. ; executive editor, Paul Price ; senior editors, Kevin Frey, Teri L. Junge.-- 2nd ed.
p. ; cm.
Includes bibliographical references and index.
ISBN-13: 978-1-4018-3848-5
ISBN-10: 1-4018-3848-0
1. Surgical technology. 2. Operating room technicians.
[DNLM: 1. Surgical Procedures, Operative. 2. Operating Room Technicians. WO 500 S96187 2004] I. Price, Paul, CST/CFA. II. Frey, Kevin B. III. Junge, Teri L. IV. Association of Surgical Technologists. RD32.3.S866 2004
617'.917--dc22

2003023512

DEDICATION

This book is dedicated to the late Dr. Bob Caruthers, whose vision brought forth this project and whose dedication saw it through.

Brief Table of Contents

Contents

CHAPTER 15

CHAPTER 16

CHAPTER 17

CHAPTER 23
Peripheral Vascular Surgery 927

CHAPTER 24
Neurosurgery 965

List of Tables

Introduction to the Second Edition

An all new, full-color design improves text readability and accessibility to the various chapter elements. The learner benefits from the ease with which content can be viewed in the tables and procedures. A consistent color palette applied to the anatomical drawings and surgical procedure drawings makes it easier to identify anatomical landmarks and to distinguish tissues. It is also easier to view the correct placement of instruments for specific procedures.

For this edition, chapters from the previous edition were expanded and improved according to feedback from instructors, and certain procedures were added. Certain chapter portions were rearranged and moved for better flow of information. Figures were updated for relevancy, and black-and-white figures were replaced with full-color figures for more detail, depth, and clarity.

This edition of the textbook is divided into three primary sections:

- Introduction to Surgical Technology
- Principles and Practice of Surgical Technology
- Surgical Procedures

For the third section of the textbook, it is important enough to repeat that, due to limited space, we feel that the best way to present surgical procedures is not to present every procedure listed in the core curriculum in an abbreviated fashion, but to instead present fewer but illustrative procedures with more detailed information. By illustrative, we mean that if students can perform the necessary steps for one procedure that is outlined in this textbook, it is assumed that they would be able to do another procedure that required the same basic steps; therefore, only the first procedure is outlined. Future Delmar publications will address other procedures not included in this edition.

New chapters were added for compliance with the *Core Curriculum for Surgical Technologists,* 5th edition, and include:

Chapter 2 Standards of Conduct, with the following elements:

- Ethical and Moral Issues
- Legal Issues
- Risk Management and Liability

Chapter 4 Special Populations, with the following elements:

- Pediatric Patient
- Geriatric Patient

- Immunocompromised Patient
- Pregnant Patient
- Diabetic Patient
- Disabled Patient
- Obese Patient
- Trauma Patient

Chapter 6 Biomedical Science, with the following elements:

- Computer Skills
- Electricity
- Physics
- Robotics

These new chapters further reflect the new content of the core curriculum and further enhance the educational experience of the surgical technology student in preparation for entry-level practice.

Additional changes for the second edition include the following:

- A Select Key Terms list was added to each chapter; terms appear in boldface within the chapter and are defined in the glossary.
- The Questions for Further Study at the end of each chapter have been expanded.
- Techniques were added in various chapters to aid in learning basic skills applicable to surgical procedures.
- For basic patient positions for surgery, a table was added for each position to highlight the potential hazards of the position and precautionary actions.

Many new topics were also added, including:

- Minimally invasive surgery
- Bispectral Index™ monitor
- Surgical instrument care and handling
- Suction systems
- Electrical shock and burn
- Hazards of vaporized tissue plume
- Sequential compression devices
- Surgical case management: preoperative, intraoperative, postoperative
- Glaucoma
- Ophthalmic medications
- Iridectomy
- Intraocular lenses
- Dermabrasion
- Scar revision
- Hydrocelectomy
- Varicocelectomy
- Hypospadias repair
- ACL repair
- Above-the-knee amputation
- Triple arthrodesis
- Achilles tendon repair
- Shoulder joint arthroscopy
- Repair of hip fracture
- Total knee arthroplasty
- Advances in neurosurgery

SUPPLEMENTS

LEARNING SUPPLEMENT

The *Study Guide to Accompany Surgical Technology for the Surgical Technologist,* 2nd edition, offers a variety of exercises to reinforce learning of vocabulary, anatomy, pathology, and surgical procedures. In addition, the exercises further aid in developing critical thinking skills.

Each chapter of the *Study Guide* includes objectives to focus the student's study, a list of Select Key Terms to be defined to build vocabulary, and two clinical Case Studies with questions to continue the development of critical thinking skills that began with the main text. Selected chapters in Chapters 1 through 12 contain Skill Assessment sheets that are used to evaluate the learner in the completion of basic skills. Beginning with Chapter 9, exercises are introduced. In the surgical procedure chapters (Chapters 13 through 24), the exercises cover anatomy, pathology, operative procedures, and specific variations. For this exercise, the instructor provides basic patient information that the learner will use to complete a case study report. A template for the report is provided in each chapter. This exercise continues the process by which the surgical technologist is learning to predict the surgeon's and patient's needs during the procedure.

TEACHING SUPPLEMENTS

INSTRUCTOR'S MANUAL

The *Instructor's Manual to Accompany Surgical Technology for the Surgical Technologist,* 2nd edition, contains a number of aids to simplify the instructor's course management tasks and evaluation of learner progress. The manual includes a correlation chart that relates the text content to the requirements of the *Core Curriculum for Surgical Technology,* 5th edition. Also provided is a list of Skill Assessments and their location in the *Study Guide*. This is followed by a complete set of Skill Assessment sheets that can be copied as needed. Minimum requirements for the completion of the Student Case Study Report in the *Study Guide* are provided, as well as a master of the report form. Each chapter of the manual includes the text objectives and suggestions for the following learning activities: reports, classroom discussion topics, activities, and variations on the activities as may be required by facility policies.

For the *Study Guide,* the following information is provided: answers to the exercises, definitions of all Select Key Terms, responses to the Case Study questions, and Skill Assessment sheets with the required competencies. For the main text, answers are given for the Case Studies and Questions for Further Study. For the surgical procedure chapters and the Student Case Study Report exercise, suggested variations on procedures are provided as report topics.

ELECTRONIC CLASSROOM MANAGER

The *Electronic Classroom Manager to Accompany Surgical Technology for the Surgical Technologist,* 2nd edition, provides a number of tools for course management and testing and evaluation:

- **PowerPoint**® presentations by chapter of key concepts help the instructor organize lectures and reinforce learner understanding of critical content.
- An **Exam***View*® Computerized Testbank with more than 1,100 questions and answers organized by chapter allows instructors to select questions for quizzes, create questions, and monitor learner progress.
- An **Image Library** provides electronic files of text figures: anatomical and surgical procedure line drawings, equipment, and surgical instruments. These figures can be used to enhance the PowerPoint® presentation.
- The complete *Instructor's Manual* is included for the instructor's convenience (in addition to the print version of the *Instructor's Manual*).
- A comparison grid simplifies the transition from the 1st edition of *Surgical Technology for the Surgical Technologists* to the 2nd edition.
- Conversion grids assist in moving from your current textbook to *Surgical Technology for the Surgical Technologist,* 2nd edition.

WebTUTORS

Delmar Learning's WebTUTORS are content-rich, web-based teaching and learning aids that clarify difficult concepts and help reinforce learning. In addition, they provide valuable communication tools for instructors and learners, including a class calendar, chat, e-mail, threaded discussions, web links, online class notes, and exercises with automatic feedback and scoring. WebTUTORS are available on the WebCT and Blackboard platforms.

Preface

INTRODUCTION

Surgical Technology for the Surgical Technologist represents a significant change in the field of surgical technology education. Surgical technology faculty and students have long depended on textbooks prepared by and for the nursing student or nursing graduate to serve as the foundation text for surgical technology education. These prior textbooks, although excellent texts for their primary audience, contained a significant amount of information not related to the role of the surgical technologist. More significantly, these texts lacked the subtle observations and nuances that come from years of experience in the role of surgical technologist. *Surgical Technology for the Surgical Technologist* is written by surgical technologists and surgical technology educators with many years of experience and commitment to the field of surgical technology.

Surgical Technology for the Surgical Technologist approaches the surgical technology student and instructor in a fresh and innovative manner. First and foremost, this surgical technology textbook focuses on the knowledge and cognitive skills required of the surgical technologist. Many specific practices and techniques are described, but all are placed in the context of the *A POSitive CARE Approach*. This approach provides a consistent and reliable way for students to learn and instructors to teach the knowledge and skills required of the surgical technologist.

The *A POSitive CARE Approach* focuses on the cognitive process used by the surgical technologist who is serving in the traditional role called "first scrub." The *A POSitive CARE Approach* for the surgical technologist finds its foundations in the following assumptions:

- The surgical technologist serves the patient's interest primarily by providing assistance to the surgeon.
- The surgical technologist's primary task during an operative procedure is to *predict* the intraoperative needs of the surgeon and surgical patient.
- To accomplish the primary task efficiently and effectively, the surgical technologist must learn to "think like the surgeon" intraoperatively.
- To accomplish the primary task efficiently and effectively, the surgical technologist must be well grounded in the basic sciences, especially anatomy, microbiology, and pathophysiology.

- The surgical technologist contributes to global patient care by serving as a team member who monitors the surgical environment along with the other team members.

The intraoperative team commonly makes these same assumptions and uses them to judge the competency of surgical technologists. Educators struggle to get students to predict the surgeon's next move or the effects of a given surgical action. Surgical technology graduates suddenly feel at home in the operating room when they begin to plan many steps ahead during an operative procedure. More importantly, the surgical technologist can be observed time and again to follow a specific sequence of cognitive steps. The cognitive steps require an adequate preparatory education. The surgical technologist must be well grounded in anatomy and microbiology. These studies are the foundation of all practices in the OR. Normal physiology and a basic understanding of pathology come next. This information is the springboard to the cognitive activity of the surgical technologist.

The basic steps of the cognitive process are easy to define. The surgical technologist

- has a mental image of normal anatomy,
- makes a mental comparison of the idealized anatomy with the actual anatomy of a specific patient,
- knows an idealized operative procedure used to correct the pathological condition,
- makes a mental comparison of the idealized procedure with the actual procedure being performed,
- allows for a particular surgeon's variations to the idealized procedure,
- allows for variances in anatomy, pathology, and surgeons' responses to the variances, and
- predicts and prepares to meet the needs of the surgeon and surgical patient prior to the need being verbalized.

The cognitive sequence described is a predictive model. Its basis is the scientific method, and it differs only by type and depth of information from other predictive models. The more information the surgical technologist has the better she or he will be able to predict needs in the surgical setting and to contribute to better patient care.

AUTHORS

The executive editor (Paul Price), senior editors (Kevin Frey and Teri Junge), and writer (Ben Price) are staff members of AST, the professional association for surgical technologists. Senior editor Teri Junge was formerly an AST staff member. Of the AST staff writers, four are past surgical technology program directors. The nonstaff writers are either current faculty members or practicing surgical technologists. *Surgical Technology for the Surgical Technologist* represents a clear and concerned effort to produce an educational text for surgical technology students and faculty that is precise, focused, and helpful.

PHILOSOPHY, ISSUES, AND PRESUMPTIONS

All books have philosophical underpinnings that include the nature of the topic, the expected audience, and the intent and use of the book. This textbook is no different.

THE SURGICAL TECHNOLOGIST

Surgical Technology for the Surgical Technologist is written by surgical technologists and for surgical technologists. More specifically, it is written with the surgical technology student and instructor in mind, and it is focused on the surgical technologist in the scrub role. Some of the underlying beliefs about the role of surgical technologists are:

- Surgical technologists are allied health professionals in a paramedical field.
- Surgical technologists primarily render care to the patient by providing assistance to the physician.
- Surgical technologists primarily work in the role traditionally referred to as "first scrub."
- Surgical technologists work within a synergistic team to provide care to the patient.
- Surgical technologists' knowledge, skills, and tasks sometimes overlap with the scope of practice of other health care providers in the OR.
- Surgical technologists best serve the patient when they have as much knowledge as possible to serve as an "extra pair of professional eyes and ears" in the OR environment.
- Surgical technology students (and their future patients) are worthy of the best educational program that can be provided.

SURGICAL TECHNOLOGY EDUCATION

Surgical technology programs vary in format, length of time, and type of educational institution. Surgical technology programs are found in community colleges, vocational-technical schools, and the military. They vary, excepting the military programs, in length from 11 to 24 months. The programs award certificates, diplomas, and degrees. In spite of the differences, there is a *Core Curriculum for Surgical Technology,* common accreditation standards, and considerable curriculum stabilization in terms of what topics are covered. Educationally, *Surgical Technology for the Surgical Technologist* is written with the following beliefs in mind:

- The necessary scope and sequence for surgical technology education are best delivered via an associate degree curriculum.
- The necessary scope and sequence for surgical technology education require a *minimum* of 12 months to execute properly.
- Students are best served when introductory anatomy and physiology and microbiology courses, with attendant lab sections, are taken as full-credit college-level courses, preferably as prerequisites.

- A separate introductory pharmacology course is preferred.
- Surgical technology students are best served when they have a solid background in the basic sciences.

PRESUMPTIONS

Given the beliefs mentioned above, several presumptions were exercised in the writing of the book:

- Students will have at least one basic anatomy and physiology course that focuses on systemic anatomy.
- Surgical anatomy must be taught within the context of surgical procedures without regard for the number of systemic anatomy courses that are taken.
- Due to the variance in surgical technology programs, some basic microbiology should be included in the chapter on asepsis. (The authors do not suggest that it is inclusive.)
- Due to the variance in surgical technology programs, some basic pharmacology should be included in the chapter on anesthesia and pharmacology. (The authors do not suggest that it is inclusive.)

ESTABLISHING A COGNITIVE MODEL

To date, one question remained unasked and unanswered, namely, what is the cognitive process used by the surgical technologist to perform her or his role during the surgical procedure? Physicians, for example, are educated according to what is commonly called the *medical model.* In other words, physicians are educated to think about health and health care in a certain way. Thinking this way does not guarantee a proper solution to a medical problem or exclude an error in judgment. Thinking this way does provide for a consistent method for approaching every medical question. Likewise, nursing has established a model for approaching nursing diagnoses and the planning of nursing care. This model is commonly referred to as the *nursing process.* These models serve the instructor because they allow for educational material to be organized in a reasonable and consistent manner. The models serve the student because they provide a way of thinking that can be used in every situation. The models serve the patient not by guaranteeing right solutions but by reducing errors in thought processes. To this point, surgical technologists have had no model, no systematic way, for describing how a surgical technologist approaches the kinds of problems faced daily in the operating room. Therefore, this book establishes and uses a cognitive model for the surgical technologist performing the scrub role. The cognitive model is based on the fact that the primary task of the surgical technologist in the scrub role is to predict a series of events and needs given specific kinds of information.

SURGICAL PROCEDURES

Every textbook is limited in terms of space. With that limitation, what is the best way to present surgical procedures? Two options present themselves:

(1) Present as many procedures as possible with brief outlines of the steps or (2) present fewer but illustrative procedures with more detailed information. The second option is exercised in this book.

THE *A POSITIVE CARE* APPROACH

This book will use a memory tool to reinforce the principles of the cognitive model discussed previously. The memory tool is **"A POSitive CARE Approach."** The A POSitive CARE Approach was developed in two phases: The **A POS** phase came directly from the review of the cognitive model—Anatomy, Pathology, Operative Procedure, and Specific Variations. This phase directly relates to operative procedures. However, even technical information and skills serve a higher purpose. Logically, the psychological and philosophical desire to care for others precedes the development of knowledge and skills.

This logic is reflected in the format of the book. The first 12 chapters reflect the **CARE** acronym. It helps the student organize information into basic units and is a reminder of the moral obligation to the surgical patient. **A POS,** as used in chapters 13–24, is a specific educational pattern that is intended for use by the educator and student. This pattern reinforces in the student's mind that caring attitudes and behaviors are a prerequisite to being a professional health care provider, but in the surgical environment, care is given through the application of technical knowledge and skills.

USING THE *A POS* ACRONYM

This systematic approach to intraoperative problem solving focuses on the ability of the surgical technologist to predict the surgeon's and patient's needs. **A POS** is defined as follows:

A Anatomy

P Pathology

O Operative procedure

S Specific variations

Each category has specific components. For instance, the surgical technologist is concerned with the following:

- Anatomy
  - Incision options
  - General topographic anatomy
  - Critical anatomy (safety features)
  - Positioning
- Pathology
  - Diagnostic procedures
  - General pathology
  - Intended surgical outcomes
  - Potential morbidity

- Operative procedure
  Procedural steps
  Nonsterile equipment needed
  Sterile equipment and instrumentation
  Suture and needles
  Dressings
  Immediate postoperative considerations
  Trouble-shooting of equipment problems
- Specific variations
  Common patient variations (examples: age, size, sex, other conditions)
  Common equipment and instrumentation variations
  Most common emergency conditions

Both the instructor and student will have the best results if they reinforce this format every time a procedure is addressed. The student guide and the instructor's manual will assist you in this effort.

USING THE *CARE* ACRONYM

CARE is intended to remind the surgical technologist that all of his or her activities affect the care given to the patient. Caring behavior for the surgical technologist is primarily exhibited by consistent and professional concern for the technical tasks for which the surgical technologist is responsible. An improperly monitored surgical environment that leads to a contaminated surgical field resulting in a wound infection is inherently uncaring. The very nature of surgical intervention requires a heightened awareness of the effects of given behaviors.

C Care directed toward the patient and/or team

A Aseptic principles and technique

R Role of the surgical technologist

E Environmental awareness and concern

In the nonprocedural chapters, objectives will be oriented to the CARE acronym. For instance, the physical environment might have objectives such as these:

C 1. Discuss the relationship between physical environment and safety procedures and patient care outcomes.

A 2. Explain the relationship between asepsis and OR design.

3. Discuss the relationship between proper OR attire and asepsis.

R 4. Discuss the role of the surgical technologist in the maintenance of the operative environment.

E 5. Describe the physical layout of the operating room.

6. Describe the piped in systems and the electrical outlets in an operating room.
7. State the proper ranges for temperature and humidity.
8. Explain the air ventilation system in the operating room including laminar flow.
9. Discuss principles of environmental safety procedures.

Both the instructor and the student should be aware that the highly variable topics of these chapters do not allow for a simple one-to-one correlation of the CARE memory tool, but that it is a conceptual tool intended to help organize the information.

FORMAT OF THE BOOK AND SUGGESTIONS FOR STUDY

Surgical Technology for the Surgical Technologist is divided into two major divisions. These divisions correspond to the *A POSitive CARE Approach*. The first 12 chapters are related to the CARE acronym. The CARE division itself is divided into two sections: Introduction to Surgical Technology and Principles and Practice of Surgical Technology. The last 12 chapters relate to the APOS acronym and focus on operative procedures by surgical specialty. A brief introduction to diagnostics precedes the specialty sections. This is intended to provide a standard background for all specialties. Surgical procedures will be taught using the APOS approach: anatomy, pathology, operative procedure, and specific variations.

CARE DIVISION

The CARE division establishes a broad context in which the student will be able to place the more specific and technical information that dominates surgical technology.

The division begins with a general orientation to the field. We review the history of surgery and surgical technology and discuss health care facilities and their organization. Inside the hospital we narrow the focus to the organization of surgical services and discuss how it relates to other hospital departments. Inside the OR we look at the surgical team and the specific role(s) of the surgical technologist. We discuss some of the responsibilities that come with being a health care professional and specifically with being a surgical technologist.

Having established a broad setting and some role definitions, our focus turns to the surgical patient. We discuss the events that bring patients to the operating room, some of their needs, ways of identifying those needs, and examples of responding to patients' needs as a surgical technologist. The surgical patient is both the primary and ultimate focus of the surgical team. We discuss the Patient's Bill of Rights, the relationship between the Bill of Rights and informed consent, and the principles of documentation. Some basic ethical and legal concepts are explored within the context of the needs and rights of the surgical patient.

We look next to certain principles and procedures that are followed in order to provide for patient care and safety. Some emergency situations and attendant procedures are reviewed. These principles and procedures are prerequisite to the step of anesthetizing the patient. A brief introduction into modern anesthesia and commonly used medications follows.

The role of the surgical technologist is initially placed within the context of history, then the modern hospital. The surgical technologist's reason for existence and the unique responsibilities that have evolved are discussed in relation to the surgical patient. For the surgical technologist, care of the patient quickly becomes technical in orientation. One does not have long philosophical conversations in the OR with a surgical patient. The typical patient is unconscious most of the time, and under any conditions, the patient's safety and return to health are heavily dependent on the surgical team. The focus of the book turns to this technical side of the surgical technologist's role. We look at the physical environment, asepsis, case preparation, instrumentation and equipment, and sutures and supplies. The text then turns to the principles, skills, and procedures that finally bring the surgical technologist, physician, patient, and surgical team to the critical juncture, the surgical intervention. The classic skills and tasks of the surgical technologist are covered sequentially: scrubbing, gowning, gloving, establishing and maintaining a sterile field, instrumentation, draping, intraoperative case management, wound protection and care, and case termination procedures and preparation for the next surgical patient.

A POS DIVISION

Surgical procedures are presented by surgical specialty. In each specialty area the following items are covered:

- Relevant anatomy
- Pathological conditions
- Diagnostic procedures and tests (Chapter 13, also)
- Special preoperative preparation procedures
- Special instrumentation, supplies, equipment, and drugs
- Patient preparation in the OR
- Typical procedural sequence
- Case management tips and predictive information
- Prognostic information and postoperative considerations

This information will be identified as fitting the *A POSitive CARE Approach* to surgical procedures. Because a significant amount of the learning that a surgical technologist student must accomplish is related to surgical procedures, we spend some time discussing a recommended way to accomplish this task. The student handbook contains support materials to assist with your learning (see "How to Use This Book" at the end of the preface).

ILLUSTRATIVE PROCEDURES

As mentioned earlier, space constraints dictate certain questions. One question was, How does one best present procedures to an entry-level student? Upon review of current textbooks and discussion with educators, two ideas seemed especially important:

- Current books did not provide adequate insight into the intraoperative thinking or tasks of the surgical technologist in the scrub role.
- Some procedures have more instructive value than others.

An example illustrates both points. In the first instance, listing of procedural steps focuses on the tasks of the surgeon only. These are important to know, but the surgical technology student should be directed to a line of thinking and sequence of tasks related to each step of the procedure. In the second instance, a procedure such as an abdominal hysterectomy with bilateral salpingo-oophorectomy requires the knowledge of skills used in many gynecologic procedures. A procedure such as a tubal ligation, on the other hand, may not require the same expanse of knowledge and skills. This book uses the illustrative procedure format.

In each specialty section, a select number of procedures is used. These are presented in detail in a specified format. This format is used time and again to help the student habituate a pattern for learning procedures.

GUIDELINES FOR THE STUDENT: LEARNING SURGICAL PROCEDURES

Surgical procedures are important to the surgical technologist for several reasons:

- Surgical procedures are the medical intervention taken to restore health to the surgical patient.
- Surgical procedures are the event around which most of the knowledge and skills of a surgical technologist are focused.
- Surgical procedures provide the best educational experience for learning "to think like the surgeon."
- Learning to think like a surgeon is the best way to organize the knowledge and skills required.

So how does one learn to think like the surgeon? You learn it by systematic practice. In this case, the practice is intellectual. Surgeons "see" their activity in a certain way. They spent many years in school gaining a foundation in the basic sciences on which to build. A surgeon also spent many years in a surgical residency program learning how to think and act like a surgeon. As you will learn in this textbook, the process of becoming a health care professional, at every level, involves intellectual, psychological, and physical development. The process includes developing specific knowledge, attitudes, perspectives, and physical skills. One of the ways to begin to understand the approach taken by the surgeon is to listen to the dictation of the surgical procedure postoperatively. The pattern of presentation is one that encapsulates a specific mindset. The information included follows a rather predictable pattern:

- Patient identification
- Preoperative diagnosis

- Surgical procedure performed
- Postoperative diagnosis
- Report of surgical procedure (step-by-step actions, including notations of anatomical conditions or variances)
- Report concerning drains, dressings, or other relevant information
- Initial status of patient following completion of the surgical procedure.

The surgical technologist should organize her or his mental approach following this pattern with variations that reflect the needs of the first scrub role. (See the student handbook for sample forms.) The student, in particular, should mimic this organizational style until it becomes habituated. For each surgical case, the student should provide the following information in the order given:

1. Patient identification (Use case number not name, age, sex, and other identifier)
2. Surgeon and other team members
3. Preoperative diagnosis
4. Preoperative tests or diagnostic studies required
5. Preoperative routines required
6. Anesthesia type and any difficulties
7. Positioning information including all devices used
8. Incision
9. Procedure (step-by-step as witnessed by you)
10. Closure
11. Drains, dressings, or other relevant information
12. Status of patient following the surgical procedure.

The student should notice that this process provides a consistent format for remembering information. It also allows the student to compare anesthesia, positioning, anatomy, procedure, and postoperative results with the idealized version learned from the classroom. The student will discover that he or she remembers more information as experience grows. As cases accumulate, the student will be able to identify variables such as different surgeons, anatomical situations, pathological conditions, and environmental conditions that resulted in variances from the idealized case. This helps the student to account for the variables and make better predictions about the patient's and surgeon's needs on the next similar case.

CORE CURRICULUM COMPLIANCE

The *Standards and Guidelines for an Accredited Educational Program in Surgical Technology* state that a program that is accredited by the Commission on Accreditation of Allied Health Education Programs (CAAHEP) must demonstrate by comparison that the curriculum designed for the program meets or exceeds the content demands of the latest edition of the *Core Curriculum for Surgical Technology,* published by AST. This textbook offers the essential elements of the core curriculum (with the exception of the in-depth basic sciences that we believe require full-length courses for proper introduction to the core surgical technology courses, as described above).

BIBLIOGRAPHY

NEUROLOGICAL FOUNDATIONS TO COGNITION

Alkon, Daniel L. (1989). Memory Storage and Neural Systems. *Scientific American*. 261:42–50.

Aoki, Chiye, and Siekevitz, Philip. (1988). Plasticity in Brain Development. *Scientific American*. 259:56–64.

Black, James E., Greenough, William T., Anderson, Brenda J., and Isaacs, Krystyna R. (1987). Environment and the Aging Brain. *Canadian Journal of Psychology*. *41*:111–130.

Boss, Barbara J. (1986). The Neuroanatomical and Neurophysiological Basis of Learning. *Journal of Neuroscience Nursing*. *18*:256–264.

Brodal, Per. (1992). *The Central Nervous System: Structure and Function*. New York: Oxford University Press.

Brody, Betty Ann, and Pribram, Karl H. (1978). The Role of Frontal and Parietal Cortex in Cognitive Processing. *Brain*. *101*:607–633.

Calvin, William H. (1989). *The Cerebral Symphony*. New York: Bantam Books.

Caruthers, B. L. (1993). The Frontal Lobes: Key to Moral Thinking. *The Surgical Technologist*. *25*:8–13.

—. (1995). Perceptions of Care Received During Childhood: A Constraint on Moral Stage Attainment. Dissertation. Ann Arbor, MI: UMI Dissertation Information Service.

—. (1997). The Frontal Lobes: Movement and Morality, Part I: Basic Anatomy and Function. *The Surgical Technologist*. *29*(3):10–15.

—. (1997). The Frontal Lobes: Movement and Morality, Part II: Neuroanatomy and Neuropsychology Converge. *The Surgical Technologist*. *29*(4):25–29.

Churchland, Patricia Smith. (1989). *Neurophilosophy: Toward a Unified Science of the Mind-Brain*. Cambridge, MA: MIT Press.

Cicerone, Keith D., and Lazar, Ronald M. (1983). Effects of Frontal Lobe Lesions on Hypothesis Sampling During Concept Formation. *Neuropsychologia*. *21*:513–524.

Edelman, Gerald M. (1987). *Neural Darwinism*. New York: Basic Books.

—. (1988). Topobiology: *An Introduction to Molecular Embryology*. New York: Basic Books.

—. (1989). *The Remembered Present: A Biological Theory of Consciousness*. New York: Basic Books.

—. (1992). *Bright Air, Brilliant Fire: On the Matter of Mind*. New York: Basic Books.

Fuster, Joaquin M. (1984). Behavioral Electrophysiology of the Prefrontal Cortex. *Trends in NeuroSciences*. *7*:408–414.

Fuster, Joaquin M., Bauer, Richard H., and Jervey, John P. (1985). Functional Interactions Between Inferotemporal and Prefrontal Cortex in a Cognitive Task. *Brain Research*. *330*:299–307.

Goldstein, L. H., Canavan, A. G. M., and Polkey, C. E. (1989). Cognitive Mapping After Unilateral Temporal Lobectomy. *Neuropsychologia*. *27*:167–177.

Lhermitte, F. (1986). Human Autonomy and the Frontal Lobes. Part II: Patient Behavior in Complex and Social Situations: The "Environmental Dependency Syndrome." *Annals of Neurology*. *19*:335–343.

—. (1983). "Utilization Behaviour" and Its Relation to Lesions in the Frontal Lobes. *Brain*. *106*:237–255.

Lhermitte, F., Pillon, B., and Serdaru, M. (1986). Human Autonomy and the Frontal Lobes. Part I: Imitation and Utilization Behavior: A Neuropsychological Study of 75 Patients. *Annals of Neurology*. *19*:326–334.

Milner, Brenda. (1968). Disorders of Memory After Brain Lesions in Man. *Neuropsychologia*. *6*:175–179.

—. (1969). Visual Recognition and Recall After Right Temporal-Lobe Excision in Man. *Neuropsychologia*. *6*:191–209.

—. (1982). Some Cognitive Effects of Frontal-Lobe Lesions in Man. *Philosophical Transcripts of the Royal Society of London*. *298*:211–226.

Pribram, Karl H. (1969). The Primate Frontal Cortex. *Neuropsychologia*. *7*:259–266.

Pribram, Karl H., and Luria, A. R., Eds. (1973). *Psychophysiology of the Frontal Lobes*. New York: Academic Press.

Purves, Dale. (1988). *Body and Brain: A Trophic Theory of Neural Connections*. Cambridge, MA: Harvard University Press.

Shepherd, Gordon M. (1988). *Neurobiology,* 2nd ed. New York: Oxford University Press.

—. (1990). *The Synaptic Organization of the Brain,* 3rd ed. New York: Oxford University Press.

Smith, Mary Lou, and Milner, Brenda. (1984). Differential Effects of Frontal-Lobe Lesions on Cognitive Estimation and Spatial Memory. *Neuropsychologia*. *22*:697–705.

Stuss, Donald T., and Benson, D. Frank. (1986). *The Frontal Lobes*. New York: Raven Press.

COGNITION

Churchland, Paul M. (1984). *Matter and Consciousness*. Cambridge, MA: MIT Press.

Dennett, Daniel C. (1981). *Brainstorms: Philosophical Essays on Mind and Psychology*. Cambridge, MA: MIT Press.

Ellis, Henry C. (1972). *Fundamentals of Human Learning and Cognition*. Dubuque, IA: William C. Brown Co.

Flanagan, Owen J., Jr. (1984). *The Science of the Mind*. Cambridge, MA: MIT Press.

Glass, Arnold L., and Holyoak, Keith J. (1986). *Cognition,* 2nd ed. New York: Random House.

Goldman, Alvin I. (1986). *Epistemology and Cognition*. Cambridge, MA: Harvard University Press.

Gregory, Richard L., Ed. (1987). *The Oxford Companion to the Mind*. New York: Oxford University Press.

Hahlweg, Kai, and Hooker, C. A., Eds. (1989). *Issues in Evolutionary Epistemology*. New York: SUNY Press.

Ingram, Rick E., Ed. (1986). *Information Processing Approaches to Clinical Psychology*. New York: Academic Press.

Klatzky, Roberta L. (1975). *Human Memory: Structures and Processes*. San Francisco: W. H. Freeman and Co.

Meichenbaum, Donald. (1977). *Cognitive-Behavior Modification: An Integrative Approach*. New York: Plenum Press.

Posner, Michael I., Ed. (1989). *Foundations of Cognitive Science*. Cambridge, MA: MIT Press.

Sternberg, Robert J., Ed. (1984). *Mechanisms of Cognitive Development*. San Francisco: W. H. Freeman and Co.

Contributors

Bob L. Caruthers, CST, PhD
Chapter 1: Orientation to Surgical Technology
Chapter 2: Standards of Conduct
Chapter 3: The Surgical Patient
Chapter 12: Surgical Case Management
Chapter 14: General Surgery
Chapter 15: Obstetric and Gynecologic Surgery

Paul Price, CST, MBA, Association of Surgical Technologists, Englewood, CO
Chapter 2: Standards of Conduct
Chapter 4: Special Populations
Chapter 6: Biomedical Science
Chapter 10: Instrumentation, Equipment, and Supplies
Chapter 11: Wound Healing, Sutures, Needles, and Stapling Devices
Chapter 13: Diagnostic Procedures
Chapter 16: Ophthalmic Surgery
Chapter 22: Cardiothoracic Surgery
Chapter 23: Peripheral Vascular Surgery
Chapter 24: Neurosurgery

Teri L. Junge, CST/CFA, San Joaquin Valley College, Fresno, CA
Chapter 8: General Patient Care and Safety
Chapter 9: Surgical Pharmacology and Anesthesia
Chapter 12: Surgical Case Management
Chapter 17: Otorhinolaryngologic Surgery
Chapter 19: Plastic and Reconstructive Surgery
Chapter 20: Genitourinary Surgery

Kevin Frey, CST, MA, Association of Surgical Technologists, Englewood, CO
Chapter 4: Special Populations
Chapter 5: Physical Environment and Safety Standards
Chapter 6: Biomedical Science
Chapter 7: Asepsis and Sterile Technique
Chapter 21: Orthopedic Surgery

Ben D. Price, CST, BS, Association of Surgical Technologists, Englewood, CO
Chapter 5: Physical Environment and Safety Standards
Chapter 7: Asepsis and Sterile Technique
Chapter 8: General Patient Care and Safety
Chapter 12: Surgical Case Management
Chapter 16: Ophthalmic Surgery
Chapter 24: Neurosurgery

Gary Allen, CST, Ludlow, MA
Chapter 14: General Surgery
Chapter 15: Obstetric and Gynecologic Surgery

Ann Marie McGuiness, CST, RN, CNOR, Charles H. McCann Technical School, Adams, MA
Chapter 9: Surgical Pharmacology and Anesthesia

Amy Croft, CST, BS, South Plains Community College, Lubbock, TX
Chapter 18: Oral and Maxillofacial Surgery

Jim Swalley, CST, Redmond, WA
Chapter 16: Ophthalmic Surgery

Reviewers

Jeffrey Lee Bidwell, CST/CSA, BS, MA
Instructor, Surgical Technology
Madisonville Community College
Madisonville, KY

Toni Crowley, BSN, RNFA, CNOR
Program Specialist, Surgical Technology
Palm Beach Community College
Lake Worth, FL

Katherine L. Gill, BSN, RN, CNOR
Coordinator/Instructor, Surgical Technologist Program
Hutchinson Community College
Hutchinson, KS

Terri Grell
Kirkwood Community College
Cedar Rapids, IA

Pamela J. Kittner, RN, MEd, CNOR
Coordinator/Instructor, Surgical Technology Program
Davis Applied Technology Center
Kaysville, UT

Connie Martin, RN, MSN, CNOR
Director and Instructor, Surgical Technology Program
Metropolitan Community College
Fort Omaha Campus, Omaha, NE

Mary Jane McClain, RN, MSN, CNOR
Director/Instructor, Surgical Technology and Medical Assistant Programs, and Coordinator/Instructor, RN Perioperative Course
Fresno City College
Fresno, CA

Lu Ann Peralta
Formerly Program Director of Surgical Technology
U.S. Army Medical Center
Ft. Sam Houston, TX

Lora Plank, RN, CNOR, CST

Department Chairperson, Health & Human Services
Program Chairperson, Surgical Technologist
Ivy Tech State College
Michigan City, IN

Emily Rogers, CST, RN, BS, CNOR

Surgical Technology Department Head
Spartanburg Technical College
Spartanburg, SC

Tracey A. Ross, MEd, CST

Staff Development Instructor, Surgical Services Department
The Lancaster General Hospital
Strasburg, PA

Kimberly A. Shannon, RN

Coordinator, Surgical Technology
Moore Norman Technology Center
Norman, OK

Dina Speicher, RN

Instructor, Surgical Technology
Iowa Western Community College
Council Bluffs, IA

Julie Vasquez, CST, CRCST

U.S. Army Medical Department Center and School
Surgical Technologist Program
Ft. Sam Houston, TX

Katherine J. Wolfer, RN, BSN, CNOR

Surgical Technology Faculty
Cincinnati State Technical and Community College
Cincinnati, OH

How to Use This Book

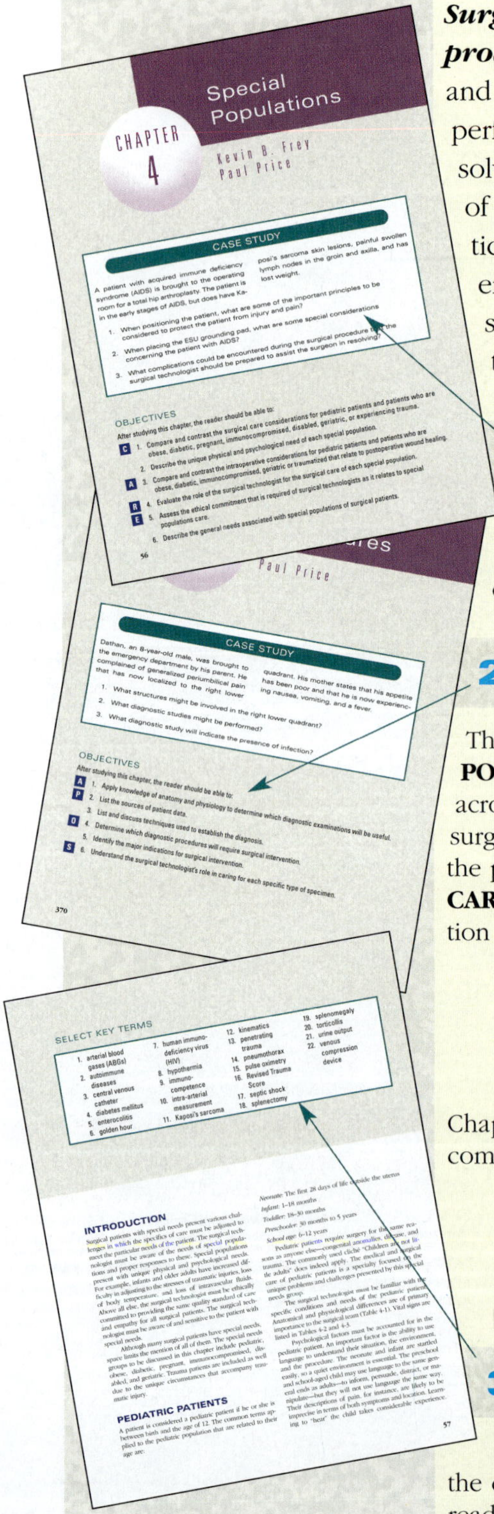

***Surgical Technology for the Surgical Technologist: A Positive Care Approach,* 2nd Edition**, presents the core physical and biological concepts and technical surgical information needed for the surgical technologist to perform efficiently and effectively in the surgical environment. A problem-solving methodology is used consistently throughout the text. The purpose of the methodology is to develop the surgical technologist's ability to anticipate the surgeon's and patient's needs and to plan ahead during the operative procedure to achieve the best possible outcome. The features shown on these pages are integrated throughout the text and all contribute to the development of the surgical technologist.

1 CASE STUDY

Two case studies are presented in each chapter. They describe clinical situations with related questions that require the learner to apply information presented in the chapter. Their intent is to help the learner develop critical thinking skills.

2 OBJECTIVES

The text uses a systematic approach to problem-solving using the **CARE** and **A POS**itive acronyms. The objectives are identified by the components of these acronyms. Chapters 1–12 apply the **CARE** components. These chapters introduce surgical technology and its principles and practices. They emphasize that the care of the patient in the operating room is the surgical technologist's highest priority. The **CARE** components provide a framework for placing the specific technical information presented in these chapters. **CARE** represents:

- **C** Care (directed toward the patient and/or surgical team)
- **A** Aseptic Principles (guiding the practice of sterile technique)
- **R** Role (of the surgical technologist during the preoperative, intraoperative, and postoperative phases)
- **E** Environmental Awareness (and concern)

Chapters 13–24 on operative procedures by surgical specialty apply the **A POS**itive components, as follows:

- **A** Anatomy
- **P** Pathology
- **O** Operative Procedure
- **S** Specific Variations

3 SELECT KEY TERMS

Each chapter contains a list of terms to be learned. Each term is emphasized in the chapter in bold face type. Definitions of these terms appear in the glossary for ready reference.

4 ART

Full color illustrations are used throughout the text. Illustrations and photos used in the **CARE** chapters show steps used in specific skills and identify general equipment and supplies common to many operative procedures.

Illustrations in the **A POS** chapters (operative procedures) show the anatomy of the surgical field for specific operative procedures. The correct placement of instruments during the procedure is also illustrated. Equipment and supplies specific to a surgical specialty or procedure are also shown.

5 TECHNIQUES

Techniques represent skills required in most operative procedures, such as the surgical scrub, donning and removing surgical attire and personal protective equipment, and setting up the OR. Each technique lists the necessary steps in sequence.

6 ILLUSTRATIVE PROCEDURES

The illustrative procedure format is based on the concept that allows one procedure to highlight several important steps that appear in related procedures. Rather than presenting many procedures with brief outlines of the steps, fewer procedures are presented in detail with information organized by Equipment, Instruments, Supplies, Operative Preparation, Practical Considerations, Operative Procedure with Technical Considerations, and Postoperative Considerations.

7 PEARL OF WISDOM

Following each procedure, these tips are based on the authors' years of experience as surgical technologists. They offer practical suggestions and cautions to be observed during the procedure.

8 QUESTIONS FOR FURTHER STUDY

These questions at the end of each chapter encourage you to seek and apply additional related information.

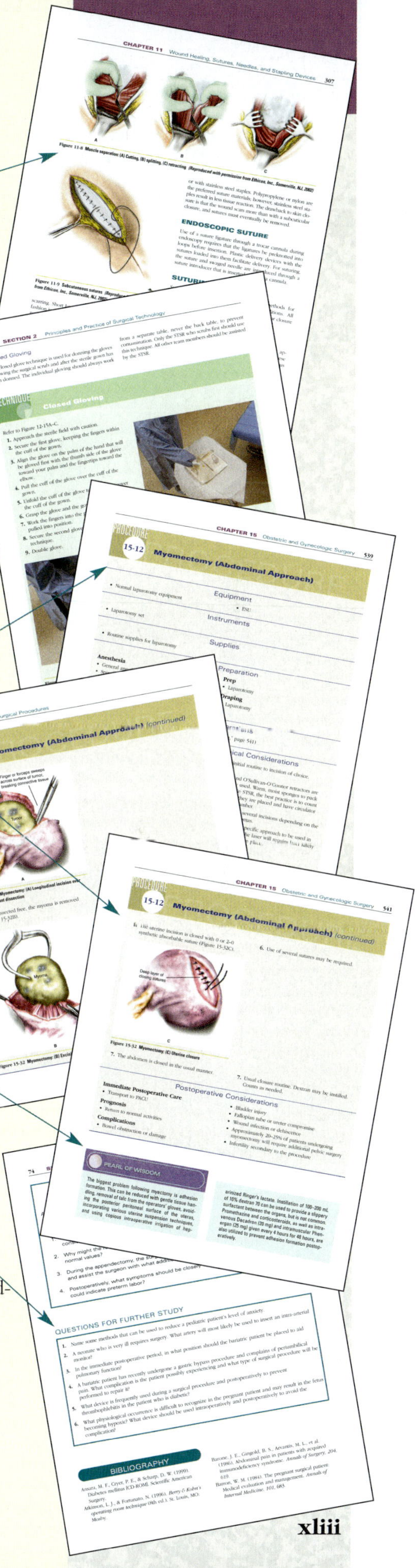

SECTION 1

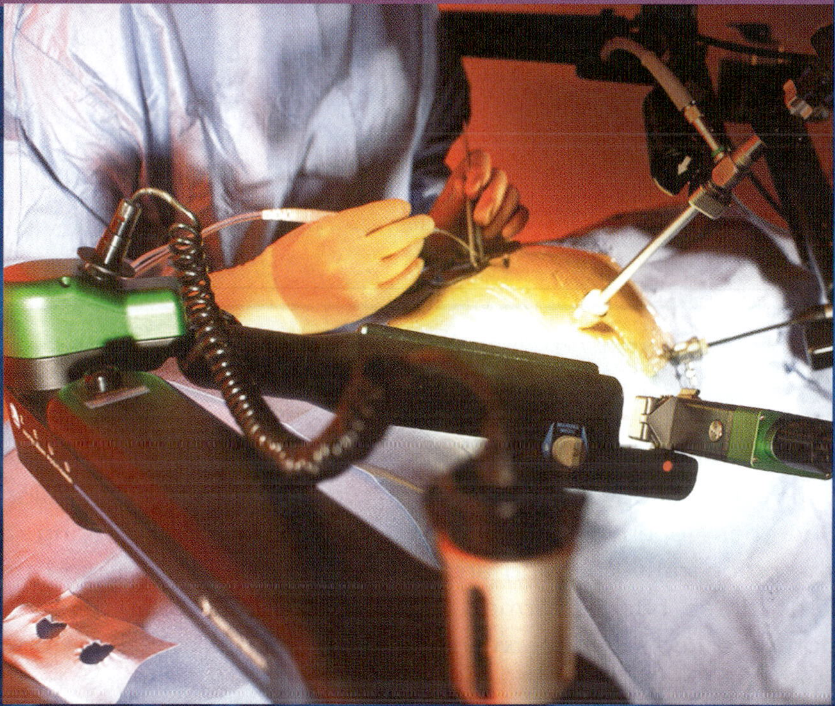

Introduction to Surgical Technology

CHAPTER 1

Orientation to Surgical Technology

Bob Caruthers

CASE STUDY

Gloria is a 43-year-old female. She is scheduled for diagnostic laparoscopy for chronic pelvic pain. She has been resting for 30 minutes in the preoperative holding area where a registered nurse has performed a nursing evaluation, checked her paperwork, history and physical, allergies, special needs, and informed consent, and provided emotional support. The anesthesia provider has reviewed the steps that will be taken and started an IV. A registered nurse and an OR nursing assistant maneuver a gurney with Gloria on it into OR 5. Gloria notices an individual who is wearing a surgical gown, gloves, cap, mask, and protective eyewear. This strangely clad person is moving surgical instruments into place on a large, flat table. The individual steps back from the table, turns slightly toward Gloria, and says, "Hello, I'm Sarah. I'm a surgical technologist and I'll be assisting Dr. J. today."

1. The registered nurse is functioning in a classic OR nursing role. This role is referred to by what common term?
2. The surgical technologist who is gowned, gloved, and working at the back table is functioning in the classic role of the surgical technologist. This role is commonly referred to by what term?
3. What is the recommended educational background for the surgical technologist according to the *Recommended Standards of Practice?*
4. What entity is responsible for verifying that the school attended by the surgical technologist meets national standards?
5. What entity is responsible for the examination taken by the surgical technologist to verify that she has an adequate entry level of knowledge to perform in the role of a certified surgical technologist?

OBJECTIVES

After studying this chapter, the reader should be able to:

C 1. Identify and demonstrate principles of communication in the surgical setting.

A 2. (No objectives focused on asepsis in this chapter; however, the student should demonstrate an awareness that the principles of asepsis are a vital component of the surgical technologist's role in surgical patient care.)

R 3. Trace the historical development of surgery and surgical technology.

4. Identify members of the surgical team and their roles.

5. Identify the various roles of the surgical technologist.

6. Identify and interpret a job description for the surgical technologist.

E 7. Identify different types of health care facilities.

8. Describe a typical hospital organizational structure.

9. Identify hospital departments and their relationship to surgical services.

SELECT KEY TERMS

1. acronym	7. Core Curriculum	14. LCC-ST	21. proprietary
2. ambulatory surgical facility	8. DO	15. optional	22. STSR
	9. elective	16. Pasteur	23. urgent
3. ARC-ST	10. emergent	17. postoperative	24. Vesalius
4. AST	11. HMO	18. preceptor	
5. circulator	12. intraoperative	19. preoperative	
6. competency	13. JCAHO	20. professional	

HISTORY OF SURGERY

The history of surgery in the Western world is closely tied to the broader history of medicine, science, and intellectual development. The earliest records indicate some amazing insights into the nature of certain illnesses and some unbelievably inaccurate observations and theories. The Classical Period revolutionized thinking in the Western world. Hippocrates, Aristotle, and Galen were insightful and influential; however, their scientific thought was subservient to their philosophical and theological biases. The so-called Dark Ages comprised a long period of arrested development in many areas of thought. The human mind is never content to ignore what it does not know, and the Renaissance issued in a new era of thought and development. **Vesalius**, almost single handedly, overthrew 1,500 years in which anatomical teaching was made to serve theological and philosophical interests. Others rose to

Table 1-1 Select History of Surgery Time Line (Dates are approximations)

Date	Person/Source	Contribution
4000 B.C.	Cuneiform script, tablets from Nineveh	First anatomical descriptions of human organs
2500 B.C.	Imhotep	Revered Egyptian physician (declared divine); wrote an early "book" on surgery
2000 B.C.	Code of Hammurabi	Medical practices of the day described; some reflect real insight into disease; most are religious in nature
	Moses	Desert community rules of cleanliness
1500 B.C.	*Papyrus Ebers* (Egypt)	Discusses polyuria and treatments
	Egyptian hieroglyph	Depicts clinical signs of paralytic poliomyelitis
	Vedas (Hindu)	Correlates "sweet smell" of urine with a specific disease
1000 B.C.	Homer	Early Greek history/myth provides a view of military medicine of the day
	Susruta	Father of medicine in India
500 B.C.	Alkmaion	Sensory nerves dissected
	Aristotle	Established an early "scientific" mindset; founder of comparative anatomy
	Herophilos	Father of anatomy; developed the Doctrine of the Pulse (diagnostic value)
	Erasistratos	Contributed to a remarkable increase in understanding the anatomy of the brain;noted difference in sensory and motor nerves
	Nei Ching	Chinese writing on acupuncture
250 B.C.	Paul of Aegina	Refined diagnosis of diabetes
0	Celsus	Described the signs of inflammation
	Galen	First great anatomist; controlled thought, unchallenged, for 1,500 years; biology made to serve theology
A.D. 500	Alexander	Described the pump-like function of the heart
A.D. 1000	Avicenna	Persian philosopher, wrote *The Canon of Medicine;* revived Aristotle's theories
	Ibn Rushd (Averroes)	Wrote a medical encyclopedia; correlated exercise to health
1400	Linacre	Translated Galen from Greek to Latin; Galen's authority still unquestioned
1500	Paracelsus	Broke with Galen and Avicenna but provided no better system
	Pare	Greatest surgeon of the 16th century; began to ligate arteries after amputation; stopped cauterizing wounds with hot irons and oil

the task and the development of science began. In many instances, the observations remained inaccurate because modern scientific tools were not available, but the attitude with which the observations were made was remarkably different. Slowly but surely, physicians began to understand and control the mechanisms of pain, hemorrhage, and infection. Except in the crudest of forms, surgery is not possible without the control of pain, hemorrhage, and infection. Parallel and correlated discoveries in microbiology, anatomy, and physiology were necessary to reach the period of modern surgery. In fact, surgery as we know it today is a 20th-century phenomenon. Given the rapid development of technology, surgical intervention will be radically changed in the next quarter century. The quest for better and safer patient care will ensure that change is a constant in surgical practice. A select review of the history of surgery is presented in Table 1-1.

SURGERY TODAY

Not even the greatest of the Renaissance minds would have envisioned the kind of surgical services available today. The surgical procedures available to the pa-

Table 1-1 *(continued)*

	Vesalius	Father of modern anatomy; challenged Galen openly and correctly; performed dissections on human cadavers himself; used illustrators to create permanent records; changed the whole approach to anatomical studies
1600	Harvey	Detailed cardiovascular anatomy; demonstrated basic functions of the circulatory system
	Willis	Responsible for development of brain anatomy, especially circulation
1700	Morgagni	Responsible for beginnings of clinical pathology
1800	Jenner	Inventor of the vaccination for smallpox
	Laennec	Developed clinical evaluation of the chest
1850	**Pasteur**	Father of microbiology, virology, and immunology
	Lister	Developed technique of antiseptic surgery
	Billroth	Responsible for advances in surgical procedures; best known for gastrectomy procedures
	Halsted	Developed meticulous closure of wounds
	Iwanowski	Demonstrated the existence of entities smaller than bacteria; beginning of virology
	Biejerinick	Developed the concept of a virus
	Horsley	Early British neurosurgeon
	Roentgen	Developed the X-ray machine
1900	Cushing	Father of neurosurgery; reduced mortality rate for meningiomas from 96% to 5%
	Reed	Demonstrated that malaria was caused by a mosquito-transmitted virus
	Kocher	Advanced knowledge of thyroid function
	Enders	Propagated the poliovirus in primary human cell cultures
1950	Cooley	Perfected the heart-lung machine; performed first U.S. heart transplant and first totally artificial heart implant
	DeBakey	Developed the first ventricular assist pump
1980s		Technological revolution begins; endoscopic surgery becomes routine
1990s		Computer age changes surgery; stereotactic approach to neurosurgery; virtual reality offers promise for education and clinical practice

tient are classified into broad categories that cross specialty areas:

- **Emergent**: Surgical pathology threatening life or limb within a relatively short time period (e.g., ruptured aneurysm of the abdominal aorta)
- **Urgent**: Surgical pathology requiring treatment within a relatively short period of time (e.g., unruptured ectopic pregnancy with stable vital signs)
- **Elective**: Surgical intervention that does not have to be performed immediately or within a short period of time (If the surgical intervention can be scheduled at a future date, it is elective; e.g., a torn meniscus in the knee.)
- **Optional**: Surgical intervention that does not have to be performed in order to preserve life or function (e.g., rhytidectomy).

SURGICAL SPECIALTIES

Medicine today is a field of specialization and subspecialization. The same is true for modern surgery. The field called "general" surgery is actually a specialty (Chapter 14). It is general only in the sense that it is not exclusively focused on one body system. General surgeons typically perform surgery on the digestive system, including the hepatobiliary system, thyroid and parathyroid glands, general skin lesions, and breast lesions (may vary by region). Some general surgeons may subspecialize, only performing surgery on the hepatobiliary system or gastrointestinal system. Other specialty areas include obstetrics and gynecology (Chapter 15), orthopedics (Chapter 21), cardiothoracic (Chapter 22), peripheral vascular (Chapter 23), genitourinary (Chapter 20), otorhinolaryngology (Chapter 17), neurosurgery (Chapter 24), ophthalmologic surgery (Chapter 16), oral and maxillofacial (Chapter 18), and plastic and reconstructive surgery (Chapter 19). Each specialty has subspecialties (e.g., pediatric cardiovascular, orthopedics, and neurosurgery). No body system is immune to surgical intervention, and each represents a specialization in modern surgery. Each specialty must account for specific variations in the population, such as age in pediatric and geriatric patients. Trauma presents variations to normal procedures and specific patient care demands. Finally, the procurement of donated organs and their transplantation into other humans affects many specialties and produces some variations in patient care.

HISTORY OF SURGICAL TECHNOLOGY

The definitions, education, roles, and job descriptions related to surgical technology are current. However, surgical technology has a history, too. The history of surgical technology is difficult to trace with certainty. Surgeons have had nonphysician and non-nursing assistants since the beginning of surgical history. The military, in particular, used nonphysician and non-nursing assistants in various roles, partly because females were excluded from the battlefield. The more modern version of surgical technology, that is, an allied health specialist serving predominantly in the scrub role, began to develop in Britain and the United States following World War II. The history of surgical technology is presented in a table format. Key examples of surgical technology history have been selected to demonstrate general themes, key issues of the day, and general development (Table 1-2). By necessity, these do not tell the whole story of surgical technology but should provide the student with a general overview.

Table 1-2 Select History of Surgical Technology—Time Line

DATE	PLACE OR ACTOR	EVENT OR INFORMATION
Late 19th century	London Hospital	Mr. Rampley employed in the OR as "surgery beadle" (theater technician)
1948	Britain	Formation of the Operating Theater Technicians
1952	Britain: situation	Five hundred men known to be employed in hospital theaters
Early 1950s	Britain: early problem identified	Education: no system of training for this field
Early 1950s	United States	Early development parallels Britain: • Many operating room technicians educated in the military • Civilian education predominant on the job and widely varying in expectations
1954	American Hospital Association	Publication of first book focused on OR technicians: *Surgical Technical Aide—Instructor's Manual* (Ginsberg)
1959	Association of Operating Room Nurses (AORN) Board of Directors	Forms survey group to study the needs of OR technicians
Dec. 1967	AORN Manual Committee	A new publication: *Teaching the Operating Room Technician*

Table 1-2 *(continued)*

DATE	PLACE OR ACTOR	EVENT OR INFORMATION
Feb. 1969	AORN House of Delegates	A critical proposal: "The Association of Operating Room Nurses, Inc. (AORN), shall structure an associated organization for Operating Room Technicians, under the auspices of AORN. This organization will be known as the Association of Operating Room Technicians (AORT) and the two associations shall relate to each other through an Advisory Board at both the Local and National levels."
July 19–20, 1969	New York Conference 1	Formal Organization: Association of Operating Room Technicians (AORT)
Dec. 1970	AORT Board of Directors and Advisory Committee	• Certification selected over licensure • First examination given
1972	American Medical Association House of Delegates	Essentials of an approved education program for the OR technician adopted
1972	AORT	First edition of *O.R. Tech* magazine
1973	AORT and AORN	National Advisory Board dissolved "as AORT was able to assume the responsibilities of managing its own association."
1974	The Liaison Council on Certification for Surgical Technology (LCC-ST)	LCC becomes arm of AST responsible for certification
1974	Accreditation Review Committee for Education in Surgical Technology (ARC-ST)	ARC on Education for the ORT appointed (Commission on Accreditation of Allied Health Education Programs [CAAHEP] system)
1978	AORT National Conference	AORT changes name to Association of Surgical Technologists (AST); *O.R. Tech* magazine changes to the journal *The Surgical Technologist*
1981	AST	*Core Curriculum for Surgical Technology* (1st ed.) published
1985	AST	Code of Ethics published
Nov. 1986	*The Surgical Technologist*	Claire Olsen: introduces associate degree discussion
May 1988	AST House of Delegates	Standards of Practice adopted
Nov. 1990	AST	Job description for Surgical First Assistant (SFA) published
Mar. 1992	AST	SFA core curriculum published
1997	AST	Workforce shortage of surgical technologists becoming apparent

FIELD OF SURGICAL TECHNOLOGY

Surgical technology is a thriving and developing allied health profession in the United States. This section provides the student with introductory information about the field of surgical technology and the surgical environment.

Surgical technology is part of the allied health field in the United States. The Joint Commission on Accreditation of Healthcare Organizations (**JCAHO**) defines *surgical technologist* in its *Lexikon: Dictionary of Health Care Terms, Organizations, and* ***Acronyms*** *for the Era of Reform* as follows:

> An allied health **professional** who works closely with surgeons, anesthesiologists, registered nurses and other surgical personnel delivering patient care and assuming appropriate responsibilities before, during, and after surgery.

The JCAHO defines the term *profession* in several different ways. It is clearer in its use of the term *paraprofessional:*

> Occupations requiring successful completion of a training program at or above the college level or its equivalent, typically lasting one to two years; the program resembles that of the profession to which it corresponds, except that the paraprofessional program is shorter and more limited in content. Members of the occupation work under the direction and supervision of the professionals whose service capabilities they extend and to whom they are responsible.

In the formative years of the professional association, surgical technology was referred to by the Association of Operating Room Nurses (AORN) and the Association of Surgical Technologists (**AST**) as a paramedical field. This term effectively communicated the same meaning as the JCAHO term *paraprofessional* but specified that the relationship was between the paraprofessional and the physician. Each of these terms contributes to our understanding of surgical technology and the role of the surgical technologist.

This textbook accepts the definition of paraprofession and paraprofessional as defined by the JCAHO as the most precise descriptors for the field of surgical technology and the broad role of the surgical technologist. For the purposes of this textbook, any use of the term *profession* or *professional* (such as *health care professional*) refers to the common use: an individual who has special education and training in a given field and who meets certain **competency**-based and ethical criteria in his or her vocational arena.

WORKING CONDITIONS

The surgical environment is brightly lit, relatively quiet, and temperature controlled. Most of the duties of the surgical technologist require standing for extended periods of time and the ability to lift and move heavy objects. Attention must be focused. The surgical technologist can be exposed to communicable diseases, unpleasant sights, odors, and hazardous materials. Most surgical procedures are carried out during the day, and a 40-hour workweek is common. The surgical technologist may be required to work the evening or night shift, weekends, and holidays and to periodically take "call" (be available to work on short notice in case of emergency).

PERSONAL CHARACTERISTICS

As part of the surgical team, the surgical technologist must be able to work quickly and accurately, with a commitment to detail. A number of activities must be integrated according to priority when under pressure in stressful and emergency situations. Therefore, a stable temperament and a strong sense of responsibility are qualities essential to the surgical technologist. Considerable patience and concern for order are required. Manual dexterity and physical stamina are vital. Sensitivity to the needs of the patient as well as other members of the surgical team must be demonstrated. Individuals who practice this profession have a strong desire to help others and make a valuable contribution to society.

SURGICAL TEAM MEMBERS

A surgical technologist works as a member of the surgical team to ensure that the operative procedure is conducted under optimal conditions (Figure 1-1). Surgical

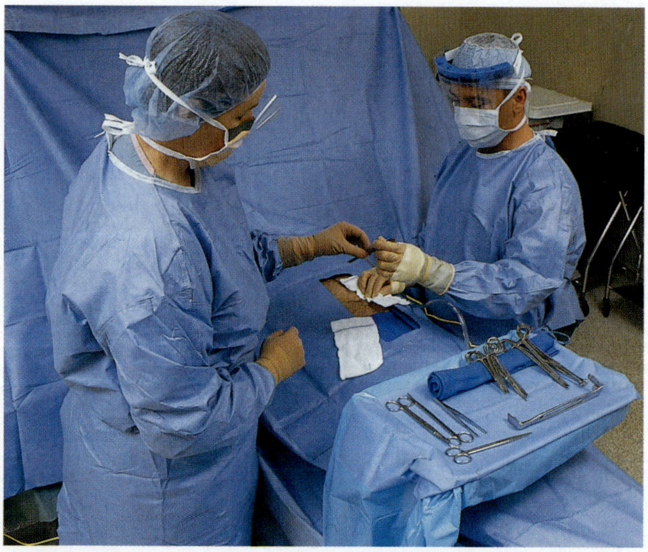

Figure 1-1 STSR passing a scalpel to the surgeon

team members are responsible for the three phases of surgical patient care (surgical case management; discussed next) and function in two capacities—nonsterile and sterile. All surgical team members must adhere to the principles of asepsis and the practice of sterile technique (refer to Chapter 7). Honesty and moral integrity are necessary to uphold these standards. While the surgical technologist in the scrub role (**STSR**) is the focus of this textbook, an overview of the roles of the other surgical team members is provided.

THE THREE PHASES OF SURGICAL CASE MANAGEMENT

The three phases of surgical case management are the **preoperative**, **intraoperative**, and **postoperative** phases.

1. **Preoperative**: The preoperative case management phase occurs prior to initiation (creation of the incision or insertion of an endoscope) of the surgical procedure.
2. **Intraoperative**: The intraoperative case management phase occurs while the surgical procedure is being performed.
3. **Postoperative**: The postoperative case management phase begins when the surgical procedure is terminated (application of the dressing or extraction of the endoscope).

NONSTERILE SURGICAL TEAM MEMBERS

The nonsterile team members are the **circulator** and the anesthesia provider. Additionally, other personnel, such as the radiology technologist or pathologist, may also be present in the operating room (OR).

The circulator is a registered nurse (RN), licensed practical or vocational nurse (LPN or LVN), or a surgical technologist. Some of the duties of the circulator include:

- Preparing the operating room
- Conducting the preoperative patient interview
- Transporting the patient to the OR
- Transferring the patient to the operating table
- Positioning the patient
- Assisting the anesthesia provider
- Prepping the patient
- Assisting with draping the patient
- Connecting various cords and tubings
- Providing additional items to the sterile field during the surgical procedure
- Maintaining the patient's operative record
- Caring for specimens
- Affixing dressings
- Transferring the patient from the operating table
- Transporting the patient to the postanesthesia care unit (PACU)
- Preparing the OR for the next patient

The anesthesia provider may be either a physician (medical doctor [MD] or doctor of osteopathy [**DO**]) or a certified registered nurse anesthetist (CRNA). Some of the duties of the anesthesia provider include:

- Assessing the patient preoperatively
- Determining the type of anesthetic to be administered
- Discussing the risks and benefits of the planned anesthetic and obtaining informed consent
- Offering alternative anesthetic options, if necessary
- Managing all phases of the anesthetic (refer to Chapter 9)
- Monitoring the patient's vital signs
- Providing any supportive measures (e.g., fluid and airway management)

STERILE SURGICAL TEAM MEMBERS

The STSR, the surgeon, and the surgical assistant (also referred to as the first assistant) are the sterile team members. Traditionally, the surgical technologist functions in a sterile capacity during the surgical procedure, but also performs many nonsterile duties (known as circulating duties) throughout the course of the workday. Some of the duties of the STSR include:

Preoperative Case Management

- Donning OR attire and personal protective equipment (PPE)
- Preparing the OR
- Gathering necessary equipment and supplies
- Creating and maintaining the sterile field
- Scrubbing and donning sterile gown and gloves
- Organizing the sterile field for use (Figure 1-2)
- Counting necessary items
- Assisting team members during entry of the sterile field
- Exposing the operative site with sterile drapes

Intraoperative Case Management

- Maintaining the sterile field
- Passing instrumentation, equipment, and supplies to the surgeon and surgical assistant as needed
- Assessing and predicting (anticipating) the needs of the patient and surgeon to provide the necessary items in order of need
- Preparing and handling medications
- Counting necessary items
- Caring for the specimen
- Preparing and applying the dressing

Postoperative Case Management

- Maintaining the sterile field until the patient is transported from the OR
- Disassembling the sterile field
- Removing used instruments, equipment, and supplies from the OR

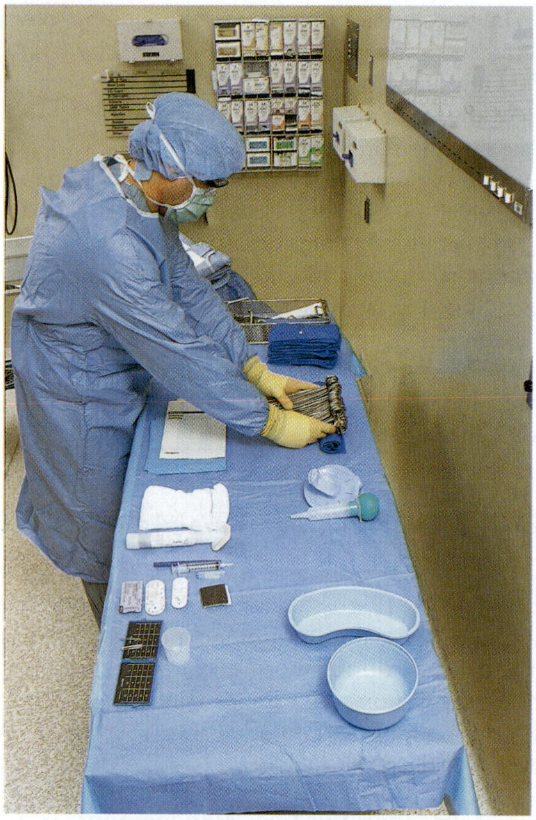

Figure 1-2 **STSR organizing the back table**

- Caring for and maintaining instruments (instrument cycle), equipment, and supplies following use
- Preparing the OR for the next patient (OR cycle)

The surgeon may be an MD, DO, doctor of podiatric medicine (DPM), or a doctor of dental science (DDS). Some of the duties of the surgeon include:

- Determining the necessity of surgical intervention and the type of procedure to be performed
- Discussing the risks and benefits of the planned procedure
- Offering alternative treatment options, if necessary
- Performing the surgical procedure
- Providing follow-up patient care

The surgical assistant may be a physician (MD or DO) or a nonphysician (physician assistant [PA], certified registered nurse first assistant [CRNFA], or a surgical technologist/surgical assistant [ST/SA]). Some of the duties of the surgical assistant include:

- Positioning the patient
- Draping the patient (Figure 1-3)
- Providing visualization of the surgical site through retraction of tissue, suctioning, and sponging
- Assisting with achieving temporary or permanent hemostasis
- Participating in volume replacement or autotransfusion techniques
- Closing body planes
- Selecting and applying wound dressings

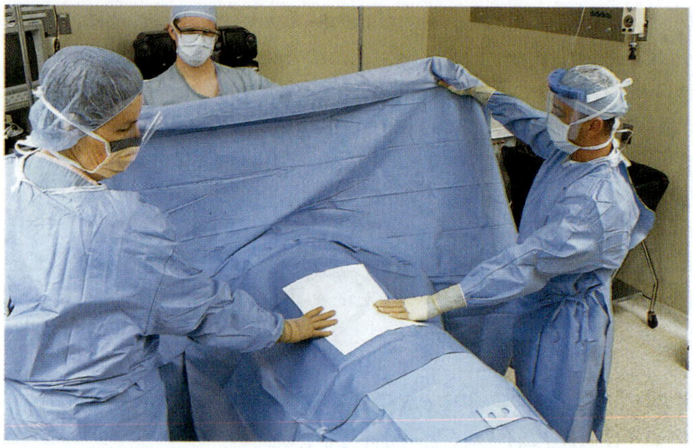

Figure 1-3 **Surgical assistant helping to drape the patient**

SURGICAL TECHNOLOGY EDUCATION AND CERTIFICATION

Educational programs for surgical technologists are accredited by the Commission on Accreditation of Allied Health Education Programs (CAAHEP) (Table 1-3). The Accreditation Review Committee for Education in Surgical Technology (**ARC-ST**) directly oversees academic accreditation for the field of surgical technology. The Liaison Council on Certification for Surgical Technology (**LCC-ST**) is responsible for the credential (Certified Surgical Technologist [CST] and Certified Surgical Technologist/Certified First Assistant [CST/CFA]) and the national certification examination for both credentials.

Surgical technology education has grown and developed in a relatively short time. Curriculum development and educational stabilization for the "operating room technician" were clearly concerns of the British as early as 1952 and for the AORN in 1959. Education was a major concern of the Association of Operating Room Technicians (now the Association of Surgical Technologists—AST) in its early period. It has not been easy to stabilize surgical technology education, but beginning in March 2000, the educational components were implemented to accomplish this task. Admission to the certification examination is restricted to graduates of accredited programs (and currently or previously certified surgical technologists). Program accreditation requires compliance with the ***Core Curriculum*** *for Surgical Technology*.

The final component for educational stability lies outside the educational arena. This will occur when certification is required as a condition for employment. While more and more employers are requiring certification as a condition of employment, this requirement is still voluntary and facility based. Speaking for the profession, the AST has affirmed the following principles:

- Certification through the process and procedures established by the LCC-ST should be required as a condition of employment in the field of surgical technology.

Table 1-3 Surgical Technology Education: Related Agencies

Association of Surgical Technologists (AST) (303-694-9130; www.ast.org)
- Responsible for *Core Curriculum for Surgical Technology*
- Responsible for *Core Curriculum for Surgical Assisting*
- Provides general services and educational products

Accreditation Review Committee for Education in Surgical Technology (ARC-ST) (303-694-9282; www.arcst.org)
- Part of the CAAHEP system of program accreditation
- All specific accreditation questions should be directed here

Commission on Accreditation of Allied Health Education Programs (CAAHEP) (312-553-9355; www.caahep.org)

Liaison Council on Certification for Surgical Technology (LCC-ST) (800-707-0057; www.lcc-st.org)
- Responsible for all aspects of individual certification, including *recertification*
- All specific certification questions should be directed here

- Candidacy for certification is properly linked to graduation from a surgical technology program that is accredited by the Commission on Accreditation of Allied Health Education Programs (CAAHEP) and is the required standard.
- The associate degree is the preferred academic credential for surgical technology.
- The *Core Curriculum for Surgical Technology* shall be considered the appropriate educational guide for curriculum design and statement of the expected base of knowledge for entry level into the field of surgical technology.
- Expanded practice role qualifications presume that the CST meets all competencies required for the specific role.

ROLES AND COMPETENCIES

The AST developed a list of roles and levels to serve as guidelines for the surgical technologist in career planning and for employers looking for appropriate criteria to develop a clinical ladder. Roles and competencies are discussed in Chapter 2. The student should focus on the broadly stated competencies to develop a plan for career development. Entry into the profession anticipates (1) graduation from an accredited program in surgical technology and (2) successful completion of the certification examination. Three critical principles serve as the foundation for all role descriptions and competencies:

1. All surgical technologists should hold the certification appropriate to each role.
2. All surgical technologists should meet the educational, competency, and legal requirements expected of all health care professionals.
3. State law and hospital policy should be followed without exception.

THE SURGICAL TECHNOLOGIST AS A PROFESSIONAL

The JCAHO definition of a professional indicates that the surgical technologist is educated and trained in a specific field of health care service. Many health care professionals believe that their profession represents a true *vocation,* that is, a calling. The surgical technology student is entering a different world. Entering that world will change the individual. The student should be aware that the terminal goal of a surgical technology program is not to "get one a job" but to make one a surgical technologist. The molding process is physical, intellectual, social, psychological, and spiritual.

This section looks at some of the expectations that will be placed on a surgical technologist. Some are professional and some are predominantly personal.

PROFESSIONALISM

Professionalism begins with competency and commitment in the workplace. Both employers and patients deserve a dependable health care professional. Some important professional traits include:

- Conscientiousness
- Consistent attendance
- Punctuality
- Understanding of policies/procedures
- Skills competency
- Ability to obey rules
- Spirit of cooperation
- Being a team member
- Commitment to continuing education
- Suggestions and problem solving
- Willingness to serve on committees

Being a health care professional entails more than competency in the workplace. Professionals are obligated to support and develop their profession.

PROFESSIONAL ORGANIZATION

The Association of Surgical Technologists is the professional organization for surgical technologists. For three decades, the primary purpose of AST has been to ensure that surgical technologists have the knowledge and skills required to administer patient care of the highest quality.

The AST's mission statement summarizes this obligation well: "Enhancing the profession to ensure quality patient care." Obviously the role of a professional organization is to enhance the profession it represents; however, there is a qualifier when it is a health care profession. The actions must be intended to provide better patient care. Being an active health care professional means many things for the surgical technologist. Since certification is voluntary at this time (although it may be required as a condition of employment), a professional chooses to take the national examination. Development of a profession requires time, energy, and money. Many activities require year-round attention and specialists working outside the OR. For instance, journal publication, interaction with other health profession associations, governmental relations, public relations, and educational activities require significant effort on an ongoing basis. The surgical technologist receives the benefits of the activities of the professional organization. Membership in the AST and participation in the activities of the professional association offer support. Continuing education is important to the surgical technologist for two reasons: (1) Continuing education is necessary for continued personal development and improved patient safety and (2) continuing certification requires demonstration of continuing education. The professional is also willing to be a role model to others in the profession and for students entering the profession. Community service outside the OR is another feature of professional responsibility. The surgical technologist should take opportunities to help serve and educate the public on health care issues. Finally, professionals must always behave in an ethical manner.

The AST logo features the roles that the surgical technologist performs within the operating room (Figure 1-4). The circles that are filled represent common roles. The filled circle in front of the dark rectangle represents the STSR (the term *STSR* arises from the fact that the STSR performs a surgical scrub prior to entering the sterile field). The two filled circles placed side by side opposite the STSR represent the surgical assistants. The filled circle with the arc extending from it represents the circulator (the term *circulator* arises from the fact that this individual can move about the OR). The large rectangle represents the operating table and the three empty circles represent the patient, the surgeon, and the anesthesia provider.

ASSOCIATION OF SURGICAL TECHNOLOGISTS

AEGER PRIMO— THE PATIENT FIRST®

Figure 1-4 **Association of Surgical Technologists logo** ***(Courtesy of the Association of Surgical Technologists)***

SURGICAL TECHNOLOGIST'S LIFESTYLE

As a surgical technologist, life is about to change in ways that the student probably has not considered. To understand this, consider that the surgical technologist:

- Is entering an environment that most of the population knows little about
- Knows more about the human body than almost anyone who lived before the 20th century and more than 95% of those living today
- Will participate in surgical procedures that the population sees as miraculous
- Spends everyday life in a world alien to non-health care friends and family
- Will have moral, ethical, legal, and professional obligations that most others do not have
- Will have to deal psychologically with events and outcomes that most seldom have to face
- Will be expected to perform well whenever called on

In the ethical and legal section of Chapter 2, the student will learn more about the concepts of duty and obligation. For the purposes of this chapter, it is enough to understand that health care professionals have duties and obligations that differ from the general population. There is a moral and legal duty and obligation to the patient. In day-to-day discussion, the words *duty* and *obligation* are not heard often, but surgical technologists will be held accountable for their actions. This means that each individual's actions are counted or evaluated against a standard of practice. Accountability for the surgical technologist extends beyond the OR and interacts with one's personal life.

Some simple illustrations demonstrate how the surgical technologist's professional obligations affect her personal life. We will list a few of these so the student can see the obvious effects and then discuss a few more subtle effects. Consider the following:

- The ST may be leaving the family at inconvenient times because of "on call" responsibilities.
- The ST cannot have a cocktail with friends because of "on call" responsibilities.
- The ST has a greater obligation to protect him or herself from communicable disease than the general population.
- The ST will know details of other people's lives that cannot be shared with family and friends.
- The ST may find that most of the exciting "world of the OR" cannot be shared because others do not want to know about it.

These obvious examples of the interaction between personal and professional life illustrate two key principles:

1. Professional obligations take precedence over personal freedom in many instances.
2. The nature of the OR results in some isolation from the general population.

The first principle is easy to understand. The surgical technologist cannot act in such a way that increases the chance of injury to a patient and cannot afford to be mentally or physically impaired in any way. The surgical technologist must think about this and make adjustments to account for this obligation to be prepared to provide the best patient care possible. Generally, the adaptations are simple and easy to accept, but they can be problematic at times. Occasionally, the surgical technologist may not be able to do something with family or friends due to the nature of the profession.

JOB DESCRIPTIONS FOR THE SURGICAL TECHNOLOGIST

Role descriptions are by their very nature broad in scope. Job descriptions, however, are produced and approved by the facility for which one works. Depending on the type of job, they may be written fairly broadly but are usually quite specific. There is seldom a directly related statute that applies to the surgical technologist's job description. The job description is typically the work and property of the given facility in which the surgical technologist works. The surgical technologist should be familiar with the job description in the facility of employment.

Job descriptions provide a job title and definition, specified requirements for the job, duties and tasks to be performed, and designation of one's immediate supervisor and to whom one is accountable. Job descriptions are placed within the context of a facility's mission and a department's role in accomplishing that mission. Surgical technologists have traditionally been assigned to the nursing department when employed by a facility such as a hospital or ambulatory surgical center. With the increased use of private surgical technologists and the "traveling" surgical technologist, the employer may be a physician, a physician's group, or an agency. In some locales, a surgical technologist who is employed outside the facility is required to seek permission to function through the medical credentials committee. No matter the employment situation, the surgical technologist must be aware of the conditions of employment, the nature of the job, and the required tasks and specified limitations. The job description may establish the criteria by which the surgical technologist will be judged in a case concerning alleged negligence or malpractice.

The surgical technologist should identify the following components of the job description:

- Job title (e.g., surgical technologist level I)
- Requirements (e.g., graduation from an accredited program and national certification)
- Nature of position (e.g., the surgical technologist is a member of the intraoperative surgical team)
- Duties (e.g., the surgical technologist, level one, shall perform in the scrub role and shall be responsible for. . . .)
- Accountability (e.g., the surgical technologist shall be directly accountable to the director of surgical services)
- Immediate supervisor (e.g., the immediate supervisor for all surgical services personnel is the OR charge nurse)

Surgical technologists should keep a copy of the job description in their personal files and update it as necessary. Should the surgical technologist find any of the components of a standard job description to be missing from the institution's job description, it should be reported to the supervisor and included in the formal job description.

CAREER OPPORTUNITIES

Most surgical technologists are employed in hospital surgery departments, obstetric departments, and ambulatory care centers to perform in the scrub role. The roles of circulator and surgical assistant have also been introduced as career opportunities for the surgical technologist. In addition, the following employment options are also available to the experienced surgical technologist, some of which will require further education:

- Specialization in an area of interest (e.g., cardiac, orthopedic, pediatric)

- Private employment by a surgeon
- Employment as a traveling surgical technologist—to fill temporary staffing needs for health care facilities nationally and internationally
- Employment by a veterinary surgeon or animal care facility
- Employment by a medical corporation to represent its products
- Research and product development
- Employment in the material management or sterile processing areas (Figure 1-5)
- Assumption of supervisory responsibilities
- Surgical technology instructor (Figure 1-6)

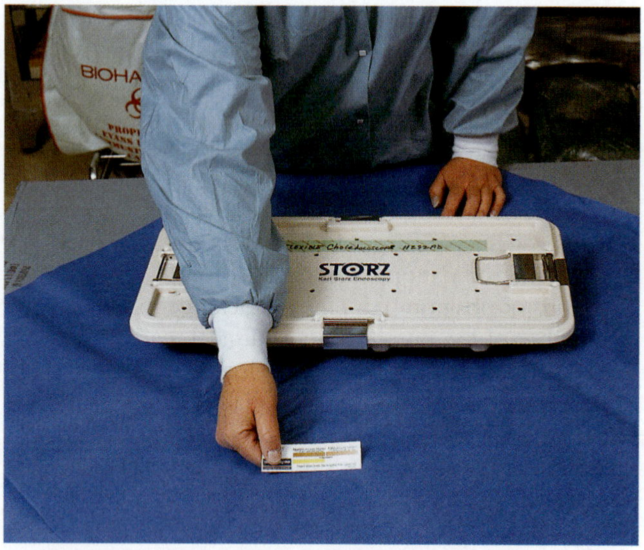

Figure 1-5 Surgical technologist preparing supplies for sterilization in the sterile processing department

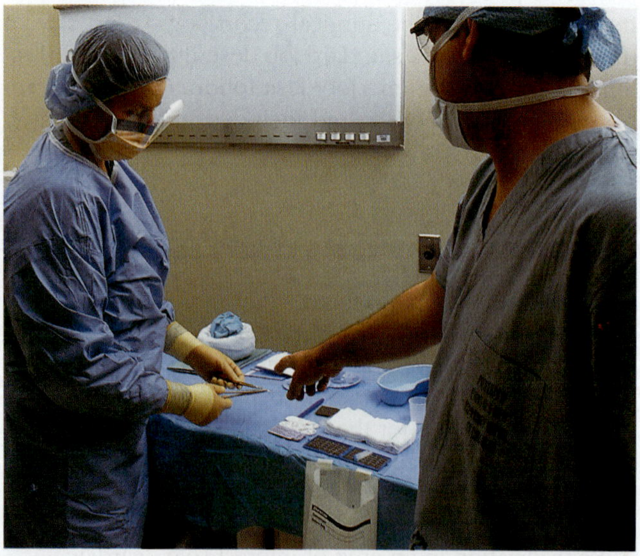

Figure 1-6 Surgical technology educator demonstrating the technique for placing a scalpel blade on a scalpel handle

- Military service
- Volunteer opportunities (e.g., Peace Corps)
- Technical writing, illustration, and photography
- Employment as a consultant

HEALTH CARE FACILITIES

Traditionally, surgical care was provided in a hospital, that is, a facility that provided many medical services. The types of hospitals were relatively few and their roles were clearly defined. These hospitals treated patients within the walls of their buildings. Health care has changed dramatically; even hospitals that still provide the traditional style of services look outside their walls to provide wellness care, education, home health care, and follow-up care. Surgical services, once restricted to a defined area within the hospital, are now provided in many different settings, including traditional ORs, free-standing **ambulatory surgical facilities**, free-standing specialty centers, doctor's offices, doctor's clinics, and labor and delivery units.

There are several ways to describe a hospital: ownership, profit philosophy, sources of revenue, and relationship to community needs. Some combination of these descriptors is needed to properly identify a given facility.

Commonly, reference has been made to three general types of hospitals: nonprofit (not-for-profit), **proprietary** (for profit), and tax supported.

A hospital is an organization with a governing body, medical staff, professional staff, and in-patient facilities. Hospitals provide medical, nursing, and related services on a permanent, around-the-clock basis. States may have varying legal definitions of a hospital as distinct from another health care organization for licensing purposes.

Not-for-profit hospitals are general, acute-care hospitals defined as nontaxable by the federal government. A private corporation owns these facilities. Profits are turned back into maintenance and improvement of the hospital, both its physical facilities and services. A community, church, or other organization that views its primary purpose as community service usually owns these facilities. Tax revenues may support some of them. In that case, the hospital is both tax supported and not-for-profit. A federal, state, county, or city hospital is an example.

Proprietary or investor-owned hospitals are owned and operated by an individual or corporation. The primary intent of these facilities is to provide good patient care. However, they differ from the nonprofit hospitals in that profits are returned to the investors. The profits are also taxable.

As mentioned above, any tax-levying entity might provide support for a hospital. These are less common in the current environment as governments at all levels are attempting to divest themselves of hospital ownership. Community agencies and organizations provide financial support through dispersal of private funds or grants.

In many hospitals, surgery may be performed in more than one setting. It is not uncommon for a hospital to have a traditional OR to serve in-patient needs, a free-standing surgical facility for out-patient surgery, separate rooms for cesarean sections, dilatation and curettage, and tubal ligation in the labor and delivery unit, and possibly a separate area for pediatric surgery. Even then surgical services are not limited to hospitals. Several other types of facilities provide surgical services.

The free-standing ambulatory surgical facility (ambulatory care center/"surgicenter") is physically or geographically separate from a hospital. It provides surgical services to patients who do not require hospitalization.

A health maintenance organization (**HMO**) is a health care organization that acts as both insurer and provider of medical services. The services provided are comprehensive but specified. A group of physicians, defined by contractual arrangement, provides services to a population of clients who are enrolled in the program. The HMO may require the clients to use a primary care physician for all referrals. This practitioner is sometimes called the *gatekeeper.*

A clinic is a facility or part of a facility designed for diagnosis and treatment of out-patients. Some clinics may perform a limited range of procedures. Some increase has been seen in clinics that specialize in one type of surgery. They are often exceptionally efficient and effective for their limited specialty. Like the clinic, certain procedures may be performed in the physician's office. Typically, a room is set aside within the office space for a limited range of procedures.

The surgical technologist should also remember that veterinarians provide a range of surgical services, too. Many veterinary colleges and animal care facilities are highly sophisticated in their surgical settings.

HOSPITAL ORGANIZATION

While recognizing that surgical services are provided outside the traditional hospital setting, most continue to have some features that resemble the traditional hospital organizational structure. With that in mind, we now look briefly at the way in which hospitals typically organize themselves.

Hospital philosophy and broad policy are typically established by a board of directors or a board of trustees. Given the type of hospital, these positions may result from election, appointment, or position. The board will hire a chief executive officer (CEO), whose job it is to put the philosophy and broad policy into practice (Figure 1-7).

Hospitals typically have several layers of administration. At the top administrative level, several vice presidents oversee broad areas. For example, each of the following areas might have a vice president assigned to it: administration, medical affairs, patient services, legal services, finances, and building and environment. Depending on the size of the hospital, these areas may be subdivided.

Typically, under medical affairs one finds a second division—medical staffing and nursing services. The physicians are organized under medical staffing. Frequently, all other nursing and allied health activities are organized under nursing services. However, there is considerable variance in this structure. The chief physician in the hospital for a given length of time is called the chief of staff. Medical services are also subdivided. Often there is a chief of medicine and a chief of surgery. These divisions are organized by specialty. In the case of surgery, one may find the surgical staff committee composed of one representative from each surgical specialty at the hospital. The representative of the specialty for a designated time is called, for example, the chief of orthopedics.

One of the functions of the medical staff committee is to verify the credentials of the physicians and specified health care personnel. The surgical technologist who is a CST/CFA may be required to submit an application for privileges to this committee.

Most hospitals place surgical technologists under nursing services. The director of nursing (DON) oversees nursing services. Nursing services is large and divided into subunits. Surgical services is one of those units, commonly referred to as a department. The director of surgical services represents the surgical nurses and allied health personnel at the nursing services meetings.

The surgical services department may also be divided into units. A head nurse oversees the day-to-day activity in the unit. Surgical specialty areas may have a coordinator. Sterile processing may be a separate unit with its own coordinator. These coordinators communicate needs, concerns, and decisions in their assigned areas.

In its day-to-day activities, surgeons, nursing personnel, anesthesia personnel, allied health personnel, and ancillary personnel staff the surgical services department.

Surgeons are medical doctors or doctors of osteopathy or podiatry who have completed a designated course of education and training and have surgical privileges. The surgeons have 4 years of college, 4 years of medical school, and 4–8 years of residency training in a surgical specialty. Most of the surgeons the surgical technologist works with are or will become board certified in their specialty.

The nursing staff a surgical technologist may work with consists of graduate nurses (GN), licensed practical/vocational nurses (LPN/LVN), associate degree registered nurses (ADN), bachelor's degree registered nurses (BSN), or registered nurses holding a master's or doctoral degree. Some of the nurses may hold a voluntary credential, CNOR (Certified Nurse Operating Room). The AORN awards this certification to applicants who meet its criteria, which include the passing of a certification examination. Today, one may see the credential CRNFA. This credential is awarded to the registered nurse who has passed prescribed criteria as a surgical assistant.

The anesthesia staff may include anesthesiologists (MD/DO), certified registered nurse anesthetists (CRNA), an anesthesiologist's assistant (AA), and anesthesia technicians. The anesthesiologist is a physician who has been through a residency program in anesthesia. Like the surgeon, the anesthesiologist may be board certified. The CRNA is a

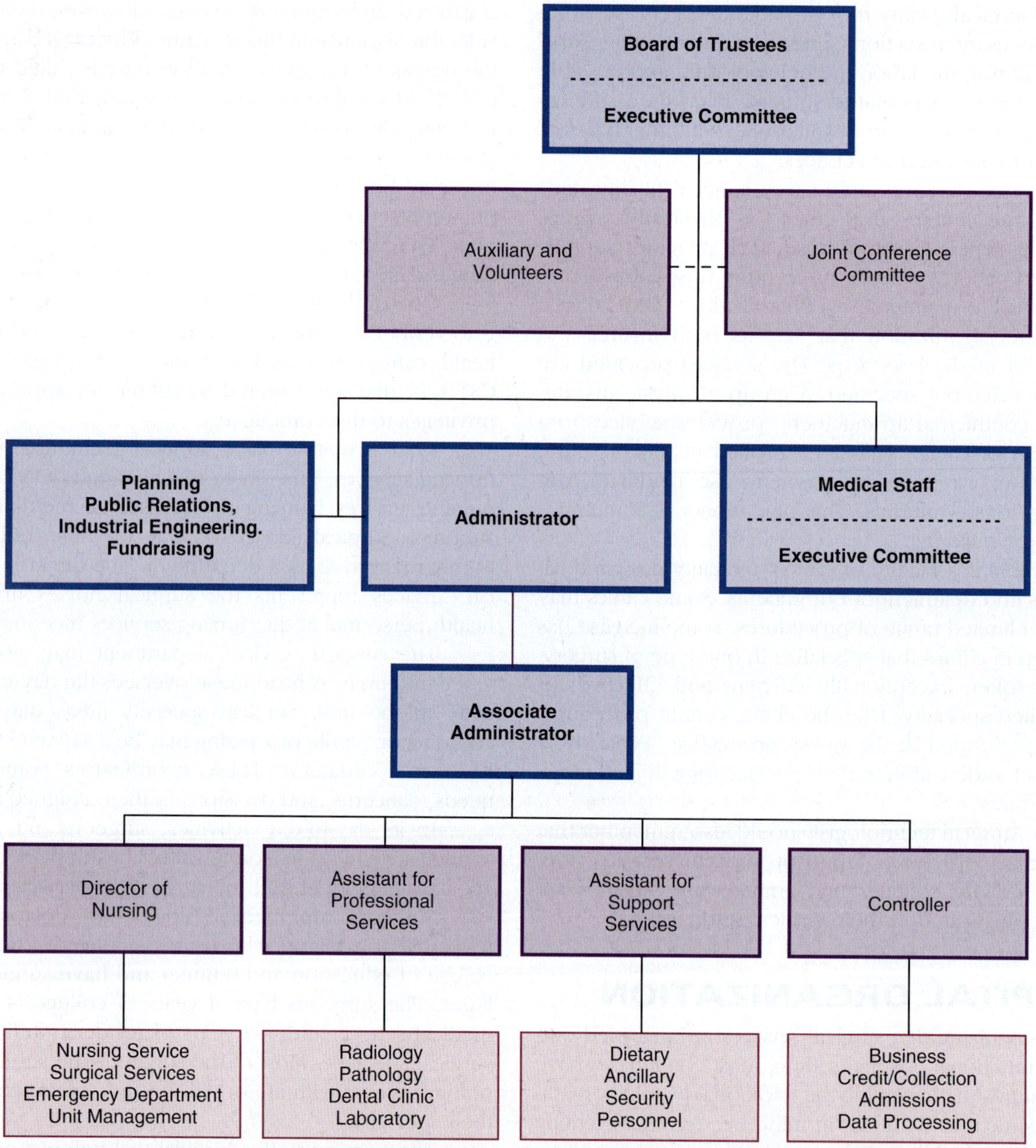

Figure 1-7 Sample hospital organization chart

registered nurse with several years of experience in critical care nursing and specialty training in anesthesia. The anesthesiologist's assistant is an allied health professional who works under the direction of an anesthesiologist. The tasks performed vary but may include collecting preoperative data, assisting with the insertion of intravenous (IV) and arterial catheters, assistance with airway management, and other tasks for which the AA is approved. The anesthesia technician supports the anesthesiologist and CRNA by caring for equipment and supplies. The anesthesia technician may be trained to assist in certain specified procedures performed by the anesthesiologist or CRNA.

A growing number of physician assistants (PA) are seen in the operating room. These are allied health personnel who have bachelor's or master's degrees. PA programs are usually 20–24 months long and often are affiliated with a medical school. The PA is a physician extender. One may see the PA in the role of surgical assistant or communicating with the physician about other patients under the physician's care.

There may be representatives of several different allied health fields in the OR. The various roles performed by the surgical technologist have been discussed above. It is not uncommon to see the following allied health personnel in the OR: diagnostic imaging technician, perfusionist, cell saver technician, bioelectrical technician, medical laboratory technician, and orthopedic and ophthalmic technician.

HOSPITAL DEPARTMENTS AND INTERDEPARTMENTAL COMMUNICATION

The surgical services department and the operating room team do not work in a vacuum. Many related departments and personnel are involved in patient care and safety in a modern hospital. There are several ways one might organize this information. The most common method is to categorize the hospital departments as having direct or indirect patient care responsibilities. The following departments have direct patient care responsibilities:

- Nursing care units (e.g., medical-surgical units, critical care units)
- Diagnostic imaging (e.g., radiology, computerized axial tomography, magnetic resonance imaging, and sonography)
- Medical laboratory (includes clinical laboratories, pathology, and blood bank)
- Pharmacy
- Physical and occupational therapy

Departments that contribute to patient care through secondary means include:

- Hospital administration
- Hospital maintenance services
- Housekeeping services
- Food services
- Purchasing and central supply
- Medical records

Tables 1-4 and 1-5 may help the student understand the position of the departments in the hospital and their service to the patient.

The department of surgical services has daily contact with most, if not all, departments of the hospital.

Table 1-4 Direct Patient Care Departments

DEPARTMENT	HOSPITAL ADMINISTRATOR	DIRECT OVERSIGHT	CONTRIBUTION
Nursing care units	Director of nursing	Charge nurse	Direct nursing care
Diagnostic imaging	Contracted physician, contracted company	Radiologist	Diagnostic support for all departments
Medical laboratory	Contracted physician, contracted company	Pathologist	Diagnostic support for all departments
Pharmacy	Hospital administrator	Pharmacist	Chemical intervention advice and control for all departments
Physical/occupational therapy	Varies	Therapist	Rehabilitation services

Table 1–5 Indirect Patient Care Departments

DEPARTMENT	HOSPITAL ADMINISTRATOR	DIRECT OVERSIGHT	CONTRIBUTION
Administration	Chief executive officer	Vice president of area	Fiscal and policy oversight
Maintenance	Vice president of physical environment	Shift supervisor	Care and maintenance of the physical plant
Housekeeping	Vice president of physical environment	Shift supervisor	Daily upkeep of rooms and furniture, including patient rooms
Food services	Vice president of food services	Chef/dietitian/ supervisor	Food preparation for patients, family, and staff
Purchasing/central services	Vice president of finances	Purchasing agent	Control, purchase, storage, and dispersal of equipment and supplies
Medical records	Varies	Supervisor	Maintains all legal records of patient care

Table 1-6 Special Relationships

DEPARTMENT	SURGICAL SERVICES INTERACTIONS OR RELATIONSHIP
Nursing care units	Patient preparation Informed consent Transportation of patient to and from unit to OR Coordination of information for family Postoperative recovery and care (Several units may be specialty units, such as orthopedics.)
Diagnostic imaging	Preoperative diagnostic studies Communication of studies and diagnostic findings to OR Intraoperative studies Stereotactic assistance Postoperative studies
Medical laboratory	Preoperative diagnostic studies Communication of studies and diagnostic findings to OR Intraoperative studies (e.g., blood gases, electrolytes) Blood replacement Pathological studies (e.g., frozen section) Postoperative studies
Pharmacy	Control of routine medication stock Response to special needs Response to emergency needs
Physical/occupational therapy	Rehabilitation (may begin in the postanesthesia care unit)
Maintenance and biomed	Control of physical environment Repair of broken equipment Safety checks
Housekeeping	Typically has personnel assigned only to the OR General housekeeping tasks
Purchasing/central services	Execution of surgical services equipment and supply needs Typically has a central sterile supply unit Oversees sterilization needs May perform basic case cart preparation Restocking of basic supplies for OR
Medical records	Transcription of history and physical Maintains and verifies all patient records Requires proper signatures May provide past medical information when needed
Administration	Budget Human resources Policies and procedures

Some special relationships may exist based on the type of service supplied by the department or their relationship to the patients in surgery. Typical interactions are defined in Table 1-6.

Each department must communicate with the other departments. Patient safety and hospital efficiency and effectiveness are related to the consistency and clarity with which these communications are carried out. Each department will have needs specific to its activities. Hospital departments communicate through several means: medical records, requisitions for services, computer records and requisitions, verbal communication (telephone and individual to individual), and through hospital education sessions. Surgical technologists must be familiar with the systems, policies, and procedures of the hospital in which they are employed. They must know the forms that are used daily in surgical services and their role and responsibility in relation to each.

FINANCIAL CONSIDERATIONS AND REIMBURSEMENT

Surgical intervention is expensive. In some instances, surgical intervention is provided free of charge. These instances invariably represent special cases. For instance, it has become a fairly common practice for a group of surgeons in a related field to give a portion of their time to treating children whose families lack the resources to secure treatment otherwise. By far, the most common situation is that surgery is performed on a fee-for-service basis. Given the nature of federal and state assistance in the United States, some funding is available most of the time for even the least financially prepared patient. The most common situation exists when both the patient and his or her insurer contribute payment for the services rendered.

Insurance designates a contractual relationship and mutual benefit that exists when one party or entity agrees to pay another for a specified loss or condition. In an insurance situation, the first party is the insurer and the second the insured. The contract is the agreed-on insurance policy. The insured pays a fee to the insurer on an ongoing basis, and the insurer covers an agreed amount of loss should the contingencies described in the policy occur. For our purpose, health insurance covers the insured when disease or trauma results in the use of medical services for which there is a fee. For many years, the most common type of insurance policy was an agreement between a private citizen and a private company. The company agreed to pay for medical and surgical intervention under certain specified conditions. This was called *private insurance*. Sometimes this same arrangement was negotiated between a business and an insurer for the benefit of the employee. The employee may or may not have paid the insurance premium directly, but the mechanism for payment for medical or surgical services was essentially the same as for private insurance.

Private insurance still exists and reimburses hospitals, physicians, and other health care professionals for their services. However, most health care coverage today comes from a different type of agreement (e.g., HMO, preferred provider organization [PPO]) than that used for the traditional private insurance. A number of different types of programs are available, but all seek to control costs through contractual arrangements with the health care providers (hospitals and physicians), limiting payment to an agreed-on amount. Furthermore, the aging culture and the availability of government-sponsored funding in the form of Medicare and Medicaid have significantly changed the way health care is financed in the United States today.

Medicare is a program administered by the federal government through the Centers for Medicare and Medicaid Services (CMS). Medicare provides reimbursement to both hospitals and physicians for the following categories:

- Qualifying people 65 years of age and older
- People eligible for Social Security disability payments for at least 2 years
- Certain workers and their families who require kidney dialysis or transplantation

In Medicare terminology, Part A refers to the hospital insurance, and Part B is supplemental and covers physicians and other services.

Medicaid is a government assistance program that is funded jointly by the state and federal government. Medicaid reimburses hospitals and physicians for services rendered to low-income persons who cannot finance their own medical care. Medicaid requires that the insured meet a means test.

HMOs and PPOs provide both the insurance coverage and a designated range of medical services. They work with a system called *capitation payments*. A set of contracted physicians provides services to the enrollees. The fees charged for the physician's services are predetermined and established in the contract. Access to some providers, medications, and procedures may be restricted. Most commonly, a family physician serves as a *gatekeeper*, that is, a first-level practitioner who determines whether or not a referral to a specialist or use of a given diagnostic test will be authorized.

In 1983, the federal government created a system under the Social Security Amendments that established a different model by which reimbursements to hospitals would be calculated. This system was called the *diagnosis-related groups* (DRGs). Prior to this, hospital reimbursement was calculated on a system referred to as *reasonable cost*. This system essentially allowed a fee to be set if the hospital could justify it based on reasonable cost. The new model was based on a *prospective payment system*. Under this system the amount paid is based on the average cost for treating a given condition and the DRG into which the patient is discharged. For example, if the average cost of treating acute cholelithiasis is $5,000, then the hospital is reimbursed $5,000 for patient A and patient B even if patient B is in the hospital 5 days longer. The DRG system is mandated for Medicare payment.

The impact of governmental financial assistance, DRGs, and the HMO type of coverage has changed health care significantly in the past decade. The cost of health care is high. Americans demand high quality and high technology. The surgical technologist and every member of the surgical team must develop both a cost awareness and a quality conscience in order to guarantee every patient the best care possible.

ORGANIZATIONS RELATED TO HOSPITALS, HEALTH CARE, AND SURGICAL SERVICES

There are many organizations, agencies, associations, and businesses that affect hospitals and health care service providers, including these:

Governmental

- Department of Health and Human Services (DHHS)—a department of the executive branch of the federal government with broad responsibility in the area of health care
- Public Health Service (PHS)—a component of DHHS that promotes physical and mental health
- Centers for Medicare & Medicaid Services (CMS)—formerly known as Health Care Financing Administration (HCFA), a component of DHHS that administers the Medicare and part of the Medicaid program
- Social Security Administration (SSA)—a component of DHHS that administers a national program of contributory social insurance involving employers, employees, and the self-employed
- World Health Organization (WHO)—a division of the United Nations that promotes health activities worldwide
- Various state, county, and city health departments—government groups that administer health policy for the political unit it oversees

Private Volunteer Agencies

- American Cancer Society—volunteer organization supporting research and education in cancer prevention, diagnosis, and treatment
- American Diabetes Association—volunteer organization supporting research and education in the field of diabetes
- American Heart Association—volunteer organization supporting research and education in the prevention, diagnosis, and treatment of heart disease
- American Red Cross—a humanitarian organization that provides relief to victims of disaster and other emergencies

Accrediting Agencies

- Joint Commission on Accreditation of Healthcare Organizations (JCAHO)—an independent, nonprofit national organization that develops standards and performance criteria for health care organizations, including hospitals, psychiatric facilities, substance abuse programs, long-term care facilities, and hospice care

Professional Associations

- American College of Surgeons (ACS)—a professional organization dedicated to the improvement of surgical care by elevating standards of surgical education and practice
- Association of Surgical Technologists (AST)—a professional organization of surgical technologists dedicated to the improvement of quality patient care in the surgical setting by elevating the standards of surgical technology education and practice
- Association of Operative Registered Nurses (AORN)—a professional organization of OR nurses dedicated to the improvement of patient care by elevating educational standards and practice for surgical nurses

The student should be aware that each surgical specialty has its own representative organization. All of these organizations work together through various joint committees and efforts to promote quality care for the surgical patient.

CASE STUDY

Ian is a surgical technologist at a busy metropolitan hospital. He has several years of experience and often serves as a **preceptor** (a surgical technologist employed by the hospital or surgery center that trains the students during their clinical rotation) for surgical technology students from the local community college. A new student is observing Ian. On this day, he is assisting the registered nurse in a room dedicated to orthopedic surgery. They have just completed positioning the patient, and the registered nurse asks Ian if he will "prep" the patient's leg while she performs the final checks of the video monitors.

1. What role is being performed by Ian? Are there any restrictions to the role?
2. Describe the various roles of the OR team members and state how they interrelate.

QUESTIONS FOR FURTHER STUDY

1. What is the difference between a job description and the role description?
2. How does health care financing affect the services that health care professionals provide?
3. List several reasons why a surgical technologist might need to communicate with the diagnostic imaging department, medical laboratory department, or a medical-surgical floor nurse.
4. Describe a "typical" workday for the surgical technologist.
5. Define the term *competency* as it relates to the role of the surgical technologist.
6. In addition to the traditional role of the surgical technologist in the surgical setting, list at least two other related employment options.

BIBLIOGRAPHY

Bell, J., Caruthers, B. L., Hunter, M. A., Kalush, S., May, M., Olmsted, J., & Santaniello, N. (2002). *Core curriculum for surgical assisting*. Centennial, CO: Association of Surgical Technologists.

Bilchik, G. (1998, May 20). When the saints go marching out. Is American health care losing its religion? *Hospitals and Health Networks*, pp. 37–42.

Caruthers, B. L. (1999). *History of surgery* [CD-ROM]. Centennial, CO: Association of Surgical Technologists.

Clendening, L. (1942). *Source book of medical history*. New York: Dover.

Cragg, G. R. (1960). *The church and the age of reason 1648–1789*. New York: Penguin Books.

Eiseley, L. (1961). *Darwin's century*. New York: Anchor Books.

Ginsberg, F. (1983, January/February). *Surgical technical aide—instructor's manual reference journal*.

Greene, J. (1998, April 20). Blue skies or black eyes? Hedis puts not-for-profit plans on top. *Hospitals and Health Networks*, pp. 27–30.

Haugh, R. (1998, June 5). Who's afraid of capitation now? *Hospitals and Health Networks*, pp. 30–37.

Holmes, G. (1962). *The latter Middle Ages, 1272–1485*. New York: W. W. Norton.

Lyons, A. S., & Petrucelli, R. J. (1978). *Medicine: An illustrated history*. New York: Abradale.

Mayr, E. (1982). *The growth of biological thought*. Cambridge, MA: Belknap.

McGuiness, A. M., et al. (2002). *Core curriculum for surgical technology* (5th ed.). Centennial, CO: Association of Surgical Technologists.

McKeon, R. (Ed.). (1947). *Introduction to Aristotle*. New York: Modern Library.

Nichols, M. L. (Ed.). (1995). *Surgical technologist certifying exam study guide*. Centennial, CO: Association of Surgical Technologists.

Nuland, S. B. (1989). *Doctors: The biography of medicine*. New York: Vintage Books.

O'Leary, M. R. (1994). *Lexikon: Dictionary of health care terms, organizations and acronyms for the era of reform*. Oakbrook Terrace, IL: Joint Commission on Accreditation of Healthcare Organizations.

Reaves, R. P. (1984). *The law of professional licensing and certification*. Charlotte, NC: Publications for Professionals.

Serb, C. (1998, July 20). Is remaking the hospital making money? *Hospitals and Health Networks*, pp. 32–33.

CHAPTER 2

Standards of Conduct

Bob Caruthers
Paul Price

CASE STUDY

Bret, a surgical technologist, has been asked by the surgeon to inject contrast medium into the cystic duct during an open cholecystectomy.

1. What scope of practice issues can you identify?
2. Is this act any different from injecting a medication into an IV? If so, how?
3. What do you think Bret should do in this situation?
4. How do you think the surgeon may respond if Bret refuses?
5. How can Bret know if he should perform this act?

OBJECTIVES

After studying this chapter, the reader should be able to:

C
1. Analyze major concepts inherent in professional practice law.
2. Interpret the legal responsibilities of the surgical technologist and other surgical team members.
3. Analyze the American Hospital Association's Patient's Bill of Rights.
4. Describe the need for professional liability insurance policies.

A
5. Analyze the key elements related to developing a surgical conscience.

R
6. Assess the resources that aid the surgical technologist in interpreting and following professional standards of conduct.
7. Develop an increased sensitivity to the influence of ethics in professional practice.
8. Analyze the role of morality during ethical decision making.

9. Cite examples of ethical situations and problems in the health professions.
10. Analyze scope of practice issues as they relate to surgical technology.
11. Evaluate the role of the risk management department in the health care facility.

E 12. Apply principles of problem solving in ethical decision making.

13. Assess errors that may occur in the operating room and devise a plan for investigation, correction, and notification.

SELECT KEY TERMS

1. abandonment
2. accreditation
3. advance directive
4. affidavit
5. bioethics
6. clinical ladder program
7. code of ethics
8. credentialing
9. deontological approach
10. ethics
11. formalism
12. incident report
13. informed consent
14. job description
15. liability
16. malpractice
17. moral principles
18. negligence
19. Patient's Bill of Rights
20. risk management
21. Safe Medical Device Act
22. scope of practice
23. surgical conscience
24. tort law
25. utilitarianism

LEGAL ISSUES

In the health care environment, there is considerable agreement over basic values and their applications for patient care. The laws, standards, and guidelines developed for health care practice reflect these basic values. As one becomes more specific (e.g., a given law or a given case) disagreement may grow, but the general intent of health care legislation has been accepted for many years, and is reflected in the **Patient's Bill of Rights**, which is discussed later in the chapter. These rights reflect a generally accepted view of the patient as an autonomous individual who is in need of a service that he or she cannot provide for himself or herself.

This chapter explores legal aspects of health care and the ethical and moral behavior necessary for proper patient care. **Risk management** procedures and scope of practice concepts are also explored. To understand some of the concepts related to legal aspects in medicine, the surgical technologist should be familiar with basic legal terminology and procedures.

DEFINITIONS OF GENERAL LEGAL TERMS

Accountability—the obligation to disclose details for evaluation; commonly used to mean "to be held responsible for"

Affidavit—voluntary statement of facts sworn to be true before an authority

Allegation—a statement one expects to prove true

Assault—intentional act intended to make another person fearful

Battery—intentional nonconsensual touching

Bona fide—in good faith or innocently

Case law—all legal decisions reported on a given legal subject

Complaint—first pleading filed by plaintiff's attorney in a **negligence** action

Defamation—injury to an individual's reputation or

character caused by false statements to a third party (inclusive of libel and slander)

Defendant—in criminal cases, the person accused of the crime; in civil matters, the person or organization that is being sued

Deposition—a method of pretrial discovery in which questions are answered under oath

Federal law—jurisdiction is given to federal courts in cases involving the interpretation and application of the U.S. Constitution, acts of Congress, and treaties

Guardian—court-appointed protector for an individual incapable of making his or her own decisions

Iatrogenic injury—an injury resulting from the activity of health care professionals

Indictment—formal written accusation from a grand jury

Jury—a group of citizens who decide the outcome of a criminal or civil trial

Larceny—taking another's property without consent

Law, common—principles that have evolved and continue to evolve on the basis of court decisions

Law, statutory—any law prescribed by the action of a legislature

Liability—an obligation to do or not do something; also, an obligation potentially or actually incurred as a result of a negligent act

Liability, corporate—an obligation to do or not do something that falls on the corporate body

Liability, personal—an obligation to do or not do something that falls on the individual

Malpractice—professional misconduct that results in harm to another; negligence of a professional

Negligence—omission (not doing) or commission (doing) of an act that a reasonable and prudent individual would not do under the same conditions; may be associated with the phrase "departure from the standard of care"

Negligence, criminal—reckless disregard for the safety of another; willful indifference

Perjury—intentionally providing false testimony under oath

Plaintiff—the person who initiates a lawsuit

Precedent—legal principle, created by a court decision, which provides an example or authority for judges deciding similar issues later

Standard of care—description of conduct that is expected of an individual or professional in a given circumstance

State law—state statutes, regulations, and principles and rules having the force of law

Subpoena—court order to appear and testify or produce required documents

Tort—a civil wrong; may be intentional or unintentional

Tort-feasor—one who commits a tort

Trial—consists of the following steps:

1. Opening statements by both sides
2. Plaintiff's presentation
3. Cross-examination by defendant's attorney
4. Defendant's presentation
5. Cross-examination by plaintiff's attorney
6. Closing statements by both sides
7. Jury instruction by judge
8. Jury deliberation
9. Verdict
10. Appeal (possible)
11. Execution of judgment

DEFINITIONS OF TRADITIONAL PRINCIPLES

Ager primo—"The patient first" (motto of the AST).

Doctrine of borrowed servant—The one controlling or directing the employee has greater responsibility than the one paying the employee. Courts frequently found that the surgeon was liable for any negligent act committed in his or her presence in the operating room under the *captain of the ship* doctrine. However, recent rulings have found that the surgeon, under the *borrowed servant* rule, is not always responsible if a surgical technologist or registered nurse on the surgical team fails to carry out a routine procedure that he or she was properly educated to perform.

Doctrine of corporate negligence—A health institution may be negligent for failing to ensure that an acceptable level of patient care was provided. This means that potential employees and medical staff should be screened in accordance with standards set by the accrediting body, and that competent staff should be maintained and monitored for proper performance.

Doctrine of foreseeability—Foreseeability is the ability to see or know in advance; the ability to reasonably anticipate that harm or injury may result because of certain acts or omissions. Some would say that the courts do not demand that you possess mind-reading skills but they do expect you to anticipate risks to participants reasonably.

Doctrine of personal liability—Each person is responsible for his or her own tortuous conduct, even though others may be liable as well; for example, an authority figure such as a physician assures the medical professional that he or she will take responsibility for an action; the health professional is still responsible.

Doctrine of the reasonably prudent man—A person should perform an action as would any reasonable person of ordinary prudence. In law, the reasonable person is not an average person or a typical person but a composite of the community's judgment as to how the typical community member should behave in situations that might pose a threat of harm to the public. A standard of conduct is not established simply because the majority of people in the community behave in a certain way.

Primum non nocere—"Above all, do no harm."

Res ipsa loquitur—"The thing speaks for itself;" harm obviously came from a given act or thing of which the defendant had sole control.

Respondeat superior—"Let the master answer;" employer is responsible for the actions of his or her employees.

TORTS

Tort law evolved in the Middle Ages (*tort* is from the Latin *tortus*, meaning "twisted") and describes any civil wrong independent of a contract. Tort law provides a remedy in the form of an action for damages. Most actions against operating room personnel are civil actions rather than criminal and may be either intentional or unintentional.

INTENTIONAL TORTS

Intentional acts are willful and violate the civil rights of a patient. These types of torts include:

Assault—an act that causes another person to fear that he or she will be touched in an offensive, insulting, or physically injurious manner without consent or authority to do so

Battery—the actual act of harmful or unwarranted contact with a person, including contact without proper consent

Defamation—slander (oral statement) or libel (written statement) that damages a person's reputation or good name

False imprisonment—illegal detention of a person without consent (e.g., use of restraints), or forcing a person to stay in an area by not allowing him or her to leave

Intentional infliction of emotional distress—disparaging remarks made about a patient that result in emotional distress

Invasion of privacy—disclosure of private information concerning a patient or photographing a patient without consent

An intentional tort requires proof of the willful action of the following three elements:

1. The defendant's action was intended to interfere with the plaintiff or plaintiff's property.
2. The consequences of the act were also intended.
3. The act was a substantial factor in bringing about the consequences.

UNINTENTIONAL TORTS

In spite of the surgical team's best efforts, individuals make mistakes. Unintentional torts are the most common types of patient indiscretions committed by operating room personnel, and include negligence and malpractice. *Malpractice* is the term used to describe the behavior of a professional person's wrongful conduct; in fact, a negligent act committed by surgical personnel is called *malpractice*.

Negligence is a breach of duty. It is defined as an omission (not doing) or commission (doing) of an act that a reasonable and prudent individual would not do under the same conditions. It may be associated with the phrase "departure from the standard of care." To establish negligence, a plaintiff must prove that the defendant had a duty to the plaintiff, the defendant breached that duty by failing to conform to the required standard of conduct, the defendant's negligent conduct was the cause of the harm to the plaintiff, and the plaintiff was, in fact, harmed or damaged.

If an individual engages in an activity requiring special skills, education, or experience, such as working in an operating room, the standard by which his or her conduct is measured is the conduct of a reasonably skilled, competent, and experienced person who is a qualified member of the group authorized to engage in that activity. In other words, the hypothetical reasonable person is a skilled, competent, and experienced person who engages in the same activity.

The following lists some of the errors and incidents that occur in the operating room:

- *Patient misidentification*—Check and cross-check procedures should be in place to prevent patient misidentification. All patients that enter the OR should have an identification (ID) band firmly attached to their wrists. Transportation personnel should always check the ID band before the patient leaves the unit. The preoperative holding area nurse should check the ID band and compare it to the chart when the patient arrives (the patient should be asked to repeat his or her name to verify identification with the wristband). The circulator and anesthesia provider are the next to verify patient identity in the same manner before taking the patient to the operating room, and the surgeon should do the same as he enters the room. Each cross-check ensures that the patient undergoing the surgical procedure is the correct patient.

- *Performing an incorrect procedure (often related to limbs)*—The surgical team must take great precautions to prevent the removal of the wrong body part or to prevent performing any surgical procedure on the wrong side or area. Identification of the correct limb and/or surgical site should be verbally confirmed by the patient. Some facilities even ask the patient to mark the correct extremity or area with a permanent marker. (All parties should agree that the mark made indicates the affected side and not the unaffected side to avoid confusion.) Information in the patient's chart should be checked by the circulator, anesthesia provider, and surgeon to verify the correct area or side. Diagnostic tests (especially X-rays, CT, or MRI scans) should be checked by the surgeon and surgical assistant and the proper area or side confirmed before the incision is made.
- *Foreign bodies left in patients secondary to incorrect sponge/instrument counts*—The circulator and STSR should count instruments, sponges, needles, tips for the electrosurgical pencil, blades, and any other items that hospital policy specifies for counting before the procedure begins, at the time that wound closure begins, and during skin closure. Although the surgeon, circulator, and surgical technologist each play an equal role in the counting procedure and share that responsibility, any one or all of them can be held liable for a foreign object left in a patient postoperatively because of an error.
- *Patient burns*—Burn wounds occur when there is contact between tissue and energy sources, such as heat, electrical current, radiation, or chemicals. Burns in the operating room can occur from the following situations:
  - Hot instruments from a steam autoclave (The surgical technologist is responsible for cooling the instrument with cool sterile water before use.)
  - Improper placement of the dispersive electrode for the electrosurgical unit (Placement is typically the responsibility of the circulator.)
  - Malfunctioning of the electrosurgical unit (The unit should be tested for proper functioning before the procedure begins.)
  - Other electrical device malfunctions (Electrical equipment must be properly grounded to reduce the risk of burns and should be tested frequently.)
  - Improper use of lasers (Special endotracheal tubes are required to prevent laryngeal injury. Wet towels may be placed around an operative area to prevent burns from an improperly discharged laser beam.)
  - Pooled flammable prep solutions
  - Flammable anesthesia gases
  - Irrigation fluid that is too hot

  Liability for malfunctioning equipment typically lies with the institution, whereas liability for improper procedures with the equipment lies with specific surgical personnel.
- *Falls or positioning errors resulting in patient injury*—Unattended patients can fall from a stretcher that has its side rails down, and patients can also fall when being transferred to the operating table from the transportation stretcher if safe procedures for transfer are not followed. A safety strap should be applied as soon as the patient is moved to the operating table to prevent a fall. Nerve, skin, joint, and vascular injuries can occur due to incorrect positioning or padding after the patient is anesthetized. Adequate support is necessary and pressure points should be properly padded. The anesthetized patient cannot report to the team that a position is causing pain, so constant vigilance and an understanding of proper positioning techniques with proper support are imperative. Each member of the team can be charged with negligence if an injury occurs due to improper positioning, although many negligent cases have been decided against the surgeon, who should supervise the positioning personally. The anesthesia provider and the surgeon may both be responsible for positioning that compromises respiration or circulation and results in injury.
- *Improper handling, identification, or loss of specimens*—Negligence occurs if a specimen is lost, improperly prepared or "fixed" for analysis, or inaccurately labeled. Loss of a specimen would prevent diagnosis and may require another surgical procedure, as could improper specimen preparation for lab analysis. The surgical team must understand the difference between frozen and permanent specimen preparation and handling, and the surgical technologist should always accurately report the specimen location and type to the circulator.
- *Incorrect drugs or incorrect administration*—To reduce the risk of incorrect administration or use of

an incorrect drug, the circulator and STSR must follow hospital policy for transfer of drugs to the sterile field (refer to "Transfer of a Medication to the Sterile Field" in Chapter 9). If the STSR has more than one drug on the back table, the drugs should be separated and labeled, preferably in two different types of containers. The surgeon is seldom liable for an incorrect drug handed to her during the procedure (the STSR should announce to the surgeon the name and strength of the drug as it is passed), but the STSR and the circulator share equal responsibility for transfer of a drug to the sterile field.

- *Harm secondary to use of defective equipment/instrument*—Malfunctioning equipment and instrumentation can cause injury to a surgical patient. Manufacturer's recommendations for service and operation should always be followed. Many facilities have biomedical engineering departments that maintain surgical equipment. Instrumentation and power equipment (e.g., saws, drills, reamers) are maintained by the surgical staff (many facilities have instrument rooms for inspection and assembly) and sterile processing department staff. Electrical equipment must be properly grounded to reduce the risk of burns, and must be tested and maintained on a regular schedule. Liability for malfunctioning equipment and instrumentation typically lies with the institution if it can be proven that the equipment was not properly maintained and tested (refer to the later section in this chapter on the **Safe Medical Device Act** of 1990).
- *Loss of or damage to patient's property*—Surgical personnel can be held liable for the loss of a patient's personal property. A patient occasionally makes it to the surgical services department from the unit with personal property or prostheses, such as dentures, hearing aids, or glasses. Each item must be removed by the circulator or holding area nurse and placed in a protective container that is clearly marked as property of the patient. The container should be placed with the patient's chart and sent along with the chart and patient to the postanesthesia care unit after completion of the procedure. The holding area nurse may want to send the property back to the patient's room before the patient is anesthetized and should follow proper hospital procedures for return of the item to the unit.
- *Harm secondary to a major break in sterile technique*—Improper practice of sterile technique can lead to a postoperative infection that can cause debilitation and even death. Because the source of an infection is difficult to establish without a given pattern (e.g., 15 postoperative infections have occurred in patients operated on during the day shift in OR 12), negligence is difficult to prove. Infections can also be caused by improper cleaning techniques or malfunctioning filtering mechanisms, also established through patterns of infection in specific areas. Malfunctioning sterilization units that are not properly sterilizing instruments and causing infections can be traced through recorded cycles and tested with biological indicators. Liability for malfunctioning equipment lies with the institution that did not properly service or test the items that caused the infection. The surgical technologist, through the application of a strong surgical conscience, should apply all principles of asepsis and should report any breaks that may occur to reduce the risk of postoperative infections.
- *Exceeding authority or accepted functions; violation of hospital policy*—Surgical technologists are negligent if they exceed the scope of practice that is defined by their education and experience and enforced through hospital policies designed to prevent malpractice. The surgical technologist should be aware of state medical practice acts, hospital policies, and scope of practice limitations. If the surgeon delegates a task to be performed by the STSR that is clearly within the **scope of practice** for surgical technology and is not prohibited by hospital policy or state law, then the surgeon accepts the responsibility for the correct performance of that task.
- *Abandonment of a patient*—If a member of the surgical team leaves a patient who is dependent on their presence as a caregiver, then the caregiver can be held liable for **abandonment**. The danger that harm could befall a patient who is not closely monitored is great because patients are often under the effects of medication and dependent on the caregiver for their safety. A confused patient could fall from an operating table or transportation stretcher or could suffer a seizure or cardiac arrest.

Prevention is truly the best medicine, and a vigilant surgical conscience would prevent every one of the incidents listed here. It is the moral and legal responsibility of everyone on the surgical team to render the best and safest care possible to the patient.

CONSENT FOR SURGERY: A BASIC RIGHT

The JCAHO's definition of a patient is as follows: "A person who receives health services from a health care provider and who gives *consent* for the provider to provide those services." Inherent in the definition of *patient* is the concept of personal decision. The right to make personal decisions extends from the concept of autonomy, and autonomy is central to the understanding of the patient in the Patient's Bill of Rights. Autonomy is the state of having control over one's life.

Consent is a term that refers to permission being given for an action. Proper consent requires that the party granting permission have the capability and authority to do so. Consent presumes that at least two individuals are involved. One is the proposed recipient of an action; the other will perform the action. Under the circumstances with which we are concerned, the authorized party is typically the patient. This may vary according to certain legal situations. In the case of a minor, for instance, the authorized party may be the parent. The individual performing the action is the health care provider. Consent, then, is a voluntary and informed act in which one party gives permission to another party to "touch." Given the nature of surgical intervention, surgical procedures are not performed without the written and **informed consent** of the patient except in a narrow range of legally defined situations. *Battery* is a legal term that refers to nonconsensual touching. To perform surgery without consent is to be liable to the charge of battery.

Consent may be given in either of two formats: express and implied. *Express consent* is a direct verbal or written statement granting permission for treatment. *Implied consent* is consent manifested by some action or inaction of silence, which raises a presumption that consent has been authorized. In health care, express consent in written form is the desired kind of consent.

INFORMED CONSENT

The requirement to obtain written, informed consent for all invasive procedures is an example of an action taken by the health care industry to protect both the patient and the health care provider. The JCAHO defines informed consent as "agreement or permission accompanied by full notice about what is being consented to." Expanding the definition to its use in tort law, the JCAHO says that informed consent refers to "the requirement that a patient be apprised of the nature and risks of a medical procedure before the physician or other health professional can validly claim exemption from liability for battery or from responsibility for medical complications and other undesirable outcomes."

Written, informed consent protects the patient in that it guarantees that the patient is aware of his or her condition, the proposed intervention, the risks, and variables that may occur. It is difficult to guarantee the concept of "informed" if one requires an *absolute* understanding of the condition, intervention, risks, and variables. Patients may be psychologically or educationally ill prepared to understand this information. Language and cultural differences may affect the understanding. Nevertheless, the best option exists when the health care providers follow the guidelines precisely. They can then verify an honest, good-faith effort to inform the patient, answer questions, and allow a free decision.

Two categories of consent are used in the hospital setting: general and special. On admission to the hospital, every patient signs a general consent for treatment. In this case, the patient consents to all routine services, general diagnostic procedures, medical treatment, and other normal and routine "touching" that may be expected to result from any hospitalization. The general consent is for treatment defined in its broadest form. General consent cannot be substituted for special consent. To do so is to sidestep the patient's right to make informed decisions. Special consent must be given for any procedure that entails a higher than normal risk—surgical procedures, fertility procedures, anesthesia, transfusion, chemotherapy, and participation in experimental programs. Special consent is the consent of the patient, preferably in written form, that relates directly to the subject of surgery. Note that verbal consent is as legally binding as written consent, but it is more difficult to prove in cases of disagreement.

The responsibility for securing written, informed surgical consent belongs to the surgeon. In practice, the surgeon will discuss the condition, proposed treatment, and risks with the patient and possibly family. Once agreement is reached, this communication is relayed to the nursing staff on the unit and the proper documents are prepared. The documents are then signed by the patient and witnessed and made part of the patient's record.

The physician's responsibility for securing an informed consent requires that the following conditions be met:

- Information must be given in understandable language.
- There can be no coercion or intimidation of the patient.
- The proposed surgical procedure or treatment must be explained.
- Potential complications must be explained.
- Potential risks and benefits must be explained.
- Alternative therapies and their risks and benefits must be explained.

Two of these items require brief elaboration. Because surgical patients vary in age, condition, psychological makeup, language usage, and cultural background, the amount and type of information supplied may vary from patient to patient.

A critical feature of informed consent is the language used. Even highly educated patients may have little experience with medical terminology. *Cholecystitis* may be meaningless to the patient, whereas *inflamed gallbladder* is understood clearly. All health care providers should accustom themselves to responding to patients with clear and understandable language.

More subtle, but equally important, is the tone of the presentation. Patients should not be made to feel as if they have no choice. This may become a critical factor if the patient is elderly, for instance, or if there is some disagreement within the family about a prospective treatment plan. The physician must carefully present the plan he or she thinks best but must not present it in such a way as to make the patient feel as if there are no other options.

A proper written, informed consent should contain the following information:

- Patient's legal name
- Surgeon's name
- Procedure to be performed
- Patient's legal signature
- Signature of witness(es)
- Date and time of signatures

The patient for whom a procedure is planned usually gives consent. In some instances, the patient may be physically unable or legally incompetent to give permission. If this situation arises under nonemergency conditions, another properly authorized individual must provide consent. The same guidelines for an informed consent apply to this individual.

The patient must be of legal age or a legally declared emancipated minor, mentally alert, legally competent, and not under the influence of drugs. The surgical consent must be signed prior to entry into surgery or the treatment area. Special circumstances such as illiteracy, sensory impairment, and emergency considerations may allow variances in procedure.

Informed consent may be given by any of the following under specific circumstances:

- A competent adult speaking for himself or herself
- Parent or legal guardian of a minor
- Guardian in the case of physical inability or legal incompetence
- Temporary guardian
- Hospital administrator
- The courts

In any situation resulting in a variance from the normal procedure for securing a consent, the consenting party or the witnesses required are determined by hospital policy. Emergency circumstances, for instance, may alter the consent process. Hospital policy dictates the methods for securing consent under these conditions, some of which include:

- Telephone
- Telegram
- Agreement of two consulting physicians (not to include the operating surgeon)
- Administrative consent

In each case, facility policy will dictate how many witnesses are required and how the verification will take place and be documented.

Under any conditions, facility policy may dictate the personnel within the facility who are authorized to witness a patient's consent. Typically, two witnesses are preferred. Witnesses may include:

- Physician/surgeon
- Registered nurse
- Other hospital employee

Implied consent is never the preferred option in a health care environment, but the law allows for implied consent in emergency situations when no other authorized person may be contacted. Implied consent may apply when conditions are discovered during a surgical procedure. Unconscious patients are presumed to have consented to appropriate medical treatment. For example, if the procedure performed extends beyond what is in the informed consent, the surgeon can be held liable for assault and battery unless it can be proven that good judgment was used when unexpected conditions were encountered. This is covered by the extension doctrine, which implies that the patient has given implicit consent for correction or treatment of pathologic conditions that were not expected or anticipated by the surgeon.

Once given, consent can be taken away. Patients have the right to change their minds and withdraw consent.

Any refusal to consent to a procedure or withdrawal of consent should be noted in the patient's medical record. If possible, a form releasing the hospital and the health care team from responsibility for the decision should be signed and placed in the patient's medical record.

DOCUMENTATION

In the health care field, the term *documentation* is used broadly to refer to the placing of information into a patient's medical record (chart). The medical record is the combined account of the interaction between the patient and the health care providers during a given incidence of illness or treatment. The medical record will typically include:

- Identification of the patient
- Identification of the physician(s), nurse(s), and other health care providers involved in the patient's care (e.g., the OR record will name each member of the surgical team)
- Patient's medical history and physical examination
- Diagnosis
- Treatment plan, details, and results
- Medication record
- Physical findings during the hospital stay
- Discharge condition
- Possible follow-up treatment plan

Anything of clinical significance should be recorded in the chart so that anyone who is involved with patient care can provide for continuity. Events should only be recorded after the fact. For legal purposes, the chart can be used to discover the source of a negligent act.

The hospital has a medical records department. The personnel there are involved with transcribing, collecting, reviewing, and verifying the medical records.

In the case of the surgical patient, special documentation is required that is focused on the surgical intervention and recovery. Prior to surgery, every patient must have a history and physical record in his or her medical record and an informed consent for the surgery. All of the patient's personal physical data, the surgical procedure, anesthetic procedure, responses to these, and postanesthesia care are placed in the patient's medical record. There are different styles of operative patient records, but the record always includes information about the surgical team, patient's condition before, during, and after surgery, time of initiation and termination of the procedure, documentation of counts, information concerning drains and dressings, and so forth. Some facilities may use separate count sheets for monitoring sponges, sharps, and instruments. If so, these sheets may become part of the record. Since most procedures produce a specimen of some sort and/or require intraoperative clinical laboratory studies, pathology and laboratory forms will be used for interdepartmental communication and will become part of the medical record. The anesthesia team will maintain an anesthesia record.

Most hospitals have a mechanism for reporting incidents related to any adverse patient occurrence. The effectiveness of **incident reports** is somewhat limited because of fear of punitive action aimed at the reporter, lack of understanding, and lack of time. Incident reports constitute much of the information used by the hospital in risk management. Risk management is the effort by the hospital to collect and utilize data to decrease the chance of harm to patients and staff or damage to property.

Hospitals are mandated to report certain items to other authorities, such as the following:

- Diseases of the neonate
- Child abuse
- Elder abuse
- Communicable diseases
- Births and deaths
- Any suspicious death
- Any known criminal act
- Professional misconduct
- Incident reports

Other records are part of the patient's medical record and may require reporting to other governmental agencies. The hospital provides a legal record of all births and deaths that take place there. Patient charges are made part of the record, and both patient and insurance provider receive detailed reports of charges. Department order forms are used to secure items for patient care and to verify the accuracy of the response and the proper charges. Other hospital forms may be part of the record depending on hospital policy and procedure.

As mentioned earlier, proper medical record keeping protects both the patient and the hospital and its employees. Proper documentation and record keeping are used for legal, accounting, and quality assurance purposes. For legal purposes, several rules for proper documentation exist. All reports, notations, and summaries are to be written using standard terminology and abbreviations. Spelling is to be correct. Information presented in medical documents should be factual in nature and not subjective.

Of course, errors occur in initial documentation. These can be corrected following a proper legal procedure. Errors are to be marked through with a single line, never erased. The correct information is placed immediately above the error. The correction is verified with the initials of the reporter. The individual who made the initial error must make the correction. All reports, notations, and summaries include the legal signature of the reporter.

EVENT/INCIDENT REPORTS

Incident reports are used by surgical personnel to describe an unusual event that has occurred that may have legal ramifications for the staff or patient. Falls, medication errors, intraoperative burns, loss of specimen, etc. are examples of incidents that would require reporting. If the behavior of any member of the surgical team is such that a lawsuit could result (e.g., sexual harassment, aggressive behavior toward other team members), then an incident report would be required before the perpetrator is confronted.

Most surgical services departments channel the incident reports to the risk management department, where representatives from various departments attempt to identify the factors that caused the incident and what can be done to prevent it from happening again.

ADVANCE DIRECTIVES

In health care, an **advance directive** is a written instruction dealing with the right of an incapacitated patient to self-determination. This directive carries the weight of state law and expresses a patient's wishes about the kinds and amount of medical treatment provided in the event that the patient can no longer make those types of decisions.

ETHICAL AND MORAL ISSUES

Surgical technologists are constantly challenged by important decisions that require an understanding of the concepts of right or wrong for matters involving the operative patient. In philosophy, **ethics** defines what is good for the individual and for society and establishes the nature of duties that people owe themselves and one another. The word *ethics* is derived from the Greek word *ethos* (meaning "character"), and from the Latin word *mores* (meaning "customs"). Ethics is an attempt to define these concepts and their relationship to beliefs, morals, and personal values. Ethics is the *system* of moral principles and rules that becomes standards for professional conduct, and should not be confused with morality, which results in *codes of conduct* that are put forward by a society and used as a guide to behavior by the members of that society.

MORAL PRINCIPLES

Basic **moral principles** are the guides for ethical decision making, the principles that we try to instill in our children (such as benevolence, trustworthiness, and honesty). These principles include the concern that we have for the well-being of others and respect for their autonomy. The principles also include those that deal with basic justice and the prevention of harm, as well as the refusal to take unfair advantage.

Individuals acting in a professional capacity take on an additional burden of ethical responsibility. The codes of ethics of professional associations (described in detail later in this chapter) provide rules of conduct and standards of behavior that include impartiality, objectivity, duty of care, confidentiality, and full disclosure.

The basic moral principles often override those at the professional levels in most situations. For example, surgical technologists should be trustworthy and honest, the basic tenets of a sound surgical conscience found at the professional level of ethical behavior.

BIOETHICS

Bioethics is the study of the ethical implications of biological research and applications, especially in medicine. It involves examination of the benefits and the risks of biotechnology, and offers a system that raises questions about medical care that can lead to answers about what is right and what is wrong.

Philosophically, bioethical principles are very different from those of traditional medical ethics that focus on the health care provider's duty to the individual patient. The focus of bioethics is essentially a utilitarian concept designed to maximize total human benefits (the good of society may sometimes outweigh the good of the individual patient or patient's family).

AHA PATIENT'S BILL OF RIGHTS

The American Hospital Association (AHA) Patient's Bill of Rights was adopted in 1972 and was revised and approved in October 1992. The AHA Patient's Bill of Rights makes several assumptions that are important to understand its context and intent. Some of these assumptions are stated in the introduction and are summarized in the following list:

- Health care requires collaboration between patients, physicians, and other health care professionals.
- Open and honest communication is essential to optimal patient care.
- Mutual respect for personal and professional values is essential to optimal patient care.
- Hospitals must provide a foundation for respecting the rights and responsibilities of all involved.
- Hospitals must respect the patient's rights and role in health care decision making.
- Hospitals must be sensitive to cultural, racial, linguistic, religious, age, gender, and other differences, including disabilities.

These general assumptions or concepts were turned into a series of 12 rights to form a "Bill of Rights." They are summarized as follows. The patient has the right to:

- Receive considerate and respectful care.
- Obtain relevant, current, and understandable information concerning diagnosis, treatment, and prognosis.
- Make decisions about care received before and during treatment or to refuse a course of treatment or plan of care.
- Prepare an advance directive concerning treatment or designating a surrogate decision maker and to the expectation that the intent of the advance directive will be honored.
- Expect every consideration of privacy.
- Expect that all communications and records pertaining to his or her care will be treated as confidential (except when otherwise determined by law).
- Review records concerning medical care and receive an explanation or interpretation
- Receive appropriate and medically indicated care and services within the capacity and policies of the hospital.
- Ask and be informed about the existence of business relationships among any and all of the care providers.
- Consent or decline to participate in research studies or human experimentation.
- Expect a reasonable continuity of care.
- Be informed of hospital policies and practices related to patient care.

(Refer to the American Hospital Association's website for further information: Go to *www.aha.org* and click on "Patient's Bill of Rights.")

The intent of the Patient's Bill of Rights was reinforced in *The Patient Self-Determination Act of 1990.* This act says that each patient has a right under state law to make decisions concerning his or her care, including the right to refuse treatment.

The Patient's Bill of Rights ushered in a new era of understanding of the relationship between hospitals and patients. A more subtle change has also affected the way in which health care is provided in the United States. Prior to the Patient's Bill of Rights, patients were a special category of persons who were placed in a highly dependent position because they had a special need (health care) but had neither the knowledge nor the ability to meet that need. This reality is one of the primary factors in understanding medical ethics. Without the Patient's Bill of Rights, however, there existed the danger that patients could be conceptually reduced to the status of things and control of their life removed by the health care professional. The Patient's Bill of Rights established the patient as a consumer of goods, that is, the knowledge and abilities of the health care provider. This move also established the patient as the primary decision maker.

ELEMENTS OF ETHICAL DECISION MAKING

Ethics has deep roots in our legal system; in fact, legal doctrines are often used to interpret ethical concepts. However, there is no necessary relationship between moral values, ethical principles, and the law. But if one can presume the adequacy of the ethical position, then the laws of the land should reflect that position. Health care facilities and professionals tend to prefer a type of procedural solution to ethical dilemmas.

One of the strongest ethical principles ever stated reads something like this: "We hold these truths to be self evident that all men are created equal"; yet for decades the law excluded African-Americans and females from voting. The moral value and ethical principle were stated as equality while the law was often the opposite.

Ethics can be difficult to define. The JCAHO defines ethics as "the branch of philosophy that deals with systematic approaches to moral issues, such as the distinction between right and wrong and the moral consequences of human actions. Ethics involves a system of behaviors, expectations, and morals composing *standards of conduct* for a population or a profession." Pozgar says that ethics is concerned with the *decision-making process* of determining the ultimate values and standards by which we judge our actions.

The health care practitioner needs consistent ethical guidelines. The lawyer knows that the guidelines may be challenged in court. The philosopher knows that all moral and ethical values are complicated interactions of human intellect, affect, social order, and spirituality.

Since this is a textbook for surgical technologists, we will give more time to the needs for practical guidelines and standards. This is done with the cautionary note that all health care providers must be aware that the standards of conduct are liable to both error and change as individual, societal, scientific, and spiritual values evolve.

In spite of the difficulties, some aspects of ethics can be agreed on. From a practical point of view, we can form functioning definitions and a somewhat systematic approach to answering questions that concern those in the health care community.

At its philosophical beginning, ethics must answer five basic questions:

1. What makes a "right act" right?
2. To whom is moral duty owed?
3. What "kinds" of acts are right?
4. What is the relationship between specific situations and ethical principles or guidelines?
5. What action is to be taken in the situation at hand?

Ethics begins with a debate about *right* and *wrong*. How do we know which is which? Many answers have been offered. There are many subtleties and subcategories in the literature, but we can consider some broad approaches that have occurred throughout history:

- *Universalism/absolutism:* Some principle or principles exist that are beyond individual and societal variance.
- *Social relativism:* Society determines the principles in order to protect and maximize its welfare.
- *Personal relativism:* The individual determines the principles in order to protect and maximize personal welfare.
- *Situational relativism:* All of the above must be applied to a given circumstance, and the circumstance dictates the rightness of the action.

Each approach illuminates some positive arguments, and each fails to account adequately for other arguments. Nevertheless, all philosophical and practical ethicists have a preference for one or the other basic approach. This preference determines how they proceed in their thinking and decision making. The question of moral duty is of critical importance in medical ethics. Medical ethics often prefers a **deontological approach**. This approach is associated with the ideas of obligation and duty. Deontology pursues the previous question of "rightness" with regard to duty in preference to outcome. If you look at the Patient's Bill of Rights, it is easy to see that the health care community believes that its primary obligation and moral duty is to the patient as an individual. This is a crucial distinction because of the power gradient that exists in health care. The patient has a need, potentially life threatening, for the services of the health care community. However, the patient has neither the medical knowledge nor the practical ability to provide these services for himself or herself.

Consent for treatment is also a type of surrender to the touch of another. A heavy duty is placed on the health care provider not to violate the trust implicit in this action. In medical ethics, the individual patient's needs are considered primary to the family, society, and state. For example, a potential felon who may receive the death penalty in the legal system will still be treated without bias by the medical system. In the area of broader ethical concerns, this question of duty is not agreed on, but in the health care field, general agreement has been reached.

The ethicist must also ask "What kinds of actions are right?" This question is central to the part of ethics called *normative ethics*. In the Western world, two basic approaches to this question have dominated the discussion. The first approach argues that there is an inherent right or wrong in a given act. This general approach is often called **formalism**. In other words, an act is not judged by its consequences. The act itself is either in accord with what is right or it is wrong. In this argument, the decisions made concerning the first question (what makes a "right act" right?) determine the answer to this question.

The second approach focuses on consequences. This approach is often referred to as **utilitarianism**. One form is well known by the principle "Do what produces the greatest good for the greatest number." For the student to understand this debate, the question is often framed as follows: "Do the ends justify the means?" One who believes that the end result is a necessary condition for evaluating an action holds a utilitarian point of view. One who believes that the action itself is good or bad and the result is secondary holds the formalist position.

Here is an example of how to use these two positions to argue about the rightness of informed consent. In both approaches, individual autonomy is important and the health care providers have an obligation toward the patient. The formalist argues that the action of informing the patient is good because it is an act intended to protect autonomy and honor obligation. The utilitarian argues that an informed consent is only good if the patient is better off having been given all the information. For example, consider a patient who is psychologically unstable and the information could result in the patient's refusing the procedure even though there is no medical doubt of the need. The formalist says the informed consent is right. The utilitarian says it is wrong if the patient refuses treatment and is damaged because of that action.

Now one can see why ethics is difficult. In the case above, everyone agrees that moral obligation is owed the patient, but there is disagreement as to which act actually benefits the patient. The physician, in particular, must try to combine these two intentions for the best result.

Ethically, it is a question of how much to tell and when to tell in order to do what is right. Neither law nor policy can draw this line, although both can criticize it.

The third question about what kinds of acts are right leads directly to the fourth question: What is the relationship between specific situations and ethical principles or guidelines? Fletcher, a well-known medical ethicist, argued that the situation dominates. He argued that good intentions in medicine are highly dependent on biological information and that there is not enough time to do an ethical exploration in every case. The proper relationship between principles and specific cases is judged relative to the case. The physician must act on the best biological data available with the understanding that the intent is to serve the patient.

Ramsey agreed that medical practice must incorporate the best biological data available into its decision making. However, Ramsey argued that certain acts had to be valued prior to and outside the influence of a specific case. The judgment needed to be made on the basis of principle and not data.

Those in Ramsey's camp might argue that Fletcher's situational ethics is not ethics at all since there are no defined principles. Those in Fletcher's camp might argue that Ramsey's followers live in an ivory tower where actions never have severe consequences.

Every health care provider will have to wrestle with this issue at some time in his or her career.

Finally, one reaches the final question of what to do in the case at hand. This is the point at which intuition, formal thought, values, and judgment must be translated into action. The behavioralist Thomas Alexander argued that action always results from an ethical decision. The choice not to act is an act of a specific sort. One might say that ethical decisions are known by what is done and not by what is said.

How then can one summarize what a health care professional should do in the complicated world of medical ethics? The following practical guidelines will help when faced with ethical dilemmas: Spend some time thinking about the five major questions listed previously so that you can identify your own value system. Pay attention to illustrative arguments in society and read broadly about them, and mentally play out scenarios in which various decisions are made. (Ask what the outcomes might be for the patient, family, physician, surgical technologist, nurse, and so forth.)

Decide under what situations you cannot participate and act on that decision. (If this involves a procedure, for instance, you need to talk to the supervisor before a patient is present and needs your services.)

Be aware that other well-intentioned individuals will have different viewpoints. The surgical technologist will be exposed to many issues that may create personal or vocational discomfort. These are just some of the issues that arise today:

- Elective sterilization
- Various fertilization procedures
- Elective abortion
- Human experimentation
- Animal experimentation
- Organ donation/transplantation
- Quality versus quantity of life
- Substance abuse
- Gender reassignment
- Care of individuals with human immunodeficiency virus (HIV) and acquired immunodeficiency syndrome (AIDS)
- Newborn with a severe disability
- Good Samaritan law
- Assisted suicide
- Genetic engineering
- Refusal of treatment (especially for a child)
- Termination of care and right to die

A wealth of information is available on these subjects. The health care professional should be well informed about these topics and others that may require ethical decision making.

PROFESSIONAL CODES OF CONDUCT

Most professions have adopted highly detailed codes of conduct for their respective memberships, along with methods for enforcement of breaches of those codes. In some cases, these codes are spoken of as *professional ethics* or, in the case of law, *legal ethics*. The American Medical Association has the Principles of Medical Ethics, and nurses often refer to the International Code of Nursing Ethics and a code established by their own professional association.

Many professional codes have been incorporated into law, and all codes can have some effect on judgments about professional conduct for litigation. Failure to comply with a code of professional conduct often results in expulsion from the profession.

In 1985 the AST established a **Code of Ethics** that provides guidelines for the surgical technologist:

1. To maintain the highest standards of professional conduct and patient care
2. To hold in confidence, with respect to the patient's beliefs, all personal matters
3. To respect and protect the patient's legal and moral rights to quality patient care
4. To not knowingly cause injury or any injustice to those entrusted to our care
5. To work with fellow technologists and other professional health groups to promote harmony and unity for better patient care
6. To always follow the principles of asepsis
7. To maintain a high degree of efficiency through continuing education
8. To maintain and practice surgical technology willingly, with pride and dignity
9. To report any unethical conduct or practice to the proper authority
10. To adhere to the Code of Ethics at all times with all members of the health care team

SURGICAL CONSCIENCE

A surgical technologist must have a **surgical conscience** that allows him or her to keep a patient's confidence, avoid discrimination against any patient based on the technologist's personal values, and be committed to cost control.

A surgical technologist must have the personal moral authority to accept responsibility for his or her own actions, be willing to be held liable for those actions, and to give the information needed for evaluation of those actions. The surgical technologist must be committed to maintaining the confidentiality of information associated with patient care. Confidence means having faith in another individual. Patients must never question whether their care will be in the hands of individuals of good faith, who handle information properly. A surgical conscience dictates a nondiscriminatory treatment of all patients. Personal values, feelings, and principles take a secondary position to the patient's need for the highest quality of treatment. Both the patient and hospital should be committed to cost control. Modern medicine is very expensive and cost containment is part of everyone's job. Patients and hospitals can save great sums of money each year with the careful management of resources.

Finally, for the surgical technologist, a surgical conscience is rooted in the fundamental understanding of the principles of asepsis and commitment to practice sterile technique. Of all the tasks and roles that a surgical technologist may play during his or her career, the most important is as a guarantor of sterile technique in the OR. A surgical technologist committed to professional honesty, patient confidentiality, nondiscriminatory treatment, cost consciousness, and sterile technique will provide the greatest level of safety to the patient that can be expected.

SCOPE OF PRACTICE

The scope of practice is a statement that identifies the knowledge and skills required for the profession in order to provide effective and reliable services. For the surgical technologist, the scope of practice identifies the disciplines and processes that define the field and the ways in which surgical technology is different from other allied health fields (i.e., how we are unique in the practice of patient care).

Scope of practice refers to our core accountabilities. For the health care provider, this refers to those services for which the provider is accountable, based on education, experience, national credentialing, and state licensure. For those in health care support roles, these accountabilities may be based on formal education or job-related training.

Several years ago, the American Nurses Association and the National Council of State Boards of Nursing developed criteria to determine scope of practice limitations. The algorithm entitled "Is This Task Within My Scope of Practice" that was developed for nursing can also be applied to the field of surgical technology (with a few minor changes). When faced with tasks that the surgical technologist may not feel are within the scope of practice, the person should ask these questions to make a final determination:

1. Was the skill/task taught in your accredited surgical technology program?
2. If it was not included in your basic surgical technology education, have you since completed a comprehensive educational program, which included clinical experience?
3. Has this task has become so routine in surgical technology practice that it can be reasonably and pru-

dently assumed within scope? Does the professional literature and/or research support this activity as being within the scope of practice?

4. Is the skill/task prohibited by hospital policy or state law? Does it require a state license to perform?
5. Does carrying out the duty pass the "reasonable and prudent" standard? That is, is this practice within an acceptable standard of care which would be provided by a reasonable and prudent person with similar education and experience?
6. Are there professional association standards or position statements that support this activity with additional education and experience?
7. Are you prepared to accept responsibility and accountability for performing the activity competently and safely?

From "Is This Within My Scope of Practice?" available at: *www.dora.state.co.us/nursing/scopeofpractice/ScopeofPracticeAlgorithm.pdf*

In the absence of specific statutory or regulatory prohibition, it is within the scope of practice for surgical technologists to perform generally accepted intraoperative activities for which they have been prepared through basic education, appropriate continuing education, and experience *and* for which they have demonstrated competence to perform safely and effectively.

To a very large extent, surgical technology and surgical assistant scope of practice is determined by the delegatory decisions made by the supervising surgeon. The surgeon has the ability to observe the surgical technologist's competency and performance and to ensure that the surgical technologist is performing tasks and procedures in the manner preferred for proper intraoperative patient care.

JOB DESCRIPTIONS AND COMPETENCIES

Job descriptions are descriptions of the tasks, functions, and responsibilities of a position within an organization. Job descriptions are usually developed by conducting a job analysis, which examines the tasks and sequences of tasks necessary to perform the job, and they typically include to whom the position reports, specifications such as the qualifications needed by the person in the job, and salary range. Note that a *role* is defined as the set of responsibilities or expected results associated with a job. A *job* usually includes several roles.

Competencies are general descriptions of the abilities needed to perform a role in the organization, and are described in terms that allow for measurement. Whereas job descriptions typically list the tasks or functions and responsibilities for a role, competencies list the abilities needed to conduct those tasks or functions. Consequently, competencies are often used in education after they have been converted to learning objectives (Table 2-1).

Table 2-1 Surgical Technologist: Nature of the Position

The surgical technologist must be able to:
• Stand, bend, stoop, and/or sit for long periods of time in one location with minimum/no breaks
• Lift a minimum of 20 pounds
• Refrain from nourishment or rest room breaks for periods up to 6 hours
• Demonstrate sufficient visual ability to load a fine (10–0) suture onto needles and needle holders with/without corrective lenses and while wearing safety glasses
• Demonstrate sufficient peripheral vision to anticipate and function while in the sterile surgical environment
• Hear and understand muffled communication without visualization of the communicator's mouth/lips and within 20 feet
• Hear activation/warning signals on equipment
• Detect odors sufficient to maintain environmental safety and patient needs
• Manipulate instruments, supplies, and equipment with speed, dexterity, and good eye–hand coordination
• Ambulate/move around without assistive devices
• Assist with and/or lift, move, position, and manipulate, with or without assistive devices, the patient who is unconscious
• Communicate and understand fluent English both verbally and in writing
• Be free of reportable communicable diseases and chemical abuse
• Demonstrate immunity to rubella, rubeola, tuberculosis, and hepatitis B, or be vaccinated against these diseases, or be willing to sign a waiver of release of liability with regard to these diseases
• Possess short- and long-term memory sufficient to perform tasks such as, but not limited to, mentally tracking surgical supplies and performing anticipation skills intraoperatively
• Make appropriate judgment decisions
• Demonstrate the use of positive coping skills under stress
• Demonstrate calm and effective responses, especially in emergency situations
• Exhibit positive interpersonal skills in patient, staff, and faculty interactions

Source: From *Core Curriculum for Surgical Technology,* 5th ed., by A. M. McGuiness et al., 2002, Centennial, CO: Association of Surgical Technologists. Adapted with permission.

CREDENTIALING

The surgical technologist works in an environment in which each of the listed entities affects the understood standard of care. The AST has both Recommended Standards of Practice (an evolving document) and a Code of Ethics, a statement of basic principles. The *Core Curriculum for Surgical Technology* and *Core Curriculum for Surgical Assisting* establish a knowledge and skills base that is used in determining a standard of care.

One of the ways in which the public is protected from unqualified health care professionals is through the process of **credentialing**. Credentialing does not verify competency because competency is an ongoing evaluation. One can be competent today and incompetent tomorrow. Credentialing does establish a minimum knowledge basis for a given health care profession. Many types of credentials are used in the health care community. Some types of credentialing that apply to an individual are (in order of restriction):

- *Registration:* Formal process by which qualified individuals are listed in a registry
- *Certification:* Recognition by an appropriate body that an individual has met a predetermined standard
- *Licensure:* Legal right granted by a government agency in compliance with a statute that authorizes and oversees the activities of a profession

Surgical technologists may sit for a national certification examination on graduation from an accredited surgical technology program. Although *certification* is a term that is sometimes used to refer to facilities and educational programs, surgical technology programs that are verified by the CAAHEP as meeting minimum standards are said to be *accredited*. Although credentials of various sorts indicate a certain level of verbal or practical competency, the best assurance of safe and professional behavior for a surgical technologist is a well-developed *surgical conscience,* which as described earlier is a term used to refer to an inner motivation and character that drives one to perform at the very highest level.

All surgical technologists should be aware of the limitations of their education and should carry out their duties in the operating room in accordance with standards of practice established by their professional organizations, federal statutes, state practice acts, or regulatory agencies. Hospital policies are designed to reflect state practice acts and federal statutes, and they should be understood and followed to the letter to prevent liability for malpractice.

ACCREDITATION

Most surgical technology programs are accredited through the Commission on Accreditation for Allied Health Education Programs (CAAHEP) from recommendations provided by the Accreditation Review Committee on Education in Surgical Technology (ARC-ST). CAAHEP accredits programs representing many allied health professions, recognizing more than 1,900 allied health education programs in more than 1,300 institutions. In addition to this programmatic accreditation, each of the sponsoring organizations for the surgical technology programs is institutionally accredited.

Accreditation is a process of external quality review used by higher education to scrutinize colleges, universities, and educational programs for quality assurance and quality improvement. The ARC-ST ensures that each of its accredited surgical technology programs is engaged in an ongoing quest for quality and can demonstrate how well it fulfills its stated purpose through annual reporting of outcomes. The quality and effectiveness of education provided by each program are major considerations in accreditation decisions. Each accredited program is expected to document quality and effectiveness by employing a comprehensive system of planning and evaluation in all major aspects of the institution.

Accreditation ensures academic quality to students and the public and also ensures access to federal funds (accreditation of institutions and programs is required for student access to grants and loans and other federal support). Accreditation status also allows for smooth transfer of courses and credits among colleges and universities. Most importantly, the accredited status of an institution or program is an important indicator for employers who are evaluating the credentials of job applicants and providing financial support to current employees seeking additional education.

CORE CURRICULA FOR SURGICAL TECHNOLOGY AND SURGICAL ASSISTING

A *core curriculum* is a document designed by educators that sets a specific standard for curriculum development. It is a template for instruction that seeks to control curriculum quality and attempts to standardize the educational process for the field of surgical technology and the field of surgical assisting. The Accreditation Standards and Guidelines for Surgical Technology require that programs follow the current edition of the *Core Curriculum for Surgical Technology* template for curriculum development.

CAREER DEVELOPMENT

The surgical technologist, with additional education or experience, can assume challenging careers outside of the primary scrub and/or circulator roles, within or outside of the surgical services department. The basic education for a surgical technologist, provided by a CAAHEP-accredited program, provides a solid platform for eventual career development. These peripheral careers include:

- Sterile processing department manager
- Educator
- Surgical assistant (self-employed)
- Materials manager
- Medical salesperson
- Organ and tissue procurement/preservation technician
- Physician's/surgeon's assistant
- Research assistant
- Veterinary assistant
- Labor and delivery staff
- Medical office manager
- Surgery scheduler
- Anesthesia technologist

CLINICAL LADDER PROGRAM

Clinical ladder programs allow a surgical technologist to ascend to positions of increased responsibility within an organization. They offer employers a long-term strategy for employee retention and the enhancement of department morale, and they also serve as incentive for surgical technologists to continually improve their knowledge, skills, and competencies.

Clinical ladder programs (Table 2-2) allow the surgical technologist to become more directly involved in decision making, broadening the role for proper surgical patient care. Once involved, surgical technologists experience great pride and satisfaction in their work. The programs also offer new staff a clear picture of advancement within the organization, so that the perception of a "dead-end job" is minimized. The result is a well-educated and knowledgeable employee with diverse skills, both surgical and nonsurgical.

The goals of the clinical ladder programs are to:

- Enhance quality surgical patient care.
- Encourage employer recognition and rewarding of advanced competency.
- Promote the accountability and responsibility of the surgical technologist toward the patient.
- Encourage the professional growth of the surgical technologist.
- Increase the visibility of the role of the surgical technologist in the hospital and other facilities.

Table 2-2 AST Recommended Clinical Ladder for the Surgical Technologist
Level I: Entry Level Practitioner
The Level I practitioner is a recent graduate of a CAAHEP-accredited surgical technology program who has been employed as a surgical technologist for one year or less.
1. Has graduated from a CAAHEP-accredited surgical technology program.
2. Independently scrubs basic surgical procedures.
3. Demonstrates ability to problem solve in relation to the procedure being performed.
4. Applies base knowledge of anatomy and physiology, medical terminology, microbiology, and pharmacology for optimal surgical patient care.
5. Applies basic knowledge of physics, electricity, computers, and robotics.
6. Demonstrates knowledge and practice of patient care concepts.
7. Applies the principles of asepsis during surgical procedures.
8. Participates in orientation program to attain competency in complex cases and achieve Level II: Proficient Practitioner.
9. Becomes certified within 1 year of graduation.
10. Maintains certification by participating in continuing education activities.
Level II: Proficient Practitioner
The Level II practitioner is a certified surgical technologist who has been employed as a surgical technologist for 1 year or more and who takes on greater responsibility in providing patient care than a Level I practitioner. Level II practitioners demonstrate higher level critical thinking and problem-solving skills than do Level I practitioners.
1. Meets the criteria stated in Level I.
2. Demonstrates advanced knowledge and proficient practice in the scrub role in a majority of surgical procedures.
3. Applies knowledge of advanced surgical techniques.
4. Applies knowledge related to emergency situations and surgical procedures.

(continues)

Table 2-2 *(continued)*

5. Demonstrates critical thinking skills in relation to anticipating the perioperative needs of the patient and surgeon.
6. Exhibits a higher level of collaboration with peers in making decisions related to surgical patient care.
7. Assists in performing circulating skills and tasks.
8. Participates in program to achieve Level III: Expert Practitioner.
Level III: Expert Practitioner
The Level III practitioner is an advanced practitioner who thinks on a more global level and is more involved in endeavors related to, but outside of, the surgery department.
1. Meets the criteria stated in Level II.
2. Demonstrates superior knowledge of the various surgical equipment and advanced surgical instrumentation.
3. Demonstrates superior knowledge and expert practice in the scrub role in advanced surgical procedures.
4. Performs the preceptor role for surgical technology students.
5. Demonstrates leadership abilities.
6. Serves as a mentor and role model.
7. Member of at least one department or hospital committee.
8. Involved with community health promotional efforts and other related community services.
9. Demonstrates knowledge of department fiscal requirements.
10. Participates in decision-making activities related to evaluating and acquiring surgical equipment, instruments, and supplies.
11. Collaborates with other health care professionals in the development of surgical budgetary requirements.
12. Demonstrates skills in organizing and coordinating the effective use of personnel and materials.
13. Develops, organizes, and delivers continuing education topics and/or courses.

RISK MANAGEMENT AND LIABILITY

Risk management is an integrated system developed by hospitals for the prevention and control of areas of potential liability. Risk management programs are designed to enhance the safety of patients, visitors, and employees and to minimize the financial loss to the hospital through risk detection, evaluation, and prevention.

Identification of hazards is the most critical aspect of every risk management process, because all subsequent phases of risk management depend on it. After the risk is identified, it should be assessed for severity and frequency. Possible risk scenarios can be analyzed and assessed in reference to past and present history.

Risk management objectives for a hospital are to:

- Minimize risks to patients and hospital employees.
- Avoid or control financial loss.
- Identify actual or potential causes of patient and employee accidents.
- Implement programs, policies, and procedures to eliminate or reduce occurrences.
- Collect and utilize data to decrease harm to patients and staff or damage to property.

MEDICAL ERRORS

In-patient error reduction in medicine began to gain attention in the second half of the 1990s with the release of the Institute of Medicine's (IOM's) *To Err Is Human: Building a Better Health System*. The IOM claimed that more people die each year from medical errors than from car accidents, AIDS, and breast cancer combined (making medical errors the country's eighth leading cause of death). The IOM identified a number of strategies to reduce the incidence of such errors during the next 5 years.

Medical errors have become such a serious problem over the years because of the myth of physician infallibility and physicians' fears of being sued for malpractice. A general reluctance to report another physician's errors also conspires to keep medical errors hidden. If the errors are not brought into the light for inspection, they cannot be prevented.

Technology has become the best weapon for the reduction of medical errors. New technologies include bar-coded medications and identification strips, handheld wireless devices, and computer drug order-entry systems. A study at two Veterans Administration (VA) hospitals in

Kansas found that these devices reduced medication error rates by 70% over a 5-year period.

Error-reducing technologies can generally improve patient outcomes, but even simple solutions can make drastic differences: Anesthesia errors were significantly reduced after specially engineered safety devices were developed to prevent gas hoses from being improperly installed.

In the operating room, the surgical technologist can help prevent medical errors by closely following written policies and procedures and by obeying standard precautions related to the use of personal protective equipment. The surgical technologist should be aware of the location and proper use of all emergency equipment. Prevention practices include routine preventive maintenance for all surgical equipment (faulty or malfunctioning equipment or devices should be removed from service) and professional development/continuing education programs for employees.

The surgical technologist should report unsafe conditions immediately. Any patient or employee injury should be reported and medical attention sought as soon as possible, with proper documentation of the incident.

SAFE MEDICAL DEVICE ACT

The Safe Medical Device Act of 1990 requires that medical device users report to the manufacturer and/or the Food and Drug Administration (FDA) incidents that reasonably suggest the probability that a medical device has caused or contributed to the death, serious injury, or illness of a patient.

A medical device includes, but is not limited to, electronic equipment such as ventilators and monitors, implants, syringes, needles, catheters, disposables, components, parts, and accessories. In accordance with the act, hospitals should establish methods for reporting injuries caused by these medical devices as described in a risk management plan.

MALPRACTICE INSURANCE

Hospital employees who commit negligent acts are typically covered by insurance polices provided by the facility, as long as the negligent act was committed within the scope of the institution's policies and procedures. If the surgical technologist is sued as an individual, however, personal malpractice insurance (professional liability) will be required to cover any discrepancy between the hospital's and the individual's policies. All practicing surgical technologists and surgical assistants should carry professional liability insurance because the odds that they will be sued for malpractice are greater than in the past.

Some health care practitioners have argued that carrying this extra personal malpractice insurance invites patients to sue them. But extra insurance coverage does not make the practitioner any more or less likely to be included in a lawsuit. When a negligent suit is filed, all those who may have had a part in the injury or death will be named in the suit. If there is a settlement against a specific health care provider and there is no malpractice insurance to cover the settlement, the judge may attach a lien on property owned by the defendant, or the money may be obtained from future earnings.

CASE STUDY

A 5-year-old child presents to the hospital emergency room after a motor vehicle accident. She is hypotensive and in shock. The physician suspects that her spleen is ruptured. He recommends to the parents that she undergo an emergency exploratory laparotomy for possible splenorrhaphy or splenectomy, and he writes orders to type and crossmatch blood for possible replacement. The parents refuse all treatment on religious grounds.

1. What legal and ethical issues can you identify?
2. Could the parents be charged if the child were to die?
3. How could the physician resolve this situation?

QUESTIONS FOR FURTHER STUDY

1. Describe the difference between case law, common law, and statutory law.
2. Under what principle are most health care providers usually sued and what are the two terms most often associated with this principle?
3. Explain the fundamental change the Patient's Bill of Rights introduced as related to the patient.
4. Explain the difference between certification and licensure.
5. A surgical technologist believes that genetic engineering is wrong and bad for society. What belief does the surgical technologist hold: formalism or utilitarianism? Explain why.
6. Discuss in the classroom if it is within the scope of practice of the surgical technologist to administer medications to the surgical patient under the supervision of the surgeon using the seven questions stated on pp. 34–35 as a guide. Things to consider include irrigating a cavity with antibiotic solution, applying hemostatic chemical agents to tissue, and parenteral injection.

BIBLIOGRAPHY

Adler, M. J. (1985). *Ten philosophical mistakes.* New York: Macmillan.

Albert, E. M., Denise, T. C., & Peterfreund, S. P. (1984). *Great traditions in ethics* (5th ed.). Belmont, CA: Wadsworth.

Anonymous. *Is this task within my scope of practice?* Retrieved March 3, 2003, from http://www.dora.state.co.us/nursing/scopeofpractice/ScopeofPracticeAlgorithm.pdf

Anonymous. *Scope of practice.* Retrieved March 5, 2003, from http://www.dora.state.co.us/nursing/scopeofpractice/scopeofpractice.htm

Anonymous. AST code of ethics. Available Interet: www.AST.org

Aquinas, T. (1980). *On politics and ethics* (P. E. Sigmund, Ed.). New York: Norton.

Aristotle. (1947). In R. McKeun (Ed.), *Introduction to Aristotle.* New York: Random House.

Atkinson, L. J., & Fortunato, N. (1996). *Berry and Kohn's operating room technique* (8th ed.). St. Louis, MO: Mosby.

Baier, K. (1965). *The moral point of view.* New York: Random House.

Berger, F. R. (1989). Classical Utilitarianism. In W. C. Starr & R. C. Taylor (Eds.), *Moral philosophy: Historical and contemporary essays.* Milwaukee, WI: Marquette University Press.

Colero, L. *A framework for universal principles of ethics.* Crossroads Programs Inc. Retrieved April 1999, from http://www.ethics.ubc.ca/papers/invited/colero.html

DeLaune, S. C., & Ladner, P. K. (2002). *Fundamentals of nursing: Standards and practice* (2nd ed.). Clifton Park, NY: Delmar Learning.

Dewey, J., & Tufts, J. H. (1932). *Ethics.* New York: Holt.

Frankena, W. K. (1963). *Ethics.* Englewood Cliffs, NJ: Prentice Hall.

Husted, G., & Husted, J. (1991). *Ethical decision making in nursing.* St. Louis, MO: Mosby Year-Book.

Irving, D. (2001). *The bioethics mess.* Washington, DC: The Morley Institute. Available from http://www.petersnet.net/browse/4123.htm

Kant, I. (1969). *Foundations of the metaphysics of morals: Text and critical essays* (R. P. Wolff, Ed.). Indianapolis: Bobbs-Merrill.

Kohlberg, L. (1958). *The development of modes of moral thinking and choice: Years 10–16.* Dissertation, University of Chicago.

MacQuarrie, J. (1967). *Dictionary of Christian ethics.* Philadelphia: Westminster Press.

Maguire, D. (1979). *The moral choice.* New York: Doubleday.

McGuiness, A. M., et al. (2002). *Core curriculum for surgical technology* (5th ed.). Centennial, CO: Association of Surgical Technologists.

McNamara, C. Employee staffing: Specifying jobs, roles, and competencies. Available from http://www.mapnp.org/library/staffing/specify/cmptncys/cmptncys.htm

Mill, J. S. (1987). *Utilitarianism.* New York: Prometheus.

O'Leary, M. (1994). *Lexikon: Dictionary of health care terms, organizations, and acronyms for the era of reform.* Oakbrook Terrace, IL: Joint Commission on Accreditation of Healthcare Organizations.

Outka, G. (1972). *Agape: An ethical analysis.* New Haven: Yale University Press.

Pieper, J. (1965). *The four cardinal virtues.* New York: Harcourt, Brace and World.

Pozgar, G. D. (1996). *Legal aspects of health care administration* (6th ed.). Gaitherburg, MD: Aspen.

Ramsey, P. (1970). *The patient as person: Explorations in medical ethics.* New Haven, CT: Yale University Press.

Ramsey, P. (1978). *Fabricated man: The ethics of genetic control.* New Haven, CT: Yale University Press.

Rawls, J. (1962). Justice as fairness. *In Philosophy, politics, and society* (2nd series). New York: Barnes and Noble.

Tokarski, C. (2000). Medical error-prevention strategies face barriers to acceptance. *Medscape Money & Medicine,* Medscape, Inc. Retrieved March 3, 2001, from http://www.ahcpr.gov/news/medscap2.htm

Veateh, R. M. (1977). *Case studies in medical ethics.* Cambridge, MA: Harvard University Press.

White, L. (2001). *Foundations of nursing: Caring for the whole person.* Clifton Park, NY: Delmar Learning.

CHAPTER 3

The Surgical Patient

Bob Caruthers

CASE STUDY

Following an automobile accident, Juan, a 37-year-old male, was in the OR with a fractured left femur and left tibia and fibula. He also had a severe compound fracture of the right tibia and fibula with a near amputation. While the anesthesia personnel were starting intravenous lines, two surgeons and the circulator were standing near the patient's right leg. The surgeons were laying out their operative approach to the circulator and the surgical technologist in the scrub role (STSR). Juan asked three consecutive times, "What is wrong with my left leg?" The first two times the anesthesia provider said, "Your left leg will be fine." Upon the third asking, the STSR said, "Juan, your left leg is severely injured, but it is not as severely injured as your right leg. We will operate on both legs tonight." Juan noticeably relaxed and said, "Thank you."

1. What do you think Juan was concerned about when he asked, "What's wrong with my left leg?"
2. At age 37, what is Juan's developmental stage?
3. Juan's first nonphysical concerns will probably focus on what area of his life?
4. The surgical team's first obligation to Juan is to care for which of his needs?
5. What spiritual issue may be raised by this incident for Juan?

OBJECTIVES

After studying this chapter, the reader should be able to:

C 1. Assess the patient's response to illness and hospitalization.

A 2. Demonstrate awareness that all surgical patients have the right to the highest standards and practices in asepsis.

R **E** 3. Distinguish and assess the physical, spiritual, and psychological needs of a patient.

4. Distinguish and assess cultural and religious influences on the surgical patient.

SELECT KEY TERMS

1. Maslow's hierarchy of needs	2. patient 3. physical need	4. psychological need	5. social need 6. spiritual need

THE STSR AND THE SURGICAL PATIENT

In Chapter 1, the surgical technologist was described using the common definition of a professional, that is, an individual who has special education and training in a given field and who meets certain competency-based and ethical criteria in the vocational arena. Surgical technology was also described as a paramedical field. The primary role of the surgical technologist in rendering care to the surgical **patient** is related to assistance provided for the physician—the establishment and protection of a sterile field, the care and handling of surgical instrumentation, and assistance with technical tasks throughout the surgical procedure. When surgical technologists refer to the tasks they perform as preoperative, intraoperative, or postoperative, they typically mean tasks performed within the surgical environment and mostly within the environment of a specific OR. The surgical technologist commonly has only a short period of contact with the conscious surgical patient. This fact is true to some degree for all surgical personnel. The transportation aide may actually have more contact with the conscious patient than any team member other than the surgeon or anesthesia provider. In emergency surgery, neither the surgeon nor the anesthesia provider may have had more than momentary interaction with a conscious patient. In facilities where surgical technologists assist with circulating, the surgical technologist does not perform any of the tasks related to nursing diagnosis or creation of a patient care plan. Even with this limited amount of time spent with the conscious patient, every surgical team member can relate stories in which the short but intense interactions were important to patient care and safety. No matter what role the surgical technologist is performing, an awareness of the surgical patient, surrounding environment, other team members, and care and safety issues must exist. Every health care professional is morally obligated to be as educated and aware as possible, given their level of experience. No one is excused from failure to notice a dangerous condition, failure to hear a patient's stated need, or failure to provide as safe an environment as possible.

The information provided in this chapter is designed to help the entry-level surgical technologist to become an "extra pair of eyes and ears" in the OR. Select material has been taken from the fields of psychology and ethics, to establish a general understanding of concerns and issues related to these areas. The role of the surgical technologist is to help magnify the awareness of the surgical team of conditions affecting the patient.

PHYSICAL, PSYCHOLOGICAL, SOCIAL, AND SPIRITUAL NEEDS OF THE SURGICAL PATIENT

The surgical patient is first and foremost a person. This is a biological, psychological, and social reality. Surgical intervention is a narrowly focused activity. A review of **Maslow's hierarchy of needs** demonstrates that this focus is appropriate for the surgical environment. Yet, one must not "lose sight" of the total person. To do so is to violate the ethical and moral obligations that every health care professional has to every patient. For the patient, surgical intervention is also a psychological, social, and spiritual event. Imagine for a moment the questions that pass through the mind of a young woman who is about to undergo a hysterectomy: Who will I be as a woman following this surgery? Who will I be as a wife and mother? Why did God let this happen to me? These are profound questions: one psychological (Who am I?), one social (Who am I in my social role of wife and mother?), and one spiritual (What does this say about my belief system?). The patient may presume good physical care because she knows the surgeon who delivered her babies, has a history of success relative to the hospital, and trusts the surgical team implicitly. It may be the questions of her inner self that haunt her the most before and after the surgical procedure.

The surgical patient has a whole life outside the role of patient. That life is at risk with every surgical intervention. The person who is brought to your OR is not "the hysterectomy in room 5" but Jane Doe, single mother of three, in middle adulthood, bank executive, aspiring vocalist, Episcopalian, African-American, Democrat, practical jokester, and a lot more. The health care professional who cannot or chooses not to care for the total individual does not belong in health care, even in an area with a narrow focus.

Humans are unique and complex. The following definitions will be used when referring to the components that make up an individual:

- **Physical need**: Any need or activity related to genetics, physiology, or anatomy
- **Psychological need**: Any need or activity related to the identification and understanding of oneself
- **Social need**: Any need or activity related to one's identification or interaction with another individual or group
- **Spiritual need**: Any need or activity related to the identification and understanding of one's place in an organized universe (Expressions may involve theology, philosophy, mythology, and intuition.)

None of these human features exists alone. They function in a dynamic state. For instance, psychological states are, at some point, merely the observable results of complex brain activity. On the other hand, the way an individual feels at one moment will affect the biochemical activity of the brain at the next moment. The caregiver, however, must make distinctions in order to respond appropriately.

UNDERSTANDING THE SURGICAL PATIENT

As one discusses the surgical patient, one must switch back and forth between generalizations and specifics. All patients are individuals but not all patients are surgical patients. The surgical technologist must comprehend concepts that apply to all individuals and must consider their impact on the surgical patient. The format will discuss the basic nature of the surgical patient first. The student should keep these features in mind when reading about the more general features illustrated later.

CAUSES OF SURGICAL INTERVENTION

Every surgical patient is a unique individual; however, all surgical patients have something in common. Given all options, they would elect not to be having surgery. Even when a surgical procedure is selected for cosmetic reasons, it is selected because the patient is dissatisfied with his or her body as it is. If the patient could have had the body desired without surgery, surgery would not be elected. Most are having surgery because genetic factors, trauma, or disease have presented them with a condition that can only or can best be corrected with surgical intervention.

Common factors that result in surgical intervention are:

Factor	Example
Genetic malformation	Atrial septal defect
Trauma	Anterior cruciate ligament tear
Nonmalignant neoplasm	Uterine fibroid
Malignant neoplasm	Colon cancer
Disease	Cholecystitis
Condition	Kidney stone
Psychological state	Rhytidectomy

The surgical patient, then, is an individual who became a patient because of an illness, disease, or condition. The patient became a surgical patient because surgical intervention offers the hope of a cure or correction.

THE SURGICAL PATIENT, A HUMAN BEING

Individuals are comprised of an interactive mix of physical, psychological, social, and spiritual needs and possibilities. In spite of genetic, cultural, and familial similarities, each individual represents a unique combination of features that exists as a single and unique entity. The surgical technologist must recognize and honor the uniqueness of each individual who comes to the OR. The uniqueness of each patient establishes guidelines for meeting needs, sets boundaries that may not be crossed, and may create ethical dilemmas for the health care provider.

There are libraries full of books that contribute to our understanding of individuals. The Bibliography at the end of the chapter lists a number of classic works. For the purposes of the surgical technologist, three types of information seem most helpful for a basic understanding of individuals and for quick recognition of concerns for a patient:

- Maslow's hierarchy of needs establishes a means of prioritizing needs.
- Life stage development concepts allow for quick recognition of the psychosocial concerns of a given patient.
- A basic understanding of cultural and religious influences helps in communication and understanding.

PRIORITIZING NEEDS: MASLOW'S HIERARCHY

Maslow (1968, 1971) constructed an elegant humanistic model of human development. The developmental stages for human progression are expressed in terms of a hierarchy. Physiological needs form the base of the hierarchical structure and self-actualization forms the pinnacle (Figure 3-1). The simple but powerful point of the hierarchical structure is that all the requisite needs of each prior level must be met in order to achieve the next level. Between the foundation and the pinnacle, the progressive steps are safety, love and belonging, and esteem. These needs can be briefly described:

- *Physiological needs:* The most basic needs are biological needs like water, oxygen, food, and temperature regulation.
- *Safety needs:* These needs refer to the perception on the part of the individual that his or her environment is safe.
- *Love and belonging needs:* These are basic social needs—to be known and cared for as an individual and to care for another.
- *Esteem needs:* This level of need refers to a positive evaluation of oneself and others, a need to be respected and to respect others.
- *Self-actualization:* This is the need to fulfill what one believes is one's purpose.

If physiological needs are not being met, the individual must spend all his energies meeting the basic needs of

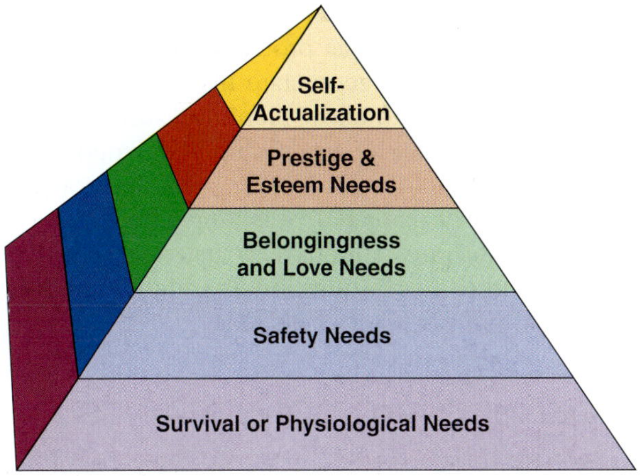

Figure 3-1 Maslow's hierarchy of needs

food, water, and temperature regulation. Without these needs being met the individual dies. One must exist for safety to be an issue. Likewise, it is easy to see that an individual who is consumed with survival will not have the time and energy required to develop the emotional and intellectual pursuits necessary for higher level development. The individual who believes that his environment is inherently dangerous cannot trust. Without trust, one cannot experience or give love and affection. If physiological and safety needs are met but an individual cannot find love and affection within their social group, he will not be able to generate positive self-regard. It is only when physical, safety, affective, and self-esteem needs are effectively met that the individual can turn his thoughts and energy to become all that he is capable of being.

While there may be theoretical issues that are questionable in Maslow's theory, he has expressed a significant truth concerning persons: Lower level needs must be met in order to meet higher level ones. This hierarchy is especially important in the field of health care. The nature of surgery requires that the surgical team concentrate on physiological needs first, followed by environmental, then affective, then self-esteem, and then self-actualization needs.

A SAMPLE APPLICATION OF MASLOW'S HIERARCHY

Think back to the opening case study. Juan has serious injuries. Both his right foot and his life are at risk. Everyone in the room must focus their attention on Juan's physical needs: blood volume, oxygenation, pain relief, anesthetic state, stabilization of the fracture, revascularization, and infection control. At the moment of Juan's question, everyone was concerned with taking care of the physical need. In this case the STSR, who had completed the case setup, was protecting the sterile field, and listening to the surgeon state his plan for the procedure, had the time to allow Juan's question to sink in and to reflect on what he was asking. It dawned on him that Juan was afraid that his left leg, a leg that was hurting and obviously damaged, was amputated. Why? No one was paying any attention to that leg. The STSR could respond to Juan's question at a higher level than the physical—at the level of his fear.

GUIDELINES AND CONSTRAINTS

Maslow's hierarchy provides both guidelines and constraints for organizing care. These guidelines and constraints are both moral and clinical. As previously discussed, medical ethics presumes a certain moral duty to the patient. Maslow's hierarchy helps us to organize that duty when emergencies or value conflicts arise. The surgical team must respond first to the physical needs of the patient in terms of clinical care, but the surgical team must also recognize that the patient's self-esteem and autonomy give the patient certain rights, even the right to refuse the most basic level of intervention.

LIFE STAGE DEVELOPMENT: SELECT BASIC CONCEPTS

There are many ways to approach a study of individuals and many theoretical designs that propose to explain all or part of the mystery of being human (Table 3-1).

Individuals age and change. The study of human development attempts to identify, quantify, and describe these changes. There are many theories of human development, and various theorists place emphasis in one area or another. Some theories are philosophically oriented and others psychologically oriented. However, all developmental theories must account for changes in physical, social, and cognitive domains. The psychologist must also explain specific cognitive changes in self-concept. Self-concept is the image of oneself. A self-concept defines who and what one truly believes about oneself. While theories vary, some basic developmental components and concepts are agreed on by most.

DEVELOPMENTAL CHANGE

One of the best approaches to understanding individuals is to study human development. One way to organize this information begins with understanding the concept of developmental change. Developmental change begins with significant observable changes in the human body that result in new social interaction. The change in social interaction and feedback from that which has become the previous norm forces a revolution in thinking, feeling, and behavior. This revolution is first felt as confusion. However, the internal revolution is most clearly characterized by a renewed asking of the question, "Who am I?" The steps involved in developmental change are:

A significant observable change occurs in the body.

The observable change results in a change in social feedback.

The change in social feedback issues in a period of confusion.

The confusion leads to a reasking of the question, "Who am I?"

The change is completed with the new response to the question.

The steps in developmental change are clearly seen in the move from late childhood to adolescence. Puberty ushers in a whole new physical potential, the potential of reproduction. The emerging adolescent does not understand this, but the parent does. The parent begins to relate to the adolescent as an adult and not as a child. In effect, the parent changes all the rules, because he or she knows what adolescence is like and what its peculiar dangers are. This confuses the new adolescent, who still sees himself as a child. The confusion creates an identity crisis. To resolve the crisis, the adolescent must accomplish several developmental tasks. When the tasks are accomplished, a young adult will emerge and begin the process of adjusting to the new stage.

LIFE TASKS

The developmental psychologist is interested in the individual. The social psychologist is interested in the individual's relation to others. The social psychologist is interested in the development of the individual's understanding of the self, as is the developmental psychologist, but the social psychologist adds to our understanding of individuals mostly by focusing on the self as it takes on social roles. In other words, one has a self that is highly personal. A Freudian psychologist focuses on that self in therapy. However, in our day-to-day interactions, most are defined by role interactions. An individual recognizes that I, myself, am not the same when I am in the role of mother as I am when in the role of surgical technologist. Most interactions revolve around our understanding of the rules related to certain roles. Human development must account for both the highly personal, core self, and the social self. When combined, we get a rather complete view of the developing person.

Table 3-1 Summary of Ages and Stages of Developmental Theories

STAGE/AGE	PIAGET'S COGNITIVE STAGES	FREUD'S PSYCHOSEXUAL STAGES	ERIKSON'S PSYCHOSOCIAL STAGES	KOHLBERG'S MORAL JUDGMENT STAGES
1. *Infancy:* Birth to 1 year	*Sensorimotor* (birth to 2 years): begins to acquire language Task: Object permanence	*Oral:* pleasure from exploration with mouth and through sucking Task: Weaning	*Trust vs. Mistrust* Task: Trust Socializing agent: Mothering person Central process: Mutuality Ego quality: Hope	
2. *Toddler:* 1–3 years	*Sensorimotor* continues *Preoperational* (2–7 years) begins: use of representational thought Task: Use language and mental images to think and communicate	*Anal:* control of elimination Task: Toilet training	*Autonomy vs. Shame and Doubt* Task: Autonomy Socializing agent: Parents Central process: Imitation Ego quality: Self-control and willpower	*Preconventional Level:* 1. *Morality Stage:* Avoid punishment by not breaking rules of authority figures
3. *Preschool:* 3–6 years	*Preoperational* continues	*Phallic:* attracted to opposite-sex parent Task: Resolve Oedipus/Electra complex	*Initiative vs. Guilt* Task: Initiative and moral responsibility Socializing agents: Parents Central process: Identification Ego quality: Direction, purpose, and conscience	2. *Individualism, Instrumental Purpose, and Exchange Stage:* "Right" is relative, follow rules when in own interest
4. *School age:* 6–12 years	*Preoperational* continues *Concrete Operations* (7–12 years) begins: engage in inductive reasoning and concrete problem solving Task: Learn concepts of conservation and reversibility	*Latency:* identification with same-sex parent Task: Identify with same-sex parent and test and compare own capabilities with peer norms	*Industry vs. Inferiority* Task: Industry, self-assurance, self-esteem Socializing agents: Teachers and peers Central process: Education Ego quality: Competence	*Conventional Level:* 3. *Mutual Expectations, Relationships, and Conformity to Moral Norms Stage:* Need to be "good" in own 'and others' eyes, believe in rules and regulations
5. *Adolescence:* 12–18 years	*Formal Operations* (12 years to adulthood): engage in abstract reasoning and analytical problem solving	*Genital:* develop sexual relationships Task: Establish meaningful relationship for lifelong pairing	*Identity vs. Role Confusion* Task: Self-identity/concept Socializing agents: Society of peers	4. *Social System and Conscience Stage:* Uphold laws because they are fixed social duties

(continues)

Table 3-1 *(continued)*

STAGE/AGE	PIAGET'S COGNITIVE STAGES	FREUD'S PSYCHOSEXUAL STAGES	ERIKSON'S PSYCHOSOCIAL STAGES	KOHLBERG'S MORAL JUDGMENT STAGES
	Task: Develop a workable philosophy of life		Central process: Role experimentation and peer pressure Ego quality: Fidelity and devotion to others, personal and sociocultural values	
6. *Young adult:* 18–30 years	*Formal Operations* continues		*Intimacy vs. Isolation* Task: Intimacy Socializing agent: Close friends, partners, lovers, spouse Central process: Mutuality among peers Ego quality: Intimate affiliation and love	*Postconventional Level:* 5. *Social Contract or Utility and Individual Rights Stage:* Uphold laws in the interest of the greatest good for the greatest number; uphold laws that protect universal rights
7. *Early middle age:* 30–50 years			*Generativity vs. Stagnation* (30 to 65 years) Task: Generativity Socializing agent: Spouse, partner, children, sociocultural norms Central process: Creativity and person–environment fit Ego quality: Productivity, perseverance, charity, and consideration	
8. *Late middle age:* 50–70 years			*Generativity vs. Stagnation* continues	6. *Universal Ethical Principles Stage:* Support universal moral principles regardless of the price for doing so
9. *Late adult:* 70 years to death			*Ego Integrity vs. Despair* (65 years to death) Task: Ego integrity Socializing agent: Significant others Central process: Introspection Ego quality: Wisdom	

The life stage approach combines physical, psychological, social, and spiritual concerns. It is one of the best ways to assess a patient's probable needs in these areas. This approach is powerful because it is practical and does not require advanced levels of education to apply.

Sample Application: Using Life Tasks Information

Think back to Juan. Look at the life stage tasks listed for middle adulthood in Table 3-2. Juan will be actively involved in adjusting to normal physiological changes in his body. The injury will force him to adapt to unexpected changes. Depending on his job, the injury may affect it directly, but certainly Juan will be concerned about his ability to make a living. He will be fearful of the effects of this on his children. What if he "doesn't make it"? What will they do? Who will care for them? He and his spouse will also be adjusting to changes in their relationship. This injury will change the relationship in the short term and affect the issues they have to deal with in the long term. For one thing, Juan will leave the hospital more childlike and will require his spouse to take care of him in ways neither expected. Juan may doubt his ability to care for his own aging parents. He has various responsibilities. He may have to surrender some of those responsibilities in the short term, which could have long-term effects. Finally, he may be unable to continue participating in some leisure activities. Juan will have a lot to worry about as a result of this injury. Most significantly, his role as a provider will be at risk. All these factors will affect Juan's mental state both prior to and following surgery.

What Can the Surgical Technologist Do?

The STSR seldom has the time or opportunity for lengthy contact with a conscious patient. Nevertheless, the surgical team should establish an environment that communicates care and concern to the patient. Some steps to take are:

- Discuss with the circulator any specific issues or concerns that exist.
- Plan for simple actions that may help the patient.
- Introduce yourself professionally.
- If the patient asks what you do, explain in simple factual language.
- Do not make light of the situation or the questions the patient has.
- Move quietly and professionally about the sterile field.

Good psychological and spiritual care begins with thinking about the patient. The life tasks scheme provides one a way to do that quickly and effectively.

The surgical technologist works with the registered nurse to provide directly for the patient's care and comfort prior to the surgical procedure or throughout the procedure if the patient is awake. Several actions may prove helpful:

- Introduce yourself in a professional manner.
- Communicate with the registered nurse throughout.
- A simple touch or squeeze of the hand may help calm a fearful patient before induction.
- Explain everything you are going to do.
- Pay attention to the language you use.
- Speak calmly.
- Move patients carefully.
- Be aware of every item in the environment that can potentially cause harm.
- Perform tasks efficiently and effectively.

CULTURAL AND RELIGIOUS INFLUENCES

Every culture expresses different value orientations. Basic cultural beliefs and value issues are presented in Table 3-3. The surgical technologist should be aware of these fundamental values and beliefs. Maslow's hierarchy establishes guidelines for responding to patients' needs. The life tasks approach establishes a broad context for understanding surgical patients' needs and fears in some detail. Cultural values will specify the way the patient thinks and feels about these issues.

Religious values are always expressed within a culture, but they reach across cultures, too. Religious values can easily conflict with modern medicine. More dramatically, religious values may create conflicts in moral values. These create both ethical and legal problems for patients and health care providers. The patient population in the United States is both multicultural and multireligious. The surgical technologist should have a basic understanding of various faith statements and their relationship to surgical care (Table 3-4).

Table 3-2 Life Tasks Approach

AGE	TASK TO BE ACCOMPLISHED
0–2	Gain foundational control of body
	Develop basic perceptual skills
	Establish basic language skills
	Bond to mother
	Perceive self as a member of a family
2–6	Achieve physiological stability
	Take solid foods
	Learn to talk
	Learn to walk
	Form simple concepts of social and physical reality
	Relate emotionally to others
	Learn a basic set of rights and wrongs
	Learn to control the elimination of body waste
	Learn basic sex differences and modesty
6–12	Develop skills and use of tools
	Distinguish sex-role differences
	Adjust to new school environment
	Moral training begins in a new way
	Learn to relate to a peer group
	Increase number of relationships outside the family
	Begin to acquire appropriate social behavior
Adolescent	Adjust to changes in body structure and size
	Separate from parents emotionally
	Establish sex-role behavior with peers of both sexes
	Begin to plan for a career
	Begin to plan for marriage or lifelong relationship
	Form a new sense of identity
	Develop formal operations in the cognitive realm
Early adult	Selection of lifelong partner
	Learn to live with lifelong partner
	Start family
	Begin role as parent
	Learn to manage a home
	Early stages of career
	Beginning of civic responsibility
	Find a congenial social group
Middle adult	Accept and adjust to physiological changes
	Attain and maintain a satisfactory occupation
	Assist children with becoming adults
	Learn to relate to lifelong partner as a person (not role)
	Adjust to aging or death of parents
	Take on a new level of civic and social responsibility
	Develop adult leisure time activities
Late middle adult	Let children become fully responsible for themselves
	Deepen relationships with lifelong partner
	Develop relationship with children as adults
	Develop relationships with grandchildren
	Develop new relations with parents (if still living)
	Reach pinnacle of power in career
	Continue to develop adult leisure time activities
Late adult, (over 70)	Review life as you have lived it
	Accept help from adult children
	Deepen relationship with lifelong partner
	Accept bodily changes in self and partner
	Develop relationship with older grandchildren
	Prepare for death event

Table 3-3 Basic Cross-Cultural Values, Value Orientations, and Beliefs

VALUE	VALUE ORIENTATION AND BELIEFS
Time	
What is the time orientation of human beings?	*Past* focus: Reverence for long-standing traditions.
	Present focus: Live in "here and now," perceive time in a linear fashion.
	Future focus: Willing to defer gratification to ensure they can meet a future goal; tend to be disciplined in scheduling and using time.
Human Nature	
What is the basic nature of human beings?	Human beings are *basically good.*
	Human beings are *evil but* have a *perfectable* nature.
	Human beings are a combination of *good and evil* requiring *self-control to perfect* nature; *lapses* occasionally occur and are *accepted.*
	Human beings are *neutral, neither good nor evil.*
Activity	
What is the primary purpose of life?	*Being* orientation: Human beings' value resides in their *inherent existence* and spontaneity.
	Becoming-in-being orientation: Human beings' value is inherent but they must engage in *continuous self-development* as integrated wholes.
	Doing orientation: Human beings exist to be *active* and to *achieve.*
Relational	
What is the purpose of human relations?	*Linear* relationships: Welfare and goals of the *hereditary and extended family* are emphasized. Goals of the family take precedence over the individual's.
	Collateral relationships: Welfare and goals of *social and family group* are emphasized. Group goals take precedence.
	Individual relationships: Individual goals and accountability for own behavior emphasized.
People to Nature	
What is the relationship of human beings to nature?	Human beings *dominate nature* and have control over their environment.
	Human beings *live in harmony with nature* and must maintain that balance.
	Human beings are *subjugated to nature* and have no control over their environment.

Source: Compiled from information in *Variations in Value Orientations,* by K. Kluckhorn and F. Strodtbeck, 1961, New York: Row, Peterson; and *Transcultural Nursing: Assessment and Interventions,* 2nd ed., by J. N. Giger and R. E. Davidhizar, 1995, Baltimore, MD: Mosby.

SAMPLE APPLICATION: USING RELIGIOUS AND CULTURAL INFORMATION IN THE OR

Think about Juan again. His concerns about life and death, family responsibility, amputation, and so forth will be expressed in a specific language and context. His cultural and religious beliefs will determine these. For instance, Juan may believe that his existence is the result of a universal action organized by a central mind and power. What he calls this universal action will depend on his cultural background, the religious story he believes, and his personal life experiences. Whether he understands the accident as ordained, punishment, or something else will arise from this foundation. Guilt will be determined by it. Postoperatively, his family and friends, clergy and counselors, physicians, and other health care providers will hear all his needs and concerns and his solutions expressed in this form.

Table 3-4 Religion and Religious Values

ITEM	JUDAISM	ISLAM	ROMAN CATHOLIC	PROTESTANT
Leaders	Rabbi	Imam	Bishop, priest	Bishop, priest, minister, pastor
Holy text	*Torah, Bible, Talmud*	*Koran, Shari'a Hadith*	*Bible*	*Bible*
Weekly holy day	Friday sundown to Saturday sundown	Friday	Sunday	Sunday
Dietary restrictions	Complex rules	Pork, alcohol, other rules	Fish on Fridays, fasting during Lent	Generally none; some variance
View of medical treatment	Encouraged	Encouraged (privacy very important)	Encouraged	Generally encouraged; sect variance
Birth control	Allowed	Allowed	Not allowed	Allowed
Infertility treatment	Allowed with some rules	Allowed with some rules	Allowed with some rules	Allowed
Abortion	Some circumstances	Some circumstances	Not allowed	Some circumstances
Removal of life support	Specific conditions	Specific conditions	Specific conditions	Specific conditions
Organ donation	Permitted	Permitted	Permitted	Permitted

ITEM	CHRISTIAN SCIENCE	JEHOVAH'S WITNESS	BUDDHISM	HINDUISM
Leaders	None	Elders	Priest/nun	Priest/guru/sadhu /yogi
Holy text	*Bible,* Mary Baker Eddy	*New World Bible*	*Book of the Dead, Buddha Dharma*	*Vedas, Upanishads, Bhagavad Gita*
Weekly holy day	None	None	None	None
Dietary restrictions	None	No blood-containing food	Varies	No beef; other rules vary
View of medical treatment	Negative view	Encouraged; no blood transfusion	Encouraged	Encouraged
Birth control	Allowed	Allowed	Discouraged	Discouraged
Infertility treatment	No	Allowed	Controversial	Allowed
Abortion	Rare	Not allowed	Specific conditions	Not allowed
Removal of life support	Personal choice	Specific conditions	Specific conditions	Specific conditions
Organ donation	No	Allowed	Controversial	No

Table 3-4 (continued)

ITEM	MORMON	UNITARIAN	SHINTO	AMERICAN INDIAN
Leaders	Bishop	Minister	Priest	Medicine man/elder
Holy text	*Bible, Book of Mormon,* other writings	Many texts used	*Kojiki, Nibongi*	Oral tradition
Weekly holy day	Sunday	Sunday	None	None
Dietary restrictions	Drugs, alcohol, tea, coffee, tobacco	None	None	Varies
View of medical treatment	Encouraged	Encouraged	Encouraged	Varies
Birth control	Allowed	Allowed	Allowed	Discouraged
Infertility treatment	Allowed	Allowed	Allowed	Allowed
Abortion	Specific conditions	Allowed	No position	Not allowed
Removal of life support	Personal choice	Allowed	No position	Not necessary
Organ donation	Allowed	Allowed	No position	Discouraged

CASE STUDY

Chandra is a 13-year-old who was involved in an automobile accident. She has a severe facial laceration but was not rendered unconscious and has no negative neurological signs. She is coming to the OR where a plastic surgeon will repair her facial laceration.

1. What psychological concerns might Chandra have? Which concerns may take priority?
2. How can the surgical team help ease Chandra's experience?

QUESTIONS FOR FURTHER STUDY

1. Are there any differences in the Roman Catholic and American Indian views of transplant surgery?
2. During a surgical procedure in which general anesthesia is being administered, which level of Maslow's hierarchy is the surgical team meeting, and why?
3. As surgical technologists, we are taught to treat every operative patient the same, without regard to background, past history, culture, or reason for surgery. Does this hold in every situation? For example, compare and contrast the type of conversation that the surgical technologist might have when transporting a female patient who will be undergoing a mastectomy, and the conversation with the female patient who will be undergoing a rhinoplasty for cosmetic reasons. Would a prisoner that has killed a police officer and is brought to the OR to repair a gunshot wound be treated any differently than a 12-year-old girl that is to have a tonsillectomy?

4. Alternative therapy treatments have been on the rise for the last few years. Should a physician consider consulting with (and possibly employing the therapies advocated by) a healing priest from a patient's nontraditional religion? What factors would prevent a physician from doing so, even at the patient's request? Could the physician's refusal affect the outcome of the treatment he prescribes?
5. Why is positioning so important to the geriatric surgical patient?
6. Discuss how physical developmental change affects the social interaction of the individual and how this relates to the care of the surgical patient.

BIBLIOGRAPHY

Anonymous (a monk of the Eastern Church). (1978). *Orthodox spirituality*. Crestwood, NY: St. Vladimir's Seminary Press.

Baldwin, J. M. (1906). *Social and ethical interpretations in mental development* (4th ed.). New York: Macmillan.

Bandura, A., & McDonald, F. J. (1963). The influence of social reinforcement and the behavior of models in shaping children's moral judgments. *Journal of Abnormal and Social Psychology, 67*, 274–281.

Bell, J., Caruthers, B. L., Hunter, M. A., Kalush, S., May, M., Olmsted, J., & Santaniello, N. (1993). *Core curriculum for surgical assisting*. Centennial, CO: Association of Surgical Technologists.

Brehm, S. S., & Kassin, S. M. (1993). *Social psychology* (2nd ed.). Boston: Houghton Mifflin.

Chapman, M. (1988). *Constructive evolution: Origins and development of Piaget's thought*. Cambridge: Cambridge University Press.

Coleman, N., Davis, T., Donley, D., Fleming, D., Keegan, C., Olson, C., et al. (1996). *Core curriculum for surgical technology* (4th ed.). Centennial, CO: Association of Surgical Technologists.

Commons, M. L., Richards, F. A., & Armon, C. (1984). *Beyond formal operations*. New York: Praeger.

Coopersmith, S. (1967). *The antecedents of self esteem*. San Francisco: W. H. Freeman.

Elkind, D. (1970). *Children and adolescents: Interpretive essays on Jean Piaget*. New York: Oxford University Press.

Elkind, D. (1981). *The hurried child: Growing up too fast too soon*. Reading, MA: Addison-Wesley.

Elkind, D. (1984). *All grown up and no place to go: Teenagers in crisis*. Reading, MA: Addison-Wesley.

Elkind, D., & Flavell, J. H. (Eds.). (1969). *Studies in cognitive development: Essays in honor of Jean Piaget*. New York: Oxford University Press.

Erikson, E. H. (1950). *Childhood and society*. New York: Norton.

Erikson, E. H. (1968). *Identity: Youth and crisis*. New York: Norton.

Erikson, E. H. (Ed.). (1978). *Adulthood*. New York: Norton.

Estes, M. E. Z. (1998). *Health assessment and physical examination*. Albany, NY: Delmar.

Flavell, J. H. (1963). *The developmental psychology of Jean Piaget*. New York: Van Nostrand Reinhold.

Flavell, J. H. (1977). *Cognitive development*. Englewood Cliffs, NJ: Prentice Hall.

Ford, R. D. (Ed.). (1990). *Diagnostic tests handbook*. Springhouse, PA: Springhouse.

Fowler, J. (1981). *Stages of faith: The psychology of human development and the quest for meaning*. New York: Harper & Row.

Frankena, W. K. (1989). The naturalistic fallacy. *Mind, 48*, 464–477.

Gilligan, C. (1982). *In a different voice: Psychological theory and women's development*. Cambridge: Harvard University Press.

Goulet, L. R., & Baltes, P. B. (Eds.). (1970). *Life-span developmental psychology: Research and theory*. New York: Academic.

Guyton, A. C. (1991). *Textbook of medical physiology* (8th ed.). Philadelphia: Saunders.

Hartshorne, H., & May, M. (1928–30). *Studies in the nature of character. Vol. 1: Studies in deceit, Vol. 2: Studies in self-control, Vol. 3: Studies in the organization of character*. New York: Macmillan.

Kagan, J. (1984). *The nature of the child*. New York: Basic Books.

Kane, R. L., Ouslander, J. G., & Abrass, I. B. (1989). *Essentials of clinical geriatrics* (2nd ed.). New York: McGraw-Hill.

Kaplan, L. J. (1974). *Adolescence: The farewell to childhood*. New York: Simon and Schuster.

Kegan, R. (1982). *The evolving self*. Cambridge, MA: Harvard University Press.

Kohlberg, L. (1987). *Child psychology and childhood education: A cognitive-developmental view*. New York: Longman.

Livingston, E. A. (1977). *The concise Oxford dictionary of the Christian church*. London: Oxford University Press.

MacQuarrie, J. (1971). *Twentieth-century religious thought: The frontiers of philosophy and theology, 1900–1970*. London: SCM Press.

MacQuarrie, J. (1972). *Existentialism*. New York: Penguin Books.

Maslow, A. H. (1968). *Toward a psychology of being* (2nd ed.). Princeton, NJ: Van Nostrand.

Maslow, A. H. (1971). *The farther reaches of human nature*. New York: Penguin Books.

Mayeroff, M. (1971). *On caring*. New York: Harper & Row.

McCance, K. L., & Huether, S. E. (1990). *Pathophysiology: The biologic basis for disease in adults and children*. St. Louis: CV Mosby.

McGaa, E. (1990). *Mother earth spirituality*. San Francisco: Harper.

McLuhan, T. C. (1971). *Touch the Earth: A self-portrait of Indian existence*. New York: Simon and Schuster.

Mead, G. H. (1934). *Self and society*. Chicago: University of Chicago Press.

Ortiz, A. (1969). *The Tewa world: Space, time, being, and becoming in a Pueblo society*. Chicago: University of Chicago Press.

Piaget, J. (1952). *The origins of intelligence in children* (M. Cook, Trans.). New York: Norton.

Piaget, J. (1962). *Play, dreams and imitation in childhood* (C. Gattegno & F. M. Hodgson, Trans.). New York: Norton.

Piaget, J. (1969a). *The child's conception of time* (A. J. Pomerans, Trans.). New York: Ballantine.

Piaget, J. (1969b). *The language and thought of the child* (M. Gabain, Trans.). New York: World.

Piaget, J. (1970). *The child's conception of movement and speed* (G. E. T. Holloway & M. J. Mackenzie, Trans.). New York: Ballantine Books.

Piaget, J. (1973). *The child and reality* (A. Rosin, Trans.). New York: Grossman.

Piaget, J. (1980). *Adaptation and intelligence: Organic selection and phenocopy* (T. A. Brown & S. Eames, Trans.). Chicago: University of Chicago Press.

Piaget, J. (1983). *The child's conception of the world* (J. Tomlinson & A. Tomlinson, Trans.). Totowa, NJ: A Helix Book.

Plato. (1967). *The symposium* (W. Hamilton, Trans.). Baltimore: Penguin Books.

Plato. (1974). *The Republic* (2nd ed.) (D. Lee, Trans.). Baltimore: Penguin Books.

Scott, A. S., & Fong, E. (1998). *Body structures and functions* (9th ed.). Albany, NY: Delmar.

Skinner, B. F. (1974). *About behaviorism*. New York; Vintage Books.

Suzuki, B. L. (1972). *Mahayana Buddhism*. New York: Macmillan.

CHAPTER 4

Special Populations

Kevin B. Frey
Paul Price

CASE STUDY

A patient with acquired immune deficiency syndrome (AIDS) is brought to the operating room for a total hip arthroplasty. The patient is in the early stages of AIDS, but does have Kaposi's sarcoma skin lesions, painful swollen lymph nodes in the groin and axilla, and has lost weight.

1. When positioning the patient, what are some of the important principles to be considered to protect the patient from injury and pain?
2. When placing the ESU grounding pad, what are some special considerations concerning the patient with AIDS?
3. What complications could be encountered during the surgical procedure that the surgical technologist should be prepared to assist the surgeon in resolving?

OBJECTIVES

After studying this chapter, the reader should be able to:

C 1. Compare and contrast the surgical care considerations for pediatric patients and patients who are obese, diabetic, pregnant, immunocompromised, disabled, geriatric, or experiencing trauma.

2. Describe the unique physical and psychological need of each special population.

A 3. Compare and contrast the intraoperative considerations for pediatric patients and patients who are obese, diabetic, immunocompromised, geriatric or traumatized that relate to postoperative wound healing.

R 4. Evaluate the role of the surgical technologist for the surgical care of each special population.

E 5. Assess the ethical commitment that is required of surgical technologists as it relates to special populations care.

6. Describe the general needs associated with special populations of surgical patients.

SELECT KEY TERMS

1. arterial blood gases (ABGs)
2. autoimmune diseases
3. central venous catheter
4. diabetes mellitus
5. enterocolitis
6. golden hour
7. human immunodeficiency virus (HIV)
8. hypothermia
9. immunocompetence
10. intra-arterial measurement
11. Kaposi's sarcoma
12. kinematics
13. penetrating trauma
14. pneumothorax
15. Revised Trauma Score
16. septic shock
17. splenectomy
18. splenomegaly
19. torticollis
20. urine output
21. venous compression device

INTRODUCTION

Surgical patients with special needs present various challenges in which the specifics of care must be adjusted to meet the particular needs of the patient. The surgical technologist must be aware of the needs of special populations and proper responses to these. Special populations present with unique physical and psychological needs. For example, infants and older adults have increased difficulty in adjusting to the stresses of traumatic injuries, loss of body temperature, and loss of intravascular fluids. Above all else, the surgical technologist must be ethically committed to providing the same quality standard of care and empathy for all surgical patients. The surgical technologist must be aware of and sensitive to the patient with special needs.

Although many surgical patients have special needs, space limits the mention of all of them. The special needs groups to be discussed in this chapter include pediatric, obese, diabetic, pregnant, immunocompromised, disabled, and geriatric. Trauma patients are included as well due to the unique circumstances that accompany traumatic injury.

PEDIATRIC PATIENTS

A patient is considered a pediatric patient if he or she is between birth and the age of 12. The common terms applied to the pediatric population that are related to their age are:

Neonate: The first 28 days of life outside the uterus

Infant: 1–18 months

Toddler: 18–30 months

Preschooler: 30 months to 5 years

School age: 6–12 years

Pediatric patients require surgery for the same reasons as anyone else—congenital anomalies, disease, and trauma. The commonly used cliché "Children are not little adults" does indeed apply. The medical and surgical care of pediatric patients is a specialty focused on the unique problems and challenges presented by this special needs group.

The surgical technologist must be familiar with the specific conditions and needs of the pediatric patient. Anatomical and physiological differences are of primary importance to the surgical team (Table 4-1). Vital signs are listed in Tables 4-2 and 4-3.

Psychological factors must be accounted for in the pediatric patient. An important factor is the ability to use language to understand their situation, the environment, and the procedure. The neonate and infant are startled easily, so a quiet environment is essential. The preschool and school-aged child may use language to the same general ends as adults—to inform, persuade, distract, or manipulate—but they will not use language the same way. Their descriptions of pain, for instance, are likely to be imprecise in terms of both symptoms and location. Learning to "hear" the child takes considerable experience.

Members of the surgical team must also be aware of their personal and communal psychological response to the pediatric patient. Almost every individual feels protective of a child. The surgical team will and should feel protective of all patients. In spite of that emotional response, the surgical team cannot explain to the neonate, infant, and toddler the nature of the condition, the procedure, or the complications. The surgical team can only explain some small portion of these to the preschool and school-aged child. These issues are, however, appropriately conveyed to the parents of the child.

In pediatric surgery, the surgical team is forced to focus on the physiological needs of the patient in a more dramatic way than it is with any other age group. In most cases, it is the role of the surgical team to efficiently and effectively achieve a state of anesthesia, complete the surgical procedure, and return the child to his or her family as quickly as possible.

Table 4-1 Pediatric Anatomical and Physiological Considerations

ISSUE	ADULT	CHILD
Temperature regulation	Shivers at reduction of ambient temperature	Child less than 6 months of age cannot shiver; therefore at risk for hypothermia, bradycardia, and acidosis Comparable to adult at age 4
Pulse and respiration	Adult norms established	Rates decline with age, reaching adult norms at adolescence
Blood pressure	Adult norms established	Child of 1 year and older: systolic pressure in mm Hg = 80 + (2 × age) and diastolic = ⅔ systolic
Head	Adult norms established	Suture ridges palpable until 6 months of age Posterior fontanel closes by 3 months Anterior fontanel closes by 19 months
Eyes	Adult norms established	Visual acuity 2/200 at birth No tears produced until 2–3 months of age
Ears	Adult norms established	Shorter external auditory canal is positioned upward Eustachian tube more horizontal, wider, and shorter, leading to more infections
Sinuses	Normal anatomical structures	Only ethmoid and maxillary sinuses present at birth Frontal sinuses develop at 7 years Sphenoid sinuses develop after puberty
Mouth	All teeth in place	Systematic development of teeth Salivation starts at 3 months
Breasts	Adult norms established	Breast tissue develops between 9 and 13 years Mature adult tissue achieved between 13 and 16 years
Thorax and lungs	Adult norms established	Chest is circular and does not reach adult ratios until age 6 Chest wall is thin in infants Ribs are horizontally displaced in infants Trachea is short in the newborn and only reaches adult length near end of adolescence Infant to 3–4 months dependent on breathing through their noses Infants and toddlers prefer abdominal breathing
Abdomen	Adult norms established	Liver proportionately larger in abdominal cavity in the infant
Bone growth	Epiphyses closed at age 20	Epiphyses not closed
Neurological	Neurological system fully developed	Neurological system not developed
Genitalia (male)	Adult norms established	Testes descend by 1 year of age

Table 4-2 Normal Heart Rate Ranges for Children

AGE	HEART RATE RANGE	AVERAGE HEART RATE
Infants to 2 years	80–130	110
2–6 years	70–120	100
6–10 years	70–110	90
10–16 years	60–100	85

Table 4-3 Normal Respiratory Rate Ranges for Children

AGE	RESPIRATORY RATE PER MINUTE
1 year	10–40
3 years	20–30
6 years	16–22
10 years	16–20
17 years	12–20

An overwhelming feeling that most pediatric patients feel is that of anxiety due to separation from the parent(s). A feeling of permanent abandonment can occur. The challenge for the surgical technologist who greets and cares for the child is to form, in a very short period, a bond of trust to allay some of the child's fears. The following are suggestions to help reduce the anxiety level of the child:

- Let the child bring a favorite toy or stuffed animal into surgery.
- During the preoperative visit, introduce the child to all of the individuals who will be involved in the surgical care.
- Take the child into the front part of the surgery department to see how it looks.
- Let the parent(s) walk alongside while transporting the patient to the surgery department. They can accompany the child into the preoperative area.
- Allow the parents to come into the PACU after the child arrives and the first set of vital signs has been recorded.

Another primary fear of the pediatric patient is fear of anesthesia. Children do not understand the meaning of unconsciousness and may fear that they are going to sleep and will never wake up. Again, the preoperative visit is helpful; it allows the anesthesia provider to show the child the equipment, and even let the child hold a mask on her face so she knows ahead of time what will be occurring. Just as with the adult surgical patient, the child should be dealt with in a truthful manner, and questions concerning needles used for injection and postoperative pain should be truthfully answered. Children are generally very quick to recognize deception, and the caregiver can quickly lose the trust of the child by trying to deceive.

Since the development of rapid induction, the child no longer has to be subjected to long induction times. Patients who are 2 years of age and younger are usually held by the anesthesia provider during induction. The circulating surgical technologist should stand nearby to assist the anesthesia provider by holding the mask on the face of the child or by holding the child's hand or arms, and by making sure that the room is kept very quiet during the induction.

MONITORING THE PEDIATRIC PATIENT

The pediatric patient must be closely monitored during the surgical procedure, and distinct differences exist for measurement between the pediatric patient and adult patient. The critical parameters to monitor for the pediatric patient include temperature, **urine output**, cardiac function, and oxygenation.

TEMPERATURE

In comparison with adults, pediatric patients, in particular neonates, have little subcutaneous fat and therefore poor thermal insulation. They also have less lean body mass, which is required for retaining and generating heat. Newborns lose heat through radiation, convection, and evaporation. Incubators aid in minimizing heat loss by radiation and convection by decreasing the airflow across the skin of the newborn.

Temperature is monitored by measuring the rectal and skin temperature. In the OR, skin temperature is the primary means of monitoring the temperature. Maintaining proper body temperature is critical in the OR, so the temperature of the room is increased prior to the patient entering. An overhead radiant heater is often used for patients 2 years and younger. However, the most effective means for maintaining body temperature is to keep the infant's extremities wrapped and covered.

URINE OUTPUT

For fluid management, urine output measurement is highly useful for all patient age groups. Neonates and infants are not usually catheterized due to the high risk of trauma to the small urethra; a collection bag is just as useful in obtaining an accurate measurement. An appropriate urine output is 1 to 2 mL/kg/hr.

CARDIAC FUNCTION

The use of the sphygmomanometer and stethoscope has disadvantages with pediatric patients due to the reliance on cuff size, which varies considerably among children. For very ill infants and children who require constant ECG monitoring, **intra-arterial measurement** is recommended. In infants and children, a cutdown approach to the radial artery is most commonly used. In neonates, the umbilical artery is most commonly used due to easy accessibility.

When no cardiac abnormalities are present, a **central venous catheter** is inserted percutaneously into the subclavian or internal jugular vein in older children. In neonates and infants, a cutdown approach to the external jugular vein is preferred. Due to higher incidences of contamination when procedures are performed in the groin region, the saphenous vein is the route least used.

OXYGENATION

The standard for monitoring oxygenation for all age groups of surgical patients is measuring the **arterial blood gases** (**ABGs**). However, with the introduction of pulse oximetry, the monitoring of oxygenation has been made considerably easier. Its advantages include immediate blood oxygen saturation information and low cost. The elimination of the necessity for an indwelling probe also decreases the possibility of infection. In surgery, it can be difficult to obtain a blood specimen from the small artery of a neonate or infant; consequently, pulse oximetry has reduced the waiting time for collecting monitoring data.

SHOCK

The two common types of shock seen in all age groups are septic and hypovolemic shock. In infants and children, **septic shock** is most commonly seen. It is highly important for the surgical technologist to be aware that the neonate and infant respond to shock differently from the older child and adult. For the neonate affected by hypovolemic shock, bradycardia is a physiological response, whereas tachycardia is the typical adult response. Neonates' blood pressure is normally low, so shock does not significantly decrease the blood pressure. However, hypovolemia does result in decreased venous return that lowers cardiac output and leads to poor tissue perfusion with eventual lactic acidosis.

Septic shock is usually caused by gram-negative bacteria. Peritonitis due to intestinal perforation is a common cause of shock in neonates and infants. Other causes of septic shock include urinary tract infection (UTI), upper respiratory infection (URI), and a contaminated intravascular catheter.

In infants, dehydration is the most common cause of hypovolemic shock; therefore, the main treatment of hypovolemic shock is quick fluid and blood replacement. As a rule of thumb, more water is lost than electrolytes. Emergency treatment is the infusion of a hypotonic solution of sodium chloride.

Septic shock also presents with reduced circulating blood volume, therefore initial treatment is the infusion of colloid solutions. Clinical research supports the infusion of colloid solutions as preferable to crystalloid solutions for treating septic shock in all age groups. In addition, the infection is treated with broad-spectrum antibiotics. If the infusion of fluids has achieved its purposes of elevating the central venous pressure (CVP), but hypotension is still present, dopamine is the agent of choice to increase cardiac output.

FLUIDS AND ELECTROLYTES

The management of fluids and electrolytes in neonates and infants requires an understanding of the changes in body fluids that occur before and after birth. The normal physiological processes presented in Table 4-4 are interrupted in premature neonates who must eliminate

Table 4-4 Changes in Body Fluids Before and After Birth

TRIMESTER OR AGE	PERCENT OF TOTAL BODY WATER	PERCENT OF EXTRACELLULAR FLUID VOLUME
First trimester	95% of body weight	
32 weeks' gestation	80%	
Term	78%	
First postnatal week	75%	
Next 1 to 2 years	60%	
Second trimester		60%
Birth		45%
Year 2		20%

excess fetal and postnatal total body water in a very short period of time after birth. This has a significant effect on the premature neonate who must undergo surgery. An increased extracellular fluid (ECF) volume in a "preemie" is a stimulus for the release of prostaglandin E_2, which will maintain the patency of a ductus arteriosus.

Newborns and infants do not tolerate dehydration well. In addition, their immature kidneys cannot excrete water as effectively as mature kidneys. Combined with the decreased renal concentrating ability of the immature kidney, fluid management can be difficult in a surgical setting.

A major concern in the OR is insensible water loss (usually transepithelial). Reasons for insensible water loss include water loss through the skin and lungs caused by overhead radiant heaters and phototherapy. The insensible water loss from the skin in the OR is decreased by covering the extremities; water loss from the lungs is decreased by the humidification of the inspired gases.

INFECTION

Immediately after birth, bacterial colonization of the newborn's skin and gastrointestinal tract begins. By the 10th day after birth, newborns have the same common aerobic and anaerobic bacteria as that found in the GI tract of adults. However, the normal microbial barriers, skin and GI tract, are still underdeveloped in the newborn, as are the host defense mechanisms.

The initial sign of postoperative infection is fever. The most common sites of postoperative infection are the lungs, surgical wound, urinary tract, and vascular access sites. Treatment for infected surgical wounds includes incision, debridement, and placement of antibiotic-impregnated packing. Frequent dressing changes are required until the wound has healed. Vascular access site infections and urinary catheter infections are treated by removing the catheter and administering antibiotics.

Generally, the indications, uses, and choices of antibiotics are the same for neonates, infants, and children as they are for adults. For clean-contaminated elective surgical procedures, such as a colon operation, the antibiotics of choice are penicillin in combination with aminoglycoside or third-generation cephalosporin. The first dose of antibiotics is given just before the skin incision is made, and they are continued postoperatively for 24–48 hours. The side effects are similar to those seen in adults, except for three important differences:

1. Sulfonamides (such as Bactrim or Septa) are associated with an increased incidence of kernicterus in neonates. Sulfonamides should *not* be administered to newborns.
2. Chloramphenicol (Chloromycetin) is the synthetic form of an antibiotic originally isolated from *Streptomyces venezuelae* and is associated with the cause of "gray syndrome" in which the infant's skin turns gray from drug toxicity. Chloramphenicol should *not* be administered to newborns.
3. Tetracycline causes staining and hypoplasia of the enamel of the developing teeth; therefore, it should *not* be administered to children.

Practically every antibiotic has been associated with the development of pseudomembranous **enterocolitis**, most likely from the overgrowth of *Clostridium difficile* due to antibiotic suppression of the growth of normal bacteria in the colon. One treatment consists of discontinuing the antibiotic that contributed to the cause of the enterocolitis (infection of the small and large bowel), and oral administration of vancomycin.

METABOLIC AND NUTRITIONAL RESPONSES

The caloric requirements of infants are much higher than those of children and adults. Surgery increases the caloric requirements (a 20% to 30% increase with a major operation). Since the work of feeding (sucking and swallowing) accounts for a large portion of the infant's caloric use in the first few months of life, gastrostomy tube feedings are often used postoperatively for procedures of the GI tract.

TRAUMA

Accidents are the number one cause of death in children ages 1–15. Each year, approximately 20 million childhood injuries result in death or permanent disability. Obviously, the emphasis should be on prevention, such as the design of better restraint devices in automobiles and the wearing of helmets when riding a bike.

The causes of trauma in children are more often the result of blunt trauma. Head trauma is much more common in children than adults and accounts for the majority of morbidity and mortality in pediatrics. Motor vehicle accidents are the major cause of trauma in children. Other causes seen more often in children than adults include falls, bicycle accidents, drowning, burns, and poisonings. Childbirth trauma and child abuse are also unique trauma circumstances.

KEY DIFFERENCES IN TREATMENT

Children's emotional reactions to trauma differ from those of an adult. They experience communication barriers in which to indicate the origin of pain. They may give misleading information, such as exhibiting signs that their abdominal region hurts when there is no abdominal injury. Children also often display signs of developmental regression, especially if the parents are not present.

A second key difference is the metabolic and nutritional differences of children as compared to adults:

- Postoperative metabolic management of the pediatric patient is important, especially if the patient is being treated for trauma.
- What seems to be an insignificant loss of blood can result in marked hemodynamic changes in the child.
- Water and heat loss can occur quickly in children, who lack insulating subcutaneous fat.
- **Hypothermia** intensifies the effects of acidosis.
- Vomiting due to gastric dilatation is common in children who experience trauma and/or surgical procedures; consequently, aspiration is of concern.
- Increased nutritional requirements that were previously discussed must not be forgotten.

General Principles of Pediatric Emergency Treatment

As with all trauma patients, the first priority is to make sure that the patient has an open airway and that it is maintained. The airway should be cleared of any obstacles, such as blood or broken teeth. If the patient is having breathing difficulties, the best treatment is to intubate the child immediately by placing an uncuffed endotracheal tube. If a neck injury is suspected, the cervical spine must be stabilized with a collar or sand bags.

If breathing continues to be difficult, **pneumothorax** (accumulation of air in the pleural cavity) can be a possibility. It is difficult to diagnose pneumothorax in children, but a chest X-ray will aid in diagnosis. A pediatric chest tube is placed to treat the pneumothorax. Hyperventilation is a common response by children to injury, resulting in gastric dilatation. This is easily resolved by inserting a nasogastric tube.

An intravenous (IV) catheter should be placed next. If it is difficult to place a needle in a peripheral vein, it is recommended that a cutdown be performed to the greater saphenous vein at the ankle. Fluids can then start to be infused to treat the pediatric patient for shock. The insertion of a central venous or arterial line may be considered.

Bleeding must also be controlled to prevent severe hypovolemia. Pressure placed on lacerations as soon as possible is important in the management of blood and body fluid loss.

TRAUMA DURING BIRTH

A small percentage of births result in a traumatic injury to the neonate (Figure 4-1). The use of prenatal ultrasonography has greatly reduced the incidence of birth trauma. The injuries typically seen are bone fractures; injuries to the liver, spleen, and adrenal glands; and nerve injuries.

The most common bone fracture is of the clavicle, usually as a result of shoulder dystocia. Upper brachial plexus palsy can occur secondary to shoulder dystocia or breech presentation. Peripheral facial nerve paralysis occasionally occurs due to direct pressure on the infant's face by the mother's pelvis or from the use of forceps. Complete recovery most often occurs by 1 year of age.

Injuries to the liver, spleen, or adrenal gland are caused by direct pressure on the infant's abdomen from the mother's birth canal. However, this rarely requires surgical intervention. Birth trauma can injure the sternocleidomastoid muscle, which leads to the formation of a hematoma and **torticollis** (a contracted state of the muscle). Surgery is necessary if the injury is not recognized in time to correct the condition.

CHILD ABUSE

Child abuse is a tragic event that often presents with multiple traumatic injuries, some of which that may have already healed, especially in the case of fractures. The abuse takes the form of physical and/or mental injury, sexual abuse, nutritional neglect, verbal abuse, and delayed treatment of disease and injuries. Surgery is often required to treat soft tissue injuries, fractures, burns, and head trauma. Visceral injuries include internal liver and splenic lacerations, internal pancreatic damage, and duodenal hematomas.

PATIENTS WITH OBESITY

Patients who are obese, that is, patients whose body weight is 100 pounds greater than ideal body weight, have an increased susceptibility to morbidity and mortality caused by the physical difficulties of carrying extra weight. The number of complications and morbidity varies according to how severe the obese condition is. Physiological and disease conditions as related to obesity include:

- Myocardial hypertrophy due to the increased demands placed on the heart, leading to congestive heart failure
- Coronary artery disease
- Hypertension and vascular changes in the kidneys, affecting elimination of protein wastes and the maintenance of normal fluid and electrolyte balance
- Varicose veins and edema in extremities due to poor venous return (Venous pooling can lead to thromboembolism)

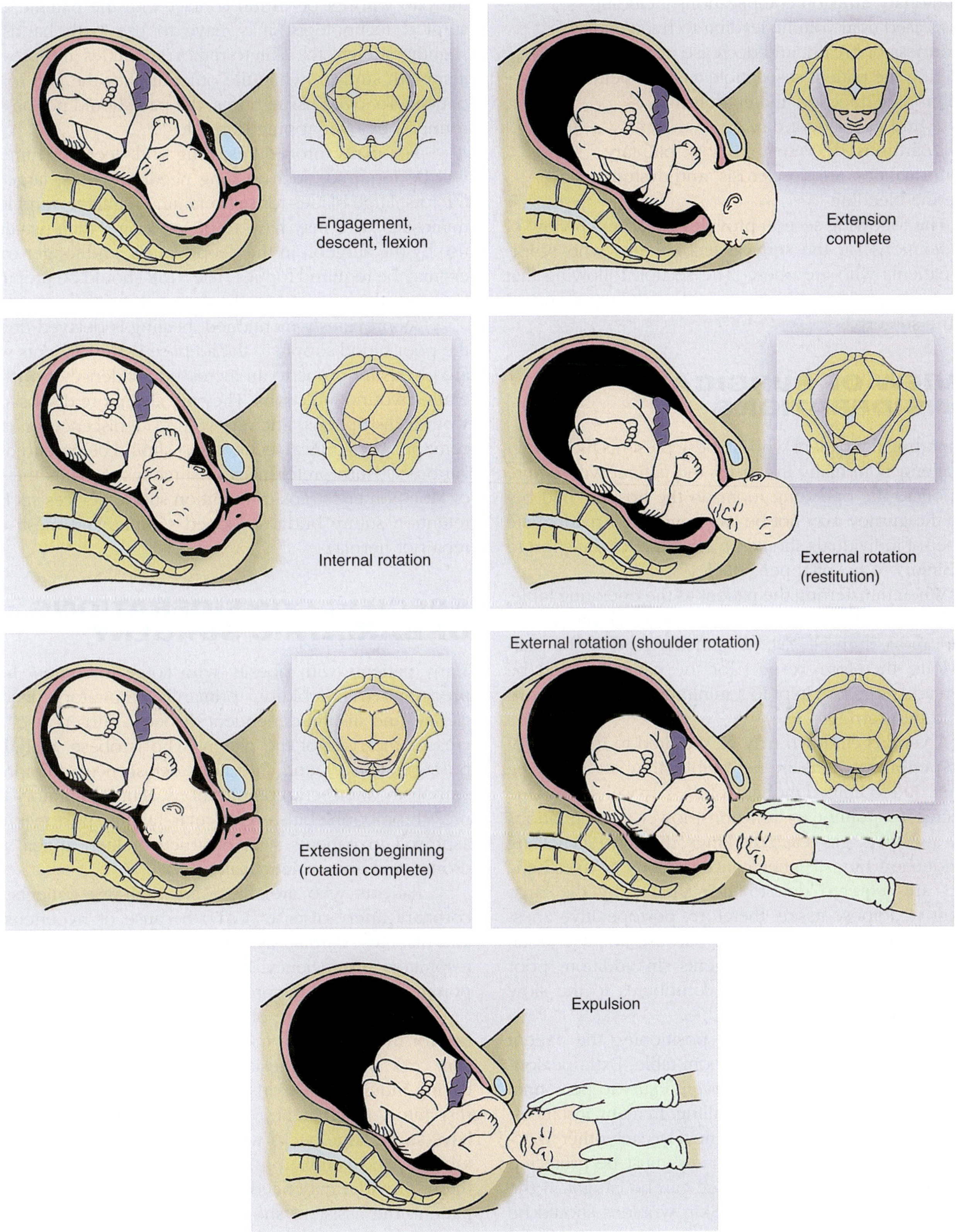

Figure 4-1 Birth of an infant

- Pulmonary function complications including decreased tidal volume leading to hypoxemia, shortness of breath, and decrease in lung expansion, making the patient susceptible to postoperative pulmonary infection and embolism
- Liver and gallbladder disease
- Osteoarthritis, **diabetes mellitus**, pituitary abnormalities, arteriosclerosis, and dysfunctional uterine bleeding

The following section provides an overall review of considerations for the surgical technologist who works with patients who are obese. The section following that focuses on specific issues to consider when performing bariatric surgery.

REVIEW OF SURGICAL CONSIDERATIONS

Transporting the patient who is obese presents the first set of challenges. In many instances, the patient will require transport to the operating room on the hospital bed because the gurney may not be large enough. An adequate number of individuals should be available for transport to avoid injury to hospital personnel.

When transferring the patient to the operating table, a mechanical lifting device may be required if the patient cannot move himself. Obese patients tend to be self-conscious; therefore, respect for the patient should be shown and exposure kept to a minimum when transporting and transferring.

A venous cutdown may be required to insert an IV line if peripheral veins are not visible. Intubation may be difficult due to limited mobility of the cervical spine. Due to decreased pulmonary functions, lower concentrations of the anesthetic gas reach the lungs, therefore increasing the induction time. Higher concentrations of anesthetic agents are required due to their uptake by the large amount of adipose tissue; therefore, postoperative anesthesia recovery time is increased because adipose tissue retains fat-soluble anesthetic agents. In addition, poor blood supply to adipose tissue contributes to the slow elimination of these agents.

Care must be taken when positioning the patient who is obese on the operating room table. Extra personnel should be present to help prevent injury to personnel and to prevent the patient from falling. In many instances, two operating tables are situated next to each other to accommodate the larger patient. Tissue must be protected from injury because folds of tissue can be caught in the crevices of the operating table. Skin wrinkles should be smoothed out when positioning to avoid cutting off the blood supply to the tissue, possibly causing skin ulcers and tissue necrosis. Areas of concern should be padded to prevent bruising and pressure injuries.

The proper principles of grounding pad placement must be followed. Avoid skin wrinkles when placing or the pad will not be in full contact with the patient. One surgical technologist may have to use both hands to slightly "stretch" the skin to remove wrinkles and provide a smooth surface, while the other applies the pad to the patient. To avoid tissue burns, the pad should not be surrounded by overlapping skin folds.

For many procedures, long and deep instruments will be required, such as long needle holders, large retractors, large blades for self-retaining retractors, and long hemostats. Ties may have to be cut longer than usual for use by the surgeon in the deep wound, and longer carriers may be required for ties. The STSR should be prepared for a lengthier procedure than normal.

As previously mentioned, healing is delayed due to the poor blood supply to the adipose tissue. Patients who are obese are prone to an increased incidence of postoperative wound infections. They are also more disposed to wound disruptions, such as wound dehiscence or evisceration. The surgical technologist should be prepared for various closure preferences of surgeons, such as the use of Montgomery straps or retention suture devices such as retention suture bridges, looped sutures, and mesh (for repair of hernia).

SPECIFIC CONSIDERATIONS OF BARIATRIC SURGERY

Many patients with obesity who come to surgery have preoperative morbidity, primarily respiratory insufficiency, and insulin-dependent diabetes. Surgery itself increases the risks of the patient who is obese, including postoperative wound infection, dehiscence, pulmonary embolism, anesthetic complications, acute respiratory failure, thrombophlebitis, ventricular failure, postoperative asphyxia in patients with obstructive sleep apnea syndrome, and anastomotic leaks.

Patients who are obese are high-risk patients for coronary artery disease (CAD) because of hypertension and diabetes. Cardiac dysfunction is also associated with respiratory insufficiency. Perioperative ECGs are very important throughout the process of caring for these patients.

Patients who are obese present numerous difficulties for the anesthesia provider. The patient is at significant risk for anesthesia complications, in particular during induction. This risk is increased for patients with respiratory insufficiency. Patients who are obese tend to have short, large necks with limited mobility, making intubation and ventilation more of a challenge. The anesthesia provider may need assistance when intubating the patient; the assistant should elevate the jaw and hyperextend the neck while the anesthesia provider performs the intubation. Placing the patient in reverse Trendelenburg's position expands total lung volume and aids in ventilation. However, this leg-down position predisposes the patient to venous stasis and thrombophlebitis. Therefore, when setting up the room prior to the procedure, the surgical technologist should make sure that a **venous compression device** is in the room and that the patient is fitted with intermittent venous compression boots.

As previously mentioned, patients who are obese are at risk for deep-vein thrombosis. This risk increases with a prolonged surgical procedure or postoperative period in which the patient is immobile and when the patient is in the supine position during surgery. Heparin is typically administered subcutaneously 30 minutes before the procedure and at intervals for at least 2 days postoperatively. As mentioned, the reverse Trendelenburg position significantly improves pulmonary function, but intermittent venous compression boots must be utilized to reduce the incidence of deep-vein thrombosis. The patient should also attempt to walk as soon as possible postoperatively to aid the prevention of thrombosis.

Postoperatively, the patient who is obese should be kept in the reverse Trendelenburg position. When respiratory insufficiency is not present, most patients can be extubated in the OR or PACU and returned to their hospital rooms. Encouragement is provided for early postoperative ambulation.

COMPLICATIONS AFTER GASTRIC SURGERY

The three most common complications after gastric bypass or gastroplasty surgery are abdominal catastrophes, internal hernia, and acute gastric distention. It can be difficult to diagnose an abdominal catastrophe in patients who are obese. The symptoms and the complaints of the patient are of great importance, and signs of infection may not be present. Often acute respiratory failure indicates peritonitis. If visceral perforation is suspected, an exploratory laparotomy will be performed.

Gastric bypass patients are at risk for internal hernia with a closed-loop obstruction leading to bowel strangulation. Left untreated, necrosis can result. The primary symptom is periumbilical pain, and again, exploratory laparotomy will be performed for repair.

Postoperatively, gastric bypass patients can develop severe gaseous distention in the distal bypassed stomach. This can lead to gastric perforation or can damage the gastrojejunostomy. Symptoms include hiccups, bloated feeling, severe left shoulder pain, and shock. Diagnosis is made by taking an upright abdominal radiograph that will show the dilated stomach. An emergency laparotomy with insertion of a gastrostomy tube is performed along with examination of the jejunostomy.

GALLSTONES

During abdominal procedures on patients with obesity, gallstones are often found (in addition to the original pathology) and the gallbladder is removed. Therefore, when performing an abdominal procedure on these patients, the STSR should have the instrumentation and other supplies available for a cholecystectomy with possible cholangiography.

DEGENERATIVE OSTEOARTHRITIS

Degenerative osteoarthritis of the back, hips, and knees is common in individuals who are obese. Weight reduction may help reduce the pain and increase the mobility of the patient, but often the damage is extensive, requiring a total joint arthroplasty. However, in very large patients (250 pounds or more), loosening of the prosthesis is common. Often, the surgeon requires the patient to lose a sufficient amount of weight before the arthroplasty is performed.

PATIENTS WITH DIABETES

Diabetes mellitus is a disorder of the endocrine system. It affects the production of insulin in the pancreas and glucose tolerance in the body. Insulin is the hormone that aids in breaking down sugars and carbohydrates. The origin of the disorder is most often genetic. There are two types of diabetes mellitus:

1. *Type I—insulin-dependent diabetes mellitus (IDDM):* The pancreas produces little or no insulin, and the individual must have daily, regular doses of insulin.
2. *Type II—non-insulin-dependent diabetes mellitus (NIDDM):* The pancreas produces different amounts of insulin. The individual is not required to take insulin.

When performing surgery on patients who are diabetic, the following conditions must be prevented:

- Ketonuria
- Hyperglycemia
- Ketoacidosis
- Acetonuria
- Hypoglycemia and hypoglycemic shock (can occur during major operations due to omission or delay of oral intake of insulin)

Preoperative preparation of the patient includes:

- Fasting
- Urinalysis to determine presence of sugar and acetone
- CBC
- BUN
- Postprandial blood sugar level
- Serum electrolyte level
- Chest X-ray
- ECG

COMPLICATIONS ASSOCIATED WITH DIABETES

Surgery affects the normal caloric intake of the patient and daily dosage of insulin. Anesthesia also affects the normal metabolic and physiological processes of the patient with diabetes. Blood glucose can increase while the serum insulin levels decrease. NIDDM patients usually go through surgery without any difficulties. Perioperative metabolic control of the IDDM patient presents the surgery team with unique challenges and difficulties, especially when the operation is lengthy and involves a large amount of tissue trauma. The patient with diabetes is at a higher risk for the following:

- Infection (Ulcers that develop on the extremities, particularly the foot, heal slowly or not at all and are prone to infection. Many elderly patients with diabetes must undergo extremity amputation to control an infection of the extremity that is not responding to antibiotics or other surgical interventions.)
- Dehydration
- Poor circulation combined with vascular disease
- Myocardial infarction
- Delayed wound healing
- Nephropathy
- Control of postoperative blood glucose level
- Neuropathic skeletal disease resulting in severe bone destruction
- Neurogenic bladder resulting in frequent UTI
- Retinopathy resulting in blindness
- Coronary artery disease
- Thrombophlebitis and peripheral edema
- Tachycardia

CARE OF THE PATIENT WITH DIABETES IN SURGERY

Patients with diabetes require specific preoperative, intraoperative, and postoperative procedures to ensure their safety:

PREOPERATIVE

- A blood sample for the fasting serum glucose test is taken to provide data for postoperative care of the patient.
- The normal dosage of preoperative medication is decreased since narcotics can induce vomiting, which predisposes the patient to fluid and electrolyte imbalance causing a hypoglycemic reaction.
- The preoperative insulin dose is reduced to prevent intraoperative hypoglycemia or insulin shock.
- When positioning the patient, bony prominences and other areas of concern must be adequately padded to prevent pressure sores and ulcers, particularly if the operation will be lengthy.

INTRAOPERATIVE

- IV access is accomplished by the anesthesia provider to monitor insulin and glucose levels. Electrolytes can be added to the IV fluids to maintain balance. Insulin can be added to the IV fluids or given as a subcutaneous injection.
- Monitoring, especially during long procedures, is important to avoid a metabolic crisis. Monitoring is necessary to determine the patient's needs for insulin, glucose, or both. A glucometer is used to measure the blood glucose level. Urine specimens are monitored for the presence of ketones.
- Antiembolic stockings are worn by the patient during surgery to prevent thromboembolism.

POSTOPERATIVE

An increased rate of infection is one of the most common postoperative complications of diabetes, primarily due to diminished levels of blood flow to the affected area. Postoperative stress hormone levels predispose the patient to hyperglycemia, as do changes in activity level and some medications or their interactions with other drugs administered postoperatively. In addition, glucose-lowering agents used to control hyperglycemia preoperatively should influence decisions regarding perioperative glucose management.

Postoperatively, the patient should be:

- Provided with proper nutrients (either intravenously or orally) for healing and glucose control
- Administered the proper type and dose of antihyperglycemic medications
- Fitted with intermittent venous compression boots to prevent thromboembolism or thrombophlebitis

PREGNANT PATIENTS

There are approximately 3.6 million live births per year in the United States. Approximately 1% to 2% of pregnancies require surgery for reasons other than cesarean section or spontaneous abortion. When planning surgery on the pregnant patient, two patients must be taken into consideration: the mother and the fetus. Immediate operative intervention is done for emergencies, such as ectopic pregnancy, appendicitis, trauma injury, or incompetent cervix. Urgent surgical procedures are delayed until after the second or third trimester, or until the mother delivers. Elective procedures are definitely delayed until after delivery and the mother has had some time to recover from the ordeal of pregnancy and delivery.

Surgical procedures performed in the first trimester should be postponed if possible, due to the increased chances of abortion. Abdominal procedures are best performed in the second trimester. In the second trimester, the fetus is stable and the tissue of major organs is well differentiated. In addition, since the uterus has not greatly enlarged, the abdominal organs have not been displaced from their normal position to any great degree, making it easier to expose the wound, retract, and manipulate the organs. For procedures performed in the third trimester, there is a 40% risk of premature labor, and further difficulties are encountered due to the displacement of organs by the enlarged uterus.

CONSIDERATIONS WHEN CARING FOR PREGNANT PATIENTS

Due to the size of the uterus, the abdominal organs are displaced from their normal anatomical location; additionally, anatomical landmarks are difficult to locate. This can make trauma and disease diagnoses difficult. When surgery is being contemplated, the anatomical changes must be considered. For example, a pregnant patient with appendicitis may initially be thought to have cholecystitis since the appendix is displaced to the lower region of the upper right quadrant (appendicitis and acute cholecystitis are the two most common nonobstetric emergencies in the pregnant patient). Results of laboratory tests are skewed by the hormonal changes and other physiological changes of pregnancy, and the results vary according to the gestational stage.

Physiological assessment is difficult since pregnancy alters vital signs. The pulse rate increases to compensate for the increase in circulatory volume. The arterial blood pressure is lower as compared to prepregnancy levels. The diagnosis of hypovolemic shock is especially challenging. The pregnant patient may not immediately display the classic physiological signs of shock (such as cool and clammy skin) because of decreased peripheral vascular resistance. Circulating blood volume may decrease as much as 30% before the patient has signs of hypovolemic shock (such as decreased blood pressure and increased pulse rate). By that time, blood is being shunted away from the placental circulation and the fetus becomes hypoxic. The intraoperative and postoperative use of the electronic fetal heart monitor (EFM) is vital for prevention of hypovolemic shock.

Postoperatively, the patient must be observed for vaginal bleeding, ruptured membranes, or uterine irritability. These symptoms can indicate preterm labor. Bladder distention can also cause uterine irritability and preterm labor; therefore, the indwelling catheter should be left in place for monitoring fluid status. The EFM should continue to be used as well.

ANESTHESIA

The three important items to remember are the increase in preterm labor, fetal death, and low birth weight when general anesthesia must be used. With this in mind, the following are considerations for the safe delivery of anesthesia to the pregnant patient.

Anesthetic agents cross the placental barrier and enter the fetal circulation. The fetal liver is not developed; therefore, it slowly metabolizes narcotics and tranquilizers. Preferably, only short-acting drugs should be used. Drugs that have an adverse effect on the fetus in the first trimester include sedatives, tranquilizers, halogenated agents, and nitrous oxide (also a consideration for the pregnant surgical technologist who breathes in these scattered fumes). Clinical research has shown that nitrous oxide and halogenated agents have been administered in the second and third trimesters with no adverse effects on the fetus. However, fetal respiratory depression is a common occurrence with the use of any of these drugs. Other adverse effects of drugs on the fetus include bradycardia (bupivacaine) and central nervous system depression (lidocaine).

The most important consideration in the delivering of anesthetic agents is to prevent preterm labor. Halogenated agents decrease the uterine tone and aid in preventing uterine contractions. On the other hand, vasopressors and neostigmine (reversed muscle relaxation) can stimulate preterm labor.

INTRAOPERATIVE CONSIDERATIONS FOR THE SURGICAL TECHNOLOGIST

The surgical technologist must be prepared to assist the surgeon in intraoperative monitoring activities and be prepared for any untoward events. The following are important considerations for the STSR to remember:

- Without compromising patient care or violating the principles of asepsis, the STSR should move as quickly as possible when assisting the surgeon to keep general anesthesia time to a minimum.
- The STSR should aid the surgeon by palpating the uterus during the surgical procedure to detect contractions.
- The circulating surgical technologist should be available to assist the anesthesia provider by providing cricoid pressure during induction.
- When positioning the patient in the supine position, the circulating surgical technologist should place a small rolled sheet or pad under the right hip to slightly laterally shift the uterus to the left. This takes the weight of the uterus off the vena cava and abdominal aorta to aid in maintaining a normotensive level.
- If irrigation is used during the procedure, the circulator should accurately document the amount used so that the anesthesia provider can estimate blood loss.
- Before the patient enters the OR, the circulator should raise the temperature of the room to prevent maternal hypothermia. Plenty of warm blankets should be available to cover the patient.
- The STSR should have the instrumentation, supplies, and equipment immediately available in the event that an emergency cesarean section must be performed.

- The STSR should be aware that the transducer of the Doppler ultrasound scanner for fetal heart rate monitoring has been placed on the maternal abdominal wall away from the operative site.

IMMUNOCOMPROMISED PATIENTS

Immunocompetence is the degree of function for an immune system that is designed to keep a patient from infection by pathogens. The immunocompromised status of a patient can be influenced by many factors. Typically, the old or very young have immune systems that are compromised to a certain degree. Certain diseases, especially chronic ones that target the immune system, can decrease the body's ability to fight off infection by pathogens. The immune system can be intentionally suppressed by specific drugs to combat an overactive immune system that is attacking the body's own tissues instead of the foreign invaders for which it was intended. These **autoimmune diseases** include multiple sclerosis, lupus erythematosus, or rheumatoid arthritis. Immunosuppressant drugs are also administered to recipients of organ transplants to prevent the recipient's immune system from rejecting the newly transplanted organ.

ACQUIRED IMMUNODEFICIENCY SYNDROME

Patients with AIDS have tested positive for the **human immunodeficiency virus** (**HIV**) and are symptomatic, usually of an opportunistic disease that the compromised immune system has allowed to take hold. In fact, AIDS patients are often inflicted with several opportunistic infections, many of which were not commonly seen until AIDS arrived, including **Kaposi's sarcoma**, severe psoriasis rash of the body, *Pneumocystis carinii* pneumonia (PCP), and other fungal and parasitic infections. HIV is grouped in the family of retroviruses and may remain inactive and undetected for a long period of time before causing disease. Once active, the virus disrupts the normal functions of the T-lymphocytes of the body, thus impairing the patient's immune system. However, during the time of inactivity in which there are no outward signs of infection, the individual can transmit the virus through blood or body fluids.

At one point in time, HIV/AIDS was considered an exclusive disease of homosexuals, intravenous drug users, or recipients of transfused blood containing HIV. We now know that anyone is susceptible to transmission, especially during unprotected sex or through the sharing of contaminated needles. In addition, infected pregnant females can transmit the virus to the unborn fetus.

COMPLICATIONS

As previously mentioned, surgical patients with AIDS may present with multiple opportunistic infections by parasites, fungi, viruses, or bacteria; malignancies; and overall general poor health that demands special care of the patient. The patient often experiences pain from various complications and should be carefully handled and made as comfortable as possible.

A common complication is the presence of multiple external and internal lesions due to Kaposi's sarcoma and/or herpesvirus, or white patches due to candidiasis infection. The external Kaposi's sarcoma lesions are often painful, open infectious wounds, so care must be taken not to aggravate these lesions when transporting patients and positioning them in surgery. Painful swollen lymph tissue masses are present in the neck, groin, and axilla, again requiring careful handling of the patient. Internal Kaposi's sarcoma can cause the following complications, providing additional challenges to the surgery team:

- If located in the esophagus, the lesions can make it difficult for the patient to swallow or can prevent swallowing altogether.
- Intestinal lesions can cause bowel obstruction and prevent the normal absorption of nutrients. Constant anorexia and diarrhea are common symptoms of the AIDS patient, contributing to overall wasting of the body.

CONSIDERATIONS FOR THE SURGICAL TEAM MEMBERS

STSRs must keep in mind how poor the physical condition of the AIDS patient will be. Most systems of the body will be involved either directly or indirectly in the disease process, requiring a comprehensive plan of care that addresses all concerns.

Even though the patient may present with extreme muscle and tissue wasting, additional personnel should be available to move the patient from the hospital bed to the gurney and from the gurney to the operating table. The patient may not be able to move due to weakness, pain, and skin lesions. The use of extra personnel will ensure a smooth transfer of the patient, causing as little pain as possible for the patient.

Many routine procedures are going to be difficult to perform. The following are examples of the difficulties encountered by the surgical team members:

- The anesthesia provider may have difficulties intubating the patient who has internal Kaposi's lesions in the trachea. The patient may have to be "masked" throughout the procedure.
- IV placement is going to be difficult because of lack of a suitable vein. Kaposi's lesions or candidiasis skin

patches may cover large areas of normal access, or veins may be "used up" due to repeated sticks during previous treatments.

- Placement of the ESU grounding pad will be difficult due to lesions and skin wrinkling (as a result of wasting). Removal of the grounding pad can injure the patient for the same reasons. Placement of adhesive monitoring devices (such as ECG leads) may also be difficult.
- Bony prominences and areas in which muscle and tissue wasting have occurred must be adequately padded and protected.
- Blankets and drapes must be carefully placed and not moved around to avoid rubbing and aggravating painful lesions.

COMMON SURGICAL PROCEDURES

The role of surgical care of the AIDS patient primarily involves diagnostic biopsies (such as bronchoscopy) and treatment of complications of malignancies and infections. Cryptosporidiosis and cytomegalovirus infections frequently occur in the biliary tree, causing acute cholecystitis and cholangitis and requiring emergency repair (a choledochoenteric bypass may be performed). *Candida* infection and Kaposi's sarcoma have also been documented as causing cholangitis, requiring bypass surgery.

Acute perforations of the GI tract from cytomegalovirus infection, cryptosporidiosis, and candidiasis have been documented, requiring bowel resection, bypass, or colostomy. GI obstruction due to Kaposi's sarcoma lesions also requires bowel surgery. A study of AIDS patients requiring an abdominal operation described four clinical syndromes that require surgical intervention:

1. Peritonitis secondary to cytomegalovirus infection
2. Non-Hodgkin's lymphoma of the GI tract resulting in obstruction and/or bleeding
3. Kaposi's sarcoma lesions of the GI tract
4. Mycobacterial infection of the retroperitoneum or spleen

Thrombocytopenia is another complication of AIDS patients. **Splenectomy** (removal of the spleen) obtains very good results in these patients and for those experiencing **splenomegaly** (enlargement of the spleen). Debilitating fevers are associated with splenomegaly, and the patient experiences positive palliative effects after splenectomy.

A frequent procedure performed by the general surgeon is placement of an indwelling catheter. The primary care physician will request the surgery in order to have long-term access for the treatment of fungal infections and for nutritional support of AIDS patients with debilitating diarrhea.

PATIENTS WITH DISABILITIES

Often, surgical technologists must deal with patients who have various disabilities that can cause increased levels of anxiety for the patient preoperatively and postoperatively. Patients may be physically, developmentally, or mentally impaired, and surgical technologists should be aware of the psychosocial and physical needs of these patients.

Patients with hearing impairments may be totally deaf or simply impaired to varying degrees. Patients who are partially deaf are typically required to remove their hearing aid devices during surgery, so they may not be able to understand spoken commands. In this case, or if the patient is totally deaf, the surgical team may be required to communicate via hand signals or sign language (an interpreter may be necessary). Occasionally, written commands may be necessary. Nonverbal communication is very important, and a gentle touch goes a long way in the transmission of a comforting emotion. It is often helpful for a surgical team member to make a preoperative visit to the unit while the patient still has a hearing aid in place, or while family members are available to translate for the totally deaf, and give details of what will transpire in the operating room. This will relieve some anxiety on the part of the patient.

Patients with visual impairments may be blind or simply have a visual impairment that can be corrected with eyeglasses. Glasses are typically not allowed to accompany the patient to the OR. Contact lenses are removed in the unit because they can cause corneal damage if the surgical team forgets to remove them before anesthesia is administered. Patients with visual impairments can usually hear verbal commands, but may require assistance (and possibly extra personnel) in carrying out those commands. An explanation of their surroundings (especially a description of who is in the room) will ease anxiety about unfamiliar areas.

Physical disabilities, such as the absence of an extremity or severe arthritis, may require the surgical team to take extra precautions when moving the patient from the gurney to the operating table, and when positioning the patient after the administration of anesthesia. Extra personnel and positioning/padding devices that protect the patient may be necessary. The surgical team should be aware of any chronic disease that could affect respiration or circulation and thus require extra precautions during positioning to protect those systems and the tissues that they serve.

A paralyzed patient will require extra personnel for transport from the gurney to the operating table, and should be carefully positioned due to chronic wasting of muscles that can lead to skin injury or compression of nerves or vessels.

GERIATRIC PATIENTS

Geriatric patients are those in a specific age group (usually over the age of 65 years), although the label is meaningless

Table 4-5 Physiological Changes in the Elderly Patient

SYSTEM	NORMAL PHYSIOLOGICAL CHANGES
Integumentary	Loss of skin elasticity
	Loss of subcutaneous fat
	Skin more prone to damage from pressure and shear forces
Musculoskeletal	Loss of bone mass
	Skeletal instability
	Curvature of the spine
	Arthritis
	Decreased range of motion
Cardiovascular	Decreased coronary artery blood flow
	Increased blood pressure
	Decreased ability to tolerate insult
Respiratory	Decreased lung elasticity
	Increased rigidity in the chest wall
	Reduced tidal exchange
Digestive	Decreased salivary and digestive gland secretion
	Decreased peristalsis and gastric motility
	Decreased body water and plasma volume
Genitourinary	Decreased nephron function
	Decreased tone in ureters, bladder, and urethra
	Decreased bladder capacity
Nervous	Decreased cerebral blood flow with accompanying psychological changes
	Decreased position sense in extremities
	Increased tolerance to pain
	Numerous sensory changes related to both central nervous system and sensory organ change

as the only indicator for surgical risk because many patients over the age of 65 are healthier than some young adults. However, for the typical older patient, some form of chronic debilitation or decreased physiologic status (especially cardiovascular and respiratory) is present that requires special consideration and precautions by the surgical team (Table 4-5). Preoperative assessment and planning that takes this status into consideration are imperative for proper surgical outcomes, as is evidenced by the fact that emergency procedures on geriatric patients are associated with much higher mortality rates than elective ones, primarily because proper planning was not possible (Figure 4-2).

Geriatric patients may come to the operating room with visual and hearing impairments that require the considerations discussed in the previous section. In addition, elderly patients are often arthritic and suffer from restricted movements of extremities that require special consideration when transporting and positioning. Cardiovascular and respiratory impairments must be considered during anesthesia and positioning. Elderly patients can easily become hypothermic in an operating room, so warm blankets are imperative. A forced air warming blanket may be applied to the patient during anesthesia.

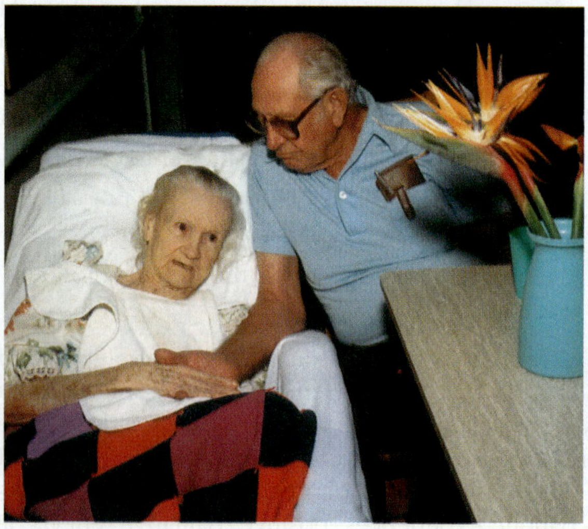

Figure 4-2 Geriatric patient

Watters and McClaran list the following eight critical factors for obtaining the best outcomes from surgical treatment in geriatric patients:

1. Careful preoperative preparation of the patient and optimization of medical and physiological status

2. Appropriate anesthesia and physiological monitoring
3. Recognition of alterations in clinical pharmacology
4. Minimization of the postoperative stresses of hypothermia, hypoxemia, and pain
5. Prevention of alterations in blood pressure and heart rate
6. Avoidance of perturbations of fluid, electrolyte, and acid–base status
7. Careful surgical technique
8. Optimization of functional level

Convalescence issues for the elderly are influenced by the possible lack of immediate family to provide postoperative care, which can increase the length of hospital stays. Nursing home or home health care may need to be arranged by hospital personnel.

TRAUMA PATIENTS

Trauma is one of the primary health care issues in the world. Approximately 160,000 Americans die from traumatic injuries each year. Treating the trauma patient is a challenge due to the multiple injuries that can be sustained by the individual. A single bullet or a car accident can injure several body structures, requiring the efforts of several surgeons and more than one surgical team to report. The surgical technologist must be prepared to assist on any type of surgical procedure when treating a trauma patient.

THE "GOLDEN HOUR" AND TRAUMA SYSTEM

Military physicians became aware, when treating those injured during war (e.g., World Wars I and II, the Korean War, and Vietnam), that the shorter the response time the greater the chance for survival of the trauma patient. Recent studies have also shown that the sooner CPR is begun for a heart attack victim, the greater the percentage of heart rhythm that will return to normal, with less damage. This concept, when applied to the civilian population, is classically referred to as the **golden hour**, meaning that reaching the trauma victim and providing treatment within the first hour following injury is critical in determining the patient's outcome. The time immediately after an injury has been sustained is the best time for rapid and aggressive interventions to effectively reduce morbidity and mortality.

The emergency medical services (EMS) system has also greatly facilitated the treatment of trauma patients by providing a system for rapid transportation to a facility designated as being able to provide optimal treatment. Facilities that are designated as trauma centers have met certain criteria indicating that they can meet the specialized treatment needs of the various types of trauma injuries. Trauma centers are designated as one of four trauma levels:

- *Level I trauma center:* Can meet all needs required for treating trauma patients, including qualified personnel and equipment on a 24-hour basis.
- *Level II trauma center:* Can treat seriously injured or ill patients, but does not have all of the resources that a Level I facility would have.
- *Level III trauma center:* Most often a community or rural hospital in an area that does not have a Level I or II facility. The trauma patient, particularly in rural areas, is stabilized and then transported to a Level I or II hospital.
- *Level IV trauma center:* Can provide advanced trauma life support to stabilize the patient before the patient is transported to a Level I or II hospital.

KINEMATICS

Compared to elective surgical procedures, little information is usually available to the health care team about the trauma patient and preparation time can be short. What does provide valuable information is the **kinematics** or *mechanism of injury (MOI)*. MOI is the action and effect of a particular type of force on the human body. By knowing the types of injuries caused by certain types of forces, the health care team can be better prepared to treat the trauma patient. For example, a bullet wound will produce a different action and effect on the body than a knife wound.

Three factors are important when considering the resulting injury the patient will sustain due to these various forces. These include:

1. Velocity of the injuring force
2. Flexibility of the tissue
3. Shape of the injuring force

For example, bones have little flexibility, resulting in fractures and shattering; whereas a soft-tissue injury due to blunt trauma often results in organ damage and bruising.

BLUNT TRAUMA

Blunt trauma results from forces such as deceleration, acceleration, compression, and shearing, and breaks in the integrity of the skin are often not present, making diagnosis difficult. Examples in which blunt trauma is sustained include motor vehicle crashes (MVCs), falls, assaults (hit with a fist or blunt object), and sports injuries. MVCs account for a large percentage of blunt trauma injuries. The spleen is the number one organ injured in a MVC. Three types of collisions can occur during a MVC:

1. Car collides with another object.
2. Person inside car collides with objects such as steering wheel or dashboard.

3. Internal body structure collides with a rigid bony surface. For example, a motorcyclist is thrown from the motorcycle and hits a tree. The brain is accelerating forward and when the person hits the tree, the brain tissue rapidly decelerates by colliding with the frontal portion of the cranium, causing severe blunt trauma.

PENETRATING TRAUMA

Penetrating trauma results when a foreign object passes through tissue. The most common foreign objects are bullets and knives. The extent of the injury depends on the:

- Type of foreign object
- Size of foreign object such as the caliber of the bullet, or a pocket knife versus a Bowie knife
- Distance the victim was from the foreign object
- Body structures that were penetrated
- Amount of energy (velocity) of the penetrating foreign object

Bullet injuries are classified as being low velocity (bullet travels 1,000 feet per second or slower) or high velocity (3,000 feet per second; commonly seen with military weapons). Factors that affect the extent of the injury include:

- High-velocity bullets, obviously, will cause more damage to tissue.
- The closer the victim is to the bullet as it leaves the weapon, the more damage that will result due to the increased speed of the bullet.
- Different bullets result in different types and severity of injury. For example, a hollow-point bullet mushrooms on impact, causing more tissue damage than other types of bullets.

If the bullet travels completely through the body (referred to as a *through and through*), the entrance wound tends to be smaller than the exit wound. For example, the bullets fired from an M-16 gun have a tumbling motion that produces a small entrance wound, but the exit wound is usually very large.

Stab wounds are low-velocity wounds. The width and length of the penetrating object influence the extent of the traumatic injury. The penetrating object must not be removed at the scene or in the Emergency Department; removal is done in the operating room. The retained object provides a tamponade effect for bleeding. In addition, if removed at the scene, the course of entry cannot be exactly followed upon removal and additional damage to body organs and tissue can occur.

TRAUMA SCORING

Injuries are scored using the **Revised Trauma Score** (RTS) to assess the severity of the trauma. Assigning an RTS assists in the triage process and provides a standardized method of communicating between facilities if, for instance, the patient has to be transported. The RTS involves the Glasgow Coma Scale as well as other physiological factors; refer to Table 4-6.

CONSIDERATIONS FOR THE SURGICAL TECHNOLOGIST

Severely injured patients most likely will require multiple procedures, performed simultaneously or in succession. For example, a patient who has sustained severe fractures of the right leg and head trauma may have a neurosurgeon performing a craniotomy at the same time as an orthopedic surgeon is repairing the fractures. This presents a challenge to the surgical technologist as far as preparation. The surgeon(s) will communicate to the surgical technologist the order of procedures, which is based on treating those injuries that are life threatening or possibly permanently debilitating before other, lesser injuries. The typical order of priority is head, chest, abdomen, and extremities.

PRESERVATION OF EVIDENCE

If the patient is a victim of a violent crime, many items will need to be preserved for the law enforcement officials as evidence against the perpetrator of the crime. All physical evidence must be carefully handled and facility policy

Table 4-6 Revised Trauma Score

GLASGOW COMA SCALE	SYSTOLIC BP	RESPIRATORY RATE	CODED VALUE
13–15	>89	10–29	= 4
9–12	76–89	7–29	= 3
6–8	50–75	6–9	= 2
4–5	1–49	1–5	= 1
3	0	0	= 0

Source: From "A Revision of the Trauma Score," by H. R. Champion, et al., 1989, *Journal of Trauma, 29*(5), pp. 623–629.

must be followed for purposes of documentation. Evidence includes the patient's clothes, bullets and bullet fragments, knife fragments, trace evidence (hair), and biologic evidence (blood and body fluids).

As previously mentioned, the policies and procedures of the surgery department and law enforcement agency must be followed. The following are some general recommendations:

- Remove clothing by cutting along the seams and around bullet or stab wound holes. The shape of the hole can provide evidence as to the type of weapon that was used. The clothes should be placed in a paper bag or wrapped in a clean sheet and given to the law enforcement officials.
- Hair, tissue, and gunpowder residue may be found on the hands of the victim. If the hand(s) does not require surgery, a bag should be placed around the hand(s) and taped in place.
- Bullets must be carefully handled since the lead can be easily scratched. They should not be handled with metal forceps or clamps. After removal, the surgical technologist should place the bullet(s) on a clean, gauze sponge and pass it from the sterile field to the circulator for placement in a specimen cup.
- A chain of custody of evidence must be documented in writing. This accounts for the identification of all individuals on the surgical team who handled the evidence and the order of handling. The anatomical site from which the evidence is retrieved must be documented and the time. The documentation will serve as legal documents.

HYPOTHERMIA

Often trauma patients have been exposed to the environment for a prolonged period and become hypothermic at the scene. Hypothermia is typically defined as a core body temperature that is below 35°C. Upon arrival in surgery, the patient should be kept as warm as possible by using warm blankets and by increasing the temperature in the operating room. The surgical technologist should only use warm irrigating solutions both externally when performing the skin prep and internally when the surgeon is irrigating the surgical wound.

INFECTION

The wounds of trauma patients are frequently contaminated with debris, dirt, grass, and, if penetrating trauma, the foreign object that was used to cause the injury is contaminated. If the stomach, gallbladder, or intestines are perforated, they will spill their contents into the abdominal cavity, putting the patient at a high risk for peritonitis.

If time permits, the STSR may be able to perform a skin prep to decontaminate the skin using sterile scrub brushes or pulse-lavage. However, the surgical technologist must be careful not to cause further damage to the traumatic wound. When presented with life-threatening circumstances, the only thing there may be time for is to quickly pour or spray some povidone-iodine solution over a large area.

PREPARATION OF THE CASE

The majority of Level I trauma centers will have two or more operating rooms designated for trauma surgery. The facility will also have preassembled emergency instrument sets such as craniotomy, abdominal and chest sets. The trauma operating rooms are stocked with necessary supplies and equipment such as sponges, catheters, sutures, a crash cart, and monitoring devices.

Many facilities have a fluoroscopic operating table to facilitate taking X-rays during surgery. The table also aids in positioning the patient. Positioning is always a concern in surgery, but for trauma patients it is of utmost concern, particularly if they have been involved in a situation such as a MVC in which the spine may have been injured. Before the patient is removed from the backboard to the operating table, the surgical technologist must confirm that the surgeon has communicated that the spine is either injury free or is injured, requiring extra positioning precautions. However, any time the patient's position is changed, the anesthesia provider will direct the team effort. The anesthesia provider is also responsible for moving the head and neck of the patient and keeping the cervical spine stable and in-line during positioning. If multiple procedures are to be performed, the patient position may be changed, again requiring the guidance of the anesthesia provider.

When performing multiple procedures, the surgical technologist will be required to organize several setups. If possible, the surgical technologist should have more than one Mayo stand and back table on which to set up the different procedures, time allowing. In addition to proper instrumentation and equipment, the surgical technologist must have an adequate supply of sponges, suture, and ties opened onto the back table, especially when the patient has sustained abdominal trauma. In such a case, more than the usual number of hemostatic clamps will most likely be needed. Hemostatic agents such as gelatin sponges and topical thrombin should be available if the need arises. In life-threatening situations in which there is not much time for preparation, the surgical technologist may not be able to perform the initial sponge, instrument, and sharp counts. The circulator should document this on the patient's operating room record and postoperative X-rays may have to be taken to confirm that nothing was inadvertently retained within the patient.

CASE STUDY

A female in the third trimester of pregnancy is brought to the operating room for an emergency appendectomy. It will be necessary for the patient to receive general anesthesia in order to perform the procedure.

1. Anatomically, what changes have taken place in the patient that must be taken under consideration for the surgical procedure?
2. Why might the results of laboratory tests be abnormal when the patient actually has normal values?
3. During the appendectomy, the surgical technologist should be ready to quickly set up and assist the surgeon with what additional emergency procedure?
4. Postoperatively, what symptoms should be closely watched for in the patient that could indicate preterm labor?

QUESTIONS FOR FURTHER STUDY

1. Name some methods that can be used to reduce a pediatric patient's level of anxiety.
2. A neonate who is very ill requires surgery. What artery will most likely be used to insert an intra-arterial monitor?
3. In the immediate postoperative period, in what position should the bariatric patient be placed to aid pulmonary function?
4. A bariatric patient has recently undergone a gastric bypass procedure and complains of periumbilical pain. What complication is the patient possibly experiencing and what type of surgical procedure will be performed to repair it?
5. What device is frequently used during a surgical procedure and postoperatively to prevent thrombophlebitis in the patient who is diabetic?
6. What physiological occurrence is difficult to recognize in the pregnant patient and may result in the fetus becoming hypoxic? What device should be used intraoperatively and postoperatively to avoid the complication?

BIBLIOGRAPHY

Ansara, M. F., Cryer, P. E., & Scharp, D. W. (1999). Diabetes mellitus [CD-ROM]. Scientific American Surgery.

Atkinson, L. J., & Fortunato, N. (1996). *Berry & Kohn's operating room technique* (8th ed.). St. Louis, MO: Mosby.

Barone, J. E., Gingold, B. S., Arvantis, M. L., et al. (1986). Abdominal pain in patients with acquired immunodeficiency syndrome. *Annals of Surgery, 204,* 619.

Barron, W. M. (1984). The pregnant surgical patient: Medical evaluation and management. *Annals of Internal Medicine, 101,* 683.

Battistella, F. (1999). Emergency department evaluation of the patient with multiple injuries [CD-ROM]. Scientific American Surgery.

Bell, E. F., Weinstein, M. R., & Oh, W. (1980). Heat balance in premature infants: Comparative effects of convectively heated incubator and radiant warmer with and without plastic heat shield. *Journal of Pediatrics, 96,* 460.

Brooks, D. C., & Sznyter, L. A. (1999). Pregnancy [CD-ROM]. Scientific American Surgery.

Champion, H. R., Sacco, W. J., Copes, W. S., et al. (1989). A revision of the Trauma Score. *Journal of Trauma, 29*(5), 623–629.

Coran, A. G. (1999). The pediatric patient [CD-ROM]. Scientific American Surgery.

Davis, J. M. (1999). Acquired immunodeficiency syndrome [CD-ROM]. Scientific American Surgery.

Friis-Hansen, B., Holiday, M., Stapleton, T., et al. (1951). Total body water in children. *Pediatrics, 7,* 321.

Frisenda, R., Roty, A. R. Jr., Kilway, J. B., et al. (1979). Acute appendicitis during pregnancy. *American Surgery, 45,* 503.

Kanne, A. F. (1999). Trauma surgery. In M. Meeker & J. Rothrock (Eds.), *Alexander's care of the patient in surgery* (11th ed., pp. 1301–1330). St. Louis, MO: Mosby.

McGuiness, A. M., et al (2002). *Core curriculum for surgical technology* (5th ed.). Centennial, CO: Association of Surgical Technologists.

Potter, P. A., & Perry, A. G. (1989). *Fundamentals of nursing: Concepts, process, and practice* (2nd ed.). St. Louis, MO: Mosby.

Robinson, G., Wilson, S. E., & Williams, R. A. (1987). Surgery in patients with acquired immunodeficiency syndrome. *Archives of Surgery, 122,* 170.

Rutledge, R., & Fakhry, S. M. (1993). Injury severity scoring in trauma patients. In K. Maull (Ed.), *Advances in trauma and critical care* (Vol. 8, pp. 117–143). St. Louis, MO: Mosby-Year Book.

Sanerkin, N. G., & Edwards, P. (1966). Birth injury to the sternomastoid muscle. *Journal of Bone Joint Surgery, 48B,* 441.

Sugerman, H. J. (1999). Obesity [CD-ROM]. Scientific American Surgery.

Trunkey, D. (1983). Trauma. *Scientific American, 249,* 28–35.

Watters, J. M., & McClaran, J. C. (1999). The elderly surgical patient [CD-ROM]. Scientific American Surgery.

Wilson, S. E., Robinson, G., Williams, R. A., et al. (1989). Acquired immune deficiency syndrome (AIDS): Indications for abdominal surgery, pathology, and outcome. *Annals of Surgery, 210,* 428.

CHAPTER 5

Physical Environment and Safety Standards

Kevin B. Frey
Ben D. Price

CASE STUDY

Larry is a surgical technologist who works in the general surgery unit of a local OR. One night he was serving as the STSR on a trauma case in which the patient had suffered several gunshot wounds to the abdomen. The patient was known to be an IV drug user. The case went well and the patient was stabilized. The count began as the peritoneum was being closed. As the case was nearing its end, a surgeon tossed a loaded needle holder onto the Mayo stand, without warning. The needle holder landed near Larry's hand, and as he turned, the needle punctured his single glove and skin.

Larry immediately reported the needle stick injury and the circulator helped him remove the glove to assess the wound. Another team member scrubbed in and replaced Larry at the Mayo stand. Larry washed the wound with soap and water. Since it was late at night and the occupational health office was not open, he reported to the emergency department for treatment. All appropriate reports were filed.

1. What should be done with the needle and the needle holder that have become contaminated by piercing Larry's glove and skin?
2. Should Larry have waited until the end of the case to "break scrub" and wash his hand?
3. What could Larry have done to afford himself extra protection from this needle stick injury?

OBJECTIVES

After studying this chapter, the reader should be able to:

C 1. Identify and describe hazards to the patient in the operative environment.

2. Identify support services that work with the OR team in the care of the patient.

A 3. Understand the type of air-handling system required in the OR and the temperature and humidity required to maintain a sterile field.

4. Identify cleaning procedures, traffic patterns, and routines required in the operative environment.

R 5. Identify the role of the surgical technologist in the protection of self, patients, and others from hazards in the operative environment.

E 6. Identify the design types of the OR.

7. Identify hospital departments that relate to surgical services.

8. Understand the working environment of the OR.

9. Identify the physical components of the OR.

SELECT KEY TERMS

1. airborne bacteria
2. back table
3. decontamination room
4. electrosurgical unit
5. hamper
6. high-efficiency particulate air (HEPA) filter
7. hypothermia
8. ionizing radiation
9. laminar air flow
10. Mayo stand
11. methyl methacrylate (MMA)
12. Occupational Safety and Health Administration (OSHA)
13. pathology department
14. perfusionist
15. personal protective equipment (PPE)
16. plume
17. postanesthesia care unit (PACU)
18. prophylaxis
19. restricted area
20. Standard Precautions
21. suction outlet
22. surgical site infection (SSI)
23. triboelectrification
24. Universal Precautions

PHYSICAL DESIGN OF THE SURGERY DEPARTMENT

When a hospital is designed, the location of the surgery department is usually such that it is easily accessible to and from the various surgical patient support departments, such as ICU, labor and delivery, and central sterile supply. Obviously, the size of the hospital will determine location and it may not be feasible to locate every department close to the surgery department. However, a key factor is locating the surgery department in an area where traffic is limited and the general public does not have access. Many surgery departments are located on the first floor or underground area.

Several basic design types are used in surgical services departments, depending on the age of the facility and the physical design of the areas outside the department.

All surgery departments are designed with the idea of controlling traffic patterns and quickly providing each OR with the necessary supplies, during, and after each case, while keeping clean and dirty traffic patterns separate. Among these designs are:

- Race track plan
- Hotel plan
- Specialty grouping plan

The "race track" plan, recently favored by many facilities, involves a series of ORs around a clean central core (Figure 5-1). In this design, the front entrance to each OR is from the outer corridor, and supplies are retrieved through a rear entrance to the room leading to the central-core storage and work areas. The soiled entrance areas are situated outside this central-core area, to allow for separation of the two areas and related traffic. Scrub sinks are also situated in the outer corridor, with easy access through the main entrances to the OR.

The "hotel plan" is a variation of this, in which the ORs are situated along a central corridor, with separate clean core and soiled work areas. The primary difference in this plan is that all traffic enters and exits the surgery department through a single entrance or a primary entrance and holding area entrance situated along the same corridor.

The "specialty grouping" plan is simply a variation on the hotel or race track plan, in which operating rooms are grouped by specialty (e.g., neurosurgery, general surgery), each with its own closely associated clean storage areas and, in some cases, each with its own soiled instrument work area.

Each department, regardless of design type, is equipped with a supply room in a restricted area. This room contains sterile supplies either for the entire department or for an entire specialty area if multiple storage rooms are used. Supplies stored within this area include towels, linens, sponges, gloves, and supplies used on a daily basis in every case. These areas also contain special prefabricated sterile case packs and instrument sets. Proper storage techniques should be followed in these storage areas, such as not placing sterile packs too close to ceilings or floors (see Chapter 7). As in the OR, temperature should be controlled between 65 and 75°F. Humidity should be maintained at no higher than 50% to help protect the sterility of packaged items. Separate storage rooms are used for large equipment such as special OR tables and attachments and endoscopic carts.

The design of any surgery department revolves around environmental control, traffic control, and the desire to prevent **surgical site infection (SSI)**. Such factors as the separation of clean and soiled work areas and areas of the department specified as restricted and unrestricted assist in the promotion of this idea. Efficiency is increased with strategic placement of computers, preparation areas, and staff areas.

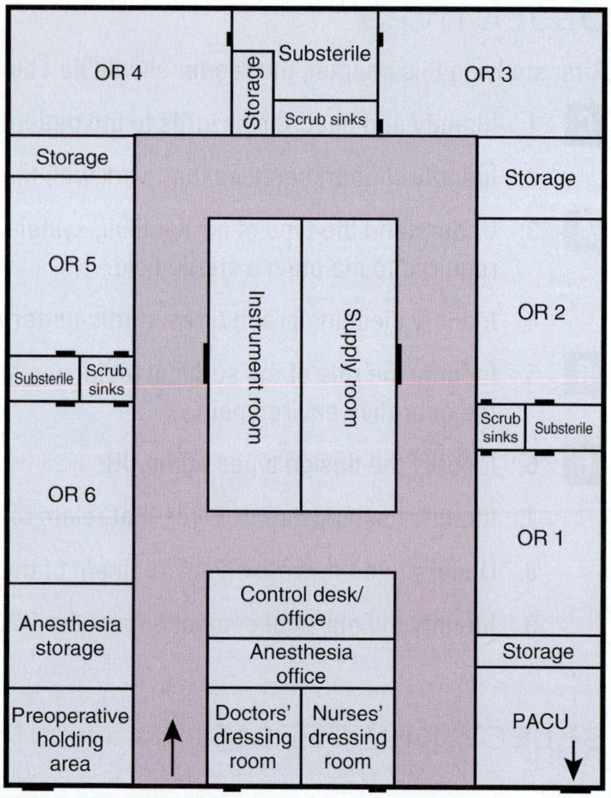

Figure 5-1 Standard surgery department plan

AREAS OF THE OR

Regardless of the design chosen by the facility, certain principles apply universally. Traffic control follows predetermined traffic patterns that all persons entering the department are expected to follow. The department is divided into unrestricted, semirestricted, and **restricted areas**, with particular attire required for each.

The unrestricted area is usually located near the entrance and is isolated from the main hospital corridor by doors. This area often contains dressing rooms for physicians and support staff, an anesthesia office, a main office, and a main desk. In this area, street clothes are allowed.

Operating room attire is required in the semirestricted and restricted areas (see Chapter 7). Surgical scrub suits as well as hats are required. Because there are often no doors to separate these areas, many hospitals designate the restricted area from the unrestricted area with the use of signage and/or a red line painted on the floor. Anyone passing this line is expected to be in proper OR attire and to observe the rules of the semirestricted area. Many hospitals have specific "clean" stretchers for use in this area to which patients are transferred on arrival, but as a cost-containment measure and for patient comfort, other hospitals have abandoned this idea.

The restricted area usually includes the inside areas as well as the sterile storage areas of the department. In addition to proper OR attire, masks are required in this area. Some hospital policies require masks to be worn in the OR only when a sterile procedure is in progress, meaning sterile supplies are being opened or have been opened or the patient is in the room.

INSTRUMENT ROOM

A separate room for storage of nonsterile equipment and instrumentation is necessary. Single instruments are stored in this room and can be pulled for use as needed. In some hospitals, the area where instruments are reassembled into sets after decontamination and prior to sterilization may also be referred to as the *instrument room*.

UTILITY AND DECONTAMINATION ROOM

The department is also equipped with a separate utility and **decontamination room** with sinks for gross decontamination of instrumentation. This room often contains an ultrasonic washer for cavitation of instruments prior to sending them to central sterile for processing. In some cases this area is divided by a wall into a cleaning area and a separate preparation area. In this setup, a washer sterilizer is used to wash the instruments, and they are removed to the other side of the wall in the preparation area. The preparation area may be used to reassemble and wrap instrument sets, basin sets, and trays prior to sending them to central sterile for final processing.

PHYSICAL COMPONENTS OF THE OPERATIVE SUITE

The individual rooms where operative procedures are performed are referred to as *operating* or *operative rooms* or sometimes *suites*. (We will restrict the use of *suite* to refer to the physical location of the entire surgical department. *Operating room,* or *OR,* will refer to a single room.) The standard size of an OR has traditionally been at least 400–600 ft^2, but as technology progresses and new equipment has been put into use, there has been an increasing need in some specialties to increase the size of the room (Figure 5-2).

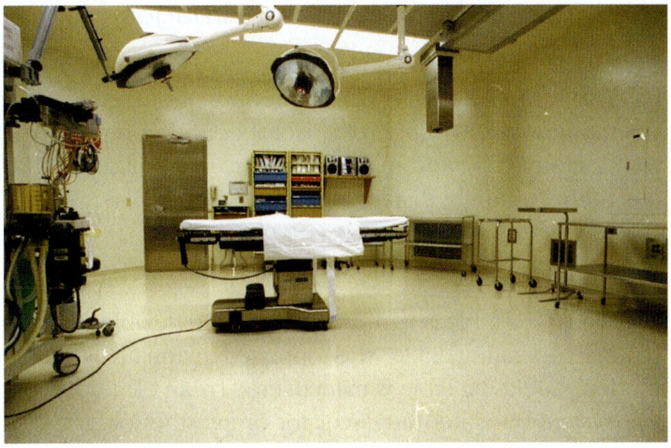

Figure 5-2 Operating room

EQUIPMENT

Each OR will be equipped with certain standard equipment plus whatever equipment and supplies are necessary for the specialty use of the room. Most ORs are relatively standardized.

Electrical Outlets

Electrical outlets are mounted well above the floor and must be on a monitored electrical system. All outlets must have ground-fault interrupters and be explosion proof. Emergency outlets are designated in red and are connected to the hospital's backup generator system in case of power outage. These outlets should be used for such equipment as anesthesia equipment and other equipment vital to the procedure and the safety of the patient.

Suction Outlets

Each OR must have at least two **suction outlets**. In some cases more suction outlets are present or required. At least one outlet is used by the surgical team for suctioning in the sterile field and one is used by anesthesia.

Gas Outlets

In addition to suction outlets, each room is provided with several banks of gas outlets, including outlets for air, oxygen, and nitrous oxide. These outlets are placed on walls or ceilings within the OR. Emergency shut-off valves must be located in the outside corridor.

Lights

Each OR is equipped with regular overhead lighting as well as surgical lights. Surgical lights should be designed to provide a range of intensity and focus with a minimum of heat and should be freely moveable. Track lights are no longer recommended because of the danger of fallout contamination. Surgical lights should be freely adjustable in both the horizontal and vertical planes and should provide a light color approximating normal sunlight. The focus point of the surgical lights should not leave a dark center spot on the surgical field. The lights must be easily accessible for cleaning, and accumulated dust on the suspension system must be easily removed. Surgical lights should be equipped with handles that adjust intensity or focus of the lights and that also may be used when covered with sterile handles or handle covers to reposition the lights intraoperatively.

Viewing Box for Diagnostic Images

A viewing box for diagnostic images is positioned at eye level so it can be seen by the surgeon without leaving the operating table. Radiographs, isotope, and computerized tomography (CT) and magnetic resonance imaging (MRI) scans are routinely displayed on the view boxes.

Operating Table

The operating table is narrow, padded, and flexible. The traditional operating table was operated manually, but the modern operating table is maneuvered by an electrical control system by either the circulator or anesthesiologist. The table has *breakpoints,* or bendable points, at the knee, waist, and head. In addition, the operating table has removable sections at the waist point and at the footboard for use in procedures where the legs are placed in stirrups. The height of the table may be adjusted preoperatively and intraoperatively to provide the surgeon with the most advantageous operative angle. The table should be constructed in such a manner that all surfaces are easily cleaned between cases. Small parts must be removable for terminal cleaning.

The operative table has a wide base to prevent tipping under uneven weight distribution and rails along the side for attachment of arm boards and other accessories (Figure 5-3). The table is always well padded prior to patient positioning, and additional padding is added when necessary.

Special operating tables are used for specific procedures. The Wilson frame operating table is used for procedures in which the patient may need to be repositioned from supine to prone position intraoperatively, such as anterior-posterior spinal fusions. Special fracture tables are used in some orthopedic procedures. In addition, many accessory attachments, such as the Mayfield headrest, are available for use in specialized procedures, such as craniotomies.

Other Items

Many procedures are time critical. Each OR should have a wall-mounted clock with an easily readable face and a sweep second hand for the timing of certain procedures and for the timing of cardiac or respiratory arrests. Many are equipped with an additional start/stop timer.

An intercom system allows for communication by the surgical team with areas outside the OR and within the surgical department without going out of the room. This can also be used for discussions with the pathology department or for calling for diagnostic imaging. Some rooms are equipped with foot-activated intercom switches so that a scrubbed member of the surgical team may operate the device.

Increasingly, ORs are equipped with one or more computer terminals to be used by the circulator and/or the anesthesiologist. The circulator may use this terminal in some cases to do all patient chart data entry, to view previous or current laboratory work values, and to order supplies for the room, X-rays, or further tests for the patient. Further, the computer may provide access to reference information such as surgeon's preference cards, the daily schedule, and common laboratory values and inventory control. The computer may also be used to monitor operating times and room turnover times. As technology increases, systems within the hospital are increasingly integrated into computer networks, decreasing the paper load and the speed with which vital patient information may be shared within the facility.

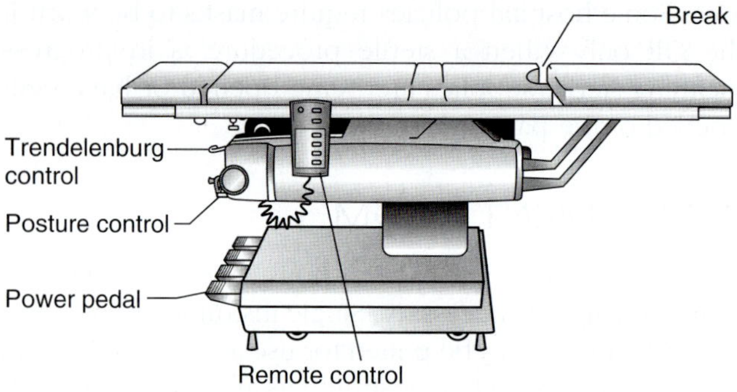

Figure 5-3 Operating table

Many ORs are now equipped with permanently installed closed-circuit television capability. This may be used to assist members of the team in viewing laparoscopic or endoscopic procedures and in some cases is connected to the pathology department so that the surgeon may have discussion with the pathologist without leaving the OR.

STANDARD OPERATING ROOM FURNITURE

Each OR should be equipped with a standard set of furniture and equipment, including the operating table, a **back table**, one or more **Mayo stands**, ring stands, and a kick bucket. Each room will also be equipped with accessories particular to the specialty or the procedure to be performed in that room, such as a Mayfield headrest for neurosurgical procedures.

A Mayo stand is the stand that is moved closest to the operative field. The STSR works from this stand to supply immediately necessary instrumentation to the surgeon. Prior to the procedure, a separate small table or Mayo stand is used to set up gowns and gloves for the sterile members of the operative team entering the sterile field (Figure 5-4).

Back tables are larger tables that are used for storage of sterile instruments and larger items before and during the procedure (Figure 5-5). The term *back* is used because these tables are usually positioned to the side of the OR opposite the door.

Ring stands are four-wheeled stands with a metal ring at the top (Figure 5-6). They are used to hold basins and are covered with a sterile drape prior to the procedure. These basins hold the various fluids to be used during the procedure, including saline and/or sterile water

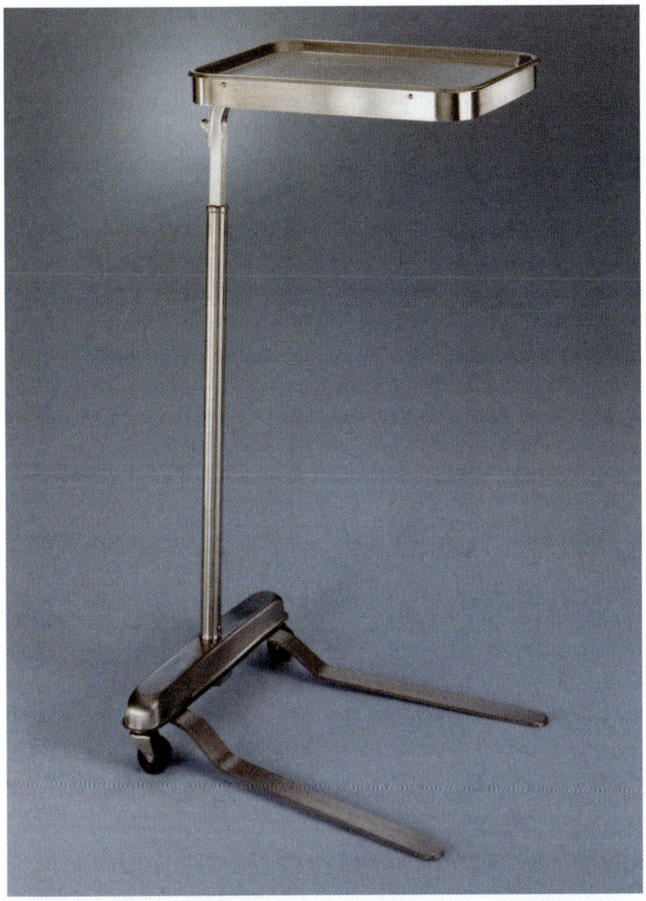

Figure 5-4 **Mayo stand** *(Courtesy of Blickman Health Industries)*

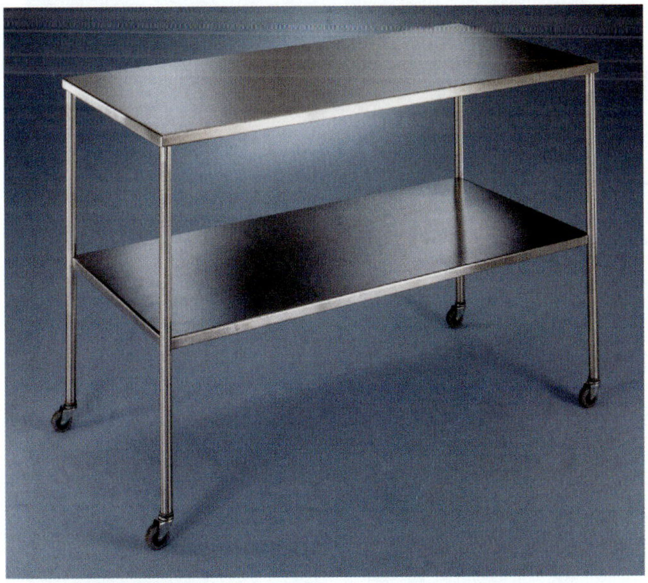

Figure 5-5 **Back table** *(Courtesy of Blickman Health Industries)*

for rinsing instruments and for irrigation. In some cases, such as cardiac cases, these basins may be used to hold a sterile ice/slush solution for hypothermia in the absence of a *slush machine.*

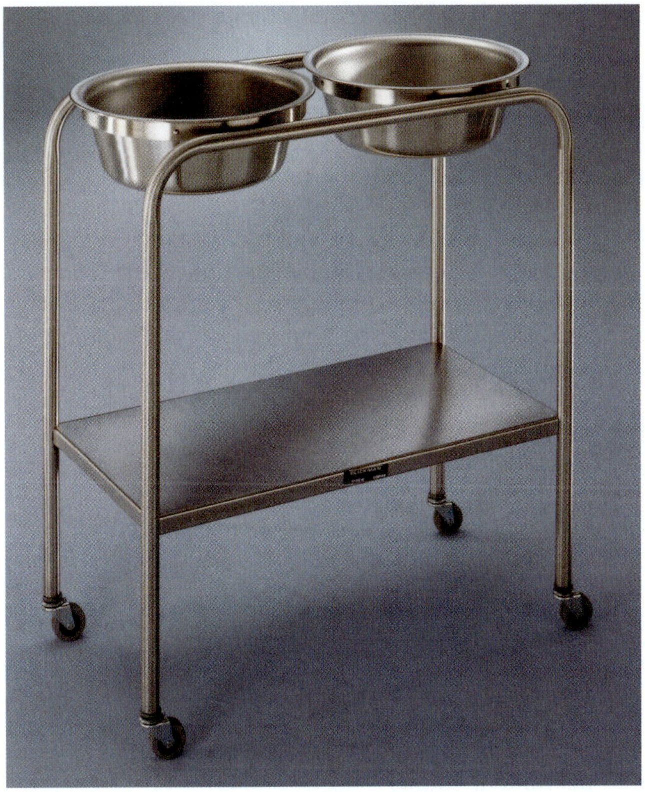

Figure 5-6 **Double ring stand** *(Courtesy of Blickman Health Industries)*

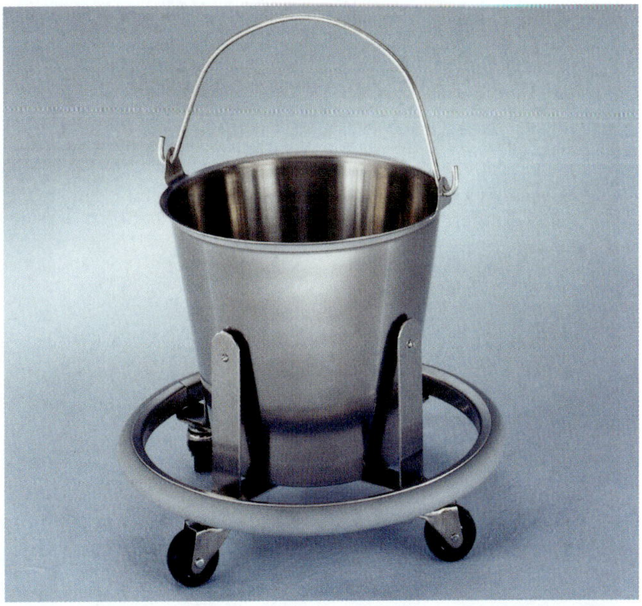

Figure 5-7 **Kick bucket** *(Courtesy of Blickman Health Industries)*

Kick buckets are also four-wheeled stands, but they are very low to the floor and can be maneuvered with the foot (kicked) (Figure 5-7). These are buckets lined with biohazard trash bags. The sterile team member tosses soiled counted sponges into these buckets. (The kick bucket is not for paper waste but for counted sponges only.)

A linen **hamper** and trash containers are typically four-wheeled stands but are large enough that soiled linens and trash from the sterile field may be placed into them by the STSR. They too may be lined with biohazardous designator bags.

Suction sets are low-wheel-based stands on which the suction canisters rest. Sterile suction tubing from the field may be attached to the canister by the circulator (Figure 5-8). The canisters are connected to the suction outlet by another plastic tube. They may be lined with plastic liners and have measurement marked on the side to help estimate fluid use or loss.

In addition to this equipment, each OR is equipped with an *anesthesia cart* and supplies. This will include patient monitoring equipment to keep the surgical team aware of the patient's physiological status and it is primarily used by the anesthesiologist. A writing surface is provided on the wall within easy view of the sterile members of the surgical team. This surface is used to provide the team with vital information about the patient, such as age, weight, name, etc., as well as to provide a surface on which to write and maintain sponge and instrument counts.

SURFACES IN THE OR

The walls of the OR should be nonporous, easy to clean, fireproof, and waterproof. Floors should also be nonporous, and tile floors are undesirable (though often seen in older ORs) because the grout tends to harbor bacteria. Walls and floors should be constructed so that they may be easily washed with antimicrobial solutions. Walls should be a nonglare, nonreflective, pleasant color. All floor surfaces should be nonporous and waterproof for cleaning and wet vacuuming. Many new ORs are using cushioned flooring systems to decrease personnel fatigue. If cushioned rubber standing mats are used around the table, they should be of the solid and smooth type with no grooves to allow for easy and complete cleaning.

CABINETS AND DOORS

Cabinets and doors within the OR should be recessed into the wall when possible to avoid dust accumulation on their top surfaces. Storage cabinets should be provided with doors when possible to lower dust accumulation on supplies and for ease of terminal cleaning of the room. Doors on cabinets should be of the surface-mounted sliding type when possible, because swinging doors move air

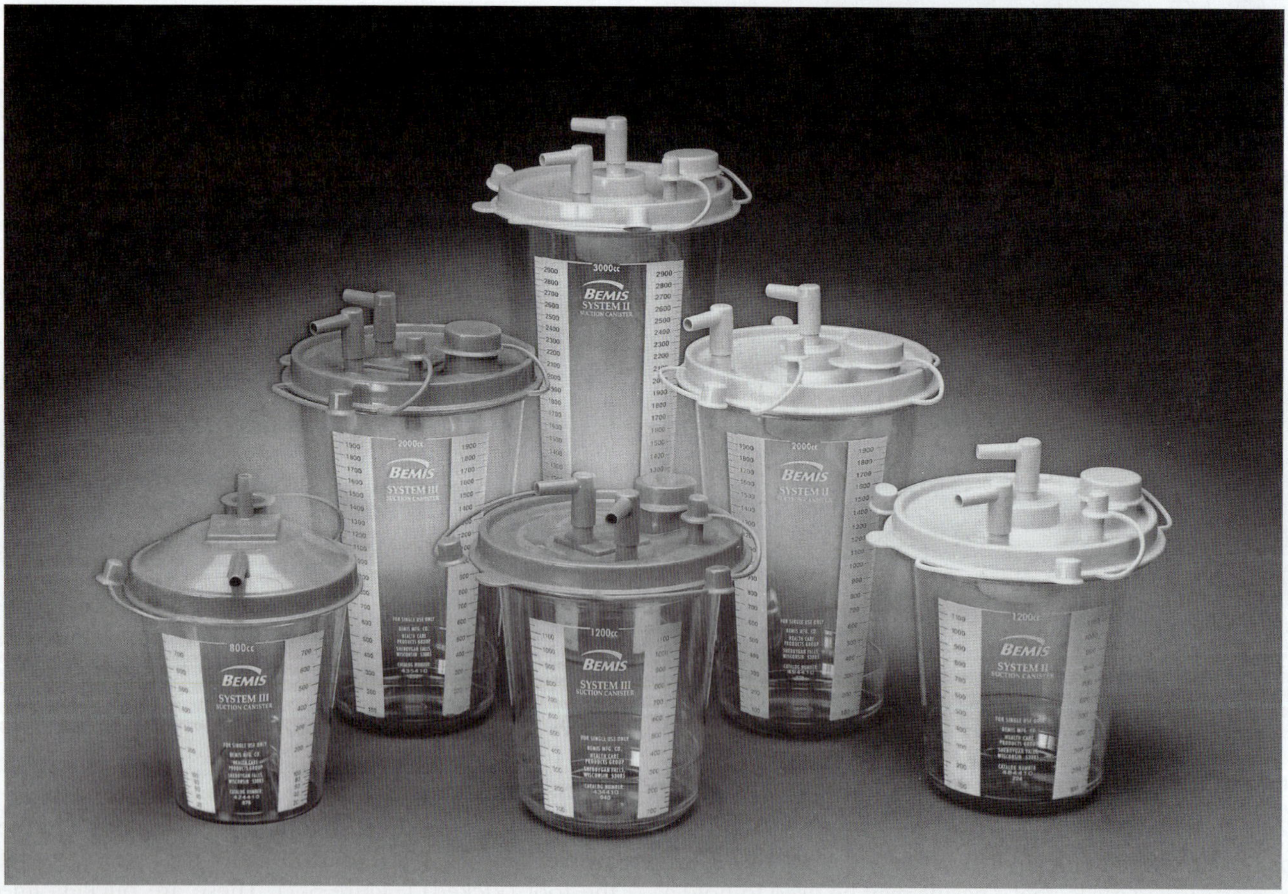

Figure 5-8 Suction system ***(Courtesy of Bemis Health Care Products)***

within the room and disturb microorganisms that have settled on floors and surfaces within the room into the operative field. Cabinets and doors, like walls and floor, should be nonporous and waterproof for easy cleaning.

DOORS

Access doors to the OR should be kept closed during all procedures to protect the room from outside contamination. When possible, surface-mounted sliding doors that can swing open in an emergency situation should be used. Sliding doors lower the incidence of swinging-door air disturbance in the room, which can redistribute contaminant microbes onto the surgical field. Traffic into and out of the OR should be limited during any procedure for this purpose; and particularly during open-joint orthopedic procedures, many ORs place signage to this effect on the doors.

VENTILATION SYSTEM

The ventilation system in the OR should provide a supply of clean air, remove airborne contamination that is produced within the room, and provide a comfortable working environment for health care personnel.

Studies in the 1940s showed that when air for the ORs was brought in through intakes in the corridors and other areas of the hospital, bacteria could be introduced into the OR. These findings led to the practice of creating a *positive-pressure* air supply for each OR. This means that the air pressure in the OR itself is kept by ventilation at a higher level than that of the surrounding corridors. When a door is opened out to the corridor, air from the room rushes outward into the corridor rather than from the corridor into the room. This process helps keep **airborne bacteria** from entering the room. To keep air movement into the OR at a minimum, no windows that may be opened are allowed in the OR.

Air Changes in OR

Studies have shown that an air exchange rate of 20 air changes per hour helps keep the amount of airborne contamination in the OR to a minimum. The Centers for Disease Control and Prevention (CDC) guidelines recommend that ORs be ventilated with at least 20 air changes per hour and that this air be filtered. **High-efficiency particulate air (HEPA) filters** are usually the filter of choice. These filters are capable of removing bacteria as small as 0.5–5 μm. The guidelines also recommend that at least 20% of the air change per hour be fresh outside air.

Temperature and Humidity

The temperature in the OR is kept between 65 and 75°F, and humidity levels are kept between 50 and 55%, but should not go below 45%. These levels provide comfort for the patient, operative team, and also provide infection control. Care should be taken to prevent patient **hypothermia**, however, because studies have shown decreased incidences of SSI and shorter recovery times in patients who were kept at a normal body temperature intraoperatively.

SUBSTERILE AREA

Each OR or group of ORs is provided with a scrub sink area and a *substerile room*. This substerile area is a workroom for that particular OR or group of adjacent rooms and contains a sink and a steam sterilizer. The substerile room may also contain blanket and solution warmers. The circulator or scrub person uses this room for cleaning and sterilization of instruments. It may be utilized in emergent situations to flash sterilize instruments or sets and can be used to flash sterilize dropped or contaminated instruments intraoperatively for return to the sterile field. This room is situated so that the circulator or STSR is able to remove instruments directly from the sterilizer and will not have to transport these instruments through the "nonsterile" corridors. This room not only provides for easy flash sterilization and transport but also provides a small storage area that allows the circulator to remain in or close to the OR at all times. Doors to this room should remain closed during the operation to prevent cross-contamination from adjacent rooms. Positive air pressure is defeated in this case because adjacent rooms also are under this same system.

DIRECT SUPPORT SERVICES

As mentioned in Chapter 1, many departments of the hospital interact with surgical services. Some are directly related to surgical services and some indirectly. Some departments may have a physical presence in the operating suite, for instance, diagnostic imaging. Others may communicate by other means from a distant location.

PREOPERATIVE OR "SAME-DAY" CHECK-IN UNIT

Many hospitals have established a preoperative "same-day" check-in unit, when separate same-day surgery facilities are not used. This is an area the patient is directed to on arrival at the hospital. The patient is admitted to this area and then is provided with a private dressing room facility to change clothes. Lockers are provided for the patient to safeguard personal items, although any jewelry or money should either be left with a family member or turned over to hospital security for safekeeping. In this area, a designated family waiting area is provided. After admission and any necessary preoperative laboratory work, the patient is taken to the preoperative holding area.

PREOPERATIVE HOLDING AREA

The *preoperative holding area* is a designated room where patients wait within the department area before entering the OR. Depending on design, this may be a large area where all patients are held until transport to the specific OR or a small room just outside the OR. Regardless of the location, this room or area should be shielded from noise and particularly from views into the OR. Patients should not be held in the main corridor, because this is typically noisy and quite frightening to the surgical patient. Ideally, the patient is held in a small room just off the main corridor and immediately adjacent to the OR. Often, this room is referred to as an *induction room*. It is better for this room to have separate doors rather than curtains. This helps alleviate patient anxiety prior to surgery. In this area, IV lines and invasive monitoring devices may be inserted. The anesthesiologist often uses this room for a preoperative interview and assessment of patient status, and regional blocks such as epidural anesthesia may be administered while the OR is being cleaned or "turned over" from the previous case. For pediatric cases, this room is often equipped with a rocking chair, and a parent is allowed to sit and wait in the room with the child to assist in the alleviation of both parent and child anxiety.

POSTANESTHESIA CARE UNIT

Postoperatively, the patient is usually transported to the **postanesthesia care unit**, or **PACU**. This area is similar to the preoperative holding area and is used to "recover" patients just after surgery, until transport to a regular patient room or discharge in the case of same-day surgery patients is possible. This area should also be quiet and at least provide the privacy of curtains. This room is equipped with appropriate emergency care equipment such as suction and a crash cart, and staff is able to closely monitor patients with electronic monitoring devices for a period of time following anesthesia. For cases in which the patient has not yet been extubated, this is usually performed at the appropriate time in the PACU. Some hospitals provide separate recovery areas for cardiac patients, because they require a higher level of postanesthesia care.

LABORATORY DEPARTMENT

The laboratory department provides the surgical team with both preoperative and postoperative laboratory values used when monitoring the patient. Certain laboratory procedures may be performed within the surgery department, such as blood gas monitoring, which is often performed by **perfusionists** during cardiovascular procedures. Other laboratory work is sent out of the OR to the laboratory, where it is assigned a value of time importance (critical, noncritical, and stat), and values are returned to the OR on completion of laboratory work. This may be accomplished by phone or by intercom and increasingly by computer. When the laboratory and OR are linked by computer network, values may be posted online as they become available and may also be compared with previous values to help in identifying a trend.

RADIOLOGY DEPARTMENT

The radiology department provides the OR with radiologic patient studies including plain X-ray films and intraoperative techniques such as fluoroscopy, which provides real-time X-ray monitoring for orthopedic and other cases. Larger hospitals often provide the surgery department with a dedicated radiology technician staff for ease and speed, and each department is usually equipped with mobile X-ray equipment and a C-arm (fluoroscope). The radiology department is usually contacted by phone or intercom system and X-rays are returned to the room as soon as they have been developed. The radiology department is often called on to take X-ray films to assist when a sponge or needle count has been found to be incorrect.

The surgical technologist in the scrub role (STSR) must always oversee any activity around the patient while radiological studies are being performed. Radiology personnel may have little awareness of aseptic principles and sterile technique and it is therefore the duty of the surgical technologist to supervise his or her movement around the field. It is also important for STSRs in cases utilizing X-ray or fluoroscopy to wear protective shields to prevent exposure to **ionizing radiation**.

PATHOLOGY DEPARTMENT

Specimens are sent to the **pathology department** for testing and processing. This department is not located within the surgery department, but communication systems such as closed-circuit television, computer networking, and direct intercoms link them closely to communicate quickly and directly. Pathology results, like laboratory results, are easily accessible by computer. Care should be taken by the STSR when sending specimens to pathology that they are placed in the proper type of containers and fluids for the specific type of specimen. The STSR should always double check with the surgeon and circulator to ensure proper labeling and handling of the specimen. Permanent specimens are usually sent to the pathology laboratory in formalin solutions, and frozen sections are sent dry. For a better understanding of the handling of specimens, refer to Chapter 13.

ENVIRONMENTAL SERVICES

Environmental services is the ancillary department charged with cleaning the surgery department. In some cases, this includes room cleaning for turnover between cases, but increasingly, the surgical team is being utilized for this purpose for speed and efficiency. In many cases, the environmental services department is charged primarily with terminal cleaning of the rooms at night and between particularly dirty cases. This department is also in charge of the removal of soiled linens and regular as well as biohazard classified trash. These workers should be well versed in **Standard Precautions** and **Universal Precautions**, because they will be in a position to potentially have contact with blood or other body fluids and dangerous operating room waste. They should also be trained in decontamination and terminal cleaning of rooms and equipment.

CENTRAL STERILE SUPPLY AND PROCESSING

The central sterile supply and processing department is usually located somewhere outside the surgical services department. Many hospitals place this department a floor above or below the ORs and utilize a dumbwaiter system to transport sterile and dirty supplies (in separate dumbwaiters) between departments. While primary decontamination of instruments (removal of gross blood and debris) is usually the responsibility of the surgical team or special OR staff, final wrapping of instrument sets and sterilization usually takes place in this department.

In addition to sterilization, the central sterile department is used for storing and distributing supplies and equipment and often for processing supplies as they arrive from the manufacturers. Supplies are maintained in the surgery department storage areas at a particular level, and the materiels management staff orders supplies from central sterile as these levels reach a preset level or time schedule. Increasingly, computers are being used between the two departments for use in patient charging and inventory control. Other hospitals have implemented a computerized storage cabinet system that automatically tracks supplies as they are used and reports stock levels within the surgery department to ancillary departments such as materiels management and central sterile supply. Some hospitals have begun using a "case cart" system, in which a cart of dirty supplies is sent to the decontamination room and then on to sterile supply and exchanged for a cart containing the same supplies preprocessed to replace the dirty ones.

The design of the central sterile supply department must be such that traffic flow patterns will allow for a separation of clean or sterile instruments and supplies and dirty or contaminated equipment to be reprocessed.

HAZARDS AND REGULATORY AGENCIES

The surgical department is an environment containing hazards to the patient and surgical team. Of utmost concern is the safety of patients, but equally important is the safety of the surgical team. For a safe environment to exist:

1. Equipment must be properly handled and operated.
2. Surgical technologists must be educated and trained in safety measures in the OR.
3. The surgical team must have knowledge of the possible hazards that exist in the OR and the methods of ensuring a safe surgical environment.

Potential safety hazards in the surgery department can be placed in one of the following categories:

Physical hazards: Noise, ionizing radiation, electricity, injury to the body, fire, and explosion

Biological hazards: Laser and/or electrosurgical **plume**, pathogens found in body fluids, latex sensitivity, and injuries from sharps

Chemical hazards: Disinfecting agents, waste anesthetic gases, and vapors and fumes from chemical agents

Surgery department policies and procedures for reducing the risks of the above three hazards are based on standards and guidelines established by numerous local, state, and federal agencies. The following is a short description of six key agencies:

National Fire Protection Agency (NFPA): Organization whose mission is to reduce the frequency of fires through the establishment of fire prevention standards, research, and public fire safety education.

***Occupational Safety and Health Administration* (*OSHA*)**: Federal organization that is dedicated to protecting the health of workers by establishing standards that address issues related to safety in the work place. The standards are legally enforceable in order to protect workers, and many of the standards are based on the findings of other agencies such as NFPA, ANSI, and NIOSH. Areas of OSHA regulation include noise levels, exposure to ionizing radiation, laser safety standards as established by ANSI, and fire safety standards for health care facilities as established by NFPA.

National Institute for Occupational Safety and Health (NIOSH): Organization whose responsibilities are similar to OSHA but tends to be more research oriented in establishing permissible exposure limits (PELs) for chemical vapors and gases. NIOSH is an arm of the CDC that falls under the Department of Health and Human Services.

American National Standards Institute (ANSI): Organization of industry experts who promote and facilitate voluntary consensus standards in technical fields. An example is the laser safety standard that is intended for use by all health care facilities that use lasers in the treatment of patients.

American Society for Testing and Materials (ASTM): Similar to ANSI, it is also an organization of industry experts who develop and provide voluntary consensus standards for medical equipment by testing the equipment.

Association for the Advancement of Medical Instrumentation (AAMI): Organization that establishes standards that reach across the spectrum of the health care field, including sterilization, electrical safety, levels of device safety, and use of medical devices.

SAFETY CONSIDERATIONS

The modern OR exists in and is itself a complex and technologically sophisticated environment. Each of the systems involved in creating a modern surgical environment also creates safety considerations.

AIR-HANDLING SYSTEM

Air-handling systems in the OR should be able to remove waste anesthetic gases, toxic fumes and vapors, and other odors. Temperature should be maintained between 65 and 75°F to prevent hypothermia in the patient, and humidity levels should be maintained no higher than 55% to reduce growth of bacteria. The air-handling system should provide for positive **laminar air flow**, a unidirectional positive-pressure flow of air that captures microbes to be filtered. HEPA filters are used to reduce the microbial count. Exceptions to the rule are made, such as with pediatric or debilitated patients, who require the room temperature to be warm.

SURGICAL LIGHTS

The beam from surgical lights should be nonglare to prevent eye fatigue (Figure 5-9). Most manufacturers of surgical lights have placed emphasis on trying to produce lights that emit a blue-white beam that still adequately illuminates the surgical site yet produces little glare and approximates the color intensities of normal sunlight. Some surgical instruments are manufactured with a satin or ebony finish to decrease surgical light reflection and glare off the instrument. Drapes and towels are designed in nonreflective colors such as blue or green in order to reduce glare.

NOISE IN THE OPERATING ROOM

Noise can be irritating to patients and the surgical team. Noise from a combination of sources can lead to interference with communication or prevent the ability to hear monitor alarms. Sources of noise include music, suction, power instruments, clattering of surgical instruments, and conversation. The circulator must make sure the door to the

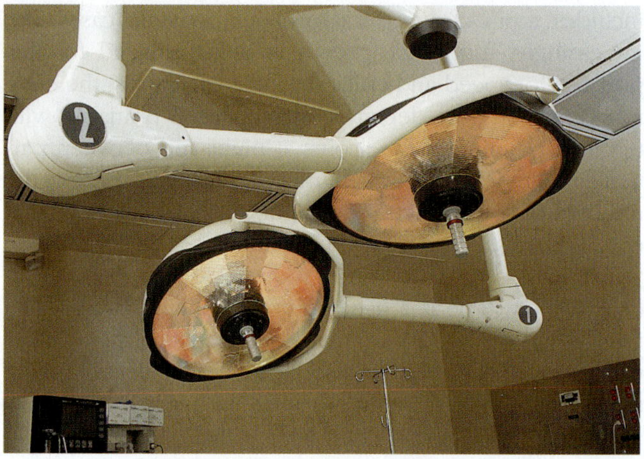

Figure 5-9 **Surgical lights**

OR is closed to eliminate external noise. Conversation should be kept to a minimum and, if necessary, carried on in a low to normal tone of voice. Music can be relaxing to the patient and may serve as a stimulant for the surgical team. For patients undergoing local anesthesia, it can be of particular benefit. However, much like conversation, it should be played in a low tone and the type of music should be appropriate for the environment and not be distracting to the surgical team.

ERGONOMICS AND SAFETY CONSIDERATIONS

Proper posture and body mechanics can help protect the body, especially the lumbar region of the back. Back injury and/or pain is usually the result of a number of factors that may include:

1. Lifting with the back bowed out
2. Bending and reaching with the back bowed out
3. Jerking or twisting at the hips
4. Obesity
5. Loss of strength and flexibility
6. Poor nutrition

The nature of the surgical technologist's job places abnormal strains on the body, in particular the lower back, knees, and feet. Proper body mechanics help prevent injury and discomfort. The following are guidelines to aid in preventing pain and injury due to poor body mechanics:

1. Stand with legs approximately shoulder width apart. This allows the ligaments of the hips and knees to naturally support the body and the wider stance is less fatiguing for the surgical technologist.
2. Avoid weight bearing on one foot for a prolonged period of time. The wide stance will prevent this from

happening. If weight bearing on one foot is necessary, shift the weight as often as possible.

3. The STSR should stand next to the OR table in an erect manner with arms relaxed from the shoulder down. The use of a standing stool(s) may be necessary.
4. For surgical procedures that require sitting, the surgical technologist should sit in an erect fashion with the spinal column straight. Do not lean forward from the shoulders, but from the hips.
5. Push, do not pull, heavy equipment such as microscopes, OR tables, gurneys, and laser equipment.

Most of the lifting done by the surgical technologist is relatively light. However, instrument sets can be quite heavy. One of the more difficult tasks for the team is moving an anesthetized or incapacitated patient. Teamwork and proper mechanics are important to the safety of the patient and the surgical team members. Proper lifting technique is summarized below:

1. Squat to lift and lower. Do not bend at the waist.
2. Lift with the legs and abdominal muscles, not the lower back.
3. Keep the weight as close to the body as possible.
4. Bow your back in and raise up with the head first; heels flat; lift with a smooth, even motion.
5. If a turn must be made while holding the weight, turn the whole body, not at the waist
6. Keep the lower back bowed in when lowering the object.
7. Keep the feet shoulder's width apart.

FIRE HAZARDS AND SAFETY

The danger of fire in the surgery department has been reduced with the introduction of halogenated anesthetic agents and the elimination of flammable cyclopropane. However, nitrous oxide, which itself is nonflammable, supports combustion in the presence of oxygen. Combined with a source of ignition, the potential for explosion and fire in the OR is an issue of significant importance.

A combination of three components can result in a fire and/or explosion:

1. Source of ignition such as a spark from metal hitting metal
2. Oxygen
3. Flammable chemical gas, vapor, or liquid such as ethyl alcohol

Standards established by the NFPA and AAMI aid in the prevention of fires in the OR. One of the NFPA standards of particular importance to health institutions is the *Standard for Health Care Facilities*.

SOURCES OF IGNITION

The nature of modern surgery creates many potential sources of ignition. Specific procedures and guidelines are in place for many of these.

Lasers

One of the newer technologies to be incorporated in surgery is the use of lasers. Often used with endoscopic procedures, the laser has contributed to the advancement of minimally invasive surgery. *Laser* is an acronym for "light amplification by the stimulated emission of radiation." This refers to (1) the process in which light energy is produced and also (2) the device that generates the laser energy or beam. However, as with most technology, the laser light presents hazards that must be understood in order to protect the patient, not the least of which is the potential to cause a fire.

Fire prevention is critical during laser surgery. The surgical team and especially the STSR must be aware of the precautions to follow to prevent a fire.

Sterile water must be available for the surgical team to use in dousing a small fire. The sterile water is also used to keep the sponges and towels wet during the procedure to prevent them from igniting.

Portable fire extinguishers must be immediately available. The *halon fire extinguisher* is recommended for laser fires due to its low toxicity and because residue is not produced.

The laser beam can ignite surgical drapes, but laser-retardant drapes are available commercially. To decrease the chance of fire, wet towels can be placed on the drapes around the surgical site.

The anesthesiologist must use a nonexplosive anesthetic agent.

Special caution should be used when laser surgery is performed in the head and neck area. Nitrous oxide and oxygen can build up beneath the surgical drapes, presenting an environment conducive to fire or explosion. Flammable preparation solutions (alcohol based) should not be used. Excess solution may pool under the patient causing vapors to be trapped beneath the surgical drapes. The volatility of these vapors increases the risk of surgical drape fires. The patient's hair should be covered with wet sponges or towels to prevent ignition if close to the laser site. The patient should be given preoperative instructions not to use hair spray that can easily ignite. During oral or laryngeal surgery, the anesthesiologist must use a flame-resistant type of endotracheal (ET) tube. Special ET tubes for laser surgery are commercially available. The ET tube balloon must be inflated with sterile water instead of air, and wet sponges placed around the tube and cuff.

During laser procedures in the anorectal area, the rectum must be packed with a sterile-water-soaked sponge to prevent a methane gas explosion or fire.

Finally, it is important to remember that a fire can be started by a reflected beam as readily as by a direct-beam impact. Nonreflective instrumentation must be used in the vicinity of the laser site.

Electrosurgical Unit

The **electrosurgical unit** generates considerable heat. If inadvertently activated, the electrosurgical pencil may burn or smolder the surgical drapes. When not in use, the handpiece should be placed in a holder attached to the drapes or positioned so that the handpiece will not be inadvertently activated.

Fiber-Optic Beam

The fiber-optic beam from the end of endoscopes must not be focused on the drapes. The heat from the beam can burn or smolder the drapes.

Static Electricity

Static electricity can ignite a flame under the right conditions. The humidity of the operating room should be no higher than 55%. Humidity lower than 50% is conducive of spark transmission.

Other Safety Guidelines

A full range of items must be considered in an environment such as the OR. Some general guidelines are used to further reduce the chance of ignition:

- Extension cords and power strips (multiple-outlet strip) are prohibited from use in the OR.
- Electrical cords should be rubber coated. The cords must be checked before use. Frayed or damaged cords are discarded; electrical tape should not be used to repair the cord.
- All electrical power equipment should be checked prior to use and plugged in before anesthetic delivery has begun.
- Electrical cords should be unplugged by pulling on the plug only.
- Movement around the patient's head should be kept to a minimum when general anesthesia is being used.
- Only cotton blankets should be used to cover the patient. Wool or blankets manufactured from other material tend to produce static electricity.
- The patient's hair should be covered to prevent static discharge.
- Never attach active electrode cord to the drapes with a metal device.

FIRE SAFETY GUIDELINES

The surgical technologist should be familiar with the health institution's fire policy and procedure. The technologist should know the procedure for reporting a fire, where the fire alarms and fire extinguishers are located, and routes of evacuation. Surgical technologists should know how to operate a fire extinguisher and know the three classes of extinguishers:

1. *Class A:* water
2. *Class B:* dry chemical for fires involving flammable liquids and gas
3. *Class C:* halon for electrical or laser fires

The three main concerns if a fire should occur in the OR are (1) protect the patient, (2) contain the fire if possible, and (3) move the anesthesia equipment as far away as possible from the fire source. The patient should be moved from the room as quickly as possible. Surgery personnel must be available to assist the anesthesia person in moving the patient. Use the proper fire extinguisher and extinguish the fire if possible.

ELECTRICAL HAZARDS

The use of electrical equipment in the surgical environment has dramatically risen with the advent of minimally invasive surgical techniques, the use of lasers, and electrosurgical equipment. Surgical technologists must be trained in the use of the equipment, safety measures, and equipment troubleshooting methods.

The manufacturer's instructions should always be followed when operating electrical equipment. The AAMI and JCAHO have developed safety standards for electrical equipment used in the OR. These instructions and standards are helpful in training surgical technologists to avoid human error or equipment malfunctions that may cause injury to the patient and staff.

ELECTRICAL CURRENT

When an *electrical charge* is in motion, it is referred to as an *electric current*. Electric current can be described as a flow of electric charge along a conductor, usually metal. The electric charge consists of electrons flowing along a path with an opening for its escape, such as the motor of an electric power saw. This is comparable to the flow of water through a pipe: To maintain a continuous flow, a supply of water must be provided at one end of the pipe and an opening at the other end into a receiving device of some sort. In other words, electric current is the flow of electrons. To ensure the electrons flow in one direction, it is necessary for electrical pressure or voltage to be present. The more electrons in motion, the stronger the current and the higher the pressure between the electrons. The greater the pressure (voltage), the greater the flow of electrons.

To prevent harm to the surgical patient, *grounding* of the electrical equipment is critical. Grounding prevents the passage of the electrical current through the patient by directing the current to the ground, therefore bypassing the patient. A common example of a grounding system is the three-prong plug. Electricity is supplied through the two upper prongs and the third prong is the grounding prong. This allows the current to have a return path to ground. Manufacturer's instructions emphasize that this third prong should not be removed in order to make it fit a nongrounded outlet. If this is done, ground protection will not be provided.

ELECTRICAL BURNS

Electrical current that is not diverted from the patient can result in first-, second-, or third-degree electrical burns usually involving a focused area of the patient's skin. The surgical technologist should be alert to the hazards of using electrical equipment.

An electrosurgical unit (ESU), also called the cautery or Bovie machine, produces an electrical current that is converted into thermal heat for cutting or coagulating tissue. To complete the circuit, a grounding pad is placed on the patient to create a pathway for the electrical current back to the ESU. The active electrode of the ESU is the tip of the pencil-like handle and the dispersive electrode is the grounding pad. If the grounding pad is not making complete contact with the skin of the patient, a burn can occur at the site. Burns could occur at the site of rings, such as wedding bands, and ECG electrodes.

It is important that the grounding pad be in place prior to the beginning of the procedure. It should be affixed firmly to the buttock or upper part of the thigh of the patient. If the grounding pad is not firmly affixed, the patient could suffer electrical burns in the area of the pad, or in other areas of the body that come into contact with metal parts of the table or equipment. Care is taken in positioning the patient so that the body does not come into contact with the operating table or other metal or conductive surfaces.

STATIC ELECTRICITY

Static electricity can be a source of ignition leading to explosion, especially in the presence of oxygen and anesthetic gases. There are two processes by which static charge buildup can occur. The first is by friction between two surfaces, called **triboelectrification**, the second is by proximity to an electrostatic field, referred to as *induction charging*. Triboelectrification is the concern of the OR. Triboelectrification is described as follows. (Simco 1998):

> When substances become charged by triboelectrification, electrons migrate from the surface of one material to the surface of the other. Upon separation of the two surfaces, one surface loses electrons and becomes positively charged. The other surface gains electrons and becomes negatively charged. As the friction increases, the amount of static buildup increases. Separating the two surfaces causes a spark(s) from the production of heat. Sparks can ignite flammable gases or substances.

Sterile surgical drapes are made of static-resistant material. Care must be taken to avoid static buildup, especially if the surgery site is in the head and neck region where waste anesthetic gases can accumulate. Towels and plastic draping materials are sources of static electricity. The surfaces of draping materials should not be rubbed together.

IONIZING RADIATION

Ionizing radiation can have therapeutic as well as harmful effects. When used in therapeutic doses, it can be used in the treatment of cancer, causing the death of cancer cells. Surgical technologists must be aware of the harmful effects of ionizing radiation, specifically X-rays.

Surgical technologists and patients are exposed to radiation during surgical procedures that require the use of the C-arm (fluoroscopy) and/or intraoperative X-rays. Ionizing radiation can cause changes in the cell membrane, enzymes, protein, and genetic material. These changes can lead to the development of bone cancer, cataracts, spontaneous abortion, and thyroid and testicular or ovarian cancer. Safety measures should be taken to protect the surgical patient as much as possible from the X-rays. The surgical technologist should utilize protective lead-lined gloves, aprons, thyroid collars, and glasses to minimize exposure to radiation.

PROTECTION OF THE SURGICAL PATIENT

The following guidelines aid in reducing the patient's exposure to X-rays and fluoroscopy:

- When possible, shield the patient's body with a lead apron. The lead shield should always be used for pregnant patients to protect the fetus. Low levels of ionizing radiation can also be harmful to the fetus.
- When fluoroscopy is not being used, it should be turned off. When fluoroscopy is turned on, the patient is continuously being exposed to the radiation.
- Cover the patient's thyroid and/or reproductive areas with lead shields made specifically for those areas.

PROTECTION OF THE SURGICAL TECHNOLOGIST

The three most important factors to remember concerning the safety of the surgical technologist and ionizing radiation are time, shielding, and distance. Surgical technologists who constantly work in surgical specialties in which X-rays and the use of fluoroscopy are routine, such as orthopedics, need to be aware of the safety precautions. Ionizing radiation can be the cause of mutagenic changes in cells leading to cancer, genetic defects that can be passed on to future offspring, or harm to the fetus of a pregnant surgical technologist. OSHA has established maximum levels of exposure with recommendations from NIOSH, ANSI, and AAMI. JCAHO guidelines must also be followed in order for the facility to retain accreditation.

The following guidelines aid in reducing the surgical technologist's exposure to X-rays and fluoroscopy:

- Pregnant surgical technologists should avoid exposure. Staff assignments should be made accordingly to allow the surgical technologist and fetus to be protected. If exposure must occur, the surgical technologist should either leave the room or wear a lead shield that adequately covers the body and fetus.
- When not in use, make sure the fluoroscope is turned off.
- Avoid overexposure to ionizing radiation. The shorter the time of exposure, the less amount of radiation absorbed.
- If possible, whether sterile or nonsterile, leave the room during exposure of X-rays.
- Surgical technologists who are a part of the sterile team and cannot leave the room should stand as far away as possible (6 ft or more) from the patient, avoiding the direct beam of ionizing radiation. Stand behind the X-ray machine if possible or behind someone wearing a lead shield.
- All members of the sterile surgical team should wear lead aprons, especially if fluoroscopy will be used throughout the surgical procedure. The lead apron is worn under the sterile gown and must be donned prior to scrubbing.
- Sterile and nonsterile lead gloves are available to protect the long bones of the hand. The gloves should be worn if it is necessary to hold an X-ray cassette for a single X-ray exposure or during the surgical procedure if an extremity must be held or manipulated during the use of fluoroscopy.
- Lead thyroid shields should be worn during fluoroscopy.
- Lead aprons should be laid flat or hung on the apron rack when not in use. Allowing the apron to fold or bend can cause cracks in the lead, rendering the lead apron inefficient.
- Surgical technologists exposed to ionizing radiation on a frequent basis or during a long surgical procedure should wear an X-ray-monitoring device. The most popular type is the film badge. The badge measures the accumulated exposure to ionizing radiation. Where the monitor is worn determines the area of the body being monitored. Individual data are collected weekly or monthly.

BIOLOGICAL HAZARDS AND SAFETY CONSIDERATIONS

Surgical technologists should be aware of the biohazards that exist in the surgical environment and their ability to cause infectious diseases. Hospital policy and procedures and federal regulations must be followed to protect patients, the public, and health care providers. OSHA has established policies to govern the disposal of infectious wastes and prevention of blood-borne diseases. The CDC established Universal Precautions and body substance isolation rules in 1985 and 1987 and have since updated these with Standard Precautions for the protection of patients and personnel from the hazards associated with exposure to blood or other potentially infectious body fluids.

UNIVERSAL PRECAUTIONS

Universal Precautions were defined in 1985 by the CDC and were designed to prevent the transmission of human immunodeficiency virus (HIV), hepatitis B virus (HBV), and other blood-borne pathogens to health care providers. Universal Precautions stated that blood and certain body fluids from *all* patients should be considered potentially infectious for HIV, HBV, or other blood-borne pathogens. Universal Precautions apply to blood, other body fluids that contain visible blood, semen, and vaginal secretions. Universal Precautions do not apply to feces, nasal secretions, sputum, sweat, tears, urine, and vomitus unless blood is visible and do not apply to saliva unless blood is present. Based on Universal Precautions, hospitals developed exposure control protocols that include the use of **personal protective equipment** (**PPE**) such as gloves, masks, and protective eyewear to prevent exposure.

STANDARD PRECAUTIONS

Standard Precautions were defined by the CDC in 1996 and combine Universal Precautions and body substance isolation rules that had preceded Universal Precautions. Body substance isolation rules had been developed to reduce the risk of transmission of pathogens from moist body substances. Standard Precautions apply to blood and *all* body fluids, secretions, and excretions (except sweat). Whether they contain visible blood or not, all body fluids should be treated as if they were potentially infectious, and the skin and mucous membranes of health care workers are to be protected from these fluids in order to reduce the risk of transmission of microorganisms. Gloves should be worn at all times when working with all body fluids. A description of potential pathogen hazards in the operating room is included in Chapter 7. These include HBV, hepatitis C (HCV), HIV, hepatitis D (HDV), tuberculosis, and other infectious diseases. Anyone in the operative environment is at risk.

Because workers in the operative environment, and especially those in the sterile field, often pass sharp instruments contaminated with blood, the likelihood of accidents is increased.

CAUSES OF INJURY LEADING TO EXPOSURE IN THE OPERATIVE ENVIRONMENT

The majority of sharps injuries in the hospital occur in the OR, and most of these are from scalpel and suture needle injury. Davis has outlined other commonly used devices that have caused percutaneous injuries leading to exposure to blood. These include all sharp and moderately sharp instruments and items used in operative procedures. Injuries occur in common situations such as the following:

- Positioning and passing a needle in a needle holder
- Suturing
- Manual tissue retraction
- Leaving needle on field which contacts worker's hand
- Dropping needle on worker's foot
- Reaching for device that is sliding off drapes
- Placing a sharp in the disposal container
- Poorly designed or overfilled container

In summary, any handling of a sharp or semisharp instrument or item is potentially dangerous. Proper technique and vigilance are required at all times. The strategies of Standard Precautions, including the proper use of PPE, and other strategies and behavior patterns will help to minimize risk.

STRATEGIES FOR EXPOSURE PREVENTION

Personal protective equipment must be provided by every facility for all workers, and OR professionals should assume a share of the responsibility for their own protection. Individual concerns and needs as to adequate protection and fit of items provided should be addressed.

In response to the increasing numbers of exposures to health care workers, an increasing number of safety devices have been and are being developed, including blunt suture needles, a suturing device to avoid manual handling of needles, double-gloving, and "no-touch" techniques during wound closure. In addition, safety syringes, IV catheters, lancets, and needleless IV connection systems have been developed. A general safety checklist is presented in Table 5-1.

Table 5-1 General Safety Checklist

ABSOLUTE PREREQUISITES
Complete hepatitis B vaccination series.
Use Standard Precautions with all patients.
Use personal protective equipment—appropriate choices.
Wear fluid-resistant head wear when appropriate.
Use adequate eye and face protection.
Use appropriate neck protection. Consider recently shaved skin nonintact.
Wear fluid-resistant or fluid-impervious gowns as appropriate to expected exposure risk.
Choose gloves appropriately.
Wear appropriate footwear or shoe covers.
Remove gloves carefully to avoid splatter.
Wash hands with antiseptic soap after removing gloves.
Remove eye protection last.
Remove contaminated PPE before leaving the room.
Carefully remove and discard mask following each procedure.
SAFETY TECHNIQUES
Wear gloves when handling surgical specimens.
Wear eye protection if container is opened or splashing is anticipated.
Apply dressings and handle drains or packs with clean gloves.
Avoid touching any surface with contaminated gloves.
Avoid touching existing contaminated surfaces.

Numerous strategies and procedures are used by every hospital to assist the employee with safety issues. These must be taught and reevaluated on an ongoing basis. Some of these strategies are:

- Have extra PPE readily available should replacement be needed.
- Position sharps disposal containers at point of use.
- Have a plan for sharps management.
- Discourage unauthorized entry into the room.
- Secure a signed preoperative consent for HIV testing, in case of exposure.
- Store a tube of blood preoperatively for all surgical patients to be held in the laboratory for possible HIV testing should an exposure occur.

Neutral Zone

In addition to the above safety practices and devices, a "neutral zone" strategy should be deployed in each procedure. Because many puncture injuries occur during hand-to-hand transfer, we recommend the use of a neutral zone in which sharps may be safely placed by one person and retrieved by another. This may be any of a number of devices, such as magnetic mats, trays, basins, an instrument stand, or a designated area on the sterile field. Small basins are not recommended because items are deep within the basin and hard to pick up and the basin may tip over.

The neutral zone is selected and agreed on prior to the beginning of the procedure by the surgeon and the STSR. This zone is a "sharps-only" zone, and all other instruments are passed directly hand to hand. It is suggested that the STSR announce the sharp by name when placing it in the neutral zone so that the surgeon is aware that a sharp object occupies that space. The sharp object is placed in the neutral zone in a position such that the surgeon may pick up the instrument with the dominant hand and use it without repositioning it, much as with hand-to-hand instrument transfer. The surgeon returns the instrument in like fashion to the neutral zone, rather than passing it back directly. Above all, a team approach should be taken with the neutral zone, and communication is key.

Other Sharps Safety Techniques

Hypodermic needles should never be recapped. In the rare occasion where recapping is unavoidable, a safety device or one-handed technique should be used.

Sharps on the Mayo stand should be kept in a central location and always in the same place. A small magnetic sterile sharps container should be used to store used needles for safety and for counting, and loaded needles should be placed at a position as far as possible from the hands of the STSR. Load needles just prior to use to avoid open needles on the Mayo stand.

Hazardous Waste Disposal

Two basic microbiological concepts govern the transmission of disease:

1. A sufficient number of microorganisms must be present in order to cause infection.
2. The microorganisms must have a path for entry into the host.

Health care providers are at risk of contracting infectious disease presented by infectious wastes and from exposure to blood or other body fluids from patients. Local, state, and federal government regulations address the issues of how infectious waste material is to be disposed of by health institutions. Infectious waste includes but is not limited to blood and body fluids and disposable surgical supplies contaminated by blood such as gloves, gowns, sponges, drapes, and sharps. These blood-contaminated items must be disposed of separately from routine surgery department waste material. Sharps must be placed in containers that are resistant to puncture and can be tightly sealed. Blood-contaminated disposable items may be placed in bags, and it may be necessary to double-bag the contaminated items. The bags should also be of a color, usually red, that distinguishes the waste material as separate from routine waste.

Universal Precautions states that all surgical patients are considered a source of infection. Therefore, surgical technologists must follow the biohazard exposure control plan that the surgery department has established as mandated by OSHA and the Standard Precautions outlined earlier in this chapter. By enforcing the policies, such as hand washing after removing surgical gloves, surgical technologists' exposure risk should be reduced.

MANAGEMENT OF EXPOSURE

Despite the best efforts of everyone in the operative environment, accidents do happen. Health care professionals should know how to respond to exposure incidents immediately. Appropriate postexposure measures including HIV postexposure **prophylaxis** (PEP) are important for the prevention of occupationally acquired HIV and other diseases. The CDC has published updated guidelines and recommendations for the care of occupationally exposed health care workers. These were published in May 1998, and further updates will follow as more information becomes available. Each institution should have a PEP protocol, and a list of names of readily available resources for consultation should be available. Some individual on this list should be available 24 hours per day, and some PEP treatments should be started within hours of an injury.

When an exposure occurs, medical personnel should immediately assess the severity of the exposure. If a needle stick or sharps injury has occurred to a person in the sterile field, the glove should be removed to assess the injury. The exposure site should be treated immediately (see following page). As soon as the wound is treated, the exposure should be reported, and assessment of the risk of infection should be made by the appropriate clinical personnel, usually the occupational health department of the hospital and the OR supervisor. When indicated, PEP should be initiated within 2 hours of exposure. In high-risk and HIV risk situations, appropriate counseling as to the risk factors should be provided.

Treatment

If the skin is broken, the wound should be washed with soap and water or a suitable scrub solution. If the exposure is to the oral or nasal mucosa, the area should be flushed with water. Eye exposures are treated by flushing with water or saline.

Risk Assessment

After exposure, the patient and the exposed health care worker are evaluated to determine the need for HIV PEP. Newer rapid HIV tests are helpful as the health care worker may need to make a decision within hours as to whether to initiate HIV prophylaxis (drug treatment). The exposure is evaluated based on a set of "risk factors" for potential to transmit HIV, which is determined by the body substance that was involved in the exposure and the route of the exposure (e.g., hollow needle stick, solid needle stick). The patient is evaluated for HIV infection, viral load, and risk factors for infection. When this information is not available, PEP should not be delayed while information is gathered. It is better to start PEP and stop it later than not to have started it within the time window recommended. Each hospital should have a well-established system of risk assessment based on CDC recommendations.

Prophylaxis for HIV

If prophylactic drug therapy is indicated based on the risk factors involved, the treatment should be explained to the health care worker exposed. The exposed surgical technologist or health care worker is informed that:

1. Knowledge is not yet complete about the effectiveness or toxicity of the drugs used for PEP.
2. Only zidovudine (ZDV) has been shown to prevent HIV transmission in humans (as of this writing).
3. Although the data are inconclusive, combination drug regimens are recommended at this time because of increased potency.
4. All PEP drugs may be declined, and health care workers must be informed of the possible side effects and toxicity of the drugs.

If PEP is to be utilized, it should be begun as soon as possible after the exposure. Health care workers exposed to HIV or HBV should receive follow-up counseling and postexposure testing and evaluation. Further testing should be performed at 6 weeks, 12 weeks, and 6 months postexposure.

LASER AND ELECTROSURGICAL PLUME

When a laser beam strikes tissue, tissue is coagulated, or a powered surgical instrument such as a saw cuts bone, a plume of smoke is produced depending on the power, duration of exposure, and tissue type. Research has been conducted over the years on the plume emitted during surgical procedures. Experiments have documented the content of the plume, particulate matter size, and toxicity of such plumes when inhaled by surgical personnel.

Electrosurgical plume causes an offensive odor and may produce watery eyes and respiratory irritation in surgical personnel. The main area of concern is the viability of the cells in the plume. Many studies have been conducted to answer the question of viability of the cellular contents, especially in the area of laser plume. Studies have not been conclusive but have proved that the laser plume contains water, carbonized particles, and intact strands of DNA. In 1998, Garden and associates discovered intact DNA strands of human papilloma virus in laser plume after using a CO_2 laser at low and high settings to vaporize plantar warts. The study concluded that target tissue can become aerosolized and could possibly be infectious.

Recommendations for protection from plume is the wearing of specially manufactured laser masks that can filter particles as small as 0.1–0.3 μm in size, proper eye protection such as face shield, goggles, or eyewear that has side shields, and a smoke evacuator.

Currently, electrosurgical plume is evacuated with regular suction often held by the STSR, a practice that may change as increasing attention is given to the possible hazards posed to the surgical team by electrosurgical plume. Special evacuator units are required for laser surgery and may soon be required for electrosurgical plume. Units available on the market filter laser plume from 0.1 to 0.5 μm in size. Usually the unit has a HEPA or ULPA (ultra-low-penetration air) filter combined with a charcoal filter. The charcoal absorbs hydrocarbons and the offensive odor produced by the plume.

When the filter needs changing, it should be done as soon as possible. The individual changing the filter should treat it as contaminated infectious waste, wearing gloves and a mask and using clean technique in discarding the biohazardous contaminated filter into a biohazardous waste container.

Positioning the evacuation wand or tip is the duty of the STSR during a laser procedure. The tip must be held very close to the laser tissue impact site in order to efficiently remove the smoke. When the tip is held within 1 cm of the impact site, approximately 98% of the plume is removed. If the distance from the impact site is doubled to 2 cm, the efficiency rate of plume removal is reduced by half.

In summary, the optimal methods to control laser or electrosurgical plume and decrease the surgical team's hazard of inhaling the plume are to:

1. Use an evacuation unit.
2. Change the filter when required.
3. Use filters that evacuate plume particulate matter a minimum of 0.3 μm in size, but ideally 0.1 μm in size.
4. Ensure the STSR holds the evacuation wand or suction tip as close as possible to the tissue impact site.
5. Wear gloves, masks, and proper eye guards.

LATEX ALLERGY

Latex is made from the natural rubber harvested from trees found in warm tropical climates. It was first discovered by the British in the mid-18th century but did not come into wide use until about 50 years ago. William Halstead introduced natural rubber latex gloves into surgery in 1890. In 1979 a British medical journal reported the first case of latex allergy—a woman had reacted to the rubber in household gloves.

About 1% of the general population is reported to have allergic reactions to latex, but of that percentage, health care workers represent the largest number of individuals who are known to be latex sensitive. Many of the items used in surgery contain latex, and surgical team members who are exposed on a daily basis can become sensitized. Some of the items containing latex even though it is not indicated as an ingredient on the packaging include tape, shoe covers, and electrode pads.

Two types of latex allergic responses have been identified, Type I and Type IV. Type IV is the less serious, more localized reaction characterized by skin irritation and discomfort. Type I is immunoglobulin E (IgE) mediated and is the most serious reaction, possibly leading to respiratory arrest. Rubber contains proteins, resins, and sugars. Many latex proteins are allergenic. Clinical research has shown that water-soluble proteins in the latex itself appear to be the primary cause, attaching to the skin from glove powder absorption, or the allergic reaction may also result from inhalation of airborne allergens bound to the glove powder.

Individuals at risk include health care providers, patients who have had multiple surgeries, and children with spina bifida. Surgical technologists should know and recognize the signs and symptoms of possible allergic reaction so immediate action can be taken by the surgical team.

Important points to remember include:

1. All high-risk patients and health care providers should be latex allergy tested.
2. A latex-safe environment should be provided for latex allergic patients. Only nonlatex products should be used.
3. Latex allergic patients should be scheduled in the OR as the first surgical procedure. This allows latex dust from the previous day's surgeries to be removed during end-of-day cleaning.
4. All departments involved in the care of the patient, such as the pharmacy and central sterile supply, should be notified so precautions will be taken.
5. The patient's chart should be properly marked signifying latex allergy, and red ID bracelet should be worn.

Examples of items used in surgery that have latex include disposable face masks, Yankauer suction tip, oral airway, nonsterile and sterile gloves, and tourniquets of all types. The types of manufacturing materials used in place of latex to produce items such as those listed above includes Nitrile, neoprene, vinyl, nonpowdered low-protein gloves, polyvinylchloride, and styrene ethylene butylene.

CHEMICAL HAZARDS AND SAFETY CONSIDERATIONS

Many important chemicals used in medical care, such as ethylene oxide and formaldehyde, are potentially hazardous. The chemicals are capable of causing effects ranging from mucous membrane irritation to cancer and adverse genetic damage.

Surgical technologists should be familiar with the chemicals used in the OR and general information concerning the chemicals. Information can be gained from the Material Safety Data Sheets (MSDS) that the surgery department must have available to the workers.

WASTE ANESTHETIC GASES

Waste anesthetic gases are vapors that escape from the anesthesia machine and tubing. Studies have indicated that chronic exposure to the gases could pose health hazards such as cancer, hepatic and renal complications, nerve and brain damage, and spontaneous abortion. OSHA enforces NIOSH recommendations for setting the standards determining the occupational limits of exposure for surgical team members.

In addition to good anesthetic techniques employed by anesthesia personnel, an effective gas-scavenging system should be used. The gas-scavenging system, which should be connected to every anesthesia machine used in the surgery department, removes waste anesthetic gases to be filtered and then dispersed to the outside atmosphere. Combined with the scavenger system, the OR ventilation system should aid in preventing the buildup of waste anesthetic gases.

METHYL METHACRYLATE

Methyl methacrylate (MMA) is a chemical compound composed of a mixture of liquid and powder. The common name of MMA used in surgery is bone cement. It is used for cementing metal prostheses in place during total joint arthroplasties. The liquid and powder components are combined by the STSR at the sterile back table. The vapors released from the mixture are noxious and irritating to the eyes and mucous membranes of the respiratory tract and can damage soft contact lenses, thus damaging the eyes. MMA has potential health effects that have not been proven. They could include mutagenic effects and carcinogenic and hepatic disorders. The liquid portion of the mixture can permeate through the sterile latex gloves, causing contact dermatitis. Self-contained vapor evacuation systems are available on the market to contain the fumes while mixing the cement.

FORMALIN

Formalin is a commonly used preservative for tissue specimens to be sent to the pathology department. The vapors from the liquid are an irritant to the mucous membranes of the respiratory tract. It is known to be a mutagen, a carcinogen, and toxic to the liver. Both OSHA and NIOSH have established standards for the PEL in the surgery department. If exposure to formalin is necessary, it should only be handled in a well-ventilated area with mask and gloves worn.

ETHYLENE OXIDE

Ethylene oxide (EtO) is a liquid chemical converted to a gas for sterilization purposes. Surgical equipment and instruments that are heat sensitive may be sterilized with the use of EtO. The hazards associated with the use of EtO are as follows:

1. Residual by-products are toxic and direct contact with the skin must be avoided.
2. Exposure to the gas can cause nausea, vomiting, and vertigo.
3. Ethylene oxide is known to be highly mutagenic and carcinogenic.
4. If EtO combines with water, the toxic by-products ethylene glycol and ethylene chlorohydrin will form. (Ethylene glycol is easily absorbed through the skin to cause systemic difficulties.)

GLUTARALDEHYDE

Glutaraldehyde is a liquid disinfectant and sterilizing agent. Commercially known as Cidex,® the fumes can be irritating to the eyes and mucous membranes. When not in use, glutaraldehyde must be kept in a covered container system. It must be used in a well-ventilated area, and many health facilities have installed commercial ventilation systems for the removal of the fumes.

CASE STUDY

Johanna is scheduled to be the STSR on a procedure at 8:00 A.M. in which a laser will be used to obliterate abnormal tissue in the larynx. She is preparing for the case.

1. What specific safety issues should she consider in preparing for this case?
2. What procedures should be in place to ensure the patient's safety?
3. Are there any anesthetic concerns?

QUESTIONS FOR FURTHER STUDY

1. What is the primary difference between Standard Precautions and Universal Precautions?
2. Name four ancillary departments in the hospital that directly support the OR.
3. At what temperature and humidity levels should the OR be maintained?
4. What agency is dedicated to protecting the health and safety of the workers in the OR?
5. Should a latex-sensitive patient be scheduled in the OR as the first patient or the last patient of the day?
6. What are the three important safety factors for surgical technologists to consider when exposed to ionizing radiation?

BIBLIOGRAPHY

American National Standards Institute (ANSI). (1996). Standard Z136.3-1996: Safe use of lasers in health care facilities [Online]. Available from *http://web.ansi.org*

Ansell Health care. (1998). Management of the latex-sensitive patient & health care workers [Online]. Available from *http://www.ansell.com/america/usa/latex/*

Atkinson, L. J., & Fortunato, N. (1996). Berry & Kohn's Operating Room technique (8th ed.). St. Louis. Mosby.

Ball, K. A. (1990). *Lasers: The perioperative challenge.* St. Louis, MO: Mosby.

Davis, M. S. (1999). *Advanced precautions for today's O.R.: The operating room professional's handbook for the prevention of sharps injuries and bloodborne exposures.* Atlanta: Sweinbinder.

Evans, W. J. (1994). Decontamination and disinfection. In *Central service technical manual* (pp. 73–90). Chicago: International Association of Healthcare Central Service Materiel Management.

Garden, J. M., O'Bannon, K., & Shelnitz, L. (1998). Papillomavirus in the vapor of carbon dioxide laser-treated verrucae. *Journal of the American Medical Association, 8,* 1199–1202.

Harris, H. R. (1994). Anesthetic gas: Danger in the OR. *The Surgical Technologist, 26* (10), 14–15.

Kanich, D. G., & Byrd, J. (1996, July/Aug.). How to increase OR efficiency. *OR Reports, 5*(4), 3–8.

Kruger, D. A. (1994). Ethylene oxide sterilization and aeration. In *Central service technical manual* (pp. 103–109). Chicago: International Association of Healthcare Central Service Materiel Management.

Kurz, A., Sessler, D. I., & Lenhardt, R. (1996). Perioperative normothermia to reduce the incidence of surgical-wound infection and shorten hospitalization. *New England Journal of Medicine, 334,* 1209–1215.

Marquette University (1997). Lifting and proper body mechanics [Online]. Available from *http://www.mu.edu/dept/pt/lift.htm*

McGuiness, A. M., et al. (2002). *Core curriculum for surgical technology* (5th ed.). Centennial, CO: Association of Surgical Technologists.

Mercy Hospital Medical Center. (1997). Are you allergic to latex? [Online]. Available from *http://www.mercydesmoines.org/health/articles/latex.htm*

National Fire Protection Agency (NFPA). (1990). Standard for health care facilities [Online]. Available from *http://www.nfpa.org/codehome/html*

Occupational Safety and Health Administration (OSHA). (1992). Bloodborne pathogens and acute care facilities [On line]. Available from *http://www.osha.gov*

Occupational Safety and Health Administration (OSHA). (1998). Hazardous medications [Online]. Available from *http://www.osha.gov*

Patterson, P. (1993). OSHA steps up action on waste anesthetic gases; OR exposure to electrosurgical smoke a concern; efficiency of evacuators depends on filtration system. *OR Manager, 9*(6), 1, 6–11.

Primary Electrical Circuits [Online]. Available from *http://www.innerbody.com*

Schaechter, M., & Frederick, N. C. (1997). *An electronic companion to beginning microbiology.* New York: Cogito Learning Media.

Simco (1998). Introduction to static electricity [Online]. Available from *http://www.simco.nl/statico.htm*

Stehlin, D. (1992). Latex allergies: When rubber rubs the wrong way [Online]. Available from *http://www.fda.gov/bbs/topics/CONSUMER/CON00165.htm*

Taylor, L. S. (1996). What you need to know about radiation [Online]. Available from *http://www. sph.umich.edu/group/eih/UMSCHPS/1st.htm*

Wenzel, R. P. (1997). *Prevention and control of nosocomial infections* (3rd ed.). Baltimore: Williams & Wilkins.

SECTION 2

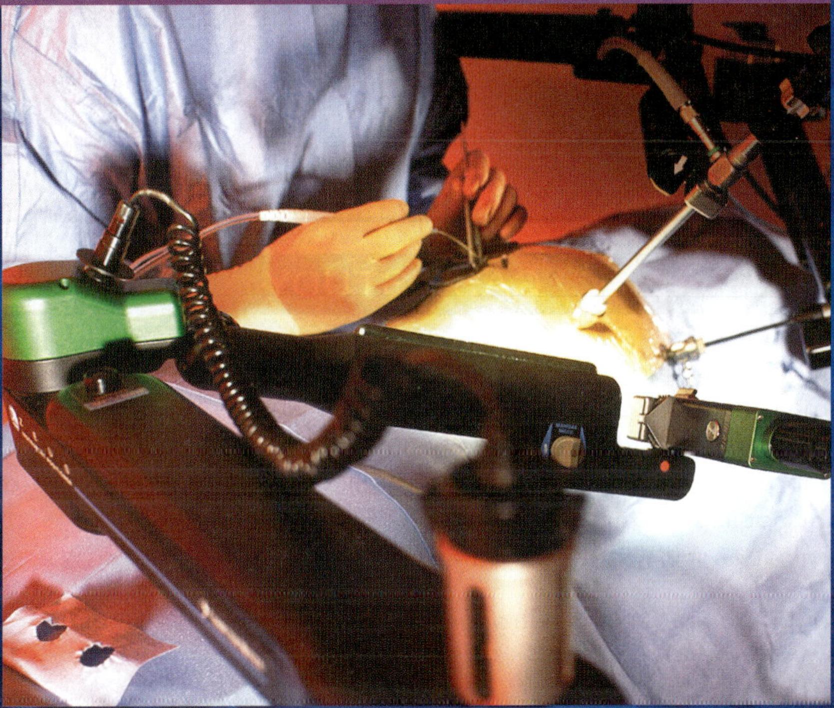

Principles and Practice of Surgical Technology

CHAPTER 6

Biomedical Science

Paul Price
Kevin B. Frey

CASE STUDY

During an open colon resection, the surgeon encounters a small bleeding vessel. A Crile hemostat is applied to occlude the vessel. While the surgeon is holding the clamp, the surgical assistant applies the tip of the activated electrosurgical pencil to the hemostat to coagulate the vessel and stop the bleeding. Suddenly, the surgeon pulls her hand away, yelling aloud. Upon examination, she discovers a pinpoint third-degree burn on her right index finger.

1. Where should the tip of the electrosurgical pencil be placed in relation to the surgeon's hand to reduce the risk of injury?
2. List two possible causes for the burn suffered by the surgeon. Explain both principles.
3. What complications may result from the burn?
4. What is acting as the insulator in this situation?
5. What three factors contributed to the outcome of this situation?

OBJECTIVES

After studying this chapter, the reader should be able to:

C 1. Identify basic components of a computer system.
2. Describe electrical safety precautions.
3. Define terms related to physics.
4. Describe the basic concepts of robotics.

A 5. (No objectives focused on asepsis in this chapter; however, the practice of sterile technique will be necessary when using related equipment in the OR.)

R 6. Perform basic word processing, Internet, and e-mail functions.

7. Apply computer knowledge to safe patient care.

8. Describe the geometrical concepts of robotics and the mechanisms of the robotic system.

E 9. Describe the basic principles of electricity and their application in the OR.

10. Apply the principles of robotics to safe patient care practices in the OR.

11. Apply the principles of physics to safe patient care pratices in the OR.

SELECT KEY TERMS

1. active electrode
2. Cartesian coordinate geometry
3. central processing unit (CPU)
4. circuit
5. degrees of freedom
6. dispersive (inactive) electrode
7. electrons
8. font
9. free electrons
10. generator
11. ground wire
12. hydraulic pressure
13. inertia
14. infrared waves
15. insulator
16. load
17. mass
18. modem
19. monitor
20. mouse
21. neutrons
22. periodic table
23. plasma
24. power
25. pressure
26. protons
27. quarks
28. refraction
29. resistance
30. switch
31. volume
32. weight
33. X-rays

INTRODUCTION

This chapter provides a broad base of knowledge for the entry-level surgical technologist in the areas of computers, electricity, physics, and robotics. As surgical equipment becomes more sophisticated, understanding the fundamental principles of these technologies is essential.

COMPUTERS

In this section a desktop version of the IBM-PC (or compatible) and the widely used Windows operating system are used to demonstrate basic computer skills. Many other platforms, operating systems, and software programs are available; however, due to space limitations, it is not possible to cover all of them in this chapter.

SURGICAL APPLICATIONS

Advanced application of computer technology in the hospital setting adds a new dimension to surgical patient care.

SCHEDULING SURGICAL PATIENTS

Scheduling of surgical patients has been streamlined because of computer technology. Communication via e-mail or fax from the physician's office instantly provides necessary patient information. The information saved in the computer is easily updated and can be printed prior to surgery in order to disseminate the information to surgical personnel and to other pertinent hospital departments.

SURGEON'S PREFERENCE CARD

In the past, surgeon's preference cards were handwritten, with additional notes scribbled in the margins, and often became illegible. In addition, if the surgeon had privileges at more than one hospital, it was difficult to get copies of the cards or, if the surgeon moved, the cards would be left behind at the previous hospital. Now, the majority of surgical facilities develop and save preference cards electronically. Consequently, it is easier to update the cards and obtain an accurate copy when preparing for a surgical procedure (preoperative case management).

PATIENT CHARTS

Computers facilitate storing, updating, and sharing patient information among hospital departments and the physician's office. The patient's chart is easily accessed to confirm results of diagnostic studies or other information vital to providing quality care to the surgical patient.

SURGICAL RECORDS

Many facilities install a computer in each OR to facilitate completion of the OR record and save it to the patient's hospital record (chart). The computer can also be used to send laboratory or radiology requisitions and receive the results of the tests in the OR. Other requests and orders can be e-mailed to various related departments (e.g., sterile processing, oncology).

STERILE PROCESSING

Computers have substantially reduced the paperwork of the sterile processing department. Supplies can be ordered online, inventory records maintained electronically, and records related to the sterilization of supplies and equipment saved on the computer. Additionally, just as with the surgeon's preference cards, the instrument list/count sheet for the assembly of instrument trays can be entered, saved, updated, and printed.

ROBOTICS

Robotics is quickly becoming a reality in the OR and is considered one of the major technological advances of the near future. Surgical technologists will be responsible for sterilizing the robotic equipment, setting up the robot, and running the computer programs and operating equipment during the surgical procedure.

HARDWARE

Hardware is the overall term used to describe the components of a computer, such as the central processing unit, **monitor**, **modem**, and memory storage devices.

CENTRAL PROCESSING UNIT

The **central processing unit** (**CPU**) is the silicon chip located within the computer case that is either a tower case (vertical) or desktop case (horizontal). It is one of the most important components of the computer system that is responsible for coordinating the operations of the computer, manages the computer systems, and facilitates the exchange of data with the computer memory. The monitor, keyboard, mouse, and printer cables all insert into ports on the computer case. If the computer operates as part of a network, the network line also connects to the computer case.

- *Ports*—specialized openings, typically found on the back of the computer case, for attaching various computer components such as the keyboard, speakers, printer, and external modem.
- *Expansion slots*—allow a computer to be upgraded with additional memory or features. When purchasing a computer, one important consideration is the number of expansion slots that are included.
- *Network or Ethernet card*—Necessary for communicating over a network. The optional network card is either built into the computer case or installed in an expansion slot (Figure 6-1).

Hard Drive

The hard drive, often designated the *C drive,* is located within the CPU. This drive has the most storage (memory) space and stores computer programs and files. Increased memory improves performance.

Memory

Floppy disks, ZIP drives, CDs, and DVDs have different storage capacities. The computer's memory is measured

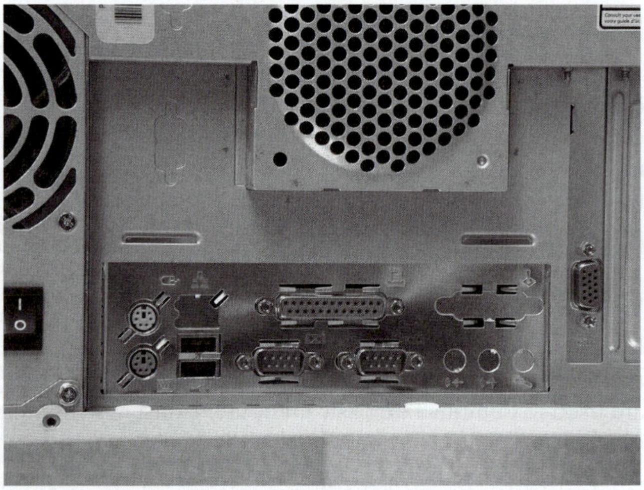

Figure 6-1 Expansion slots and ports *(Copyright © 2002 Technological Sciences for the Operating Room, Association of Surgical Technologists)*

in bytes. One byte of memory holds one character. One page of text averages 1,024 bytes. The prefix *kilo* is used to mean 1,000. Now one page contains 1,024 bytes and requires 1 kilobyte (KB) of memory. One thousand pages of text equals about 1,024 KB, or 1 megabyte (MB). One thousand and twenty-four megabytes equals 1 gigabyte (GB). One thousand and twenty-four gigabytes equals 1 terabyte (TB), which is the equivalent of one trillion characters. The newest unit of measurement for storage is *googlebytes*. One googlebyte is equal to 1,000 TB.

Floppy Disk Drive. The floppy disk drive, often designated the *A drive,* is typically located on the front of the computer case and allows information to be saved and retrieved on a disk, sometimes called a floppy disk. Floppy disks are a common method of transporting and exchanging files. They are also used to save or "back up" files to a separate location in the event of an error in the hard drive.

As a floppy disk is inserted in the drive, the drive automatically accepts and positions the disk. A clicking sound indicates the disk is fully seated in the drive. To eject the disk, depress the button next to the drive.

ZIP Drive. The optional ZIP drive can be either an internal or an external device. ZIP disks hold substantially more information than floppy disks. The ZIP disk is inserted into the ZIP drive in a similar fashion to a floppy disk.

CD-ROM Drive. Usually located on the front of the computer, the CD ROM drive reads CD ROMs that contain everything from music to encyclopedia volumes or computer software for installation. To operate, depress the button on the CPU to open the drawer and insert the CD. Push the same button to close the drive and start the CD. Like the floppy disk, a CD-ROM also offers convenient, portable storage but with a much larger capacity. Another benefit is that the information on a CD-ROM is "read only," which prevents an unintended deletion of files and information. However, a type of CD called read/write CD (CD-RW) is available for recording purposes. A CD recorder is required to transfer, or "write," files to a disk. This process is often referred to as "burning the CD."

DVD-ROM Drive. The latest method to provide convenient, removable data is the DVD, which is powered by an internal DVD-ROM drive. The DVD offers superior storage capacity that exceeds CD-ROM technology, and as of 2003 DVD-RW drives could archive up to 7 GB on one disk. These larger capacities are practical when working with video and sophisticated graphics programs. DVD drives are also capable of reading CD-ROMs.

Modem

The modem is a communications device that enables computers to send information over a telephone line, cable network, or satellite system to other computers for Internet connections and the exchange of e-mail. The modem is either an internal device built into the computer or an external unit with a cable that plugs into the back of the computer case. The telephone cord or cable is connected into the back of the computer or external modem and then connected into the telephone jack.

MONITOR

The monitor is the screen that displays the output of the computer. One of the most important features of a monitor is the amount of "viewable" space, which is measured diagonally; the larger the actual screen, the better. The term *resolution* refers to the clarity of the screen image and is another crucial consideration. Standard resolutions are 640 × 480, 800 × 600, and 1024 × 768.

KEYBOARD

The keyboard is used to enter characters (letters and numbers) and commands into the computer. The keyboard is divided into four areas: alphabet keys, function keys, number keys or keypad, and cursor control keys.

- *Alphabet keys*—These keys are similar in configuration to the keys of a typewriter, with the addition of specialty keys, such as the Control key and Backspace key.
- *Shift key*—Used to create uppercase letters or generate specific symbols.
- *Control key (Ctrl)*—Used in conjunction with other keys, such as the function keys, to accommodate a wider range of options.
- *Backspace key (←)*—Used to delete the characters to the left of the cursor.
- *Enter key*—Used to create spaces between sentences or paragraphs. There is no reason to strike the Enter key at the end of every line, because the word processing program automatically "wraps around" and advances the text to the next line.
- *Caps Lock key*—When activated, all letters are typed in uppercase without having to hold down the Shift key. This function only works for letters; to type punctuation symbols that are listed above other characters, depress the Shift key.
- *Function keys*—These keys begin with an "F" and are followed by a number, such as F1. They are shortcuts to commands and help in maneuvering within programs.
- *Number keys*—To activate, press the Num Lock key. If the Num Lock key is not activated, the numeric keys on the right will act as cursor-directional keys.

Most keyboards also have a second set of directional keys next to the numeric keypad.

- *Cursor control keys*—Located on the extended keyboard above the second set of directional keys, the cursor control keys include Delete, End, Home, Page Up, and Page Down.
- *Delete key*—Used to delete characters to the right of the cursor.

MOUSE

The handheld mouse moves the cursor to different areas on the screen and can be used to select commands. A popular model is the wireless mouse, which employs infrared technology. (Wireless keyboards are also available.) Many have a "roller" in the middle for quickly scrolling through a document.

When the mouse's cursor is placed over an icon or word in the Task Bar, the cursor changes to an arrow. The arrow indicates that the icon or word is a function that can be activated.

Pressing a button on the mouse is called *clicking*. Usually, the left click performs the majority of general functions and the right click performs specialized functions. Two left clicks on a document name will open it; two left clicks on a word will highlight it.

SCANNER

The scanner is a hardware component that converts printed text or pictures into digital information that can be used by the computer (Figure 6-2). It reproduces the image electronically rather than generating a printed version. Many scanners also function as copy and fax machines.

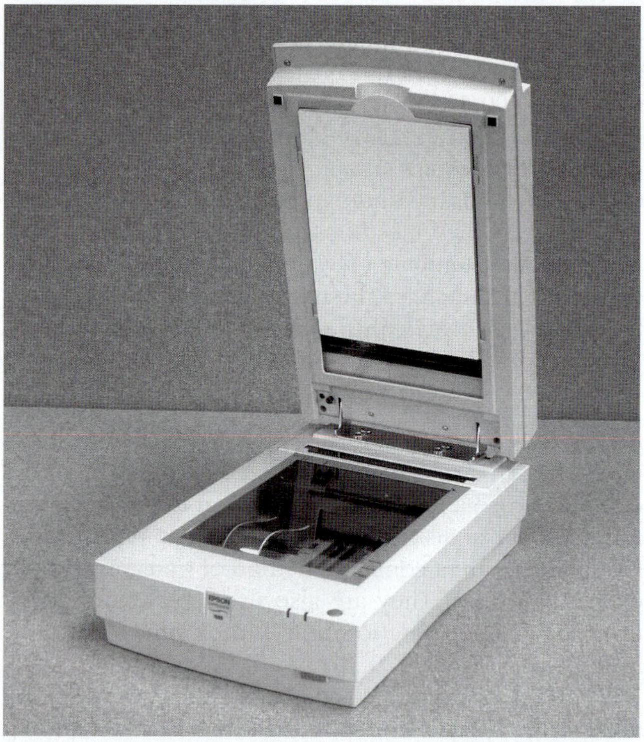

Figure 6-2 Scanner *(Copyright © 2002* **Technological Sciences for the Operating Room,** *Association of Surgical Technologists)*

SPEAKERS

Speakers, which accommodate the audio functions of many programs and CD-ROMs, are connected to the back of the computer case and require a sound card. It is cost effective to purchase a computer that already contains a sound card.

PRINTER

The printer produces paper versions (hard copies) of documents (e.g., e-mail) and images (e.g., photographs). Printers have black-and-white and/or color capabilities. The necessary software is included or can be downloaded from the website of the manufacturer.

SURGE PROTECTOR

Surge protectors provide a buffer against damage from high-voltage surges and are a highly recommended option to safeguard the computer and all of its components and accessories. An electrical power strip accepts several of the computer plug-ins and centralizes the outlet to the electrical power source.

USING THE COMPUTER

The first step is to switch on the computer and the related hardware. Typically, a power button located on the front of each item must be depressed. Once the power is turned on, the CPU goes through a start-up process (sometimes referred to as "booting") and opens the desktop. For security purposes, a log-in screen that requests the user's name and password may be required. Passwords can be easily changed and updated.

Desktop

The first thing that will pop up on the monitor screen is the desktop, the general background on which windows, dialog boxes, and icons appear. Shortcuts to programs can be placed on the desktop, the screen background (called *wallpaper*) changed, and the Task Bar customized.

Task Bar. Along either side or the top or bottom of the desktop is a gray bar called the Task Bar. It shows all applications or documents that are currently "open" or running and enables the user to switch between applications or have multiple applications open on the desktop.

In the lower left-hand corner of the Task Bar is the Start Button. Left click once with the mouse to open a box with various options, called the Start menu. The user can access additional submenus by moving the mouse over any of the words on the menu. This menu allows the user to access many areas and functions of the computer. Typically, one left click of the mouse will activate (open) the selected program.

Opening a Program. From the Start menu, move the mouse over the word Programs. A larger submenu appears that lists all programs currently installed on the user's computer. To open a program, place the mouse arrow over the desired program to highlight it and left click the mouse to open it.

Opening a Document. As the user creates and saves documents, the computer tracks these and makes them easy to access by showing them in the Start menu under Documents. The user can easily access a particular document without opening the program by looking in the Documents submenu.

Changing the Desktop. The Settings menu gives the user easy access to the Control Panel, the system software that controls the desktop options, time and date settings, sound, printers, and so on.

Searching the Computer. The Search menu allows the user to search for programs, documents, or to access the Internet quickly.

Getting Help. The Help menu can be used to find information about the computer system itself and for individual programs. Move the arrow of the mouse up to Help and left click once. Three items are listed near the top of the Help window that pops up: Contents, Index, and Search. Click on Contents and several topics appear; when one is clicked, another menu of subtopics appears. When the user clicks on a subtopic, directions appear in the box to the right. There may even be shortcut directions and words that are printed in blue that can be selected for more information. Click on Index and detailed topics appear. Look for the cursor blinking on and off in an empty box above the list. Type in a key word to retrieve specific help topics.

Shutting Down the Computer. To turn off the computer without losing files, the user must go through a shutdown process. Click on the Start menu and scroll to Shut Down. When the mouse arrow is used to highlight Shut Down, a submenu will pop up asking how the user would like to continue. To end all programs safely, choose Shut Down and press OK.

This menu can also be used to restart the computer, which is often required after installing programs or updates. If the computer is connected to a network, the user can choose Log Off to disconnect from the network.

Maneuvering Through the Desktop. Before discussing software, the user must be able to maneuver through the desktop environment, including minimizing and maximizing a window and using the mouse.

Minimizing and Maximizing a Window. Whenever a window is opened, the following icons appear in the upper right-hand corner: — (used to minimize the window), 🗗 (used to maximize the window), and X (used to close the window). These icons are located in the blue Title Bar that contains the title of the open window.

Opening Multiple Windows. Opening two windows simultaneously can be helpful to view or compare information saved in two different documents.

Scrolling. *Scrolling* refers to moving up and down within a document or window. Within a document, the cursor can be moved around with the aid of the direction arrows. More often, the roller on the mouse is used for scrolling. On the right-hand side of the screen in a Word® document or in the Help window, a light gray vertical bar, called the Scrolling Bar, features arrows pointing up and down. To move one line at a time, move the mouse arrow over the ▲ or ▼ and click. Keep clicking to move up and down the document. Even though the screen is showing a different part of the document, please notice that the blinking cursor has not moved with the screen. To make changes or insert new copy in a different area of the document, click on the screen to insert the curser on the page being viewed. If the user begins to type before inserting the cursor on the current page, the screen will return to the area of the document containing the cursor.

SOFTWARE

Computer software refers to the programs that operate the computer system and its individual hardware components, as well as the user's programs, such as word processing, games, or Internet access. Software or computer programs are available on floppy disks or CD-ROMs to facilitate loading (installation) on the computer.

Many varieties of software are on the market. Some computer systems are factory equipped with more software programs than others. One popular word processing program is Microsoft Word®. The word processing sections of this chapter are based on Microsoft Word 97 software.

INSTALLING SOFTWARE

To install a program, simply insert the first floppy disk or CD-ROM in the correct drive, and a message will appear with directions, such as when to insert the next disk or CD-ROM, to complete the installation of the program. The computer is simply copying (downloading) the information onto the hard drive.

WORD PROCESSING

Word processing is a term that simply means creating a document. Word processing is described here using the Windows '98® program and Office '97® program, which includes Microsoft Word, Excel® (a spreadsheet application), and PowerPoint® (an application that allows users to create presentations for groups). This section concentrates only on the use of Microsoft Word.

The first step is to click on Start in the Task Bar at the bottom of your screen. Next click on Programs and a large menu will appear. Find Microsoft Word (the "W" icon). Click on it to open the program.

The Title Bar at the top of the screen will indicate a new document by displaying "Document 1," and the cursor will automatically appear on the first line. The Title Bar, Menu Bar, Standard Tool Bar, and Formatting Tool Bar are useful when maneuvering through this program.

- *Title Bar*—Appears at the top of the monitor and displays the title of the document in the open window.
- *Menu Bar*—Appears below the Title Bar and includes functions such as File, Edit, View, and Insert. As the name indicates, when a word is clicked on, a menu of functions appears.
- *Standard Tool Bar*—Appears below the Menu Bar and uses symbols (icons) to indicate various functions. Move the arrow of the mouse over one of the symbols and a tool tip appears to indicate the function.
- *Formatting Tool Bar*—Appears below the standard Tool Bar and displays examples to indicate functions such as setting the font size, italicizing words, underlining words, and aligning words, titles, or paragraphs.

If the desired Tool Bar does not appear on the screen, perform the following steps:

1. Click View on the Menu Bar.
2. Use the mouse arrow to highlight Toolbars. A submenu appears.
3. If a check mark (✓) does not appear next to Standard and/or Formatting, click on the word; the check mark will appear next to the word and the toolbar will appear at the top of the screen.

MENU BAR

As indicated by the name, different menus are accessible to perform various functions. Some of these functions are duplicated between the Menu Bar and the Standard Tool Bar.

- *File*—Lists many functions that may also be performed using the Standard Tool Bar including Open, Close, Print Preview, and Print.
- *Edit*—Cut/Copy/Paste functions are found in this menu.
- *View*—Provides options to display various Tool Bars, including the Ruler.
- *Insert*—Two important functions on this menu are Page Numbers and Footnote. Footnotes are especially important for documenting sources without interrupting the flow of the text.
- *Format*—Functions in this menu include changing the spacing in a document and creating a hanging indent. Number and bullet functions create hanging indents automatically.
- *Tools*—The most important function in this menu is Options, which allows the user to change various aspects of how the program functions.
- *Other Menu Bar functions*—The Table menu facilitates the creating and editing of tables within documents. The Window menu allows the user to switch between documents or split the screen to view two documents at once. The Help menu is similar to the one in the Start menu, but is customized for the particular program open at the time (e.g., the word processing program).

STANDARD TOOL BAR

The following options from the tool bar are only available when a word document is open:

- *Creating a Document*—Each time the user opens the word processing program a new document (clean sheet of paper) is automatically created. Click on the white paper icon to manually create a new document.
- *Opening a Document*—To locate and open a previously saved document (the Save function is discussed next), click on the yellow folder icon, then select the desired document from the window that appears and click on the document title to open it.
- *Saving a Document*—While typing a document, the user must frequently save the work, so that entered information is not lost in case of a power outage or computer malfunction. Additionally, a document must be saved prior to closure. Use the File command on the Menu Bar and click on Save on the submenu. The operating system automatically stores saved files in the "My Documents" folder on the hard drive (C drive). When saving a file from e-mail, the user may have to tell the computer where to save the file. To change the location of the file being saved, use the File command on the Menu Bar then choose the Save As option to display the options.

Use the down arrow in the window to reveal a submenu.

- *Printing a Document*—Click on the icon that represents a printer. To print part of a document or change the print parameters, use the File command in the Menu Bar and click on Print in the submenu. Another menu with various options will appear.
- *Previewing a Document*—The Print Preview function is used to see how each page of a document will look before printing it. Click on the icon that resembles a sheet of paper with a magnifying glass or use the Print Preview command found in the File menu.
- *Spell Checker*—This function is used to search for spelling, grammatical, and sentence structure errors. Activate the Spell Checker function by clicking on the icon that displays the letters ABC followed by a check mark. Be aware that the Spell Checker may not catch a word that is spelled correctly, but is not the correct word (e.g., *patience* instead of *patients*). Always proofread the document for these kinds of errors.
- *Cutting/Copying/Pasting*—This feature provides the ability to move words, sentences, or whole portions of a document to another place within the document. In addition, the user can repeat a phrase instead of having to retype it or move it using the cutting/copying/pasting functions. To select the text to be copied, depress the left mouse button and drag the cursor over the text to highlight the area of text to be moved. Then click the right mouse button to display the menu options. Click on the desired function. Position the cursor in the new location where the text should be displayed and again click the right mouse button to display the options. Click on the desired function.
- *Correcting a Mistake*—Use the Undo icon (backwards arrow) after making a mistake and the computer will "undo" the user's most recent action. To use this function, the user must recognize the mistake immediately after making it (for instance, deleting an entire sentence instead of one word).

The Redo icon (clockwise arrow) will "redo" the user's most recent action. For example, type "hhhh;" click the Undo icon and the h's disappear. To bring the h's back, click the Redo icon.

FORMATTING TOOL BAR

Some of the basic functions found in the Formatting Tool Bar are as follows:

- *Bold*—Darkens the character for emphasis.
- *Italics and underlining*—Also used for emphasis. Click on *I* to italicize or U to underline selected text.
- *Fonts*—Refers to the style of lettering. Click on the arrow next to the **font** to display the options and make a selection.
- *Font size*—Refers to the size of the letters. Click on the arrow next to the font size to display the options and make a selection.
- *Font color*—Used to change the font color (black is automatically selected). This option is located to the right on the Formatting Tool Bar—it appears as an A with a black (or the color selected) bar underneath.
- *Center/align*—Commands for text alignment are located in the section of the Formatting Tool Bar to the right of the U command. Text or images may be aligned to the left, centered, aligned to the right, or set to fill the width of the document.
- *Numbering and bullets*—Used to number sequential items or emphasize items in a list. A numbered list may be manually or automatically created by the word processing program. The steps for automatically creating a numbered list follows:
  1. Type the number one (1) followed by a period (.) and then a space. Type in the word *student* and press Enter.
  2. The number 2 automatically appears. Type another word and press Enter.
  3. Now the number 3 appears. Continue as needed.

GRAPHICS

Two methods are used to import graphics (e.g., photographs or drawings) into a Word document: importing clip art or importing images from the Internet.

IMPORT FILES FROM CLIP ART

Typically, a graphics program is included with the purchase and installation of Microsoft Office®. The clip art provided with the Office program features all sorts of drawings categorized according to subject areas. The Copy/Paste function is used to move graphics from one program to another. The size and location of the graphic can easily be manipulated. Left click on the imported graphic to display several small squares around the perimeter of the picture. To change the length, width, and diagonal size of the picture, double-click on the picture. A menu box will appear that will allow the user to change its size or wrap text around the picture.

To move the picture around on the screen, place the cursor over the picture. The cursor will change to two criss-crossed arrows. Depress the left button of the mouse, move the arrows and the picture will move. Release the mouse button and the picture is now placed in a different location.

IMPORTING IMAGES FROM THE INTERNET

Photographs and drawings can be imported into a document from the Internet in the same manner described for clip art. Be aware, however, that material placed on the Internet, in particular documents and photographs, are often copyrighted. Unless a website specifically states that copying is permitted, it is always advisable to write the author, photographer, or artists for permission to use their article or image.

INTERNET BASICS

Just as a single computer in a hospital is one of many computers connected via cables to the same server creating a network, the Internet is a gigantic international network connected via millions of servers (including providers for thousands of individual computers). E-mail began as a form of communication on the Internet. Now, much e-mail exchange is done through World Wide Web-based software.

The World Wide Web is an easy-to-navigate, user-friendly format for browsing Internet pages. Unlike the Internet, the web features computer graphics, text formatting, and even some programming functions that make a logo flash or a word spin. Each photo or article stored on the web has a different address where the information is stored. These addresses usually start with *http://* and usually contain the letters *www*. (*Note:* Many Internet software programs no longer require the user to type in the *http://* part of the address.) The address ending typically tells the user what type of organization owns the information. Addresses ending in *.com* are corporations, those ending in *.org* are nonprofit organizations, and those ending in *.gov* are governmental agencies. For example, the web address for the Association of Surgical Technologists is *http://www.ast.org*. Addresses ending in *.edu* typically signify educational institutions. E-mail addresses are similar to Internet addresses and are discussed later in this chapter.

ACCESSING THE INTERNET

To access the Internet, users must set up an account with an Internet service provider (ISP) directly or through their school or library. There are many Internet providers, local and national. Some national Internet providers include AT&T, AOL, Earthlink, and Microsoft. Each requires the user's computer to contain Internet browser software, such as Microsoft Explorer® or Netscape Navigator®. This section describes Internet access using Microsoft Explorer.

The home page appears on the screen whenever the user accesses the Internet. Additionally, the user can always click on the icon that looks like a house with the word "Home" underneath to return to the designated home page.

The phrase *surfing the Internet* refers to looking at many different web pages and jumping from one to another. This is similar to browsing through a magazine; therefore, software for accessing the web is often referred to as a *browser*. Surfing or browsing is made possible using *hyperlinks*—the bold or underlined words on a particular web page. Clicking on one of these words (sometimes an icon) immediately takes the user to a different page. Notice that when a mouse points to a link, the arrow changes to a hand with the index finger pointing to the item.

Favorites and History Features

Several methods are available to archive website addresses for easy referencing, such as the Favorites and History features. The Favorites feature stores addresses permanently for easy access. The History feature displays sites that have been accessed within the period of time selected.

Forward and Back Buttons

To move back and forth among pages of a website, use the Back and Forward Buttons in the Standard Tool Bar. After surfing through several websites, the user can return to previously viewed pages by clicking these buttons. These buttons only access very recently viewed websites. If the user closes the Internet for any reason, these buttons lose the stored memory of recent pages. In this case, the user can access the History function to return to a particular page.

INTERNET RESEARCH

The World Wide Web contains so much information that the user would quickly be frustrated if he or she could not search for a specific topic. Research is conducted by means of a *search engine* (the user's Internet browser always contains a Search function with instant access to one of these engines). Some of the more popular search engines are Google, Alta Vista, and Yahoo.

The biggest challenge to doing research on the web is helping the search engine understand what exactly to look for. It takes the word or phrase you type in and finds any links associated with the subject. Consequently, many items will be useless for research purposes, since the link may lead to an advertisement or an unrelated article. As a rule of thumb, the first 20 to 30 articles listed pertain directly to the subject area.

When performing a search, keep the subject to one word or a short and succinct phrase. More words result in a larger search and leads to many unrelated articles and documents being listed. Use quotation marks around the phrase to tell the search engine to search only for those exact words. For instance, a search for "laparoscopic cholecystectomy" would produce a listing of web pages that contain those exact words.

USING E-MAIL

Individuals who communicate by e-mail are assigned an e-mail address similar to a home street address. The e-mail address always employs the symbol @ within the address. The first portion of the address is usually personalized by the user and the last portion indicates the Internet/e-mail provider, for example, johndoe@msn.com or janedoe@aol.com (msn represents Microsoft Network; AOL denotes America On-Line).

Internet providers often include an e-mail software program. Other types of e-mail programs are also available via certain websites. These include Hotmail, Yahoo, and Juno. The Microsoft Outlook® e-mail program is used in the following examples.

Several functions can be performed within the e-mail program including saving the message and replying to, forwarding, printing, or deleting it.

- *Saving*—To save the message, use the File function as previously described for saving other types of files.
- *Replying*—To reply to the sender, simply click on Reply in the Standard Tool Bar, type your reply, and click Send in the Standard Tool Bar.
- *Forwarding*—To send a particular message to others, click Forward on the Standard Tool Bar. The cursor will appear in the To line. This allows the user to input the e-mail addresses of the individual(s) who should receive copies of the e-mail.
- *Carbon Copy (cc)*—The term *carbon copy* is from the days of manual typewriters. It indicates to the persons being copied that they do not need to reply, but they should read the message. The appropriate address is typed in the cc box.
- *Printing*—To print the message, use the Print icon as previously described.
- *Deleting*—To delete an e-mail click the X in the Standard Tool Bar with the message open. The message is sent to the Delete box and the next new message is automatically opened. Alternatively, close the message by clicking the X in the upper right-hand corner of the screen. Click once to highlight the message, and then click the X in the Standard Tool Bar.
- *Address Book*—Used to avoid typing the same addresses repeatedly. The address is entered into the Address Book and can then be accessed automatically for all future use.

ELECTRICITY

Physicians have long recognized the benefits of using heat on wounds, with electrocautery, which utilizes a heated wire in direct contact with tissue, eventually being developed to accelerate blood clotting. In the 1920s, the physicist W. T. Bovie developed the first spark-gap tube generator, which culminated in the electrosurgical generator now commonly used in surgery to coagulate or cut tissue. Although the electrosurgical unit (ESU) is completely different from the original machine developed by Bovie, many facilities still refer to the ESU as the *Bovie*.

To ensure patient safety, it is crucial to study the basic terminology and principles of electricity and examine its applications as they relate to the OR. Ultimately, the surgical technologists of the future must be comfortable with theories relating to electricity and its usage. Medicine in the 21st century will increasingly be electronic and, in many cases, robotic.

SURGICAL APPLICATIONS

Electricity is employed in numerous ways in the OR environment. The following examples represent just a few applications encountered while working in the OR.

ELECTROSURGICAL UNIT

The electrosurgical unit generates current that is used to cut or coagulate tissue. Current flows from a generator to a device (**active electrode**) that delivers electric current to the surgical site through the patient or tissue and is channeled back to the generator via the **dispersive** (**inactive**) **electrode** (also referred to as a grounding pad). Several types of ESUs are available and are employed in many surgical specialties.

X-RAY MACHINE

The X-ray machine utilizes electromagnetic radiation to view internal structures. In the OR, X-rays are used to determine the presence of abnormalities and foreign bodies, to locate retained sponges or sharps, to verify the presence of fluid or air, to confirm correct location of the surgical site, to assist in bone realignment, to aid in prosthesis placement, and to identify the placement of catheters, tubes, and drains.

ENDOSCOPES

An endoscope is a viewing instrument that is used for diagnosis, biopsy, visualization, repair, retrieval of an object, and hemorrhage control in a hollow structure, such as the abdomen, thorax, heart, ureters, and ventricles of the brain. Endoscopes may be flexible or rigid, are frequently attached to a camera and light cord to produce images on a video monitor, and are used in conjunction with an ESU for coagulation and dissection or paired with a laser for better coagulation and treatment of tumors.

LASERS

Initially used in the OR in 1960, the laser is now utilized in almost all surgical specialties and its technology is based on the conversion of some type of energy into a form of light energy. Surgeons choose the type of laser beam based on several factors, including power, wavelength, color, duration of exposure, and type of tissue. Lasers are classified by the type of active media and are categorized as gas, solid, liquid, or semiconductor crystals.

ROBOTICS

Robotics seeks to extend and enhance human capabilities by using powerful computers and robots. Traditional surgery will soon be replaced by the "intelligent OR." Surgical technologists will be encountering the robotic arm, the voice-activation control system, and the remote surgical manipulator. Robotics is discussed in more detail later in this chapter.

BASIC PRINCIPLES OF ELECTRICITY

The principles that govern the behavior of tiny particles known as **electrons** are called the *electron theory,* which helps to explain electricity and serves as the basis for design of all electrical equipment.

ATOMS, ELECTRONS, AND MATTER

Matter is anything that has mass and occupies space. All matter consists of atoms and all atoms are composed of small particles: protons, electrons, and neutrons. The center of the atom is called the *nucleus* and contains **protons**, positively charged electric particles, and **neutrons**, neutral particles. Electrons are negatively charged particles that travel in concentric paths or orbits around the nucleus.

Electrons revolve around the nucleus in paths called *shells* or *orbits.* Electrons located closer to the nucleus demonstrate a stronger attraction to the nucleus; whereas, electrons moving in the outer orbits are less attracted. In certain atoms, if these outer electrons are exposed to light, heat, or electric energy, they will speed up and leave the atom. These outer electrons are referred to as **free electrons**, and it this movement of free electrons that creates electric current. The term *electricity* describes the free electrons moving or flowing from the ring of one atom to another. This principle of electricity is based on Bohr's theory.

Materials that allow the flow of free electrons are called *conductors.* Examples of conductors are silver, copper, aluminum, zinc, brass, iron, saltwater, carbon, and some acids. Copper is the most commonly used conductor because it is the most economical. Examples of devices that use copper wire as a conductor in the OR include surgical lamps, electrosurgical units, and power drills.

INSULATORS

Materials that inhibit the flow of electrons are called **insulators**. Insulators are simply poor conductors. Conductors, such as copper and other metals, are wrapped with an insulating material that does not conduct electricity in order to prevent leakage of electrons while the current flows to the device that will use it. Examples of insulators in the OR are the rubber and plastic casings around the cords of the ESU or X-ray machine.

Because water is a conductor of electricity, the amount of humidity in the air within an environment is important to consider. High humidity often results in static charge leakage and low humidity results in the formation of sparks; therefore, humidity in the OR should be maintained between 50% and 55%, but not less than 45%.

ELECTRICAL CHARGE

Electrical charges can be either negative or positive and are simply defined as too many or too few electrons on an atom respectively. One important rule to remember is the law of electric charges: Like charges repel each other; unlike charges attract each other. In other words, two negative charges (materials that have more electrons than protons) or two positive charges (substances that have more protons than electrons) will repel each other. Conversely, unlike charges are attracted to each other. Just remember: opposites attract!

ELECTRICAL CURRENT

Electric current is movement of the electrical charge (Figure 6-3). For example, a light bulb illuminates because the electrons move through the conductor and the tungsten filament in the bulb. The filament heats up and brightens. The electrical current travels through conductors by movement of the free electrons that migrate from atom to atom inside the conductor.

MAGNETISM AND ELECTRICITY

Electricity and magnetic fields share an important relationship. Today, generators depend on this relationship to produce most of our electricity. Other methods of producing electricity include heat, gas, solar, photoelectric, and thermocouples.

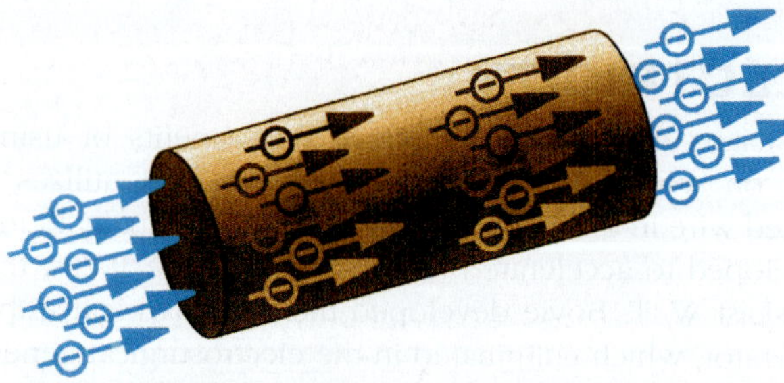

Figure 6-3 Electrical current *(Copyright © 2002* Technological Sciences for the Operating Room, *Association of Surgical Technologists)*

Magnetic Fields

In all atoms, electrons create a magnetic field or electric charge as they orbit the nucleus. In most substances, the effect is neutral since electrons are traveling in different directions. However, in some materials, they line up in the same direction and their magnetic fields are combined and strengthened. Naturally, occurring magnetic substances include iron, nickel, and cobalt. Even the earth is one super-size magnet.

Like the earth, magnets have two ends or poles. The north pole of a magnet is located at the end that would point north if the magnet could swing freely. The opposite end is the south pole. A magnetic field is the lines of magnetic force that flow between the north and south poles on a magnet. If two like poles are placed together (north to north), the magnetic force will push the two apart. Conversely, if two unlike poles are placed near each other, the two would move quickly together. Remember, opposites attract!

The magnetic field also causes metallic objects, such as paperclips, to be attracted to the magnet or to follow the magnet when it is moved in a certain direction. Another familiar item is the needle in a compass that rotates to align with the magnetic north of the earth.

Two principles are briefly discussed that have important applications in the OR: (1) Magnetism can generate an electric current and (2) electricity is used to generate magnetism.

Electromagnets

Electromagnets are metals that become magnetic when a conductor, such as copper wire, is wrapped around it. Current flowing through the wire creates a magnetic field in the metal. A magnetic field can also create electricity. Remember, electricity does not produce power; it is only the means for transporting it. The interaction between the wires and magnets is what produces the power. An example is a rotating magnet that creates an electrical current in a wire conductor. This is how a power plant works. In a coal- or oil-powered hydroelectric plant, water from a dam or waterfall is heated to form steam that is used to turn the turbines. Turbines are simply generators—devices that convert mechanical energy (from steam or water) to electric energy. The turbines rapidly spin magnets that create the electricity used by hospitals and clinics, businesses, and homes.

VOLTS

The term *volt* defines electrical potential. Voltage is the potential energy of electrons (or the electric charge) at any given time between two points. An electric system uses a battery or generator to create a force or voltage to move the electricity from one point to another. The path that electricity travels from the energy source to a device and then back to the energy source is defined as a **circuit**. A simple electrical circuit is comprised of a source of **power**, conductor, **load**, and **switch**.

CURRENT

Current is measured in amperes (amps). *Current* is the flow of electric charge or the rate of flow of electrons. For example, a single strand of copper wire is laid on a table: One end of the wire is negative, and the other is positive. All free electrons in the wire will be attracted to the positive end and consequently flow in the same direction. Free electrons will always be attracted from a point of excess electrons to a point that lacks them.

OHM'S LAW

The scientific law that pertains to electricity is called *Ohm's law*. Ohm's law is a mathematical equation that shows the relationship between voltage, current (amps), and **resistance**. Resistance refers to restricting the flow of the current and is measured in ohms. Ohm's law states that more voltage will produce more current if resistance remains constant, but higher resistance will cause the current to decrease if the voltage remains constant. A battery generates a force or voltage to move the electrons (current). Current flows from a power supply and equals the voltage divided by the resistance. Ohm's law represents the rate of flow of electrons, and voltage represents the electric charge or potential between two points. Mathematically, this relationship is represented by the following equation:

Ohm's law: $V = I \times R$,

where V = voltage, I = amps (current), and R = resistance.

POWER, LOAD, AND SWITCH

Power is defined as "the rate at which work is done, expressed as the amount of work per unit time." Remember that current is the flow of electric charge and voltage is the electrical charge (potential) between two points. The product of voltage and current is power or

$$P \text{ (power)} = I \text{ (amps or current)} \times V \text{ (voltage)}$$

Power is measured in watts (W), and to facilitate usage, watts are converted to kilowatts (kW). One kilowatt equals 1,000 watts. If a DC (direct current) circuit is 12V and 20 amps, the power is calculated as follows:

$$\begin{aligned} P &= 20 \times 12 \\ &= 240 \text{ W} \\ &= 0.24 \text{ kW} \end{aligned}$$

In a simple electrical circuit, the device that transforms the electrical energy into a useful function, such as heat or light, is the load. The load is the device that uses the electricity to perform some type of function. The load can also change the amount of energy that is delivered from the power source. Examples of loads are surgical lamps, electrosurgical units, surgical power drills, surgical robots, and video monitors.

Surgical lamps are resistive energy loads. The conductor material, such as the filament in a light bulb, has a high resistance to the flow of electricity. The electricity has to force its way through the resistance and the energy causes the conductor to glow or heat up. When the load increases or decreases, the power source is delivering more or less power.

A switch is the device used to open or close a circuit and controls the flow of electricity. Examples in the OR include switches for the surgical lights, operating table, endoscopic camera, and computer monitor.

A flashlight is another common example of a simple electrical circuit (Figure 6-4). The source of power for the flashlight is the batteries. Wires (conductors) are connected to the battery, which is connected to a switch activated by the user. The bulb at the end of the flashlight is the load. The bulb must have voltage in order to work. The voltage is carried by the conductor, and the switch controls the flow of the current to the load. When the switch is "open," there is no flow and the flashlight is not on. When the switch is "closed," the flashlight is on.

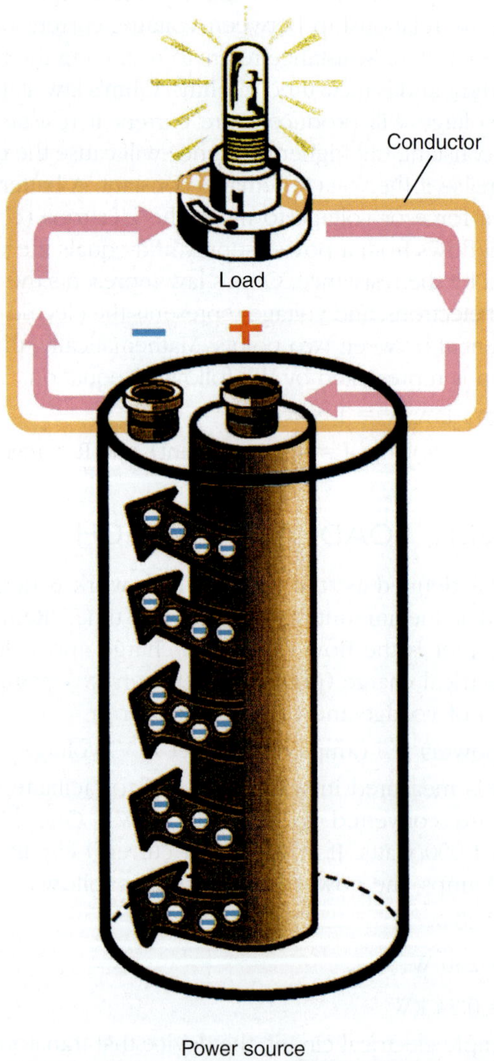

Figure 6-4 **Electrical circuit** ***(Copyright © 2002*** **Technological Sciences for the Operating Room,** ***Association of Surgical Technologists)***

When a surgical lamp burns out, the resistance to the current flow will increase and prevent the flow of current. When the voltage remains constant, resistance increases, and the watts decrease. When the current ceases, the bulb is not lit.

HOT WIRE, NEUTRAL WIRE, AND GROUND WIRE

In a simple electrical circuit, the wire that connects to the switch is the *hot wire*. The second wire, called the *neutral wire,* serves as the pathway for the electrons to return to the energy source, and it completes the circuit. The **ground wire** is a separate wire that safely conveys any leaking electrons to the ground and prevents injury to the patient and personnel. A ground wire is essential for prevention of electric shock.

WALL OUTLETS

In the OR, wall outlets are usually 110V, excluding the outlet for the mobile X-ray unit, which is 220V. Plugs used in surgery have three prongs. Components of the three-prong plug are

- First prong (positive)
- Second prong (negative)
- Third prong (ground)

If an electrical short occurs, the electrical current will flow through the grounded plug, reducing the risk of current passing through the surgical team or the patient.

RESISTORS

Insulators provide resistance to current flow. However, every material has some degree of resistance to the flow of electrons. Devices that are made of materials chosen for their resistance properties are known as resistors and designated with the letter "R."

DIRECT CURRENT AND ALTERNATING CURRENT

There are two types of electrical systems: direct current (DC) and alternating current (AC). Direct current (DC) indicates electrical current that flows in one direction from the negative pole to the positive pole. Batteries are a common example of DC current. Batteries have a negative (−) terminal and a positive (+) terminal. When the switch is closed, current flows from one terminal to the other. Current ceases when the switch is open.

The four components of a DC circuit are:

- Source of electricity (e.g., battery)
- Conductor (e.g., wire from source to load)
- Control device (e.g., switch)
- Load (e.g., bulb, heater, or other load)

Alternating current (AC) describes the flow of current that reverses direction periodically. A complete AC cycle occurs when current moves in one direction and then reverses its course. The cycle represents one AC cycle called a hertz (Hz). The number of cycles per second is called *frequency* and is indicated by the symbol *f*. The most commonly used power in the United States is 60 cycle AC, meaning there are 60 AC cycles per second. Typical home voltage in the United States is 110V or 120V.

Alternating current is characterized by its ability to change the voltage. AC can be delivered at a high voltage and then "stepped down" (reduced) to a lower voltage at the point of use. Consequently, smaller conductors can be used so that the cost of delivering power is lower.

Transformers are devices that step down or step up (increase) the exiting voltage and only work with alternating current. Power lines are a common example. Utility companies deliver electricity through power lines at a very high voltage. However, before the voltage can be safely used by a hospital, it must be reduced or stepped down to a lower voltage.

RADIO FREQUENCY

All radio and television signals are electromagnetic waves, which are discussed in detail in the physics section. However, for now, an important concept to remember is that the number of wave cycles (remember, one cycle is called a hertz) per second is called frequency.

The radio or TV transmitter output is connected to the antenna system located at a distance from the transmitter. The energy travels through a transmission line from the transmitter to the antenna. Transmission lines can be cables, hollow tubes called waveguides, or parallel-wire transmission lines that are similar to the cable used for consumer TV receiving antennas. The spectrum of the radio frequency (RF) begins at 9 kHz or less and increases to more than 3 GHz. Depending on the frequency, the waves travel through the atmosphere or space in varying ways.

ISOLATED CIRCUIT

One of the least understood concepts in electricity is protection against electric shock from an isolated or floating circuit. The energy source, or AC **generator**, is grounded. The secondary circuit contains hazardous current due to the isolated circuit. The secondary circuit is isolated from other circuits by the transformer insulation. However, if a person touches both poles of the isolated circuit in the area where insulation is absent, current will flow through the body to the ground, producing an electrical shock or burn.

Two simple methods are used to prevent shocks from isolated circuits. In the first, a person is prevented from access to all parts of the circuit by the placement of a barrier of basic insulation, usually solid insulation. The second method involves a conductive barrier of insulation between the isolated circuit and conductive barrier that prevents access to all parts of the circuit. The conductive barrier does not require grounding.

ELECTROSURGERY

One of the occupational hazards of working in the OR is electrical burn or shock during electrosurgery. The surgeon or surgical technologist who experiences a shock or burn usually attributes it to a hole in the surgical glove. However, other causes exist for shocks and burns during electrosurgery.

As mentioned earlier, electrosurgery is the application of electrical current through tissue to coagulate or cut tissue. The electrosurgical generator is the device that provides the power for electric current to travel to the tissue. Components of the electrosurgical unit include the generator, optional foot pedal, cords, an active electrode, and a dispersive (inactive) electrode.

ESU Circuit

The circuit of the ESU consists of

- Generator (power source)
- Active electrode (electrosurgical pencil)
- Patient
- Dispersive (inactive) electrode (also called a *grounding pad*)

Current flows from the generator through a conductor cord to the active electrode. The active electrode channels the flow of current to the surgical site. When the electrical current passes through the active electrode, the concentrated energy is converted into thermal energy (heat) that is used to desiccate (dry out) the tissue or provide hemostasis. Results at the surgical site are dependent on the size of the active electrode, amps, and duration for which the ESU is activated.

Monopolar and Bipolar Electrosurgical Units. Electrosurgical units fall into two main categories: *monopolar* (or unipolar) and *bipolar*. A surgeon will utilize bipolar electrosurgery for very delicate procedures, at sites where moisture is nearby or to prevent nerve damage. Monopolar electrosurgery is chosen when large surgical areas are involved.

In bipolar units, the active and inactive electrodes are the tips of a two-prong forceps. Current travels from one tip, passes through the tissue grasped by the forceps and disperses to the other tip. No dispersive electrode (ground pad) is required.

In monopolar units, current travels from the generator to the active electrode. The tip of the active electrode is applied to the tissue, generating heat. Current passes from the surgical site, through the patient, to the inactive electrode back to the generator through a cord (Figure 6-5). The inactive electrode is usually a grounding pad or plate that is in direct contact with the patient's skin.

It is critical that the dispersive electrode be properly placed to avoid electrical burn to the patient. The grounding pad must be completely in contact with the designated area of the patient's skin. If the pad is pulled up and part of the skin is not in contact, burns can result due to the inability of the heat to disperse over the entire pad.

Electrical Shock and Burn. One of the dangers with electrosurgery is electrical burn. These burns may be very deep, causing extensive tissue necrosis and deep thrombosis. Often, debridement may be necessary. In addition to the patient, surgical team members may be at risk. Possible causes for shock or burn are RF capacitive coupling and high-voltage dielectric breakdown.

RF capacitive coupling occurs when alternating current travels from the active electrode, across intact insulation, and into the skin. For example, a surgeon clamps a Crile hemostat onto a bleeding vessel. While holding the Crile, the surgeon's skin and metal Crile hemostat act like two conductors. During electrosurgery, the alternating current travels down the hemostat from the active electrode. The surgeon's rubber glove normally functions as the insulator. However, if the glove is composed of thin rubber, current can possibly travel from the Crile to the surgeon's skin.

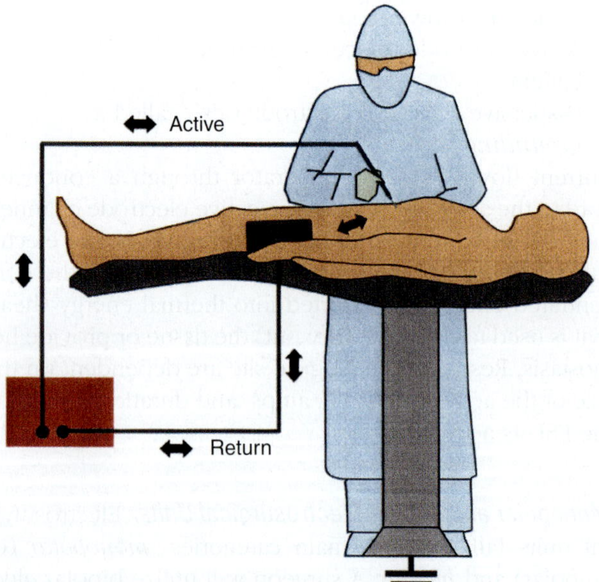

Figure 6-5 Monopolar electrosurgery ***(Copyright © 2000, 2001, 2002, 2003 Valleylab, a division of Tyco Healthcare Group LP: Principles of Electrosurgery, Boulder, CO. All rights reserved.)***

Dielectric breakdown occurs when high voltage breaks down some insulating material, such as sterile gloves. During electrosurgery, it may result when the material in the gloves is unable to withstand the leakage of current generated by the ESU. A high voltage can produce a hole in the glove and consequently the surgeon will sustain a burn. The size of the active electrode, duration of activation, and amps are contributing factors that will influence the outcome.

Hazards of Vaporized Tissue Plume. Certain surgical procedures involving electrosurgery, lasers, and power drills can produce a potentially dangerous plume of vaporized tissue. Research has found the plume to contain hazardous ingredients such as carcinogens, blood-borne pathogens, and mutagens.

To minimize exposure to vaporized tissue plume, use of a smoke evacuator is recommended. The tip of the evacuator is positioned as close as possible to the surgical site to allow maximum removal of the plume.

PHYSICS

Why should the surgical technologist study basic physics? Principles of physics are observed in virtually all aspects of the OR: needles, endoscopes, microscopes, lasers, washer-sterilizers, autoclaves, electrosurgical units. It is no longer adequate for the surgical technologist simply to have the ability to turn this sophisticated equipment on and off. The basic concepts for design of OR equipment must be understood according to the principles of physics that provide the foundation for them. As the OR evolves to include advanced computer systems and robotics, surgical technologists will also evolve into technical experts who understand these complex systems well enough to prepare, operate, and troubleshoot them. The first step to understanding these complex systems is to understand basic physics.

MEDICAL AND SURGICAL APPLICATIONS

Physicists have been enhancing the practice of medicine for the past 100 years through the development of complex measuring machines and surgical devices. Although this section deals with basic physics as it is applied to surgical equipment, the student should also know that the human body can also be better understood through the study of physics. The human body is a physical object that can be measured just like any other physical object. Many basic physical principles that are applied to machinery—such as principles of light, sound, waves, mechanics, energy, and heat—can also be applied to the motions and perceptions of the human body.

MEDICAL (DIAGNOSTIC) APPLICATIONS

Physicians requested noninvasive methods for observing and measuring internal structures, and physicists responded. Wilhelm Conrad Röntgen discovered X-rays (and Thomas Edison further developed the technology) to peer inside the human body without changing its physical structure. Electrocardiograms were developed to study the electrical activity of the heart, and electroencephalograms were later devised to study the electrical activity of the brain.

Computerized axial tomography (CAT) and ultrasound were invented as noninvasive diagnostic methods that allowed even greater access to details of the body's inner tissues than X-ray. Magnetic resonance imaging (MRI) and positron emission tomography (PET) technology soon followed. While CAT scans employ X-rays for imaging, the MRI uses radio frequencies to excite the protons in tissue. Once these protons return to a state of equilibrium, they emit energy as an RF signal that can be analyzed as an image. By varying the sequence of the RF pulse as it is applied and collected, radiologists can create different types of images.

Ultrasound imaging is a noninvasive diagnostic tool that transforms sound waves into images. The basic requirements for ultrasound imaging are an ultrasound source, a medium (e.g., tissue) that will reflect or scatter the source signal, and a detector. The image created is a result of acoustic reflectivity of the tissue at various locations in space. These "echoes" from the tissue are reconstructed to provide an ultrasound image.

PET is a medical imaging technique that reveals dynamic activities within the body, such as blood flow and glucose uptake in tissues. In preparation for a PET, the patient ingests a radiopharmaceutical agent that emits a positively charged electron called a *positron* (a form of antimatter). When the positron meets a normal electron, the two annihilate each other, emitting a pair of gamma rays in opposite directions. A circle of detectors pinpoints the location of each annihilation event and creates a colored image that indicates levels of activity.

SURGICAL APPLICATIONS

Minimally invasive surgical techniques significantly reduce time spent under anesthesia and recovery time for patients. The implanted pacemaker and defibrillator are used to overcome electrical conduction problems of the heart. Implantable devices are used to replace or augment defective or failing organs within the body. Lasers and surgical robots are increasingly used in the OR to provide greater surgical precision. Telesurgery, the use of robots to perform surgical procedures from a distance, is poised to become the next important surgical application. Advances in fiber optic technology have enabled the use of smaller, more precise flexible scopes for peering into the body to diagnose and treat disease. High-intensity sound waves (ultrasound) will soon be used as a noninvasive method for treating certain brain tumors and will also be used to treat internal bleeding at accident scenes and on battlefields. Gamma knife radiosurgery has allowed surgeons to destroy small, deep brain tumors, and vascular malformations without affecting healthy brain tissue.

MECHANICS

Mechanics is the study of objects in motion and is normally limited to the study of a small number of rather large, slow objects. We discuss classical mechanics in this section, specifically *dynamics* (the study of motion and the forces that cause it) and *kinematics* (the study of objects in motion without much concern for the forces that produced the motion).

SPEED

Speed simply describes how fast something is moving without consideration of the object's direction. An instrument designed to measure speed also describes motion (100 miles per hour). But the instrument will not describe the direction in which the object is traveling, an important distinction.

Average speed is the distance that is traveled by an object divided by the time it took to actually travel that distance; therefore,

$$\textit{Average speed} = \frac{\textit{Distance traveled}}{\textit{Time taken to travel that distance}}$$

VELOCITY

Whereas speed is not dependent on direction, *velocity* involves both direction and speed. To solve a problem related to an object's velocity, the object's speed as well as its direction must be known. For velocity to be constant, an object's speed and its direction must not change. Velocity is expressed as

$$v = d/t$$

ACCELERATION

Acceleration is defined as the change in velocity over time. In physics terms, acceleration involves any change in velocity—changing direction, speeding up, or slowing down.

PROJECTILE AND SATELLITE MOTION

Projectile motion refers to the motion of an object launched into the air at an angle, such as when a football is kicked or a baseball is thrown. In fact, any object thrown at an arbitrary angle relative to the horizontal is considered a projectile.

Without air resistance, a projectile is launched vertically and is brought back to the launching level in an accelerated motion. The vertical motion controls the time the object will remain aloft. The horizontal motion (range) is a constant motion laterally from the point that it was launched.

An orbiting earth satellite is considered a projectile because gravity acts on the object after it is launched and accelerates it toward Earth, preventing it from moving in a straight-line trajectory into space. A satellite does indeed fall toward the earth, but never completes the fall because of the curvature of the earth. The projectile's trajectory will match the planet's curvature and will fall "around" the earth, accelerating toward it under gravity's influence but never crashing into it.

NEWTON'S LAWS OF MOTION

Isaac Newton's three laws of motion are the basis for what is referred to as classical mechanics, or Newtonian mechanics. The three laws are as follows:

> **Law 1**: An object that is at rest will remain at rest unless a total force is exerted on it. All objects will remain at rest or in uniform motion unless acted on by some outside force.

This law expresses the physical concept of **inertia**. Inertia is a property of matter that causes matter to resist change in motion. **Mass** is the measure of the amount of inertia an object possesses.

The first part of this law states simply that an object will not move unless an outside force acts on it in some way. The second part of the law states that an object moving at a constant velocity will continue to move at a constant speed and in a straight line unless a force acts on the object (Figure 6-6).

> **Law 2**: An object's acceleration is in the same direction as the force exerted on it.

This law basically states that an external force causes an object to accelerate. Objects move in straight lines and at constant speeds unless a force acts on them, causing them to change velocity. For an object to accelerate at a specific rate, the amount of force applied depends on the mass of the object. In other words, if the mass of the object to be moved is twice that of another object, then twice the force is required to achieve the same rate of acceleration.

Mathematically, the relationship between force, mass, and acceleration in Newton's second law of motion can be expressed by the following formula:

$$a = F/m$$

where a = acceleration, F = force, and m = mass.

> **Law 3**: For every action there is an equal and opposite reaction.

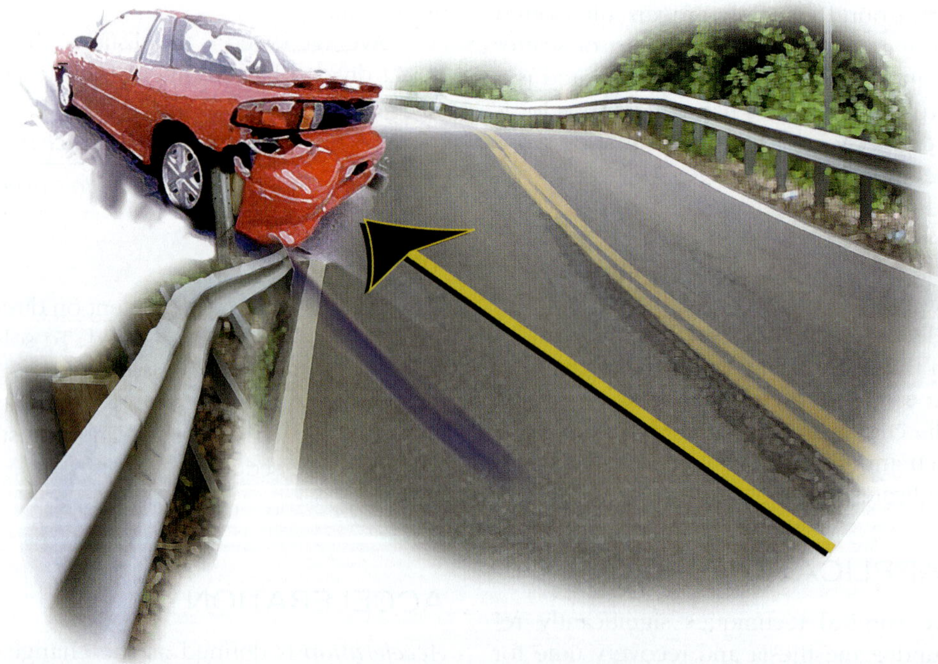

Figure 6-6 **Newton's first law of motion: an object moving at a constant velocity will move in a straight line** ***(Copyright © 2002 Technological Sciences for the Operating Room, Association of Surgical Technologists)***

Newton's third law, also known as the *law of conservation of momentum,* states that whenever a force is exerted, an equal and opposite force arises in reaction.

MOMENTUM

Since Newton's third law states that for each action, there is an equal and opposite reaction, then it is not possible to exert a force on an object without exerting a force on another object in the opposite direction. A cannon recoils (rolls backward) when it propels a cannonball, and a ship moves forward because its propeller throws water away from the ship.

Newton defined the *momentum* of a body as mass multiplied by linear velocity:

$$M = mv$$

where M = momentum, m = mass, and v = velocity. Momentum is, in essence, the propulsive force of a body.

A rocket is propelled upward by discharging burning gases downward from its engine. The velocity of this gas creates a forward momentum for the rocket that is equal to the backward momentum of the discharged gases. Therefore, the momentum of the rocket (M) is equal to the mass of the discharged gases (m) times the velocity of the gases (v).

The law of conservation of momentum states that in an isolated system the total momentum before any event is equal to the total momentum after the event. Before a cannon fires a cannonball, both the cannon and the cannonball are at rest, so their total momentum is zero. After the cannon fires, the cannonball gains momentum (mass of the cannonball times its velocity). If momentum is to be conserved, something must gain momentum in the opposite direction of the cannonball's forward direction. The recoil of the cannon does that, equalizing momentum (Figure 6-7).

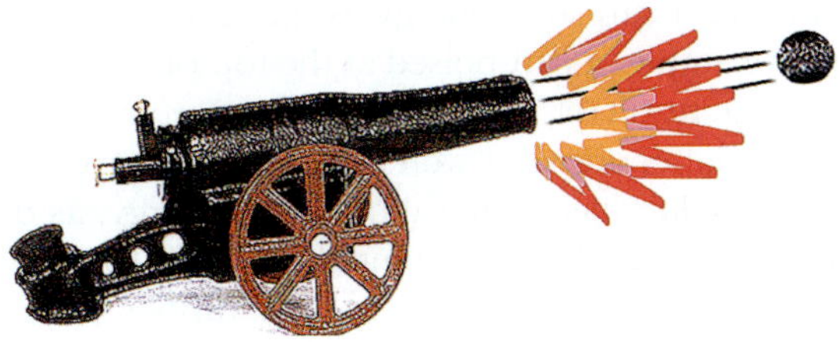

Figure 6-7 **Law of conservation of momentum: cannonball gains momentum, recoil of cannon equalizes momentum** ***(Copyright © 2002*** **Technological Sciences for the Operating Room,** ***Association of Surgical Technologists)***

SIMPLE HARMONIC MOTION

Simple harmonic motion is one of the most common types of motion found in nature. If any object is displaced slightly from equilibrium, it will oscillate about its equilibrium position in what is called *simple harmonic motion.* Common examples are a mass on a spring, a plucked guitar string, and a simple pendulum. Coiled springs are said to be elastic since they return to their original position after a force is applied and removed. The following definitions help explain this concept:

- *Period (T)*—The time it takes for the oscillator to execute one complete cycle of its motion.
- *Amplitude (A)*—The maximum distance that an object moves from its central position (equilibrium).
- *Frequency (f)*—The number of cycles (or oscillations) the object completes per unit time. The simple relationship between period and frequency is defined as $f = 1/T$.

Hooke's law states that a force will cause a mass to move with simple harmonic motion if the friction is zero. As the mass moves through the equilibrium position, it reverses direction. If the mass is displaced a small amount from its equilibrium position and then released, it will vibrate back and forth through the equilibrium position with constant amplitude and a constant well-defined period (the time taken for one complete oscillation). For this reason, the motion is said to be simple harmonic.

WORK

In physics, *work* is defined as a force acting on an object to cause a displacement. Work only occurs only when a force succeeds in moving the object it acts on, such as when a horse pulls a buggy down a dirt road. The amount of work done is equal to the amount of force multiplied by the distance the object moves in the direction that the force is acting. Therefore,

$$W = fd$$

where W = work, f = force, and d = distance.

ENERGY

Light, electricity, sound, and heat are not forms of matter. They are forms of energy that produce changes in matter. For example, electrical energy can run an electric motor and atomic energy can power an atomic bomb. The most common form of energy is *mechanical energy,* the type of energy that makes objects move or change course. The mechanical energy of an object is measured by the amount of work it can do.

POTENTIAL ENERGY

Potential energy is the energy that an object has stored due to its position relative to some zero position. An object possesses gravitational potential energy if it is positioned at a height above (or below) zero.

An object can store energy as the result of its position. For example, a cart poised at the top of a hill stores energy as a result of its position. The cart would not have potential energy if it were sitting at the base of the hill. A firecracker has chemical potential energy, as does the battery of a car. Elastic potential energy is the energy stored in elastic materials, such as a rubber band or bungee cord, as the result of their stretching or compressing.

KINETIC ENERGY

Kinetic energy is the energy of motion. The cart at the top of the hill expends its potential energy as it speeds down the hill. Just before it began to move, the cart had only potential energy; just before it reached the bottom of the hill, it had only kinetic energy.

The mechanical energy of an object can be the result of its motion (e.g., kinetic energy) and/or the result of its stored energy of position (e.g., potential energy). The total amount of mechanical energy is merely the sum of the potential energy and the kinetic energy where TME = total mechanical energy, PE = potential energy, and KE = kinetic energy. Therefore,

$$TME = PE + KE$$

POWER

Power is the rate at which work is done (the work/time ratio). Power is defined as work divided by the time used to do the work:

$$P = W/t$$

where P = power, W = work, and t = time. If engine A does the same amount of work faster and more efficiently than engine B, then engine A has a greater power rating than engine B, meaning that the more powerful engine can do the same amount of work in less time. The standard metric unit of power is the watt.

The expression for power is work/time ($P = W/t$), and the expression for work is force times distance ($W = fd$), and the expression for speed (velocity) is distance divided by time ($v = d/t$); therefore, a formula for power that represents a machine that is both strong and fast, or powerful is

$$P = fv$$

where P = power, f = force, and v = velocity. A powerful machine can use a force to displace an object in a relatively short amount of time.

PROPERTIES OF MATTER

Objects that have mass and take up space are referred to as *matter*. **Weight** and mass are different; weight represents the pull that the earth's gravity has on an object (an object has weight relative to its distance to a large object), and mass is the amount of matter an object contains.

All matter is the same in that it is all is made up of atoms. But different types of atoms make up different types of matter, giving each individual object distinct properties.

STRUCTURE OF THE ATOM

The Bohr model of the atom describes its structure as electrons circling the nucleus at different levels, or orbitals, much like planets circle the sun. Atoms are composed of three types of particles: protons, neutrons, and electrons. Protons and neutrons are responsible for most of the atomic mass because the mass of an electron is very small.

Both the protons and neutrons reside in the nucleus of the atom, but protons have a positive charge, while neutrons have no charge. The orbiting electrons are negatively charged. For any element, the electrons in the outermost energy level/shell are the most important. Called *valence electrons,* these determine an element's chemical properties—how it will react in a chemical reaction.

The number of protons determines the atomic number of the atom, and is typically equal to the number of orbiting electrons. The number of protons in an element is constant (e.g., H = 1, Ur = 92) but neutron number may vary, so mass number (protons + neutrons) may vary. In fact, varying numbers of neutrons within an element form *isotopes*. The chemical properties of isotopes are the same, although the physical properties may be different. For example, oxygen has an atomic number of 8 but may have 8, 9, or 10 neutrons.

ELEMENTS

All matter is made up of fundamental elements that cannot be broken down by chemical means. There are 92 elements that occur naturally (and a few more synthetic varieties). Hydrogen, carbon, nitrogen, and oxygen are the elements that make up most living organisms. Other elements found in living organisms include calcium, magnesium, sodium, phosphorus, and potassium.

Elements are sorted by chemical properties, listed horizontally in order by atomic number on the **periodic table** of elements. Living organisms require chemically reactive gases; therefore, the noble gases, such as helium, are not found in living organisms.

Atoms constantly seek stable electron configurations, like the noble gases, and can obtain stability by losing, sharing, or gaining electrons. For a stable configuration, each atom must fill its outer energy level, but the maximum number that can exist at any level is strictly limited:

- First level: 2 electrons
- Second level: 8 electrons

- Third level: 8 electrons
- Fourth level: 8 electrons

Atoms that have one, two or three electrons in their outer levels will tend to lose them in interactions with atoms that have five, six, or seven electrons in their outer levels. Atoms that have five, six, or seven electrons in their outer levels will tend to gain electrons from atoms with one, two, or three electrons in their outer levels. Atoms that have four electrons in the outermost energy level will neither totally lose nor totally gain electrons during interactions. *Ionization* is the gain or loss of electrons. The loss of electrons converts an atom into a positively charged ion, while the gain of electrons converts an atom into a negatively charged ion.

MOLECULES

Molecules are groups of atoms joined by chemical bonds (created by electron attraction and interaction). For example, two hydrogen atoms and one oxygen atom combine to form a water molecule (H_2O).

Molecular weight equals the sum of the atomic weights of the atoms in the molecule. A salt molecule (NaCl) contains one sodium and one chlorine atom. The atomic weight of sodium is 23 and the weight of chlorine is 35; therefore, 23 + 35 = 58, the molecular weight of NaCl.

SOLIDS, LIQUIDS, GASES, AND PLASMAS

Matter takes three basic forms, called *states of matter:* solids, liquids, and gases. A solid form of matter has definite shape and **volume**; a liquid has volume but no shape (it takes on the shape of whatever contains it); and a gas has neither definite shape nor volume. **Plasmas**, or ionized gases, are sometimes considered a fourth type of matter.

Matter is constantly in a state of flux given the conditions that surround it (usually a change in temperature). Physical changes in matter allow it to change states but still keep its identifying characteristics. For example, ice is water in the solid state, but if the ice is dropped into a liquid, it begins to melt because the temperature is higher than that of the ice cube. If the water is heated it changes to a gas form (steam).

Unlike physical changes, chemical changes in matter are irreversible and alter the identifying chemical characteristics. Spoiled milk is an example of a chemical change that cannot be reversed.

Plasmas are a super high-energy form of matter. Their properties are similar to gases, except that their atoms are made up of free electrons and ions from the element. If enough energy is infused into almost any gas, the energy will pull the electrons off of the gases' neutral atoms, breaking the electrons apart into positively and negatively charged ions and free electrons. These positively and negatively charged particles reach almost equal concentrations, causing the charge of the entire plasma to be close to neutral.

The universe is primarily composed of this form of matter. On earth, a fluorescent light bulb is an example of plasma. The glass tube encloses a gas that is charged by electricity flowing through it. The energy from electricity excites the atoms in the gas, and creates plasma inside the bulb. The plasma's energy glows, giving off light.

PRESSURE

The amount of force that acts on a given object does not completely describe its physical condition. **Pressure** exerted on an object as a result of force must also be considered. Pressure can be evaluated for solids, liquids, and gases.

As mentioned, force is used to move matter and is measured in terms of work. A solid object lying on a surface exerts a downward (gravitational) force that is equal to the weight of the object. The pressure exerted by the object against the surface depends on the area of contact and is measured by dividing the force by the area on which it acts:

$$p = f / A$$

where p = pressure, f = force, and A = area.

Liquid exerts pressure on the sides of the object that contains it, and also presses against an object that is placed within it. Pressure within a liquid at rest is the same in all directions, but increases in all directions with depth. To find the amount of pressure within a liquid at any given depth (**hydraulic pressure**), its density must be considered. Density is proportional to weight. Doubling the density of a column of liquid would therefore double its weight:

$$p = hD$$

where p = pressure, h = height or depth of liquid in a container, and D = density of the liquid. If h is given in feet, then D must be given in pounds per cubic foot.

Gases also exert pressure against the sides of a container because they have a small amount of mass and, therefore, a small amount of weight. Gases also exert pressure on anything immersed in it, including objects within the earth's atmosphere (air contains a number of gases). At sea level, air pressure exerted on a human body is about 14.7 lb/in.^{2} Pressure decreases as altitude increases.

In addition to pressure, gases have other properties that can be measured, including temperature, mass, and the volume (V) which contains the gas. Each of these variables is related to one another, and their values determine the state of the gas.

To force a gas into a smaller space, pressure must be applied; the more pressure applied, the smaller the space the gas can be forced into. Robert Boyle studied the relationship between the pressure and the volume of a confined gas held at a constant temperature, and noticed that volume is inversely proportional to pressure. If pressure is doubled, the volume is halved. This is known as Boyle's law.

HEAT

The temperature of any object, in physical terms, is how its degree of heat or cold (or intermediate degrees in between) feels on contact. When two objects with different temperatures make contact, the object with the higher temperature (e.g., the object with the faster moving molecules) cools and the cooler object warms until a point is reached after which no more change occurs. When touched they feel the same. Physicists describe this state as *thermal equilibrium*.

Heat Transfer

Molecules carry thermal energy in the form of motion. Some energy is transferred to molecules of a second object when they collide. This mechanism for transferring thermal energy by contact is called *conduction*. The conduction capacity of substances is measured with assigned numbers that compare their rates to that of silver, which has been arbitrarily assigned a coefficient of heat conduction of 100. Copper is close to silver with a coefficient of 92. Iron has a coefficient of 11, while glass is 0.20. Liquids and gases are poor conductors. They transfer the heat through convection, which involves the bodily movement of the more energetic molecules in a liquid or gas.

The third way that heat energy can be transferred from one body to another is by thermal radiation, which does not require contact for the transfer of heat. The sun warms the earth through thermal radiation that flows to the earth, where some of it is absorbed.

Greenhouse Effect

The glass panes of a greenhouse and the earth's atmosphere are both transparent to sunlight—they let in the sun's energy. Both also trap heat. Sunlight passes through the atmosphere and warms the planet's surface. Heat rising from the surface warms the atmosphere; gases in the atmosphere absorb some of the heat and reflect it back to the ground. This warming process is called the *greenhouse effect* and is worsened by a higher amount of carbon dioxide in the atmosphere. The burning of fossil fuels contributes more carbon dioxide to the atmosphere. The planet will continue to warm until we develop alternative fuel sources.

GENERAL PROPERTIES OF WAVES

A wave is a disturbance or variation that travels through a medium and transfers energy from point to point. The medium through which the wave travels may experience some local oscillations as the wave passes, but the particles in the medium do not travel with the wave. The repeating and periodic disturbance that moves through a medium from one location to another is referred to as a *wave*.

A *medium* is a substance or material that carries the wave (or disturbance) from one location to another. In the case of a wave in the ocean, the medium through which the wave travels is the water. In the case of a sound wave moving from a singer to the audience, the medium is the air in the room.

The interactions of one particle of the medium with its adjacent particles allow the disturbance to travel through the medium. In the case of a sound wave in air, the particles of the medium are the individual molecules of air. In the case of a wave in the ocean, the particles are the molecules of water (H_2O).

When a wave is present in a medium, the individual particles of the medium are only temporarily displaced from their resting position; they seek restoration to their original position. In a water wave, each molecule of the water always returns to its original position. As a disturbance moves through a medium from one particle to its adjacent particle, energy is being transported from one end of the medium to the other without transporting the medium (matter) through which it moves. This property of the wave—the ability to transfer energy without transporting matter—is unique.

ELECTROMAGNETIC WAVES

Visible light is just one of the waves that originate in electric and magnetic fields (Figure 6-8). The electromagnetic spectrum includes radio waves, microwaves, infrared waves, visible light, ultraviolet light, **X-rays**, and gamma rays. Each of these is placed on the spectrum in the order of their vibration (slower to faster).

The human eye can perceive light with a wavelength between 1/30,000 and 1/60,000 of an inch. Other similar waves are shorter or longer than these are. For example, shorter waves that fall beyond the violet end of the spectrum make up the ultraviolet region (used in sunlamps), and the longer waves beyond the red end of the spectrum are called **infrared waves**.

X-rays

Waves that are shorter than ultraviolet and about one-thousandth the wavelength of visible light are called X-rays. X-rays were discovered in 1895 by a German physicist named Wilhelm Conrad Röntgen. Because of

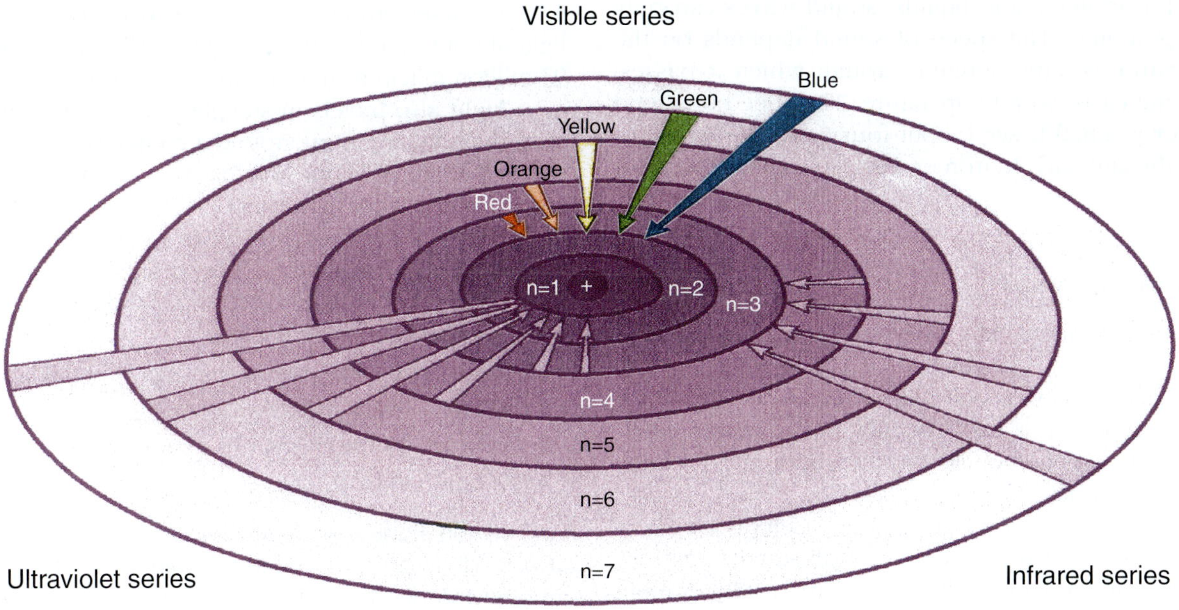

Figure 6-8 Electromagnetic spectrum of light *(Copyright © 2002* **Technological Sciences for the Operating Room,** ***Association of Surgical Technologists)***

their short wavelength, X-rays can pass through objects that can be made visible on a fluorescent screen coated with barium platinocyanide.

Thomas Edison began researching better materials than barium platinocyanide for the fluorescent screen and concluded that calcium tungstate was far more effective. By 1896, Edison had incorporated this material into a device constructed from a tapered box with a viewing port and a calcium tungstate screen (later called a *fluoroscope*). Edison's version of the fluoroscope quickly became the tool that physicians used to view X-ray images.

A modern X-ray machine consists of a cathode tube (Coolidge tube) in which highly accelerated electrons are aimed at heavy atoms (a tungsten filament) heated to a high temperature. When this stream of high-energy electrons strikes the metallic electrode (anode), the electrons are slowed down, and some of them penetrate the metal. The sudden "braking" of the electrons produces the electromagnetic radiation of very short wavelength, called X-rays.

Sounds and Vibrations

A sound wave is produced by vibrating objects that set surrounding air molecules into vibrating motion. For example, when strummed, a guitar string creates a frequency in the surrounding air molecules that is equal to the frequency of the vibration of the string.

As the air molecules oscillate (move back and forth along a center), they create a pressure wave consisting of compressions and rarefactions that travels away from the source. The compressions are regions of high pressure, where the air molecules are compressed into a small region of space. The rarefactions are regions of low pressure, where the air molecules are spread apart. This alternating pattern of compressions and rarefactions is known as a *sound wave.*

The human eardrum (tympanic membrane) receives sound waves that cause it to compress, creating a higher pressure that moves it inward. This resulting inward motion causes a rarefaction that pushes it outward, and the resulting vibrations are converted to electrical energy that are interpreted by the brain as specific sounds.

The number of waves produced in one second is equal to the number of vibrations per second sent out by the vibrating object. One wavelength on a sound wave is defined as the distance between two successive spots in the same state of compression (from one crest to the next) and is equivalent to one cycle.

The frequency of sound is stated in hertz (Hz), a unit referring to wave cycles per second (1 hertz = 1 cycle per second). The human ear can perceive sounds ranging from about 20 to 20,000 Hz. Frequencies above this are called *ultrasonic* frequencies, usually expressed in megahertz (MHz); 1 MHz equals 1 million cycles per second.

Sounds travel through all states of matter (but not in a vacuum like light waves), although they move through some media better than others. In solids, sound can exist as either a longitudinal or a transverse wave, but in gases and liquids, sound waves can only be longitudinal. The speed of sound depends on the temperature of any medium through which it passes. Speed increases with temperature. The speed of sound in water is 4,820 ft/sec (about four times the speed of sound through air). In iron or steel, sound travels about 16,800 ft/sec.

Vibrating Strings

A string instrument can make a variety of different sounds, depending on whether it is plucked like a guitar, bowed like a violin, or struck like a piano. The difference in relation to pitch is the frequency of the string's vibration, which depends on its characteristics and the way that it is manipulated.

Although a vibrating guitar string itself disturbs very little air when plucked (due to its small surface area), its attachment to the large, hollow wooden box allows more air to be disturbed as the guitar string forces the sound box to vibrate. The sound box, in turn, forces surrounding air molecules into vibrational motion.

Doppler Effect

In 1842, Christian Doppler explained the sudden change in pitch of a passing train's horn. His theory, called the *Doppler effect,* involves the shift in frequency and wavelength of waves that results from a source moving with respect to the medium, a receiver moving with respect to the medium, or even a moving medium.

As the train approaches, the sound waves from its horn are compressed toward the observer. The intervals between waves diminish, which is heard as an increase in frequency or pitch. As the train recedes, the sound waves from the horn are stretched (relative to the observer), resulting in a decrease in pitch. By the change in pitch of the train's horn, an observer can determine if the train is approaching or moving away, and can even determine its rate of speed.

The Doppler effect is also observed when electromagnetic radiation, which is emitted by a moving object, moves away from or toward an observer. The radiation emitted by an object moving toward an observer is squeezed, and its frequency appears to increase ("blue shift"). Radiation emitted by an object moving away is stretched ("red shift").

BEHAVIOR OF LIGHT

Light is a very mysterious phenomenon to physicists, who have been studying it for hundreds of years. Just from observing lightning and listening to thunder in a thunderstorm, anyone can observe that the speed of light is greater than the speed of sound. The speed of light is 3×10^8 m/sec (about 186,000 miles per second). It takes light about 9 minutes to travel 140 million kilometers (or 93 million miles) from our sun to the earth.

Light also travels in straight lines. People can hear each other talking from around a corner, but they cannot see each other. This means that sound waves can bend around corners but light cannot.

Visible light waves consist of a continuous range of wavelengths or frequencies. When a light wave with a single frequency strikes an object, any of the following could happen. The light wave could be:

1. Absorbed by the object; its energy would be converted to heat
2. Reflected by the object
3. Transmitted by the object

When light strikes an object, it interacts with its atoms. The manner in which visible light interacts with an object depends on the frequency of the light and the nature of the object's atoms. For example, when light hits transparent objects, the electrons vibrate and slow the light waves so that no energy is left behind. Nontransparent objects either reflect or absorb light. The light waves do not slow down, and light energy is converted into heat energy.

Reflection

A light from a flashlight shined into a mirror will be reflected from the mirror at a specific angle, depending on the angle of entry (incidence). The law of reflection states that the angle of reflection equals the angle of incidence (the angle between an incident ray and the normal to a reflecting surface). These angles are measured from the normal, the direction perpendicular to the mirror.

For objects with smooth surfaces, such as mirrors, the law of reflection applies on a large scale. Light that travels to the mirror in one direction reflects from the mirror in one direction; reflection from such objects is known as *specular reflection*. However, most objects exhibit *diffuse reflection,* that is, the sending of light in all directions.

Refraction

Refraction is the bending of a light ray as it passes from one substance to another. Light travels at different speeds when it moves through certain substances, such as water or glass. The speed of light in a given material is related to a quantity called the index of refraction, n, which is defined as the ratio of the speed of light in vacuum to the speed of light in the medium:

$$n = c / v,$$

where c = speed of light and v = velocity.

Color

Within the spectrum of visible light, each individual wavelength that comprises light is representative of a particular color. Isaac Newton proved this when he used a prism to separate light into different wavelengths showing the various colors of visible light (a process known as *dispersion*).

Dispersion of visible light produces the colors red, yellow, orange, blue, green, indigo, and violet. The red wavelengths of light are the longer wavelengths and the violet wavelengths of light are the shorter wavelengths. Between red and violet, there is a continuous range or spectrum of wavelengths.

White is perceived when all wavelengths of the visible light spectrum strike the eye at the same time. White is not really a color because it is a combination of all colors of the visible light spectrum. Black is not really a color, either; it is the absence of the wavelengths of the visible light spectrum.

Wave-Particle Duality

The mysterious nature of light is related to how it behaves, in terms of how physicists can define that behavior. Robert Hooke, in the early 1600s, proposed that light was a wave. Sir Isaac Newton, a contemporary of Hooke's, thought that if light were a wave, it would bend around corners.

After observing that light breaks up into colors when passed through a prism, Newton described light as tiny particles that he called corpuscles. The two brought up a classic problem in physics: Does light behave like a wave or a particle? In 1801, the British scientist Thomas Young performed experiments on the interference of light passing through a double slit, which unequivocally proved that light was a wave.

In 1905, Albert Einstein explained details of the photoelectric effect, which required that light be a collection of particles that he called *photons*. The photoelectric effect seemed to clearly prove that light is a particle, yet Young's experiments proved that light was a wave. Physicists at the time knew that particles and waves were very different things.

Niels Bohr of the University of Copenhagen described this paradox as the *complementarity principle*, a new theory that stated that light could be described as behaving as both a wave and a particle (the two complemented each other). In other words, it was suggested by Bohr that these two models were both sufficient and insufficient, but it was the best way to describe the nature of light. This principle is also referred to as the *wave-particle duality of nature*.

LASERS

A *laser* (*l*ight *a*mplification *s*timulated *e*mission of *r*adiation) is a special type of light that contains atoms whose electrons radiate in synchronous vibration. In principle, the laser is a device that transforms energy from other forms into electromagnetic radiation.

The components of a laser can be divided into three main parts: the energy pump source, the gain medium, and the resonator cavity. The specifics of these components depend on the gain medium and whether it is pulsed or a continuous beam.

The source of a laser's energy can come from any energy form: electromagnetic radiation, electrical energy, chemical energy, and so on. A pump source, such as an electrical discharge, sets the particles in motion. Energy is always emitted from the laser as electromagnetic radiation (which includes light beams). When the gain medium of a laser is excited, it may be stimulated by a photon to release its stored energy and emit another, identical photon.

The gain medium amplifies the light as it passes through and can be made from a solid, liquid, or gas. The gain medium determines the type of laser: solid state, gas, semiconductor, and liquid. Solid-state lasers have the most power output.

The resonator cavity consists of mirrors that direct and redirect the particles through the gain medium to achieve the desired charge.

Gas lasers can be composed of pure gas, a mixture of gases, or metal vapors. The gas is contained in a cylindrical glass. Two mirrors are located outside the ends of the tube to form the laser cavity.

Semiconductor lasers usually consist of a junction between layers of semiconductors with different electrical conducting properties. The laser cavity is confined to the junction region by means of two reflective boundaries. Common uses for semiconductor lasers include CD players and laser printers.

Liquid lasers are comprised of inorganic dyes contained in glass vessels. The frequency on tunable dye lasers can be adjusted with the help of a prism inside the laser cavity.

How Lasers Work

When an electron of an atom is stimulated to an outer orbit (excitation), it spontaneously falls back to an inner orbit (de-excitation), simultaneously emitting a photon of light. This is called *spontaneous emission* and is basically the same process that accounts for the glow of a neon sign. It is unpredictable and uncontrolled.

Einstein proved that if one of these photons encounters an excited atom in just the right way, it will drop down to a lower energy state and emit a photon with properties that are the same as the original photon. The new photon will:

- Be of exactly the same wavelength
- Have exactly the same phase
- Be emitted in exactly the same direction
- Have exactly the same polarization

The lasing medium spontaneously emits these photons in all directions at random times. For a laser light to be generated, a photon must be emitted parallel to the long direction of the resonator. The photon will travel down to one of the mirrors (laser mirrors reflect light through the gain medium 18 times) and begin to bounce back and forth many times. Along the way, the photon encounters excited atoms and forces them to give up their photons, creating a cascade of more and more synchronous photons. The resulting beam is almost entirely one wavelength (monochromatic), and all the waves are in step (coherent).

The electromagnetic light wave from a laser can be either continuous, with billions of oscillations, or pulsed with as few as two oscillations. Laser light ranges in color from the far infrared to the deep ultraviolet.

NUCLEAR PHYSICS

Nuclear physics is the study of the properties of the atomic nucleus, a very tiny object at the center of every atom. The protons (positively charged) and neutrons (no charge) of an atom's nucleus are collectively known as *nucleons*. The nucleons themselves are made of subatomic particles called **quarks**.

A very strong force pulls nucleons toward each other, and an even stronger repulsive force keeps them from overlapping. The result is that a nucleus appears as a closely packed set of spheres that are almost touching. When these are forced apart with what is known as *binding energy*, a tremendous amount of energy is released.

Nuclear physics is concerned with the fundamental nature of matter, and its central focus has been on the relationship between energy and mass. Einstein's famous equation, energy (E) is equivalent to mass (m) times the speed of light (c) squared ($E = mc^2$), stated that mass and energy are essentially the same thing. A very small amount of mass holds an enormous amount of energy.

Nuclear physicists have also been interested in the fact that matter can be converted from one form (energy) to another (particles) in particle accelerators and nuclear reactors. The results of particle accelerator experiments have led scientists to postulate the existence of three types of nuclear forces that account for all types of interaction found in matter:

1. The strong force, not charge related and only effective at very short distances
2. The weak force, 100 times weaker than the strong force
3. The electromagnetic force, thought to be exerted through the exchange of photons

The fourth force found in nature, but not in the nucleus, is the gravitational force. These forces are believed to be generated by the exchange of particles between the interacting pieces of matter.

GRAVITY

For situations near the surface of the earth, gravity causes objects to accelerate downward at 9.81 m/sec for each consecutive second they fall. We usually associate the letter g with acceleration due to gravity (g = 9.81 m/sec/sec. In other words, the force of gravity would cause an object to accelerate 9.81 m/sec downward the first second, 19.62 m/sec the next second, 29.43 m/sec the third second, and to progressively speed up at a rate of 9.81 m/sec until stopped by impact.

Gravity causes all objects to accelerate downward regardless of size, shape, or mass. This means that without air resistance (passing through air and encountering many air molecules that slow the object dropped), a feather dropped from a cliff will fall at the same rate as a rock and will hit the ground at exactly the same time.

SURGICAL ROBOTS

A *robot* is a sophisticated machine developed to perform specific tasks. Most robots are used in factories, but with advances in technology, robots are functioning in agriculture, construction, retailing, and other services. This section deals with surgical robots and their applications in the OR.

A machine is defined as a robot if it features some degree of mobility and, once programmed, operates automatically and performs a large variety of tasks.

Robots are classified by generations. First-generation robots are simple mechanical arms without artificial intelligence (AI). They perform precise repetitive motions at high speeds for industrial applications and require consistent oversight.

Second-generation robots incorporate a level of artificial intelligence. Characteristically, these machines may include pressure or tactile sensors and some type of vision and hearing. While not requiring constant supervision, occasional monitoring is necessary.

Third-generation robots include autonomous and insect robots. An autonomous robot works independently, without supervision by human controllers or an overseeing computer. The insect robots are controlled by a larger central AI computer.

Fourth-generation robots are not yet fully developed, but will be distinguished from the other generations by their ability to learn, reproduce, and evolve. Eventually, the intelligence of these robots will exceed the collective computing power of every human brain on the planet.

Surgical robots improve surgical patient care by helping to overcome limitations in human precision and reliability. Although surgical robots are increasingly complex, they still require surgeon control and input, primarily by remote control and voice activation. In the future, autonomous robots will operate on people without human interaction. Experts believe that a robot can be designed that will be able to diagnose and surgically correct a disease without human intervention before the end of this century.

Robots will help control the cost of health care not only by replacing expensive surgical personnel but also by enabling surgeons to perform surgical procedures from a distance. Another cost-saving benefit is the shorter period of convalescence resulting from the minimally invasive procedures performed by robots. Robots can also mitigate the surgeon's hand tremors that can result from fatigue. The da Vinci™ Surgical System ignores hand tremors and keeps the manipulator steady. The most popular technology currently available is AESOP 3000™ (Automated Endoscopic System for Optimal Positioning) manufactured by Computer Motion. As the first widely used robotic arm, AESOP is used to position a surgical camera inserted into the patient (an endoscope). Foot pedals or voice-activated software permits the physician to position the camera, leaving his or her hands free to continue operating on the patient.

The da Vinci and ZEUS™ robotic systems both share similar design elements. Each has a computer workstation (where the surgeon sits and engages the hand manipulators), a video screen, and a robot that is stationed next to the patient and equipped with three manipulators for the camera and instruments.

With advances in robotic technology, the surgeon may perform a surgical procedure from miles away. The surgeon can remotely control the robotic arms at a computer station in Washington, D.C., for a patient and robot located in Las Vegas. Performing a surgical procedure in real time at a distance is termed *telesurgery*. A major obstacle of telesurgery has been the time delay between the surgeon's hand movements and the robotic arms' responses.

TERMINOLOGY

Before a discussion can take place concerning the clinical applications of robotics in surgery, basic robotic concepts must be understood. The robotic "language" presented next will be frequently used by OR personnel:

- *Articulated*—Broken into sections by joints. Many robot arms have articulated geometry and the versatility is measured in **degrees of freedom**.
- *Binaural hearing*—The ability of humans and robots to determine the direction from which sound is coming. Humans have two ears that provide this ability; robots are given two sound transducers that provide the ability.
- ***Cartesian coordinate geometry*** —Derived from the Cartesian system used for graphing mathematical functions. The axes are always perpendicular to each other. Also called rectangular coordinate geometry.
- *Cylindrical coordinate geometry*—Refers to the plane that is used in combination with a plane coordinate system and elevation in conjunction with a robotic arm.
- *Degrees of freedom*—The number of ways that a robot manipulator can move. The majority of manipulators move in three dimensions, but have more than three degrees of freedom.
- *Degrees of rotation*—The extent that a robot joint or a set of joints can move clockwise or counterclockwise about an axis. A reference point is established and the angles of the joint are stated in degrees.
- *Expert systems*—A method of reasoning in AI used to control smart robots. The expert system consists of facts or data supplied to the robot about the robot's environment; also called rule-based system.
- *Machine hearing*—Advanced "hearing" by a robot that can pick up a sound, amplify it, and determine from which direction the sound is coming.
- *Manipulators*—Technical term for robot arms.
- *Resolution*—The extent to which a machine, microscope, human, or robot can differentiate between two objects.
- *Revolute geometry*—Refers to a robotic arm that can move in three dimensions resembling the movements of a human arm such as rotating through a full circle (360 degrees).
- *Sensitivity*—Ability of a machine or robot to see in dim light or detect weak impulses at invisible wavelengths.
- *Telechir*—Name given to remotely controlled robots.
- *Telepresence*—Refers to the operation of a robot at a distance, meaning the operator is situated in one location, usually miles apart, and the robot is on-site with the patient.

DESIGN

Robots are ultimately designed to deliver better patient care through more precise and accurate surgical intervention. The components of a surgical robotic system include manipulators, instrumentation, remote consoles with micromanipulators and computers, and voice-activation control systems.

ROBOTIC ARM (MANIPULATOR)

Robotic arms are the workhorse elements of the robotic system and may provide simple functions, such as holding an endoscope for operative site viewing, or complex manipulation of minimally invasive instrumentation (Figure 6-9).

The robotic arm is an automated device that is attached to the rail of the OR table. The distal end of the arm attaches to minimally invasive instrumentation or an endoscope. The robotic arm is connected by cables to a computer that sends messages to the arm for guidance of its movements.

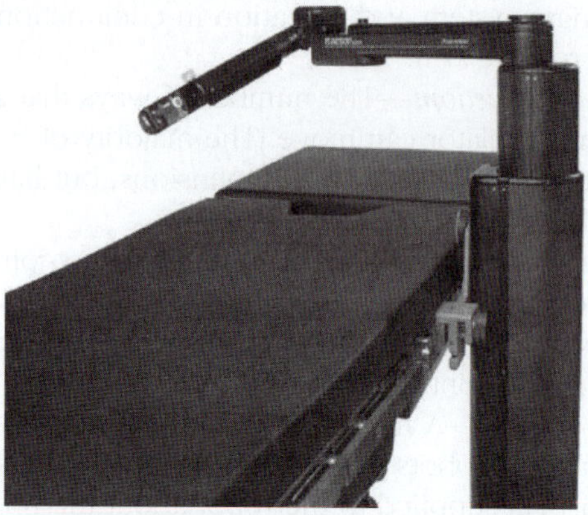

Figure 6-9 Manipulator attached to an operating table ***(Courtesy of Computer Motion, Inc.)***

REMOTE MANIPULATION

A single robotic arm can hold an endoscope while the surgeon manipulates instruments at the operative field. Several manipulators (remotely controlled) may be necessary for more complex simultaneous functions, such as holding an endoscope and manipulating an array of surgical instrumentation. The instruments are similar to minimally invasive instruments, but are designed to articulate with and be manipulated by robotic arms.

The computer translates messages received from micromanipulators on the remote console that are controlled by the surgeon's hands. The micromanipulators translate the surgeon's hand movements to the robotic arms and instrumentation. The surgeon watches the activity on a three-dimensional screen in the console.

Advantages of Remote Manipulation

- Eliminates hand tremor for more precise surgical technique and fewer errors.
- Allows the surgeon to effectively perform complex interventions within a confined space via small access portals (1.5 mm).
- Affords better visualization of the operative site through 3D imaging.
- Fosters telesurgery, which is a benefit to small rural hospitals.

VOICE-ACTIVATED CONTROL SYSTEM

Another component of the surgical robotics system is the voice-activated control system. It is a master control unit that is activated by the surgeon's hand or voice via a headset and microphone. The unit controls the manipulator and other surgical applications, such as the shaver and fluid pump in arthroscopic surgery, the light controls in the OR suite, or the printer and computer for storage of intraoperative photographic documentation. It is programmed to ignore casual conversation.

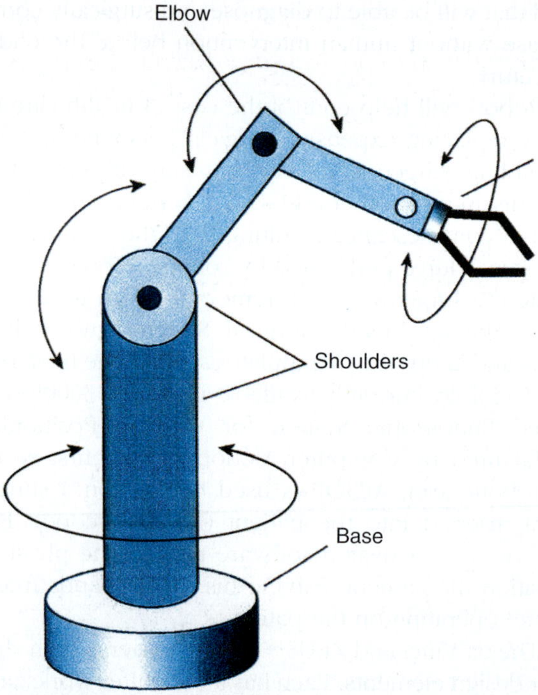

Figure 6-10 Rotation of the manipulator ***(Copyright © 2002 Technological Sciences for the Operating Room, Association of Surgical Technologists)***

GEOMETRY

Manipulators are categorized by their geometrical design. The joints are referred to as shoulders, elbow, and wrist. Cartesian coordinate geometry, or rectangular coordinate geometry, is a manipulator design derived from the Cartesian system for graphing mathematical functions. An arm with Cartesian geometry moves along *x, y,* and *z* axes (up-down, right-left, and front-back).

The manipulator has a definite number of degrees of freedom and rotation (Figure 6-10). Degrees of freedom refer to the number of dimensions in which a manipulator can move (most have three dimensions). An up-and-down movement is known as *pitch,* while right and left movements are called *yaw.* A rotating movement is a *roll.* By comparison, the human arm has seven degrees of freedom. Degrees of rotation relate to a manipulator's clockwise and counterclockwise movements around an axis.

Other manipulator geometry designs include cylindrical coordinate geometry, a manipulator design that incorporates a plane polar coordinate system with an elevation dimension added; and revolute geometry, a design that allows an arm to move in three dimensions with 360-degree rotation and 90-degree elevation from the shoulder. An elbow joint moves through 180 degrees (from a straight position to double back on itself), and a wrist joint revolves and flexes like the elbow.

HEARING AND VISION

Machine hearing is analogous to human hearing. A robot can distinguish from which direction sound originates and the actual type of sound, such as a human voice. To accomplish this, robots are built with binaural hearing, the same type of hearing humans possess. To provide a robot with binaural hearing, robots, particularly voice-controlled units employed in surgery, are equipped with two sound transducers. This makes it possible for the robot to determine the source of the sound and its origin. Each human voice produces a unique waveform. A recording of the voice (waveform) can be made. The robot will be able to analyze the waveform and interpret commonly spoken commands issued by specific individuals.

Two important concepts must be understood when discussing robotic vision: sensitivity and resolution. *Sensitivity* is the ability of the robot to see in dim light. In some instances, a high level of sensitivity is necessary. For example, during endoscopic procedures, the lights in the OR, including the surgical overhead lights, are either dimmed or turned off. A robot would require a level of sensitivity designed to see in such dim lighting. *Resolution* is the ability to differentiate between two objects and resolution capabilities vary. Obviously, the better the resolution, the better the vision.

However, sensitivity and resolution have a negative effect on each other. If the resolution is improved, the vision function of the robot will decrease in dim light, and vice versa: Improved sensitivity causes a decrease in resolution.

Just as binaural hearing is analogous to human hearing, binocular machine vision is analogous to binocular human vision, also referred to as stereo vision. Binocular vision permits depth perception. In surgery, if vision is ever realized for robots, a high-resolution camera will need to be developed that can be used in conjunction with a powerful robot controller, computer, and an advanced AI robot.

DECONTAMINATION AND STERILIZATION OF ROBOTIC COMPONENTS

The sterile instruments and endoscope (with camera and light cord) held by the robot's manipulators are cleaned and sterilized in the same way that any other minimally invasive components are cleaned and sterilized. The manipulators of the robot that hold the endoscope and instruments are not sterilized, but are covered with special sterile sleeves.

CLINICAL APPLICATIONS

Robotics in the OR would not have been possible if it were not for the evolution of endoscopic surgery. During the last 15 years, the progression of minimally invasive surgery has been explosive. Advances in endoscopic technology have allowed the development of safe, efficient, and advanced surgical techniques that have resulted in decreased morbidity, length of hospital stay, and costs.

The primary systems used in the OR are the AESOP and da Vinci systems, which have been used on humans and lab animals for experimental purposes to perfect surgical techniques. Surgical specialties that have either investigated the use of robotics or currently apply the systems in the OR include cardiovascular, neurosurgery, general, orthopedic, and maxillofacial.

THE OR OF THE FUTURE

Ten years from now, the OR will be a vastly different place than exists today. The changes that will transform the surgical environment are occurring now, and identifying the core knowledge needed to incorporate these changes is important for surgical technology education. Robots are already being utilized for minimally invasive surgical procedures, and virtual reality simulations for surgical training are also occurring more frequently. The OR of the future will involve the following technologies:

- Surgical planning and rehearsal
- Surface-based registration

SURGICAL PLANNING AND REHEARSAL

Image-based planning and rehearsal for surgical intervention consist of three segments: patient imaging, creating a satisfactory three-dimensional model of the imaging data (modeling), and planning and rehearsing the procedure with the information obtained. Imaging is achieved via MRI or CAT for the generation of two-dimensional images. These images will eventually be transformed into three-dimensional models through deformable modeling.

Deformable modeling provides realistic mechanical simulations of bones and tissue using computational models of the behavior of human joints and tissue. This technology will aid surgeons in predicting potential complications through computerized manipulation during rehearsal. Essentially, images obtained through noninvasive methods are transformed into three-dimensional models that can be manipulated with virtual instrumentation. Before the actual procedure begins, the surgical team deploys this technology, thereby avoiding potential errors and resolving unforeseen complications. For example, deformable modeling enables the surgeon to deal with a large vessel that is not where it should have been or the variations in normal anatomy during rehearsal and thereby begin the procedure with accurate information.

The goal of deformable modeling is to achieve realistic three-dimensional simulation of soft tissue behavior under the effect of external simulation. Before the first incision is made, the surgeon utilizes a customized, computer-generated model of the patient to diagnose the condition, evaluate treatment options, and practice the personalized surgical procedure. The key word here is *customized.* Surgeons are not rehearsing on general models of probable tissue—they have obtained these images from the actual patient (e.g., the patient's virtual tissues). This imagery almost exactly simulates the circumstances that will be encountered during the actual procedure.

SURFACED-BASED REGISTRATION

After the completion of the planning and rehearsal phase that produced the three-dimensional model of the patient's tissues and pathology associated with the surgical procedure, the biomechanical control system must be able to register (determine the orientation of) tissues in the real-time environment of the OR. Harvard University uses a surgical navigation system consisting of laser scanners and video cameras. This equipment produces composite images of the actual patient and magnetic resonance images of the surgery site before and during the procedure.

The surgical site, for instance the patient's brain, is scanned using MRI or CAT technology. This scan produces a large number of slices through the brain. Computer analysis of the data highlights the various structures and types of normal and abnormal tissue. For example, the normal tissue of the brain and the ventricles can be color contrasted with the abnormal tissue of a brain tumor.

After abnormal tissue is differentiated from normal, a computer algorithm generates three-dimensional images of the surfaces of the structures. The surfaces are displayed by selecting a virtual-viewing camera location and orientation in the magnetic resonance data using computer graphics techniques. This process removes hidden portions of the surface, shades the surface, and can vary opacity to allow glimpses into internal structures.

In the OR, the scan-based images must be superimposed precisely on the actual head of the patient. This is accomplished by scanning the patient's head with a laser to obtain a set of three-dimensional coordinates for points on the skin. The magnetic resonance image is now combined with images of the patient recorded by video cameras in the OR. Registration optimizes the combined magnetic resonance and laser data.

Surgeons can now see exactly where the magnetic resonance points are positioned in the patient, both internally and on the surface. In other words, the patient's virtual head is superimposed on his real one. The image can then be manipulated so that the surgeon can literally peer inside the patient's head before the initial incision is even made. The surgeon now has "X-ray vision." During surgery, the imaging system tracks the position of the instruments (internal probes), because their tips may not be visible.

ROLE OF THE SURGICAL TECHNOLOGIST

The OR of the future will be staffed by surgical technologists with an in-depth understanding of

- Physics
- Biomechanics
- Computer science
- Software
- Electronics
- Robotics

Surgical technologists with training in these subjects can assume the future technological roles in tomorrow's OR, as well as responsibilities in emergency care. With this specialized training, surgical technologists can maintain, troubleshoot, and operate the complex machinery related to robotics.

Despite these futuristic considerations, surgical technologists will still require basic traditional training in order to respond when a patient needs to be opened during the procedure. However, the combined training adds further value to the surgical technologist's roles and responsibilities. Hospitals will no longer need to bring in outside specialists for this technology in the OR, because properly trained surgical technologists are cost-effective alternatives. Consequently, members of the profession will be functioning in prominent positions in the OR for years to come.

CASE STUDY

Endoscopy involves the insertion of a scope into various regions of the body for preoperative, intraoperative, or postoperative diagnosis and treatment. The endoscope may be rigid or flexible, and it is equipped with lenses and a light source for illumination. The endoscope is used for such procedures as laparoscopy (viewing of abdominal organs), thoracoscopy (viewing of organs of the thoracic cavity), arthroscopy (viewing of joint spaces), and ventriculoscopy (viewing of the ventricles of the brain). Rigid endoscopes use an optical system called a *rod lens system.* The rod lens system is a series of lenses that reflect the image through a straight tube to the eyepiece. Flexible endoscopes use fiber optics, thin strands of pure glass that are arranged in bundles to transmit the light signals. Flexible endoscopes are equipped with controlling wires to allow for a wider range of motion. Fiber-optic endoscopes work through a physics principle called *total internal reflection.* The light in a fiber-optic cable travels through the endoscope core by bouncing (reflecting) from the glass cladding along its walls. The cladding does not absorb any light from the core, so the light wave can travel great distances.

1. List two surgical procedures that would most likely require the use of a rigid endoscope.
2. List two surgical procedures that would most likely require the use of a flexible endoscope.
3. In terms of physical principles, how is a laser similar to an endoscope?
4. Given the similar physical principles, why does the light emitted by a laser create different results than a light emitted by an endoscope?

QUESTIONS FOR FURTHER STUDY

1. Briefly describe the function used to move up and down within a document.
2. What are some of the consequences of high humidity in the OR?
3. Why might a patient's jewelry be hazardous in the OR?
4. Name two applications for the principles of light in surgery
5. What is binding energy?
6. Briefly describe Newton's law of gravity.

BIBLIOGRAPHY

Atkinson, L. J., & Fortunato, N. (1996). *Berry & Kohn's OR technique* (8th ed.). St. Louis, MO: Mosby.

Baaea, I., Schultz, C., Grzybowski, L., & Gotzen, V. (1999, March). Voice-controlled robotic arm in laparoscopic surgery. *Croatian Medical Journal, 40*(3), 409–412.

Basic electricity. Retrieved August 22, 2002, from *http://www.actechelp.com/Electrical/basic_electricity_lesson.htm*

Computertime technologies. Retrieved July 29, 2002, from *http://www.computertim.com/howto*

Cosgrove, D. M., & Sabik, J. F. (1996). Minimally invasive approach for aortic valve operations. *Annals of Thoracic Surgery, 62,* 596–597.

Cosgrove, D. M., Sabik, J. F., & Navia, J. L. (1998). Minimally invasive valve operations. *Annals of Thoracic Surgery, 65,* 135–138.

Donnelly, S. (1998). Solids, liquids, and gases, oh why? Retrieved October 16, 2002, from *http://www.cpo.com/Weblabs/solig.htm*

Felger, J. E., Nifong, L. W., & Chitwood, W. R. (2001, March). Robotic cardiac valve surgery: Transcending the technologic crevasse! *Current Opinions in Cardiology, 16*(2), 146–151.

Feynman, R. P. (1995). *Six easy pieces.* Cambridge: Perseus Books.

Freeman, I. A., & Durden, W. J. (1990). *Physics made simple.* New York: Doubleday Dell Publishing.

Geis, W. P. (1995). Efficiency & outcomes improve with AESOP. *Computer Motion Review, 1*(1).

Getting results with Microsoft Office 97. (1997). Redmond, WA: Microsoft Press.

Gibilisco, S. (2002). *Teach yourself electricity and electronics* (3rd ed.). New York: McGraw-Hill.

Goldwasser, S. A. (1998). A practical guide to lasers for experiments and hobbyists. Retrieved October 16, 2002, from *http://www.eio.com/repairfaq/sam/laserfaq.htm#faqwil*

Gussow, M. (1983). *Schaum's outline of theory and problems of basic electricity.* New York: McGraw-Hill.

Harada, K. (2002). Basic electrical principles. Retrieved October 7, 2002, from *http://www.harada-sound.com/sound/handbook/basicelec.html*

Henderson, T. (1996). The physics classroom: Work, energy, and power. Retrieved October 7, 2002, from *http://www.glenbrook.k12.il.us/gbssci/phys/Class/energy/energtoc.html*

INT Media Group, Inc. (2002). Webopedia. Retrieved July 29, 2002, from *http://www.webopedia.com*

Intuitive Surgical, Inc. (2000). da Vinci surgical system. Retrieved November 14, 2000, from *http://www.intuitivesurgical.com/html/index.html*

John Hopkins University Office of News and Information. (1998). John Hopkins University launches research center to expand role of computers. Retrieved September 24, 1998, from *http://www.hopkinsmedicine.org*

Karney, J. A. (2001). *A + certification training kit* (3rd ed.). Redmond, WA: Microsoft Press.

Kasser, B. (1998). *Using the Internet* (4th ed.). Indianapolis: Que Corporation.

Konecny, C. (1995). Laparoscopic cholecystectomy setup. *Computer Motion Preview, 1*(1).

Konecny, C. (1995). Scrub nurse (tech) considerations for laparoscopic cholecystectomy. *Computer Motion Preview, 1*(1).

Kozierok, C. M. (2002). The pc guide. Retrieved July 29, 2002, from *http://www.PCGuide.com*

Kuhn, K. F. (1996). *Basic physics: A self-teaching guide* (2nd ed.). New York: John Wiley & Sons.

Law, C., Taralekar, C., & Wang, J. (2002). Basic electricity and magnetism. Retrieved October 7, 2002, from *http://www.library.thinkquest.org/16600/beginner/electricity.shtml*

Lawson, P. (1996). Laparoscopic Nissen fundoplication. *Computer Motion Preview, 1*(2).

Lehrman, R. L., (1998). *Physics the easy way* (3rd ed.). Hauppauge, NY: Barron's Educational Series.

Marion, J. B. (1979). *General physics with bioscience essays.* New York: John Wiley & Sons.

Massillon, O. H. (2001). *Understanding the relationship between surgical gloves and electrosurgery.* Red Bank, New Jersey: Ansell Healthcare Products, Inc.

McGuiness, A. M., et al. (2002). *Core curriculum for surgical technology* (5th ed.). Centennial, CO: Association of Surgical Technologists.

Medical Robotics at University of California-Berkeley. (2002). Surgical robotics. Retrieved November 14, 2000, from *http://robotics.eecs.berkeley.edu/medical*

Meeker, M. H., & Rothrock, J. C. (Eds.). (1995). *Alexander's care of the patient in surgery* (10th ed.). St. Louis, MO: Mosby.

Meyer, L. A. (1995). *Basics of electricity.* Hayward, CA: LAMA Books.

MIT Medical Vision Group. (2001). Project on image guided surgery: A collaboration between the MIT AI Lab and Brigham and Women's Surgical Planning Laboratory. Retrieved November 14, 2000, from *http://www.ai.mit.edu/projects/medical-vision*

Nute, R. (2002). Floating circuits—protection against electric shock. Retrieved October 7, 2002, from *http://www.ewh.ieee.org/soc/emcs/pstc/TechSpk/floating.html*

Oman, D. M., & Oman, R. M. (1999). Physics for the utterly confused. New York: McGraw-Hill.

Padwick, G., et al. (1997). *Using Microsoft Outlook 97.* Indianapolis: Que Corporation.

Person, R., & Rose, K. (1995). *Using Word for Windows 95.* Indianapolis: Que Corporation.

Sullivan, L. (1993, July). Autoclaves. Safe Science Newsletter. Lansing: Office of Radiation, Chemical and Biological Safety, Michigan State University. Retrieved October 16, 2002, from *http://www.orcbs.msu.edu/newsletters/July1993/autoclave.html*

Tusczynski, J. A., & Dixon, J. M. (2002). Biomedical applications of introductory physics. New York: John Wiley & Sons.

Valkenburgh, V., & Nooger, N. (1992). *Basic electricity* (4th ed.). Indianapolis: PROMPT Publications.

Valley Lab. (2002). Principles of electrosurgery. Retrieved October 7, 2002, from *http://www.valleylab.com*

Woods, J., Yong, W. J., Sutton, A., & Hopkins, W. (1999). Light and lasers: Behavior of light. Retrieved January 12, 1999, from *http://www.ece.utexas.edu/projects/k12-fall98/14540/Group7/Behavior.html*

CHAPTER 7

Asepsis and Sterile Technique

Ben D. Price
Kevin B. Frey

CASE STUDY

It was a Thursday morning in operating room 10. The room, instrumentation, and patient were prepared for a left frontal craniotomy for the removal of a meningioma. The neurosurgeon had just made the skin incision when the unit charge nurse opened the door and said, "Stop where you are! Central processing just called. There was a malfunction of the sterilizer during the night shift. The chart does not confirm that the instruments went through a complete cycle. All the external indicators are turned and, thus far, all the internal indicators have turned."

1. What steps should be taken at this point?
2. If all the indicators are "turned," why is the unit charge nurse concerned?
3. What mistake or mistakes were made that allowed the instruments to reach the OR?

OBJECTIVES

After studying this chapter, the reader should be able to:

C 1. Discuss the relationship between the principles of asepsis and practice of sterile technique and surgical patient care.

2. Define and discuss the concept of surgical conscience.

A 3. Discuss the principles of asepsis.

4. Define the terms related to asepsis.
5. Discuss the sterile practices related to the principles of asepsis.
6. Identify the principles and procedures related to disinfection and sterilization.
7. **R** Demonstrate competency related to the practice of sterile technique.
8. Demonstrate competency in the procedures related to disinfection and sterilization.
9. **E** Discuss the surgical environment and the application of the principles of asepsis to the environment.

SELECT KEY TERMS

1. asepsis
2. autoclave
3. bioburden
4. biological indicator
5. Bowie-Dick Test
6. chelation
7. chemical indicator
8. colonization
9. contaminated
10. emulsification
11. endoscope
12. event-related sterility
13. flash sterilization
14. immersion
15. integrity
16. intermediate-level disinfection
17. Julian date
18. Lister
19. lumen
20. pathogen
21. permeability
22. sterile field
23. sterile technique
24. sterilization
25. surgical conscience
26. ultrasonic washer

HISTORY OF STERILIZATION

A brief review of the history of **sterilization** will help the student appreciate the long struggle to find and prevent the causes of surgical site infections (SSIs). This review is select and short but will provide a historical setting for the principles of **asepsis** and practice of **sterile technique**.

Even in ancient times some forms of disinfection were practiced, but, of course, there was not a developed understanding of why disinfection practices prevented disease. The ancients were well acquainted with the use of burning chemicals to allow the fumes to deodorize and disinfect. Sulfur in the form of sulfur dioxide is the first chemical disinfectant to be reported, and the individual responsible for its mention is the Greek poet Homer. In the *Odyssey,* Odysseus killed his wife's suitors and after disposing of the bodies the following passage can be found:

> To the nurse Eurycleia then said he:
> "Bring cleansing sulfur, aged dame, to me
> And fire, that I may purify the hall."

The Bible is filled with many passages suggesting purification by fire and strict rules of cleanliness. Moses was the first to advise purification by fire. The books of Leviticus and Deuteronomy report that he developed the first system for purification of infected premises. His commands laid the groundwork for the first sanitary code established by the Hebrews, and the various systems of purification were based on Mosaic law.

Aristotle understood the need for soldiers to avoid disease and instructed Alexander the Great to require his soldiers to boil drinking water and bury their waste. Hippocrates advocated the use of boiled water for irrigating wounds, a definite precursor to later sterile technique. Galen, a Greek physician, boiled the instruments used in the care of Roman gladiators who were wounded.

The Middle Ages, specifically the period A.D. 900–1500, showed little progress or contribution toward the development of sterilization. The only notable exception was an Italian, Girolamo Fracastorius, who was the first to recognize that disease could be spread by direct contact, from fomites (he first used the word), and through the air.

The following are brief descriptions of individuals whose contributions advanced the science of sterilization.

1775: Lazzaro Spallanzani, an Italian naturalist, demonstrated that boiling microbes in a sealed flask for 1 hour killed microbes.

1832: William Henry, an English chemist, demonstrated that heat could be used to sterilize infected clothing. He designed an early jacketed dry heat/hot air sterilizer.

1847: Ignaz Semmelweis, a Hungarian obstetrician, proved that puerperal fever was transmitted from health care providers to patients. Advocated handwashing and scrubbing fingernails between patient contact.

1862: Louis Pasteur, a French chemist and bacteriologist and "father of bacteriology," developed principles that contributed to the founding of modern sterile technique. His greatest contribution to the development of sterilization was his establishment of the germ theory of disease.

1867: Joseph **Lister**, an English surgeon and "father of antiseptic surgery," applied Pasteur's principles to surgical practice. His contributions led to the establishment of the principles of asepsis and practice of sterile technique in the operating room.

1876: John Tyndall, an English physicist, discovered the heat-resistant phase (spore stage) of bacteria and originated a process of fractional sterilization by intermittent heating later called *tyndallization*.

1880: Charles Chamberland, a French bacteriologist and pupil and assistant to Pasteur, developed the first pressure steam sterilizer, called *Chamberland's autoclave*.

1881: Robert Koch, a German bacteriologist, along with his associates, developed the first non-pressure-flowing steam sterilizer.

1885: Curt Schimmelbusch, a German surgeon, was the first to use steam sterilization in the sterilization of surgical dressings.

1885–1900: Germans made the most noteworthy contributions to the principles of steam sterilization and disinfection. Unfortunately, the adoption of these principles on a universal scale did not take place until some 30 years later when the modern temperature-controlled sterilizer was invented in America.

1888: Ervin Von Esmarch recommended the use of bacteriological tests as proof that sterilization of materials occurred.

1888: J. J. Kinyoun, an American bacteriologist, was the first to recommend that the vacuum process be used to enhance the steam penetration of items to be sterilized.

1915: American hospitals were introduced to the concept of gravity sterilizers.

1933: The first pressure- and temperature-controlled steam sterilizer was introduced. Weeden Underwood was an American engineer whose contributions in design and applications led to the development of the modern **autoclave**.

1963: Glutaraldehyde was first introduced and subsequently was the first liquid chemical agent approved by the Environmental Protection Agency (EPA) for use as a sterilant for heat-sensitive instruments.

BASIC TERMINOLOGY

The terminology related to the principles of asepsis and sterile technique is essential to all practices in the OR. Table 7-1 is provided to establish clear definitions of terms and to assist the student with more productive reading time.

PATHOGENS AND INFECTION

Microorganisms, minute life forms invisible to the naked eye, are a natural part of the world in which we live. They include both free-living and parasitic life forms. In nature, microorganisms serve to convert complex organic compounds such as animal and plant matter into more simple forms through the process of decay. Some microorganisms take inorganic compounds and convert them to higher forms that can be used as nutrients by plants and animals. These organisms are used beneficially by humans in the production of food products such as yogurt and cheese, in nutrient compounds, and even in antibiotics.

Certain microorganisms have come to rely on a parasitic relationship with plants and animals. Usually, the growth of these life forms in the host is damaging. These microorganisms are referred to as **pathogens**. This chapter attempts to give only an overview of the basic information about the primary microorganisms encountered in the OR.

INFECTION

The multiplication of organisms in the tissues of a host is called *infection*. Any infection that develops while a patient is in the hospital or is produced by microorganisms acquired during hospitalization or in any health care setting is termed a *nosocomial infection*. These infections may affect not only a patient but also any individual who has contact with the hospital or health care setting, including health care workers and visitors. Many nosocomial

Table 7-1 Terminology of Asepsis and Sterile Technique

Term
Antiseptic: substance commonly used on living tissue to inhibit the growth and reproduction of microbes to prevent infection
Asepsis: absence of microbes, infection
Bacteriocidal: substance that destroys/kills bacteria
Bacteriostatic: substance that restrains the further development or reproduction of bacteria
Bioburden: the number of microbes or amount of organic debris on an object at any given time
Contamination: the presence of pathogenic materials
Cross-contamination: the contamination of a person or object by another
Decontamination: to reduce to an irreducible minimum the presence of pathogenic material
Disinfectant: chemical agent that kills most microbes, but usually not spores; usually used on inanimate objects because these compounds are too strong to be used on living tissues
Fomite: an inanimate object on which pathogens may be conveyed
Fungicide: agent that destroys fungus
Infection: the invasion of the human body or tissue by pathogenic microorganisms that reproduce and multiply, causing disease
Nosocomial: an infection acquired within a health care setting
Pathogen: any microbe capable of causing disease
Resident flora: microbes that normally reside below the skin surface or within the body
Sepsis: infection, usually accompanied by fever, that results from the presence of pathogenic microorganisms
Spore: a resistant form of certain types of bacteria, able to survive in adverse conditions
Sporicidal: substance that kills/destroys bacteria in the spore stage
Sterile: item(s) that has been rendered free of all living microorganisms, including spores
Sterile field: specified area, usually the area immediately around the patient, that is considered free of microorganisms
Sterile technique: methods used to prevent contamination of the sterile field by microorganisms; protection of the patient against infection causing microbes preoperatively, intraoperatively, and postoperatively
Sterility, event related: sterility determined by how a package is handled rather than time elapsed; package is considered sterile until opened or integrity of packaging material is damaged
Sterilization: the destruction of all microorganisms, including spores, on inanimate surfaces; the destruction of all microorganisms in or about an object, as by steam (flowing or pressurized), chemical agents (alcohol, phenol, heavy metals, ethylene oxide gas), high-velocity electron bombardment, or ultraviolet light radiation
Strike-through contamination: contamination of a sterile field that occurs through the passage of fluid through or a puncture in a microbial barrier
Surgically clean: items mechanically cleaned and chemically disinfected but not sterile
Terminal disinfection: to render items safe to handle by high-level disinfection
Terminal sterilization: to render items safe to handle by sterilization
Transient flora: microbes that reside on the skin surface and are easily removed
Vector: a living carrier that transmits disease
Virucide: agent that destroys viruses

infections become apparent while the patient is still hospitalized; however, onset of disease may occur after the patient has been discharged. As many as 25% of nosocomial infections acquired perioperatively do not become evident until the patient has been discharged from the hospital. The primary goal of the surgical technologist in the scrub role (STSR) is the use of proper sterile technique to prevent the transmission of microbes perioperatively and thus to prevent SSIs.

PATHOGENS ASSOCIATED WITH SURGICAL SITE INFECTION

In this chapter, we describe only the most commonly occurring pathogens associated with SSI. The types of microorganisms that may cause infection are numerous, and for a more in-depth look, the reader should refer to a standard microbiology text.

BACTERIA

Many bacteria reside naturally within the human body and cause no disease unless the opportunity arises. For example, *Escherichia coli* resides in the **lumen** of the intestine in humans. This bacterium is capable of causing infection when released into the peritoneal cavity.

Bacteria are classified according to the environment that sustains their life. They are either *aerobic* (must have oxygen to survive) or *anaerobic* (live without oxygen). Additionally, bacteria are classified as gram positive or gram negative. A Gram stain is a laboratory process in which gentian violet is placed on bacteria. If the bacteria stain blue, it is gram positive; if not, it is gram negative. Bacteria are also identified by shape:

- *Cocci:* Generally spherically shaped bacterium
- *Bacilli:* Generally rod-shaped bacterium

Table 7-2 lists common bacterial pathogens. Table 7-3 provides an overview of pathogens most commonly associated with surgical site infections. In addition to bacterium, fungi, such as *Candida albicans,* and viruses, such as the hepatitis virus and human immunodeficiency virus, may cause infections.

As shown in Table 7-3, the most commonly transmitted pathogen in the operating room is *Staphylococcus aureus,* a gram-positive cocci. This bacterium is common in the flora of the skin, and this is probably the source of the organisms in most ORs. Not only are most patients carriers of the bacterium, but the surgical staff may also carry the bacteria on their skin and in their nares. *Staphylococcus aureus* thrives in the nose, and 25% of all people are colonized with this organism. Studies have shown that the nares and hair of personnel may be the source when the infection that develops is not from the patient's own skin. We will explore the transmission modes of infection further following an overview of microbial viability.

VIABILITY

To survive in any environment, microorganisms must have adequate time to reproduce. They must also be supplied with food, moisture, and the proper temperature for that particular species. In addition, bacteria must be in an environment with the correct amount of oxygen for survival. Aerobic bacteria thrive in oxygen-rich environments, while anaerobic bacteria thrive in oxygen-free environments. With the removal of any of these factors, viability is lost in a fairly short period of time, although some bacteria are able to remain dormant while transferred from one host to another. This dormancy period, however, is usually short. Because of the necessity for all of the above factors to be present in order to support microorganism life, most bacteria, viruses, and fungi are destroyed easily in the sterilization process. Bacterial spores, however, are not that easily destroyed.

TUBERCULOSIS

Tuberculosis (TB), caused by *Mycobacterium tuberculosis* and transmitted through airborne droplet nuclei, usually

Table 7-2 Common Bacterial Pathogens

TYPE OF BACTERIA	CLASSIFICATION	SPECIFIC BACTERIA
Aerobic bacteria:		
These bacteria require oxygen to sustain life.	Gram-negative bacilli	*E. coli, Enterobacter cloacae, Pseudomonas aeruginosa, Proteus, Salmonella, Haemophilus influenzae, Serratia marcescens, Legionella pneumophila*
	Gram-positive bacilli	*Bacillus, Mycobacterium*
	Gram-negative cocci	*Neisseria gonorrhoeae*
	Gram-positive cocci	*Staphylococcus aureus, S. epidermidis, methicillin resistant S. aureus, Streptococcus* group B
Microaerophilic bacteria:		
These bacteria require an oxygen level lower than that in normal air.	Gram-positive cocci	*Streptococci*
Anaerobic bacteria:		
These bacteria grow in an oxygen-free environment.	Gram-negative bacilli	*Bacteroides fragilis*
	Gram-positive bacilli	*Clostridium tetani, C. welchii*
	Gram-positive cocci	*Peptostreptococcus*

Table 7-3 Pathogens Commonly Associated with Surgical Site Infection

PATHOGEN	PERCENTAGE OF INFECTIONS
S. aureus	17
Enterococci	13
Coagulase negative staphylococci	12
E. coli	10
P. aeruginosa	8
Enterobacter spp.	8
Proteus mirabilis	4
Klebsiella pneumoniae	3
Streptococcus spp.	3
C. albicans	2
Other	20

Source: Adapted from *Prevention and Control of Nosocomial Infections,* 3rd ed. (Table 37.3), by R. P. Wenzel, Ed., 1998, Baltimore: William and Wilkins.

infects the lungs but may also infect kidneys, joints, or skin. Elective operations on patients with TB are postponed until drug therapy is effective. Surgical procedures performed on known TB carriers require the use of special filter masks, which are provided along with other available personal protective equipment (PPE).

SPORES

Some bacteria, especially *Bacillus* and *Clostridium,* develop a very tough shell within the bacterial cell during its resting stage that is resistant to environmental changes. In this stage, a bacterium can survive extremes in temperature as well as drying and the total lack of a source of food. When the proper conditions for bacterial growth are restored, the bacterium returns to its vegetative state and is able to grow and reproduce once again. Although only about 150 types of bacteria produce spores, they are universal, and not only must the bacteria be destroyed in the sterilization process, the difficult-to-destroy spores must be destroyed as well.

VIRUSES

Unlike bacteria, which are living cells, viruses are nonliving small particles that are completely reliant on the host cell for survival. These pathogens may be transmitted via fluids from or contact with the respiratory, intestinal, urinary, or genital tract as well as through blood and blood products. Each virus has a particular mode of transmission, and some have multiple modes. Human immunodeficiency virus (HIV), for instance, may be transmitted through blood, semen, mother's milk, and potentially other body fluids.

A virus invades a host cell and then combines with the DNA or RNA of the cell and changes the cell's metabolism in order to accommodate the replication of the virus. The replication of the virus causes an antibody defense in the host.

Most viruses are destroyed by high-level disinfection and/or sterilization. Many viruses found in the operative environment pose risk to health care personnel, and therefore PPE should be worn and Standard Precautions should be followed. Table 7-4 lists viral pathogens common to the OR.

OTHER INFECTIOUS DISEASES

Tuberculosis and other infectious diseases have been transmitted in the operative environment, and the emergence of drug-resistant strains of tuberculosis is reason for additional concern. Rarely seen infectious agents such as malaria and Ebola virus could also be spread within the operative environment, as could any of a number of bacteria, viruses, fungi, and other pathogens. The use of such protective strategies as sterile technique along with Standard Precautions is necessary for the protection of patient and personnel from all pathogens.

MICROBIOLOGY IN THE OPERATING ROOM

As previously stated, the source of most surgical site infections is the patient's own flora (endogenous flora), which contaminate the wound at the time of surgery, usually by direct contact. This occurs most often in clean-contaminated, **contaminated**, and dirty procedures (refer to Chapter 11). In addition, the patient is at risk of infection from personnel, inanimate objects (e.g., contaminated instrumentation), and airborne contaminants.

Table 7-4 Viral Pathogens Common to the Operating Room

VIRUS	TRANSMISSION	DESCRIPTION
Hepatitis B (HBV)	Percutaneous or permucous in blood, serum, and other body fluids	Causes inflammation of the liver, jaundice, cirrhosis, and in some cases liver carcinoma
Hepatitis C	Blood-borne RNA; health care workers at particular risk; transmitted through blood and blood products	Asymptomatic when acute, may be carried for 25 years, chronic hepatitis, cirrhosis, liver cancer
Hepatitis D (Delta)	Coexists with HBV	Liver disease, superinfection of HBV, death
Human immunodeficiency virus (HIV)	Blood or other body fluids	Compromises immune system
Herpes simplex virus (HSV)	Contact with fluid from lesions	Causes localized blister-like eruptions; can also cause keratoconjunctivitis, acute retinal necrosis, meningoencephalitis
Cytomegalovirus (CMV)	Direct contact with body fluids	Infects salivary glands or viscera, opportunistic infection in patients with HIV or hepatitis
Creutzfeldt-Jakob disease (CJD)	Exact mode of transmission unknown; thought to be by percutaneous inoculation with brain tissue or cerebral spinal fluid from infected persons; transmission has been associated with use of contaminated instruments; longer sterilization times (1 hour at 132°C) required	Rapidly progressive fatal central nervous disease characterized by dementia, myoclonus

In clean surgical procedures, entry into the gastrointestinal, genital, urinary, or respiratory tract is avoided, and the incidence of endogenous infection is decreased.

METHODS OF TRANSMISSION

Any infection requires a primary agent, such as a bacterium, virus, fungus, or parasite. In the hospital setting, most infections are caused by bacteria and viruses, although fungi and parasites occasionally are involved in nosocomial infection. Frequent hand washing helps to eliminate transient microbes from the skin, thereby reducing the risk of nosocomial infection. SSIs are the second most frequent nosocomial infections and are acquired almost exclusively in the OR itself and not in the postanesthesia care unit (PACU) or general patient care areas.

Surgical site infection facts to remember include these:

- The primary mode of airborne bacteria in the operating room is the surgical team. Team members may disperse microorganisms from their own skin.

TECHNIQUE: Basic Hand Washing

1. Turn on the faucet and adjust the water temperature.
2. Inspect hands and wrists.
3. Wet hands and wrists.
4. Apply soap; lather.
5. Use moderate friction and circular motions.
6. Interlace fingers to facilitate cleaning of the web spaces.
7. Continue washing for 30 seconds to 1 minute.
8. Rinse.
9. Turn off the water.
10. Dry hands and wrists.
11. Discard the towels.

- Most SSIs are caused by the patient's own flora contaminating the wound by direct contact. Meticulous preoperative skin preparation renders the skin surgically clean, decreasing the number of microorganisms near the surgical site.
- Most SSIs in the OR occur because of contamination during the procedure.

Since most SSIs are acquired at the time of surgery, rather than at some point after surgery, the major sources of microbes causing these infections must be located within the surgical suite. These sources can be divided into two groups, environmental and endogenous. Environmental sources include personnel, the environment, and contaminated instrumentation. The other primary source is the patient's endogenous flora. Modes of transmission are shown in Table 7-5.

PERSONNEL

Although the surgical technologist will focus on the hands during the surgical scrub and a large part of surgical awareness focuses on the hands, they have been shown to be of little importance statistically in the development of SSI. This is directly related to proper preoperative scrubbing and the proper wearing of intact surgical gloves to prevent skin-to-skin contact intraoperatively.

The skin and hair of operative personnel are reservoirs of bacteria, which may be shed in particle form into the air and therefore pose a risk of surgical site infection to the patient. Bacteria thrive in the hair and nares, *S. aureus* in particular. It is therefore proper OR practice for the scrubbed members of the surgical team to don OR attire, protective attire, and scrub attire prior to the procedure not only to protect the patient from any shed bacterial particles but also to protect personnel from contact with the patient's blood or body fluids (refer to Chapter 12).

Table 7-5 Modes of Transmission

TRANSMISSION MODE	EXAMPLES
Direct contact	Oral–fecal hepatitis transmission, postoperative cholecystectomy wound infection from contact with patient's own gallbladder
Indirect contact	Infection spread by contaminated surgical instruments
Airborne spread	Infection through the air, from sneeze droplets
Common vehicle spread	Infection carried in blood products

Gowns on personnel and drapes on the patient cover the skin on areas of the body other than the hands. The use of caps and masks in the operating room is based on observations of increased infection rates when members of the surgical team were carriers of *S. aureus.* Since such a high percentage of the populace are carriers of this organism, the threat is considerable enough to warrant the use of caps and masks. A recent random study, however, has shown that the surgical wound infection rate was unaffected by whether the operative team wore masks intraoperatively. Further studies should be performed before a definite conclusion may be drawn about this practice. The primary purpose of wearing gowns around the operating table is to provide a barrier to contamination, both from personnel to patient and from patient to personnel. The gown should be constructed of a breathable material, but one that will not allow blood and other fluids from the outside to penetrate scrub attire and possibly the OR attire of the sterile team members. Barrier gowns are available, but have thus far been uncomfortable to wear. Gowns should be selected based on the level of protection from fluid strike-through and the type of procedure planned but also on the level of comfort of the product.

The hair of operative personnel should be covered prior to entry into restricted or semirestricted areas of the surgical site. If the team member has a beard or long sideburns, various types of hoods are available for full coverage. The patient is also asked to don a cap prior to surgery.

In addition to the above, Standard Precautions dictate the use of additional protective items such as protective eyewear. The reader is referred to Chapters 5 and 12 for further information about proper attire and PPE. Some authorities have recommended the use of ventilated space suits and helmets during ultraclean implant procedures and open-joint procedures. These suits serve to totally isolate the surgical team from the operative environment during the procedure.

In addition to the role served by surgical attire in protecting the patient, surgical attire serves to protect the surgical technologist and other sterile team members from potential infection by the patient. The potential for exposure to such blood-borne diseases as the hepatitis virus or the HIV is high in the OR. Inadvertent sharp injuries and splashing of body fluids on the skin or mucous membranes occurs often in the operative environment. Studies have shown that simply knowing whether the patient is infected does not in itself decrease the instances of accidental exposure of fluid-borne pathogens to operative team members. The best protection, therefore, appears to be the use of Standard Precautions, including double-gloving, use of face shields, careful use of sharps, and the use of gowns, which provide a level of protection from strike-through contamination. Both Standard Precautions and its predecessor, Universal Precautions, are more clearly defined in Chapter 5 of this text.

Finally, personnel contribute to surgical site infection through human error or lapses in sterile technique. When breaks in sterile technique occur, for whatever reason, the patient is exposed to a preventable risk. Errors, therefore, should be noted, communicated, and corrected immediately; this practice is commonly termed **surgical conscience**

ENVIRONMENT

A second source of microbial transmission is environmental, both from fomites (pathogens on inanimate objects) and through the air. A safe, clean, and spacious OR helps to provide a lower level of microbes in the environment. For example, ORs designed with a clean zone, filtered, controlled air systems, and the use of soil-resistant building materials have become routine in surgical services. The OR has become a sort of sacred place where strict cleanliness rituals are followed, and this has been effective.

Within the operative environment, the patient is at risk of infection from airborne pathogens, and ORs are designed to minimize this by using laminar air flow systems (see Chapters 5 and 8). The aforementioned attire assists in the prevention of pathogen transmission from personnel to patient, and vice versa.

Surgical site infections have also been documented from such environmental sources as contaminated antiseptic solutions, contaminated wound dressings, and contaminated or improperly sterilized surgical instrumentation as well as a variety of other sources. Patients may be infected by direct contact with carriers, infected personnel, by droplets, or by shedding from personnel within the OR environment.

Fomites include walls, floors, cabinets, furniture, and nonsterile supplies. Contamination may also result from the improper cleaning/decontamination of anesthesia or surgical equipment, IV lines, and fluids. The use of nonsterile medications also poses a risk of infection to the patient.

THE PATIENT

As previously stated, most surgical site infections are contracted through the patient's own endogenous flora. One common example is a surgical site infection resulting from removal of the contaminated appendix through a skin incision during an appendectomy. This is certainly true for contaminated procedures, in which the gastrointestinal tract or other contaminated areas are opened and exposed to the surgical wound. Preoperative prophylaxis with antibiotics has been shown to reduce surgical site infections. Studies have shown that patients who are carriers of *S. aureus* are at particular risk for SSI, even in clean procedures. Carriers have colonies of these bacteria living in the deeper layers of their skin, making preoperative skin preparation less effective. As time passes after preoperative skin preparation, these bacteria reach the surface, where they may be shed and contaminate the surgical incision. Patients who have infections at other body locations are also at increased risk for SSI. Also, patients with urinary tract infections have been shown to be at higher risk of postoperative SSI. The two primary sources of risk to the patient of SSI are the endogenous flora encountered in contaminated procedures and the resident flora of the skin.

FACTORS THAT INCREASE RISK OF SURGICAL SITE INFECTION

The risk to the patient of developing an infection postoperatively may be influenced by several factors:

- *Age:* Geriatric and pediatric patients have lower immunological defenses.
- *Obesity:* Diminished blood flow, larger wound sizes, and the difficulty of handling adipose tissue mark these patients as more susceptible to infection.
- *General health:* Patients in poor health generally have a predisposition to infection.
- *Nasal carriers of* S. aureus: These patients are at greater risk of infection from their own endogenous flora.
- *Remote infections:* Infections at other body sites increase the chance of SSI. Bacteria in the bloodstream enter and infect the surgical site.
- *Preoperative hospitalization:* Infection rates are higher with increase in duration of preoperative stay. Patients are exposed to higher numbers of antibiotic-resistant strains of bacteria within the hospital.
- *Preexisting illness and related treatment:* Infection rates are higher in patients with compromised immune systems from preexisting illness, who have been treated with certain medications including steroids or chemotherapy agents, or who have recently undergone radiation therapy.

Other factors that may contribute to an increased likelihood of SSI include malnutrition, cigarette smoking, diabetes, malignancy, and immunosuppression.

Certain procedure-related risk factors also increase the danger of SSI:

- *Preoperative hair removal:* Although hair removal has been standard and considered an important part of surgical practice, studies have shown that hair removal is a risk factor for the development of SSI. The risk is greater when the preoperative shave is performed the day before surgery, and the use of razors carries greater risk than the use of clippers. Razor blades leave many small cuts, nicks, and scrapes on the skin, allowing bacteria easier access for **colonization**. If the patient is not allergic, use of depilatory creams is less traumatic and is therefore a safer alternative.

- *Type of procedure:* Clean-contaminated (Class II), contaminated (Class III), and dirty (Class IV) cases carry a higher risk of infection (refer to Chapter 11), as do cases that compromise blood flow to a particular area, such as coronary artery bypass procedures, where one or both internal mammary arteries are used.
- *Duration of procedure:* Longer anesthetic and operative times have an accompanying increase in time for bacterial contamination to occur, increased tissue damage, and greater immunosuppression. Team members become more fatigued, which may lead to breaks in sterile technique.

PRINCIPLES OF ASEPSIS

The safety of the patient depends on strict adherence to the practice of sterile technique by the surgical technologist. Advances in the control of pain, bleeding, and infection have made surgery a viable branch of medicine. Sterile technique was born out of the desire to control postoperative SSI. The surgical technologist must not only practice sterile technique, but must also be constantly aware of the sterile technique of others on the sterile surgical team to identify breaks in technique as well as the position and activities of nonsterile team members within the OR. Adherence to the principles of asepsis reflects the surgical technologist's surgical conscience and ability to aid in preventing SSI and will result in lower SSI rates. Here we have narrowed the concept of asepsis to three basic principles, supported by several applications or practices called sterile technique:

1. A **sterile field** is created for each surgical procedure.
2. Sterile team members must be appropriately attired prior to entering the sterile field.
3. Movement in and around the sterile field must not compromise the sterile field.

There are many applications to the above principles, and many "rules of thumb" are followed in order to keep in compliance with these principles. All are designed to protect the sterile field and thus keep microbial counts within the sterile field to an irreducible minimum, protecting the patient from infection. Achieving the goal of an irreducible minimum of microbes is the basic intent of all three principles of asepsis, and every practice of sterile technique is based on this concept.

PRINCIPLE 1: STERILE FIELD

A sterile field is created for each surgical procedure.

The primary method through which microbes are kept to an irreducible minimum in the OR is through the creation of a sterile field for each procedure. The sterile field is a separate, sterile area that in a larger sense consists of the surgical site itself, the draped portions of the patient and operating table, the sterile portions of the gowns and gloves of the sterile team members, and the draped ring stands, Mayo stand, and back table. The reality is that in this setup, many small separate sterile fields exist: the surgical site and draped portions of the patient, the individual draped ring stands, back table, and Mayo stand, and the sterile portions of the gown of sterile surgical team members. Within this sterile field are all sterile instruments, sutures, and equipment to be used during the procedure (Figure 7-1).

TIME

As time passes, the likelihood that a sterile field has become contaminated by error or by airborne contaminants increases. Therefore, the sterile field should be created as close as possible to the time of use. Components of the sterile field should never be covered with sterile drapes, because it is almost impossible to remove the drape without contamination resulting.

INSTRUMENT SETS, PEEL PACKS, AND WRAPPERS

- The use of **chemical indicators** as well as biological monitoring of the sterilization process must ensure the sterility of all instruments used during the procedure.

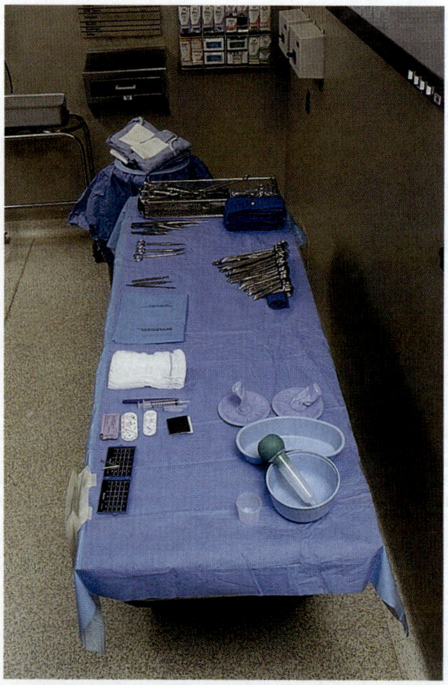

Figure 7-1 Sterile back table

- Instruments, such as scalpel blades, that come into contact with the skin of the patient should not be reused.
- For clean-contaminated and contaminated procedures, such as cases where the bowel is opened, separate setups should be used for the clean and dirty portions of the procedure. Personnel should not reuse the instruments used during the open bowel or dirty portion of the procedure and should regown and reglove before returning to the use of sterile instruments from the clean setup.
- When removing contents from the autoclave, the surgical team member must not touch the edge of the sterilizer with the instrument or tray. Sterile transfer handles may be used.
- The inner edge of a heat-sealed peel pack is considered the line between sterile and nonsterile. The flaps of the peel pack should be pulled back upon opening with no tears in the pack itself. The contents should then be transferred onto the sterile field or the STSR should grasp only the edge of the inner contents without touching the peel pack, lifting upward. The contents must never be allowed to slide over the edge of the peel pack.
- The inside of paper wrappers containing linens or other sterile items is considered sterile except for a 1-in. perimeter around the outside edge of the wrapper.
- When opening a sterile package, the circulator opens the top flap away from the body, grasping it in the hand holding the package. The side flaps are then opened downward, securing them in the same hand, and the last flap is pulled toward the body, exposing the sterile contents while covering the nonsterile hand. The item is then transferred onto the sterile field (refer to Chapter 12) or is taken from the package by the STSR.
- The top of a sterile, draped table is the only portion that is considered sterile. Any part of the drape extending below the top of the table is considered nonsterile.
- Any item extending or falling over the top of the table edge is considered nonsterile. Examples are suction tubing or the cord to a power instrument hanging below the table edge. The portion hanging below the table edge must not be brought onto the sterile field.
- Once sterile drapes have been applied, they should not be repositioned. The portion of the drape that falls below the table edge is considered nonsterile, and repositioning the drape exposes the sterile field to contaminated portions of the drape.

QUESTIONABLE STERILITY

If the sterility of any item or the integrity of packaging is in question, the item should be considered contaminated.

- If in doubt about the sterility of an item, consider it nonsterile and do not use: "If in doubt, throw it out."
- The **integrity** of sterile packages must be checked before opening. There must be no evidence of strike-through, tears, or punctures; all seals must be intact; and chemical indicators must have correct appearance.
- Sterile packages found in storage areas commonly used for storage of nonsterile items must not be used.

CAUSES OF CONTAMINATION

Destruction of the integrity of microbial barriers by puncture, tear, or strike-through results in contamination.

- Punctures, tears, or strike-throughs compromise the sterility of packages or drapes.
- If a permeable drape covers a table or sterile field and any liquid penetrates the drape either from above or below, the drape must be considered contaminated.
- Sterile packages and drapes should be stored on smooth, clean, dry surfaces to prevent damage to packaging materials.
- Sterile packages should be stored in a designated sterile supply storage area.
- Sterile packages should be handled only with clean, dry hands.
- If towel clips used on the sterile field puncture any draping material, the tips of the instrument must be considered contaminated and should be left in place until the end of the procedure.

PRINCIPLE 2: STERILE TEAM MEMBER ATTIRE

Sterile team members must be appropriately attired prior to entering the sterile field.

The attire worn by sterile individuals, including gown, gloves, mask, and hair cover, aids in preventing wound contamination. The surgical team members don gown and gloves using proper technique to maintain the sterility of the outer surfaces (see Chapter 12).

- The surgical gown is considered sterile from the waist to the mid-chest line in front and to 2 in. above the elbows on the sleeves. The upper chest area on the front of the gown is considered nonsterile because it cannot be directly viewed by the wearer and because of the possibility of the chin coming into contact with this part of the gown.
- When standing at a table, the gown should be considered sterile to the top of the operating table or the back table's top surface. Areas below this level may contact nonsterile surfaces and should be considered contaminated.
- The arms should not be folded with the hands in the axillary region. This region is considered nonsterile

because it cannot be viewed by the wearer and because strike-through contamination from perspiration can occur in this area.
- Hands should never be allowed to fall below waist or table level. The team member should avoid raising the hands above the mid-chest line or over the head to prevent contamination. A few exceptions exist, such as reaching for sterile light handles to adjust lights. This should be done at the beginning of the case and should not be repeated unless absolutely necessary.
- The back of the sterile gown is considered nonsterile.
- When wearing a sterile gown, the nonsterile back should never be turned toward the sterile field.
- A separate sterile surface should be used for gowning and gloving to avoid contamination of the back table. The gown and gloves may be opened in sterile fashion on a separate Mayo stand or small table prior to the surgical scrub.
- The stockinette cuffs of the surgical gown are considered nonsterile and should be covered by the cuff of the sterile gloves at all times.
- Members of the surgical team should sit only when the entire surgical procedure will be performed sitting down, and while seated, the hands must not be allowed to fall into the lap.
- If a member of the sterile team must stand on a platform, the platform should be positioned before the individual approaches the field, when practical. Members of the team should avoid as much as possible changing levels at the sterile field. Moving from a lower position to a higher position within the field exposes contaminated areas of the gown to the field.

PRINCIPLE 3: MOVEMENT IN AND AROUND STERILE FIELD

Movement in and around the sterile field must not compromise the sterile field.

STERILE TO STERILE

Only sterile items and individuals may contact sterile areas, and only sterile items may be placed within or moved within a sterile field:

- Only sterile members of the surgical team may touch sterile surfaces and items.
- The circulator and other nonsterile personnel must not touch or come into contact with sterile surfaces or items and should never walk between two sterile areas.

STERILE INDIVIDUALS KEEP WITHIN STERILE AREA

- Scrubbed personnel should stay close to the sterile field throughout the procedure.
- Movement within the sterile field should be kept to a minimum to avoid airborne contamination.
- Sterile surgical team members should either pass while facing one another or back to back by rotating 360°.
- The STSR should turn her or his back to a nonsterile individual or area when walking past.
- Talking, especially at the sterile field, should be kept to a minimum to prevent contamination from airborne moisture droplets.
- The STSR must always face the sterile field or area to avoid contamination.
- A nonsterile individual must maintain a minimum of 12 in. from any sterile item, area, or field to prevent contamination.

NONSTERILE TO NONSTERILE

Nonsterile items and individuals may only contact nonsterile areas.

- Nonsterile individuals never extend over a sterile field to transfer sterile items to a sterile individual. Items should be opened by the nonsterile individual using sterile technique and transferred onto the back table. Extending the hands over a sterile area could lead to contamination of that area by skin fallout.
- To avoid reaching over a sterile basin, the circulator should hold only the lip of a bottle over the sterile basin or container and should maintain a 12- to 18-in. distance above the sterile container while pouring. Sterile fluid bottles should never be recapped and reused, because replacing the cap contaminates the fluids within the bottle.
- The STSR must place basins and/or medicine glasses to be filled near the edge of the sterile table to allow the circulator to pour fluids without extending over the table.
- When draping a nonsterile table to create a sterile field, the nonsterile individual should cuff the hands in the underside folds of the drape or table cover to avoid contaminating the top surface. The drape should be opened away from the body toward the far side of the table first and then toward the body to avoid contamination.

SURGICAL CONSCIENCE

Surgical conscience is the basis for the practice of strict adherence to sterile technique by all surgical team members, including the surgical technologist. It involves a level of honesty and moral integrity that every surgical technologist must uphold in order to deliver quality patient care. Surgical conscience is a responsibility toward the patient and oneself that seeks to ensure consistent delivery of quality care to the patient.

The surgical technologist must be conscientious enough to be able to recognize and correct breaks in sterile technique, whether they were committed in the presence of others or alone. There should be no reluctance on the part of the surgical technologist or any member of the surgical team to admit to a break in technique. The surgical technologist who hesitates or cannot carry through with this duty has no place in the OR. There can be *no compromise of sterile technique.* Surgical conscience requires practice that puts the safety and well-being of the patient first, avoiding any lapse in technique that puts the patient at risk of immediate physical harm or future SSI.

The reader is encouraged to read Chapter 12 for a more thorough examination of the applications of the principles of asepsis and practice of sterile technique, including gowning, gloving, the surgical scrub, and the creation of a sterile field.

Standard Precautions covered in Chapters 5 and 12 should be used when handling used instruments, sharps, and specimens and when cleaning and sanitizing the OR, to prevent personnel exposure to infection from pathogens in blood or other body fluids on surfaces, instruments, or equipment.

CLEANING, DISINFECTION, AND STERILIZATION

Proper cleaning, disinfection, and sterilization provide an environment and equipment that are conducive to the ability to follow the principles of asepsis and the practice of sterile technique. These practices could be drawn into an endless circle, which begins with the cleaning (decontamination) of the OR. A sterile field is then created within the OR, and following the principles of asepsis and utilizing sterile technique, a procedure is performed on a patient. After the patient has left the OR, instruments are cleaned of any gross contamination and covered for safe transport to the decontamination area. Equipment and furniture in the room are cleaned (decontaminated) and disinfected, and waste is removed in the proper manner and placed in the proper receptacles (covered below). Instrumentation and equipment are then taken to the decontamination room (Figure 7-2), where they are further cleaned and then disinfected manually or by the use of **ultrasonic washers** (Figure 7-3) and/or washer-sterilizers (Figure 7-4). After decontamination and disinfection, these instruments are taken to the clean processing area, sorted, reassembled, and wrapped for sterilization (Figure 7-5). The instruments are taken to the sterilization area (Figure 7-6) and sterilized for use in the future and then are placed in the sterile equipment storage area of the OR. The OR itself is prepared for the next procedure, and new sterile supplies are brought in for the next case. The above is repeated for each successive procedure of the day, and at the end of the day, daily,

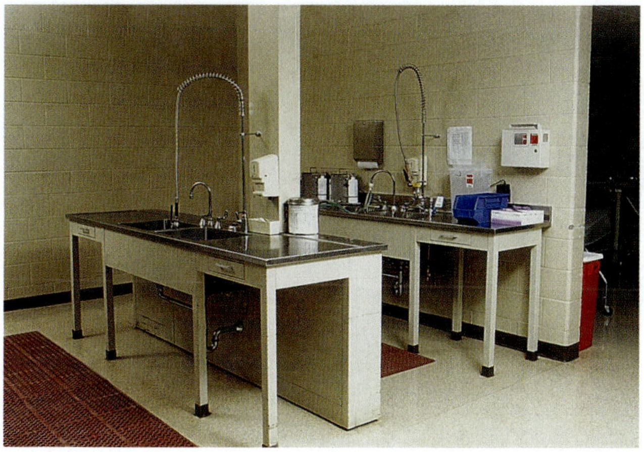

Figure 7-2 **Decontamination room**

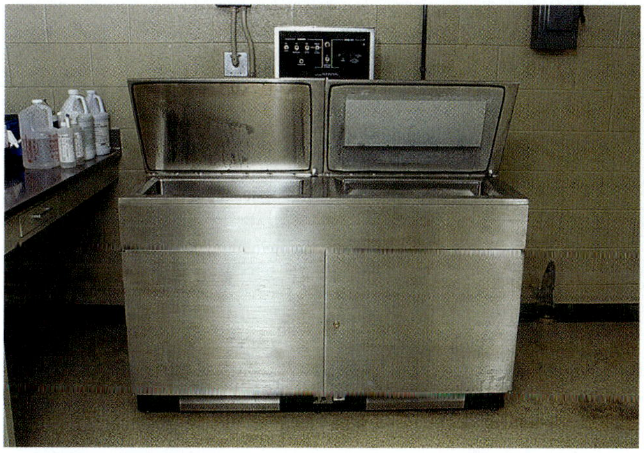

Figure 7-3 **Ultrasonic washer**

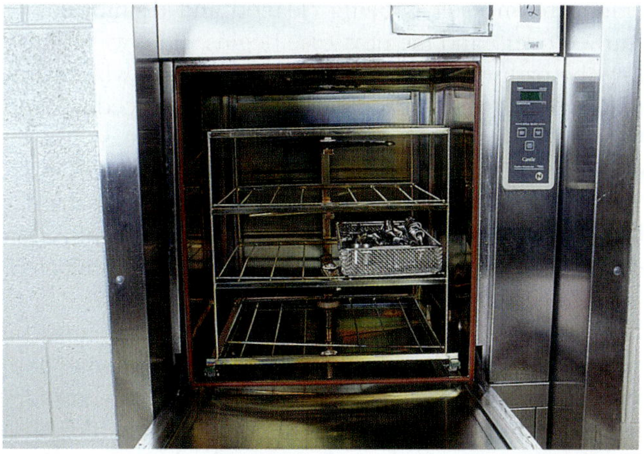

Figure 7-4 **Washer-sterilizer**

weekly, or monthly cleaning routines are followed. Obviously, certain parts of the above "circle" happen simultaneously. After initial cleaning of the instruments in the OR, the STSR usually delivers the instruments to the decontamination, or "dirty instrument," room, where they

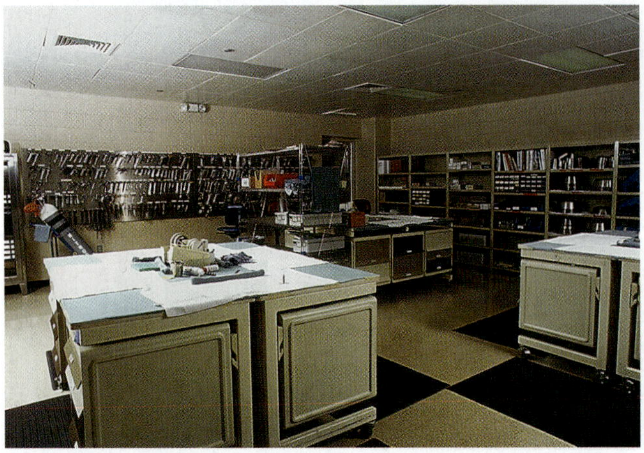

Figure 7-5 **Clean processing area**

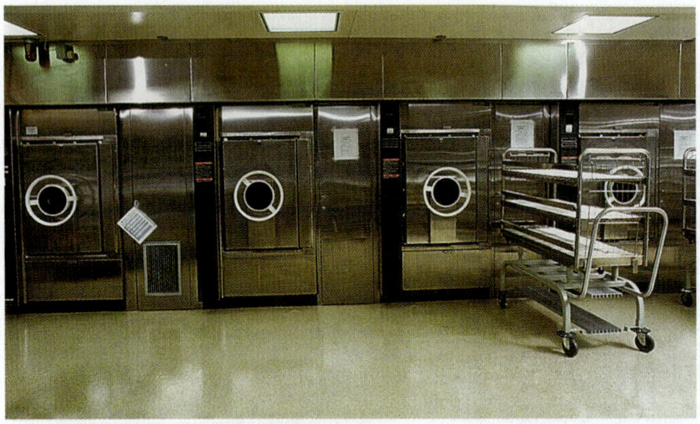

Figure 7-6 **Steam sterilization area**

may be processed by other personnel. While the instruments are being decontaminated and reprocessed, the operating room itself is being cleaned and disinfected, or "turned over," and the next case begins. Here we will follow the pathway of a typical case, beginning with instrument cleaning and disinfection after a procedure and following them through the sterilization process, finally ending with the cleaning and disinfection of the OR itself. To understand this flow, one must first understand the differences between cleaning, disinfection, and sterilization and which items in the OR must be cleaned, disinfected, sterilized, or all of the above prior to use.

Any item that will be used on open tissue must be sterile. All items that will be used in the sterile field should be sterilized, although certain instruments are heat sensitive and cannot withstand thermal sterilization. For these instruments, an alternative method of sterilization such as the hydrogen peroxide plasma (Sterrad) or peracetic acid (Steris) systems may be used (Figure 7-7). Some **endoscopes** and other sensitive equipment are disinfected (high level) in order to render them surgically clean. The OR itself is cleaned and furniture and floors are disinfected before and after each surgical procedure and according to a daily, weekly, and monthly schedule.

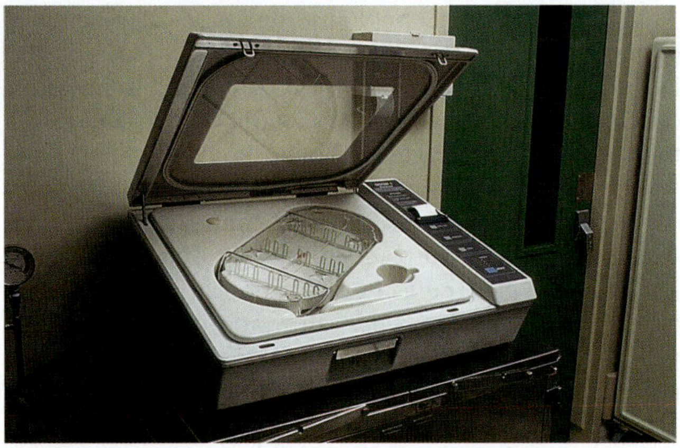

Figure 7-7 **Peracetic acid (Steris) sterilization system**

In this chapter we discuss cleaning, disinfection, and sterilization and the appropriate uses of each. Cleaning and decontamination involve removal of gross blood, debris, soil, and body fluids from an item:

- *Cleaning:* The physical removal of blood, body fluids, and/or gross debris (**bioburden**) from an inanimate object.
- *Disinfection:* Destruction of pathogenic microorganisms or their toxins or vectors by direct exposure to chemical or physical agents. Disinfection is discussed on three levels:
    - *High-level disinfection:* Kills all microorganisms except spores and may kill certain spores with sufficient contact time. Only sterilization assures that all spores are killed.
    - ***Intermediate-level disinfection***: Kills most microorganisms except spores.
    - *Low-level disinfection:* Kills fungi, bacteria, and hydrophilic viruses but is not effective against some viruses and is also ineffective against spores such as *M. tuberculosis.*
- *Sterilization:* Destruction of all microorganisms in or about an object, as by steam (flowing or pressurized), chemical agents (alcohol, phenol, heavy metals, ethylene oxide gas), high-velocity electron bombardment, or ultraviolet radiation.

CLEANING AND DISINFECTION

Cleaning is the physical removal of soil, debris, blood, and body fluids from instruments, furniture, or any item. Cleaning is necessary before disinfection, because organic debris decreases the effectiveness of disinfectants. Cleaning is an ongoing part of the environmental routine of the operative environment.

Prior to use or reuse in the OR, instruments are cleaned of gross contaminants, washed, and disinfected. They are then lubricated and inspected for damage and proper functioning prior to being assembled into sets and packaged for sterilization. The majority of surgical instruments are sterilized with steam, so here we focus on steam sterilization. However, because new instruments have been developed that are unable to withstand the heat and pressure of steam sterilization, alternative methods of sterilization have been developed.

Before the used instruments leave the OR, the surgical technologist should remove any gross contaminants. Some facilities use a spray disinfectant in the OR that neutralizes and breaks up blood and other gross contaminants.

During OR turnover between cases, and as part of daily, weekly, and monthly routine, cleaning is accomplished along with disinfection when floors, furniture, and equipment are decontaminated using mechanical cleaning and disinfecting agents. *Decontamination* is the process that combines cleaning and disinfection, such as the washing and disinfection of instruments after a case or the cleaning of the floor with a disinfecting agent.

Instruments are further cleaned in the decontamination, or dirty instrument, area, where they are taken after each case. Instruments should either be transported in a case-cart system or carefully covered according to hospital protocol prior to transport from the operating suite to the decontamination area.

Decontamination of instruments is accomplished by manual cleaning of instruments or by manually cleaning instruments of gross debris and cycling them through an ultrasonic washer and in some cases a washer-sterilizer. Decontamination is the first step in the prevention of transmission of microbes from instruments to patient or from instruments to personnel and renders the instruments safe for handling by OR and sterile processing personnel.

The decontamination room is a separate area, usually in proximity to the clean sterile processing area. The design of the decontamination area environment should follow these principles:

- Filtered air is exhausted to the outside of the health care facility.
- The minimum air exchange rate is 10 times per hour.
- Temperature should be maintained between 64 and 70°F with a humidity of 35% to 72%.
- Negative air pressure is maintained.

Cleaning of items manually or mechanically is the first step when instruments arrive in the decontamination area. Various detergents, enzymes, and cleaning agents are used to lower surface tension, break down fat, oil, and grease, break soil into fine particles, and suspend particles during the cleaning process to aid in soil removal. After initial cleaning, instruments are disinfected.

A direct relationship exists between the number (bioburden) and type of microbes present on an item and the length of time necessary to achieve proper disinfection. It is important for contaminated items to be thoroughly cleaned prior the decontamination process. By reducing the number of microbes, less time is required for the disinfectant to kill the remaining microbes. Thorough cleaning before disinfection cannot be overemphasized. The presence of organic material and debris such as blood and tissue will prevent direct contact of the disinfectant solution. The presence of gross contaminants can also inactivate disinfectant solutions.

DETERGENTS

Detergents are selected according to the type of instrument to be cleaned. The manufacturer's instructions must always be followed for correct dilution, temperature, and use. A neutral-pH detergent should be used for the manual cleaning of surgical instruments because strong detergents may damage instruments. A slightly more alkaline detergent is usually used when using automatic machines. This compensates for the lack of friction achieved with manual cleaning. Low-sudsing detergents must be used in mechanical equipment to avoid damage to the equipment.

The pH scale is used to indicate the acidity or alkalinity of a substance. Levels of pH are measured on a scale from 0 (highly acidic) to 14 (highly alkaline). Distilled water is considered neutral and has a pH of 7. The scale from 0 to 14 is logarithmic, meaning that a pH of 8 is 10 times more alkaline than a pH of 7 and a pH of 9 is 100 times more alkaline than a pH of 7. Cleaning agents with either a high pH or a low pH are damaging to metals, rubber, and plastics and may cause pitting and staining of metal instruments, leading to corrosion. Instruments should be rinsed with distilled or demineralized water and then dried. The use of distilled water (neutral pH) for rinsing adds years to the life of surgical instruments and prevents mineral residue buildup.

The following are general guidelines and concepts for use when cleaning items and using disinfectants:

1. Items must be thoroughly rinsed and/or cleaned before disinfectant is used. Blood, tissue, soil, and other body fluids interfere with the action of disinfectants.
2. Items with multiple parts must be disassembled before cleaning.
3. The foundation of manual cleaning is friction. Friction will loosen the organic material to allow its removal during the rinsing process.
4. The steps of the cleaning process are as follows:
   a. Transport from the point of use to the decontamination area.
   b. Sort instruments by type and weight so large instruments do not damage small, delicate ones during cleaning.
   c. Disassemble (if necessary).
   d. Soak with H_2O plus enzymatic solution followed by disinfectant solution.
   e. Sterilization—manual or mechanical washing (e.g., ultrasonic and washer-decontaminator or washer-sterilizer)—takes place in

washer-sterilizer, if used, or instruments are soaked in disinfectant to decontaminate.
f. Rinse.
g. Lubricate (milking).
h. Dry.
i. Inspect and reassemble.
j. Package and prepare for sterilization.

5. When cleaning stainless steel instruments, a back-and-forth motion should be used to follow the grain of the instrument, rather than a circular motion, which can scratch the surface of the item.
6. To avoid spotting on the instruments, the items should be immediately dried after rinsing.

The first step in the decontamination process actually begins at the point of use. The individuals who used the instruments and equipment are responsible for keeping the items moist to prevent the drying of organic material. They are also responsible for placing the items in some type of closed container for safe transport to the decontamination area. The following solutions may be used for soaking the instruments:

1. Tap water; do not use saline. The salt will pit the stainless steel finish on the instrument, permanently damaging the instrument and leading to the formation of rust.
2. Enzymatic solution:
   a. Proteolytic enzymatic cleaner: Facilitates the removal of protein materials such as blood.
   b. Lipolytic enzymatic cleaner: Facilitates the removal of fatty materials such as adipose tissue and bone marrow.
3. Detergent solutions.

As with most situations, there are advantages and limitations to the use of presoaking solutions (Table 7-6).

When cleaning instruments, organic and inorganic soil may be removed through one of the following methods, depending on the type of cleaning solution used:

- ***Chelation***: The process of binding ions, such as iron and magnesium, in the solution to prevent their deposit on the surface of surgical instruments, causing spotting.
- *Enzymatic:* Enzymes are catalysts that aid in breaking down organic soil such as blood and tissue into solution.
- ***Emulsification***: The action of dispersing two liquids that are not capable of being mixed.
- *Solubilization:* The action by which the solubility of a substance is increased within a solution.

Table 7-7 shows the common types of chemical cleaners.

CLEANING/DISINFECTION (MACHINES NOT AVAILABLE)

If mechanical methods of cleaning and decontamination are not available, the items must be manually or hand cleaned. PPE must be worn for this process. It is recommended that delicate instruments always be manually cleaned and decontaminated to preserve the integrity of the instruments. The purpose of manual cleaning is to physically remove debris that was not removed or softened during the presoak. Ideally, a three-sink arrangement is utilized as follows:

- *First sink:* Wash sink with water and detergent or disinfectant detergent solution.
- *Second sink:* Intermediate rinse with distilled water.
- *Third sink:* Final rinse with distilled water.

The manual cleaning of instruments is a three-step process:

1. Instruments are immersed in a solution of water, detergent, and/or enzymatic cleaner with a neutral pH. The enzymatic cleaner is to aid in the removal of bioburden. Each instrument must be individually cleaned with a soft-bristled brush in order to apply friction to loosen the organic debris. The instrument and brush must be kept submerged in the solution while cleaning to avoid contaminated water droplets from aerosolizing. Particular attention must be directed toward serrations on jaws, ratchets, box locks, and teeth of forceps. Instruments with lumens may be cleaned with a tube brush, pipe cleaner, or hand-held water pressure gun. The cleaning solution should be changed frequently to avoid buildup of microbes and soil.

Table 7-6 Advantages and Limitations of Presoaking Solutions

SOLUTION	ADVANTAGES	LIMITATIONS
Tap water	Keeps organic debris moist.	Ineffective in softening or removing dried debris.
Enzyme	Removes moistened and dried debris without the need for mechanical action.	Efficiency depends on concentration of solution, temperature, and contact time.
Detergent	Keeps organic debris moist while loosening dried-on debris.	Mechanical action necessary to completely remove soil.

Table 7-7 Common Chemical Cleaners

TYPE	CHARACTERISTICS
Enzymatic	Organic substance that aids in the chemical reaction of breaking down organic debris. As previously stated, enzymes are specific to the type of debris to be removed. Enzymes are usually used as a soaking solution. They require dilution and are more effective in warm water than cold because the temperature of the warm water increases the speed of the chemical reaction.
Ultrasonic	Cleaning solutions are manufactured specifically for use in ultrasonic cleaners. The solution may contain a surfactant to enhance wetting ability and chelating agents.
Manual detergent	Products usually used for hand cleaning of items and/or for presoaking. Some of the manual cleaners are high foaming and therefore should not be used in mechanical cleaning equipment. They must be diluted for use but are safe to use on most materials, including stainless steel. Mechanical action is required to assist in removing the soil. Surgical instruments must be thoroughly rinsed after being placed in the detergent.
Washer-decontaminator	Liquid solution that is available in three different pH levels. *Neutral-pH product:* Least corrosive to surgical instruments but less effective at removing substantial amount of organic soil. *Moderate-pH product:* Low level of alkaline and may be combined with surfactant and chelating agents. Safe for use on stainless steel instruments but could be harmful to the chromium oxide layer that protects the instruments from corrosion. *High-pH product:* Most effective for removing heavy amounts of soil. Can be corrosive to stainless steel. If used, it must be neutralized by a neutralizing rinse to prevent damage to the instruments.

2. Cleaning should be repeated using a disinfectant agent. The instruments should have wet contact with the disinfectant for the length of time recommended by the manufacturer (see disinfection sections of this chapter).
3. The last step is to rinse the instruments in distilled water. Do not use tap water due to the presence of minerals that can stain and form a film on the instruments when the tap water evaporates.

MACHINE DECONTAMINATION

To protect individuals responsible for the decontamination of surgical instruments and equipment, some health care institutions have purchased mechanical cleaning equipment to eliminate manual cleaning. The types of cleaning equipment include washer-sterilizer, washer-decontaminator, and ultrasonic washer. Instruments must be placed into a perforated or wire mesh tray to prevent interference with the cleaning action of the machine. Heavier instruments should be placed on the bottom of the tray to avoid damage to the lighter, more delicate instruments. Hinged instruments must be left in an open position to allow water, cleaning agent, and steam to contact the total surface area. Instruments with attachments must be disassembled. Instruments with concave surfaces should be placed upside down to allow proper cleaning, rinsing, steam contact, and drainage.

Ultrasonic Washer

The ultrasonic washer (UW) is utilized to remove small organic particles and soil from areas of instrumentation that manual or mechanical cleaning cannot reach. These areas include box locks, serrations, and ratchets. Before items are placed in the UW, gross soil must be removed or the large particles of soil will absorb the energy generated by the machine. The UW utilizes the process of cavitation for cleaning instruments. Cavitation works as follows:

- The machine works by using high-frequency sound waves that are converted to vibrations in the solution.
- As the ultrasonic waves travel through the cleaning agent, the energy causes the molecules to be set in rapid motion, forming microscopic bubbles on the surface of the instruments.
- The bubbles enlarge, become unstable, and implode (collapse inward). The implosion creates a vacuum dislodging minute particles of soil and organic material from the instruments.

Ultrasonic washing is not considered a true disinfecting process but rather a method of cleaning instrumentation. The cleaning solution must be frequently changed due to the increase of bioburden with each use. The UW process creates fine aerosols that may contain microbes harmful to personnel. Whenever the UW is in operation, the lid must be closed.

Various types of UWs are on the market. Models consist of one, two, or three chambers. For the three-chamber unit, the first chamber is for cleaning, the second chamber is for spray rinsing the instruments, and the third is for hot air drying. The rinse and dry cycles are combined in the second chamber in a two-chamber UW. Each cycle lasts approximately 4–5 minutes.

Two theories exist concerning when the UW should be used. Some support the use of the washer-sterilizer prior to placement of instruments in the UW in order to remove microbial contaminants that might be aerosolized and present a hazard to personnel. However, the use of the washer-sterilizer prior to the ultrasonic cleaner may leave some contaminants and gross soil baked on the instruments. Some facilities wash gross soil off of the instruments and then place them in the ultrasonic cleaner prior to the washer-sterilizer. Facility policy and procedure will govern when the UW should be used.

Instruments to be processed through the UW are to be placed in a metal mesh tray. The tray is immersed in a solution of warm water and a low-sudsing, free-rinse detergent with a neutral pH in the first chamber. When the solution is changed and the chamber refilled, it is necessary to run one empty cycle. Gas bubbles form during the filling and will absorb the ultrasonic energy generated by the machine, decreasing the cleaning effectiveness. Running an empty cycle degasses the chamber.

Washer-Decontaminator

The washer-decontaminator (WD) is similar to the washer-sterilizer, except the sterilizing phase is eliminated. The cycle of the WD is as follows:

1. *Prerinse cycle:* Some models allow the use of an enzymatic solution in this phase.
2. *Cleaning cycle:* Detergent solution is used in this cycle.
3. *Final rinse:* Hot water is used during this rinse. The water temperature is maintained at 180–195°F.
4. *Dry phase:* High temperature is used to dry the instruments.

Some models add an ultrasonic cleaning phase after the cleaning cycle and/or a chemical disinfectant rinse. These units allow totally hands-off processing. Instruments that are placed in perforated or mesh-bottom trays can come directly from the point of use, such as the OR, and be placed in the WD without any further handling or arranging of instruments by decontamination personnel.

At the conclusion of the cycle, items are considered clean and have been exposed to an intermediate level of disinfection. This makes the items safe for handling but not necessarily ready for immediate use.

Washer-Sterilizer

A majority of stainless steel surgical instruments and heat-tolerant items can be processed through the washer-sterilizer (WS). After gross soil is removed, the items may be processed in the WS. Always consult the manufacturer's instructions for operating the WS and for arrangement of the instrument trays inside the machine. If the soil is not removed or instruments are improperly arranged, the remaining soil may not be removed during the wash phase and could be baked on during the sterilization phase, possibly damaging the stainless steel and making the removal of such baked-on materials difficult.

Stainless steel instruments should not be placed next to instruments made of other metals, such as brass or copper (some uterine sounds are still made of copper). An electrolytic conduction reaction can occur when two different metals come into contact in a wet, hot environment such as the WS chamber. The reaction causes one metal to plate to the other and may permanently damage instruments.

A free-rinsing, low-sudsing detergent with a neutral pH should be used. High-sudsing detergent will leave residue on instruments and may cause overflow of detergent solution and decrease the efficiency of the pumps within the machine.

Some types of WSs require the detergent to be added manually with each load; others are designed with a system that automatically adds the detergent when required. A typical WS cycle is as follows:

1. *Prerinse:* A continuous spray rinse aids in removing organic and soil matter such as blood and tissue.
2. *Automatic detergent injection:* The machine injects a measured amount of detergent into the chamber.
3. *Fill phase:* Chamber is filled with water for total instrument immersion and cleaning.
4. *Wash phase:* Water is agitated inside chamber for soil removal; the machine controls water temperature.
5. *Postrinse:* Loose soil and detergent film are rinsed off items.
6. *Sterilization phase:* Steam sterilization cycle—this is usually a gravity cycle.
7. *Lubrication (milking).*
8. *Dry phase.*

Two types of WS machines are commercially available. The first type is a tunnel-like chamber with a door at each end and rotating sprayer arms that distribute the liquid detergent agent from multiple directions during the wash phase. The second type is the horizontal/cabinet type and has a door at one or both ends of the chamber. This design allows for the use of standard instrument trays that also allow easier and efficient loading/unloading of the chamber. The chamber fills with water and detergent, not relying on rotating sprayer arms. Steam and air are injected through the solution, producing a turbulent action, which loosens the soil and produces the washing action. As the heated water expands and rises within the chamber, the loose soil overflows into the waste pipe line. The automatic program control activates the steam inlet valve to open and the water outlet valve to open. The steam enters at the top of the chamber, forcing the water out, and the sterilization cycle begins. The steam sterilization cycle is a gravity cycle at 270°F.

Although a steam sterilization cycle is the last step of the WS, items still should not be considered ready for use on patients. Because this is not a monitored process, instruments must be sterilized after this cycle. Prior to final sterilization they are inspected for damage and cleanliness, lubricated, assembled into sets, and packaged for sterilization and storage. We will examine the sterilization process further, but first we will look at disinfectant and disinfectant/sterilant agents, environmental decontamination, and the care of special instruments.

DISINFECTANT AND DISINFECTANT/STERILANT AGENTS

The reader will note that several disinfectant agents have been mentioned. This section provides an overview of disinfectant agents and their actions. Manufacturer directions should always be followed, particularly when a disinfectant/sterilant agent is to be used. Additionally, the use of PPE may be necessary according to the Material Safety Data Sheet (MSDS) when utilizing various chemicals.

Disinfection is defined on page 142 at three levels: high-, intermediate-, and low-level disinfection. High-level disinfection is used when items are to be used on tissue or in body cavities. The other levels are detailed in Table 7-8.

DISINFECTANT EFFICIENCY

Certain disinfectant compounds also serve as sterilants when used in sterilization systems (e.g., hydrogen peroxide, peracetic acid) or when used according to manufacturer's directions as a sterilant when adequate exposure time is allowed (e.g., glutaraldehyde).

A number of factors influence the efficiency of disinfectants. These include

- Concentration level of disinfectant solution
- Number and type of microbes present, including gross contamination (bioburden)
- Contact time
- Physical factors (exposure time, temperature, etc.)

While high concentrations of active ingredients in disinfectants increase the level of disinfection they can provide, high concentrations may be too corrosive for use on certain items.

A direct relationship exists between the number and type of microbes present on an item and the length of time necessary to achieve proper disinfection. It is important for contaminated items to be thoroughly cleaned prior to the decontamination process. By reducing the number of microbes, less time is required for the disinfectant to kill the remaining microbes.

For a disinfectant to be efficient, it must come into direct contact with all surface areas of the item and thus into contact with all microorganisms present on the item. Instruments that have multiple parts must be disassembled to allow the disinfectant to contact all parts. All ratchets and box locks must be opened to expose all surface areas. When disinfectants are being used in environmental settings (e.g., furniture), all surfaces must be wiped with the disinfectant agent.

Thorough cleaning before disinfection cannot be overemphasized. The presence of organic material and

Table 7-8 Disinfectant Uses and Classification

LEVEL	EFFECTIVE AGAINST	INEFFECTIVE AGAINST	USE ON	EXAMPLES
High	All microorganisms except spores	Spores	Critical items—used in sterile tissue or body cavity	Surgical instruments, implants, hypodermic needles
Intermediate	Fungi, bacteria, hydrophilic viruses, *M. tuberculosis*, and HBV	Spores	Semicritical items—come into contact with mucous membranes or nonintact skin but not used in sterile tissue or body cavity	Cystoscopes, colonoscopes, laryngoscopes
Low	Fungi, bacteria, hydrophilic viruses	Some viruses, such as *M. tuberculosis*, and spores	Noncritical items—contact only environmental surfaces and unbroken skin	Blood pressure cuff, OR furniture, operating tables

debris (bioburden) such as blood and tissue will prevent direct contact of the disinfectant solution. The presence of gross contaminants can also inactivate disinfectant solutions.

Various types of disinfectants will vary in their ability to kill microbes and the types of microbes that will be destroyed. Twenty to 30 minutes of contact time is generally recommended for high-level disinfection. Low and intermediate levels of disinfection can be generally achieved in 10–15 minutes.

Physical and chemical factors that affect the efficiency include:

Physical

- Temperature
- Presence of gross debris and high concentration of microbes (bioburden)

Chemical

- pH
- Water hardness

Generally, increasing the temperature speeds up the rate of the chemical process; hence, a rise in temperature will hasten the disinfection process. However, manufacturer instructions for temperature must be strictly followed. Failure to adhere to the instructions could result in possible health hazards to the health care worker and also accelerate the degradation of the disinfecting solution. Standard Precautions, including the use of proper PPE, should always be adhered to.

HIGH-LEVEL DISINFECTANT AND STERILANT COMPOUNDS AND STERILIZATION METHODS

This section looks at high-level disinfectant solutions, which when used within a carefully designed cleaning system can be used for the sterilization of instruments. While the methods for sterilization vary, the principle is the same, and all pathogens must be destroyed. (For a more in-depth overview of the theories and practices of sterilization, see the section on steam and/or alternative sterilization techniques in this chapter.)

Glutaraldehyde

Glutaraldehyde, 2% concentration with a pH of 7.5–6.5, is a high-level disinfectant. Its common commercial name is Cidex. Glutaraldehyde has been recognized as one of the best overall sterilant/disinfectants available on the market. Glutaraldehyde has the following characteristics:

Action

- Alkylation of cell protein

Advantages

- Used as disinfectant, it is bactericidal against gram-positive and gram-negative vegetative microbes, tuberculocidal, fungicidal, virucidal; sporicidal as a sterilizing agent
- Noncorrosive to metals
- Noncorrosive to lensed and cemented items
- Noncorrosive to rubber and plastic

Disadvantages

- Noxious odor
- Has vapors that can cause irritation of the eyes and mucous membranes of the nose and respiratory tract
- Unstable, expiration date for use
- Items to be disinfected must be cleaned prior to immersion

Glutaraldehyde is used for devices that can withstand complete liquid **immersion**. The liquid must contact all surface areas of the item, including lumens. Rigid and flexible endoscopes are two examples of surgical instruments frequently decontaminated or sterilized using glutaraldehyde.

Glutaraldehyde has an established shelf life. *Shelf life* is defined as the period of time between activation, mixing of the alkaline buffer with the glutaraldehyde, and disposal. For products without a surfactant, the shelf life is 14 days; it is increased to 28 days for products with a surfactant. The concentration of glutaraldehyde must be frequently tested during the 14- or 28-day period to determine if it has reached a point of no use based on dilution by organic soil and in-use dilution. Commercially produced test strips are available to test the concentration. If concentration falls below 1%, the solution should not be used. To avoid dilution, items should be dry before immersion in glutaraldehyde. A minimum exposure of 20 minutes at room temperature is required for disinfection.

All items disinfected with glutaraldehyde must be rinsed thoroughly with sterile water before use on a patient. Failure to rinse thoroughly may lead to patient burns. Do not use tap water for rinsing because this will contaminate the item. Goggles or protective glasses and barrier-proof gloves, such as neoprene rubber gloves, must be worn when mixing or using glutaraldehyde. The use of respirators to avoid the inhalation of fumes is also recommended. Avoid placing unprotected hands in liquid. Activated glutaraldehyde must be stored in a covered container and well-ventilated room. Some health care facilities have installed fume hoods over glutaraldehyde containers to remove the vapors.

Most solutions of activated glutaraldehyde require exposure times of 10 hours for sterilization and 20 minutes for high-level disinfection.

6% Hydrogen Peroxide

Solutions of 6% hydrogen peroxide (H_2O_2) with detergents and 0.85% phosphoric acid have been proven to be sporicidal with 6 hours of exposure at 20°C and can therefore be considered a sterilant. This solution can be used on stainless steel instruments and is also safe for plastic, rubber, and glass. Skin and eyes of personnel should be protected with proper PPE, because this is an acidic solution.

Peracetic Acid (Steris) Sterilization

Peracetic acid is a strong sterilant and should be handled carefully, because this compound has been shown to promote skin tumors in mice. This sterilant is usually used in a machine (Steris) that heats the sterilant to about 50°C and can be used to sterilize endoscopes (both flexible and rigid). This cycle usually takes 30 minutes, including a rinse cycle. Water used for rinsing is filtered of all bacteria to render instruments sterile. Because the sterilant can only be used for a single sterilization cycle, this method of sterilization is more expensive, but it is useful for instruments that would be difficult to sterilize otherwise. Products sterilized with the hydrogen peroxide system cannot be stored, because they are sterilized in the system cassette itself. Therefore, items sterilized in this fashion are for immediate use only.

Chlorine Compounds

Chlorine compounds in dilute form (household bleach) are an effective disinfectant for surfaces, floors, and equipment. A 1:10 dilution of 5% bleach is sporicidal in 1 hour at room temperature and can therefore be used to render floors and equipment virtually sterile. Chlorine compounds are bactericidal, virucidal, and tuberculocidal and are effective against HIV, HBV, and other viruses.

Commercially available chlorine sterilants include chlorine dioxide and chlorous acid. These sterilant/disinfectants are corrosive to some metals, rubber, and plastics. Because of this, chlorine compounds are usually used for tabletop and floor sanitation. Because these solutions are unstable and lose their effectiveness rapidly when organic soil is present, a fresh solution should be prepared daily.

Immersion Times and Temperatures

Immersion times and temperatures vary with the different sterilants. These are summarized in Table 7-9.

INTERMEDIATE-LEVEL DISINFECTANTS

These disinfectants are not capable of killing spores and cannot kill certain types of viruses, but they do kill all bacteria. They are unable to kill certain hydrophilic viruses, but they do kill all others, and they kill all fungi. Because these compounds are intermediate-level disinfectants, they are used to disinfect countertops, OR furniture, floors and other surfaces, and instruments that only come into contact with the skin of the patient.

Phenolic Compounds

Phenolic compounds are based on modifications of pure phenol compounds. They denature enzymes and lyse cells, thus bringing about microorganism death. Phenolic compounds are usually used as a concentrate with detergent additives that is diluted 1:64 with tap water.

Phenol is a skin irritant and should be used with proper PPE for personnel safety. Phenol disinfectants are mostly odorless and can be used to disinfect large areas like floors and countertops. Because phenol disinfectants can be highly concentrated and then diluted for use, they are an economical choice for disinfectant use in the OR. Phenol is especially effective in eliminating fecal contamination.

Quaternary Ammonium Compounds

These compounds, commonly called *quats,* cause leakage in the protoplasm of some microorganisms, especially bacteria. They are bactericidal, tuberculocidal, and fungicidal but not sporicidal. They are not virucidal to hydrophilic viruses.

The use of quats is diminishing, because their biocidal effect is easily reversed with contact with organic debris, tap water, and detergents. In addition, gauze or fabrics absorb the disinfectant ingredient, minimizing their usefulness for mopping or wiping surfaces. Some facilities consider quaternary ammonium compounds low-level disinfectants because of their inability to kill TB, spores, or hydrophilic viruses and their vulnerability to inactivation.

Table 7-9 Immersion Times for Sterilization

AGENT	TIME	TEMPERATURE
Glutaraldehyde (Cidex)	10 hours	Room temperature
6% Hydrogen peroxide + 0.85% phosphoric acid	6 hours	20°C
Peracetic acid (Steris)	12 minutes exposure (machine cycle 30 minutes)	55°C

Iodophors

Iodophors are formulations of iodine complexed with a carrier molecule. When diluted, free iodine disassociates from the carrier molecule and oxidizes to kill TB, viruses, bacteria, and fungi. Some personnel and patients with iodine allergies cannot tolerate contact with these compounds.

Iodophors are used as environmental disinfectants to clean floor surfaces, OR furniture, and walls. They are also used as surgical scrub solutions, and for preoperative skin preparation of the patient. Patients with allergic sensitivity to iodine and/or shellfish may have allergic reactions to iodophors, and iodophor use should be avoided with these patients.

Iodophors are corrosive to metal, and stain fabrics, tissue, and some hard-surface materials. Organic soils, hard water, or heat inactivates them. Because of their susceptibility to inactivation, iodophor solutions should be replaced daily.

Alcohol

Isopropyl and ethyl alcohols in formulations of 50–90% alcohol concentration are tuberculocidal, bactericidal, mostly virucidal, and fungicidal. They are not sporicidal. This disinfectant is flammable and therefore is most useful for cleaning and disinfecting small noncritical surface areas. Recent studies show that these alcohol compounds may be as effective or more effective than other compounds for use in skin disinfection for surgical scrub and preoperative preparation. Further studies are warranted.

As the reader can see, disinfectants/sterilants vary widely in their effectiveness against microbes, toxicity, and chemical stability. Hospital protocols should be developed for use of these solutions, so that the proper selection and use of these compounds for cleaning ORs, equipment, and critical surgical instrumentation minimize risk of infection to patients.

These compounds are not only used in environmental and instrument decontamination but also in certain sterilization processes, such as the peracetic acid process used in the Steris sterilization system. Manufacturer's instructions should be carefully followed in these systems and in each brand of activated glutaraldehyde system to ensure sterilization. Alternative methods of sterilization are discussed after steam sterilization, including hydrogen peroxide gas/plasma (Sterrad) sterilization and EtO (ethylene oxide) gas sterilization. In addition, ionizing radiation (gamma or cobalt 60) may be used for the sterilization of surgical instruments. Ionizing radiation is usually used in mass production sterilization facilities rather than in hospital settings.

INSTRUMENTS REQUIRING SPECIAL CARE IN CLEANING

Items with lumens such as trocar sheaths, nondisposable suction tips, and endoscopic instruments require special care to ensure adequate decontamination. Blood and tissue can be difficult to remove from lumens, especially if dried. Items may have to soak in an enzymatic solution for a period of time to loosen the debris. The lumen should be flushed until the fluid emerges clear. Hydrogen peroxide is an excellent flushing agent to rid the lumen of blood. The peroxide will react with the blood by producing foam that will disappear when the blood has been thoroughly rinsed away. The lumen must then be rinsed with distilled water to flush away the hydrogen peroxide.

A number of surgical procedures, particularly orthopedic procedures, require the use of powered instruments such as saws and drills. Powered instruments must never be submerged in cleaning solution or placed in any type of mechanical decontaminating equipment. Manufacturer's instructions for cleaning must be followed. General instructions are as follows:

1. Leave the air hose attached to the power handle while cleaning. This will prevent any cleaning solution or rinsing water from entering into the cord or handle.
2. Wash off the cord (hose) with lukewarm water using a neutral detergent, cloth, or soft-bristled brush. Hold the end of the hose not attached to the power handle downward to allow water to run off and not enter the hose.
3. The handle is wiped down using a cloth or soft-bristled brush, lukewarm water, and neutral detergent.
4. All components are rinsed with distilled water and wiped dry.

There are two types of endoscopes: flexible and rigid. The following are general recommendations for the decontamination of both types.

Rigid Endoscopes

1. Channels, holes, and joints must be thoroughly cleaned and rinsed to remove blood and debris.
2. Soaking of the endoscope in an enzymatic solution is recommended.
3. A handheld water pressure gun for washing and compressed air for drying will aid in the cleaning process. The endoscope must be dry before storage to prevent bacterial growth.
4. The detergent should be one that the manufacturer recommends.
5. Care should be taken not to damage the delicate eyepiece, which can be easily scratched.

Flexible Endoscopes

1. Flexible endoscopes have many channels that require cleaning. Examples include the suction, biopsy, and air/water channels. Cleaning brushes on the end of long, thin, flexible wires are available to clean the channels.
2. If recommended by the manufacturer, soaking the endoscope in an enzymatic solution with the channel ports open will help in the cleaning process.
3. The exterior of the scope should be cleaned with a neutral detergent and a soft brush or cloth.

LUBRICATION

Surgical instruments must be lubricated to maintain optimal function. Special surgical instrument lubricants are available and should be used on a schedule developed by the facility to lubricate surfaces and box locks of instruments. This process is commonly called *milking,* since the lubricant solution is usually white in color. Instruments are lubricated prior to sterilization and usually prior to being assembled in sets.

INSTRUMENT PREPARATION AND WRAPPING FOR STERILIZATION

Instruments must be cleaned, checked for function and integrity, and prepared for sterilization. This activity takes place in a room designed for that purpose and commonly referred to as a *clean room.*

INSTRUMENTS

Preparation for sterilization of instruments begins after decontamination and involves the following steps:

1. Inspection
2. Reassembly
3. Preparation

The items to be sterilized must first be inspected for blood and soil remnants that may be left after decontamination. Traditional surgical instruments (e.g., scissors, Crile hemostats, Kocher clamps) can be easily inspected under normal lighting. More complex devices, such as endoscopic instrumentation, contain areas that are more difficult to reach while cleaning and require thorough inspection.

Instrument function must be determined for repair or replacement. The following are general guidelines to follow for functional testing:

1. The cutting edges of scissors should have no burs or cracks. The blades should close smoothly. Scissors should be sharp enough to cut two 4 × 4 sponges with little effort.
2. The instrument's ratchet must be checked to ensure that it locks properly and will not spring open. If the instrument is tapped lightly in the palm of the hand and the ratchet remains closed, then the ratchet is working properly.
3. The jaws of clamps should close evenly with no gaps and the tips should be evenly lined.
4. Forceps should close evenly with tips evenly lined. Tissue forceps' teeth should fit smoothly in the groove of the opposite side.
5. Ratchets on self-retaining retractors should be checked to make sure they remain locked in the open position and release with little effort.
6. The points on nondisposable trocars should be inspected for burs, cracks, scratches, or bends. Dull or burred trocars make insertion difficult.
7. Manufacturers' instructions must be followed for proper inspection of powered instruments. The instrument may need to be lubricated and operated for a designated amount of time for lubricant distribution. The power hose should be checked for cracks and cuts.

Reassembly of instruments with more than one piece may be necessary before sterilizing. However, most surgical instruments, such as the Balfour retractor, should not be reassembled so that the sterilant can reach all surface areas.

Items must be properly prepared for effective sterilization. Proper preparation will ensure that

- The sterilant comes into contact with all surface areas.
- The instruments are positioned in a protective manner until they are used.
- The instruments are evenly distributed.

SPECIFIC PROCEDURAL TRAYS

Surgical instruments may be prepared for procedural trays that are designated for a specific procedure. Examples include cut-down trays, suture trays, and tracheotomy/tracheostomy trays. Only a few instruments are required in the assembly of these specialty trays, and most are assembled on a stainless steel, perforated tray.

Procedural trays can be laid flat on the sterilizing cart since the trays are perforated. This also prevents the contents from scattering inside the tray.

INSTRUMENT SETS

Instruments should be placed in a mesh-bottom or wire mesh basket with an absorbent towel lining the bottom.

A nonwoven disposable wrapper should not be used to line the tray because the water-repellent nature of the wrapper will cause moisture to pool at the bottom. The instruments should be evenly distributed within the basket for balance. Instruments can be placed on a "string" (two metal rods inserted through the finger rings of the instruments) or secured with clips and pins that can be used to maintain the instruments in an open, fixed position. Some facilities still use two ring forceps inserted through the instrument finger holes and secured with towel clips.

The instruments should be placed into the tray in the open position (ratchets unlocked) so that the sterilant can reach the areas between the ratchets. Instruments of like size, shape, and function should be grouped together on the string to help the user quickly identify and retrieve the instruments needed for the surgical procedure.

Microsurgical instruments can be easily damaged if not properly arranged in preparation for sterilization. Special trays lined with molded plastic mats or pins and locking lids are commercially available to secure and protect these delicate instruments.

Instruments with lumens, such as the Frazier suction tip, require special preparation. Air trapped in the lumen may prevent steam from contacting the inner surface. To prevent this entrapment of air, a residual amount of distilled water should be left inside the lumen of the instrument. The water will boil during sterilization, turning to steam and displacing the air within the lumen. This technique is especially important if gravity displacement steam sterilization is utilized.

Instruments with concave surfaces also warrant special preparation for sterilization. Examples include bone curettes, bone rongeurs, and gallstone scoops. To prevent moisture and air from being trapped within the concave surface, the instruments should be placed on their sides for sterilization.

Loose instruments are instruments that are not on a string but are arranged in the pan's bottom and include forceps, retractors, knife handles, and suction tips. These instruments should not be grouped together in a pile and/or wrapped. Instrument grouping and excessive metal contact will inhibit the ability of the sterilant to contact all surfaces and may allow condensate to collect.

Larger loose instruments, such as Deaver retractors, Richardson retractors, and long forceps, should be arranged within the pan so that movement is minimized and should not be placed one upon the other. The heavier instruments should be placed on the bottom of the tray or at one end of the tray to avoid damaging other, more delicate instruments. In some instances, an absorbent towel can be used to separate layers of instruments within the tray to aid in absorbing moisture and drying. The two-basket system is ideal in that it not only evenly distributes the weight of the set but also increases the contact surface area.

It is important to remember that the manufacturers of instrument containers generally recommend that instrument trays not exceed 16 pounds. The instrument trays and/or containers should be laid flat on the shelves of the sterilizing cart.

PACKAGING FOR STERILIZATION AND STORAGE

Packaging refers to the various types of materials available for the wrapping and packaging of reusable items so they can be safely sterilized and stored until used. The Food and Drug Administration (FDA) lists sterilization wraps, also known as central supply room (CSR) wraps, as Class II medical devices. The Federal Food, Drug, and Cosmetic Act states that "the prime purpose and function of a packaging material (pack, sterilization wrapper, bag, or accessories) is to enclose a medical device that is to be sterilized by a health care provider. It is intended to allow sterilization of the enclosed device and also to maintain sterility of the device until it is used."

PERFORMANCE STANDARDS OF PACKAGING MATERIAL

Packaging material must meet three performance standards:

- The packaging material must be able to maintain the sterility of the items up until use.
- The packaging material should permit the package to be opened in a manner that allows for easy removal of the sterile items without contamination.
- The packaging material should allow the sterilizing agent to penetrate and reach all surface areas of the items to be sterilized.

PERFORMANCE CHARACTERISTICS

Packaging material must have the following performance characteristics when used for any sterilization method:

1. Efficiency
   a. The packaging material must be able to conform to the size and shape of the items, even when they are irregularly shaped.
   b. The packaging material must cover the contents in entirety.
   c. The packaging material should provide the maximum amount of use. For example, some wrappers are also utilized to establish a sterile field after the item is unwrapped. When used in this manner, the material must be flexible and memory free to prevent any folding back along the folding creases.

2. Ease of opening
   a. The packaging material should allow the package to be easily opened and transferred to the sterile field or point of use while maintaining sterility.
3. Sterilization suitability
   a. The material must allow air to be completely removed from the package.
   b. The material must be able to withstand the physical conditions produced by the autoclave (moisture, pressure, and high temperatures).
   c. The material must allow for the escape of the sterilizing agent at the end of the sterilization cycle.
   d. The packaging material must allow the contents and material to be dried after steam sterilization.
   e. The packaging material must allow the gas and moisture to escape during the aeration cycle after ethylene oxide sterilization.
4. Strength
   a. The packaging material should resist tears and punctures during normal handling and sterilization.
   b. The packaging material should not easily degrade when sterile packages are stored.
   c. The packaging material should not develop holes at the folds or corners after placement in storage.
   d. The packaging material seals must not deteriorate and spontaneously open when in storage.
5. Barrier efficiency
   a. The packaging material should provide a barrier to the penetration of dust and particles and should resist moisture penetration.
   b. The packaging material should be lint free to prevent contamination of the sterile items.
6. Impermeability
   a. The packaging material must not contain any toxic material or dyes that could produce a reaction during the sterilization process. This toxic residue could be harmful to the patient and individuals handling the sterile items.
   b. The packaging material must not contain dyes that could "bleed" onto the items and cause discoloration.
   c. Items to be sterilized, including rigid instrument containers, must be rinsed free of detergents or other chemicals that could react with the sterilant, causing discoloration of items.
7. Seal integrity
   a. The packaging material must permit integrity of the seal so that content sterility is maintained.
   b. Peel-pack pouches ("peel-packs") should permit self-sealing or sealing by heat or tape.
   c. Indicator tape or banding material that secures items wrapped in flat wrappers should be able to withstand the sterilization process.
   d. Broken locking devices for rigid instrument containers should be easily detected.
   e. Seals must not be able to reseal after opening to prevent mixing contaminated items with sterile items.

TYPES OF PACKAGING MATERIALS

Several standard types of packaging materials exist and are used in different facilities or within the same surgical services unit.

WOVEN TEXTILES

Woven textiles are made of either cotton or blends of cotton with synthetic materials such as polyester. Woven textile fabrics are reusable, meaning that they can be repeatedly used in the wrapping of items in preparation for sterilization. With each repeated laundering and sterilization cycle, however, the barrier quality of the fabric decreases. Fibers are lost with each laundering, increasing the space between the threads and reducing the microbial barrier.

Before use, the wrapper must undergo a lint removal and inspection process (usually over some type of large, illuminated table) to detect holes, worn areas where the fabric has thinned, and stains. If the wrapper has holes or is worn, it must be discarded. Small holes and worn spots can be repaired using heat-sealed patches. Holes must never be stitched closed because the needle and thread would create another small set of holes that can allow microorganisms to migrate to the inside of the sterile package. The advantages and disadvantages to woven materials are illustrated in Table 7-10.

MUSLIN

For many years, unbleached, double-thickness, 140-thread-count (140 TC) muslin set the standard for wrapping materials and, therefore, was the standard steam sterilization wrap. Muslin is made of cotton fibers with a minimum of 140 threads per square inch and is available as single or double ply (two muslin wraps sewn together at the edges). Single-ply muslin is not an effective barrier because the spaces between the threads are large enough to allow microbes and dust to pass through. Double-ply muslin is the best choice for steam sterilization because it helps prevent the absorption of moisture, which can create a pathway for microbes through a wicking action.

Table 7-10 Woven Materials

ADVANTAGES	DISADVANTAGES
Economical, reusable	The absorbent material may absorb the moisture in steam sterilization, inhibiting necessary contact of the moisture with all surface areas of the items.
Easily penetrated by sterilants	Least effective at providing bacterial barrier when compared to other wrapping materials.
	Not recommended for use with EtO.
	Additional personnel required for laundering.

Woven Textiles with Barrier Properties

Woven barrier fabrics are generally manufactured of a cotton/polyester fiber blend with d 180, 240, 272, or 288 TC. The higher thread count reduces the chances of bacterial and dust penetration. Some manufacturers apply a chemical treatment to the fabrics to make them moisture resistant. Barrier fabrics are manufactured as single ply; therefore, two wrappers are necessary for proper sterilization. Because the barrier fabrics do not absorb moisture, water droplets may be retained during the steam sterilization process. A towel placed between the instrument tray and barrier wrap will help absorb residual moisture.

NONWOVEN MATERIALS

Nonwoven materials are disposable wrappers that are designed for single use and are commonly referred to as *disposables*. They are made of plastic synthetic fibers that, through processes of heat and pressure, are layered together to form sheets of fabric. Nonwoven wraps are available in a variety of sizes to accommodate the various sizes and shapes of items to be sterilized. Nonwoven wrappers should be stored in a manner that eliminates folding. The advantages and disadvantages of nonwoven materials are listed in Table 7-11.

Table 7-11 Nonwoven Materials

ADVANTAGES	DISADVANTAGES
Excellent barrier properties	Cost, as they are single-use items
Lint free	Not as "memory" free as woven materials
Impervious to moisture	
Tear resistant	

Paper

Paper is actually a type of single-use, nonwoven material, but it has extreme memory characteristics and does not have the flexibility of other nonwoven materials. Paper is easily penetrated by steam, so it is particularly useful as a sterilization barrier. The advantages and disadvantages of paper materials are listed in Table 7-12.

Table 7-12 Paper

ADVANTAGES	DISADVANTAGES
Plentiful supply	Becomes brittle in dry conditions
Inexpensive	Easily torn, punctured, or ruptured
Porous	Not uniform in thickness

Peel Pack Pouches

Two types of pouch packaging are generally used by health institutions:

- Paper-plastic combinations that are used for steam and EtO sterilization
- Tyvek-plastic combination used only for EtO

Plastics

Various polymers are used as sterilization barriers. The compatibility of the plastic with the chosen method of sterilization must be confirmed. Tyvek should only be used for EtO. Steam will melt or burn the material, creating a flammable hazard and damaging the contents of the package.

Paper-Plastic Peel Packs

The combination of paper and plastic peel packs is the most commonly used type of pouch packaging in health institutions. Peel packs are manufactured with one side of the pouch as paper and the other a layer of plastic. The thickness of the plastic layer must be a minimum of 2 mm and should allow visualization of the contents. The two materials are heat sealed along the edges lengthwise, forming a pouch with one open end that allows for the placement of the item(s) to be sterilized.

The open end can be sealed either by heat or tape, or self-seal pouches may be commercially purchased with a strip of adhesive that is folded over to seal the pouch. The opposite end has been heat sealed by the manufacturer and is designated for the opening of the peel pack. Peel packs are available in a variety of precut sizes, including rolls that allow the user to cut the pouch to the desired length.

Heat sealing is the most popular method of sealing peel packs. Most heat-sealing machines have an internal timer that eliminates the need for holding the jaws closed during sealing and a dial to adjust the temperature of the heat.

Staples should not be used to close the peel pack. This increases the chance of microbial penetration of the contents. Rubber bands, paper clips, or tape should not be used to organize or "bind" package contents together for organizational purposes. Rubber bands and tape may prevent the contact of the sterilant with the surfaces underneath. The item(s) should be placed inside the peel pack so that the end of the item to be secured is presented when the pouch is opened.

It is important to select the correct size pouch. Pouches that are too small for the contents may not allow adequate air removal, penetration of the sterilant, and proper drying. Also, pouches that are too small or contain too many items may tear or the seals along the edges may rupture during sterilization and/or handling. On the other hand, too large a pouch will allow excessive movement of the contents, possibly tearing the pouch or rupturing the seals.

The ink from a felt-tip marker may leach through the paper side of a pouch, compromising the sterility of the items; therefore, felt-tip labeling should only be made on the plastic side of the pouch.

Pouches have a tendency to "bulge" outward during steam sterilization. To prevent the rupture of the pouch's seals, as much air as possible should be forced out from the pouch before sealing. Sharp edges of items to be sterilized should be protected with either sterilant-permeable tip protectors or foam sleeves to prevent the peel pack from being torn open. Latex tubing should never be used to protect the tips of instruments due to the sterilant-inhibiting property of latex.

Items that have multiple pieces or multiple items that must be kept together may be double peel packed. Double packing requires placing the items to be sterilized into a paper-plastic peel pack that is subsequently placed into a slightly larger paper-plastic peel pack. The inner peel pack should not be sealed or folded because entrapped air can prevent penetration by the sterilant.

When loading the sterilizer, plastic-paper pouches should be placed on their edges and positioned paper side to plastic side to ensure adequate air removal, sterilant penetration, and drying. Perforated baskets with support pins are commercially available to maintain the proper position of the peel packs.

RIGID INSTRUMENT CONTAINERS

Reusable rigid instrument containers with locking lids have become popular with some health institutions in the last few years. The containers are multipurpose and have the following characteristics:

- They provide containment of items during sterilization.
- They provide assurance of sterility because metal or plastic containers cannot be torn or compromised.
- They are easily opened and provide for excellent sterile presentation of contents.
- They can be used for returning contaminated items to the decontamination area.

The containers are available in a variety of sizes and designs but always feature a removable lid that is sealable with some type of locking device. The containers are generally manufactured of a sturdy anodized aluminum, stainless steel, plastic, or a plastic-metal combination that allows the stacking of the containers in storage without damaging the containers or contents.

Sterilization recommendations when using rigid containers include:

- The sterilization load should be a dedicated load (all rigid containers).
- The drying phase should be increased to allow for the revaporization of moisture/condensation on the outside and inside of the container.
- Prevacuum sterilization should be used instead of gravity displacement because of the increased difficulty of adequate air removal.
- Gaskets should be inspected and replaced if torn, cracked, or nonpliable.

GENERAL PRINCIPLES OF PACKAGING

A number of general packaging principles exist including:

- After laundering, woven fabrics should be stored at a temperature of 64–72°F and a humidity of 35–70% for at least 2 hours to rehydrate the fabrics.
- The recommended maximum size of a linen pack is 12 in. high × 12 in. wide × 20 in. long and must not weigh more than 12 pounds.
- If linen packs are sterilized, they must be packaged loosely so that steam can make contact with all surface areas.
- Double, sequential wrapping is essential for a proper bacterial barrier and sterile presentation of the contents.
- Any commercial or facility sterilized package must be inspected for holes, tears, perforations, and seal integrity before opening.

No magic number exists for governing the weight of instrument sets. Sterilizer manufacturers generally recommend that wrapped instruments sets should not exceed 16 pounds. Density is the key sterilizing factor for an instrument set: The more densely packed the set, the greater the odds that the sterilant is not contacting all surface areas and that drying will not be adequate.

Protective plastic wraps that are 2–3 mm thick ("dust covers") can be used to cover a sterile package. These dust covers provide further barrier efficiency and prolong the shelf life of the package. After sterilization, the package must be cooled to room temperature before being placed in the dust cover. The cover can be heat or tape sealed and should be clearly marked as "dust cover" to prevent the mistake of using the cover as part of the sterile field.

PREPARATION FOR STERILIZATION

After the proper materials are chosen and the guidelines for preparation understood, specific items present unique requirements or problems. The steps in preparation are discussed below.

Basin Sets

Basin sets are conducive to the formation and retention of condensate due to their density and positioning for sterilization. Basins that will be nested within each other or that may contain other metal items must have adequate air space between each item. An absorbent towel should be used to separate the basins and items.

The absorbent towel should be fully opened and placed between nested basins to absorb the condensate, to aid in air removal, and to create an adequate space for the penetration of steam. If other metal items are placed inside the basin, the towel should be used to separate the items from the bottom of the basin and from each other.

Sponges and woven fabrics should not be placed inside a basin because the material can deflect the steam, preventing proper surface contact. Hollow OR light handles should be placed into the basin with the handle down so that moisture can drain out of the handles when the basin is positioned on the sterilizing cart. Basins should be placed on the sterilizing cart with the fold down to aid in the removal of air and to prevent condensate accumulation.

PACKAGING

After an item to be sterilized is prepared, it must be placed within a rigid container or wrapped in woven or nonwoven wraps. The use of two wrappers applied in a sequential manner ensures that the contents are adequately protected. The outer wrapper is securely closed with chemical indicator tape and the tape is labeled to aid in identifying the contents.

It is important to choose the correct size wrapper. Too large a wrapper can inhibit the penetration and release of the sterilant; too small a wrapper will not adequately cover the contents and could possibly tear at the corners. If the wrapper is to be used for the establishment of a sterile field, it should be large enough to extend to a minimum of 6 in. below the four sides of a table or basin ring stand. The wrapper must also be large enough to cover the hand of the individual opening it if the package is to be handed in a sterile manner to the STSR or transferred onto a sterile field.

Before wrapping, it is advisable to place an absorbent towel between the bottom of the tray and the wrapper, especially if the wrapper is nonwoven material. If necessary, another towel may be placed on top of the instrument tray before wrapping. The towels cushion the sharp corners of the instrument trays and prevent tearing.

The two most common types of packaging methods are

- The envelope, or diagonal, fold, which is useful for smaller instrument trays and individual items
- The square fold, which is useful for large packs and instrument trays

Envelope Fold

The square wrapper is arranged diagonally on the table with a corner pointing toward the user. The item to be sterilized is placed in the center of the wrapper using imaginary lines dividing the wrapper into quarters.

Square Fold

The square or rectangular wrappers are arranged squarely in front of the user. The package is placed in the center of the wrappers.

1. The wrapper edge nearest the user is folded over the top of the item, covering the lower half of the item, and a cuff is formed.
2. The top section of the wrapper is folded down over the item and a cuff is formed that overlaps the first cuff.
3. The left section of the wrap is folded over the pack and a cuff is formed.
4. The right section of the wrap is folded over the pack overlapping the previous fold and a cuff is formed.
5. The second wrapper is applied in the same manner, except that the last cuff is folded under. The chemical indicator tape is then added.

LABELING

The user must be able to identify the contents of a package, especially when a woven or nonwoven wrap is used.

TECHNIQUE

Packaging (Envelope Fold) (Figure 7-8 A-E)

1. Items to be wrapped are prepared for sterilization.
2. Assemble all necessary supplies (e.g., internal indicator, appropriate size wrappers, external indicator, and labeling materials).
3. Place the wrapper diagonally on a flat surface.
4. Place the item to be wrapped in the center of the wrapper.
5. Place the internal indicator near the center of the package in a visible location.
6. The near corner of the wrapper is folded over the item.
7. A tab is created by folding 2–3 in. of the corner back onto itself.
8. One side of the wrapper is folded over the item as far as possible.
9. The corner is mitered, if necessary.
10. A tab is created by folding 2–3 in. of the corner back onto itself.
11. The opposite side of the wrapper is folded over the item as far as possible, overlapping the first side of the wrapper.
12. The corner is mitered, if necessary, and the tab is created.
13. The final flap is folded over the item, overlapping the wrapper sides.
14. The corners are mitered, if necessary.
15. If this is the first of two wrappers, the corner of the wrapper is tucked under the other three folds—the tab remains exposed. Otherwise, the corner of the wrapper is brought around the outside of the package and secured with the appropriate tape, which may also serve as the external indicator.
16. Repeat the process if a second wrapper is required.
17. Label the item according to facility policy.
18. The wrapped item is sterilized.

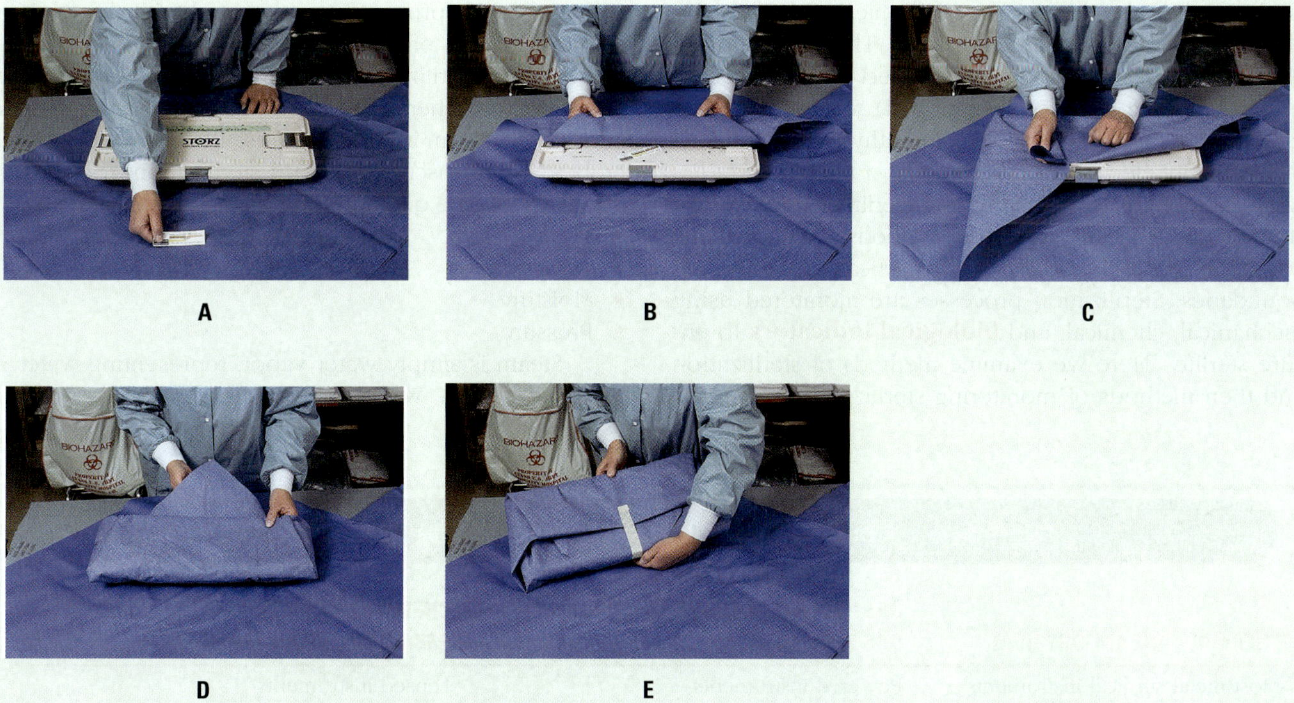

Figure 7-8 Packaging (envelope fold): (A) Placement of item on wrapper and addition of chemical indicator, (B) first fold with tab, (C) second fold with tab; repeat for third fold with tab, (D) final fold tucked, (E) package secured with chemical indicator tape

Items within paper-plastic peel packs can be seen but should still be labeled. Items are also labeled for quality assurance, inventory control, and rotation of stock.

The packages should be labeled before being sterilized. Most facilities use a felt-tip, quick-dry marker for labeling. All the information can be recorded on the chemical indicator tape or on the front, plastic portion of the peel packs.

Written label information should include:

- Package contents
- Shelf-life indication (either the expiration date or indication of **event-related sterility**)
- Date of sterilization
- Identification of the sterilizer (usually by number designation)
- Cycle number
- Initials of the employee who prepared the package
- Department to which the package is to be sent

Many institutions use a label "gun" that discharges printed labels onto the chemical indicator tape. The printed label typically contains:

- **Julian date** that indicates the date of sterilization
- Identification of the sterilizer
- Cycle number

STERILIZATION

Sterilization is the destruction of all microorganisms, including spores, on inanimate surfaces. The destruction of all microorganisms in or about an object is accomplished using steam (flowing or pressurized), chemical agents (alcohol, phenol, heavy metals, and ethylene oxide gas), high-velocity electron bombardment, or ultraviolet radiation (Table 7-13). The condition of sterility cannot be absolutely proven using scientific methods; therefore, this condition is only achieved theoretically, within set boundaries. Sterilization processes are monitored using mechanical, chemical, and **biological indicators** to ensure sterility. Here we examine methods of sterilization and then methods of monitoring sterilization processes. We focus first on thermal sterilization, primarily steam sterilization, as a dependable, inexpensive method of sterilization.

SATURATED STEAM UNDER PRESSURE

Thermal sterilization is an inexpensive, dependable method of sterilization that destroys all microbes, including spores. The most common thermal method of sterilization used in health care institutions is saturated steam under pressure. In this chapter, we focus on steam sterilization as the primary method of sterilization used in the OR and by sterile processing departments.

PRINCIPLES OF STEAM STERILIZATION

Steam sterilization utilizes moist heat in the form of saturated steam under pressure within an enclosed environment and is the most dependable method of sterilization in which all microbes, including spores, are destroyed. It is the recommended method of sterilization for items that are not heat, moisture, or temperature sensitive. Advantages and disadvantages of steam sterilization are listed in Table 7-14. Microbes are killed by the combination of two factors: moisture and heat. Heat alone can destroy microbes, but the process is accentuated with the addition of moisture and pressure. Therefore, steam alone is not sufficient for sterilization to occur. Pressure that is greater than the atmosphere is necessary to increase the temperature of the steam in order to cause the destruction of microbes. When discussing steam sterilization, four factors are critical to the outcome of the sterilization process:

- Time
- Temperature
- Moisture
- Pressure

Steam is simply water vapor, representing water in its gaseous state. When water is heated, the steam bub-

Table 7-13 Sterilization Methods and Uses

THERMAL—STEAM, DRY HEAT	GAS—ETHYLENE OXIDE, GAS PLASMA	CHEMICAL—CIDEX, PERACETIC ACID (STERIS)
Most metal surgical instruments	Powered instruments	Lensed instruments
Powered instruments (per manufacturer's instructions)	Delicate instruments	Fiber-optic instruments and cables
Microinstruments (per manufacturer's instructions)	Fiber-optic instruments Lensed instruments Plastic, rubber, porous instruments Moisture- or heat-sensitive instruments	Heat-sensitive instruments

Table 7-14 Advantages and Disadvantages of Steam Sterilization

ADVANTAGES	DISADVANTAGES
Saturated steam is many times more effective in transferring thermal energy than hot air.	Not all items can be steam sterilized. Heat- and moisture-sensitive items must be sterilized by other methods.
Any type of resistant and protective outer layer of microorganisms is softened by steam, allowing the denaturation of protein within the microbe.	Human error is a factor that can contribute to sterilizing failures.
It is the most economical and inexpensive sterilizing agent.	
It is the safest method of sterilization in comparison to other methods.	
The method is relatively quick.	
It is nontoxic and does not leave a toxic residue on items.	
Quality control/assurance methods are easy to control and maintain.	
Steam is readily available and easy to deliver to health care institutions.	

bles rise to the surface of the water, bursting and releasing the steam vapor. This steam is known as *saturated steam;* it is saturated when it contains the maximum amount of water vapor.

Moisture plays an important part in the steam sterilization of porous and nonporous items. The thermal destruction of microbes is the result of the denaturation and coagulation of the enzyme-protein system within the cells. Moisture acts as a catalyst and the coagulation can occur at lower temperatures as compared to the much higher temperatures required in the absence of moisture.

In the case of porous materials, such as woven linen towels, saturated steam heats the materials and permeates the porous material by the process of condensation. Only through *condensation*—the return of steam back into water—is the steam able to generate the heat needed for sterilization to occur. This explains why the arrangement of woven materials in a package to be sterilized is critical for steam to penetrate, heat the items through condensation, and sterilization to take place.

The same concepts apply to the sterilization of surgical instruments. Direct steam contact of all surface areas of the instrument must occur for an item to be sterile, the objective being to heat and sterilize the surface. In this instance, the condensation, which occurs due to heat contacting cold metal, liberates heat, thereby heating the instrument to the temperature of the steam and sterilization taking place.

The quality of steam entering the autoclaves must be such that it contains 2–3% liquid water. If water saturation levels are less than 3%, the steam in the chamber is known as *dry steam.* In these conditions the steam becomes superheated with a deficiency of heat transferred to the items, resulting in a sterilization failure.

The opposite occurs if excessive liquid water is present. The results are overly wet packages and items that require a longer drying time to avoid wicking action through the packaging material.

Air must be completely removed from the chamber for efficient sterilization of materials within. Unless the air is removed or steam displaces the air, the steam cannot make complete contact with the surface of items to be sterilized. Air and steam do not easily mix, resulting in

1. Temperature variations within the chamber
2. Heat not transferred to and condensation on the surface of items

Air is removed either by gravity displacement or by a prevacuum cycle. Additional information is presented in this chapter on the processes of air removal.

REQUIREMENTS AND ESSENTIAL FACTORS

In addition to the ability of steam to penetrate the wrapping material and destroy microbes, its effectiveness also depends on five other conditions:

1. Temperature, pressure, and moisture level reached in the sterilization cycle.
2. Type of microbe to be destroyed; bacteria in the spore stage are much harder to destroy than bacteria in the vegetative stage.

3. The number of microbes or bioburden on items to be sterilized. Bioburden must be low enough to ensure all microbes are killed.
4. Amount and type of soil present on items. Soil and debris, such as dried blood, acts as protection for microbes; thorough cleaning and decontamination of items are required prior to sterilization.
5. Instruments with box locks, joints, crevices, and serrations provide places for microbes to survive. Instruments must be opened to expose all surfaces to steam.

As previously stated, the four factors critical to the success of steam sterilization are time, temperature, moisture, and pressure. A fifth is added, contact.

There has been a tendency to discuss steam sterilization in terms of pressure and not temperature. It must be understood that saturated steam is the sterilizing agent and pressure only plays a minor role. Pressure is utilized to raise the temperature of the steam but has nothing to do with the microbicidal properties of steam.

CONTACT

The most frequent reason for failures during the sterilization cycle is lack of contact between steam and surface of items to be sterilized, thereby allowing viable microbes to survive the sterilization cycle. The majority of sterilization failures may be traced to human error or mechanical malfunction. Reasons for failure include:

1. Obstructed strainer. The strainer is located at the bottom front of the chamber. Its purpose is to prevent lint and objects from entering the exhaust line. If the strainer is not cleaned daily, it can become clogged and trap air in the chamber of the autoclave.
2. Containers positioned incorrectly on sterilization cart. Containers (pans, basins, etc.) must be positioned to allow air to escape. Nonperforated pans and basins should be placed upright on their sides to allow air to be displaced downward.
3. Items to be sterilized are inadequately cleaned. Soil and debris prevent the saturated steam from making direct contact with surface areas to kill microbes.
4. Wrapped packs are placed too close together on sterilizing cart. Packs should be loosely arranged on the cart or autoclave rack to allow the escape of air.
5. Instrument trays, pans, basins, etc., are wrapped too tightly. This also prevents the escape of air, which forms cool air pockets that prevent the temperature from increasing to the level needed to kill microbes.

TIME

Sterilization times are discussed in simple mathematical terms. Not all microbes die at the same time when exposed to saturated steam at a constant temperature. Some microbes are more difficult to kill than others. Sterilization time is denoted by the use of *D-values*. The *D*-value is the amount of time required at any temperature to kill 90% of the microbes. Each type of microbe has its own assigned set of *D*-values, which depend on the temperature required to destroy that particular microbe.

Bacillus stearothermophilus is a highly resistant, nonpathogenic microorganism used as the biological indicator for steam sterilization. This microorganism has a *D*-value of 2 minutes at 250°F or approximately 20 seconds at 270°F. This means it takes 2 minutes at 250°F or 20 seconds at 270°F to kill 90% of the microbes present.

To allow for a wide margin of safety, *B. stearothermophilus* has been assigned six *D*-values. This calculates to be 12 minutes sterilization time at 250°F or 2 minutes at 270°F.

Knowledge of these concepts is important, but manufacturer's recommendations must always be followed. Manufacturers of sterilizers provide recommendations for minimum exposure times according to the items to be sterilized. Manufacturers of instruments and equipment also provide similar recommendations. These recommendations should be strictly followed.

MOISTURE

The role and importance of moisture are illustrated by a comparison. *Bacillus stearothermophilus* spores are killed in 12 minutes at 250°F when saturated steam is used but require more than 6 hours when dry heat is used at the same temperature. Moisture allows the use of a lower steam temperature required to denature protein within the microbes.

A separate mechanical measuring device on sterilizing machines is not necessary to measure the moisture content in the chamber. Moisture or saturation is directly related to variations in temperature and pressure, which are mechanically measured.

BASIC COMPONENTS OF A STEAM STERILIZER

The structure of an autoclave (steam sterilizer) is based around the chamber in which items are placed for sterilization. Autoclaves range in size from small tabletop units to large industrial-sized machines.

Some autoclaves generate their own steam, while others rely on steam from an outside source. When steam is supplied to the autoclave from an outside source, the walls of the chamber are preheated before allowing the steam into the chamber. This is accomplished with a metal jacket that is built around the chamber. The space between the jacket and chamber allows steam to be introduced to preheat the chamber walls when the machine is turned on and the steam remains until the sterilizer is turned off. Preheating the chamber walls aids in maintaining a constant chamber temperature throughout the sterilization cycle and prevents the formation of condensation on the chamber walls when steam is introduced inside the chamber at the beginning of the cycle. Small sterilizers, such as the tabletop models, usually do not rely on an external steam source, and the chamber walls must be heated for every load, increasing the total cycle time.

The system of pipes to the sterilizer is relatively simple. Three main pipes exist:

1. A pipe to bring steam to the sterilizer and the chamber
2. A drain pipe for steam, air, and water from the chamber
3. A pipe to deliver filtered air to the chamber at the end of a cycle

A series of filters is placed at intervals to prevent contaminants from entering the chamber and altering the quality of steam.

Lastly, each autoclave must have a control system. The electromechanical switches of older machines have been replaced by microprocessor systems that control the sterilization process and perform operation self-diagnoses (Figure 7-9).

GRAVITY AIR DISPLACEMENT STERILIZER

Gravity air displacement sterilizers rely on gravity to passively remove air from the sterilization chamber. Steam enters at the top of the chamber and displaces the air in the chamber. Air is heavier than steam, and as the steam occupies more space, the air is pushed out the drain at the bottom front of the chamber. During this stage of the cycle, the pressure in the chamber increases until the temperature of the steam reaches a preset temperature.

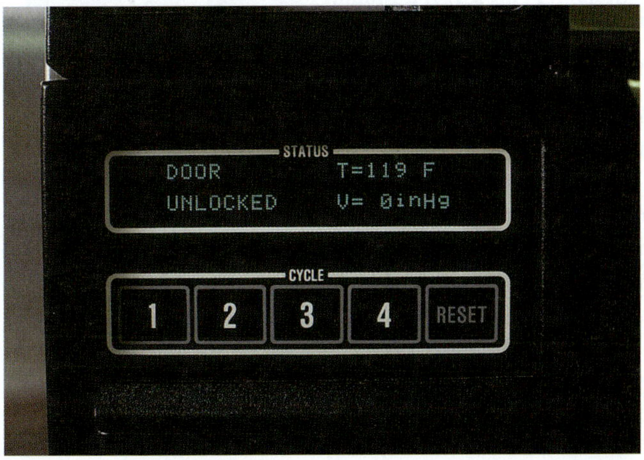

Figure 7-9 Steam sterilizer control panel

A general description of the cycle is as follows:

1. *Condition cycle:* Steam inlet valve opens and steam enters into the chamber at the top rear opening. Air is displaced; temperature and pressure increase until preset temperature is reached; timing begins.
2. *Exposure cycle:* The sterilizing temperature is maintained for the amount of time required to kill all microorganisms. Periodically, cooled steam is removed through the bottom front drain and replaced with fresh steam to maintain correct temperature.
3. *Exhaust cycle:* When the timer signals the conclusion of the exposure cycle, the steam inlet valve closes, the chamber drain opens, and the steam is removed from the chamber. Air is reintroduced into the chamber and the chamber reaches atmospheric pressure.
4. *Dry cycle:* The heated, fresh air, and heat generated by the jacket slowly revaporize and remove moisture from the packs. At the end of this cycle, an audible signal indicates the door may be opened.

PREVACUUM STEAM STERILIZER

Prevacuum steam sterilizers are similar in construction to gravity sterilizers except a vacuum pump is built into the system to remove air. Before the steam is injected into the sterilizer, air is removed from the chamber, reducing the total cycle time.

A typical cycle is as follows:

1. *Prevacuum cycle:* Vacuum pump removes approximately 90% of the air out of the chamber.
2. *Conditioning cycle:* Steam is injected into chamber to begin heating process of the load and aid in removing air.
3. *Second prevacuum cycle:* Vacuum pump removes another 90% of the air. The combination of the two vacuum cycles removes 99% of the air.
4. *Exposure cycle:* Steam inlet valve opens and steam enters the chamber. As with gravity, the temperature is held constant by the removal of cooler steam and replacement with fresh steam.
5. *Exhaust cycle:* After exposure cycle is complete, outlet drain opens and steam exits chamber.
6. *Dry cycle:* Vacuum pump turns on again and draws a 90% vacuum. This vacuum is held during the drying cycle and moisture is removed from packs by heat generated from the jacket. When drying cycle is complete, the vacuum is released as filtered air is allowed into the chamber. A signal indicates the door can be opened.

Another version of the prevacuum cycle involves up to four or five vacuum cycles instead of the two described above. Between each vacuum cycle steam enters the chamber to aid in removing air and preconditions the load by penetrating the packages.

There are several advantages to this type of system:

1. Increases speed of operation and lowers total cycle time.
2. More efficient at removing air than gravity sterilizers.
3. Not as dependent on the positioning of load contents as gravity sterilizer.
4. Condensate is produced during preconditioning phases, reducing cycle time.

STERILIZING LIQUIDS

Only the liquid cycle on gravity sterilizers is to be used on liquids, and liquids must be sterilized in a dedicated load. Liquid loads require exhaust and cooling settings that differ from a regular load.

Steam does not penetrate the liquid; rather it heats the liquid to 250°F. Several minutes are needed for the liquid to attain this temperature and the volume of liquid in the container dictates the exposure time.

The sterilization temperature is above the boiling point of water; therefore, the chamber pressure must be slowly released to allow the liquid to cool below 200°F before the autoclave door is opened. If this rule is not followed, the containers of solution may boil over or possibly explode. Because of the danger of explosion and because hospitals are not equipped to monitor each autoclave load of fluids to ensure sterility, in-hospital sterilization of fluids is discouraged by the American Institute for the Advancement of Medical Instrumentation (AAMI). In emergency situations when fluids must be sterilized, solutions should be sterilized separately, and manufacturer's instructions for exposure time and cycle setting should be followed.

A typical liquid sterilization cycle is as follows:

1. *Condition:* Steam is admitted and air is displaced. Pressure and temperature increase until preset temperature is reached. Exposure timer begins.
2. *Exposure:* Temperature is maintained for prescribed amount of time.
3. *Exhaust:* Steam inlet valve closes, outlet drain opens slightly, and steam escapes very slowly. Concurrently, the jacket pressure is slowly released to allow the temperature to drop. This process will take 30 minutes or more. An audible signal will indicate when all the steam has exited, the chamber temperature is below 200°F, and the door can be opened.

STEAM STERILIZATION MINIMUM EXPOSURE TEMPERATURES, PRESSURES, AND TIMES

The most common temperature, pressure, and time required for gravity sterilizers are 250–254°F (121–123°C), 15–17 psi, and a minimum exposure of 15 minutes, respectively. For prevacuum sterilizers the temperature is 270–276°F (132–135.5°C) at 27–30 psi with a minimum exposure time of 4 minutes for wrapped items. Refer to Table 7-15 for additional details pertaining to time and temperature standards, including liquid exposure times.

TROUBLESHOOTING WET PACKS

A wet pack or instrument set, whether the moisture occurs on the outside or within, must be considered contaminated. Moisture creates a pathway for microorganisms from the outside to the inside of a package through wicking action.

If packs are consistently wet, the cause must be identified and corrective actions performed. Various rea-

Table 7-15 Minimum Steam Sterilization Exposure Cycle Standards

CONTENTS	GRAVITY, 250°F	GRAVITY, 270°F	PREVACUUM, 270°F
Instrument sets, wrapped	30 minutes	N/A	4 minutes
Instrument set, unwrapped, no lumen instruments	15 minutes	3 minutes	3 minutes
Instrument set, unwrapped, some instruments with lumens	20 minutes	10 minutes	4 minutes
Basin set, wrapped	20 minutes	N/A	4 minutes
Solutions	Slow exhaust	N/A	Time and temperature determined by manufacturer of machine
75–250 mL	20 minutes		
250–1000 mL	30 minutes		
1500–2000 mL	40 minutes		

sons exist for moisture found on the outside and/or inside of packages:

- Condensate dripping from the shelves and/or railings of the sterilizing cart
- Condensate buildup in steam lines
- Metal items on upper shelf of cart dripping condensate onto items below

Moisture on the inside of packs may be the result of

- Too many instruments placed in tray produces more condensate than can be revaporized.
- Instrument and basin sets are assembled without using absorbent towels to absorb moisture as an aid for efficient drying.
- Woven textile packs, such as towels, are wrapped too tightly and retain moisture.
- Trays and items are improperly loaded on sterilizer cart and moisture is unable to escape the package.

FLASH STERILIZATION

Flash sterilization is the process of sterilizing unwrapped items, such as when an instrument has been dropped during a surgical procedure. Flash sterilization has become a necessity in the OR but in some instances has been misused to compensate for an inadequate inventory of surgical instrumentation. It is recommended that flash sterilization be avoided for the routine sterilization of instrument sets and its use be reserved to sterilize items that are immediately needed.

Items to be flash sterilized must be decontaminated and cleaned. Items must be disassembled and thoroughly cleaned with detergent and water to remove gross contamination. The composition of the item to be flash sterilized, not its size or shape, determines the exposure time.

Flash sterilization is primarily accomplished with the item unwrapped and placed in a perforated instrument tray. Flash sterilization containers are commercially available that totally contain the instrument during and after sterilization. Flash sterilization of implantables should not be a part of routine practice.

Flash sterilization can be performed in gravity or prevacuum sterilizers. Refer to Table 7-16 for sterilization times and temperatures.

Safety considerations to remember include:

- Caution must be used with jacketed sterilizers. After the steam enters the jacket, the chamber walls are hot and can cause burns if skin contacts them.
- Make sure door is tightly closed before starting the sterilizer.
- The door is to be opened only when the exhaust valve indicates zero pressure. To avoid hot steam, stand behind the door when opening.
- Do not touch the sterilizing cart until sufficiently cool.

GAS STERILIZATION

Gas sterilization is used to process materials that cannot be processed using steam sterilization, such as heat- or moisture-sensitive materials. Ethylene oxide has been the predominant chemical used in this sterilization process, but new technologies are emerging, including plasma and ozone sterilization processes.

ETHYLENE OXIDE

Ethylene oxide (EtO) may be used to sterilize heat- and moisture-sensitive materials and supplies. Exposure to this gas is a risk for employees. The process must be closely monitored to ensure that exposure does not occur. The process takes up to 16 hours, a disadvantage in situations where supplies are limited and quick turnover time is necessary or where an instrument may be needed in an emergency situation. Also, EtO produces chlorofluorocarbons, considered detrimental to the earth's ozone layer. These issues have caused health care providers to search for other technologies to replace EtO sterilization.

In instances where steam sterilization has been impractical, EtO has been an accepted chemical in sterilization. This chemical has long been used to sterilize plastics, rubber, and other materials that would be damaged by the high temperatures of steam sterilization.

Ethylene oxide is an organic gas, a member of the ether group. It is effective against all forms of microbes and is sporicidal. It does not corrode metal and passes

Table 7-16 Flash Sterilization: Times and Temperatures

CONTENTS	GRAVITY, 270°F (132°C)	PREVACUUM, 270°F (132°C)
Metal, nonporous and no lumens	3 minutes	3 minutes
Metal, porous or with lumens	10 minutes	4 minutes
Metal power tools or rubber hoses with lumens	Manufacturer's directions	Manufacturer's directions

through woven materials just like steam. However, it is very expensive, and the sterilization process can take up to 16 hours, because sterilized packages must be aerated, or "aired out," before use. The gas is flammable and very toxic, with effects ranging from skin irritation to respiratory difficulty, headaches, and nausea. In extreme instances, EtO has been linked to cancer, reproductive difficulties, and chromosomal alteration. Careful monitoring, adequate ventilation, and safe work habits are a must when dealing with this dangerous gas.

Because of the dangers presented by EtO gas, sterilization is performed in a closed room specifically designed for EtO sterilization. This room is designed with the ability to vent extra gas at the end of the sterilization process without releasing it to the atmosphere. Several factors are required for proper EtO sterilization:

- *EtO gas concentration:* The gas comes in cylinders, which are attached per manufacturer's instructions to the sterilization machine at the beginning of the cycle. The machine withdraws air from the chamber and replaces it with pressurized EtO gas.
- *Temperature:* Higher temperatures are used in the EtO sterilization process to increase the **permeability** of cell walls. Gas sterilizers, however, are designed to work at lower temperatures than steam sterilizers, and most operate at from 85 to 145°F.
- *Humidity:* Moisture hydrates spores and bacteria that would otherwise be resistant to the gas alone. Humidity is kept between 30% and 80% during the EtO sterilization process.
- *Time:* EtO sterilization requires less time at higher temperatures but is still a lengthy process.

Instruments must be clean, dry, and free of all lubricants for the EtO process to be effective. The gas cannot penetrate lubricating oils.

The EtO sterilizer consists of the sterilization machine in a separate vented chamber. These machines have vacuum pumps to evacuate air from the chambers and humidifiers to maintain the proper humidity levels. The most favorable setup is a combination sterilization machine aerator, which aerates the materials after sterilization. If this setup is not available, materials are removed from the sterilizer after the sterilization process and placed on shelves within the chamber for aeration.

The Environmental Protection Agency has voiced concern over the effects of EtO on personnel and the environment. Chlorofluorocarbons (CFCs) are used to reduce the flammability of EtO but are damaging to the ozone layer, and many countries banded together to eliminate the use of CFCs by the year 2000. This combined with the danger to personnel has led to the search for safer, quicker methods of sterilization for sensitive instruments.

ALTERNATIVE STERILIZATION METHODS

As awareness of the dangers of EtO sterilization has increased, new methods of sterilization for sensitive instruments and materials have emerged.

Plasma sterilization (Sterrad) uses gas at low temperature to sterilize heat-sensitive materials. This method of sterilization is safer than EtO sterilization. At this time, however, fewer items used in the OR can be sterilized because of limitations on materials that may be sterilized with this method and because of limitations on wrapping materials suitable for this method. This method cannot be used for long cannulated instruments. The most commonly used plasma sterilization system uses hydrogen peroxide in plasma form. Plasma is a fourth state of matter, different from liquid, solid, or gas. It is produced when a strong electrical current is passed through a gas, causing a cloud of plasma to be produced. This plasma destroys all microbes and spores at a low temperature.

Ozone gas sterilization oxidizes bacteria, thus destroying them. As with plasma sterilization, it is limited in the products suitable for sterilization and in the types of containers and wrappers that can be used. Ozone is destructive to rubber and plastics and corrodes some metals. This method cannot be used for long cannulated instruments. A generator converts oxygen into ozone. Ozone has the ability to penetrate cell membranes and cause them to explode. These machines use a vacuum pump to increase penetration of ozone. At the end of the sterilization cycle, the chamber of the sterilizer is purged of ozone, which is replaced with oxygen. These machines have a cycle time of up to 60 minutes and can be used with metals. This method is preferable in that it leaves no residue and aeration is not required.

Vapor phase hydrogen peroxide (VPHP), while not an effective sterilizing agent in liquid form, is effective in gas form. At concentrations of 30% in vapor phase, hydrogen peroxide sterilizes in less than 30 minutes and requires no aeration. However, VPHP cannot be used with paper wrappers or nylon or rubber products and is corrosive to certain metals.

Chlorine dioxide gas sterilizes rapidly at temperatures from 25 to 30°C. The sterilization machine generates the gas for each cycle, and the gas is exhausted at the end of the cycle. The gas is generated by the reaction of chlorine gas with sodium chlorite, a simple and inexpensive process. This method is corrosive to some metals and may not penetrate paper and certain wrappers well. Studies are ongoing as to the effects of exposure to personnel.

While the above alternative methods to EtO show promise, they do not yet have its wide-ranging application. All of the above methods have limitations that in some instances make them impractical for heavy use in the OR environment. For larger hospitals, the cost of these methods combined with their limitations as opposed to the availability and relatively low number of limitations of EtO use has led to a search for safer methods of using EtO. Gas sterilization clearly has both advantages and disadvantages (Table 7-17). In addition to these methods of gas sterilization, liquid chemical methods have been developed.

LIQUID CHEMICAL STERILIZATION PROCESSES

In addition to the above-mentioned gas sterilization processes that serve as useful alternatives to steam sterilization, liquid chemical sterilization processes have been developed. These chemical sterilants, which can also be used as high-level disinfectants, have been discussed in this chapter in the section on disinfectant solutions. The two primary liquid chemical sterilization compounds are peracetic acid, used in the tabletop Steris process, and glutaraldehyde. The peracetic acid systems are gaining widespread favor with hospitals because of their rapid processing times and the ability they give hospitals to maintain a lower instrument inventory, particularly for endoscopic instruments. Prior to the widespread use of this system, hospitals had to maintain a higher inventory of endoscopic equipment because of the longer process (up to 10 hours) required with the use of glutaraldehyde. Monitoring methods for gas and liquid sterilization are discussed below.

IONIZING RADIATION

Ionizing radiation is primarily used commercially to sterilize prepackaged products for use in the OR and hospital environment. It uses a process of irradiation to produce thermal and chemical energy, which causes the death of all microbes and spores by disrupting the DNA. These sterilization methods primarily use gamma rays or beta particles to sterilize products. Sterilization times vary depending on the source of radiation used.

METHODS OF MONITORING THE STERILIZATION PROCESS

Quality assurance is an essential component of the sterilization process. To provide safe patient care and prevent SSI, sterile surgical instruments and equipment must be used. Methods must be used to confirm the sterility of items and proper operation of the sterilizers. Three methods of monitoring the sterilization process exist:

1. Mechanical
2. Chemical
3. Biological

MECHANICAL METHODS OF MONITORING THE STERILIZATION PROCESS

Autoclaves are equipped with recorders and gauges that allow the operator to monitor the progress of the machine during the sterilization cycle. The monitors also aid the operator in confirming that sterilization parameters for time, temperature, and pressure have been met, assuring the machine is properly working.

A permanent record of the temperature is attained through the use of a cycle tracing on a chart recorder. The autoclave contains a standard electrically driven clock mechanism that slowly revolves a 6-in. recording chart once over a 24-hour period. Each sterilization cycle temperature is recorded on the chart by a tracing pen. After 24 hours, the chart must be changed. Older autoclaves use needle gauges to display the pressure. Pressure gauges reveal the performance of the sterilizer during every load. Sterilizers use two main gauges, jacket steam pressure and chamber steam pressure.

Newer autoclaves utilize digital recorders that are much easier to read. Also, a printout is produced by the machine, providing detailed information on the performance of the machine. The operator is able to initial the printout, verifying the cycle parameters were achieved

Table 7-17 Advantages and Disadvantages of Gas Sterilization

ADVANTAGES	DISADVANTAGES
Can be used to sterilize materials too heat sensitive for steam sterilization.	Aeration times required with EtO sterilization process can be extraordinarily lengthy—up to 21 days with internal pacemakers.
In some cases, these processes are significantly less corrosive to metals.	Personnel hazards are created by the use of ethylene oxide gas.
Less damaging to sensitive plastic and rubber materials.	Some of the gas sterilization processes are damaging to certain materials, requiring the availability of more than one alternative process.

and maintained, and the printout is filed for record-keeping purposes.

CHEMICAL METHODS OF MONITORING THE STERILIZATION PROCESS

Chemical indicators are used externally and internally to verify the item has been exposed to sterilizing conditions. It must be emphasized that chemical indicators only validate that a package was exposed to a specific temperature, humidity, or sterilant; they do not authenticate the sterility of the items. Chemical indicators aid in detecting potential sterilization failures that may result from

- Machine malfunction
- Incorrect assembly of the package and wrapping
- Incorrect loading of the sterilizer cart or basket

Chemical indicators consist of paper that has been chemically treated with a dye that changes color in the presence of temperature or the sterilant. The most popular type of external chemical indicator is autoclave tape (Figure 7-10). The tape is used as a package closure to keep wraps in place. Autoclave tape is available for steam and EtO. When the tape has been exposed, the ink will uniformly change color. For example, most steam autoclave tape is cream in color with diagonal lines of chemical agent evenly spaced. When the agent has been exposed to the steam sterilization process, the ink changes to a black color.

Internal chemical indicators are placed inside packages to indicate the contents have been exposed to one or more conditions necessary for sterilization. The indicators should be placed in the area of the package where there is greatest chance of entrapped air. The internal indicator is then read when the package is opened at time of use. If the indicator has not changed to the proper color, the contents of the package may not have been exposed to the correct sterilizing temperature or some other condition and should be considered nonsterile. Internal indicators are available as commercial strips of paper that have been impregnated with the thermochromic (color-changing) ink.

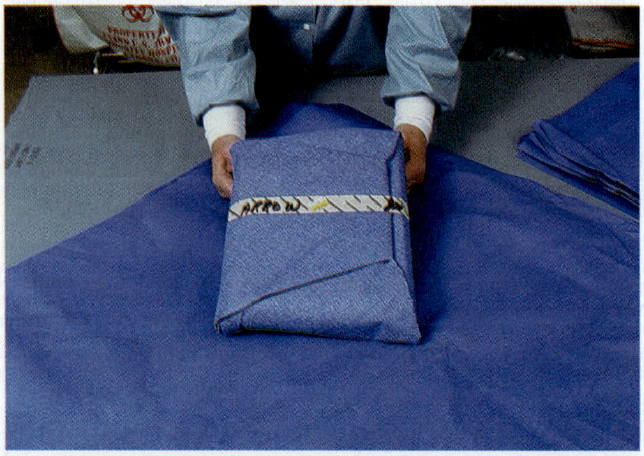

Figure 7-10 Indicator tape showing color change appropriate for exposure to the steam sterilization process

BIOLOGICAL METHODS OF MONITORING THE STERILIZATION PROCESS

A biological indicator (BI) is a device that contains a known number and specific type of microorganisms that are killed when exposed to the sterilizing conditions. The BI is the only test that ensures items are sterile and the conditions necessary for sterilization have been met.

The BI for steam sterilization contains the bacterial spore *B. stearothermophilus,* and *Bacillus subtilis* is used for EtO. These two microorganisms have been determined to be the most resistant to their respective methods of sterilization but are harmless to humans.

Most institutions purchase commercial test packs that contain a vial of the microorganism in the spore stage impregnated on a disk. Test packs can be produced in-house based on standards established by the AAMI, but production is time consuming and consistency is difficult to maintain. If the test packs are produced in-house, the components, arrangement of items, placement of the BI, and size of the pack must be the same every time, which is difficult at best. Therefore, the commercial test packs offer many advantages over the "home-made" packs.

The EtO biological test pack produced in-house consists of

- One biological indicator placed in a 20- or 30-mL syringe so that the plunger does not touch the vial when inserted into the syringe. The needle end of the syringe must be open with the guard removed.
- The syringe and a chemical indicator strip are placed within the folds of an absorbent towel.
- The towel is placed in a peel pack and sealed.

An example of a biological steam test pack produced in-house consists of

- Sixteen absorbent towels approximately 16 × 26 in. in size are each folded to approximately 9 × 9 in.
- Towels stacked with the BI vial placed in the center
- Pack that is taped together and should weigh about 3 pounds

The test pack is placed in the part of the sterilizer where it is most difficult for the sterilant to reach. This represents the "coldest" part of the sterilizer or portion where air entrapment is most likely to occur. For steam sterilization, the cold point is on the bottom front of the sterilizing cart over the chamber drain. For EtO, this point is the center of the load, and the test pack is placed on its side. After the sterilization cycle is complete, the test pack is removed and the BI vial is taken out and incubated. The vial is "crushed," releasing the growth medium that covers the spore-impregnated disk. After completion of incubation, if any microorganisms survived the sterilization cycle, the nutrient broth turns yellow as a result of a chemical by-product the bacteria produce.

For example, the nutrient broth in most commercially available vials containing *B. stearothermophilus* is red in color. After incubation, if the liquid remains red, the results are considered negative; however, if the culture turns yellow, microbes survived and grew in the culture. A positive reading indicates that conditions for sterilization were not met and the load must be considered nonsterile. The items in the load must be recalled and reprocessed.

Steam BIs are incubated for 24 hours before a reading is recorded and EtO BIs are incubated for 48 hours even though they can be read after 24 hours. The steam BI is incubated at 131–140°F (55–60°C) and the EtO BI incubated at 95–98.6°F (35–37°C). The test/experimental vial is incubated with a control vial that was not put through the sterilization process in order to validate the results of the test vial.

The recommended frequency of monitoring varies. The various organizations such as the AAMI, American Hospital Association (AHA), AORN, CDC, and JCAHO all vary in their recommendations. Only two recommendations are agreed on by all five organizations:

- Loads containing implantables must always be monitored and the BI must be read before the implantables are used. The implantables are quarantined and not released for distribution until the BI indicates negative results.
- The placement of the test pack in steam and EtO loads.

Generally, EtO is monitored more often than steam loads due to the more complex process of EtO sterilization. It is recommended that every EtO load be monitored. For steam sterilization, the recommendation varies from every load to one load per week. At a minimum, steam sterilization should be monitored at least weekly. All test results are filed as a permanent record for each sterilizer.

BOWIE-DICK TEST

The **Bowie-Dick test** derives its name from two English microbiologists who developed the test, J. H. Bowie and J. Dick. The test is used in the prevacuum sterilization cycle to check for air entrapment and is conducted daily. Usually the test is performed as the first run of the day before any loads are sterilized or after the sterilizer has undergone repairs. The test pack must be placed horizontally on an empty sterilizing cart on the front bottom shelf over the chamber drain in an empty prevacuum chamber.

Test packs may be commercially purchased or prepared in-house. Department-produced test packs consist of fan-folded absorbent towels with a Bowie-Dick test sheet placed in the center of the pack. The test sheet can be commercially purchased or three to four strips of steam autoclave chemical indicator tape can be placed in a crisscross pattern on a plain sheet of paper. The in-house produced test pack consists of

- Between 24 and 44 absorbent towels fan folded and placed in a stack that is 9 × 12 × 11 in.
- Bowie-Dick test sheet placed in the center of the pack
- Pack that is single wrapped

All test sheets are filed as a permanent record for each sterilizer.

It must be emphasized that the Bowie-Dick test is not a sterilization test but rather a test of the vacuum system in a prevacuum sterilizer. It is never performed on gravity sterilizers since these sterilizers do not rely on a vacuum system. The result that is important to the Bowie-Dick test is not the intensity of the color change of the heat-sensitive ink but the uniformity of the color change. Any machine malfunction in which air is entrapped will result in uneven color changes of the chemical ink.

EVENT-RELATED STERILITY

Event-related sterility is a concept that is replacing the older time-related system. The concept of event-related sterility means that the sterility of an item is determined by how it is handled and that contamination is "event related" rather than "time related." For years, expiration dating has been used to indicate that at the end of a prescribed number of days microbes invaded a sterile package and rendered the item(s) nonsterile. The standard time periods consisted of

- 30 days for items in peel packs and wrapped in nonwoven wrapper
- 3 weeks for muslin-wrapped items
- 9 months if items were placed in a dust cover

With improved packaging materials and a better understanding of the factors that affect sterility, the AAMI and JCAHO have changed their standards to reflect the premise that contamination is event related and items will remain sterile indefinitely until the package becomes wet or torn or the seal is broken or compromised in some way. The major difference in the new standards is that a specific expiration date is no longer required.

According to the AAMI

> The shelf-life of a packaged sterile item is event-related and depends on the quality of the wrapper material, the storage conditions, the conditions during transport, and the amount of handling. There should be written policies and procedures for how shelf-life is determined and for how it is indicated on the product.

The adoption of the practice of event-related sterility is economical for the health institution. Previous use of expiration dating meant that on a weekly basis "out-dates" must be checked and the expired items pulled from the shelf. The items had to be reprocessed, which was labor intensive and uneconomical due to the waste of disposable wrapping materials. Event-related sterility eliminates this practice, as well as many steps in the sterility assurance process, while continuing to provide the necessary sterility of items for use in the sterile field.

ENVIRONMENTAL DECONTAMINATION

An important part of maintaining asepsis is minimizing microbial counts in the OR environment itself. The operating room is designed to minimize contamination. Laminar air flow systems, washable floors and walls, and easily cleaned furniture are required in every operating room (see Chapters 5 and 8). Effective sanitation and decontamination techniques and established procedures help prevent cross-infection of patients intraoperatively. As previously stated, this takes place not only between cases but also while the patient is in the room. During a procedure, traffic should be minimized into and out of the OR, and any spills or contaminated materials should be handled using Standard Precautions. Environmental services personnel involved with OR decontamination must follow the aforementioned guidelines for Standard Precautions and the use of PPE at all times. Cleaning procedures should be established for each facility and should be followed on a per-case daily, weekly, and monthly schedule.

ENVIRONMENTAL SERVICES

A sanitary and clean, decontaminated surgery department must be ensured to control the spread of microbes to workers and patients. The hospital exposure control plan, required by OSHA, should explain the protective measures to create a safe working environment.

The following are guidelines for housekeeping, laundry, and regulated waste procedures:

- A routine schedule should be established for the cleaning and decontamination of OR surfaces, scrub sinks, cabinets, floors, walls, and ceilings.
- Contaminated work surfaces such as the OR floor should be decontaminated by the circulator with a disinfectant. When not possible to immediately decontaminate the floor, this should be done at the end of the procedure.
- Reusable contaminated linens must be handled as little as possible to prevent airborne contamination. The contaminated linen should be placed and contained in a leak-proof bag. These biohazard bags should be clearly marked with the biohazard symbol or the bags themselves should be red.
- Contaminated linen must not be rinsed or sorted in the area of use.
- When handling contaminated linen, the surgical technologist must wear gloves and other PPE as deemed necessary.
- Regulated waste must be placed in leak-proof bags that are either clearly marked with the orange biohazard symbol or are red in color. Only regulated (contaminated) waste should be put in these designated bags because they are more costly to dispose of than common hospital waste.

CASE BY CASE

The CDC recommends that all ORs be cleaned between procedures. This usually means removal of all soiled linens and waste and deposit in the appropriate bags and receptacles and "wiping down" all OR furniture, including the operating table, back table, Mayo stand, and anything that may have come into contact with patient body fluids. Floors are cleaned with an appropriate disinfectant solution.

DAILY

Each hospital designs its own daily cleaning, or "terminal cleaning," routine. This entails a more thorough cleaning of rooms after the last case of the day has been completed. Within each OR, floors should be disinfected, window ledges and shelves should be dusted or wiped with disinfectant solution, as should cabinet doors and handles. Furniture, including casters and wheels, should also be cleaned with a disinfectant. Care should be taken that suture pieces and other debris are removed from wheels of furniture and from crevices of the operating table. Because surgical lamps are near the sterile field, they should also be wiped down with a disinfectant and any blood or debris removed. Because walls and ceilings are seldom a source of airborne microorganisms, a longer cleaning interval is acceptable. They should be checked on a daily basis for gross contamination, but walls may be cleaned weekly and ceilings may be cleaned weekly or monthly according to hospital policy.

Outside the OR, corridor floors should be disinfected on a daily basis. In the substerile room, countertops and sinks should be cleaned, as should scrub sinks. Carts and stretchers used for transportation of patients or storage of equipment should also be cleaned on a daily basis.

WEEKLY AND MONTHLY CLEANING

In addition to the case-by-case and daily cleaning routines, certain cleaning and disinfection practices are scheduled on a weekly or monthly basis by the hospital.

Ceilings and walls, although spot cleaned on a daily basis, should be thoroughly cleaned and disinfected to dislodge dust and microbes on at least a weekly or monthly basis. Mounted lighting tracks and fixtures should be cleaned, as should any other fixtures on the walls or ceiling. Air vents and grills should be vacuum cleaned at this interval to remove loose dust and contaminants. Sterilizers must be cleaned according to manufacturer's instructions and intervals. Floors should be cleaned at this interval, preferably using a machine that can remove any soils or residues that are not removed with day-to-day cleaning. Finally, storage cabinets and supply areas should be cleaned to remove any dust.

Disinfectant Container Refill

Gram-negative bacilli have been reported to contaminate disinfectant solutions and soap dispensers in the OR, including surgical scrub solution dispensers. This is usually due to the practice of refilling disinfectant bottles without sterilizing them or by simply topping them off with fresh solution. This practice contaminates the solution inside. These containers should be sterilized before refilling and should not be topped off. Because the risk of this problem is higher with quaternary ammonium compounds, they should not be used for the surgical scrub. Many hospitals now use prepackaged scrub brushes with antiseptic solutions that come in sterile packaging.

Dirty Cases

The customary practice at some hospitals has been to close an OR for 48 hours if a "dirty" case has been performed in that room. This practice is no longer considered necessary. In these cases, the floor should be cleaned with a phenolic detergent and then all equipment surfaces should be wiped down with 70% alcohol solution. Rubber and plastic tubings in the room should be replaced, and if gross contamination of walls and ceiling has occurred, these should be wiped down with disinfectant solution as well.

CASE STUDY

Early one morning, Lucy is setting up a case in room 3. The patient has been brought into the room and is on the table. The anesthesia provider is about to induce anesthesia. Lucy moves her basin set from the sterile ring stand to the back table and begins to remove items from the basin and place them in the appropriate positions on the table. Just before anesthesia is induced, the circulator notices water on the paper in which the basin set had been wrapped.

1. Should the anesthesia provider go ahead with the induction of anesthesia?
2. What action should be taken by the STSR in this instance to alleviate the danger of contaminating the patient?
3. Would the basin set still be considered sterile, since the indicator inside showed that it had been sterilized?
4. Could the STSR simply replace the basin set if it is determined to be nonsterile or must the entire back table be replaced?
5. Should an incident report be filed?

QUESTIONS FOR FURTHER STUDY

1. What different information comes from a chemical indicator and a biological indicator when concerned with sterility?
2. What are the conditions necessary to guarantee sterility via steam sterilization?
3. What are the steps required to verify both contact with sterilants and sterilization of an instrument set?
4. What is a prion and why is it a concern in the operating room environment?
5. Does the term *sterile* refer to an absolute? Explain your answer.
6. What safety guidelines apply when utilizing ethylene oxide (EtO) as a sterilant?

BIBLIOGRAPHY

Alexander, D., Reichert, M., & Young, J. H. (Eds.). (1993). *Sterilization technology for the health care facility.* Gaithersburg, MD: Aspen.

Allen, D. (1998, September). Packaging for the surgical suite. *Pharmaceutical & Medical Packaging News,* No. 6, pp. 21–23.

American Hospital Association (AHA). (1997). *Training manual for central service technicians* (3rd ed.). Chicago: Author.

Association for the Advancement of Medical Instrumentation (AAMI). (1990). *Good hospital practice: Guidelines and use of reusable rigid sterilization container systems.* Washington, DC: Author.

Association for the Advancement of Medical Instrumentation (AAMI). (1993). *Good hospital practice. Draft: Steam sterilization and sterility assurance* (ANSI/AAMI ST 46). Washington, DC: Author.

Association for the Advancement of Medical Instrumentation (AAMI). (1996). *Flash sterilization: Steam sterilization of patient care items for immediate use.* Washington, DC: Author.

Bennett, J. V., & Brachman, P. S. (1992). *Hospital infections* (3rd ed.). Boston: Little, Brown and Company.

Berube, R., & Oxborrow, G. S. (1993). *Sterilization technology for the health care facility.* Gaithersburg, MD: Aspen.

Block, S. S. (1991). *Disinfection, sterilization, and preservation* (pp. 3–17). Philadelphia: Lea & Febiger.

Chobin, N. (1998). Step-by-step flash sterilization [Online]. Available from *http://www.ascrs.org/publications/ao/6-3-12.html*

Donaldson, J. (1998). An overview of the process of sterilization [Online]. Available from *http://www.nurseceu.com/cpul.htm*

Evans, W. J. (1994). Decontamination and disinfection. *Central Service Technical Manual,* 73–90. Chicago: International Association of Healthcare Central Service Material Management.

Fluke, C., Ninemeier, J. D., & Webb, S. B. (Eds.). (1994). *Central service technical manual.* Chicago: International Association of Healthcare Central Service Material Management.

Food and Drug Administration. (1976). Federal food, drug, and cosmetic act, as amended 1976 (FDA Stock #017-012-00239-1). Washington, DC: U.S. Government Printing Office.

McGuiness, A. M., et al. (2002). *Core curriculum for surgical technology* (5th ed.). Centennial, CO: Association of Surgical Technologists.

Miner, N. (1998). Chemical disinfectants in central service departments [Online]. Columbus: Purdue University.

Occupational Safety & Health Administration (OSHA). *Bloodborne pathogens and acute care facilities* [Online]. Available from *http://www.osha.gov*

Perkins, J. J. (1983). *Principles and methods of sterilization in health sciences* (2nd ed.). Springfield, IL: Charles C. Thomas.

Rieu, E. V. (1952). *Homer, the Odyssey.* London: Methuen.

Strong Memorial Hospital. (1996). Basics on processing and sterilization [Online].

Strong Memorial Hospital. (1996). Event related sterility [Online].

Taurasi, R. A. (1998). Ethylene oxide alternatives [Online]. Columbus: Purdue University.

University of Michigan. (1998). Central sterile supply [Online].

Wenzel, R. P. (Ed.). (1998). *Prevention and control of nosocomial infections* (3rd ed.). Baltimore: Williams & Wilkins.

CHAPTER 8

General Patient Care and Safety

Teri Junge
Ben D. Price

CASE STUDY

Mary is an 82-year-old female who suffers from rheumatoid arthritis. Today, she has fallen and hit her head. She was alert when she arrived at the emergency department but quickly lost consciousness. The physician feels she has a probable left ventricular myocardial infarction. She is scheduled to be taken to the OR for coronary artery bypass surgery. Her daughter arrived at the emergency room with her and has been answering basic patient history questions for the surgeons.

1. When will Mary sign the consent for her surgery? Should the surgeons wait for a moment when she is conscious, or should they use some other method to attain consent?
2. What special considerations, if any, will need to be taken in positioning this patient for surgery?
3. Will this patient be scheduled for surgery immediately, even though her daughter states that she has eaten within the last few hours?

OBJECTIVES

After studying this chapter, the reader should be able to:

C 1. Demonstrate an understanding of the process used to obtain an informed consent for a surgical procedure or treatment.

2. Describe preoperative routines.

3. Identify, describe, and demonstrate the principles of transportation of the surgical patient.
4. Discuss, demonstrate, and apply the principles of surgical positioning.
5. Understand the methods of preparation of the operative site for surgery.
6. Describe the application of thermoregulatory devices.
7. Explain the principles and demonstrate the taking and recording of vital signs.
8. Explain the principles of urinary catheterization and demonstrate the procedure.

A 9. Describe how the principles of operative site preparation and urinary catheterization are related both to patient care and to the principles of asepsis.

R 10. Discuss methods of hemostasis and blood replacement and demonstrate the preparation and use of appropriate agents or devices.

11. Identify developing emergency situations, initiate appropriate action, and assist in treatment of the patient.
12. Discuss methods and types of documentation used in the OR.

E 13. Discuss the relationship between patient safety and the surgical environment.

SELECT KEY TERMS

1. apical pulse	6. dyspnea	12. laser	18. sedation
2. autologous	7. hemolysis	13. NPO	19. shock
3. cardiac dysrhythmia	8. hemostasis	14. prep	20. suction
	9. hemostat	15. prone	21. supine
4. catheterization	10. homologous	16. pulse oximeter	22. tourniquet
5. CPR	11. informed consent	17. Rh factor	23. vital signs

PREOPERATIVE PATIENT ROUTINES

Preoperative care includes the psychological and physiological preparation of the patient before surgical intervention. No two patients are exactly the same, and each brings his or her own specific set of psychological and physiological needs. Providing for the safety of the patient requires knowledge not only of the procedure to be performed but also of any special needs, such as physical limitations or allergies that the patient may possess. Every effort should be made to make the patient as mentally and physically comfortable with the process as possible, and for the safety of the patient as well as the hospital, all prepared protocols must be followed. Knowledge of the proper techniques of patient identification, transport, and required chart documentation are essential to the surgical technologist in preparing the patient for surgery, as are proper techniques of positioning and emergency procedures. These skills prepare the surgical technologist to provide whatever level of care the individual patient may require.

In the past, almost all surgical patients were admitted several days before surgery for all required laboratory work and surgical preparation. The nurse in the physician's office did presurgical patient education, and the postsurgical stay in the hospital ranged from a few days to weeks of in-hospital recovery. In today's "managed care" environment, patients are usually admitted the day of the surgery to a "same-day surgery" unit, where final laboratory work and preoperative teaching are performed by the hospital's staff nurses. Patients with special medical conditions such as diabetes mellitus or heart disease may be admitted earlier so that these conditions can be controlled as much as possible throughout the process.

Prior to surgery, certain information and studies must be compiled into the patient's chart or record. These will include any final laboratory results, radiology reports, and the surgical consent form, along with a preoperative checklist. Along with the surgical consent form, consents for anesthesia, blood products, and any special consent forms, such as a consent to sterilization, should be placed in the chart. Any previous pathology reports and/or nurses' notes will also be included in the chart, along with a complete history and physical report. Also included should be an identification of any known patient allergies, handicaps, or limitations. When the patient arrives in the surgery department, the surgical technologist should be able to review the patient's chart for required preoperative information. For his or her own protection, the surgical technologist should review the consent-for-surgery form. The history and physical form will give important background on the patient that may help the team member anticipate necessary equipment and possible intraoperative complications. The records kept in the chart provide both information for the surgical team and an accurate record of patient care. Special needs of the patient may be easily identified from the information available in the chart. For instance, the arthritic patient will need special care to avoid pain prior to anesthesia induction and special care during positioning to prevent joint damage. It is especially important that the surgical technologist as well as other members of the team note any medicine or food allergies. These are written in bold letters on the outside of the chart to minimize danger of administration of drugs to which a patient may have an allergic reaction.

SURGICAL CONSENT

Before any surgical procedure, the patient must sign a statement indicating his or her **informed consent** to have the procedure performed (Figure 8-1). The patient has the right to refuse surgery at any time, even after the consent form has been signed. Signed consent implies that the patient has been given the information needed to understand the procedure and any possible consequences. This information must be sufficient to enable the patient to make an informed decision after weighing the risks and benefits of the proposed procedure. The form will not contain all of the information given to the patient by the surgeon prior to the procedure but should be comprehensive enough to cover the more significant information presented.

The consent forms should include the risks of any surgery as well as the risks specific to the procedure proposed. The form should mention that there is always a small chance of death and brain injury from anesthesia. The consent form should present an accurate picture of the risks of the procedure. There is no way to determine exactly which complications may arise, so it is important to list on the consent form all possible known risks and complications of the procedure. These will include bodily harm or death and in most cases will also list the common postoperative complications such as bleeding, infection, or thrombosis. One specific risk that should always be mentioned is that the surgery may not cure the underlying problem. No guarantee should be made, either implicit or explicit (Figure 8-1).

The consent form will usually contain a clause specifying permission to perform any further action if, during the course of the operation, unforeseen conditions are revealed that require an extension of or modification to the procedure. This does not generally give the physician permission to perform separate and unrelated procedures. For example, this does not permit the surgeon to perform a rhinoplasty along with a blepharoplasty, unless specified in the consent.

Generally, surgical consent forms will contain a brief note about the risks of anesthesia. The risks will be separately delineated, as will possible alternatives. The anesthesia provider should be named, just as the surgeon is named.

Patients must not be allowed to sign the consent for surgery after preoperative medications have been administered, because decision-making abilities may be impaired at this point. If an adult is judged by the surgeon to be incapable of giving informed consent, consent should be obtained from the next of kin, as prescribed by law. By most legal definitions, the succession would be spouse, adult child, parent, and sibling. In the case of a

SAMPLE

Standard Consent to Surgery or Special Procedure

Patient Name ______________________________

Attending Physician ______________________________

Surgeon or Supervising Physician ______________________________

1. (*Name of facility*) maintains personnel and facilities to assist your/the patient's physicians and surgeons in their performance of various surgical or other special diagnostic or therapeutic procedures. These operations and procedures may involve risks of unsuccessful results, complications, injury, or death, from known and/or unforeseen causes, and no warranty or guarantee is made as to results or cure.

   You have the right to be informed of such risks as well as the nature of the operation or procedure; the expected benefits of such; and any available alternatives and their risks and benefits. Except in case of emergency, operations or procedures are not performed until you have had the opportunity to receive this information and have given your consent. You have the right to consent or refuse any proposed operation or procedure any time prior to its performance.
2. Your/the patient's physician/surgeon has recommended the operation or procedure set forth below. Upon your authorization and consent, the operation or procedure set forth below, together with any different or further procedures which in the opinion of the supervising physician/surgeon may be indicated due to an emergency, will be performed on you/the patient. The operation or procedure will be performed by the supervising physician or surgeon named above (or in the event of an emergency causing his/her inability to complete the procedure, a qualified substitute supervising physician or surgeon), together with associates and assistants, including anesthesiologists, pathologists and radiologists from the medical staff of (*name of facility*) to whom the supervising physician or surgeon may assign designated responsibilities. The persons in attendance for the purpose of performing specialized medical services such as anesthesia, radiology or pathology are not agents, servants, or employees of the facility and your/the patient's supervising physician or surgeon, but are independent contractors, and therefore your agents, servants, or employees.
3. The pathologist is hereby authorized to use his/her discretion in disposing any member, organ, or other tissue removed from your/the patient's person during the operation or procedure set forth below.
4. Your signature below constitutes your acknowledgment that: you have read and agree to the foregoing; that the operation or procedure set forth below has been adequately explained to you by the above named physician/surgeon and by your/the patient's anesthesiologist and that you have received all of the information that you desire concerning such operation or procedure; and that you authorize and consent to the performance of the operation or procedure.

Procedure: ______________________________

____

____

Signature (Patient/Parent/Conservator/Guardian) Relationship (if other than patient)

____

Date Time Witness

I have been informed of the risks/benefits and alternatives of blood product infusions. I consent to the use of blood product infusions.

____

Signature (Patient/Parent/Conservator/Guardian) Relationship (if other than patient)

____

Date Time Witness

(Name of Facility
Address of Facility)

(Patient Identification–Stamp)

Figure 8-1 Sample of a standard consent to surgery or special procedure form

minor, consent is usually obtained from a parent or legal guardian. "Emancipated minors" or minors who are married may sign their own consent. In an emergency, a surgeon may operate without written consent from either the patient or the family if two physicians agree that the surgery is necessary and both sign the consent. If time permits, every reasonable effort must be made to contact a family member. In these special cases, a witnessed telephone consent would be permissible.

PREOPERATIVE EDUCATION

The patient facing surgery has many decisions to make, any of which may produce anxiety. Being given the opportunity to talk with supportive individuals who will be directly involved with the procedure at hand helps to alleviate this anxiety and has been shown to promote better postoperative outcomes. Studies have shown that patient education has a positive effect on postoperative recovery, including improvement in patients' ventilatory status and a decreased need for postoperative analgesic medications. In addition, patients who have received preoperative education have shown shorter hospital stays, some by as much as 1.3 days. In a study of 100 patients who received preoperative education, a decrease was seen in patient pain, depression, and disability, along with a significant increase in patient compliance.

Preoperative education is intended to alleviate anxiety, educate the patient about expected experiences before, during, and after the procedure, and teach preoperative and postoperative behaviors and activities that may enhance or promote healing and faster recovery. Increasingly, preoperative education is being done in the physician's office prior to admission. The advent of short-stay and same-day surgery has increased the percentages of admissions on the morning of surgery, bringing about the need for in-office patient education. In some cases, educational pamphlets or videotapes are used. The amount of information presented preoperatively should be based on the background of the patient, as well as the interest and anxiety level of the patient. Most patients will find information relating to preoperative tests and procedures and postoperative expectations helpful. The patient should also be informed about what pains and discomforts he or she may expect to experience postoperatively, along with how to deal with medications. The patient will also be educated at this point about how to deal with any body changes, immobilizations, or permanent disabilities.

Patients may benefit from information about sensations in the OR, such as the coldness of the OR or feelings of drowsiness from premedication. It is helpful to reassure the patient that little or no discomfort is to be expected prior to anesthesia, other than a small needle stick for IV insertion, and that warm blankets will be provided for comfort if desired.

Many patients are taught specific activities to help alleviate preoperative anxiety. These include deep-breathing exercises and positive imagery. One recent approach is the use of music therapy, both preoperatively and in the OR.

In the process of preoperative patient education, the need, type, and extent of the surgery should be explained to the patient and to significant others. The patient's understanding should be clarified and explanations should be given about any preoperative tests. The patient should be given the opportunity to express his or her feelings and concerns about the surgery, and significant others who may offer support should be identified.

PATIENT POSSESSIONS

The patient should be instructed to leave valuables at home. Prior to surgery, any remaining valuables and possessions should be collected and either given to a family member or significant other or locked in the hospital's safe for security purposes. The patient should be reassured that his or her possessions are safe and that they will be returned after surgery. Patients sometimes request that religious medals be brought into the OR. If the patient is to be permitted to wear a wedding ring, it should always be taped or otherwise secured to the hand to prevent loss. Generally, all jewelry should be removed prior to surgery. Dentures, prostheses, and implants are removed prior to surgery, labeled, and placed in safekeeping with the rest of the patient's possessions. Dentures must be removed because of the danger of falling into the pharynx and causing respiratory obstruction when the jaw relaxes under anesthesia. Some anesthesia providers prefer that the patient leave the dentures in until the moment of intubation, as the shape of the dentures allows for a better fit for the face mask. Wigs and hairpins must be removed as hairpins may become dislodged and injure the scalp and wigs may be lost. If the patient utilizes a hearing aid, it may be left in place. This facilitates verbal communication with the surgical team in the OR.

A common admissions process for the surgical patient in the modern hospital setting is as follows:

1. Patient arrives at hospital the evening before or morning of surgery.
2. Required paperwork is completed, including all operative and special consents.
3. Identification bracelet is affixed.
4. Vital signs are taken.
5. Patient changes clothes.

6. Any necessary IVs are started.
7. Preoperative medication is given if required.
8. Time is allowed with family.
9. Patient is transported to the OR.

EVENING/MORNING BEFORE SURGERY

Certain preoperative procedures will be scheduled the evening or morning before surgery. If the patient is being admitted on a "day surgery" or same-day basis, some of these procedures will be explained in the office to the patient, and the patient will be expected to complete them at home.

ENEMAS

The enema is no longer a routine preoperative procedure, except in the case of certain gastrointestinal and gynecological procedures. Its purpose is the prevention of injury to the colon and for better visualization of the surgical area. Any time a patient has had barium studies performed immediately before surgery, enemas are indicated because the presence of barium in the bowel will predispose the patient to postoperative fecal impactions.

If ordered, the enema should be administered 8–12 hours prior to the operation. A typical enema order will be for 500–1500 mL of warm tap water, saline, or 120–150 mL of hypertonic sodium phosphate solution. Sodium phosphate solution is readily available in a preoperative kit and can be purchased commercially at most drugstores for use at home. When full bowel cleansing is not required, the patient may be given a mild laxative to provide for successful evacuation the evening before surgery.

NAIL POLISH

Prior to surgery, nail polish should be removed. The **pulse oximeter**, a device used intraoperatively to measure blood oxygen saturation, cannot function properly with nail polish present, as it relies on a light beam focused through the skin and nail of the finger. The presence of nail polish changes the color of the light beam and causes the pulse oximeter to malfunction. Colored nail polish also prevents proper assessment of nail bed color for capillary blanching and refill.

SEDATION

In many cases, preoperative medications are administered to help alleviate anxiety and to relax the patient as well as to decrease nausea, if present. These medications are usually administered 1–2 hours prior to surgery in order to decrease anxiety and produce amnesia. Preoperative medications used to induce **sedation** are often administered by the anesthesia provider at the time of the preoperative visit. Other medications are given to decrease the secretion of saliva and gastric juices and to prevent allergic reaction to anesthetic drugs. Any delay in the administration of these drugs should be reported to the anesthesia provider. All preoperative routines should be completed prior to the administration of preoperative medications, and the patient should be allowed to relax in a quiet place after receiving the medication. During this time, side rails on the gurney should be raised, and the patient should not be left alone. The patient must not be allowed to sign an operative consent after receiving this medication.

PREOPERATIVE HYGIENE

The surgical patient should shower or bathe the night before or morning of the surgery and should be reminded to wash the hair as it may be several days or longer before this can be done again. In some cases, the physician will request the use of a special antiseptic solution. The patient should also be reminded to brush his or her teeth prior to surgery, as good oral hygiene is helpful in prevention of infection. Some studies have shown a decreased microbial count on the skin of surgical patients who have showered with an antimicrobial soap preoperatively. Surgeons may request that the patient shower with an antiseptic containing chlorhexidine or povidone-iodine in some cases where there is a particular risk of surgical site infection (SSI).

PREOPERATIVE SHAVE

If ordered, a shave may need to be performed prior to surgery. The area(s) to be shaved by the patient will be detailed by the physician and either this information should be relayed to the patient or the shave may in some instances be performed by a nurse or nurse's assistant. Personnel responsible for shaving should be skillful with the razor. Clippers are less hazardous than a razor and are the preferred method in many facilities. Care should be taken to avoid cutting or nicking the skin, as breaks in the skin surface provide an easy opportunity for bacterial entry and wound infection. Some medical facilities will choose the use of a depilatory cream. After the cream has remained on the skin for the prescribed amount of time, it is wiped off and hair is removed. This method is beneficial in that is does not cut the skin. It is preferable to shave any required areas in the preoperative holding area, as this area has brighter lighting, which helps prevent nicks and cuts. Often, patient shaves are performed in the OR, although objections have been raised to this on the grounds that the operation is delayed and loose hair is released into the operative environment and may find its way onto the sterile field. Recent studies have shown that the preoperative use of clippers is the best method for hair removal if hair is to be removed at all, and the CDC recommends not removing hair preoperatively unless it interferes with the operation, as microbial counts have been shown to be increased in preshaved areas of the skin.

DIET

The day before surgery, a normal diet is usually indicated. In the case of bowel surgery, a low-residue diet may be necessary. When general anesthesia is to be used, no food or liquid is permitted by mouth for at least 4–8 hours prior to surgery. A general rule of thumb is 8 hours, or "nothing after midnight," for patients scheduled for surgery the next morning. If a local or spinal anesthetic is to be utilized, a light meal may be permitted prior to surgery. The presence of food or fluids in the stomach during surgery increases the danger of aspiration should the patient vomit while under anesthesia, which can lead to pneumonia and death. If it is discovered prior to surgery that the patient has consumed food or fluids while ordered "nothing by mouth" (**NPO**), the surgeon should be notified immediately. The surgeon may then reschedule the procedure.

MAKEUP AND DRESS

It is best that a patient be instructed not to wear any makeup to the OR. While the danger of makeup shedding and entering the operative site is minimal, it does exist, and the use of makeup prevents the anesthesia provider in some instances from monitoring skin tone and color properly. A psychological consideration may be made, however, for the patient who is uncomfortable without the most basic makeup. The danger of SSI occurring from the use of makeup by the patient is generally considered to be low to negligible. The patient is generally required to remove all personal clothing and wear a clean hospital gown. In the case of the large patient, two gowns may be tied back to back to facilitate comfort and provide cover. In cases where the patient is allowed to keep some personal clothing items, such as the underwear under the gown, those items will need to be removed in the OR after induction of anesthesia and returned to the family or locked up for safekeeping with the rest of the personal belongings. In cases of high risk for postoperative thromboembolism, the patient will be requested to apply antiembolic stockings or elastic bandages to the lower extremities. These use pressure to help prevent venous stasis, which can lead to thromboembolism and **shock**.

CALL TO THE OPERATING ROOM

When the call has come that the OR is prepared, the patient should be notified. He or she should be instructed to void (urinate) just prior to leaving for the OR, in order to permit better visualization of the abdominal organs and to decrease the chances of injury to the bladder. If the procedure will require the bladder to be collapsed throughout the surgery, a Foley catheter may be inserted and attached to a closed drainage system. This is often done in the OR itself after anesthesia induction to ensure sterile conditions and for patient comfort. Prior to transportation to the OR, the patient's identification bracelet should be checked by the caregiver for accuracy and firmness of attachment. In addition to simply reading the identification bracelet, the patient should be asked to verbalize his or her name. A preoperative assessment including **vital signs**, consciousness and anxiety levels, skin condition, and personal information should be conducted and recorded prior to transport of the patient to the OR. This should also include personal data and any known allergies. This information provides the surgical team with a quick and concise view of the patient and his or her status prior to transport to the OR, so that any intraoperative or postoperative changes may be noted.

FAMILY VISIT

If possible, the patient should be allowed to visit with family or significant others prior to being transported to the OR. Some patients may request a visit by a member of the clergy at this time. This is psychologically important to the patient and aids in the relief of anxiety and mental preparation for surgery. Care should be taken that visitors not overstimulate the patient at this time, as premedication has usually already been given. Visitors should be informed at this time of the location of the waiting area and when and how to expect to receive information on the status of the patient.

PATIENT IDENTIFICATION

The patient identification bracelet is extremely important in that it helps ensure that the correct patient is brought to the OR, receiving the correct procedure performed by the correct physician. On admission to the hospital, the bracelet is typically affixed to the patient's wrist and should not be removed unnecessarily until the patient has been discharged. When the transportation attendant or OR personnel arrive to transport the patient to the OR, nursing personnel should be notified. The individuals transporting the patient should introduce themselves and request that the patient verbally state his or her name. The patient identification band should then be read and compared with the patient's chart and with the information on the surgical schedule. The information should also be confirmed with the patient's chart label. If any discrepancy is found, the patient should not be taken to the OR. The discrepancy should be reported immediately to the nursing unit personnel and the OR personnel, and the patient should not be transported until and unless identification can be absolutely verified.

TRANSPORTATION

Surgical patients are usually transported to the OR using a gurney or the patient's bed. In some cases, the patient may be transported in a wheelchair or may even walk to the OR. Infants may be transported in an isolette or accompanied by a parent. Some hospitals provide a wagon, which may be more comfortable and familiar to a child. Whatever the mode of transportation, care must be taken to protect the patient as well as the individual providing transportation from injury. Side rails of the gurney or bed should always be placed in the up and locked position to prevent falls. When using a wheelchair, the safety belt should be securely fastened, and the wheels should be locked before the patient sits and when the patient prepares to stand on arrival at the OR.

When a patient will need to have accessory equipment such as IV stands or traction apparatus moved along with the bed, extra personnel should be available to assist. Care must be taken not to catch such equipment on walls, doors, or ceilings, as patient injury or equipment damage could occur. The transporter should not attempt this alone, as use of improper body mechanics may result in injury to the individual moving the patient. Before the patient is moved, a check should be made that all drainage collection devices, IV tubings, and oxygen delivery devices are ready for transport. If the patient requires oxygen, a portable tank should be safely affixed to the gurney and the oxygen should be connected to the delivery device from this site. Extra assistance in transport will also be necessary if the patient requires a ventilator. The respiratory therapy department of the hospital will provide personnel to assist with ventilator transport.

The patient should be transported slowly, feet first, to maintain control of the gurney at all times. When entering an elevator with a patient on a gurney or in a wheelchair, the patient is taken in head first, so that when the elevator opens the patient is again being moved in the forward-facing position. Proper body mechanics and lifting techniques should be observed by the transportation personnel to avoid personal injury. To avoid injury, the patient should be instructed to keep hands and feet inside the guardrails at all times. Care should be taken to protect the patient's dignity as well as comfort. Blankets should be provided both for warmth and privacy. The patient's head should be raised or lowered into a position that is comfortable, unless physician orders or a patient condition will not permit this.

On arrival at the preoperative holding area, the surgical team is notified of the patient's arrival. The patient should not be left alone in the holding area. This is often the point of greatest anxiety for the patient, and feelings of abandonment may result if the patient is left alone. At the time of arrival to the holding area, the circulator will identify and interview the patient. The chart is reviewed to verify the presence of the surgical consent, history, physical assessment, radiology results, and laboratory reports. Preoperative plans for positioning should be made before the patient enters the OR, to assure that all necessary positioning aids and accessory equipment for the table are available. In addition to the type of procedure and position to be used, any preoperative neuropathies, preexisting conditions, or diseases should be considered prior to positioning. Age, physical limitations, skin condition, and height and weight must also be considered to avoid injury to the patient. Muscles and nerves are easily injured from overstretching because muscle tone is lost during anesthesia. Pressure for any length of time on any part of the body may also easily injure the anesthetized patient. Very young, obese, elderly, or debilitated patients are at increased risk of compromise to the circulatory, respiratory, and integumentary systems. Prolonged procedures without position change can lead to a decrease in tissue perfusion, as can the use of positioning devices of inappropriate size. Because of these risk factors, the proper pads and positioning devices must be available and in proper working order prior to placing the patient on the table.

TECHNIQUE: Patient Transport

1. The guardrails are in the upright and secure position.
2. The safety belt is secured, if necessary.
3. The wheels are in the correct position (straight or swivel).
4. Transport the patient slowly, feet first.
5. Enter an elevator head first and exit feet first.
6. Be certain that all parts of the patient's body are within the guardrails.
7. Use good body mechanics.
8. Never leave the patient unattended.

TRANSFER AND POSITIONING

Usually, the patient is brought into the OR from the holding area on a gurney and then transferred to the operating table. Patients who are not too heavily sedated and are ambulatory may move under their own effort onto the table. Typically, two individuals assist the awake patient capable of moving him or herself from the gurney onto the operating table. The gurney is placed next to the operating table and the wheels are locked. Then, one individual will stabilize the gurney, while another stands on the other side of the operating table to receive the patient and assist in movement.

Many patients' first complaint about the OR is often the low temperature, and the feet are often the first to feel uncomfortably cold. Booties and an additional blanket will provide warmth and comfort. A hair cover is placed on the patient's head. While the patient is moving or being moved from the gurney to the operating table, care must be taken that IV tubing, O_2 tubings, etc., do not become entangled or snagged in the bedding, on the patient, or on parts of the table causing them to be dislodged.

If the patient is too heavily sedated or is unable to move, he or she will need to be transferred onto the operating table by an appropriate number of personnel. Usually, four individuals will be required for this process: One will support the head and shoulders, one will lift the feet and legs, and one will stand on each side to lift and stabilize the patient's trunk. The movement is typically coordinated by the individual at the patient's head and should be smooth to avoid injury to the patient. If too few individuals attempt to move a patient, strained backs or other personnel injuries may occur. Always use the correct number of personnel when moving a patient to guarantee safe transfer of the patient and protection for the team members. The use of a roller or draw sheet may be helpful. Once the patient has been moved onto the operating table, he or she must not be left alone for any reason. The safety strap should be securely placed 2 in. proximal to the knees. This strap should not be tight, but just tight enough to secure the patient. The patient should be assured that this strap is only placed for safety and is not being used for the purpose of restraint. The draw sheet may be used to hold the arms at the patient's side, being careful that the elbows do not rest against the metal table, to prevent ulnar nerve damage. Often, the arms are not tucked until after induction of anesthesia to reduce patient anxiety at feelings of being restrained. If this is to be the case, operative personnel should be careful not to let the arms fall off of the table on anesthesia relaxation. Every effort should be made to make the patient comfortable on the operating table. A pillow may be placed under the head for comfort until the anesthesia provider needs for it to be removed. The patient's gown should be checked to make sure that it is not too tight and that free breathing is permitted. A warm cotton blanket may be placed over the patient for modesty and warmth. For the patient's psychological comfort, personnel around the table should introduce themselves and explain in as calm a manner possible what the patient may expect.

The patient is transferred to the operating table using one of the two following methods.

TECHNIQUE Patient Transfer

1. The mobile patient may be able to move herself to the operating table independently.
   - A minimum of two nonsterile team members should be available to assist with transfer of a mobile patient.
   - Position the gurney next to the operating table.
   - Instruct the patient not to move until you give the command.
   - Be sure that the wheels of both the gurney and the operating table are locked.
   - One individual should be positioned at the side of the gurney and the other at the side of the operating table.
   - Brace your bodies against the gurney and operating table to prevent any unexpected movement.
   - Instruct the patient to keep her blanket on and move to the operating table.
   - Assist the patient any way you can (e.g., move the pillow from the gurney to the operating table or assist by lifting an extremity that is casted).
   - Apply the safety strap, then remove the gurney.
2. The immobile patient will be unable to assist with the transfer and will have to be moved onto the operating table.
   - A minimum of four nonsterile team members should be available to assist with transfer of an immobile patient.
   - Position the gurney next to the operating table.
   - If necessary, explain the transfer procedure to the patient.

(continues)

(continued)

- One individual should be positioned at the side of the gurney, another at the side of the operating table, and one at the head and foot of the gurney.
- Brace your bodies against the gurney and operating table to prevent any unexpected movement.
- Keep the patient covered and transfer him to the operating table using the preferred method.
- Apply the safety strap, then remove the gurney.

BASIC POSITIONING FOR SURGERY

Positioning for surgery usually takes place after the administration of anesthesia. The goal of proper positioning is to provide the best possible access and visualization of the surgical site while causing the least possible compromise in physiological function and stress to joints, skin, and other body parts. Positioning should also provide access to the patient for the administration of IV fluids and anesthetic agents and provide patient safety.

When a patient is awake, physical indicators such as pain and pressure that warn when the limits of stretching and twisting are being reached maintain the range of motion of the body. Muscle tone also helps prevent strain and stress to muscle groups. Under anesthesia, these protective devices are no longer active. After anesthetic agents have been administered, the patient is completely relaxed and paralyzed and has no ability to react to movements that could potentially damage joints or stress muscle groups. This is especially important to note with the arthritic patient, who may have joint changes that will prevent even slight movement beyond the normal range of motion. For these reasons, it is important to avoid extreme exaggerated positioning for extended periods of time. Patients are at higher risk in long surgical procedures and during vascular surgery, where blood perfusion may be low or even interrupted. Patients with demineralizing bone diseases such as osteoporosis are also at increased risk for injury. When moving the legs, both extremities should be moved slowly and simultaneously, as this helps prevent muscle injury.

The pooling of blood in dependent areas is a major problem and causes sudden shifting of blood when the patient is returned to the **supine** position following surgery. This places a strain on the cardiovascular system and may cause a rapid rise or drop in blood pressure. The patient should always be returned slowly from the operative position back to the supine position. This gives the cardiovascular system time to adjust. Patients with cardiovascular conditions and the elderly are at particular risk and should be carefully monitored. Respect for the patient as an individual should be maintained at all times, and covering for modesty should be continued even after the induction of anesthesia.

Safe positioning of the surgical patient is the responsibility of the entire surgical team. Two concepts are the basis for surgical positioning:

1. Access to the surgical site, airway, intravenous line(s), and monitoring devices must be provided.
2. Compromise to the patient's integumentary, nervous, respiratory, musculoskeletal, and cardiovascular systems must be prevented.

Several factors must be considered prior to positioning the patient for a procedure:

- Basic anatomy and related physiology must be understood.
- Factors specific to each patient must be considered.
  - Planned surgical procedure
  - Primary condition
  - Underlying conditions
  - Allergy status
  - Age
  - Size
  - Nutritional status
  - Planned anesthetic
- Knowledge of positioning equipment and supplies is imperative.
- Proper body mechanics must be implemented.
- Injury to the patient and surgical staff must be avoided.
  - Chemical
  - Electrical
  - Mechanical (gravity, friction, shearing)
  - Thermal
- Surgeon and anesthesia provider preferences must be considered.

For the safety and comfort of the patient—as well as personnel safety—many basic safety measures must be followed each time the patient is transferred or positioned:

- Patient identification and assessment (including allergy status and surgical site confirmation) occurs prior to transportation to the OR.
- A minimum of two individuals should be available to assist the mobile patient.
- A minimum of four individuals should be available to assist the immobile patient.

- The patient is assessed prior to arrival in the OR and preparations to meet special needs are made in advance.
- All patient care devices (e.g., oxygen and IV administration equipment, Foley catheter, and drainage collection devices) must be protected during transfer or positioning.
- Adequately cover the patient to provide warmth and privacy.
- Provide comfort devices (such as a pillow) and adjust the head of the transport device or operating table to a comfortable level, as the patient's condition allows.
- The wheels of both the operating table and transportation device must be locked and the mattress stabilized.
- Lift, rather than slide, the patient to prevent friction and shearing injuries (transfer devices may be used).
- The patient is moved slowly to maintain control of the body and allow for circulatory changes.
- Pressure points and bony prominences should be padded to prevent gravity-related injuries.
- The patient's skin should not come in direct contact with any metallic table parts, accessories, or unpadded surfaces to prevent electrical and gravity-related injuries.
- No part of the patient may extend beyond the table surface.
- Restraints are used whenever indicated.
- The anesthetized patient is not moved without permission from the anesthesia provider. The anesthesia provider directs movement of the patient.
- The anesthesia provider is responsible for maintaining the patient's airway and may not be able to help lift the patient.
- The armboard may not extend beyond a 90° angle.
- The patient's legs may not be crossed.
- The patient must be protected from injury during movement of the operating table.
- Patient care supplies (e.g., Mayo stand) and personnel may not rest on the patient.
- The patient's eyes must be protected from drying and abrasion.
- Excessive torsion, flexion, and/or extension of any part of the patient's body must be avoided.

There are three basic surgical positions—supine, **prone**, and lateral—and each may be varied to accommodate specific patient needs. Body region(s) that may be accessed when the patient is in each position, the potential hazards to the patient, and the precautions that must be taken to prevent injury to the patient are discussed next. Keep in mind that variations may occur due to the specific patient's situation, surgeon and anesthesia provider preferences, product differences, and facility policy.

SUPINE POSITION

The *supine position* is the most natural position for the body at rest (Figure 8-2). The patient lies flat on the back with the arms secured at the sides with palms facing inward. The elbows may be protected with plastic shells or egg crate elbow padding. The legs are straight and parallel, in line with the head and spine, placing the cervical, thoracic, and lumbar vertebrae in a straight line with the hips. A safety belt is placed across the thighs 2 in. proximal to the knees. If armboards are used, they should be placed at no more than a 90° angle to the table to prevent hyperextension of the shoulder. Areas of the body that are in direct contact with the table will be under pressure during the procedure and are therefore at risk of tissue injury. These will include the occiput, scapula, olecranon, sacrum, ischial tuberosity, and calcaneus. The use of egg crate padding and gel pads on the operating table help to minimize pressure on the body.

Small pillows may be placed under the head and lumbar curvature. The heels must be protected from pressure on the table by a pillow, ankle roll, or donut. The feet must not be in prolonged plantar flexion to prevent stretch injury. A pillow or padded footboard may support the soles of the feet, and care should be taken that the ankles are not crossed to prevent pressure injury. This position is used for most procedures on the anterior surface of the body, including abdominal, abdominothoracic, cardiac, and some lower extremity procedures. Modifications of this position may be used for procedures involving specific body areas. A small pad or donut should be used to stabilize the head, as extreme rotation of the head intraoperatively can lead to occlusion of the vertebral artery.

Any one of several modifications to the supine position may be used, depending on the requirements of the particular procedure. For shoulder and neck procedures, the patient's neck may be extended by the use of a shoulder roll. For certain procedures, the arms may be extended on armboards. To avoid hyperextension injuries, the arms should not be extended at more than a 90° angle to the body.

Typically, the patient is placed in the supine or dorsal recumbent position prior to the administration of anesthesia. The patient may remain in the supine position for

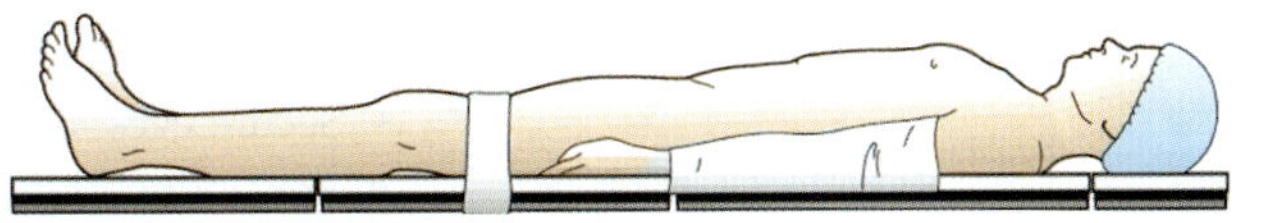

Figure 8-2 Supine position

the procedure or be repositioned, as needed, once anesthetized. Any additional procedures such as application of antiembolic stockings, insertion of a Foley catheter, or application/insertion of additional monitoring devices are performed prior to repositioning. Once the patient is anesthetized, permission must be sought from the anesthesia provider to reposition the patient. The anesthesia provider usually assumes the leadership role in positioning the anesthetized patient, giving the commands to the other team members.

Body regions that may be accessed with the patient in the supine position include:

- Anterior lower extremity
- Pelvis
- Abdomen
- Chest/breast
- Shoulder
- Head and neck
- Upper extremity

Potential hazards and necessary precautions that apply to the patient in the supine position are presented in Table 8-1.

TECHNIQUE: Supine Position

1. The patient is transferred onto the operating table.
2. Instruct the awake patient to keep her arms across her abdomen temporarily (the arms of the unconscious patient must be held by a team member).
3. Apply the safety strap snugly across the thighs approximately 2 in. proximal to the knees. Allow approximately 2 finger breadths of space beneath the strap.
4. Be sure the patient is comfortable (offer pillow and warm blanket).
5. Be sure the patient's spine and lower extremities are in alignment.

Table 8-1 Patient Safety—Supine Position

POTENTIAL HAZARD	PRECAUTIONARY ACTION(S)
Brachial plexus injury	• Position armboard at less than a 90° angle.
Ulnar nerve injury	• Pad elbows. • Place arms on armboards with palms facing upward. • Place arms next to patient's body with palms facing inward.
Pressure injury to skin, blood vessels, and nerves	• Pad all bony prominences. • Uncross ankles. • Be sure restraining devices are not restrictive. • Use egg crate padding or gel pads on the operating table. • Do not let any part of the patient's body extend beyond the padded operating table. • Avoid excessive torsion, flexion, and/or extension of any part of the patient's body.
Back and neck pain	• Legs are parallel and the spine is in alignment. • Provide lumbar support pillow. • Head is stabilized on a pillow or foam headrest.
Hypo/hyperthermia	• Adjust OR temperature. • Provide or remove blankets. • Implement use of hypo/hyperthermia unit. • Ensure solutions (IV and irrigation) are at correct temperature. • Provide warm humidified inhalation agents.
Corneal drying and abrasion	• Lubricate eyes. • Secure eyes in the closed position. • Prevent pressure on the eyelids.
Foot drop	• Use padded foot board.
Electrical injury	• Do not let any part of the patient's body contact any metal object.

6. Be sure the legs are parallel and the heels are resting on the table. Heel pads may be applied. The ankles may not be crossed.
7. There are two options for positioning the arms. Arm position will be determined by patient situation, surgeon, and anesthesia provider preference.
    - The arms may be placed on armboards, palms up, at no greater than a 90-degree angle. The elbows may be padded. A safety strap is snugly applied approximately 2 in. proximal to the wrist. Allow approximately 1 finger breadth of space beneath the strap. Be sure the strap does not interfere with IV infusion. A blanket may be placed across the arms.
    - The arms may be placed, palms facing the body, along the patient's sides. The elbows may be padded and the arms are secured with the draw sheet or other device.

TRENDELENBURG POSITION

The *Trendelenburg position* is a modification of the supine position (Figure 8-3). It is used to displace the abdominopelvic organs cephalad to provide better visualization of the surgical site. Another benefit of the Trendelenburg position is that blood flow to the lower body is reduced and venous drainage is promoted. Conversely, the position may be used to increase blood flow to the upper body, as in the treatment of shock or for distention of blood vessels to be cannulated.

Body regions that may be accessed with the patient in the Trendelenburg position include:

- Pelvis
- Lower abdomen

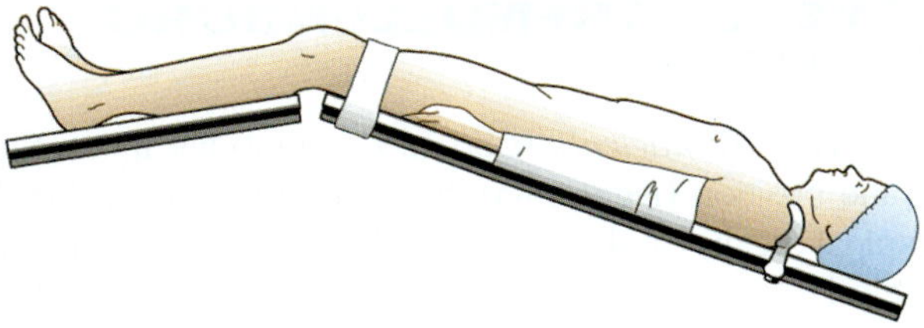

Figure 8-3 Trendelenburg position

Potential hazards and necessary precautions that apply to the patient in the Trendelenburg position (in addition to those previously listed for the supine position) are presented in Table 8-2.

TECHNIQUE Trendelenburg Position

1. Place the patient in the supine position as previously described.
2. Apply the safety strap snugly across the thighs approximately 2 in. proximal to the knees.
3. Be sure the patient's knees are over the lower break of the operating table.
4. The leg section of the operating table is lowered to the desired angle.
5. Padded shoulder braces may be applied to both sides of the operating table.
6. Secure permission to move the patient.
7. The operating table is tilted head downward to approximately 45° or to the desired angle.

Table 8-2 Patient Safety—Trendelenburg Position

POTENTIAL HAZARD	PRECAUTIONARY ACTION(S)
1. Cardiovascular and respiratory compromise	• Decrease angle of operating table.
	• Return patient to supine position as soon as possible.
2. Pressure injury to skin, blood vessels, and nerves *Note:* Special attention is given to the peroneal nerves.	• Flex leg section of the operating table.
3. Patient movement toward the head of the operating table	• Use padded shoulder braces.
4. Venous stasis	• Use antiembolic devices.
	• Raise leg section of the operating table slowly prior to leveling the table.
5. Blood pressure changes	• Level the operating table slowly.

REVERSE TRENDELENBURG POSITION

The *reverse Trendelenburg position* is a modification of the supine position (Figure 8-4). It is used to displace the abdominal organs caudad to provide better visualization of the surgical site. Other benefits of the reverse Trendelenburg position are that blood flow to the upper body is reduced, venous drainage is promoted, and respiration is facilitated.

Body regions that may be accessed with the patient in the reverse Trendelenburg position include:

- Upper abdomen
- Head and neck

Potential hazards and necessary precautions that apply to the patient in the reverse Trendelenburg position (in addition to those previously listed for the supine position) are presented in Table 8-3.

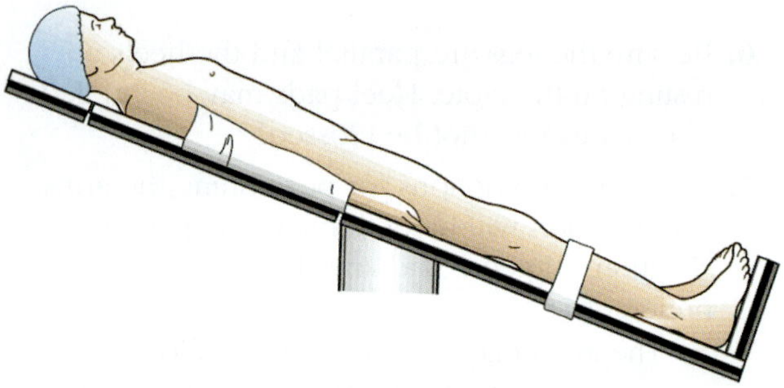

Figure 8-4 Reverse Trendelenburg position

TECHNIQUE Reverse Trendelenburg Position

1. Place the patient in the supine position as previously described.
2. Apply the safety strap snugly approximately 2 in. distal to the knees.
3. A padded footboard may be applied to the operating table.
4. Secure permission to move the patient.
5. The operating table is tilted foot downward to approximately 45° or to the desired angle.

FOWLER'S POSITION AND SITTING POSITION

Fowler's position is a modification of the supine position (Figure 8-5). Fowler's position provides improved access to the surgical site and reduces blood flow to the upper body, promotes venous drainage, and facilitates respiration. Air embolism is a potential concern when the patient is in the Fowler's position.

Body regions that may be accessed with the patient in the Fowler's position include:

- Breast
- Head and neck
- Shoulder

Potential hazards and necessary precautions that apply to the patient in the Fowler's position (in addition to those previously listed for the supine position) are presented in Table 8-4.

The sitting position is a modification of Fowler's position (Figure 8-6). The torso is in an upright position. The flexed arms rest either on a lap pillow or on an adjustable

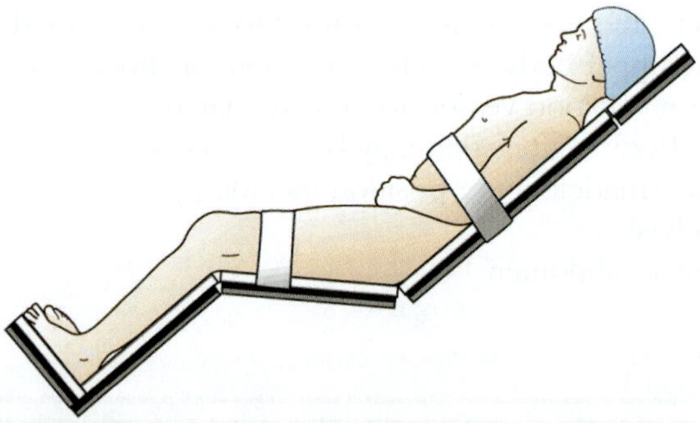

Figure 8-5 Fowler's position

Table 8-3 Patient Safety—Reverse Trendelenburg Position

POTENTIAL HAZARD	PRECAUTIONARY ACTION(S)
1. Patient movement toward the foot of the operating table	• Use a padded footboard. • Safety strap is placed approximately 2 in. distal to the knees. • Pillows or a kidney lift may be used.
2. Venous stasis	• Use antiembolic devices.
3. Blood pressure changes	• Level the operating table slowly.

Table 8-4 Patient Safety—Fowler's Position

POTENTIAL HAZARD	PRECAUTIONARY ACTION(S)
1. Blood pressure changes *Note:* Postural hypotension is of special concern.	• Make adjustments to the operating table slowly. *Note:* A pneumatic compression device may be useful in combatting postural hypotension.
2. Respiratory compromise	• If arms are not placed on an armboard, they will be placed and restrained on a pillow resting across the abdomen, **not** on the chest.
3. Venous stasis	• Use antiembolic devices.
4. Patient movement on the operating table	• Padded footrest may be used. • Upper body may be restrained. • Neurosurgical headrest may be used.
5. Pressure injury to skin, blood vessels, and nerves *Note:* Special attention is given to the sciatic nerves.	• Pad pressure points. *Note:* Special attention is given to the ischial tuberosities.

TECHNIQUE Fowler's Position

1. Place the patient in the supine position as previously described.
2. The patient's arms may be secured on armboards or across the abdomen.
3. Be sure the patient's hips are positioned at the table flex.
4. A padded footboard may be applied to the operating table.
5. The leg section of the table is lowered to the desired angle.
6. The body section of the table is raised to 45° or to the desired angle.
7. The entire operating table may be tilted head downward to achieve the desired level.

table in front of the patient. A body strap should support the shoulders, and padding should be added to prevent sciatic nerve damage. When this position is to be used for a neurosurgical procedure, the head will be in a cranial headrest.

LITHOTOMY POSITION

The *lithotomy position* is a modification of the supine position (Figure 8-7). A variety of positioning devices are available to place the patient in the lithotomy position. The use of candy-cane style stirrups is presented here.

Body regions that may be accessed with the patient in the lithotomy position include:

- Perineum
- Anus and rectum
- Vagina
- Urethra

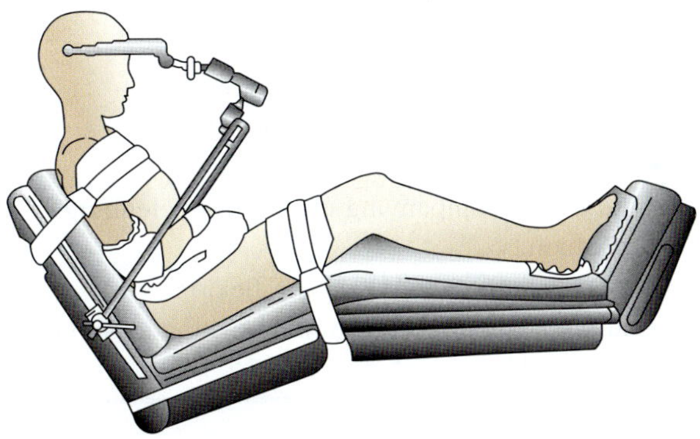

Figure 8-6 Sitting position

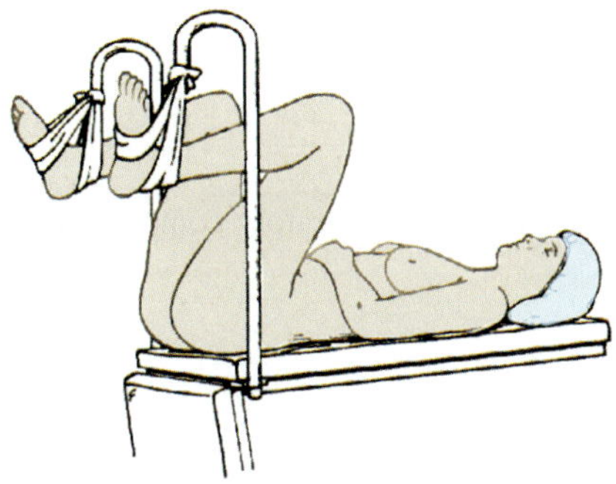

Figure 8-7 Lithotomy position

Potential hazards and necessary precautions that apply to the patient in the lithotomy position (in addition to those previously listed for the supine position) are presented in Table 8-5.

PRONE POSITION

Prior to placement in the prone *position,* the patient is anesthetized on the gurney or another operating table (Figure 8-8). All preoperative procedures, such as Foley catheter insertion, must be performed prior to placement of the patient in the prone position.

Body regions that may be accessed with the patient in the prone position include:

- Posterior lower extremity
- Dorsal body surface
- Spine
- Posterior cranium

Potential hazards and necessary precautions that apply to the patient in the prone position (in addition to those previously listed for the supine position) are presented in Table 8-6.

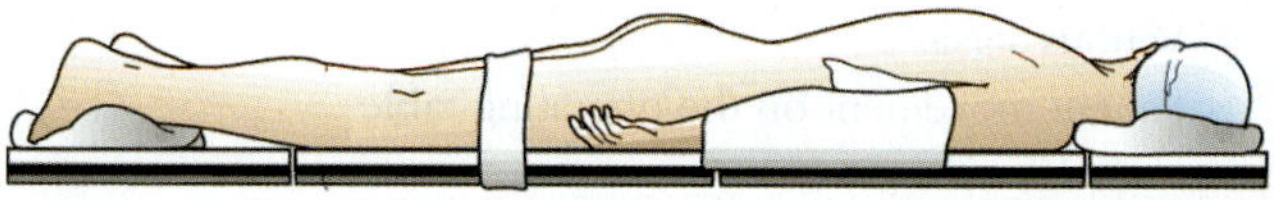

Figure 8-8 Prone position

Table 8-5 Patient Safety—Lithotomy Position

POTENTIAL HAZARD	PRECAUTIONARY ACTION(S)
1. Crushing or shearing injury to the hand	• Arms are placed on armboards. • If arms are positioned at the patient's sides, the hands must be observed during movement of the operating table.
2. Pressure injury to skin, blood vessels, and nerves *Note:* Special attention is given to the peroneal nerves.	• Pad feet and ankles. • Be sure restraining devices are not restrictive. • Avoid excessive torsion, flexion, and/or extension of any part of the patient's body. • The legs may **not** come in direct contact with the stirrups. • Stirrups are adjusted to an equal height and length. • Legs are raised and lowered slowly and simultaneously by two individuals.
3. Back, knee, and hip pain	• Buttocks rest completely on the operating table. • Stirrups are adjusted to an equal height and length. • Legs are raised and lowered slowly and simultaneously by two individuals.
4. Blood pressure changes	• Legs are raised and lowered slowly and simultaneously by two individuals.
5. Venous stasis	• Use antiembolic devices.
6. Cardiovascular and respiratory compromise	• Restrict accompanying use of Trendelenburg's position. • Decrease leg height and hip flexion. • Return patient to the supine position as soon as possible.

TECHNIQUE

Lithotomy Position

The operating table is prepared in the following manner prior to patient placement:

1. Remove the head section of the operating table and place at the foot; secure.
2. The indentation in the mattress must be positioned to allow access to the operative site.
3. The sheet and draw sheet are applied to the table.
4. An absorbant pad may be placed.

The procedure for placing the patient in the lithotomy position is as follows:

1. Place the patient in the supine position as previously described with the arms on armboards, if possible.
2. Be sure the patient's hips are positioned at the table break.
3. Pad the patient's lower extremities as needed.
4. Apply the sockets and stirrups of choice to the operating table bilaterally.
5. Adjust the height and length of stirrups as needed.
6. Secure permission to move the patient.
7. Remove the safety strap.
8. Two nonsterile team members raise the patient's legs slowly and simultaneously by grasping the sole of the foot in one hand and supporting the calf with the other. The hips are rotated externally.
9. The extremities are placed and secured in the stirrups.
10. Make any final height and length adjustments to the stirrups.
11. Release and remove the head section from the foot of the table and place in a convenient location.
12. Remove the mattress and Bakelite portion from the leg section of the table and place in a convenient location.
13. Lower the leg section of the table as far as possible.

TECHNIQUE

Prone Position

1. Necessary accessories are placed within reach.
2. Pads are applied to the ankles, knees, and elbows as needed.
3. A minimum of four nonsterile team members are required to place the patient in the prone position.
4. Align the gurney alongside the operating table and be certain that both are in the locked position.
5. Chest rolls may be positioned on the operating table at this time.
6. Secure permission to move the patient.
7. Be sure that any patient care equipment is not disrupted when moving the patient.
8. The patient's arms are positioned alongside the body.
9. The patient is rolled onto the operating table.
10. Be sure to secure the patient's arms.
11. The gurney is removed.
12. The position of the chest rolls is verified if already in position, or they may be placed at this time.
13. Breasts and external genitalia must be positioned to alleviate any pressure.
14. The head may be turned to the side and placed on a pillow or foam headrest or be placed face down on a foam headrest designed for this purpose.
15. The arms may be secured alongside the body with the palms facing upward or toward the body or the arms may be placed palms facing downward on angled armboards. This is accomplished by lowering the arms toward the floor then rotating them upward. The armboard is placed after the arm is positioned. Secure the arm on the armboard.
16. A pillow is placed under the ankles.
17. The safety strap is applied proximal to the knees.

Table 8-6 Patient Safety—Prone Position

POTENTIAL HAZARD	PRECAUTIONARY ACTION(S)
1. Pressure on abdominal contents and thoracic compression *Note:* The vena cava and abdominal aorta are of particular concern.	• Use chest rolls. • Use axillary rolls. • Use antiembolic devices. • Move breasts laterally.
2. Pressure injury to skin, blood vessels, and nerves	• Place arms on armboards, rather than at the patient's sides. • Be sure all pressure on the male genitalia is removed. • Place pillows under the knees and ankles. • Place padding under the knees. • Flex arms on armboards with the palms facing downward or along the sides of the body with the palms facing inward.
3. Venous stasis	• Use antiembolic devices. • Elevate lower portion of the legs.
4. Shoulder injury	• Lower and rotate arms for placement on armboards.

KRASKE (JACKKNIFE) POSITION

The *Kraske (jackknife) position* is a modification of the prone position (Figure 8-9). Body regions that may be accessed with the patient in the prone position include:

- Anus
- Pilonidal area

Potential hazards and necessary precautions that apply to the patient in the Kraske position (in addition to those previously listed for the supine and prone positions) are presented in Table 8-7.

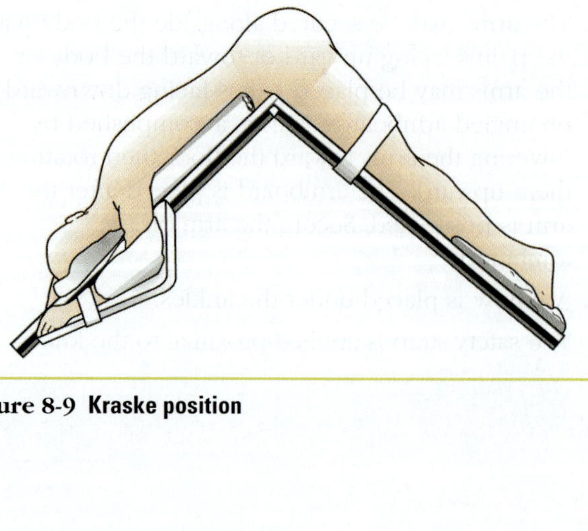

Figure 8-9 Kraske position

Table 8-7 Patient Safety—Kraske Position

POTENTIAL HAZARD	PRECAUTIONARY ACTION(S)
1. Blood pressure changes	• Return the patient to the horizontal position slowly.

TECHNIQUE
Kraske Position

1. Place the patient in the prone position as previously described.
2. Be sure the patient's hips are positioned at the table break.
3. The operating table is flexed to the desired angle.
4. The operating table is tilted head downward to elevate the hips.
5. The safety strap is applied proximal to the knees.
6. Tape may be used to expose the anal area.

LATERAL POSITION

The *lateral position* is also referred to as the lateral recumbent or lateral decubitus position (Figure 8-10). The patient in the right lateral position is placed on the operating table with the right side downward, exposing the left side of the body. The patient in the left lateral position is placed on the operating table with the left side downward, exposing the right side of the body. All preoperative procedures, such as Foley catheter insertion, must be performed prior to placement in the lateral position.

Body regions that may be accessed with the patient in the lateral position include:

- Retroperitoneal space
- Hip
- Hemithorax

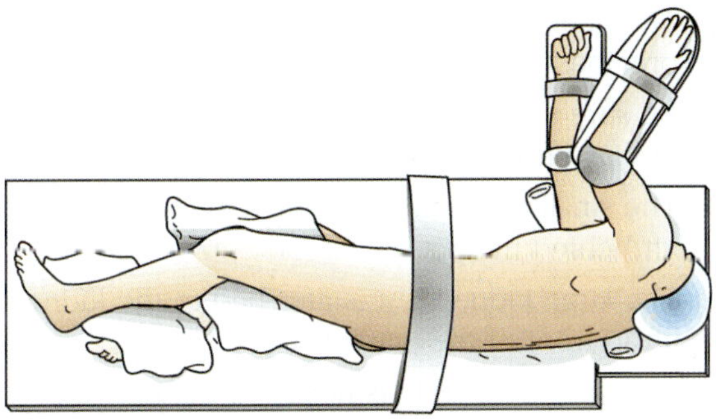

Figure 8-10 Right lateral position

Potential hazards and necessary precautions that apply to the patient in the lateral position (in addition to those previously listed for the supine position) are presented in Table 8-8.

TECHNIQUE Right Lateral Position

1. Place the patient in the supine position as previously described.
2. Pads are applied to the ankles, knees, and elbows as needed.
3. Necessary accessories are placed within reach.
4. A minimum of four nonsterile team members are required to place the patient in the lateral position.
5. Secure permission to move the patient.
6. Remove the safety strap.
7. Be sure that any patient care equipment is not disrupted when moving the patient.
8. Use the draw sheet to slide the patient as far as possible to the left side of the operating table.
9. Roll the patient onto his right side.
10. Stabilize the patient's torso.

(continues)

Table 8-8 Patient Safety—Lateral Position

POTENTIAL HAZARD	PRECAUTIONARY ACTION(S)
1. Respiratory compromise *Note:* Due to gravitational forces the lower lung is better perfused, but contains less residual air due to diaphragmatic and mediastinal compression.	• Positive pressure ventilation is implemented. • Maintain cervical alignment. • An axillary roll is placed.
2. Circulatory compromise *Note:* Arterial circulation to the lower body is restricted, as is venous return.	• Use antiembolic devices. • Avoid excessive compression of the abdomen. • Blood pressure is measured from the lower arm.
3. Movement on the operating table	• Lower leg is flexed. • Safety strap is applied over the hip, if possible. • An upper body restraint may be necessary.
4. Pressure injury to skin, blood vessels, and nerves *Note:* The peroneal nerve, brachial plexus, and the vascular structures of the axilla are of special concern.	• Pillows are placed between the knees and ankles. • An axillary roll is placed. • Arms are placed on a double padded armboard. The palm of the lower hand faces upward and the palm of the upper hand faces downward. • The head is in alignment with the spine.
5. Foot drop	• Support foot and ankle of upper leg.

(continued)

11. An axillary roll is placed.
12. A pillow or foam headrest may be used to stabilize the patient's head.
13. The lower leg is flexed.
14. Two pillows are placed between the legs.
15. The upper leg remains straight.
16. The safety strap is applied over the hip.
17. Shoulders and spine are aligned.
18. The arms are placed on a double armboard. The palm of the lower arm faces upward and the palm of the upper arm faces downward. The elbows may be slightly flexed.
19. The upper torso may be secured if necessary.

Note: An alternate method for stabilizing the patient in the lateral position is with the use of a beanbag.

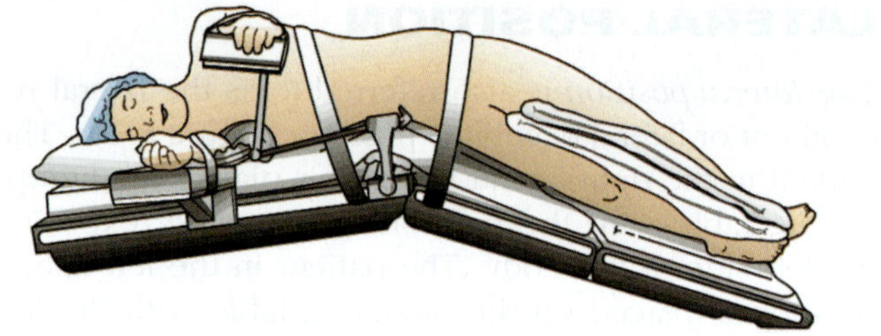

Figure 8-11 Right kidney position

KIDNEY POSITION

The *kidney position* is a modification of the lateral position (Figure 8-11). Body regions that may be accessed with the patient in the kidney position include:

- Retroperitoneal space

Potential hazards and necessary precautions that apply to the patient in the kidney position (in addition to those listed for the supine and lateral positions) are presented in Table 8-9.

TECHNIQUE Right Kidney Position

1. The patient is rolled onto her right side as previously described.
2. Be sure the patient's flank is located over the kidney lift of the operating table.
3. The small kidney rest is attached to the kidney lift behind the patient.
4. The large kidney rest is attached to the kidney lift in front of the patient.
5. The operating table is flexed to the desired angle.

Table 8-9 Patient Safety—Kidney Position

POTENTIAL HAZARD	PRECAUTIONARY ACTION(S)
1. Abdominal compression	• The large kidney rest is attached anteriorly. • Both kidney rests must be well padded. • Be sure patient is positioned correctly over the kidney lift. • Lower kidney lift as soon as possible.
2. Circulatory compromise	• Reduce table flexion as soon as possible. • Be sure patient is positioned correctly over the kidney lift. • Lower kidney lift as soon as possible. *Note:* Reducing table flexion will also facilitate tissue approximation.
3. Venous stasis *Note:* The dependent arm and leg are at greatest risk.	• Use antiembolic devices.
4. Shoulder pain	• Place a chest roll.
5. Muscle strain to the torso	• Use the least possible amount of table flexion. • Reduce table flexion as soon as possible. • Be sure patient is positioned correctly over the kidney lift. • Lower kidney lift as soon as possible.
6. Blood pressure changes	• Ensure fluid management.

6. The kidney lift is raised to the desired height.
7. The safety strap is applied over the hip.
8. Shoulders and spine are aligned.
9. The arms are placed on a double armboard. The palm of the lower arm faces upward and the palm of the upper arm faces downward. The elbows may be slightly flexed.
10. The upper torso may be secured if necessary.
11. The table is tilted head downward until the flank area is horizontal.

SIMS' POSITION

Sims' position is a modification of the left lateral position. This is the preferred position for endoscopy performed via the anus. Typically, the patient remains on the gurney (rather than being transferred to the operating table) and is awake and able to assist with positioning.

Body regions that may be accessed with the patient in the Sims' position include:

- Anus

The potential hazards and necessary precautions that apply to the patient in the supine and lateral positions apply to the Sims' position.

TECHNIQUE Sims' Position

1. Apply padding to the knees, ankles, and elbows, if needed.
2. Ask the patient to roll onto his left side using the side rail for support as necessary.
3. A pillow or foam headrest may be used.
4. Request that the left leg be kept straight.
5. Have the patient slide his left hip back and flex the right leg.
6. The arms are either flexed or placed on the gurney (a pillow may be placed between the arms) or the left arm may be placed behind the patient along the back and the right arm flexed and placed on the gurney.
7. A safety strap is not generally used; the side rail is lowered and the area exposed just prior to the start of the procedure.

THERMOREGULATORY DEVICES

Control of patient body temperature is important in the OR environment, and several devices are available to assist with providing hypothermia, normothermia, or hyperthermia intraoperatively. During operative procedures, the body core temperature tends to drop due to heat loss in the cool dry climate in the OR, the length of the operation, and the use of cold or room temperature irrigation fluids.

Most of a patient's heat loss occurs in the early stages of the procedure, when the patient is brought from a warm, humidified environment into a cold, dry one. In addition, the patient is no longer covered with clothing and bedding and is anesthetized, which further decreases ability to control core temperature. Additionally, the patient is uncovered and cold, wet skin prep solution is applied, which only adds to a rapid fall in body temperature.

Hypothermia affects up to 60% of all surgical patients. The goal for every patient should be the maintenance of a normal core temperature, unless the procedure specifically calls for the use of hypothermia. Studies have shown that the maintenance of a normal core temperature decreases the incidence of wound infection, may reduce blood loss, shortens the hospital stay, and helps decrease the incidence of fatal cardiac events.

Intraoperative heat loss occurs through the following mechanisms:

- *Radiation:* Loss of heat from the patient's body to the environment
- *Convection:* Loss of heat into the air currents (the "wind chill" effect)
- *Conduction:* Loss of heat from the patient's body into a cooler surface such as the operating table
- *Evaporation:* Loss of heat via perspiration or respiration

Radiation and convection are the major modes of heat loss to the patient, accounting for up to 80% of the total body heat lost intraoperatively.

Inadvertent hypothermia causes problems intraoperatively and postoperatively in the surgical patient. These include increased oxygen consumption due to shivering, cardiovascular and nervous system changes, and increased metabolism. Postoperative shivering is common and can cause serious cardiovascular and respiratory complications as well as discomfort, dental damage, and damage to the surgical repairs. Shivering also increases muscle metabolism, increasing oxygen consumption by up to 700%. Increased oxygen demand puts undue strain on the respiratory and cardiovascular systems. This undue stress may cause bradycardia and premature ventricular contractions.

Hypothermia also causes vasoconstriction, leading to increased blood pressure and tissue hypoxia, which increases the patient's susceptibility to wound infection.

The central nervous system depression caused by hypothermia slows metabolism of medications, which in turn slows emergence from anesthesia.

Some of the safest methods of maintenance of normothermia are noninvasive, passive methods. These methods include keeping the OR at a warmer temperature until the skin is prepped and the patient is draped in order to maintain body temperature. Additional passive methods of temperature control are the use of blankets, particularly on the extremities, including the hands and feet, and the head. Many hospitals have begun the use of thermal caps and blankets, especially in the preoperative waiting period to reduce heat loss from the head and extremities, and studies have shown that this effectively reduces the amount of heat lost after induction of anesthesia.

The most effective, albeit most extreme and invasive, means of warming core temperature is direct treatments such as the use of warmed gastric lavage, peritoneal irrigation, and fluid warmers for blood and IV fluids. Special care must be taken to avoid burning the patient when using this technique. Blood warmers may also be used to avoid the necessity of administering refrigerated blood directly to the patient.

Another method of temperature control is the active method using the application of heat to the outside of the body. These methods include the use of warmed blankets, warming blankets (water circulating), and forced-air warmers. Infants are often placed on the operating table with warming lamps overhead. When these techniques are used, care should be taken that they are only applied to the patient's head, trunk, and groin. Special care must be taken to avoid burns. The use of active warming on the extremities causes vasodilation and a shift of cooler blood to the trunk, which reduces the core temperature.

For certain procedures, such as cardiac procedures requiring cardiopulmonary bypass, hypothermia is desirable and necessary, in that it provides a lowered cellular metabolism and therefore a lower need for cellular perfusion. A warming device may then be used to return the patient to his or her normal body temperature.

Several devices are available today that will assist the surgical team in controlling patient body temperature. Among these are "forced-air" warming blankets and water-circulating blankets that may be used for either warming or cooling. Forced-air blankets are placed over unaffected parts of the patient's body prior to sterile draping and pump warmed air through channels in the blanket to warm the patient. Circulating-water or alcohol blankets are placed on the table prior to positioning the patient. Care should be taken if the blanket is to be used for warming that a sheet is placed over the warming blanket to prevent direct contact that may overheat the skin. During the procedure, the circulator is able to adjust the temperature of the blanket for either warming or cooling to help achieve the desired patient body temperature.

VITAL SIGNS

Monitoring vital signs in the OR assists the surgeon and anesthesia provider in determining patient condition at any given time and can be an indicator of pathology. Baseline vital signs including height and weight are taken prior to the start of the procedure. These give a good basis on which to monitor changes. Taking vital signs involves the mechanical or automated electronic monitoring of such life functions as pulse, respiration, temperature, and blood pressure. Intraoperatively, these functions are usually monitored electronically by the anesthesia provider.

Electronic monitoring equipment is able to monitor all of the vital functions simultaneously and to correlate the information into an easily readable format. Many of these devices are so small that they can be attached to an IV pole and transported along with the patient. Many of these devices are now commonly built in to the anesthesia machine.

When necessary, the health care provider should be able to manually monitor vital signs. This involves the use of some basic diagnostic equipment including a stethoscope, sphygmomanometer, and thermometer. Regardless of whether monitored electronically or manually, preoperative, intraoperative, and postoperative vital signs must be recorded periodically to provide trends and timed information on the status of the patient. The recording of vital signs is also a protection to the hospital and surgical team in instances of liability.

TEMPERATURE

Human body temperature is regulated by the hypothalamus, which monitors the processes of heat production and heat loss. When the hypothalamus senses a lowered body temperature, it signals the body to increase heat production through muscle contractions and increased cellular metabolism. The mechanisms of heat loss are more thoroughly described in the section "Malignant Hyperthermia." As little as a 0.04°F change in blood temperature sets the hypothalamic process in motion.

Increases in body temperature can be triggered by any of several outside factors, including infection, increased physical exertion, exposure to environmental heat, pregnancy, medication, stress, and age. Body temperature decreases can result from viral infections, decreased physical activity, depressed emotional state, exposure to environmental cold, metabolism-decreasing drugs, and age. The elderly tend to have a slightly decreased body temperature. Body temperature is also affected by the time of day, with the temperature at its lowest early in the morning. In the OR setting, body temperature can be affected by such outside factors as cold prep solutions, exposure, and anesthesia.

When temperature rises above the baseline preoperative level, the patient is said to have a *fever*. Fevers may indicate infection, drug reaction, or in some rare cases, intraoperatively and in the immediate postoperative period, malignant hyperthermia.

Preoperatively, temperature is taken to establish a baseline for the patient and to help rule out preoperative infection (Table 8-10). In the OR, temperature is closely monitored by automatic monitoring devices controlled by the anesthesia provider. It is important to monitor patient temperature carefully perioperatively to avoid undesirable hypothermia or hyperthermia.

The methods for temperature monitoring are listed in Table 8-11.

Table 8-10 Normal Temperature Values

Oral	98.6°F (37°C)
Rectal	99.6°F (37.6°C)
Axillary	97.6°F (36.5°C)

Table 8-11 Temperature-Monitoring Methods

Noninvasive	Touch Skin sticker Ear Axilla
Invasive	Oral Rectal Esophageal Bladder

TECHNIQUE Temperature Assessment

1. Wash your hands.
2. Assemble equipment and supplies.
    - Watch or clock with second hand
    - Thermometer of choice, including accessories
    - Gloves and lubricant, if necessary (*Note:* The patient's condition may require the use of gloves.)
    - Appropriate waste receptacle
3. Prepare equipment.
    - Apply gloves, if necessary.
    - Thermometer is covered or removed from package, as needed.
    - Place thermometer in ready mode, if electronic.
    - Apply lubricant, if necessary.
4. Introduce yourself, identify the patient, and explain the procedure, if necessary.
5. Position the patient, if necessary.
6. Place the thermometer according to site location.
7. Thermometer remains in position for the prescribed length of time.
8. Support the thermometer, if necessary.
9. Carefully remove the thermometer according to protocol for site location.
10. Read the thermometer.
11. Wash your hands.
12. Record or report findings.
13. Care for the equipment as needed.

PULSE

The *pulse* is composed of two phases of heart action (systole and diastole) and is measured when the health care provider palpates an artery, usually the radial artery (Table 8-12). If being measured electronically, a pulse oximeter may be used. Increased blood under pressure moves through the artery and expands the arterial wall. When the heart is in the opposite phase, the pressure is decreased in the artery. Each heartbeat consists of one contraction phase and one relaxation phase, felt as a pulse.

PULSE MONITORING

The pulse may be felt in any point of the body that has near-surface arteries and bony understructures. These

Table 8-12 Normal Pulse Values

Birth	130–160 bpm*
Infants	110–130 bpm
Children (1–7 years)	80–120 bpm
Children (over 7)	80–90 bpm
Adults	60–80 bpm

*bpm = beats per minute

TECHNIQUE Pulse Assessment

1. Wash your hands.
2. Assemble equipment and supplies.
   - Watch or clock with second hand
   - Stethoscope, if apical or fetal pulse
   - Gloves if warranted by the patient's condition
3. Introduce yourself, identify the patient, and explain the procedure, if necessary.
4. Position the patient, if necessary.
5. Locate the site by gently palpating with the first two or three fingertips (thumb may not be used).
6. Gently compress the artery or listen with the stethoscope.
7. Note the time. *Note:* For accuracy, the pulse rate should be counted for one full minute.
8. Count the pulse rate and note the rhythm, volume, and condition of the arterial wall.
9. Wash your hands.
10. Record or report findings.
11. Care for equipment as needed.

sites include the radial, carotid, brachial, temporal, femoral, popliteal, and dorsalis arteries. The pulse may also be monitored apically, or at the apex of the heart (referred to as the **apical pulse**), by using a stethoscope to listen between the fifth and sixth ribs just to the left of the sternum and just below the nipple. The most commonly utilized pulse point is the radial artery, located about 1 in. proximally to the base of the thumb. Refer to Figure 8-12 for a diagram of the location of other pulse points in the body.

In addition to the basic rate of pulse, or heart rate, several other pulse characteristics are monitored, including rhythm, volume, and strength. To measure the pulse rate, the number of pulsations is counted for 1 minute. This number of beats is the pulse, or heart rate. The pulse may also be measured for 10 seconds, and the number is multiplied by 6 to obtain the heart rate. The rate will vary with age, level of activity, pain, medication, and emotional condition. Patients entering the OR will sometimes have an elevated pulse rate due to anxiety. The rhythm of the pulse refers to the regularity of the beats.

ABNORMALITIES

Common pulse abnormalities include bradycardia (pulse rate less than 60) and tachycardia (pulse rate over 100) (Table 8-13). A dysrhythmia is an irregular pulse and may indicate heart disease. The pulse strength is noted as full, strong, hard, soft, thready, or weak. The most commonly felt dysrhythmia includes premature ventricular contraction (PVC), felt as a pulse beat earlier than expected. It can occasionally occur as a stress response or may be caused by caffeine, nicotine, alcohol, and sleep deprivation. Any pulse abnormalities should be noted and the surgeon or anesthesia provider should be alerted, as these can be serious and even fatal. An ECG may be needed prior to initiation of the surgical procedure (refer to Chapter 13).

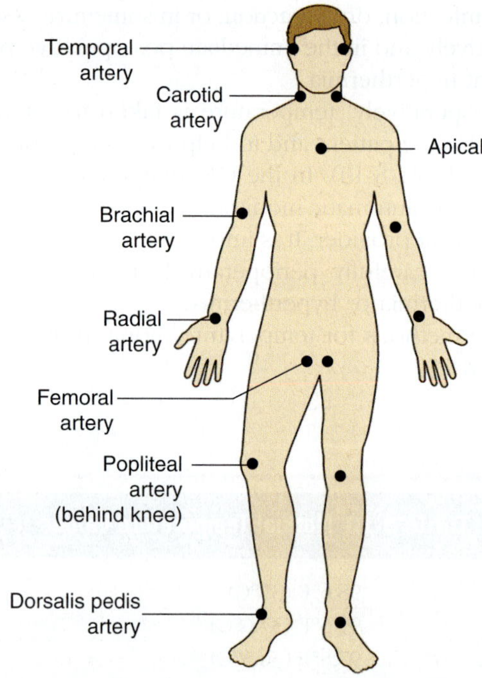

Figure 8-12 Pulse points in the body ***(Courtesy of Delmar Learning)***

RESPIRATION

Respiration is the exchange of oxygen and carbon dioxide between the atmosphere and the cells of the body. It is a two-part process that includes external atmospheric respiration as air is taken into and blown out of the lungs and cellular respiration. Atmospheric respiration includes inspiration and expiration as well as the diffusion of oxygen from the alveoli to the blood and the diffusion of carbon dioxide from the blood through the alveoli to the air. All cells of the body utilize oxygen for cellular function, and cellular function produces carbon dioxide and other wastes as byproducts of cellular respiration. The function of respiration is involuntary and is controlled by the medulla oblongata in the brain. The medulla oblongata triggers respiration whenever the CO_2 level in the blood increases. Although respiration is involuntary, it can be controlled to an extent by holding one's breath or by hyperventilation. One respiration is one inhalation and one

Table 8-13 Pulse Rate Patterns

TYPE	RATE	CAUSES
Normal	60–80 bpm*	Age, activity level, and gender variations (refer to Table 8-12)
Tachycardia	Greater than 100 bpm	Stimulation of the sympathetic nervous system by stress or drugs Exercise Congestive heart failure, anemia
Bradycardia	Less than 60 bpm	Very fit athlete Stimulation of the parasympathetic nervous system by certain drugs Physical problems such as cerebral hemorrhage and heart blockage
Irregular	Uneven beat intervals	Cardiac irritability or hypoxia Chemical or drug issues such as potassium imbalance If premature beats are frequent, this condition may indicate a serious dysrythmia

*bpm = beats per minute
Source: Adapted from Mednet (*www.sermed.com*).

exhalation. The normal respiratory rate is called eupnea and varies with age, emotions, activity level, and medication. Normal respiration is one respiration for every four heart beats, or a 1:4 ratio.

RESPIRATION MONITORING

When monitoring respiration, rate, rhythm, and depth are noted. Rhythm of respiration is a measure of the pattern of breathing. This will vary with age, with adults having a regular pattern and infants having an irregular one. The depth of respiration is the amount of air taken in and exhaled with each respiration, an amount that is easily measured by anesthesia equipment in the OR. Manually, it is measured by watching the rise and fall of the chest. The rate is recorded, along with whether respirations are shallow or deep (Table 8-14).

TECHNIQUE Respiration Assessment

1. Wash your hands.
2. Assemble the equipment and supplies.
   - Watch or clock with second hand
   - Stethoscope, if necessary
   - Gloves if warranted by the patient's condition
3. Introduce yourself, identify the patient, and explain the procedure, if necessary.
4. Position the patient, if necessary.
5. Note the time. *Note:* For accuracy, the respiratory rate should be counted for one full minute.
6. Obtain respiratory rate, depth, rhythm, and breath sounds.
7. Wash your hands.
8. Record or report findings.
9. Care for the equipment as needed.

Table 8-14 Normal Respiration Rates

Infants	30–60 respirations per minute
Children (1–7 years)	18–30 per minute
Adults	12–20 per minute

ABNORMALITIES

Respiration rate abnormalities include apnea, tachypnea, and Cheyne-Stokes breathing (Table 8-15). Apnea is the complete cessation of breathing. Apnea temporarily occurs upon induction of some types of anesthesia, hence the need for manual/mechanical ventilation during general anesthesia. Obstructive apnea occurs when there is a blockage in the airway. Tachypnea is very rapid respiration. This occurs in patients with a high fever as the body attempts to rid itself of excess body heat and also occurs when the patient is experiencing alkalosis and the body is attempting to rid itself of excess carbon dioxide. Bradypnea is the opposite of tachypnea, a decreased rate of respiration. Cheyne-Stokes respiration is a pattern of rhythmic waxing and waning of the depth of respiration. The patient breathes deeply for a short period of time and

Table 8-15 Breathing Patterns

NAME	DESCRIPTION	CAUSE
Eupnea	Normal breathing	Normal
Apnea	No breathing	Obstructed airway Disruption or damage to lateral medulla oblongata (breathing center)
Bradypnea	Slow, even respirations	Normal during sleep Depression of respiratory center
Cheyne-Stokes	Fast, deep breaths for a period of time, followed by 20–60 seconds of apnea	Intracranial pressure increase Congestive heart failure Renal failure Cerebral anoxia
Kussmaul's	Fast, deep, labored breaths over 20 per minute	Blood pressure systolic 140–160 Diastolic 70–90
Tachypnea	Rapid breaths that rise with body temperature	Pneumonia Respiratory insufficiency Respiratory center lesions

Source: Adapted from Mednet (*www.sermed.com*).

then breathes only very slightly or not at all for a period. This pattern repeats itself and can be caused by heart failure or brain damage. The term **dyspnea** refers to shortness of breath or difficulty breathing (e.g., during intense physical exercise or due to heart/lung disease).

BLOOD PRESSURE

Blood pressure is the pressure of the blood against the walls of the blood vessels, affected by several different factors. Pressure is affected and determined by the pumping of the heart, the resistance of the arterioles to the flow of blood, the elasticity of the arterial walls, the volume of blood in the body, and the blood thickness. The extracellular fluid volume also affects blood pressure. The pumping action of the heart is a measure of how hard the heart pumps, how much blood is pumped (cardiac output), and how efficiently the blood is pumped.

Blood pressure is usually expressed as two numbers, systolic and diastolic (Table 8-16). *Systole* refers to the contraction of the heart, which forces the blood through the arteries. The relaxation phase of the heartbeat is referred to as *diastole*. As the heart contracts and blood is forced into the aorta, the walls of the aorta and major arteries are forced to expand by the pressure of the blood being pumped into them. As the heart relaxes between beats, the aortic valve closes, preventing blood from flowing back into the chambers of the heart, and the arterial walls spring back from the expansion that took place during the contraction of the heart, forcing the blood through the body between contractions of the heart. This gives us two separate pressure readings during the beat of the heart, a higher pressure during contraction, called systole, and a lower pressure during the relaxation phase, called diastole. These two pressures are called the systolic blood pressure and diastolic blood pressure.

BLOOD PRESSURE MEASUREMENT

In the OR setting, blood pressure may be measured manually for a baseline and then may be measured via an automatic electronically controlled recording sphygmomanometer.

To manually measure blood pressure, an appropriately sized blood pressure cuff is placed around the upper arm. This device consists of a rubber cuff and a gauge. The rubber cuff is placed around the upper portion of the patient's arm and air is pumped into the cuff through an air inflation device. As the cuff pressure increases, the arterial blood flow is momentarily stopped. A stethoscope is placed over the brachial artery at the antecubital portion of the elbow and the air in the cuff is slowly released. The health care practitioner auscultates, or listens, for Korotkoff's sounds, which will be heard as a tapping sound that gradually increases in intensity. These sounds take place in five distinct phases, which must be recognized for proper blood pressure measurement:

Phase I: On hearing two initial tapping sounds, the gauge is read and the number is recorded as the systolic blood pressure.

Phase II: Soft swishing sound as more blood passes through the vessels as the cuff is deflated.

Table 8-16 Normal Blood Pressure Values and Classifications of Abnormal Blood Pressure

Newborn	50–52 systolic/25–30 diastolic
Child (under 6)	95/62
Child (to 10 years)	100/65
Adolescent	118/75

ADULTS

CATEGORY	SYSTOLIC (mm Hg)	DIASTOLIC (mm Hg)
Normal†	less than 120	less than 80
Prehypertension	120–139	80–89
Hypertension‡		
Stage 1 (mild)	140–159	90–99
Stage 2 (moderate)	at or greater than 160	at or greater than 100

†Optimal blood pressure with respect to cardiovascular risk is systolic less than 120 and diastolic less than 80. However, unusually low readings should be evaluated for clinical significance.

‡Based on the average of two or more readings taken at each of two or more visits following an initial screening. Thus, a reading in the OR of 140–159 would not necessarily classify a patient as clinically chronically hypertensive.

Source: From the Fifth Report of the Joint National Committee on Detection, Evaluation, and Treatment of High Blood Pressure, Oct. 30, 1992.

Phase III: Rhythmic tapping sound returns as more blood passes through the vessels as the pressure is slowly released in the cuff. If phases I and II are missed, phase III may be improperly recorded as the systolic pressure.

Phase IV: Muffled, fading tapping sounds heard as the cuff is deflated further.

Phase V: Sounds disappear altogether. The point at which these sounds disappear is recorded as the diastolic blood pressure.

Blood pressure is recorded in a fraction format on the patient's chart; location of the measurement and the position of the patient (e.g., supine) are usually noted. For example: "120/80, left arm, supine." In children and patients where the blood pressure sounds can still be heard at zero, the beginning of phase IV and zero should both be recorded. For example: "120/90/0."

In some critically ill patients, and especially in the OR setting, blood pressure will be monitored via a catheter inserted into an artery and attached to a catheter-monitor-transducer system. This pressure is displayed on a monitor at the head of the table and is usually inserted and controlled by the anesthesia provider. This is called intra-arterial blood pressure monitoring and provides constant, accurate blood pressure data.

TECHNIQUE

Blood Pressure Assessment

1. Wash your hands.
2. Assemble the equipment and supplies.
   - Sphygmomanometer
   - Stethoscope, if necessary
   - Gloves if warranted by the patient's condition
3. Introduce yourself, identify the patient, and explain the procedure, if necessary.
4. Position the patient and expose the site, if necessary. *Note:* Left upper extremity is preferred.
5. Apply the appropriate size blood pressure cuff.
6. Place the stethoscope.
   - Stethoscope is placed over the brachial artery.
   - Stethoscope is secured with fingers only (not the thumb).

(continues)

(continued)

7. Inflate the blood pressure cuff to the desired pressure.
8. Deflate the blood pressure cuff slowly, while listening for Korotkoff's sounds.
   - Listen for Korotkoff phase I; note systolic blood pressure.
   - Continue to listen for sequential Korotkoff phases.
   - Note diastolic blood pressure; Korotkoff phase V.
9. Continue deflation of blood pressure cuff and note auscultatory gap, if present.
10. Continue deflation of blood pressure cuff and remove it if the situation allows.
11. Wash your hands.
12. Record or report findings.
13. Care for the equipment as needed.

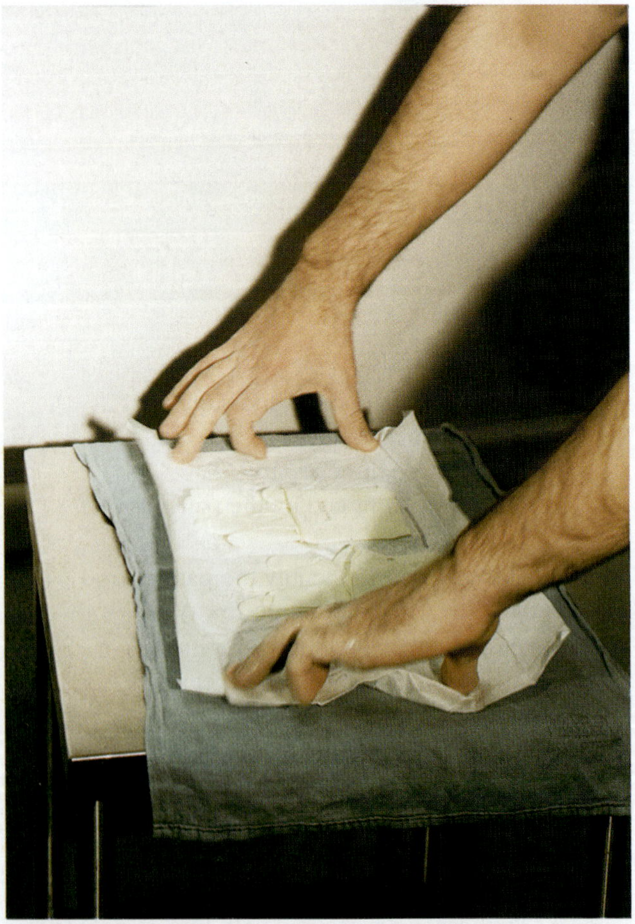

Figure 8-13A Open gloving; open inner glove wrapper

STERILE TASKS PERFORMED BY NONSTERILE TEAM MEMBERS

In preparing the patient for a surgical procedure, several sterile tasks are performed by the nonsterile team members. Two of the more common, Foley catheter insertion and the surgical skin prep, are presented, but first we discuss the gloving procedure required before these sterile tasks can be performed.

Open Gloving

Prior to the nonsterile individual performing a sterile task, sterile gloves must be applied using the open-gloving technique (Figure 8-13A–D). The open-gloving technique is not recommended when wearing a sterile gown.

TECHNIQUE

Open Gloving

1. Retrieve the wrapper containing the gloves from the outer package (e.g., outer glove wrapper, Foley catheter insertion kit, prep tray).
2. Place the glove wrapper on a suitable surface.
3. Open the wrapper to create a small sterile field by touching only the outer edges of the inside of the wrapper (1- to 2-in. perimeter).
4. Secure the first glove from the wrapper by pinching the cuffed edge and lifting the glove up and away from the wrapper.
5. Orient the fingertips of the glove downward.
6. Apply the glove to the opposite hand by inserting the fingers and pulling the glove over the palm without touching the glove exterior.
7. Unfold the cuff of the glove.
8. Secure the second glove from the wrapper by inserting the fingertips of the already gloved (sterile) hand under the cuffed edge of the glove.
9. Keep the gloved thumb tucked under the cuff or well out of the way.
10. Lift the glove up and away from the wrapper.
11. Apply the glove in the manner previously described and make any minor adjustments.
12. The gloved hands are now considered sterile and the planned task (e.g., skin prep, Foley catheter insertion) is performed.

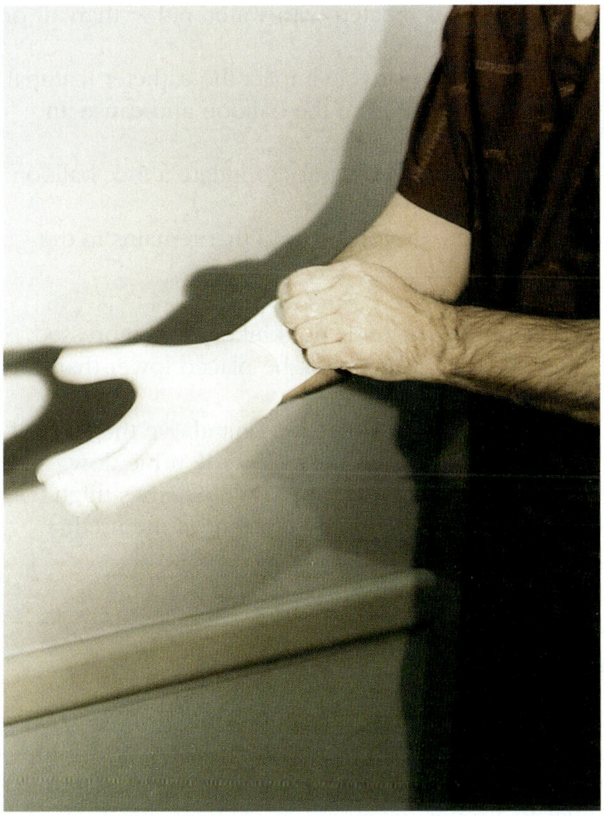

Figure 8-13B Don first glove

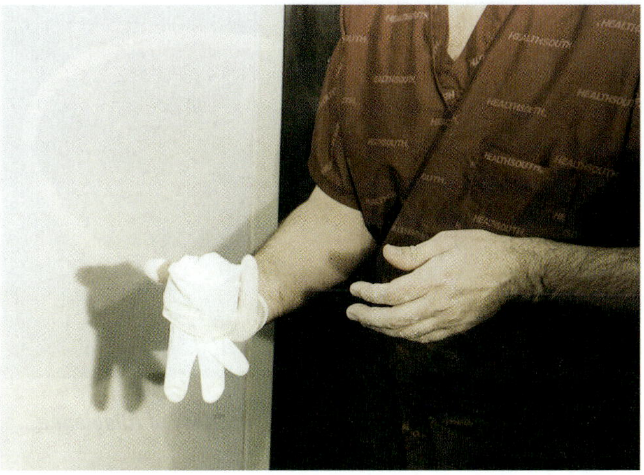

Figure 8-13C Secure and lift second glove

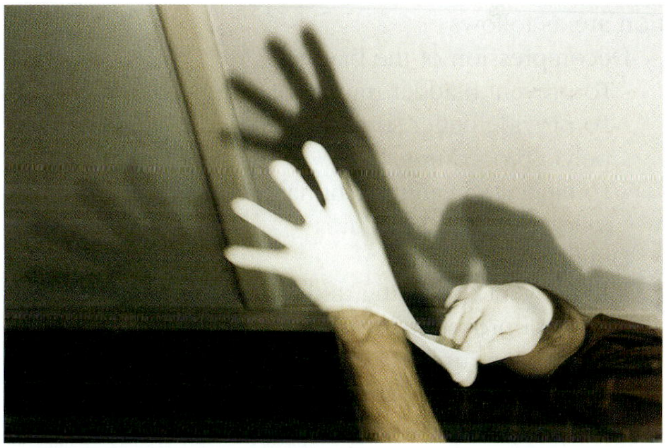

Figure 8-13D Second glove donned

TECHNIQUE Removal of Soiled Gloves

1. Grasp the palm of the glove to be removed first with your opposite hand.
2. Remove the glove by inverting it as you remove it; be sure that you do not touch your skin with your gloved hand.
3. Use slow movements to prevent snapping of the glove and splattering of debris.
4. Keep the removed glove in the hand that remains gloved.
5. Begin to remove your second glove by sliding your degloved hand between the skin of your wrist and the glove. Touch only your skin and the inner aspect of the glove.
6. Invert the glove as you remove it to contain both gloves.
7. Dispose of the gloves.
8. Wash your hands.

Soiled gloves are removed and discarded as described in the previous technique to reduce the risk of exposure and/or cross contamination.

URINARY CATHETERIZATION

The most commonly used method of draining the bladder is urethral **catheterization**. Catheterization involves the introduction of a flexible tube via the urethra into the bladder for the purpose of drainage and/or irrigation. Foley catheterization is considered an invasive procedure (Figure 8-14). A physician's order is required for catheterization. The health care provider must use strict sterile technique to prevent infection.

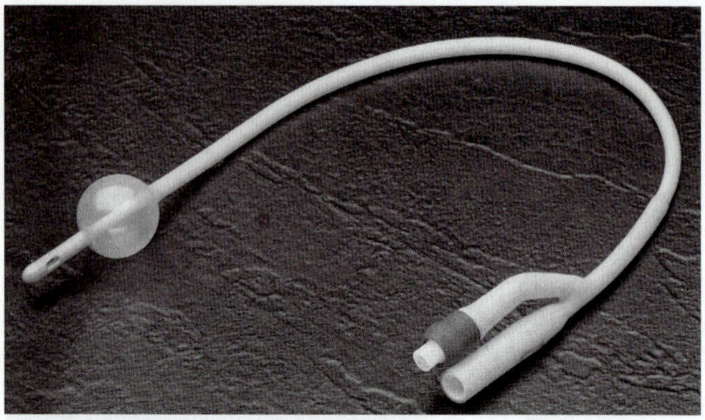

Figure 8-14 Two-way Foley catheter ***(Courtesy of Allegiance Healthcare)***

INDICATIONS

Foley catheter insertion may be indicated for one or more reasons. Some of the indications for urethral catheterization are as follows:

- Decompression of the bladder
  - To prevent bladder trauma during pelvic procedures
  - To provide better surgical site visualization during pelvic procedures
  - To facilitate healing of urinary tract structures following GU procedures
- Drainage of urine
  - To prevent overfilling of the bladder during lengthy surgical procedures
  - To measure urinary output
  - To obtain a sterile urine specimen
  - To relieve urinary retention
  - To treat incontinence
- Irrigation of the bladder
- Control of bleeding
  - Balloon may be used to place pressure on the bladder neck

CONSIDERATIONS

Several factors must be considered prior to and during catheter insertion:

- Sterile technique must be used.
- Catheter insertion may cause patient injury.
  - Urinary tract infection
  - Urethral injury
- Catheters are available in a variety of styles, materials, and sizes.
  - Use the smallest size that will drain the bladder without leakage.
  - The surgeon will order the style catheter desired.
  - The Foley catheter is the most common style.
  - Be aware of the patient's allergy status; use a latex alternative if necessary.
- The balloon is inflated with water, rather than air or saline.
  - Saline may negatively impact the catheter material.
  - Air may escape from the balloon and cause an embolism.
- 10 cc of water is necessary to inflate a 5-cc balloon completely.
  - To compensate for the fluid that remains in the inflation channel
- Drainage of urine occurs by gravity.
  - Be sure the tubing is not kinked or compressed.
  - The collection unit must be placed lower than the level of the bladder.
  - Do not raise the collection unit above the level of the bladder to prevent retrograde urine flow.
- Secure the catheter tubing to the patient's thigh.
  - To prevent unnecessary tension on the urethra
  - To prevent accidental catheter removal

PROCEDURE

The surgical technologist may be called on to insert the catheter preoperatively, intraoperatively, or postoperatively. Knowledge of the perineal anatomy is therefore essential to proper technique in catheter insertion. Sterile technique is essential, as 40% of all nosocomial infections are urinary tract infections. Urinary tract and/or kidney infections, blood infections, septicemia, or urethral injury can result from improper catheter insertion and care.

Catheters come in a large variety of sizes from 8 French (pediatric) to 12 French up to 30 French, with 30 being the largest. They are available in various materials, including latex, silicone, and Teflon, and types, including Foley, straight (Robinson), and coude tip. The smallest gauge catheter that will drain the bladder is recommended. Commonly, a size 14 French or size 16 French catheter is used. Although larger catheters are more likely to cause urethral damage, some people will require larger catheters to control leakage of urine around the catheter. Some people have developed allergies or sensitivity to latex; these people should be catheterized using the silicone or Teflon catheters.

Catheterization is usually performed after the induction of anesthesia to prevent undue patient pain and discomfort. For the male patient, the supine position is ideal. For the female patient, the legs should be spread, or "frog-legged," and may need to be held by an assistant.

The following supplies should be gathered prior to catheterization and are often available as a kit:

1. Sterile drape, one fenestrated
2. Sterile gloves
3. Lubricant (KY or other)
4. Antiseptic cleansing solution (iodine solution or chlorhexidine solution)

TECHNIQUE

Urethral Catheterization

Note: If a sterile kit with plastic tray is used, this may be placed between the patient's thighs; otherwise, work from a sterile Mayo setup specifically for catheterization.

1. Don sterile gloves using the open-glove technique.
2. Drape the patient:
   - For female patient, place sterile bottom drape just under patient's buttocks using sterile technique and taking care not to touch contaminated surfaces. Apply fenestrated drape over perineum, leaving labia exposed.
   - For male patient, place fenestrated drape over thighs below the penis and unfold up over the penis with penis exposed through the fenestration using sterile technique.
3. Prepare supplies in order of use. Test balloon.
4. Cleanse urethral meatus.
   - For female patient, use nondominant hand to retract the labia and expose the urethral meatus. This hand should remain in place for the entire procedure and should not return to the sterile setup. Using the dominant hand and forceps, pick up gauze pad soaked in antiseptic solution and use it to cleanse perineal area. This should be done with a wiping motion anterior to posterior from the clitoris toward the anus. A new gauze or cotton ball should be used for each wiping motion, cleansing along each labial fold and then along the meatus.
   - For male patient, retract foreskin (be sure to replace at end of procedure) with nondominant hand. The penis should be grasped at the shaft below the glans, and the urethral meatus retracted between the thumb and forefinger. The nondominant hand should remain in this position for the duration of the procedure and should not be placed back on the sterile setup. Using the dominant hand and forceps, pick up gauze pad or cotton ball and cleanse the penis using cotton once around the penis. Begin at the meatus and work toward the base.
5. Pick up catheter with the dominant hand and lubricate the tip. Catheter should be grasped about 5 cm (2 in.) from the tip and held with the end of the catheter coiled loosely in the palm of the hand. The distal end of the catheter should be placed in the prep tray receptacle unless it is already attached to the drainage bag.
6. Insert catheter.
   - For a female patient, slowly insert catheter through meatus. If no urine appears, it is likely that the catheter has been inserted in the vagina. If this occurs, another sterile catheter should be obtained and inserted, leaving the first one in the vagina until the second catheter insertion is complete, to prevent contamination.
   - Insert catheter approximately 5 cm (2 in.) in adult patient, 2.5 cm (1 in.) in child, or until urine is seen flowing out the end of the catheter.
   - Labial retraction may now be released and catheter held with the nondominant hand.
   - For a male patient, insert catheter approximately 17.5–22.5 cm (7–9 in.) in an adult or 5–7.5 cm (2–3 in.) in a child, or until urine is seen flowing out the end of the catheter. Catheter should not be forced against resistance. If resistance is felt, catheter should be withdrawn slightly. The catheter should be advanced another 5 cm (2 in.) after urine appears for retention catheters.
   - The penis should now be released and catheter should be held securely with the nondominant hand.
7. Inflate balloon.
   - Holding the catheter with the thumb and little finger of the dominant hand at the meatus, the end of the catheter is placed between the first two fingers of the nondominant hand.
   - With the dominant hand, the syringe should be attached (if not already attached) to the injection port.
   - Inject solution slowly. If resistance is felt, solution should be aspirated back and catheter inserted farther. Do not push against resistance, particularly in the male patient, in whom this may cause prostate damage.
   - After balloon is fully inflated, release catheter and pull gently to feel resistance, and move catheter back into bladder. Disconnect syringe.
8. Connect the end of the catheter to the drainage system, unless already connected. Drainage tube should be placed under the patient's leg and bag should be hung on the operating table so that it cannot be pulled off. The catheter may be taped to the patient's leg using hypoallergenic tape.

5. Gauze squares
6. Forceps
7. Prefilled syringe filled with sterile water (amount determined by balloon size of catheter)
8. Catheter of correct size and type
9. Sterile drainage tubing and collection bag
10. Sterile basin (bottom of sterile catheterization tray or basin containing **prep** solution may be used)

Prior to catheterization, a Mayo stand or prep stand should be set up using sterile technique. This area should contain the fenestrated sterile drape, lubricant, a basin or cup with the antiseptic cleansing solution, sterile gauze squares, and forceps. Also on the stand should be either a sterile specimen cup with sterile water and syringe for catheter balloon filling or a prefilled syringe of sterile water. Next, the catheter should be placed on the sterile setup. An alternative is to place the catheter on the sterile back table and have the STSR test the balloon and hand the catheter and syringe to the person performing the catheterization in a sterile fashion at the appropriate time. Sterile catheter trays are available, containing all of the above. With these premade setups, one need only open the tray using sterile technique and pour the antiseptic solution into the tray. Finally, the sterile urine collection bag should be placed on the setup table or given to the STSR, who will hand it off at the appropriate time.

The health care provider dons sterile gloves using the open-glove technique and then tests the balloon of the catheter by filling it with sterile water from the syringe. The balloon should fully inflate without leakage. Fluid should then be withdrawn, and the syringe left attached to the port of the catheter. The catheter is left on the sterile table at this point.

It is important that the catheter be connected to a closed drainage measurement system at all times to prevent infection. These bags generally hold 1000–1500 mL of urine and should be hung on the table so that gravity will cause the urine to flow into the bag. Most bags have a spigot at the bottom that allows the bag to be emptied if necessary. Urine output is monitored during surgery in order to help assess kidney function and fluid balance. Output is documented periodically in the patient's chart.

After catheter insertion, the setup is disassembled and drapes are removed from the patient.

SKIN PREPARATION

The surgical skin prep is performed on the surgical patient for the same reasons that the sterile surgical team members perform the surgical scrub prior to entry into the sterile field:

1. To remove transient organisms from the patient's skin
2. To reduce the number of resident organisms on the patient's skin

Living human tissue cannot be sterilized. Therefore, the goal related to the principles of asepsis is the basis for performance of the surgical skin prep: "Keep the microbial count within the sterile field to an irreducible minimum."

Several factors must be considered prior to and during the surgical skin prep. Probably the most controversial of these is hair removal from the surgical site. Hair that may interfere with electrode placement, the surgical site, wound closure, and dressing application may be removed according to surgeon preference, facility policy, age and gender of the patient, and the planned operative site. Hair removal should occur as close as possible to the time of the planned surgical procedure to reduce the risk of microbial growth in any breaks in the skin surface caused by the hair removal. Be sure that the privacy of the awake patient is ensured to avoid embarrassment during the hair removal procedure. Several techniques, including the use of razors (may incorporate the wet or dry method), clippers, and depilatories, may be used to remove the hair. Hair removal with the use of a razor is demonstrated in the video entitled "Preoperative Case Management."

Other factors related to the skin prep are as follows:

- All necessary procedures are carried out prior to performing the surgical skin prep.
  - Anesthesia administration
  - Foley catheterization
  - Positioning
  - Exposure of the surgical site
  - Hair removal
  - Skin marking
- Gross soil and skin oils must be removed from the planned operative site.
  - May require use of a fat solvent or degreaser
  - May require use of a scrub brush and/or nail cleaner
- Prep fluids may not be allowed to accumulate adjacent to or under the patient.
  - May cause chemical irritation
  - Increases the risk of electrosurgical or **laser** burn
- Consider the patient's allergy status prior to application of any chemical (an alternate antiseptic may be needed).
- Certain areas are considered contaminated and may require special attention. The general rule in prepping these areas is to prep the surrounding areas first and the contaminated area last and to use a separate sponge for each area. Exceptions to the rule may occur in specific situations.
  - Mucous membranes
  - Stomas
  - Nonintact skin
  - Sinus tracts
  - Umbilicus
- Two separate skin preps may be necessary in certain situations (e.g., skin graft—donor and recipient sites).

- The prep is initiated at the planned incision site and carried toward the periphery, using a widening circular motion.
- An assistant may be necessary to elevate a large limb that must be circumferentially prepped.
- The recommendations of the antiseptic manufacturer must be followed (e.g., exposure time).
- Preoperative skin markings are not removed during the surgical skin prep.

Note: Some of the preparatory steps (e.g., hair removal and skin degreasing) may also apply to the skin sites selected for placement of the dispersive electrode for the electrosurgical unit and the ECG electrodes.

Types of skin prep solutions used in the OR are:

- *Alcohol:* Provides a rapid and significant reduction in skin microbial counts.
- *Iodine:* Provides rapid reduction in skin microbial counts. Should be removed after 2–3 minutes to prevent skin irritation.
- *Iodophors:* Less likely to cause skin irritation and do not need to be removed.
- *Chlorhexidine:* Does not provide as rapid a reduction in skin microbial counts as alcohol, but provides a longer residual effect (5–6 hours). This effect remains active in the presence of blood and other organic material.
- *Hexachlorophene:* This agent must be used for several days prior to surgery because it builds up a cumulative antimicrobial effect.

Several products are available for use in skin preparation, including scrub soaps, scrub solutions, and single-use prep applicators. The agent used in the OR should be a broad-spectrum antimicrobial and should provide residual protection. The agent chosen for use should be based on the particular patient and skin sensitivity, and the surgical site should be taken into consideration.

SKIN PREPARATION SETUP

The items necessary for final skin preparation should be arranged on a separate sterile Mayo stand or prep stand. Prep packs are available in sterile form, containing all the necessary equipment except for the antiseptic scrub solution and "paint" solution.

SINGLE USE

Single-use applicators are available for the skin prep. These contain an alcohol-based antiseptic solution that leaves an antimicrobial film. They are self-contained units, and after activation as per manufacturer's instructions, the solution flows onto the applicator sponge. These are used in the same incision site first and in an outward circular motion and are discarded after use. These have shown to have a long-lasting antimicrobial effect and leave an antimicrobial film on the skin.

ABDOMINAL AND THORACOABDOMINAL PREPARATIONS

Abdominal and thoracoabdominal preps are the most common preoperative skin prep performed in most ORs. The area covered for an abdominal prep is indicated in Figure 8-15.

CHEST AND BREAST

For procedures in the area of the chest and breast, the arm on the affected side is elevated by an assistant during the prep (Figure 8-16). The area to be prepped will include the shoulder, the upper arm and extending down to the

TECHNIQUE: Preoperative Skin Preparation of Clean Area

Supplies

If a pack is not available, a sterile tray will need to be set up using sterile technique with the following items:

1. Two small basins for solution filled with the scrub solution and "paint" of choice.
2. Sponges: either 4- × 4- or 4- × 8-in. or foam sponges. The sponges used must not be counted radiopaque sponges but must be disposable.
3. Cotton-tipped applicators for cases where the umbilicus will need to be prepped. This is used to clean any detritus out of the umbilicus prior to applying the prep solutions.
4. Sterile towels to be used to define the area to be prepped and to soak up solutions along the sides of the patient in order to prevent pooling.
5. Forceps.

(continues)

(continued)

Steps

1. Sterile gloves are donned using the open-glove technique.
2. Sterile towels are placed around the area to be prepped in order to demarcate areas to be prepped and to absorb solutions.
3. Sponge is soaked in antiseptic and the agent is applied using forceps or the gloved hand to hold the sponge. If the sponge is held in the hand, the gloved hand must not be allowed to touch the skin, so that the hand may remain sterile.
4. Sponges used in scrubbing must be discarded as each one is used, and a fresh one is used to replace it. A soiled sponge must never be brought back over a scrubbed surface.
5. Skin is scrubbed starting at the incision site in a circular motion working in widening circles toward the outer edges of the area to be prepped. Effective cleansing requires both mechanical and chemical action, so enough friction must be applied to cleanse the skin and the pores.
6. After the periphery is reached with the first sponge, it is discarded, and a second sponge is used to start at the incision site and work outward again.
7. Again, when prepping contaminated areas, prep those areas last. If a stoma is in the area to be prepped, cover it with 4- × 4-in. gauze soaked in the antiseptic solution. At the end of the prep, this sponge is discarded.
8. This process is repeated for at least 5 minutes, or in some cases, until the counted number of prepared sponges has been used.
9. After scrubbing for 5 minutes or as prescribed with the scrub solution of choice, the antiseptic agent is applied using more sterile sponges and utilizing the same incision site outward technique until the entire area is covered with a film of the antiseptic agent, or "paint."
10. After the completion of the prep, any stomas or intestinal fistulas are covered with a plastic transparent adhesive drape.

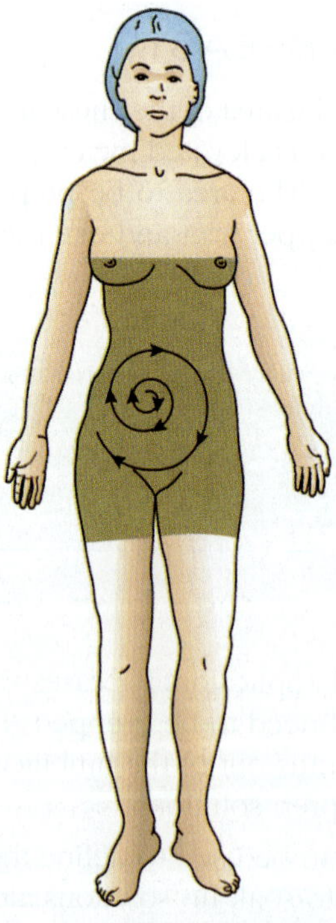

Figure 8-15 Skin prep perimeters—abdominal

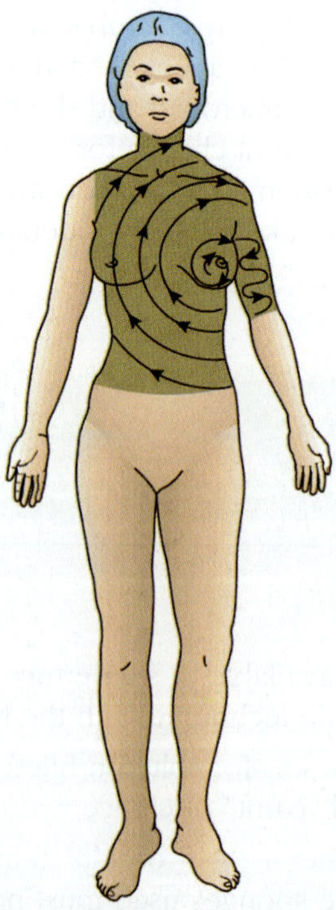

Figure 8-16 Skin prep perimeters—left chest/breast

elbow, the axilla, and the chest to the table line and to the shoulder opposite from the affected side.

EYES, EARS, FACE, AND NOSE

For preparation of these areas, a piece of sterile plastic sheeting may be used to protect the eyes. The area to be prepped will vary, but as much of the area surrounding the incision site that can be should be prepped and the prep should always extend to the hairline.

EXTREMITIES

When an extremity is to be prepped, an assistant should don sterile gloves and elevate the extremity so that it may be prepped around its entire circumference. For prep of the leg or legs, the assistant holds the extremity at the foot, and the leg is prepped around the entire circumference (Figure 8-17). A moisture-proof pad may be placed under the extremity to collect any excess solution that may drip. The pad is removed after the prep is completed and before draping.

Areas to Be Prepped: Leg and Hip Procedures

The general boundaries for leg and hip preps are:

- *Foot and ankle procedures:* Foot and entire leg from ankle to knee
- *Bilateral leg procedures:* Both legs from toes to waist level
- *Hip procedures:* Abdomen on affected side, entire leg and foot, buttocks to the table line, groin, and pubis

Areas to Be Prepped: Hand and Arm Procedures

To prep the arm, the arm is elevated by the individual performing the prep or an assistant. The arm is held by the hand so that the entire circumference may be prepped (Figure 8-18). If a pneumatic **tourniquet** is not used, the axillary area should also be prepped. The general boundaries for hand and shoulder preps are:

- *Hand procedures:* Hand and arm to 7.5 cm (3 in.) above the elbow

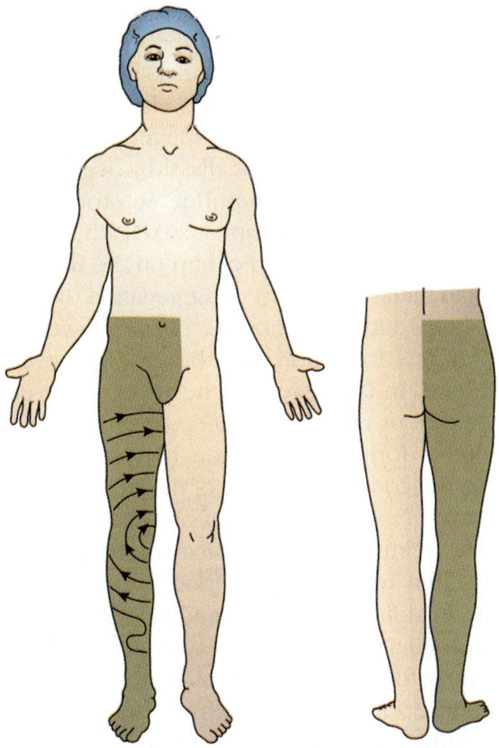

Figure 8-17 Skin prep perimeters (circumferential)—right lower extremity: (A) Anterior view, (B) posterior view

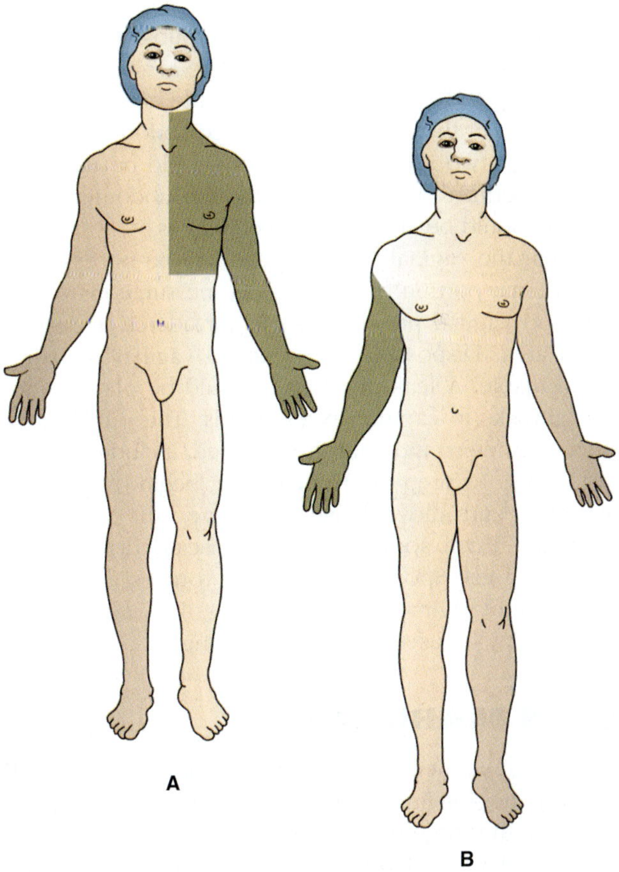

Figure 8-18 Skin prep perimeters (circumferential)—upper extremity: (A) Left proximal portion, (B) right distal portion

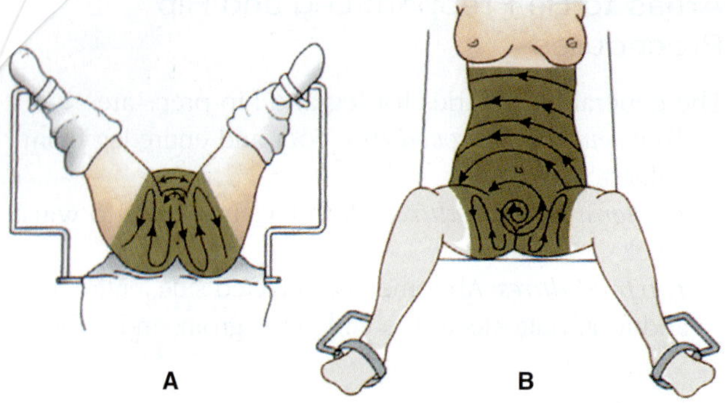

Figure 8-19 Skin prep perimeters—perineum: (A) Perineal view, (B) anterior view

- *Shoulder procedures:* Base of neck, shoulder, scapula, chest to midline, and circumference of upper arm down to the elbow
- *Arm procedures:* Entire arm, shoulder, and axilla, including hand

PERINEAL AND VAGINAL PREPS

The perineal prep should begin at the pubic area, using a downward motion toward and over the genitalia and perineum (Figure 8-19). Each sponge should be discarded after going over the anus. For combined abdominoperineal operations, two separate prep sets should be used, one for the perineal area and one for the abdominal area. Gloves should be changed between areas.

For the vaginal prep, forceps will be necessary for the internal portion of the prep. Some surgeons will require no vaginal prep, as this is considered a contaminated area. Disposable prepackaged vaginal prep trays are available. A leak-proof pad should be placed under the buttocks to capture excess fluids. The pubis, vulva, labia, perineum, and anus are prepped, including the upper thighs. To prep the vaginal area, begin over the pubic area and move downward over the vulva and perineum. Each sponge must be discarded after going over the anus. Sponges on sponge forceps are used to cleanse the vagina. After scrubbing the vagina, a dry sponge may be used for internal drying.

SKIN MARKING

Sterile skin markers are available for the surgeon's use in marking incision lines on the skin preoperatively. In some instances the surgeon may prefer to use a cotton applicator dipped in methylene blue or gentian violet. These markers may also be used intraoperatively, although the original skin marker should be discarded and a fresh sterile marker should be used.

HEMOSTASIS AND BLOOD REPLACEMENT

Because surgery is invasive, it is almost a given that some blood and fluid loss is expected. In most surgical procedures, blood loss is negligible, but it is the goal of every surgeon to absolutely minimize blood loss and to anticipate any major blood loss. **Hemostasis** is the arrest of the loss of blood or hemorrhage. This may be accomplished by either clot formation or vessel spasm, by mechanical pressure, or surgically, by ligation or the application of hemostatic agents. Intraoperative hemostasis may also be achieved thermally. Some patients in need of surgery have congenital or acquired clotting disorders, making the maintenance of hemostasis more difficult.

Blood usually flows smoothly through the vascular system without cellular adherence to the vessel walls. When vascular injury occurs following trauma or in certain vessel diseases or surgery, the endothelial cells interact with platelets and clotting factors to form a blood clot at the site of injury.

When a blood vessel is injured, such as by being incised during surgery, the hemostatic process must begin in order to stop the flow of blood. The body uses the process of *coagulation,* the formation of a blood clot, to achieve hemostasis. As soon as a vessel is injured, a period of *vasoconstriction* begins, in which the muscular walls of the vessel constrict and help to slow the flow of blood. This constriction of the vessel only lasts for a short time and slows but does not stop the bleeding. After the vasoconstriction of the vessel, platelets begin to adhere to the sides of the injured vessel walls, clumping together to form a plug at the cut end of the injured vessel. After the platelets adhere to the vessel walls, they begin to extrude their contents, including epinephrine, serotonin, and most importantly adenosine diphosphate (ADP). The release of ADP causes more platelets to clump on the first layer, resulting in an initial thrombus, or aggregation of blood factors that helps aid in hemostasis. In small vessels, this initial thrombus formation may be enough to stop the flow of blood. In larger vessels, however, a second, permanent thrombus must be formed. After the initial white cell thrombus formation, reaction between plasma and fibrin from the connective tissue of the cells activates clotting factors that cause another set of reactions. Prothrombin reacts with thromboplastin to form thrombin. Thrombin then reacts with fibrinogen and forms fibrin, which has an ability to stabilize blood clots. If any of these factors are deficient, bleeding may continue. Over time, fibrin strands form a matrix through the clot to form a stronger, more solid plug that can withstand the pressure of blood within the vessel.

The phases of the clotting process are as follows:

I: Platelets adhere to subendothelium of vessel walls.
II: Platelets release ADP.

III: Release of ADP causes further layers of platelets to adhere.
IV: Platelet aggregate forms (white thrombus).
V: Permanent thrombus forms after clotting factor reaction.

FACTORS AFFECTING HEMOSTASIS

Both preexisting hemostatic defects and acquired hemostatic disorders affect the ease or ability of the blood to clot.

PREEXISTING HEMOSTATIC DEFECTS

Some patients have congenital or preexisting bleeding disorders that will affect bleeding during the surgical procedure. Hemophilia is the most common of these and manifests itself as a clotting deficiency. Preoperative testing is useful in determining whether these conditions exist.

ACQUIRED HEMOSTATIC DISORDERS

More commonly seen in the OR are bleeding disorders caused by an outside source, or acquired bleeding disorders. Among these are liver disease, anticoagulant therapy with heparin or warfarin sodium, aplastic anemia, and alcoholic liver failure. Most commonly, drug-therapy-induced platelet dysfunctions affect hemostasis in the OR. Patients are requested not to take aspirin for 1 week prior to surgery because of its anticoagulant properties.

CONTROL OF BLEEDING DURING SURGERY

Patients generally enter the OR hemodynamically normal, and it is the goal of the surgical team that the patient leave the OR as close to hemostatically normal as possible. Fifty percent of postoperative bleeding is due to poor hemostasis during surgery. If a patient enters the OR bleeding from a traumatic injury or any other source, it is the goal of the surgical team to bring about hemostasis. While intraoperative bleeding from cut vessels is the most obvious and immediately treated, oozing from denuded surfaces and smaller vessels can eventually lead to a large-volume blood loss and must also be controlled. Also, certain procedures such as cardiopulmonary bypass and liver transplant surgery are commonly associated with large blood loss that may require transfusion or the administration of blood and blood products in order to achieve hemostasis. Key to proper hemostasis are gentle tissue handling, proper wound closure without dead space, and proper wound dressing. In addition, several methods exist to achieve hemostasis intraoperatively.

MECHANICAL METHODS

Mechanical hemostasis is achieved using any of several instruments or devices to control bleeding until a clot may form.

INTERNAL INTRAOPERATIVE METHODS

Most intraoperative methods of achieving hemostasis involve clamping and/or ligating or clipping the cut vessels with ligating clips or using electrosurgery to achieve hemostasis. Meticulous hemostasis is important to prevent postoperative bleeding. This also provides the surgeon with a dry field in which relevant structures may be clearly visualized. When the field cannot be kept completely dry, a clear field is achieved by the use of sponging or by suctioning the field. If blood loss is great, transfusion may be necessary.

CLAMPS

Clamps are used to compress the walls of vessels together and also for grasping tissue. Most commonly used is the **hemostat**, a clamping instrument with a fine point that is available with either straight or curved jaws. Special hemostatic clamps are available for different situations, such as vascular clamps designed to be noncrushing and do little damage to delicate vessels.

LIGATURE

Ligatures, or *ties* (referred to as "stick ties" when a needle is attached), are strands of suture material used to tie off blood vessels. Ligatures are made of either natural or synthetic material and are designed either to dissolve over a period of time or to remain in the body tissue. Vessels are ligated using the smallest possible diameter ligature in order to lower the amount of tissue reaction and are often placed at the base of a hemostat that has been used to clamp the end of a vessel. The hemostat may then be removed, the ligature tightened and tied, and the ends cut as close to the knot as possible. When the material used to tie off a bleeding vessel is of a monofilament type, the tails of the suture should be left approximately ¼ in. long from the knot. This enhances knot security.

CLIPS

Ligating clips are often used in place of suture ligatures when many small vessels need to be ligated in a short period of time. These clips are made of a nonreactive metal such as titanium or stainless steel or of a plastic material and come in various sizes as well as absorbable or permanent varieties. They are applied either from a manually loaded applicator or from any of several preloaded disposable applicators.

When placed on the cut end of a vessel and squeezed shut, these clips occlude the vessel and stop bleeding.

SPONGES

Sponges (also called *laps, micks, tapes,* or *Ray-Tecs*) are used to put pressure on bleeding areas or vessels and to absorb excess blood or fluid of any type. Patties (cottonoids) are smaller compressed radiopaque sponges that may be placed on the surface of brain tissue or nerves. These are always moistened with saline prior to use. All sponges are carefully counted at the beginning of surgery and have a radiopaque strand attached to them. They are recounted during closure to ensure that none have been left in the open surgical site. If a count is incorrect, X-rays may be taken, and the radiopaque strand will be visible. All sponges must be removed from the patient prior to closure to prevent infection. The surgeon may request that these sponges be moistened with saline or unfolded to provide more surface area for packing.

PLEDGETS

When bleeding might occur through needle holes in vessel anastomoses, small squares of Teflon called *pledgets* are used as buttresses over the suture line. These are sewn over the hole in the vessel along with the suture and exert outside pressure over any small needle holes to prevent bleeding and promote clotting. These are often used in peripheral vascular and cardiovascular surgery.

BONE WAX

Bone wax, made of refined and sterilized bee's wax, is used on cut edges of bone as a mechanical barrier to seal off oozing blood. This method should always be used sparingly because the body recognizes bone wax as a foreign body and this may cause tissue reaction and rejection, and bone wax is only minimally absorbed by the body. Bone wax is used in thoracic surgery when the sternum is split, in neurosurgical procedures, and for orthopedic and otorhinolaryngologic (ORL) procedures. Bone wax should be softened by kneading prior to use.

SUCTION

Suction is the aspiration of fluid by mechanical means. Suction is used intraoperatively to clear the surgical site of blood and body fluids. Several different styles of suction tips are available for different types of procedures, and many are disposable. The tip is connected to a sterile disposable suction tubing, which is in turn connected to a vacuum device by the circulator at the beginning of surgery. The circulator controls the strength of suction, and the surgeon may request it to be increased or decreased at any time during the procedure. It is important that suction always be available during surgery and until the patient has left the room, in case of an emergent bleeding situation. Both preoperatively and postoperatively, suction is used to maintain a clear airway.

DRAINS

Drains are used postoperatively to remove blood and fluid from the operative side and to aid in removing air in order to prevent dead spaces within the surgical wound. Removal of blood and fluids helps prevent edema and hematoma as well as infection. Several different types are available, each with a specific use (Table 8-17).

PRESSURE DEVICES

The application of external pressure, as with the use of a tourniquet, to a vessel occludes the flow of blood until a

Table 8-17 Drains

NAME	TYPE	DESCRIPTION
Penrose	Passive	Thin rubber tube that facilitates drainage by capillary action from a closed or partially closed area. This type of drain has no collection device.
Jackson-Pratt Hemovac	Active manual suction	Closed wound drainage system comprised of a drainage tube and collection vessel, usually of the "hand grenade" or spring-loaded active suction type.
Sump	Active mechanical suction	Double-lumen drain that allows air entering the drained area through the smaller lumen to displace fluid into the larger lumen.
Chest tube	Water seal	Active or passive chest-tube drainage device using a water seal that can be used to prevent and treat pneumothorax.

clot has time to form. Prophylactically, pressure devices, such as sequential stockings, may also be used to prevent venous stasis and deep-vein thrombosis.

Tourniquet

Tourniquets are used to stop excessive bleeding from trauma by the application of pressure to a blood vessel. They are often used on extremities to keep the operative site free of blood. The provision of a bloodless field makes visualization easier and reduces the operative time. Bleeding must be controlled prior to removal of the tourniquet, however, because the use of a tourniquet alone does not achieve hemostasis. The use of a pneumatic tourniquet is dangerous, and care should be taken in application to prevent pressure injury to the patient. The skin must be protected using soft cotton padding under the area of the tourniquet. The tourniquet must be placed around the largest circumference of the extremity to prevent nerve damage; the extremity should be elevated prior to tourniquet inflation to assist in venous drainage. The time the tourniquet is inflated should be recorded along with the pressure, and the surgeon should be notified when it has been inflated for 1 hour and should be reminded every 15 minutes thereafter. If the tourniquet is to be used for more than 1 hour on an arm or 1½ hours on a leg, it must be deflated for 10 minutes and then reinflated. The deflation times and final deflation time should be recorded in the patient's chart by the circulator.

THERMAL HEMOSTASIS

One of the most common means of obtaining hemostasis during a surgical procedure is with the use of heat. Several different types of devices are available for achieving thermal hemostasis.

ELECTROSURGERY

Electrosurgery is the most commonly used thermal hemostatic device. The electrosurgical unit is connected by the circulator to the active electrode or "pencil," which is passed off the sterile field to the circulator prior to the beginning of the case. This pencil has a small metal loop or blade tip that passes electric current through the patient to an inactive (dispersive) electrode or "grounding pad" in order to generate intense heat at the site being touched by the tip of the active electrode. The tip of the electrosurgical pencil is the active electrode, and current returns to the generator through the grounding pad, which acts as the inactive or dispersive electrode. In some procedures, bipolar electrosurgery is used. This utilizes a forceps-like tip, with one side of the forceps acting as the active electrode and the other acting as the inactive electrode. Bipolar electrosurgery provides a much more controlled and localized coagulation. Both methods of electrosurgery provide a searing heating effect that seals the tissues and provides hemostasis. Electrosurgery utilizes high-frequency alternating current, and the electrosurgical pencil may be set to cut or coagulate tissue. The use of electrosurgery produces burned tissue which causes a foreign body reaction, and must be absorbed by the body. Care should be taken not to leave excess char in the wound. To prevent patient burns, care must be taken that the grounding pad is firmly affixed to the patient prior to the start of surgery. (Refer to Chapter 10 for more information.)

LASER

Often, laser beams are utilized in much the same way as electrosurgery for cutting and coagulating tissue producing little blood loss. The laser provides an intense and concentrated beam of light that is able to cut and coagulate tissue at the same time with very little surrounding tissue destruction. Several types of lasers are available, each with a specific surgical use. Care should be taken by the surgical team that all laser protocols are followed and protective devices are used for the surgical team and the patient at all times.

PHARMACOLOGICAL AGENTS

Several pharmacological agents that aid in hemostasis are available, with more being developed each year. Each has its own method of action and preferred usage, and manufacturer's instructions should be carefully followed.

ABSORBABLE GELATIN

Gelatin is composed of collagen, a structural protein found in connective tissues. It is available in either powder form or in the form of a foam pad, which comes in a variety of sizes and can be cut. When gelatin is placed over an area of bleeding, fibrin is deposited, assisting in clot formation. In addition, the sponge is very absorbent and may be soaked in thrombin, epinephrine, or saline or used dry. This hemostatic agent may be left in the wound postoperatively, because it will be absorbed by the body in approximately 30 days.

COLLAGEN

Collagen is available in several absorbable forms and assists in activating the coagulation process. The collagen is dissolvable, and as hemostasis occurs, it disappears. Any collagen material must be kept dry or it becomes extremely sticky and difficult to use and should therefore be applied using only dry instruments and gloves. Avitene is a powdery substance composed of 100% collagen and is available in powder, sheets, and preloaded applicators and via a powered dispenser. Avitene is a hemostatic agent that potentiates the body's natural clotting mechanism and helps prevent postoperative bleeding. This product is also available in Actifoam form, which is similar to the gelatin foam but is more effective in that it is not a passive agent, but an active one that promotes the coagulation process.

OXIDIZED CELLULOSE

Available as Nu-Knit and Surgi-Cel, absorbable *oxidized cellulose* products are available in the form of pads or fabric (Surgi-Cel). Blood clots rapidly in the presence of oxidized cellulose, and the products form a gel, which aids in hemostasis as it becomes soaked with blood. These products are applied directly to the bleeding surface and held in place until bleeding stops.

SILVER NITRATE

Silver nitrate is often used to control cervical or nasal bleeding. This product is available in several forms.

EPINEPHRINE

Epinephrine is a vasoconstrictor and is often mixed with local anesthetic agents or with Gelfoam to aid in local hemostasis. It is absorbed rapidly by the body but provides good localized hemostasis.

THROMBIN

Part of the blood-clotting mechanism, *thrombin* is an enzyme that results from the activation of prothrombin, part of the chain of coagulation. In the OR, thrombin of bovine origin is used as a topical hemostatic. Thrombin may be poured directly onto a bleeding site but is usually used either in powder form or saturated into a Gelfoam pad, cottonoid, or collagen sponge to aid in hemostasis. The circulator charts thrombin use, and thrombin should be discarded if not used within several hours as it loses potency.

BLOOD LOSS

Blood loss is monitored by several means intraoperatively to aid the surgeon and anesthesia provider in making decisions regarding the patient's status and potential need for transfusion or autotransfusion.

Calibrated suction devices (canisters) are used between the suction and the vacuum source at the wall to monitor the amount of blood and body fluids suctioned from the field. The STSR should keep close track of the amount of irrigation fluids used, and this information is used to calculate the amount of blood in the calibrated suction canister. The amount of irrigation fluid used is subtracted from the total volume in the canister to give a more accurate amount of blood loss.

In addition, the circulator may weigh sponges removed from the field to give an estimate of blood lost to sponges. Either the circulator may use a scale and a predetermined sponge weight formula, or some hospitals have a bloody-sponge weight estimate that is used and multiplied by the number of sponges removed from the field. The sponges must be weighed wet as the formula is based on the dry and wet weights of the sponges. This is not an exacting method but provides the surgeon and anesthesia provider with a fairly reliable estimate of blood loss.

Any drainage from within collection devices used should be measured periodically, and this amount of blood loss is added to the total amount. Blood loss is charted by the circulator and reported to the surgeon upon request or immediately in extreme-loss situations.

BLOOD REPLACEMENT

When blood loss is too great to be controlled by intraoperative hemostatic techniques alone, blood replacement therapies are in order, but blood loss must still be controlled. Some types of surgery, such as cardiovascular or prostate surgery, will often call for blood replacement due to the high volume of blood lost during surgery. Blood replacement involves the administration of whole blood or blood components such as plasma, packed red blood cells, or platelets via an IV. This is used to increase the circulating blood volume, to increase the number of red blood cells, and to provide plasma-clotting factors that have been depleted during surgery. Blood products used may be either **homologous** (donated by another person) or **autologous** (donated previously by the patient and stored or through autotransfusion). Autotransfusion is the use of the patient's own blood, which has been processed for reinfusion. When homologous banked blood is used, blood typing and crossmatching are essential to prevent transfusion reactions.

BLOOD TYPES AND GROUPS

The four main blood types are A, B, O, and AB, based on the presence or absence of A and B red cell antigens. Individuals with A antigens, B antigens, or no antigens belong to groups A, B, and O, respectively, and individuals with both A and B antigens belong to group AB. In addition, the blood contains agglutinins, which are antibodies that work against the A and B antigens. Individuals with type A blood naturally produce anti-B agglutinins and individuals with type B blood naturally produce anti-A agglutinins. An individual with type O blood, however, naturally produces both A and B agglutinins, making the O− (negative) individual a universal donor. Type AB individuals produce neither antibody, and therefore, type AB individuals may receive any type and are called universal recipients. If mismatched blood is transfused, a transfusion reaction occurs and may range from a mild reaction to anaphylactic shock.

Also to be taken into consideration in blood matching is the **Rh factor**, which is an antigenic substance found in the erythrocytes in most people. Individuals with the factor are termed *Rh positive,* whereas individuals lacking the factor are termed *Rh negative.* If blood given to an Rh-negative individual is Rh positive, **hemolysis**, or red blood cell destruction leading to anemia, occurs.

Due to these factors, blood is carefully typed and crossmatched prior to being administered.

HANDLING OF BLOOD REPLACEMENT COMPONENTS

Blood products are usually obtained from the blood bank by a responsible individual, signed for, and brought to the OR. If the products are not to be used immediately, they should be stored in a refrigerator at a temperature between 1 and 6°C. The refrigerator may be in the OR, but most hospitals have a refrigerator placed in a convenient location for use by several ORs at one time. Prior to administration, blood products must be carefully identified, checking for both the proper product and patient. Either two licensed nurses or a nurse and a physician should perform this identification. One individual reads aloud while the other checks and verifies the information. The information for blood group, Rh type, and unit number should match both the tag on the blood bag and the patient's chart, and these should be checked by the two-individual verbal method listed above. The physician's order should also be double-checked, as should the expiration date on the blood bag. Finally, the product itself should be inspected for clots. If clots are present or any of the information does not match correctly, the blood should not be administered and should be returned to the blood bank. In addition, the patient's armband should be checked for final verification of identification. In many procedures this will be impossible, and the chart should be checked. The patient's armband should be checked upon entry into the OR.

AUTOTRANSFUSION

Autotransfusion is the reinfusion of the patient's own blood, whether donated prior to surgery or collected and reinfused perioperatively. This process is preferable to the use of homologous blood in that it uses the patient's own blood, eliminating the danger of a compatibility mismatch or disease transmission. Blood may either be donated prior to surgery or recovered during surgery and reinfused. In the latter case, blood is suctioned directly from the wound into a sterile machine (cell saver or cell salvager) that filters and anticoagulates the blood and reinfuses it intravenously with little or no damage to the red blood cells. Several machines are available for intraoperative use and all work on the same principle. Some are designed for more rapid reinfusion in emergency situations. In addition to suctioned blood, blood may be extracted from bloody sponges, drained into a basin of saline, and then aspirated into the autotransfusion machine. Blood that has been exposed to collagen hemostatic agents and certain antibiotics cannot be used with these devices, as blood may coagulate in the system. If the procedure involves blood exposed to gastric or enteric contents or amniotic fluid, it may not be salvaged, and blood may not be used when the patient has a known local or systemic infection.

When a cell-salvaging machine is not available, blood may be collected in a salvage collection bag containing an anticoagulant and reinfused through a blood filter. Another available method is a sterile blood collection canister into which blood can be suctioned. There, it collects in a reservoir. When the canister reaches capacity, it is emptied and the contents are washed in a red cell washer and reinfused. In many hospitals, this equipment is located in the blood bank and the blood must leave the OR for washing, so this method takes more time than the two previously outlined.

HEMOLYTIC TRANSFUSION REACTIONS

If blood is not properly matched prior to transfusion, a hemolytic transfusion reaction, or hemolytic anemia, may develop. This may result from Rh incompatibility from mismatched blood transfusions. Severe hemolytic reactions can be fatal and must be treated immediately.

The conscious patient may exhibit fatigue and complain of lack of energy. The patient may experience rapid pulse, shortness of breath, and pounding of the heart. The skin may appear jaundiced and pallor may be exhibited, especially in the palms of the hands.

The patient under general anesthesia will not show these signs, and the only signs noted may be a generalized diffuse loss of blood and a lowered blood oxygen saturation level due to the inability of the red blood cells to carry oxygen.

If a hemolytic transfusion reaction is suspected, the transfusion should be immediately stopped and a blood sample sent to the blood bank to rule out the mismatch. Appropriate drug therapies, usually including steroid therapy, are begun as quickly as possible. Urine output is monitored closely in these patients, as hypovolemia may hinder kidney function. In some cases, the patient will need to undergo dialysis, which will aid in the systemic removal of the mismatched blood.

CARDIOPULMONARY RESUSCITATION

Every health care professional should be familiar with the techniques of cardiopulmonary resuscitation (**CPR**), that is, manually providing chest compressions and ventilations to patients in cardiac arrest in an effort to provide oxygenated blood to the brain and vital organs and reverse the processes that lead to death. The best way for the surgical technologist to learn this technique is to obtain certification in CPR or Basic Life Support (BLS), offered in classes available in hospitals and from such organizations as the Red Cross and the American Heart Association. Hospital employees should attend this seminar every 2 years to renew their CPR/BLS certification.

CPR must be started as quickly as possible, as time is of the essence in cardiac arrest. "Clinical death" begins at the moment heart action and breathing stop; the patient has only 4–6 minutes before the cells of the brain begin to deteriorate. Therefore, it is very important that breathing and circulation be restored within this time frame to prevent "biological death" from occurring.

A "chain-of-survival" concept applies to both in-hospital and out-of-hospital cardiac arrests. Successful resuscitation requires:

- Early recognition of cardiac arrest
- Early activation of trained responders
- Early CPR
- Early defibrillation when indicated
- Early advanced cardiac life support (ACLS)

To provide these early interventions, the hospital develops written policies and procedures that the health care provider must be familiar with. In the OR, the STSR's primary function is to protect the sterile field; however, instances may arise outside the OR that could require the surgical technologist to utilize CPR skills.

According to procedures defined by the American Heart Association, the preliminary steps of CPR that apply outside the hospital are:

- Check the scene for safety.
- Call for help.
- Establish unresponsiveness by gently shaking and shouting at the individual.
- Activate the emergency medical system (EMS).

These procedures apply inside the hospital, too. The primary difference is that an internal team is activated and not the EMS.

The CPR provider or hospital team then begins providing the ABCs—airway, breathing, and circulation:

- *Airway:* Must be opened and free of foreign bodies for proper ventilation. The chest should be checked for movement and the provider should listen and feel for breath sounds.
- *Breathing:* Artificial respiration is necessary until breathing can be restored. In the hospital setting, breathing is facilitated by use of an Ambu-bag.
- *Circulation:* External chest compressions are given in the absence of a palpable pulse, at a rate of 80–100 compressions per minute for an adult victim.
- *Definitive treatment:* Definitive treatment is therapy intended to cause the cardiac function and respiration to return to normal spontaneous function.

In the monitored hospital setting, one situation that immediately overrides the use of the "ABCD" approach is ventricular fibrillation. Upon recognition of ventricular fibrillation, electrical defibrillation is immediately used, even before airway management. Another exception is the trauma patient in cardiac arrest. For these patients, it has been shown that cardiac arrest is usually caused by exsanguination or a critical thoracic injury. For these patients, the head tilt should not be used to open the airway if any suspicion of cervical spine injury exists. In trauma patients, it has been shown that chest compressions usually are not adequate to reverse the cardiac arrest and that the most critical factor is the restoration of circulating blood volume. Many of these patients will require resuscitative thoracotomy. Cardiopulmonary resuscitation is not performed without danger of injury to the patient. The technique must be performed with great care. Careful attention to proper technique helps minimize injury to the patient. Certification in CPR/BLS and biannual review help ensure that the health care provider has an adequate working knowledge of the technique.

CARDIAC ARREST IN THE SURGICAL SETTING

In the surgical setting, the "D" of the ABCs of cardiac arrest is undertaken when the physician begins to provide definitive treatment. This will include IV drugs, control of dysrhythmias by cardiac defibrillation or the use of medications, and postresuscitation care. Arterial lines are used to monitor blood pressure and blood gases. The role of the STSR in this situation is to protect the sterile field from contamination during the resuscitation efforts. In some cases, the STSR may be required to assist by providing artificial respiration ("bagging") or providing chest compressions. In most cases, roles are well defined by facility policy and each team member will have a specific function. In the OR, anesthesia personnel are available to deal with the cardiopulmonary arrest situation, or "code." They provide IV access and arterial pressure and blood gas monitoring as well as airway management respiratory and cardiac support including defibrillation. The circulating nurse is available to provide support to the patient and physicians and to bring necessary supplies, including the "crash cart" when necessary.

The primary responsibility of the STSR, as stated previously, is to protect the sterile field. The surgical technologist should remain sterile and should keep the tables and the operative area sterile. The surgical wound should be packed and covered with a sterile drape. It is also the responsibility of the STSR to keep track of all instruments, sponges, and needles on the field and to pay careful attention to the needs of the surgeon. When CPR must be accomplished through the sterile field, sterile team members should perform whatever procedures are necessary (e.g., open-chest heart massage). Sterility may become secondary to lifesaving procedures.

MALIGNANT HYPERTHERMIA

Malignant hyperthermia is a life-threatening, acute pharmacogenetic disorder, developing during or after anesthesia. This is a disorder that presents itself in some patients undergoing anesthesia and in some cases in the postoperative care unit that is characterized by a rapid increase in body temperature, unexplained tachycardia, unstable blood pressure, muscle rigidity, tachypnea, and cyanosis. The body temperature may rise to over 46°C.

Malignant hyperthermia is usually triggered by an anesthetic agent, such as Halothane, Enflurane, or Isoflurane, and may be triggered by muscle relaxants such as succinylcholine. The rapid increase in body temperature is due to an increase in the metabolic state, caused by an inherited defect in the muscles of the skeletal systems of some patients. In patients with this prior disposition, the anesthetic acts as a triggering agent to the muscle to release calcium. This high level of calcium accelerates the cellular metabolism rate, which drastically raises the body temperature. This may lead to renal failure, heart failure, or neurological damage if not controlled, and in many patients, death results. Predisposition to malignant hyperthermia cannot be absolutely determined, but a history of unclear complications related to general anesthesia, myalgia, or muscle cramps are indicators. Family history of muscle disorders may also indicate a predisposition to malignant hyperthermia crisis. Predisposition to malignant hyperthermia may also be diagnosed with a muscle biopsy taken under a local anesthetic.

The advent of modern monitoring, along with increased knowledge of malignant hyperthermia by anesthesia providers and the surgical team, has reduced the incidences of malignant hyperthermia crisis, but every member of the surgical team should be aware of the signs and treatment.

Increased body temperature is actually one of the last signs seen in a malignant hyperthermia crisis. The first indicator is an unanticipated increase in end-tidal CO_2. This increase may be very sudden or may develop over a longer period of up to 20 minutes. The most obvious sign to the surgical technologist will be total body rigidity. Chapter 9 contains additional information on MH.

PREVENTION

Control of patient anxiety is very important in the prevention of malignant hyperthermia. The use of sedative premedication may help prevent a crisis situation. When a patient is known to have a predisposition to malignant hyperthermia, nontriggering anesthetic agents are used, and all triggering agents are removed from the room. In addition, the anesthesia provider will change the anesthetic vaporizer and filter and flush the hose circuit with oxygen. The patient should be monitored with ECG, capnography, and pulse oxymetry, and blood gases, creatine kinase, and electrolytes should be checked. The strongest preventive is the use of trigger-free anesthesia agents, such as propofol or vecuronium.

TREATMENT

At the first sign of masseter spasm, or jaw muscle tightness, the anesthesia provider will stop the administration of triggering anesthetic agents and deepen the anesthesia using opioids, barbiturates, or propofol. Every hospital has its own protocol for dealing with the crisis, and the STSR should be familiar with the protocol in order to anticipate emergency needs of the surgeon. In the case of a sudden, intense, and unanticipated attack, the surgery may need to be stopped as soon as possible. The various methods of treatment include packing the patient in ice, circulating ice water through the nasogastric tube, and irrigation of the open abdominal cavity with chilled irrigation fluids. Dantrolene is the drug of choice in treating the hypermetabolism, and steroids and diuretics may also be administered. Ventilation will be adjusted to compensate for the increased end-tidal CO_2, and 100% oxygen will be administered.

Since the surgery may need to be stopped as soon as possible in order to focus attention on dealing with the malignant hyperthermia crisis, the STSR must be prepared to anticipate the needs of the surgeon for quick closure and/or actions within the sterile field to assist in cooling the patient.

EMERGENCY MEDICAL SERVICES

Almost every community in the United States now has some form of emergency medical service or prepared emergency personnel at the ready. These professionals, whether volunteer or paid, are associated with fire or police departments or are associated directly with a community's private emergency medical service.

The National Highway Safety Act authorized guidelines to be developed for emergency medical services in 1966. The act required every county in the United States to form a committee for emergency medical care. Soon thereafter, communities began forming their own emergency medical services. Through this system, such services as the now prevalent system of access to 911 were developed, through which citizens have immediate access to emergency services.

Through the established emergency medical services, emergency personnel provide on-site care and first aid to patients, some of whom will ultimately be seen in the OR. There are two basic levels of emergency personnel. Emergency medical technicians (EMTs) are providers of health care at the basic life support level. Their duties include spinal immobilization, administration of oxygen, and control of bleeding. Paramedics have had further training from the EMT level and are able to carry out tasks such as the administration of injections and IV fluids, the reading of electrocardiograms, and other advanced life support measures such as defibrillation and intubation.

Patients seen by EMTs and paramedics are brought into the hospital system through the emergency room. Certain hospitals across the nation have been designated trauma centers by the American College of Surgeons Committee on Trauma, which has also established special treatment centers for burns and other problems requiring specialized treatment. Patients are taken to the most appropriate centers for their particular injury or ailment.

In the emergency department of the hospital, nurses triage, or sort and classify patients in order of need for immediate medical attention. Emergency physicians then assess which patients may be treated in the emergency center or on the medical wards of the hospital and which need emergency surgery.

INDICATIONS OF EMERGENCY SITUATIONS

The surgical technologist is frequently called on to work in emergency surgery situations or to react appropriately when an elective surgery becomes an emergency. The surgical technologist must be able to anticipate emergency situations and to prepare for them in advance. This skill comes with experience, but the entry-level surgical technologist should be able to recognize an emergency situation when it occurs. Such indicators as rapidly dropping blood pressure, **cardiac dysrhythmia**, and any vital sign out of the normal range provide the surgical team with information about impending emergent situations. In addition, some emergencies occur suddenly, with little or no warning, such as rapid hemorrhaging, and must be immediately acted upon. It is extremely important that the entire surgical team react in a calm and quick fashion in these circumstances. Prior to surgery, the surgeon or anesthesia provider should be notified immediately if any of the indicators of emergency situation occur:

- Difficulty breathing
- Chest pain
- Changes in skin color or temperature
- Changes in vital signs
- Open bleeding wounds or visible punctures not indicated on the patient's chart
- Inability to move an extremity
- Misshapen/misaligned body part
- Disorientation or confusion

The surgeon and/or anesthesia provider will assess the situation in these cases and provide the surgical team with instructions on how they should act on the situation.

OBJECTIVES AND PRIORITIES IN EMERGENCY SITUATIONS

The objective of emergency care and emergency and trauma surgery is to preserve life, to prevent further deterioration of patient condition, and then to provide whatever care necessary to restore the patient to his or her previous lifestyle.

When providing emergency care, treatment should be prioritized to fit the objectives. As soon as an emergency patient situation is identified, the health care provider in the field or the surgical team member should signal for assistance. Treatment will then follow a pattern of priorities of care. The first priority in any emergency situation is to check for and provide a patent airway to ensure or restore respiratory status and breathing. Second, cardiovascular status should be maintained or restored and hemostasis should be provided to maintain circulatory status. Following these first two priorities, treatment is provided in the following order:

- Chest injuries
- Shock
- Wound protection/closure
- Fractures
- Vital sign monitoring
- Provision of reassurance and comfort for the patient

The following covers several of the most commonly seen emergencies in the OR.

SYNCOPE

Syncope is a sudden loss of consciousness, either without warning or with only momentary symptoms, caused by cerebral ischemia. Syncope can be caused by any of several factors, including ventricular asystole, extreme bradycardia, or ventricular fibrillation. It is also caused in some instances by disorders of arterioventricular conduction, which is mediated by the vagus nerve. Syncope indicates an underlying problem that must be diagnosed and treated by the physician.

When the surgical patient experiences an episode of syncope, the surgeon and anesthesia provider should be notified immediately. The anesthesia provider will provide immediate care and together with the surgeon will attempt to find the underlying cause of the loss of consciousness.

The unconscious patient should be protected from falls, and the head should be turned to one side to aid with airway maintenance and to help prevent aspiration. The patient having intermittent losses of consciousness should be made comfortable and reassured when conscious. Vital signs should be constantly monitored, so that an episode of ventricular fibrillation does not go untreated.

CONVULSIONS/SEIZURES

Seizures and *convulsions* are defined as "disturbances of nervous system function resulting from abnormal electrical activity of the brain." Seizures are caused by sudden overloading electrical discharges without order within the neurons of the brain and involve either the entire brain at once or a finite spot.

TYPES OF SEIZURES

The most common type of seizure is the *grand mal seizure,* characterized by loss of consciousness and convulsive body movement. These seizures follow a specific pattern, including the patient's crying out, loss of consciousness, convulsions, and incontinence. Prior to a grand mal seizure, the patient may experience symptoms of numbness, flashing lights, dizziness, arm tingling, or seeing spots before the eyes. After a grand mal seizure, the patient may be drowsy and confused and may have no memory of the seizure event.

Petit mal seizures are much shorter in duration and come about quite suddenly and without warning. Symptoms include a vacant facial expression and a cessation of all motor activity except for slight twitching of the eyelids or face and arms.

Psychomotor seizures present with a sudden change in consciousness accompanied by the patient making a series of movements or statements that seem out of place or bizarre. Following this type of seizure, the patient is usually amnesic and will often fall asleep. These seizures are often caused by temporal lobe lesions.

Focal seizures arise in the motor or sensory areas of the brain. They occur in patients with structural diseases of the brain and may occur as a symptom in persons with brain tumors or arteriovenous malformations. These seizures present with symptoms of clonic muscle spasm beginning in one muscle group that spreads systematically to other muscle groups.

Following a seizure, a patient usually feels fatigued and may be amnesic to the episode. Patients in a post-seizure state are said to be postictal.

MANAGEMENT OF SEIZURE

The primary duty of the surgical team, including the surgical technologist, is to protect a patient having a seizure from injury. As in all emergency situations, the airway should be maintained. Seizure patients sometimes have airway problems arising from aspiration, and an oral airway device should be inserted prior to mouth clenching when possible. Airway insertion should not be attempted when the mouth is clenched, as the health care provider and the patient could both be injured. The patient may be positioned on the left side to assist in drainage of secretions, and if possible, suction may be used. When the seizure has ended, the patient should be calmed and reassured. The sequence and type of events during the seizure episode should be carefully documented, as the details of the event will assist the surgeon in diagnosis of the type of seizure as well as the possible location of any cerebral lesion.

ANAPHYLACTIC REACTIONS

Anaphylactic reaction is an exaggerated allergic reaction to a substance or protein. Among the substances most likely to cause anaphylactic reaction are drugs such as local anesthetics, codeine, antibiotics, animal derived drugs such as insulin, contrast media, and in some cases the latex found in surgical gloves and Foley catheters. In some cases, patients may experience anaphylactic reactions to local anesthetic or cocaine used in surgical procedures.

A patient suffering an anaphylactic attack generally first shows only mild inflammatory symptoms such as itching, swelling, and in some cases, difficulty breathing. Hives or urticaria may be present on the skin with severe itching. These symptoms may cause apprehension in the patient and should not be ignored as these symptoms can rapidly escalate to a systemic anaphylactic attack. As the reaction progresses, the patient experiences further difficulty breathing due to bronchospasm and laryngeal edema. At the same time that these respiratory symptoms are occurring, another chain of events takes place that causes vascular collapse due to shifts in body fluid. This presents with hypotension, tachycardia, and diminished urine output.

During an anaphylactic reaction, the surgical team must maintain the airway and provide supplemental oxygen or the patient may die of respiratory failure. The symptoms of vascular collapse must also be treated to prevent death from cardiovascular failure. Because of the symptoms, the patient should also be treated for shock, which ultimately develops and could also lead to death.

Epinephrine is the first-line drug in the treatment of a severe anaphylactic reaction and causes bronchodilation, reduces laryngeal spasm, and raises blood pressure. After the administration of epinephrine, steroids are administered to stabilize mast cells and slow or stop the chain of events that caused the reaction. Intravenous fluids and plasma may also be utilized to restore fluid volume, and vasopressor agents such as Levophed are given to increase blood pressure.

Because an anaphylactic reaction occurs so quickly and can so often lead to death, it is important in the clinical setting that it be avoided altogether by identifying patients with known allergies and making this information available to the entire surgical team. This lowers the risk of provoking an anaphylactic reaction. Allergies should be clearly identified on the chart and preferably on the patient identification band, and any prior history of reactions should be carefully noted in the chart. If suspicion of reactivity exists, skin testing prior to surgery can help determine what drugs should be used intraoperatively.

CLINICAL MANIFESTATIONS OF IMPENDING CARDIAC ARREST

There are several warning signs of impending cardiac arrest, and the surgical technologist should be able to recognize these in order to anticipate emergent needs of the patient. A patient who exhibits any of the following may be in danger of cardiac arrest:

- Chest pain (in the awake patient)
- Unstable blood pressure
- Tachycardia
- Cardiac dysrhythmias
- Respiratory changes
- Hypovolemia
- Laryngospasm

CASE STUDY

Sheree is 24 years old, and she is donating a kidney to her sister who has end-stage renal disease. The procedure is scheduled to begin at 8:30 A.M. Her sister will be in the adjoining room. Sheree's kidney will be placed in her sister's right lower quadrant.

1. In what position will Sheree be placed on the operating table? Will it require any special pads or devices?
2. Sheree's skin will be prepped. What are the boundaries for the prep? What are the boundaries for her sister's skin prep?
3. Both patients will have an indwelling catheter. What is the procedure for the insertion of a urethral catheter?

QUESTIONS FOR FURTHER STUDY

1. What are three signs of malignant hyperthermia?
2. What are the indications for urinary catheterization in surgery?
3. Why is it important that all joints and surfaces of the body that come into contact with the operating table or accessories be padded when positioning the patient and during surgery?
4. What are two reasons why the limbs should be moved slowly and simultaneously during positioning?
5. What is one indication for the use of hypothermia intraoperatively?
6. Describe the auscultatory gap that may be noted during blood pressure measurement.

BIBLIOGRAPHY

Association of Operating Room Nurses (AORN). (1996). *Standards & recommended practices*. Denver: Author.

Bowen, D. R. (1997). Intraoperative thermoregulation. In J. J. Naglehout & K. L. Zagliniczny (Eds.), *Nurse anesthesia*. Philadelphia: W. B. Saunders.

Centers for Disease Control and Prevention (CDC). (1998). Draft guideline for the prevention of surgical site infection. *Federal Register, 63,* 33168–33192.

Ethicon. (1987). *Nursing care of the patient in the O.R.* Trenton, NJ: Author.

Gruendemann, B. (1987). *Positioning plus: A clinical handbook on patient positioning for perioperative nurses*. Chatsworth: Devon Industries.

Haines, N. (1992). Same day surgery—coordinating the education process. *AORN Journal, 55*(2), 60–68.

Kurz, A. (1996). Perioperative normothermia to reduce the incidence of surgical wound infection and shorten hospitalization: A randomized clinical trial. *New England Journal of Medicine, 334,* 1209–1215.

Lach, J. (1974). *O.R. nursing: Preoperative care and draping technique*. Chicago: Kendall Company.

Lawrence, P. (1992). *Essentials of general surgery*. Baltimore: Williams & Wilkins.

Mathias, J. (Ed.). (1998). Sacred cow survey—Survey finds progress in outdated OR rituals. *OR Manager, 14*(9), 1–14.

McGuiness, A. M., et al. (2002). *Core curriculum for surgical technology* (5th ed.). Centennial, CO: Association of Surgical Technologists.

Miner, D. (1987). Patient positioning—Applying the nursing process. *AORN Journal, 45*(5), 1117–1133.

Moore, S., Green, C. R., Wang, F. L., Pandit, S. K., & Hurd, W. W. (1997). The role of irrigation in the development of hypothermia during laparoscopic surgery. *American Journal of Obstetrics and Gynecology, 176*(3), 598–602.

Moss, R. (1998). Clinical issues—Inadvertent perioperative hypothermia. *AORN Journal, 67*(2).

Moss, V. (1988). Music and the surgical patient. *AORN Journal, 48*(1), 64–68.

O'Toole, M. (Ed.). (1997). *Miller-Keane encyclopedia & dictionary of medicine, nursing, & allied health* (6th ed.). Philadelphia: W. B. Saunders.

Paff, S. (1998). Vital signs and measurements. In Lindh, W., Pooler, M., Tamparo, C., & Cerrato, J. (Eds.), *Clinical medical assisting*. Clifton Park, NY: Delmar Learning.

Phipps, W., Long, B., Woods, N., & Cassmeyer, V. (Eds.). (1991). *Medical surgical nursing concepts and clinical practice* (4th ed.). St. Louis, MO: Mosby-Year Book.

Potter, P., & Perry, A. (Eds.). (1989). *Fundamentals of nursing: Concepts, process, and practice* (2nd ed.). St. Louis, MO: CV Mosby.

Shafer, D., Rush, S., & Cleary, P. (1998). Hemostasis basics programmed learner part I. Dade Behring online [Online]. Available from *http://www.dadebehring.com/hemo/tutorial.html*

Way, L. (1994). *Current surgical diagnosis & treatment* (10th ed.). Norwalk, CT: Appleton & Lange.

CHAPTER 9

Surgical Pharmacology and Anesthesia

Ann Marie McGuiness
Teri Junge

CASE STUDY

Amber, a 23-year-old female, has been scheduled for an emergency laparoscopic appendectomy. She was admitted to the emergency department at 2:03 P.M., and the surgery is expected to be performed at approximately 4 P.M. Amber states that she has increased her fluid intake the last 2 days due to the fever that she is experiencing and that she had creamy chicken noodle soup for lunch today. She was instructed by the emergency department staff shortly after her arrival not to eat or drink anything, and IV was started.

1. What type of anesthetic is Amber likely to receive and why?
2. Is Amber likely to receive any premedications? If so, what type and why?
3. Amber's NPO status is known. Are any special precautions necessary prior to administering her anesthetic?
4. What type of medications may be ordered by the surgeon and used within the sterile field intraoperatively?

OBJECTIVES

After studying this chapter, the reader should be able to:

C 1. Define general terminology and abbreviations associated with pharmacology and anesthesia.

2. Describe the action, uses, and modes of administration of drugs and anesthetic agents used in the care of the surgical patient.

3. Describe the side effects and contraindications for use of drugs and anesthetic agents.
4. Describe the factors that influence anesthesia selection for individual patients.

A 5. Demonstrate safe practice in transferring drugs and solutions from the nonsterile area to the sterile field.

6. Demonstrate the procedure for identifying a drug or solution on the sterile field.
7. Explain how sterile technique is used in relation to certain anesthesia procedures.

R 8. Convert equivalents from one system to another and accurately identify, mix, and measure drugs for patient use.

9. Explain the roles of the STSR and circulator during the administration of anesthesia.

E 10. Discuss care and precautions in identifying drugs and solutions in the OR.

11. List the equipment used as an adjunct to anesthesia.

SELECT KEY TERMS

1. agonist	9. buccal	17. iatrogenic	25. pharmaco-dynamics
2. amnesia	10. capnography	18. indication	26. pharmacokinetics
3. anaphylaxis	11. contraindication	19. induction	27. pharmacology
4. anesthesia	12. Doppler	20. intra-articular	28. prophylaxis
5. antagonist	13. drug	21. laryngospasm	29. topical
6. antimuscarinic	14. generic	22. NPO	30. volatile agents
7. aspiration	15. homeostasis	23. PACU	
8. biotechnology	16. hypnosis	24. parenteral	

PHARMACOLOGY

Pharmacology is the study of drugs and their actions. A **drug** is defined as a substance used as medicine for the diagnosis, treatment, cure, mitigation, or prevention (**prophylaxis**) of disease or a condition. Humans have been aware of the therapeutic value of natural substances since the beginning of time; this is evidenced in some of the art forms of the prehistoric era. History shows that treatment for a specific problem was developed by coincidence. The information was then passed verbally to a select few. Modern pharmacology is a progressive exact science constantly seeking new drugs for treatment of specific problems. New medications are developed/discovered almost daily. All drugs on the market today have been standardized and approved for safety, accuracy of the dose, and effectiveness by the Federal Drug Administration (FDA) after undergoing several phases of formal independent testing.

DRUG SOURCES

Drugs are derived from five main sources:

- *Plants:* At one time, most drugs originated from plants. A number of medications from plant sources are still used today. Examples include morphine and digitalis.

- *Animals:* Primarily hormones are derived from animal (including human) sources. Drugs obtained from cows are referred to as *bovine* and those from pigs as *porcine*. Heparin and thrombin are examples.
- *Minerals:* From the earth, minerals and mineral salts have a variety of applications. Minerals are available in several drug forms, and some commonly used minerals are calcium, gold, iron, magnesium, silver, and zinc.
- *Laboratory synthesis:* The majority of drugs in use today are manufactured in the laboratory. Laboratory synthesis is accomplished by one of two methods:
  - Synthetic drugs are manufactured totally from laboratory chemicals. Meperidine sulfate (Demerol) is an example of a synthetic drug.
  - Semisynthetic drugs begin with a natural substance, which is then chemically altered.
- ***Biotechnology***: The newest source of drugs from the laboratory comes to us from genetic engineering. This new technology is referred to as *recombinant DNA technology*. DNA is artificially constructed by introducing foreign DNA into the DNA of a specific organism. The two types of DNA combine and the new DNA and its specific protein are replicated in the daughter cells of the organism. Cell reproduction occurs rapidly, providing large amounts of the desired protein for use in the manufacture of certain drugs. The hepatitis B vaccine is produced as a result of recombinant DNA technology.

Key words that relate to pharmacology include:

Pharmacodynamics: The interaction of drug molecules with the target cells. The resulting action is biochemical and physiological.

Pharmacokinetics: The entire process of the drug within the body. It involves absorption, distribution, biotransformation (metabolism), and excretion.

Indication: A reason to perform a specific procedure or prescribe a certain drug.

Contraindication: A reason why a specific procedure or drug may be undesirable or improper in a particular situation.

DRUG FORMS

Drugs are prepared for administration in several different forms. The type of preparation, or form, in which the drug is available will determine the route of administration as well as the pharmacodynamics and pharmacokinetics. The forms in which drugs are prepared for administration are found in Table 9-1.

DRUG NOMENCLATURE

Three different names are assigned to each drug. Use of the **generic** name is advocated in the health care setting to avoid confusion. The names that may be assigned to a drug are as follows:

- *Chemical name:* Precise chemical composition and molecular structure of the drug. The chemical name is complex and difficult to use.
- *Generic name:* Nonproprietary name for a drug that is often a shortened version of the chemical name and may include a reference to the intended use. The

Table 9-1 Forms of Drug Preparation

CATEGORY	SUBCATEGORY	DEFINITION/EXAMPLE
Gas		Oxygen and nitrous oxide are included in this category.
Liquid		Two primary types of liquid preparations: solution and suspension.
	Solution	Drug (solute) is dissolved in a liquid (solvent).
	Aqueous	Solution prepared with water.
	Syrup	Sweetened aqueous solution.
	Tincture	Solution prepared with alcohol.
	Elixir	Sweetened alcohol solution.
	Suspension	Solid particles are suspended in a liquid. Particles may settle and must be redistributed prior to administration of a suspension.
	Emulsion	Combination of two liquids that cannot mix. Small droplets of one liquid are dispersed (suspended) throughout the other.
Solid		Powder is considered a solid form of a drug. It may be in the powdered state, contained within a capsule, or compressed into tablet form. Some powders must have liquid added (called reconstitution) prior to use. Troches or lozenges also fall into this category.
Semisolid		Creams, foams, gels, lotions, ointments, and suppositories.

generic name is often selected by the original developer.

- *Trade or brand name:* Drug name selected and copyrighted by the manufacturer for marketing (proprietary) purposes. The brand name of the drug is capitalized and may be followed by the ® symbol. A generic drug may be produced by several proprietors under as many trade names. Keep in mind that manufacturing differences may occur, making the preparation of each manufacturer slightly different.

ROUTE OF ADMINISTRATION

Each drug is designed for administration by a certain route. Some drugs are formulated in several different ways to allow administration via several routes. Some of the routes of administration have limited use in the operating room setting. Drug administration routes are:

- *Oral or enteral* (abbreviation is PO, meaning *per os* or by mouth): Through the alimentary tract.
- *Ingest:* To swallow.
- ***Buccal***: Medication is placed between the cheek and the teeth until it is dissolved or absorbed.
- *Sublingual:* Medication is placed under the tongue until it is dissolved or absorbed.

(*Note:* Buccal and sublingual administration are also considered **topical**.)

- *Topical:* Drug is applied to the skin or mucous membrane to provide a localized or systemic effect.
- *Inhalation:* Direct administration via the respiratory tract.
- ***Parenteral***: Other than enteral, by injection.
- *Dermal:* Between the layers of the skin.
- *Subcutaneous (SC or SQ):* Under the skin, into the adipose tissue layer.
- *Intramuscular (IM):* Within a muscle.
- *Intravenous (IV):* Into a vein.
- ***Intra-articular***: Within a joint.
- *Intrathecal:* Into the subarachnoid space.
- *Intracardiac:* Into the heart.

DRUG CLASSIFICATIONS

Drugs are classified in many ways for a variety of reasons; each classification may have several subclassifications. This can be confusing, as some of the classifications overlap and a specific drug may be cross-referenced in several categories.

Drugs for sale are classified in two ways: over the counter (OTC), drugs that may be sold without a prescription, and those requiring prescription. A prescription is a doctor's order that is necessary prior to dispensing a certain drug. In some states, controlled substances may require a specific type of prescription. Controlled substances are those drugs with a high potential to cause psychological and/or physical dependence and abuse. The Controlled Substances Act of 1970 designates certain drugs as controlled substances and defines five classifications, or schedules (Table 9-2).

Drugs are also classified according to chemical type (e.g., barbiturate), body system affected (e.g., neurologic agent), physiological action (e.g., central nervous system [CNS] depressant), or therapeutic action (e.g., anticonvulsant). As an example, the drug phenobarbital fits into each of these categories.

PHARMACOKINETICS

Pharmacokinetics is the term used to describe the entire process of the drug within the body. The process of

Table 9-2 Controlled Substances Act
Schedule or Class I: Includes substances for which there is a high abuse potential and no current approved medical use (e.g., heroin, marijuana, LSD, other hallucinogens, and certain opiates and opium derivatives).
Schedule or Class II: Includes drugs that have a high abuse potential and a high ability to produce physical and/or psychological dependence and for which there is a current approved or acceptable medical use.
Schedule or Class III: Includes drugs for which there is less potential for abuse than drugs in Schedule II and for which there is a current approved medical use. Certain drugs in this category are preparations containing limited quantities of codeine. In addition, anabolic steroids are classified in Schedule III.
Schedule or Class IV: Includes drugs for which there is a relatively low abuse potential and for which there is a current approved medical use.
Schedule or Class V: Drugs in this category consist mainly of preparations containing limited amounts of certain narcotic drugs for use as antitussives and antidiarrheals. Federal law provides that limited quantities of these drugs (e.g., codeine) may be bought without a prescription by an individual at least 18 years of age. The product must be purchased from a pharmacist, who must keep appropriate records. However, state laws vary, and in many states, such products require a prescription.

pharmacokinesis involves absorption, distribution, biotransformation, and excretion.

ABSORPTION

A drug must be absorbed to produce an effect. *Absorption* occurs at the site of administration; the substance is taken into the bloodstream by the capillaries. This process is referred to as passive transport. The drug substance is transferred from an area of higher concentration to an area of lower concentration until the concentration on both sides of the cell membrane is equal. Passive transport requires no energy. Most drugs are transported in this manner.

Active transport is required for a limited number of drugs, glucose, and amino acids. An energy source in the form of a cation, such as sodium, is required to carry the substance from an area of lower concentration to one of higher concentration.

The rate of absorption affects the final drug action, or pharmacodynamics, of the substance. Absorption is influenced by several factors that include the type of drug preparation, dosage, route of administration, and the patient's condition. For example, a liquid that has been injected will be absorbed more quickly than an ingested tablet that must undergo dissolution prior to absorption. Rapid absorption is not always desirable. A drug intended for local use must remain at the site of administration to be effective. A vasoconstrictor may be added to the drug preparation to slow absorption.

DISTRIBUTION

Distribution is the transport of the drug substance that occurs once it enters the circulatory system. The substance is distributed to the target cells for action or to the liver for biotransformation. Distribution of the drug is affected by the rate of absorption, systemic circulation (cardiovascular function), and regional blood flow to the target organ or tissue. The drug is carried to all parts of the body; effects other than those that are intended may be noted.

Distribution of the substance is also affected by plasma protein binding, tissue binding, and certain barriers established by the body (e.g., the placental barrier and blood–brain barrier).

BIOTRANSFORMATION

Biotransformation, or metabolism, of the drug most often occurs in the liver, but other tissues, including the intestinal mucosa, lungs, kidneys, and blood plasma, may be involved. A few drugs are converted to an active substance by the liver, but the main function of the liver in metabolism is to break down the drug molecules with enzymes for excretion. The breakdown products of metabolism are called metabolites that are smaller, less active or inactive substances. The hepatic first-pass effect must be considered when planning drug dosage and route of administration.

EXCRETION

A drug's effect continues until it is biotransformed and/or excreted. Drugs are physiologically removed from the target organ or tissue through the circulatory system in the intact or biotransformed (changed or inactivated) state. The kidneys, with subsequent elimination in the urine, are primarily responsible for excretion. Additionally, drug substances may be eliminated fecally, via sweat or saliva, or exhaled. Some medications are also eliminated in breast milk, which can pose danger to a breast-fed baby.

PHARMACODYNAMICS

Pharmacodynamics is the term describing the interaction of drug molecules with the target cells. The action of the drug substance causes an alteration in physiological activity but is incapable of initiating a new function. Types of drug actions include inhibition or destruction of foreign organisms or malignant cells, protection of cells from foreign agents, supplementation or replacement of specific hormones, vitamins, or enzymes, and increasing or decreasing the speed of a physiological function.

Drugs are administered to produce an expected or therapeutic effect. There are three time- and action-related aspects of pharmacodynamics:

- *Onset:* Time that it takes from administration of the drug for its action to become evident
- *Peak effect:* Period of time during which the drug is at its maximum effectiveness
- *Duration of action:* Time between the onset of action to the cessation of action (timing of future doses of the drug will depend on time of onset, peak effect, and duration of action)

Certain variables, such as the type of drug, dosage, route of administration, and patient condition, affect all three aspects of pharmacodynamics.

Drug action defines the effect of the substance at the target site. Three main theories have been developed to explain the ways that drugs produce their effects. The theory of drug-receptor interaction states that the active substance in the drug has an affinity for a specific chemical constituent of a cell. The interaction occurs on a molecular level with a specific receptor on the cell surface or within the cell to produce the pharmacological response. The theory of drug-enzyme interaction argues that a drug may combine with a specific enzyme to inhibit the action of the enzyme or alter the cellular response to the enzyme. A third type of interaction, nonspecific drug interaction, is related to drugs that do not act by either of the two previously described methods and are considered nonspecific in their interaction. These drugs accumulate on the cell membrane or penetrate the membrane and interfere physically or chemically with a cellular function or metabolic process.

Side effects are undesirable consequences along with the therapeutic responses to a drug. Side effects are expected, predictable, and unavoidable and are usually tolerable or treatable. Some common side effects are nausea, vomiting, abdominal distress (gas or cramping), diarrhea, constipation, dry mouth, dizziness, and drowsiness. Side effects may become evident shortly after administration of the drug or may have a delayed onset of action.

Adverse effects or reactions are also undesirable responses to drug therapy. Adverse reactions are unintended and for the most part are unpredictable and unavoidable. Some predictable adverse reactions can be avoided or altered by considering certain factors (age, weight, time of administration) when the drug is prescribed and administered. The most common unpredictable adverse or idiosyncratic response is hypersensitivity or allergic reaction, which can range from mild skin irritation to **anaphylaxis**.

An **iatrogenic** response is an unavoidable effect or disease induced by pharmacological therapy. There are five syndromes associated with iatrogenic responses: blood abnormalities, liver toxicity, kidney toxicity, teratogenic (producing a deformity in the developing embryo), and dermatologic effects.

Tolerance is a decreased therapeutic response to a drug following repeated administrations causing the dose to be increased to maintain the therapeutic effect.

Addiction refers to psychological or physiological dependence on a specific agent (drug or alcohol) with an increasing tendency to its use or abuse (Controlled Substances Act).

Drug interaction can occur when two substances are prescribed concurrently, causing a modification of action of one or both of the drugs. Drug interaction may be intentional (beneficial) or undesirable (detrimental). Drug interactions are categorized as **agonist** or **antagonist**. An agonist interaction occurs when a drug potentiates or enhances the effect of another substance. An antagonist interaction occurs when a drug blocks the action of another substance but produces no physiological effect of its own.

DRUG-HANDLING TECHNIQUES

Drug safety is of utmost concern to all involved. Medication errors can be minimized by following some basic safety guidelines:

- Know the pertinent state and federal laws.
- Know the policies of the health care facility.
- Follow the procedures set forth by the health care facility.

There are five basic "rights" for correct drug handling, which are absolute. They include:

1. The right patient
2. The right drug
3. The right dose
4. The right route of administration
5. The right time and frequency

These five items are all components of the physician's order. In the OR, the list of expected medications for a specific procedure is found on the surgeon's preference card. The final medication order is often finalized verbally. Everyone on the team is responsible for making certain that these five rights are ensured.

Safe handling and use of drugs requires knowledge of the drugs, the rules and procedures for safe handling, and the ability to recognize and use dosage-related information. This often requires converting from one system to another. The surgical team must be adept at making these conversions accurately. Basic conversion information for the metric system is included in Table 9-3.

MEDICATION IDENTIFICATION

Medications for use in the OR environment are available from the manufacturer in many types of packages. Common types of medication packaging that will be used in the OR are glass, plastic, and metal containers. Extra caution must be used when handling glass containers. Containers vary in type and require different techniques for access or use. Types of common containers are:

- *Ampule:* Glass container that requires the top to be broken off to access the contents—usually contains liquid
- *Vial:* Plastic or glass container that has a rubber stopper at the top that is held in place with a metal retaining ring—may contain liquid, powder, or compressed powder
- *Preloaded syringe:* usually contains liquid
- *Tube:* Metal or plastic—may contain cream, gel, or ointment

The surgical technologist must be able to correctly identify the necessary aspects of the drug intended for use to ensure that the five rights are protected. No matter which type of packaging is used, all drugs must be labeled by the manufacturer and the label must contain the following information (Figure 9-1):

- Drug name (trade and generic)
- Manufacturer
- Strength
- Amount
- Expiration date
- Route of administration
- Lot number
- Handling/storage precautions and warnings

Table 9-3 Metric Conversion Charts

UNIT	ABBREVIATION	METRIC EQUIVALENT	U.S. EQUIVALENT
Note: 1 milliliter (mL) = 1 cubic centimeter (cc).			
Length			
Kilometer	km	1000 m	0.62 miles; 1.6 km/mile
Meter	m	100 cm; 1000 mm	39.4 in.; 1.1 yd.
Centimeter	cm	1/100 m; 0.01 m	0.39 in.; 2.5 cm/in.
Millimeter	mm	1/1000 m; 0.001 m	0.039 in.; 25 mm/in.
Micrometer	μm	1/1000 mm; 0.001 mm	
Weight			
Kilogram	kg	1000 g	2.2 lb.
Gram	g	1000 mg	0.035 oz.; 28.5 g/oz.
Milligram	mg	1/1000 g; 0.001 g	
Microgram	μg	1/1000 mg; 0.001 mg	
Volume			
Liter	L	1000 mL or 1000 cc	1.06 qt.
Deciliter	dL	1/10 L; 0.1 L	
Milliliter	mL	1/1000 L; 0.001 L	0.034 oz.; 29.4 mL/oz.
Microliter	μL	1/1000 mL; 0.001 mL	

TEMPERATURE

Celsius (°C), Fahrenheit (°F)

Freezing point: 0°C, 32°F

Boiling point: 100°C, 212°F

To convert Fahrenheit to Celsius use the formula: °C = 5/9 (°F − 32)

To convert Celsius to Fahrenheit use the formula: °F = 9/5°C + 32

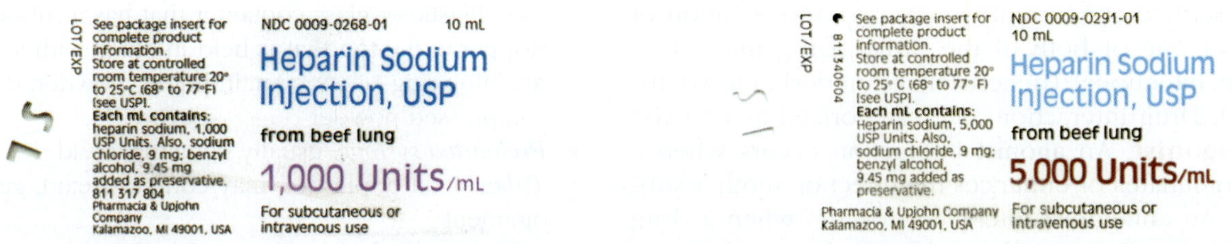

Figure 9-1 Medication label ***(Courtesy of the Upjohn Company)***

- Controlled substances classification (if applicable)

The medication name, strength, amount, and expiration date should be identified/verified a minimum of three times prior to administration:

- First identification/verification occurs when the drug listed on the preference card is obtained from the storage area or removed from the case cart for the procedure.
- Second identification/verification is done prior to preparation for use or placement on the sterile field.
- Third identification/verification is done once the medication is prepared for use or placed on the sterile field.

IDENTIFICATION OF MEDICATIONS ON THE STERILE FIELD

Immediately following transfer of a medication to the sterile field, it must be labeled. Each health care facility will have specific policies and procedures that must

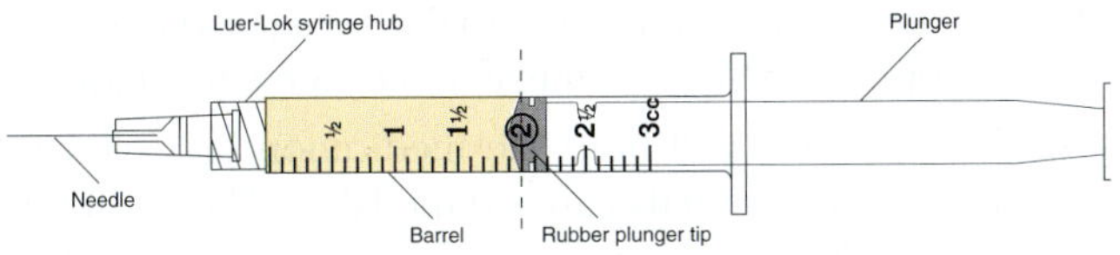

Figure 9-2 Syringe

be followed when handling medications on the sterile field. Many methods of identification are available to the STSR. Suggested methods are as follows:

- Sterile preprinted drug labels (paper stickers) are available at some facilities.
- Sterile preprinted reusable drug labels (plastic markers) are available at some facilities.
- The STSR may create a label using a sterile marking pen and a blank sterile label.
- *Note:* If blank labels are not available, a sterile skin closure tape (Steri-strip) is a possible alternative.

It may be necessary to have a medication in two locations on the sterile field. For example, the main supply of a medication may be in a medicine cup on the back table and the remainder drawn up in a syringe, ready for use on the Mayo stand. Both containers must be labeled. Be sure when labeling a syringe that the increments for measurement are not covered with the label.

It may also be necessary for more than one medication to be on the sterile field. It is imperative that all team members are quickly and accurately able to identify all medications (including irrigation solutions). If any confusion exists about the identity or strength of a medication, it **MUST** be discarded immediately (and replaced, if necessary).

SUPPLIES FOR MEDICATION HANDLING

A variety of supplies are necessary for the reconstitution, transfer, and administration of different types of medications. Medications may be placed into a medicine cup or a small basin during transfer to the sterile field or for storage on the sterile field. Most often, a syringe (Figure 9-2) and needle (Figure 9-3) are used in the OR, although a graduated pitcher and a bulb syringe may be used for irrigation fluids. Occasionally, a medication is applied from a dropper or a tube.

TRANSFER OF A MEDICATION TO THE STERILE FIELD

The method of transfer of the necessary medication to the sterile field will be situational, according to the type of medication ordered and the specified route of administration. Controlled substances may require a different type of handling, according to facility policy. Sterile technique must be employed for the transfer of medications to the sterile field and administration of the medication from the

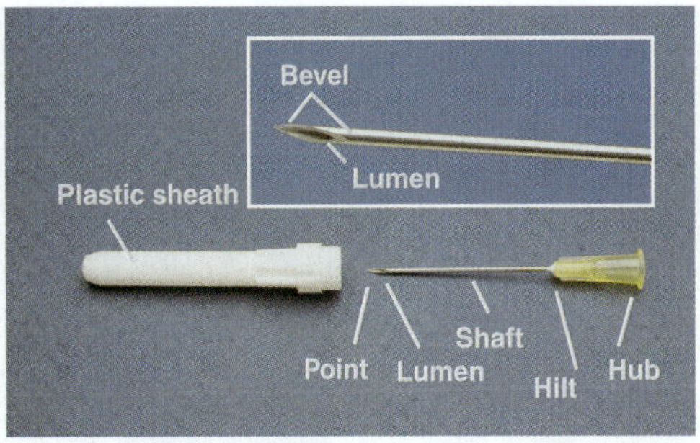

Figure 9-3 Needle

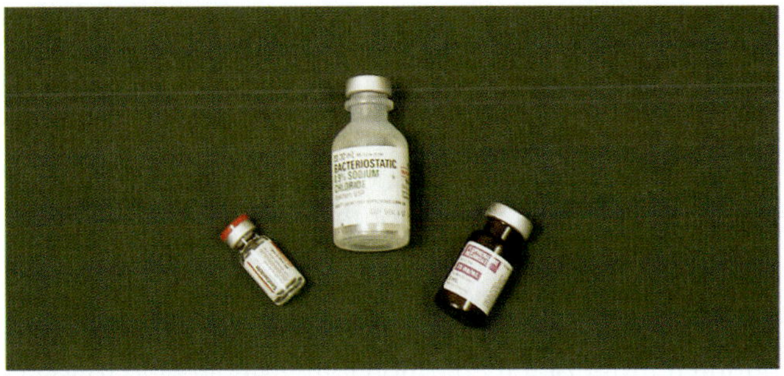

Figure 9-4 Vials

sterile field. A team effort involving the circulator, STSR, and the surgeon is required.

Medications requiring reconstitution are often mixed by the circulator, then transferred to the sterile field for use. Additional liquid may be added to the medication once it is on the sterile field to achieve the proper dilution. Medications from a vial (Figure 9-4) may be transferred to the sterile field by one of three methods:

- The circulator will remove the top of the vial and dispense the substance into the proper receptacle on the field using sterile technique.
- The circulator will clean the stopper in the top of the vial if necessary, draw the substance into a syringe with the use of a needle, and eject the medication into the proper receptacle on the field using sterile technique.
- The circulator will clean the stopper in the top of the vial if necessary and hold the vial upside down while the STSR withdraws the substance into a syringe with the use of a needle using sterile technique.

Medications from an ampule (Figure 9-5) may be transferred to the sterile field by one of two methods:

- The circulator will remove the top of the ampule, draw the substance into a syringe with the use of a needle, and eject the medication into the proper receptacle on the field using sterile technique.
- The circulator will remove the top of the ampule and hold the ampule while the STSR withdraws the substance into a syringe with the use of a needle using sterile technique.

Medications from a tube are squeezed onto the sterile field by the circulator using sterile technique.

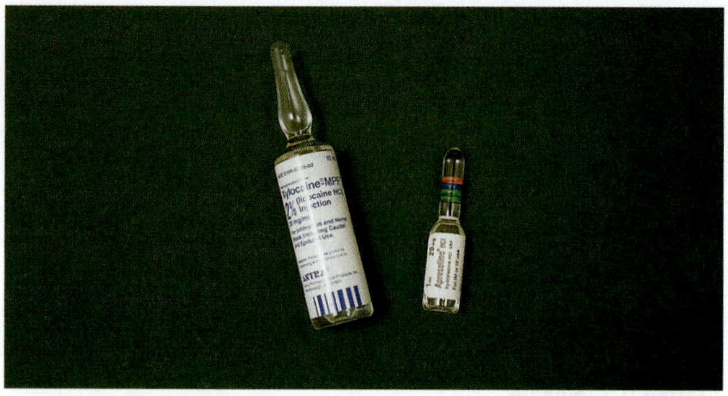

Figure 9-5 Ampules

Many medications in all of the above types of packages may be available in a form that will allow the vial, ampule, or tube to be placed directly on the sterile field. No matter what type, all medication containers, once used, are to remain visible for the duration of the procedure for reverification, if necessary.

A typical example of the steps taken and the interaction that occurs between the circulator and the STSR during transfer of a medication to the sterile field follows:

1. Both the circulator and STSR are familiar with the surgeon's preference card request and have checked all medications and supplies prior to the start of the case (first identification/verification).
2. The STSR or circulator may initiate the request to transfer a medication to the sterile field. Ideally, the transfer is made at a mutually convenient time.
3. The circulator approaches the sterile field with the medication.
4. The circulator will hold the medication container so that both individuals can see the label. The circulator will read out loud the pertinent label information, stating the name of the drug, the strength of the drug, and the expiration date (second identification/verification).
5. The substance is transferred to the sterile field using the appropriate method of transfer and sterile technique.
6. The circulator will hold the medication container so that both individuals can see the label. The STSR will read out loud the pertinent label information, stating the name of the drug, the strength of the drug, and the expiration date (third identification/verification).
7. The drug is immediately labeled on the sterile field.
8. *Every time* the STSR passes a medication to the surgeon for use, it is verbally identified. The name of the drug, strength, and amount are stated. All team members should be aware that a medication is being administered; it may be particularly important for the anesthesia provider to be informed that a particular drug (e.g., epinephrine) is in use.

Finally, before administration of any medication, *verify that the patient is not allergic to the medication.* It is important to note not only the patient's allergy status to medications, but to foods and other substances as well (e.g., a shellfish allergy could be indicative of an iodine allergy or an allergy to beets could indicate an allergy to dextrose that may be manufactured with beet sugar).

MEDICATIONS COMMONLY USED IN THE OPERATING ROOM

Table 9-4 identifies some of the commonly used drug classifications and gives selected examples for each. Remember, some drug classifications overlap and some drugs have more than one action. Drugs that fit more than one category will be repeated in this table. Drugs used to produce anesthesia will be listed in the table and discussed in detail in the following section.

(*Text continues on page 229*)

Table 9-4 Medication List

DRUG CLASSIFICATION	DESCRIPTION	EXAMPLES*
*Only generic names are given. Italics signifies emergency drugs.		
Adrenergic	Increase blood pressure Dilate bronchioles	*Epinephrine* Phenylephrine hydrochloride
Analgesic (narcotic)	Minimize perception of pain Potentiate anesthesia	Codeine Fentanyl citrate Meperidine hydrochloride Morphine sulfate
Antianxiety	Reduce anxiety May have antiemetic properties Potentiate anesthesia	Diazepam Hydroxyzine hydrochloride Promethazine hydrochloride

Table 9-4 ***(continued)***

DRUG CLASSIFICATION	DESCRIPTION	EXAMPLES*
Antiarrhythmic	Correct cardiac dysrhythmia	*Lidocaine* Procainamide hydrochloride
Antibiotic	Antibacterial	Bacitracin Cefazolin Gentamicin Kanamycin Neomycin Polymyxin B sulfate Quinupristin and dalfopristin Vancomycin
Anticoagulant	Interfere with blood-clotting mechanism	Heparin Warfarin
Antiemetic	Reduce nausea Prevent vomiting	Droperidol Metoclopramide
Antihistamine	Counteract allergic reaction	Diphenhydramine
Antihypertensive	Reduce blood pressure	Nitroprusside sodium
Antimuscarinic (anticholinergic)	Block secretions Prevent laryngospasm Prevent reflex bradycardia Increase heart rate Increase respiratory rate	*Atropine sulfate* Glycopyrrolate Scopolamine
Bronchodilator	Expand lumens of upper respiratory passages	*Aminophylline* *Ephedrine sulfate*
Cardiac glycoside	Increase cardiac output	*Digitoxin*
Cholinergic	Increase smooth muscle activity Antagonize nondepolarizing neuromuscular blocking agents	Prostigmine
Contrast media	Enhance X-rays	Diatrizoate meglumine Diatrizoate sodium Iodipamide Lothalamate meglumine Meglumine diatrizoate
Coronary artery dilator	Increase blood flow to the heart	Nitroglycerine
Cycloplegic	Paralyze ciliary muscle Usually accompanied by a mydriatic	Tropicamide (cycloplegic/mydriatic)
Diuretic	Increase urinary output Reduce edema	Furosemide Mannitol
Dye	Enhance visualization Mark intended incision lines	Brilliant green Gentian violet Indigo carmine Methylene blue
Hemostatic agents	Control intraoperative bleeding	Absorbable gelatin sponge Microfibrillar collagen Oxidized cellulose Protamine sulfate Thrombin

(continues)

Table 9-4 *(continued)*

DRUG CLASSIFICATION	DESCRIPTION	EXAMPLES*
Histamine 2 (H_2)	Decrease gastric acidity and volume	Cimetidine Ranitidine
Hormone	Supplement or replacement	Glucagon Insulin
Immunosuppressant	Reduce the body's natural immunity	Cyclosporine
Inhalation anesthetic agents	Produce systemic anesthesia Maintain systemic anesthesia	Enflurane Halothane Isoflurane Nitrous oxide
Intravenous anesthetic agents	Produce systemic anesthesia Maintain systemic anesthesia	Diazepam Droperidol Fentanyl citrate Innovar (combination of droperidol and fentanyl) Ketamine hydrochloride Propofol Thiopental sodium
Miotic	Constrict pupil	Acetylcholine chloride
Mydriatic	Dilate pupil	Atropine Cyclogyl Epinephrine Phenylephrine hydrochloride
Narcotic antagonist	Reverse narcotic effects	Naloxone
Nerve conduction blocking agents	Produce local or regional anesthesia	Bupivacaine hydrochloride Cocaine hydrochloride Lidocaine hydrochloride Procaine hydrochloride Tetracaine hydrochloride
Nerve conduction blocking agent agonist	Enhance effect of local or regional anesthesia	Epinephrine Hyaluronidase
Neuromuscular blocking agents	Produce total skeletal muscle relaxation (paralyzation)	Depolarizing Succinylcholine hydrochloride Nondepolarizing Atracurium besylate Pancuronium bromide Prostigmine Tubocurarine chloride Vecuronium bromide
Nonsteroidal anti-inflammatory drug (NSAID)	Reduce inflammation	Ketorolac tromethamine
Oxytocic	Contract uterus	Methylergonovine Oxytocin
Sedative/hypnotic	Promote sleep Reduce anxiety	Phenobarbital sodium

Table 9-4 *(continued)*

DRUG CLASSIFICATION	DESCRIPTION	EXAMPLES*
Stains	Identify abnormal tissue Usually iodine based	Lugol's solution Schiller's solution
Steroidal anti-inflammatory agents	Reduce edema Prevent swelling Treat shock	Dexamethasone Hydrocortisone Methylprednisolone
Vasodilator	Dilate peripheral blood vessels	Papaverine
Vasopressor	Vasoconstrictors Raise blood pressure	Vasopressin *Metaraminol* *Norepinephrine*
Miscellaneous drugs	Enzyme to dissolve zonules that hold ocular lens in place Skeletal muscle relaxant used to treat malignant hyperthermia	Alpha-chymotrypsin Dantrolene sodium
Electrolyte replacement	Myocardial stimulant Enhance blood clotting Prevent seizures in eclamptic patients Correct cardiac dysrhythmia Combat metabolic acidosis	Calcium chloride Calcium gluconate Magnesium sulfate Potassium chloride *Sodium bicarbonate*
Intravenous solutions	Provide hydration Enhance renal function Medications may be added Dextrose (sugar) solutions provide calories Balanced solutions similar to plasma Provide nutrition Replace blood loss Treat red blood cell deficiency Replace plasma Used when plasma not available Plasma expander for patients in shock	Dextrose 5% in water Dextrose in normal saline (NS) 0.9% NaCl 0.45 NS Lactated Ringer's solution Ringer's solution Hyperalimentation solutions that include amino acids, glucose, and water Whole blood Packed red blood cells Plasma Dextran—artificial plasma Albumin
Irrigation solutions	Surgical wound irrigation Medications may be added Corneal irrigation Intraocular irrigation	Normal saline (most common) Lactated Ringer's solution Sterile distilled water (occasionally) Balanced salt solution (BSS)

HISTORY OF MODERN ANESTHESIA

The term **anesthesia** is derived from the Greek word *anaisthesis,* meaning "lack of sensation." When the potential value of ether was recognized, Oliver Wendell Holmes suggested that the word "anesthesia" be used to describe the phenomenon. The term is now used to characterize the process used to relieve the pain and suffering encountered during and related to surgical intervention. General anesthesia was one of the three significant surgical concepts introduced in the 19th century, along with aseptic principles to combat infection and the discovery of hemostatic controls such as ligatures and electrocautery. Since its introduction in 1846, general anesthesia and its adjuncts have developed into the art and science that is the supporting cornerstone of today's surgical practice.

In the 16th century, coca leaves used for their anesthetic properties during trephination of the skull for the release of "evil humors" provided evidence of local anesthesia to relieve surgically induced pain. While crude and unrefined, medical practitioners recognized the need to address the pain management needs of the surgical patient.

In 1656, Percival Christopher Wren and Daniel Johann Major, two English physicians, demonstrated that an IV injection of opium would render an animal "stupefied." They developed the first method of medication injection, accomplished by attaching a "bladder of medication" to a quill inserted into the vein.

It was the introduction of inhalation anesthesia that brought the practice of intraoperative pain relief formally into the OR. The origins of inhalation anesthesia are fraught with controversy.

Ether was first discovered in 1275 by the Spanish chemist Raymundus Lullius. It was given the name "sweet vitriol" until 1730, when its name was changed to "ether." The first widespread use of ether was not medicinal but was instead social. In the 1800s, "ether frolics" were a source of entertainment for partygoers. In March 1842, Crawford W. Long, a dentist in practice in Jefferson, Georgia, persuaded a young man, James M. Venable, to inhale ether while undergoing excision of a neck growth. Long, unfortunately, did not publish his findings until 1848, leaving the major credit for the introduction of general anesthesia into medical practice to others. In January 1842, William Clark of Rochester, New York, first administered ether as a dental anesthetic during a tooth extraction performed by Elijah Pope on a Miss Hobbie. In nearby Connecticut, Horace Wells was promoting the use of nitrous oxide anesthesia for dental extractions. Wells and chemist Charles T. Jackson collaborated on the uses of nitrous oxide and ether. It was through this collaboration that Jackson's associate, William Thomas Green Morton, began experimentation with ether anesthesia. Morton's first administration of an inhalation anesthetic occurred on September 30, 1846, when he painlessly removed a tooth from Eben H. Frost, a city merchant. When news of the event found its way into the newspaper the next day, a surgeon at Massachusetts General Hospital arranged for the first public demonstration of this new practice. On October 16, 1846, Morton anesthetized Guilbert Abbott, a printer, while John Collins Warren, a prominent Boston surgeon, ligated a congenital venous malformation on the patient's neck. The successful event culminated in Warrens's pronouncement, "Gentlemen, this is no humbug!" The Ether Dome, preserved to this day within Massachusetts General Hospital, stands as a memorial to that fateful day that forever changed the practice of surgery as no other event has. News of the event was published in the *Boston Medical and Surgical Journal,* now the *New England Journal of Medicine,* on November 18, 1846.

Years of controversy followed, as Long, Wells, Jackson, and Morton fought over the recognition and title of "founder," an issue that carried on until their deaths. In 1905, a group of physicians formed the Long Island Society of Anesthetists to promote the art and science of anesthesia. In 1936, the name was eventually changed to the American Society of Anesthesiologists (ASA). The term *anesthesiologist* was used to designate physicians who have received formal training in the area of anesthesia administration and was accepted by the American Medical Association in 1940. The introduction of antibiotics in the 1940s and of curare as a muscle paralyzer in 1942 began the revolutionary practice changes leading to today's challenging and demanding, fast-paced, complex practice of anesthesia delivery and patient monitoring.

Anesthetic agents have developed significantly from the days of "opium and alcohol." Newer, safer, and better agents today are constantly replacing the myriad of anesthetic agents in use in an attempt to find the "ideal" anesthetic. Optimal balanced anesthesia is achieved when all of the following components are addressed:

- ***Hypnosis***: Hypnosis results from an altered state of consciousness related to the patient's perception of the surgical environment and the surgical procedure. Hypnotic drugs are classified as those that induce sleep. Many patients fear "being awake" during surgical intervention. Today's pharmaceutical agents permit varying levels of hypnosis to be achieved, from the light, more natural sleep of sedation to the full unconsciousness of general anesthesia.
- *Anesthesia:* Freedom from pain is the major focus of anesthesia practice. A patient's concern for proper and consistent pain management lies second only to the fear of anesthesia-related death. Today's OR practices deliver pain-free surgery in a variety of ways, using topical, local, regional, and general (systemic) agents.
- ***Amnesia***: Amnestic agents provide a lack of recall (amnesia) of perioperative events for the surgical patient and permit the use of safer, less toxic anesthetic agents and techniques while providing a calm and cooperative surgical patient.
- *Muscle relaxation:* Neuromuscular blocking agents in combination with inhalation agents are capable of producing profound muscle relaxation (to the point of paralysis), permitting tracheal intubation and the development of surgical interventions previously unable to be performed. Since a muscle layer overlies most surgical areas, a means of relaxing these muscles facilitates retraction and exposure of underlying organs and tissues.
- *Optimal patient positioning:* Advances in surgical procedures demand advantageous access to the surgical site. General anesthesia, patient physiological monitoring, and control of essential life processes must function in harmony to provide for an optimal patient outcome. Patient positioning must allow for surgical site access while maintaining physiological **homeostasis**.

- *Continued homeostasis of vital functions:* It is said that general anesthesia is intentionally capable of inducing a state close to death and requires maintenance of the patient at this level for the duration of the surgical procedure. This makes anesthesia administration the most dangerous component of any surgical intervention. Today's use of invasive and noninvasive monitoring devices, as well as the use of safer anesthetic agents, assists the anesthesia provider in maintaining the patient in a state of optimal homeostasis during the entire surgical experience.

METHODS AND TECHNIQUES OF ANESTHETIC ADMINISTRATION

Anesthetic agents can be administered primarily in two ways: general anesthesia and nerve conduction blockade anesthesia. *General anesthesia* focuses on altering the patient's level of consciousness, minimizing pain and awareness of the surgical environment. *Nerve conduction blockade* anesthesia involves the prevention of sensory nerve impulse transmission. Many of today's anesthetic administrations involve components of both methods.

Anesthetic choices are made on a case-by-case basis to meet the goals of maximum patient safety and optimal results while considering the following criteria:

- Anticipated procedure and estimated duration
- Patient positioning
- Age, size, and weight of the patient
- Patient status
- Emotional
- Mental
- Physical
- General health
- Current medications
- Allergies
- History of substance abuse
- Emergency conditions
- Surgeon, anesthesia provider, and patient preference

The ASA has set forth a classification system for assessing patient risk. The classes are as follows:

- *Class 1:* No organic, physiological, biochemical, or psychiatric disturbance
- *Class 2:* Mild to moderate systemic disease disturbance: controlled hypertension, history of asthma, anemia, smoker, controlled diabetes, mild obesity, age less than 1 or greater than 70
- *Class 3:* Severe systemic disturbance or disease: Angina, post-myocardial infarction (MI), poorly controlled hypertension, symptomatic respiratory disease, massive obesity
- *Class 4:* Patient with severe systemic disease, disorders that are life threatening: unstable angina, congestive heart failure, debilitating respiratory disease, hepatorenal failure
- *Class 5:* Moribund patient with little chance of survival who is operated on in desperation
- *Class 6:* Brain dead, life support provided, organ procurement intended
- *Emergency modifier (E):* Applied when doing emergency surgery

GENERAL ANESTHESIA

General anesthesia involves an alteration in the patient's perception of his environment by alterations in the level of consciousness. This is accomplished by three techniques: agent inhalation, agent injection, and less commonly agent instillation. When several methods for general anesthesia are used in combination, the technique is referred to as *balanced anesthesia.*

Agent inhalation involves the delivery of gases across the alveolar membrane to the vascular system, where the agent is able to cross the blood–brain barrier, affecting CNS function. Medication delivery relies on an adequately functioning respiratory and circulatory system. These agents are delivered via a closed anesthesia circuit connected to a vaporizer.

Agent injection involves the administration of medications directly into the bloodstream intravenously. This is accomplished by use of a venous access device, usually a peripheral intravenous catheter, or a central venous delivery system. Medication effect does not rely on adequate respiratory function, only on circulatory function. Occasionally, a medication is injected intramuscularly (e.g., Ketamine).

Agent instillation involves the administration of medication into an area such as the rectum, where the agent is absorbed via the mucous membranes and transported to the CNS by the circulatory system. This method can be used in selected cases where patient cooperation is less than optimal.

DEPTH OF GENERAL ANESTHESIA

There are four stages to describe the depth of general anesthesia:

- Stage I is referred to as the amnesia stage and begins with the initial administration of an anesthetic agent to loss of consciousness.
- Stage II consists of the period from the loss of consciousness to the return of regular breathing and loss of the eyelid reflex. This stage is often referred to as the *excitement* or *delirium stage,* due to the uninhibited movement of the patient demonstrated during this period. Vomiting, **laryngospasm**, hypertension, and tachycardia may all be seen in this stage. The activities of this stage may be reduced or

passed through rapidly by the administration of an IV **induction** agent, which carries the patient rapidly from Stage I to Stage III.

- Stage III consists of the period between the onset of regular breathing and loss of eyelid reflex to the cessation of breathing. This is known as the *surgical anesthesia stage.* The patient is unresponsive to painful stimuli and sensation, with the sense of hearing being the last sense to be obtunded. This stage is often divided into four planes, with planes 2–3 considered to be the optimum level of anesthesia for surgical intervention.
- Stage IV is referred to as the *overdosage stage.* Dilated and nonreactive pupils mark this stage, as do the cessation of respiration and marked hypotension leading to circulatory failure. If uncorrected, this stage leads to patient death.

PHASES OF GENERAL ANESTHESIA

The period prior to the induction of general anesthesia is sometimes referred to as the *preinduction period.* It is considered to begin at the time the premedication is administered and to end when the induction of anesthesia is begun. The patient may be preoxygenated during this period.

There are four phases of general anesthesia: induction, maintenance, emergence, and recovery:

Induction phase: Induction involves altering the patient's level of consciousness, from the conscious (alert) state to the unconscious ("asleep") state with depressed reflexes. During induction, loss of consciousness occurs and may be associated with respiratory depression and an inadequate airway. Induction may be carried out in two ways: the use of an IV induction agent or the inhalation of gaseous vapors. Management and maintenance of the patient's airway is critical and may involve the use of oral or nasal airways, a face mask, laryngeal mask airway (LMA), or endotracheal intubation. The patient's hearing is the last sense to be obtunded and may even be more acute during this phase of anesthesia; therefore, noise should be kept to an absolute minimum.

Maintenance phase: Surgical intervention takes place during the maintenance phase of anesthesia. Maintenance of homeostatic function of all vital organs with the provision of appropriate operating conditions is critical to a successful anesthetic and good surgical outcome. Anesthesia administration is most dynamic during this period, as the anesthesia personnel monitor the patient closely for changes in oxygen saturation, blood loss, muscle relaxant state, and cardiac status. Surgical manipulation may change any of these parameters, and it is the function of the anesthesia provider to adjust anesthetic levels accordingly.

Emergence phase: Emergence occurs as the surgical intervention is being completed. The goal of emergence is to have the patient as awake as possible at the end of the surgical intervention. The primary focus of activities during this period is the monitoring of adequate independent respiratory rate and function, with a restoration of the "gag" reflex. Extubation, if necessary, will be accomplished during this phase. Residual undesired neuromuscular blockade might require the administration of a reversal agent. As the state of consciousness increases, the patient is at risk for laryngospasm. Patients may also experience thermoregulatory changes due to the effects of the anesthetic agents and exposure of the viscera. It is common to see patient rigidity and/or tremors late in this period.

Recovery phase: Recovery is that period of time during which the patient returns to the optimum level of consciousness and well-being. It usually begins in the OR suite, carries through the patient's stay in the postanesthesia care unit (**PACU**) and may continue through the patient's discharge and initial healing stages.

ADVANTAGES OF GENERAL ANESTHESIA

The use of general anesthesia has several advantages:

- The patient is usually unaware of the activities and noises associated with the operative intervention.
- Once an adequate airway has been secured, the depth and rate of respiration can be controlled and attempts are made to protect the pulmonary tree from **aspiration** (inhalation of foreign material such as saliva or gastric contents).
- Medication dosages can be easily titrated.
- Muscle relaxation for intubation and retraction at the surgical site is easily achieved.

RISKS AND COMPLICATIONS ASSOCIATED WITH GENERAL ANESTHESIA

The risks and complications associated with general anesthesia administration are many. Fortunately, current monitoring techniques and improved pharmacological agents have lowered the morbidity associated with anesthesia administration and reduced the risk of mortality to less than one death per 200,000 anesthetics administered. The preoperative condition of the patient is a major factor when calculating anesthetic risk. Complications of anesthetic administration may occur even during "routine" surgery and must always be anticipated. Aspiration of secretions or gastric contents may occur in patients where inadequate time for gastric emptying has elapsed, in trauma patients with a full stomach, or in patients with gastric secretions present related to meal anticipation. Induction agents and neuromuscular blockade both permit relaxation of the cardioesophageal sphincter, causing the patient to vomit, permitting gastric contents to enter the esophagus. Without adequate protection of the trachea by a functioning epiglottis "gag reflex," application of cricoid pressure, use of an LMA, or use of a cuffed endotracheal tube, the gastric contents or secretions may be aspirated into the airway, resulting in a chemical pneumonitis that could become bacterial. This is referred to as *aspiration pneumonia*.

Note: The risk of aspiration is greatest during the induction and emergence phases of general anesthesia. The patient should be fasting or **NPO** (Table 9-5). The term *NPO* is from the Latin *non per os* or *nil per os,* meaning "nothing by mouth." If this is not possible, the application of cricoid pressure can reduce the risk of aspiration. Suction apparatus should be available at all times.

CRICOID PRESSURE

Sellick's maneuver, or the application of cricoid pressure, is performed to reduce the risk of aspiration (Figure 9-6). External pressure is applied to the cricoid cartilage, causing occlusion of the esophagus between the cricoid ring and the body of the sixth cervical vertebrae. This maneuver is designed to prevent the stomach contents from ejection during vomiting, thereby reducing the risk of aspiration into the respiratory tract.

Firm pressure is applied with the thumb and index finger forming a V to the cricoid cartilage, located inferior to the prominence of the thyroid cartilage. Cricoid pressure must be applied prior to the induction of anesthesia and continue until the endotracheal tube is placed, the correct position of the tube verified, and the cuff of the endotracheal tube inflated. It is generally accepted that the individual applying cricoid pressure does not release the compression without the permission of the individual controlling the airway.

Cricoid pressure is employed in the OR in situations where the patient requires emergency surgery shortly after eating, the NPO status of the patient cannot be verified, or the patient is experiencing gastrointestinal (GI) bleeding. Cricoid pressure may also be applied during basic life support (CPR) settings as needed.

LARYNGOSPASM AND BRONCHOSPASM

Laryngospasm and *bronchospasm* are reactions demonstrated by the lightly anesthetized patient. A slight trigger of the "gag" reflex results in a spasm or rigidity of the upper respiratory tract, resulting in an inability of the patient

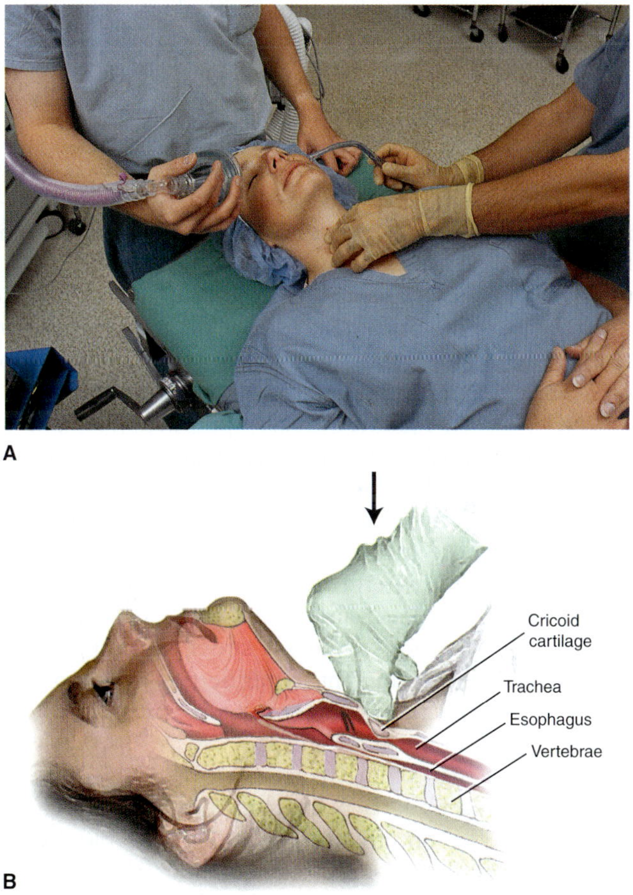

Figure 9-6 Cricoid pressure: (A) Application technique, (B) compression mechanism

Table 9-5 ASA Fasting Recommendations to Reduce the Risk of Pulmonary Aspiration (Healthy Patients, Elective Procedures)

FASTING PERIOD (MINIMUM)	INGESTED ITEM
2 hours	Clear liquids
4 hours	Breast milk
6 hours	Infant formula/nonhuman milk/light meal
8 hours or longer	Solids (meat, fried or fatty foods)

Note: The standard "rule" is NPO after midnight. Guidelines that are more liberal may be used according to the situation.

and/or anesthesia provider to move air and waste gases in and out of the lungs.

Laryngospasm and bronchospasm may be triggered by saliva in the back of the throat, stimulation of the lightly anesthetized surgical patient, or inflammation due to endotracheal tube placement. Laryngospasm and bronchospasm may occur during induction of or emergence from anesthesia and can lead to total airway obstruction, which is treated with positive-pressure breathing. If this does not provide relief, the patient will be given an ultra-rapid acting neuromuscular blocker, preferably succinylcholine, to relax the spasm. The patient will need artificial respiratory support and monitoring until independent respiratory ability returns. Supplies for dealing with a difficult airway should be readily available.

MALIGNANT HYPERTHERMIA

Malignant hyperthermia or malignant hyperpyrexia (MH) is a potentially fatal hypermetabolic state of muscle activity resulting from a defect in calcium transportation within the muscle fibers of skeletal muscles. During MH crisis, the skeletal muscles are stimulated to contract, but due to the inability of the calcium to release, the muscles cannot relax, resulting in rigidity, heat generation, and a buildup of lactic acid and carbon dioxide. An MH crisis is characterized by muscle rigidity, increased production of carbon dioxide, tachycardia, and finally, a significant, rapid increase in core body temperature.

Malignant hyperthermia is a genetically transmitted disease, more commonly seen in males than in females. Malignant hyperthermia can be triggered by the use of succinylcholine, curare, and halogenated inhalation agents. Strenuous exercise, stress, or trauma may also trigger MH. Malignant hyperthermia is diagnosed either by acute crisis symptoms or by muscle biopsy performed under local anesthesia.

The first sign of an MH crisis is unexplained tachycardia followed by tachypnea and an increased level of carbon dioxide. Shortly thereafter, an unstable blood pressure, perspiration, muscle contraction, and cyanotic, mottled skin are demonstrated. A late sign of MH crisis is a rise in temperature, sometimes as high as 107°F.

Supplies for the treatment of MH crisis should be readily available, and all staff should be familiar with the location of the supplies and the treatment protocol. The treatment interventions for a patient in MH crisis include the discontinuation of anesthesia administration and the oxygenation of the patient with 100% oxygen. A nontriggering anesthetic agent may be given. Dantrolene is the only pharmacological agent for the treatment of MH crisis. It is mixed with sterile injectable water and is given IV. A loading dose of 2.5 mg/kg is given, followed by a dose of 1 mg/kg every 5 minutes until a maximum dose of 10 mg/kg is reached. Additional interventions include the administration of chilled IV fluids of normal saline or dextrose in water.

Chilled saline lavage of body cavities is also performed, including the bladder, rectum, stomach, and peritoneum, if exposed. The patient is also packed with ice along heat transfer points, including the axilla, base of skull, and groin area. Care needs to be taken that, as the crisis diminishes, the patient does not become hypothermic.

Other treatment interventions during MH crisis include the administration of sodium bicarbonate to assist in metabolic and respiratory acidosis regulation, dextrose and insulin to provide available glucose to the cells to maintain cellular metabolism, furosemide or mannitol to promote renal clearance of waste products, and heparin to prevent intravascular clot formation.

PSEUDOCHOLINESTERASE DEFICIENCY SYNDROME

Pseudocholinesterase deficiency syndrome is a genetically transmitted trait that decreases the amount of acetylcholinesterase available in the neuromuscular junction to break down acetylcholine during muscle stimulation. Acetylcholine remains effective in the neuromuscular junction, permitting prolonged effect of depolarizing neuromuscular blockade agents. This prolonged effect can last for several hours after agent administration. There is no direct treatment for pseudocholinesterase deficiency outside of respiratory support of the patient until the body eliminates the neuromuscular blockade. Prophylactic treatment includes the avoidance of the administration of depolarizing neuromuscular blocking agents and the notification of anesthesia care providers of the deficiency prior to future anesthesia administration.

ALLERGIC REACTION

An allergic reaction may be mild (such as skin irritation) or life threatening (anaphylaxis). Anaphylaxis is an immediate hypersensitive reaction, the most severe form of allergy, resulting in life-threatening respiratory distress that leads to vascular collapse and shock. The patient's history should include any prior allergic reactions, and those substances should be avoided if possible. Treatment of the allergy will vary according to the severity of the reaction.

SHOCK

Shock is an abnormal physiological state indicated by the presence of reduced cardiac output, tachycardia, hypotension, and diminished urinary output. This state may be induced secondary to severe tissue damage, significant blood loss, or infection.

The goal in shock treatment is to promote optimal circulatory load and function. This may be accomplished by pharmacological treatment to treat toxic shock (antibiotics) or increase cardiac output, blood and crystalloid administration, and surgical intervention to limit blood loss or treat infection.

CARDIAC DYSRHYTHMIAS

Cardiac dysrhythmias involve abnormal heart rate or rhythm, evidenced by electrocardiogram monitoring. The dysrhythmias may be atrial or ventricular in origin and deadly if untreated.

Life-threatening dysrhythmias include ventricular tachycardia and ventricular fibrillation. The treatment for cardiac dysrhythmia includes the IV administration of lidocaine hydrochloride. Additionally, defibrillation and pacemaker insertion may be necessary.

CARDIAC ARREST

Cardiac arrest involves the cessation of heart pumping action and blood circulation. This, in turn, prevents the delivery of oxygen and glucose to cells for metabolism and the removal of wastes. This results in metabolic and respiratory acidosis. The initial treatment for cardiac arrest is CPR, followed up with advanced cardiac life support (ACLS).

ANESTHETIC AGENTS

Anesthetic agents are divided into three categories: inhalation agents, IV agents, and local/regional agents. The patient is provided supportive oxygen therapy with almost every anesthetic.

INHALATION AGENTS

Anesthetic agents that are inhaled and pass to the bloodstream via pulmonary function are called *inhalation agents*.

Oxygen

Although oxygen is not classified as an anesthetic agent, it is a component of most anesthetic administrations. In its pure form, oxygen provides the gas essential to the survival of the patient by promoting respiration and cellular function.

Nitrous Oxide

Nitrous oxide is a clear, colorless gas with a subtle fruity odor and is the only true gas still in use. It interacts with the cellular membranes of the CNS to produce analgesia with some amnesia. It is not sufficiently potent to be used alone for general surgical anesthesia but may be used in conjunction with other anesthetic agents in a balanced anesthesia state. Nitrous oxide alone does not produce sufficient muscle relaxation for surgical intervention and may cause a mild decrease in myocardial contractility and respiratory depression, but it has little effect on heart rate and/or blood pressure. The gas itself is not flammable, although it does support combustion when used in combination with oxygen. Nitrous oxide freely diffuses into closed spaces, such as the middle ear, the bowel, and the pleural space, causing increased pressure in those spaces, contraindicating its use in some surgical procedures (e.g., tympanoplasty). Nitrous oxide is eliminated by exhalation.

Waste Gases

All waste gases (exhaled or escaped) should be captured with a scavenger system and removed from the OR and filtered prior to release to prevent occupational exposure of health care workers.

Volatile Agents

The **volatile agents** consist of a group of liquids whose potent evaporative vapors, when inhaled, produce general anesthesia through interaction with the CNS, causing generalized CNS depression as evidenced by depressed EEG (electroencephalogram) activity. They also produce generalized myocardial and respiratory depression. Muscle tone is generally decreased, enhancing ease of exposure of the surgical site. The volatile agents are delivered to the patient via a series of tubing called the *anesthesia circuit,* with the use of a vaporizer that is a part of the anesthesia machine. Agents in use today include halothane, enflurane, isoflurane, desflurane, and sevoflurane. Halogenated anesthetic agents are considered a trigger for malignant hyperthermia, a potentially deadly condition.

Halothane (Fluothane) is a nonflammable, potent, rapid-acting inhalation agent generally considered nonirritating to the respiratory tree. It is used for both induction and maintenance of general anesthesia and is often used with other agents for balanced anesthesia. Halothane has a pleasant smell allowing for smooth induction. Its high potency allows for concomitant use of high oxygen levels, permitting adequate patient oxygenation. It causes both profound uterine relaxation and bronchodilation. It may induce bradycardia and cardiac dysrhythmia, especially when used in conjunction with aminophylline or epinephrine. Halothane is known to cause hepatic toxicity due to its metabolism by the liver and may lead to halothane-induced hepatitis in the adult population. Halothane should not be administered to patients with poor liver function, liver disease, or a recent history of jaundice and should not be readministered within a 3-month period.

Enflurane (Ethrane) is nonflammable, stable, halogenated ether similar in properties to halothane. Enflurane has a mild, sweet odor. It provides a rapid induction and recovery. Enflurane causes hypotension in the absence of surgical stimulation. It has a minimal effect on cardiac rate and output. It produces muscle relaxation adequate for surgical intervention but may be supplemented with neuromuscular blockers. Enflurane potentiates nondepolarizing neuromuscular blockade.

Isoflurane (Forane) is a mildly pungent, musty smelling halogenated inhalation agent. It provides a rapid induction and recovery. It is a profound respiratory depressant and may cause hypotension, which is reversed with surgical stimulation. Isoflurane markedly potentiates neuromuscular blockade. It also increases intracranial pressure (ICP), which is reversible with hyperventilation.

Desflurane (Suprane) is one of the newer halogenated inhalation agents on the market and requires the use of a heated vaporizer for administration. It has a pungent aroma, making it an agent not advisable for use with mask induction. It provides a more rapid onset and recovery than halothane, enflurane, or isoflurane. Because it is not biotransformed in the liver, desflurane is safe to use for patients with hepatic insufficiency.

Sevoflurane (Ultane) is an odorless inhalation agent that does not cause irritation to the respiratory tree. It has a more rapid and smooth onset and recovery than either enflurane or isoflurane. Sevoflurane causes bradycardia, hypotension, and cardiac dysrhythmias and reduces cardiac output. It may also produce nausea and vomiting in the postoperative period. Sevoflurane does not cause liver damage but may cause mild renal complications. Its use potentiates the use of neuromuscular blockers. It can be a triggering agent for MH.

INTRAVENOUS AGENTS

Intravenous agents, introduced in the 1930s, comprise the largest group of surgical pharmacological agents in use today. Delivered directly into the bloodstream, these agents act quickly, with rapid evidence of their action demonstrated. Intravenous access is commonly achieved by placement of a catheter in a peripheral vein of the upper extremity, though use of central venous access via a subclavian line or venous access port is also permitted. Higher concentrations of IV agents can be found in high-blood-flow organs, such as the liver, spleen, kidney, and brain. Intravenous agents are removed from the body through redistribution and biotransformation in the liver and kidneys. The safety of IV agents is directly related to their ease of metabolism and is dependent on the overall level of hepatic and/or renal function. Intravenous agents are grouped into induction agents, dissociative agents, opioids, sedatives/tranquilizers, neuromuscular blocking agents, **antimuscarinic** (anticholinergic) agents, and adjunctive agents.

Induction Agents

The IV induction agents are those medications used to permit a rapid and pleasant transition from a state of consciousness (stage 1) to unconsciousness (stage 3) by quickly passing through the excitement or delirium stage (stage 2). While they do not provide pain relief or motor-impulse blockade, induction agents do produce marked sedation and amnesia. Hypotension and respiratory depression are common side effects of induction agent administration, necessitating the availability of supportive and resuscitative equipment when these agents are used. Some induction agents may also be used for maintenance of general anesthesia.

Propofol (Diprivan) is a sedative-hypnotic agent introduced into anesthesia practice in the early 1990s. Due to its milky appearance, the drug has been nicknamed "milk of amnesia"; propofol is a soy-oil-in-water emulsion capable of supporting microbial growth. Strict sterile technique is used during its preparation and administration, and syringes of prepared medication must be used or discarded within 6 hours of preparation. Induction doses produce unconsciousness, but lower doses produce conscious sedation. Because of its alkaline nature, propofol is irritating to the vein and may cause patient discomfort at the IV site on administration. Lidocaine given IV just prior to propofol injection may ease the discomfort of this side effect. Propofol provides a rapid induction and emergence without the prolonged "hangover" effect of other agents. It is the agent of choice for short surgical interventions and procedures on day-admission patients. Because it causes increased ICP and marked hypotension, propofol is contraindicated for those patients with unstable hemodynamics and/or head trauma.

Etomidate (Amidate) is a nonbarbiturate hypnotic agent used for anesthesia induction. Similar to propofol in the time of induction and emergence, etomidate does not produce analgesia. Because it produces minimal cardiovascular system effects, etomidate is the preferred agent of choice for hemodynamically unstable patient indications. Postoperative nausea and vomiting as well as adrenal suppression are seen more frequently in patients given etomidate.

Thiopental sodium (Pentothal Sodium) is a short-acting, potent barbiturate that does not provide anesthesia or muscle relaxation but does have hypnotic, amnesic, and sedative effects. Given over a period, thiopental sodium has a cumulative effect, being stored in lipid-based tissues and slowly released. While less expensive to administer than propofol, thiopental sodium leaves the patient with a residual hangover effect lasting through and prolonging the patient's emergence and recovery phases. The advantages of thiopental sodium use include marked respiratory and circulatory depression immediately following injection, nonflammability, inability to cause irritation to the respiratory tree, and lack of salivary stimulation. Thiopental sodium in combination with nitrous oxide and opioids has a synergistic effect, permitting lower and safer doses of potent agents to be used. Disadvantages of thiopental sodium use are minor patient stimulation during the lighter stages of anesthesia administration, which may cause laryngospasm, and the alkaline nature of the drug, which may be locally irritating to the vein.

Methohexital sodium (Brevital) is similar in action to propofol and thiopental sodium. Methohexital sodium has an ultrashort onset and duration of action, making it the agent of choice for achieving short-term loss of consciousness during regional blockade for ophthalmology cases and electroconvulsive therapy treatment.

Dissociative Agents

The dissociative agents selectively interrupt the associative pathways of the brain. Patients may appear wide awake, yet they are unaware of their surroundings. Dissociative agents also produce amnesia and profound analgesia.

Ketamine hydrochloride (Ketalar) is the most commonly used dissociative agent. It is administered either IM or IV. It produces a rapid induction of the dissociated and amnesic state, which may be potentiated by the concurrent use of other narcotics and/or barbiturates. Ketamine hydrochloride, in and of itself, does not produce relaxation nor does it obtund the reflexes, in particular the "gag" reflex. Muscle tone is generally increased. It also increases ICP and intraocular pressure (IOP) and causes hypertension. Salivation is markedly increased with the administration of ketamine HCl. The major disadvantage of ketamine HCl use is the production of vivid imagery and morbid hallucinations during administration and recovery. Documented cases of "flashbacks" related to ketamine HCl administration limit this agent's use to children 2–10 years of age.

Opiate/Opioids

The opiate/opioids are a group of narcotics classified as analgesics, which also produce sedation. They act by binding to CNS and spinal cord receptors, producing a decrease in pain impulse transmission. Euphoria or a feeling of happiness and well-being may also be experienced, thereby incidentally reducing surgery-related anxiety. High doses of these agents may lead to a loss of consciousness and respiratory depression. Opioids do not produce muscle relaxation. Inversely, these agents are known to increase overall muscle tone. Opioids are commonly used as an adjunct to general anesthesia agents, permitting the use of lower, safer concentrations of inhalation agents. Occasionally, opioids are used as the sole anesthetic agent in cardiac surgery. They are biotransformed primarily in the liver and eliminated in urine. All opiates/opioids are Class II controlled substances (narcotics) regulated by the FDA. Drugs in this classification are the opiate morphine sulfate and the synthetic opioids, including meperidine (Demerol), fentanyl (Sublimaze), sufentanil (Sufenta), alfentanil (Alfenta), and remifentanil (Ultiva).

Morphine sulfate is used for the control of severe pain. It is given IM as a preoperative sedative/analgesic or postoperative analgesic, IV as an anesthetic agent, or intrathecally via spinal administration for intraoperative and postoperative pain control. The use of morphine sulfate permits a reduction in dosage and/or concentration of more potent agents. Side effects of morphine sulfate administration include bradycardia, hypotension, vasodilation, nausea and vomiting, confusion, and respiratory depression.

Meperidine (Demerol) is similar in action to morphine. Used to treat moderate to severe pain, meperidine may be administered IM but is given IV when used as an anesthetic adjunct. In addition to respiratory depression, side effects include increased ICP, tachycardia, and vasodilation. Meperidine should not be used for patients concomitantly using monoamine oxidase (MAO) inhibitors.

Fentanyl citrate (Sublimaze) is the first of the synthetic narcotic analgesics to be used for anesthesia administration. Its actions include inhibiting CNS ascending pain pathway stimulation, resulting in an alteration in pain perception and an increased pain threshold. Fentanyl citrate may be combined with droperidol (Inapsine) in the form of the agent Innovar. Innovar is used as a preoperative agent to produce analgesia and sedation while decreasing the potential for inducing nausea and/or vomiting. One hundred micrograms of fentanyl is equivalent in analgesic effect to 10 mg of morphine or 75 mg of meperidine. Given IV, fentanyl citrate has a rapid onset and short duration of action. Adverse reactions seen with fentanyl citrate include bradycardia, laryngospasm, and cardiorespiratory arrest. The use of fentanyl citrate for patients with myasthenia gravis is contraindicated.

Sufentanil citrate (Sufenta) is similar in nature to fentanyl but is five times more potent. Given as a primary anesthetic agent or as an adjunct, sufentanil citrate produces analgesia with marked sedation and euphoria. Sufentanil citrate is a respiratory depressant and has a rapid onset of action when given IV. It has a short duration of activity and is rapidly eliminated.

Alfentanil hydrochloride (Alfenta) is similar in action and usage to fentanyl citrate and sufentanil citrate but acts on pain receptors of the limbic system, thalamus, midbrain, and hypothalamus, altering pain perception and response. Alfentanil hydrochloride is a short-acting analgesic, but the induced respiratory depression may outlast the analgesic effect produced.

Remifentanil hydrochloride (Ultiva) is an ultrashort-acting synthetic opioid metabolized in blood and muscle tissue. It has a short duration of action, approximately 5–10 minutes. Its potency and action are similar to the other synthetic opioids. Remifentanil may cause respiratory depression, bradycardia, hypotension, and muscle rigidity. The advantage of remifentanil over other opioids is that its short duration of action allows more accurate dose titration.

Narcotic Antagonists. The opioid effect can be antagonized or reversed by the administration of naloxone hydrochloride (Narcan), which works by competing for CNS receptor sites, preventing opioid binding. Given IV at a dose of 0.4–2 mg, patient response (increased level of consciousness and respiratory effort) should be seen within 1–2 minutes. Naloxone hydrochloride administration may lead to an abrupt onset of pain as the opioid effect is reversed. This may cause tachycardia and hypertension. Because the effect of naloxone hydrochloride begins to decline after 30 minutes, prior to full opioid biotransformation and reduction in side effects, patients should be closely monitored for opioid-induced rebound respiratory depression.

Benzodiazepines

Benzodiazepines (sedative tranquilizers) are used in anesthesia in two ways: to reduce the anxiety and apprehension of the preoperative patient and as an adjunct to general anesthesia to reduce the amount and concentration of other more potent agents. Sedatives do not produce analgesia. The most commonly used agents come from the benzodiazepine group and are used for their ability to produce amnestic, anticonvulsive, hypnotic, and sedative effects. They also produce muscle relaxation. Hypotensive changes and respiratory depression may occur, especially when benzodiazepines are administered concomitantly with an opioid agent. The two most commonly used benzodiazepines are diazepam (Valium) and midazolam (Versed).

Diazepam (Valium) is a Class IV controlled substance. It acts by increasing the action of gamma-amino butyric acid (GABA) receptor sites, particularly in the limbic system and reticular formation. Its primary anesthetic use is to reduce anxiety and provide some skeletal muscle relaxation. It also provides retrograde amnesia of short duration. Given IV, diazepam has an onset of action within 5 minutes, with a 15-minute duration. It is metabolized in the liver for renal excretion.

Midazolam (Versed) is also a Class IV controlled substance. It is a rapid-onset and short-acting benzodiazepine, making it an ideal agent for patients undergoing outpatient procedures. Its action is similar to diazepam, but its memory impairment is of shorter duration. Since midazolam is twice as potent as diazepam, the IV dosage is commonly diluted with injectable dextrose/water or saline for administration.

Droperidol (Inapsine) is a butyrophenone, which produces marked sedation with a long duration of action. Droperidol provides the additional benefit of acting as an antiemetic both intraoperatively and postoperatively. Mild amnesia may also be produced. Droperidol also comes premixed with fentanyl citrate, under the trade name Innovar, providing a combination of sedation and analgesia.

Benzodiazepine Antagonists. The benzodiazepines may be antagonized by the administration of flumazenil (Mazicon). Flumazenil works by competing for benzodiazepine inhibitory receptor sites. Flumazenil has a rapid onset of action but an unknown duration. It reverses the sedative effects but may not reverse the amnesia effects. Convulsions may also occur with flumazenil administration. Patients need to be assessed and monitored for rebound sedation and/or respiratory depression.

Neuromuscular Blockers

Skeletal muscle relaxants, or neuromuscular blockers (NMBs), interfere with the passage of impulses from motor nerves to skeletal muscles, resulting in neuromuscular blockade causing muscle weakness and paralysis. Jaw relaxation is achieved for ease of endotracheal intubation, the muscles of respiration are affected allowing for mechanical ventilation, and the musculature at the surgical site is relaxed to allow retraction for surgical exposure. Administered IV, NMBs serve as an adjunct to other general anesthesia agents, permitting a decrease in dosage and concentration of other more potent agents. Depending on the agent's onset and duration, neuromuscular-blocking agents may need to be readministered throughout the surgical intervention. The blockade effect is monitored by the use of a peripheral nerve stimulator, capable of evoking a "train of four" response in patients with waning or without neuromuscular blockade. *Train of four* is a term used to describe a series of muscle contractions demonstrated by a single simulated nerve stimulation, causing a series of muscle contraction responses. Neuromuscular blockade must be naturally or pharmacologically reversed prior to airway extubation.

Neuromuscular blocking agents are divided into two major categories: depolarizing agents and nondepolarizing agents (Table 9-6).

Depolarizing Agents. Depolarizing agents work by mimicking a release of acetylcholine across the neuromuscular junction. The agent binds to the postsynaptic receptors, causing muscle contraction to occur, which is followed by a period of muscle fatigue. The contraction/relaxation in the muscle is strong enough to be visible; the

Table 9-6 Neuromuscular Blocking Agents

TYPE	GENERIC NAME	BRAND NAME
Depolarizing agents	Succinylcholine	Anectine
Nondepolarizing agents	Mivacurium chloride	Mivacron
	Vecuronium bromide	Norcuron
	Rocuronium bromide	Zemuron
	Atracurium besylate	Tracrium
	Cisatracurium besylate	Nimbex
	Tubocurarine chloride	Curare
	Pancuronium bromide	Pavulon
Nondepolarizing neuromuscular agent antagonists	Edrophonium chloride	Tensilon
	Neostigmine	Prostigmin

action is referred to as *fasciculation* and the patient may experience postoperative muscle ache because of fasciculation. As the agent is metabolized by plasma cholinesterase in the synapse, the effects of the agent are reversed. The effects of depolarizing agents cannot be pharmacologically reversed. The main depolarizing agent in anesthetic use today is succinylcholine.

Succinylcholine (Anectine) is an ultrashort-acting agent. It has a rapid onset and is useful in producing neuromuscular blockade for intubation. It causes an increase in both IOP and ICP. Succinylcholine may be given as an IV bolus or in a continuous IV drip for neuromuscular blockade maintenance. A mild nondepolarizing agent may be given just prior to succinylcholine administration to reduce or eliminate fasciculation. Succinylcholine is also a known triggering agent for MH.

Nondepolarizing Agents. Nondepolarizing agents work by competing for postsynaptic receptor sites at the neuromuscular junction. This competition prevents acetylcholine from being able to stimulate muscle contraction. Spontaneous recovery of neuromuscular blockade may occur as the agent diffuses from the receptor sites into the synapse. Nondepolarizing agents may also be reversed by the administration of agents that inhibit acetylcholinesterase, the enzyme that breaks down acetylcholine. This provides a higher amount of acetylcholine to be present for muscle stimulation. Nondepolarizing agents are preferred agents of choice for blockade induction because of the low incidence of associated cardiovascular side effects.

Nondepolarizing agents may be further divided into short-, intermediate-, and long-acting agents.

Mivacurium chloride (Mivacron) is a short-acting nondepolarizing muscle relaxant with intermediate length of onset. It should be used with caution in patients with a familial history of pseudocholinesterase deficiency and in patients with hepatic or renal insufficiency.

Vecuronium bromide (Norcuron) is a short-acting nondepolarizing muscle relaxant with an intermediate onset. It is comparable to gallamine and pancuronium in its actions. The use of succinylcholine for intubation prior to administering vecuronium for maintenance may prolong the effects of neuromuscular blockade.

Rocuronium bromide (Zemuron) is a short-acting nondepolarizing muscle relaxant with a rapid onset. It may be given by IV bolus for induction or by continuous IV drip for maintenance. It provides a rapid, spontaneous recovery, similar to succinylcholine, without the side effects of depolarizing blocker usage. Because rocuronium is metabolized by the liver, it should be used with caution in patients with hepatic insufficiency.

Atracurium besylate (Tracrium) is an intermediate-acting nondepolarizing muscle relaxant with a short onset. It provides a rapid recovery from NMB effect, making it one of the first agents to replace the commonly used succinylcholine.

Cisatracurium besylate (Nimbex) is an intermediate-acting nondepolarizing muscle relaxant with an intermediate duration of action. It is two to three times more potent than atracurium.

Tubocurarine chloride (Curare) is a long-acting nondepolarizing muscle relaxant with a rapid onset of action. It was first used by South American Indians to poison their arrows for hunting. It causes histamine release and may induce bronchospasm and hemodynamic changes.

Pancuronium bromide (Pavulon) is a long-acting nondepolarizing muscle relaxant with an intermediate onset. The action of pancuronium is enhanced by inhalation agents, requiring a reduction in dosage. It may cause an elevation of blood pressure and heart rate. It is eliminated in urine, and therefore care should be used when administering this agent to patients with renal disease.

Neuromuscular Blockade Antagonism. Antagonism of nondepolarizing neuromuscular agents is produced by two agents: edrophonium chloride (Tensilon) and neostigmine (Prostigmin). These cholinergic agents inhibit the destruction of acetylcholine, increasing its presence in the neuromuscular synapse and facilitating neuromuscular transmission of impulses. To prevent a cholinergic crisis, these agents are usually given in conjunction with an antimuscarinic agent such as atropine.

Antimuscarinic Agents

Antimuscarinic (formerly known as *anticholinergic*) agents act as blockers of the cholinergic effects. Antimuscarinic agents are used to limit undesirable parasympathetic nervous system responses such as salivation and bradycardia; these agents are given preoperatively to inhibit cholinergic responses or in conjunction with neuromuscular blockading agents to prevent undesired side effects of NMB reversal. The two most commonly used agents are atropine sulfate and glycopyrrolate (Robinul).

Nonsteroidal Anti-Inflammatory Agents

Ketorolac (Toradol) is a nonsteroidal anti-inflammatory drug (NSAID) used for moderate pain control. This agent is given IM by anesthesia personnel to aid in pain management during emergence and recovery.

Gastric Acid Management

Histamine H_2 antagonists and antacids are agents used to alter the pH of gastric secretions and reduce gastric volume and hydrogen ion concentration. They are given during the preoperative or intraoperative period. Included in this group are the oral agent citric acid (Bicitra) and the IV agents including cimetidine (Tagamet) and ranitidine (Zantac). Metoclopramide (Reglan), a cholinergic agent, promotes pyloric emptying.

Antiemetic

Antiemetic agents are used to prevent or treat nausea and vomiting. Droperidol (Inapsine), metoclopramide (Reglan), or ondansetron (Zofran) have antiemetic properties and can be given by intravenous injection.

ADJUNCTS TO GENERAL ANESTHESIA

Several revolutionary types of treatment that in the past have not been considered a traditional part of general anesthesia are now incorporated into balanced anesthesia. Some of the adjunctive treatments are discussed next.

INDUCED HYPOTHERMIA

Induced hypothermia involves the artificial, deliberate lowering of the body's core temperature below normal limits. The resulting lower temperature causes an overall reduction in body metabolism with a concomitant reduction in oxygen and glucose consumption and waste production. Induced hypothermia permits the use of lower dosages of inhalation and IV agents, providing a safer level of anesthetic agent administration.

There are four levels of cooling involved with induced hypothermia (Table 9-7). The first is light hypothermia, where the core body temperature is brought to a range of 98.6–89.6°F. At this level of cooling, the sensorium fades, resulting in an altered or reduced level of consciousness. A core body temperature ranging from 89.6 to 78.8°F marks moderate hypothermia. A core body temperature between 78.8 and 68°F marks deep hypothermia. Profound hypothermia occurs when the core temperature drops below 68°F.

Hypothermic levels are induced by several methods, including body surface cooling, internal cavity cooling, and systemic blood circulation cooling. Induced hypothermia is indicated as an adjunctive therapy for use during open-heart surgery, following cardiopulmonary resuscitation, as a treatment for MH, and during a hypertensive crisis, organ transplantation, and periods of decreased blood flow to the brain.

INDUCED HYPOTENSION

Induced hypotension is an adjunctive therapy involving a controlled decrease of arterial pressure during anesthetic administration. Hypotension results in a decrease in bleeding and overall blood loss while increasing visibility within the surgical field. Induced hypotension is an adjunctive therapy technique used as one of the components of "bloodless surgery" protocols for those patients who do not desire to receive a blood transfusion.

NEUROLEPTANALGESIA

Neuroleptanalgesia utilizes high doses of neuroleptics (tranquilizers) and narcotic analgesic agents to induce a

Table 9-7 Induced Hypothermia Levels

INDUCED HYPOTHERMIA LEVELS	TEMPERATURE RANGE (°F)
Light hypothermia	98.6–89.6
Moderate hypothermia	89.6–78.8
Deep hypothermia	78.8–68
Profound hypothermia	68 and below

state of diminished anxiety, sedation, and amnesia, allowing the patient to retain the ability to respond to commands. Two medications commonly used to induce neuroleptanalgesia are fentanyl citrate and meperidine hydrochloride.

NEUROLEPTANESTHESIA

Neuroleptanesthesia occurs when neuroleptanalgesia is reinforced with an inhalation or IV anesthetic agent.

ANESTHESIA EQUIPMENT

The primary goal during anesthesia is to keep the patient as safe as possible throughout the perioperative period. Several pieces of assistive equipment are required to deliver safe and effective anesthesia care to the patient. The most prominent piece of equipment in the anesthesia care delivery system is the anesthesia machine. Several other devices are necessary to support and monitor the patient. These devices allow the entire surgical team to promote homeostasis, readily identify any physiological change, and implement early intervention of any condition prior to it becoming life threatening. Much of the equipment described will be used for general patient care; its use is not restricted to the OR specifically.

ANESTHESIA MACHINE

Today's anesthesia machine provides a combination of inhalation agent delivery systems, including vaporizers, respiratory support equipment, and sophisticated monitoring devices (Figure 9-7). The inhalation gases and respiratory support are provided to the patient through a series of tubing that is referred to as the anesthesia circuit. Many machines also incorporate an integrated system for patient monitoring and documentation.

During the delivery of anesthesia, several assistive devices aid in the delivery of adjunct treatments and maintenance of optimal levels of patient homeostasis.

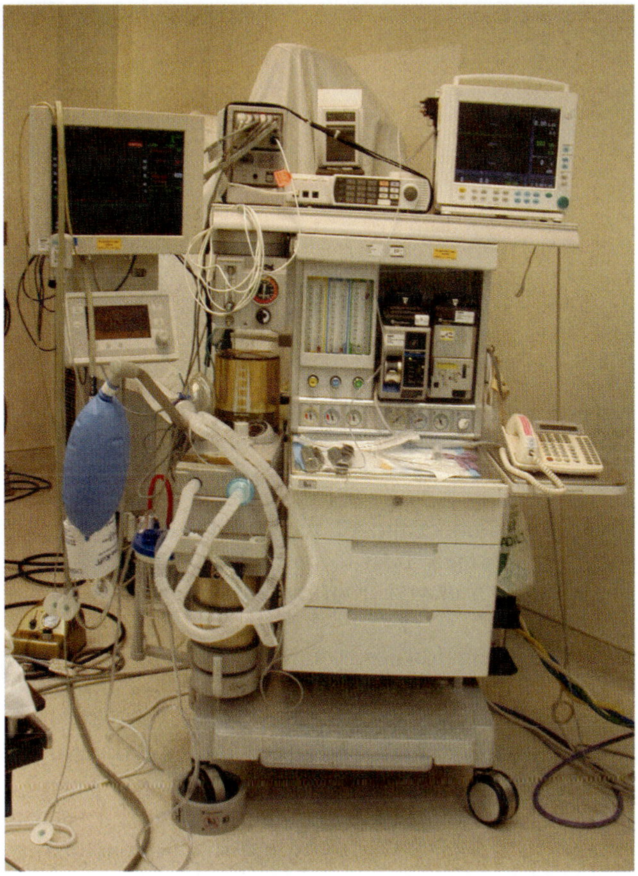

Figure 9-7 Anesthesia machine

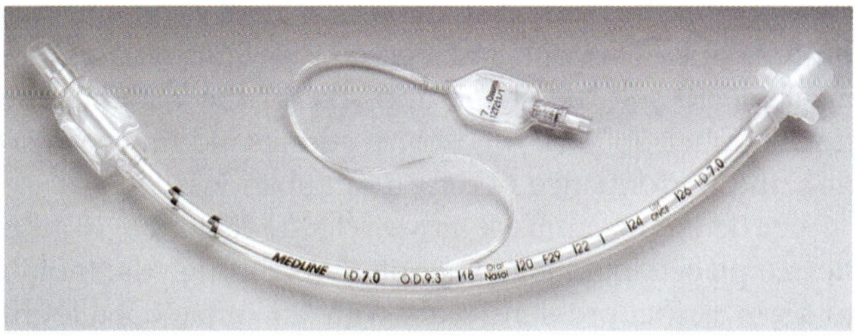

Figure 9-8 Endotracheal tube ***(Courtesy of Medline Industries, Inc.)***

AIRWAY DELIVERY/MAINTENANCE DEVICES

Ventilators are commonly used in conjunction with neuromuscular blockade during general anesthesia. Mechanical ventilation permits the anesthesia provider to control the rate and volume of respiration during the surgical intervention. Ventilators are equipped with disconnect alarms and spirometers with built-in high and low alarms. An overpressure "pop-off" valve is included.

Endotracheal (ET) tubes are devices placed through the patient's nose or mouth, between the vocal cords, and into the trachea to provide a patent airway intraoperatively or during ventilatory support (Figure 9-8). A laryngoscope is necessary to facilitate tube placement. Tubes are commonly made of polyvinylchloride (PVC) but may also be made of rubber or silicone impregnated with metal particles for use in endotracheal laser procedures. Endotracheal tubes are available in many diameters and configurations and are of a measured length, marked in millimeters. Adult-sized tubes and larger sized pediatric tubes come with inflatable (ballooned) cuffs, permitting the creation of a closed airway system when the cuff is inflated. The ET tube is connected to the anesthesia machine by a series of tubings and connectors called the anesthesia circuit.

A stylet is used to modify the configuration of or stiffen an ET tube during placement. A stylet is made of malleable metal or stiff plastic and is placed within the lumen of the ET tube. The distal tip should not protrude

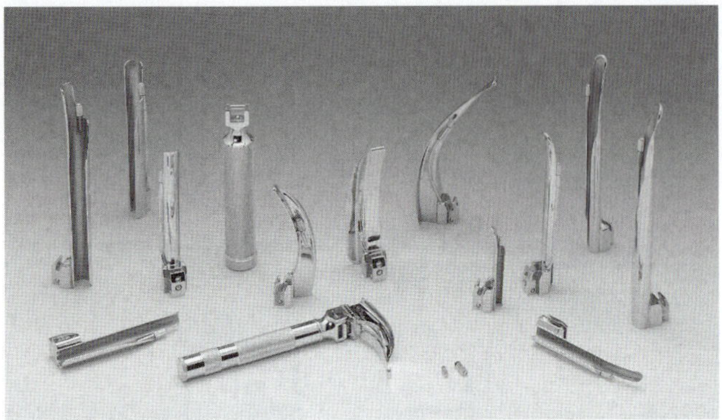

Figure 9-9 Laryngoscope and various blade attachments *(Courtesy of Armstrong Medical Instruments, Inc.)*

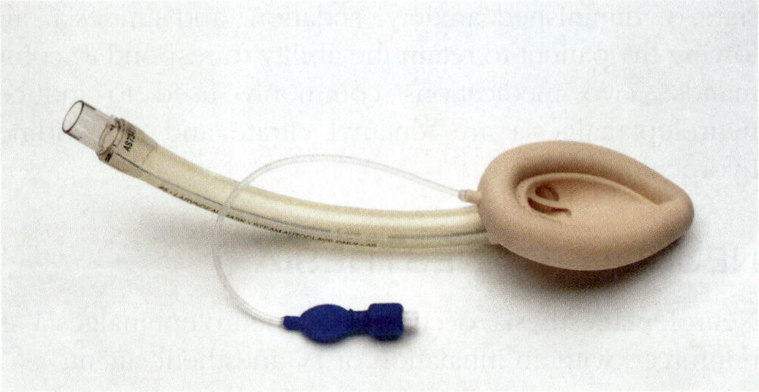

Figure 9-10 Laryngeal mask airway *(Courtesy of LMA North America, Inc.)*

beyond the end of the ET tube, and the proximal end should be severely bent to prevent accidental retention. The stylet is removed from the ET tube following tube placement.

The McGill forceps is an instrument used to aid and facilitate the placement of nasotracheal tubes and nasogastric tubes or to insert pharyngeal packing. They are used transorally to grasp the tube or packing material and deliver the item to the appropriate area for placement.

The laryngoscope (Figure 9-9) is a device used to expose the glottis to facilitate endotracheal intubation. The rigid laryngoscope consists of a handle and interchangeable blades. The handle contains batteries, which provide current to the small light bulb found on the distal aspect of the blade. Laryngoscope blades come in two basic shapes: straight and curved. Several variants are available to suit the shape and size of the patient. The flexible fiber-optic laryngoscope permits aid in visualization and performance of difficult intubations.

The laryngeal mask airway (LMA) (Figure 9-10) is a device placed into the laryngopharynx through the mouth to form a low-pressure seal (with an inflated balloon) around the laryngeal inlet, while providing minimal stimulation to the airway. It provides a simple and effective way of establishing a patent airway without the dangers and complications of endotracheal intubation. Constructed of silicone rubber, the reusable airway has three fenestrations to allow for ventilation in the distal flanged area, connected to a tube, exiting the patient's mouth. This tube is then connected to the tubing of the anesthesia machine for the delivery of inhalation agents.

The face mask is used to cover the nose and mouth area of the patient and permit the delivery of anesthetic gases and/or oxygen to the patient. Made of plastic with a molded or balloon-like ridge to facilitate the creation of an airtight seal, the face mask assists in the application of positive-pressure breathing techniques. Some face masks are manufactured of clear plastic to allow the anesthesia provider to observe the nose and mouth for secretions or emesis.

Oropharyngeal airways and nasal airways are devices used to provide a passageway around the relaxed tongue, establishing an unobstructed airway for gas exchange. Oropharyngeal airways, placed through the mouth, are rigid plastic, with a preformed curve, which lifts the tongue forward. Nasal airways, placed through the nostril, are soft, hollow tubes with a flanged end to prevent aspiration of the tube. Placed into the nostril, the nasal airway lifts the soft palate from the back of the oropharynx.

HYPOTHERMIA AND HYPERTHERMIA DEVICES

Temperature control is important to patient safety.

The Bair Hugger is a patient-warming device that utilizes warm air blown into a special blanket that is placed over the patient (Figure 9-11). The blankets come in a variety of sizes and configurations to meet the needs of the surgical patient. The blanket may be secured to the patient's skin with adhesive to prevent migration.

Warming/cooling devices utilize warmed or cooled water or isopropyl alcohol, which circulates through coils in a pad that is placed under the patient. These devices promote the maintenance of optimal body temperature during surgical intervention and minimize the induction of hypothermia related to room temperature and surgical manipulation of tissues. Alternatively, the body temperature can be manipulated for therapeutic reasons, for example, to induce hypothermia in conjunction with general anesthesia or to cool a febrile patient.

A variety of devices are available to assist with fluid delivery. These tools are designed for use along with the patient's peripheral IV system. These devices include:

- *Fluid-warming devices:* Fluid-warming devices are used to raise the temperature of blood and other IV fluids to body temperature just prior to infusion into the patient. Warming prevents induced hypothermia and concomitant metabolic acidosis.
- *Rapid infusion pump:* A rapid infusion pump is a device attached to the IV line used to rapidly deliver

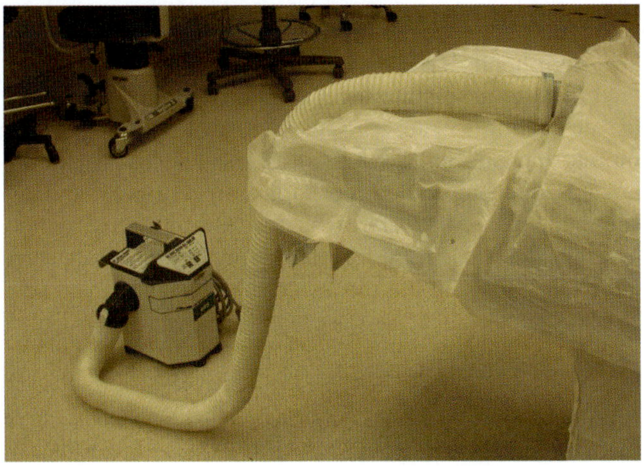

Figure 9-11 Bair Hugger surgical access blanket

a large volume of blood or other fluid to the patient. The device may be a complex computerized machine or as simple as a pressurized cuff wrapped around the outside of the fluid administration bag to exert external force. The device may also incorporate a fluid-warming device, eliminating the need for a second piece of equipment.

- *Infusion control devices:* Infusion control devices are mechanical devices that regulate the delivery of IV fluids and medications. They may involve the attachment of a monitoring device to the external surface of the IV tubing drip chamber or may hold a syringe of medication that is delivered in a prescribed and controlled manner.

MONITORING DEVICES

The surgical patient is monitored continuously prior to induction and during the anesthetic and postanesthetic states. Monitoring devices of various types and complexity are used to accomplish this task.

Electrocardiogram

The electrocardiogram is a noninvasive method used to monitor the rate, rhythm, and electrical conduction of the heart, indicating cardiac function. Detection, identification, and treatment of any dysrhythmia or arrhythmia are critical. Electrodes are placed on the patient's skin and are connected to the monitor with a series of leads.

Blood Pressure Monitor

Blood pressure monitoring is used to evaluate the patient's cardiac output and vascular status. Blood pressure measurement is commonly performed using noninvasive techniques but may also be monitored invasively with the insertion of an arterial line. Systolic, diastolic, and mean arterial pressures are monitored and tracked for trends indicating any changes. Automatic devices with adjustable time interval settings perform most blood pressure monitoring in the OR.

Arterial and Venous Catheterization

Pulmonary artery catheters are invasive monitoring devices placed into the pulmonary artery via subclavian or jugular access. The catheter is then threaded through the right side of the heart, with the ballooned tip "wedged" in the pulmonary artery. The catheter is connected via sterile tubing to a transducer and monitor, providing information in a digital format to the observer. The catheter permits monitoring of cardiac output from the right side of the heart, an indicator of overall cardiac function and fluid status. The reading is referred to as the "wedge" pressure.

Central venous pressure (CVP) catheters are invasive monitoring devices placed into the right atrium via subclavian or jugular access. The catheter is placed to monitor pressure in the vena cava and right atrium, indicating the patient's fluid status.

Temperature Monitors

Temperature monitors are noninvasive or invasive methods used to assess the patient's body temperature. A common form of monitor, the surface monitor, may be placed on the patient's forehead. The ear monitor is often used for general patient care but is impractical in the OR. Other, more invasive monitors of body core temperature include esophageal, bladder, and rectal probes and are better suited for intraoperative use. Monitoring of patient body temperature is helpful in monitoring intentional changes in the patient's temperature or for identifying hypothermia (which can lead to metabolic acidosis) and hyperthermia (an indicator of sepsis or MH).

Pulse Oximeter

Pulse oximetry involves noninvasive assessment of the hemoglobin saturation levels in arterial blood. Monitoring takes place using a two-wavelength light absorption technique, which focuses on the pulsatile absorption of light. There are several choice locations for placement of the sensor. The fingertip is commonly used; other sites include the toe, earlobe, and the bridge of the nose. Pulse oximetry permits a continuous, rapid, and easy means of monitoring blood oxygenation. The sensor is motion sensitive, giving a false reading or no reading during patient motion. Substances, such as dyes (nail polish), methemoglobin, and carbon monoxide, may affect accurate monitoring. Introduced in the 1980s, pulse oximetry monitoring enhances the safe delivery of anesthesia. Pulse oximetry monitoring is now considered an industry standard of practice.

Bispectral Index™ (BIS) Monitor

The Bispectral Index™ (BIS) monitor assists anesthesia providers in monitoring the dose of anesthesia delivered to the patient during the surgical intervention. A noninvasive sensor is placed on the patient's forehead and attached by a cable to the monitor, which continuously monitors the patient's brain waves, computing them into a number ranging from 100 to 0. The number correlates with the patient's level of consciousness, with a recording of 100 when the patient is wide awake and under 60 when the patient is unconscious. As the numbers change, the dose of anesthetic is titrated or adjusted, providing the patient with an optimal level of surgical anesthesia.

SARA

A monitoring device, System for Anesthetic and Respiratory Analysis (SARA), is incorporated into most anesthesia machines today and is used to monitor the patient's physiological respiratory and anesthetic gas levels. This device is capable of several monitoring functions, including:

- ***Capnography***: Commonly used in the anesthetic setting to provide breath-by-breath analysis of expired carbon dioxide (end-tidal CO_2).
- *Spirometry:* Gives information about the pulmonary status by monitoring ventilatory flow, volume, and pressure. This information allows for calculations pertaining to lung compliance and resistance, providing information that could indicate emphysema or adult respiratory distress syndrome (ARDS).
- *Oxygen analyzer:* Confirms the delivery of oxygen to the patient and that the concentration of oxygen is adequate.

Stethoscope

The stethoscope is used for auscultation during anesthetic delivery. Assessment of proper ET tube placement by auscultating the lung fields, assessing lung sounds, verifying placement of nasogastric tubes, and checking the stomach for inadvertent endoesophageal placement of the endotracheal tube are all uses of the stethoscope. An internal stethoscope is available in the form of an esophageal probe; incidentally, a thermometer is often included.

Doppler

The **Doppler** is an ultrasonic device used to identify and assess vascular status of peripheral arteries and veins by magnifying the sound of the blood moving through the vessel. This may assist in the identification of structures for cannulation and locating obstructions. A sterile probe is available for use within the sterile field.

Peripheral Nerve Stimulator

The peripheral nerve stimulator is a battery-operated device used to assess the level of neuromuscular blockade by attempting to cause a muscle to twitch. Train-of-four monitoring permits assessment of the level of nondepolarizing neuromuscular blockade and assists in the assessment of recovery from blockade during emergence. The most common site for placement of the noninvasive electrodes is along the ulnar nerve.

Arterial Blood Gases

Arterial blood gases (ABG) involve invasive monitoring of pH, oxygen saturation, and carbon dioxide levels. Arterial blood gases are commonly obtained by accessing the radial artery or by placement of a monitoring line into the radial artery (arterial line or a-line). Direct blood pressure monitoring may also be performed via the a-line.

NERVE CONDUCTION BLOCKADE

Nerve conduction blockade anesthesia involves the use of pharmaceutical agents to prevent the initiation and/or transmission of sensory nerve impulses. The conduction-blocking agent is absorbed by nerve sheath, decreasing nerve conduction to a point where sensory impulses are unable to be transmitted. Anesthesia is achieved for a specific region of the body. Motor impulse transmission may or may not be affected, depending on the function of the blocked nerve. Care must be taken to perform the operative intervention within tissues affected by the nerve blockade. A variety of techniques are used for nerve conduction blockade:

- Topical anesthesia
- Local anesthesia
- Regional anesthesia
- Nerve plexus block
- Spinal (intrathecal) block
- Epidural block

NERVE CONDUCTION BLOCKING AGENTS

Nerve conduction blocking agents are used to prevent initiation and/or transmission of impulses along an individual nerve pathway or at a nerve plexus providing anesthesia or lack of sensation to tissues adjacent or distal to the injection site. They act by competing for calcium sites in nerve sheaths, inhibiting sodium transportation in the sodium-potassium pump, thereby preventing impulse transmission. These agents are commonly referred to as *local* or *regional anesthetics*. Nerve conduction blocking agents are used in low concentrations (0.25–4%), with the exception of cocaine hydrochloride, which is commonly

Table 9-8 Commonly Used Nerve Conduction Blocking Agents

TYPE	NAME	BRAND NAME(S)
Amino amides	Lidocaine hydrochloride	Xylocaine, Lignocaine
	Mepivacaine hydrochloride	Carbocaine
	Bupivacaine hydrochloride	Marcaine, Sensorcaine
	Etidocaine hydrochloride	Duranest
Amino esters	Cocaine hydrochloride	
	Procaine hydrochloride	Novocaine
	Tetracaine hydrochloride	Pontocaine, Cetacaine

used in slightly higher concentrations (up to 10%). The agents are divided into two groups: the amino amides and the amino esters (Table 9-8).

AMINO AMIDE GROUP

Drugs in the amino amide group are metabolized in the liver and excreted by the kidneys and include lidocaine hydrochloride (Xylocaine, Lignocaine), mepivacaine hydrochloride (Carbocaine), bupivacaine hydrochloride (Marcaine, Sensorcaine), and etidocaine hydrochloride (Duranest). Toxicity may occur in patients with liver disease.

Lidocaine hydrochloride (Xylocaine, Lignocaine) is the most widely used local anesthetic agent with a rapid onset of action with moderate duration. Lidocaine HCl can be administered topically for application on mucous membranes, infiltrated locally for peripheral nerve block, or injected epidurally to provide regional block. The maximum dosage of lidocaine HCl for infiltration is 7 mg/kg of body weight, or 500 mg. Available in concentrations ranging from 0.5 to 5%, lidocaine HCl is prepackaged with or without epinephrine. (*Note:* Lidocaine also has properties that affect the function of the heart.)

Mepivacaine hydrochloride (Carbocaine) acts similarly to lidocaine HCl but has a longer action. It is commonly used for local infiltration. Mepivacaine HCl has a maximum dosage of 500 mg or 5–6 mg/kg. It is commonly used for patients who are hypertensive, since mepivacaine HCl does not usually produce a significant rise in blood pressure.

Bupivacaine hydrochloride (Marcaine, Sensorcaine) is an agent that is four times more potent than lidocaine HCl. It has a longer onset of action and a longer duration of effect. It is commonly administered by local infiltration or injected for regional block. In concentrations less than 1%, bupivacaine HCl also comes prepackaged without or with epinephrine. The maximum dosage of bupivacaine is 400 mg in a 24-hour period, with a maximum dosage at each administration of 175 mg plain or 225 mg with epinephrine 1:200,000. Concentrations of 0.75% bupivacaine produce complete motor blockade as well as sensory blockade; lesser concentrations may only produce sensory blockade. Lidocaine HCl and bupivacaine HCl may be combined to provide an agent for infiltration, which has a rapid onset of anesthesia with prolonged duration.

Etidocaine hydrochloride (Duranest) is an agent with a prolonged onset and long duration of action. Used in concentrations of less than 2%, etidocaine HCl is used as a topical agent in operative wounds, minimizing postoperative surgical site discomfort. The drug is highly toxic; therefore, its use is contraindicated in children younger than 12 years of age. The maximum recommended dose of etidocaine is 400 mg or 8 mg/kg.

AMINO ESTER GROUP

Drugs in the amino ester group are biotransformed by pseudocholinesterase (produced by the liver) in plasma and include cocaine hydrochloride, procaine hydrochloride (Novocaine), and tetracaine hydrochloride (Pontocaine, Cetacaine).

Cocaine hydrochloride, a CNS stimulant, is one of the oldest recorded anesthetic agents, its use being documented in the 16th century as an agent used to control pain during trephination of the skull. Cocaine HCl is still used in OR practice today, but only as a topical agent on mucosa of the upper aerodigestive tract due to its high toxicity. It is the most widely used topical anesthetic and is classified as a controlled substance. In concentrations of 4–10%, cocaine HCl produces anesthesia and vasoconstriction, causing shrinkage of mucous membranes. The maximum dose of cocaine HCl is 200 mg or 4 mg/kg of body weight. Cocaine is metabolized in the liver and excreted by the kidneys.

Procaine hydrochloride (Novocaine) has similar properties to cocaine HCl but is less toxic. Available for SC, IM, or intrathecal injection, its use in the surgical setting is limited, as newer, safer agents are developed.

Tetracaine hydrochloride (Cetacaine, Pontocaine) is an agent with a slow onset of action but prolonged duration. It is not used for infiltration or peripheral nerve block. Its primary uses are as a topical anesthetic on oropharyngeal mucous membranes and ocular mucous membranes or for intrathecal injection during spinal anesthesia administration.

ADJUNCTIVE AGENTS TO NERVE CONDUCTION BLOCKADE

Two adjunctive agents commonly associated with nerve conduction blockade agents influence the onset and duration of action of these agents. These agents include hyaluronidase (Wydase) and epinephrine (Adrenalin).

Hyaluronidase (Wydase) is an agent added to local infiltration agents to assist in their distribution into the subcutaneous tissues for contact with the peripheral nerves. This is especially useful during retrobulbar block. The usual dose is 150 units added to the anesthetic solution.

Epinephrine (Adrenalin) is a potent vasoconstrictor. Because of its vasoconstrictive properties, the use of epinephrine as an adjunctive agent to nerve conduction blocking agents provides two main benefits for the patient and the surgeon. First, the area's blood supply is limited and intraoperative bleeding is reduced. Second, also because the blood supply to the area is limited, the body is unable to redistribute the anesthetic agent effectively, prolonging the overall anesthetic effect.

Caution must be exercised in administering epinephrine to patients with hypertension or cardiac disease because of its side effects. Epinephrine use should be limited during administration of a digital or penile block, for use in tissue with preexisting vascular compromise, and in small children because of its vasoconstrictive properties.

As a convenience, epinephrine is available premixed by the manufacturer with lidocaine HCl or bupivacaine HCl in concentrations ranging from 1:1000 (1 mg/mL) to 1:200,000 (0.005 mg/mL). The label of these premixed agents is usually color coded red to indicate the addition of epinephrine.

TOPICAL ANESTHESIA

Topical anesthesia involves the placement of a nerve conduction-blocking agent onto a tissue layer (skin or mucous membrane). This method is used to provide anesthesia on mucous membranes of the upper aerodigestive tract, urethra, vagina, rectum, and skin. The tissue affected is limited to the area in contact with the topical anesthetic, onset is rapid, and duration of action is usually related to the specific agent and dose used. Topical anesthesia is usually administered by the surgeon and is achieved with either the use of cryoanesthesia and/or a pharmacological agent.

Cryoanesthesia involves the reduction of nerve conduction/transmission by localized cooling. This may be accomplished with ice or the use of a cryoanesthesia machine to produce the cooling action, or the reduced skin temperature may be a result of a pharmaceutical agent sprayed onto the skin, such as ethyl chloride. In any case, the result is a localized "freezing" of the skin and superficial nerve endings, blocking nerve impulse transmission and, therefore, eliminating pain.

Pharmaceutical agents applied directly to the skin are absorbed and come in contact with the peripheral nerve endings providing anesthesia by preventing the initiation of the nerve impulse. Lidocaine and cocaine are examples of topical anesthetic agents.

LOCAL ANESTHESIA

Local infiltration involves the injection of a nerve conduction-blocking agent into the tissues surrounding a peripheral nerve or nerves that serve only the tissue at the site of surgical intervention. The onset, depending on the agent used, occurs within 5–15 minutes. The duration of action depends on the agent used and may be prolonged by the addition of epinephrine or hyaluronidase to the anesthetic agent. The surgeon usually administers the local anesthetic, and readministration may be necessary as the surgical site is expanded or additional tissue layers are exposed.

MONITORED ANESTHESIA CARE

Monitored anesthesia care (MAC) involves a combination of nerve conduction blockade on the topical or local level that is supplemented with analgesics, sedatives, or amnesics. It is indicated for some patients with complex medical problems or as a supplement to local anesthesia to provide amnesia during local anesthesia injection. The surgeon commonly performs nerve conduction blockade, with patient monitoring and IV sedation/analgesia performed by the anesthesia provider.

REGIONAL ANESTHESIA

Regional blockade involves the administration of an anesthetic, usually by the anesthesia provider, along a major nerve tract. This technique blocks conduction from all tissues distal to the injection site. Onset of action is slower than with local infiltration, and the duration is agent dependent. Common types of regional blockade include the nerve plexus block, Bier block, spinal block, and epidural block.

NERVE PLEXUS BLOCK

Nerve plexus block is usually accomplished with the injection of an anesthetic solution in an area of a major plexus, such as the brachial plexus or at the base of a structure. The resulting anesthesia includes all tissue innervated by the plexus. Commonly used in conjunction with IV sedation, plexus blockade permits the administration of a safer, less systemically impacting anesthetic experience while permitting analgesia to continue through the immediate postoperative/recovery phase. Nerve plexus blocks have surgical, diagnostic, and therapeutic applications.

BIER BLOCK

Bier block provides anesthesia to the distal portion of the upper extremity by injecting an anesthetic agent into a vein at a level below a tourniquet. A double-cuffed tourniquet is placed on the upper arm, and venous access is obtained by the placement of a catheter close to the intended site of surgical intervention. The limb is then exsanguinated with the use of an Esmarch bandage, and the proximal cuff of the tourniquet is inflated to a level approximately 100 mm Hg above the systolic blood pressure. The inflated cuff provides a containment system for the IV anesthetic agent and provides a bloodless surgical field. Once the agent has been injected via the IV catheter, the catheter is removed. The agent is absorbed into the surrounding tissues through the vein walls. The tourniquet remains inflated for the duration of desired anesthesia, preventing normal circulation from redistributing the anesthetic agent. Should the patient experience discomfort related to the tourniquet, the distal cuff may be inflated after limb anesthesia has been established and the proximal cuff released. Bier block is used on interventions of the extremity of 1-hour duration or less. At the conclusion of the surgical intervention, the tourniquet is slowly released, permitting the agent to circulate throughout the body. Inadvertent systemic administration of the anesthetic agent could occur during injection due to tourniquet failure, or when releasing the tourniquet, and may cause adverse cardiovascular or CNS effects.

SPINAL BLOCK

Spinal anesthesia, also referred to as intrathecal block, is injection of an anesthetic agent into the cerebrospinal fluid (CSF) in the subarachnoid space between the meningeal layers of the spinal cord to provide loss of sensation to the entire body below the diaphragm. The procedure for spinal administration is as follows:

- The circulator assists the patient into the desired position and stands by to help the patient safely maintain the position and to provide emotional support.
- The lower lumbar area is cleansed (prepped) and draped with a fenestrated sheet.
- Prior to placement of the spinal needle, a small amount of local anesthetic is placed into the subcutaneous tissues along the intended needle path to maximize patient comfort and cooperation.
- Access to the subarachnoid space is achieved by the insertion of a fine-gauge, 3-in. spinal needle through the tissues of the L2–3 or L3–4 disk spaces of the vertebral column.
- Correct needle placement is confirmed by the presence of CSF in the needle hub when the needle stylet is removed.
- The syringe containing the anesthetic is gently connected to the spinal needle, ensuring that air is not allowed to enter the system.
- The agent is then slowly injected, and the needle is removed. A dressing may be applied.
- The patient is repositioned for the intended procedure.

Onset of effect is seen within 3–10 minutes. Spinal anesthesia lasts approximately 1–1½ hours, depending on the agent used. Additives to the anesthetic solution may prolong the action of the agent. (*Note:* The procedure for obtaining spinal fluid for analysis is similar to the one just described, but instead of injecting the anesthetic, spinal fluid is withdrawn. This is commonly called a *spinal tap.*)

Special Considerations

Several factors can influence the effect of the spinal anesthetic:

- *Patient cooperation:* Patient cooperation is critical to the successful administration of spinal anesthesia. Patients are commonly sedated prior to needle placement to reduce anxiety and promote cooperation.
- *Position:* The patient is usually positioned in the lateral or sitting position, depending on the administrator's preference, the patient's primary and/or secondary medical conditions, and the patient's ability to cooperate. It is possible to administer a spinal anesthetic with the patient in the prone position, but this is rarely done. Whatever the position of choice, the goal is to expose the intervertebral spaces to allow for needle placement (Figure 9-12).
- *Agent baricity: Baricity,* in spinal anesthesia, refers to the specific gravity of the anesthetic solution in comparison to CSF. Solutions with high specific gravity are referred to as hyperbaric solutions and tend to settle toward gravity. Inversely, a solution with low specific gravity is referred to as a hypobaric solution and tends to "float" or move away from gravity. Isobaric solutions are solutions with the same specific gravity as CSF.

Prior to administration, the anesthetic agent may be altered with sterile injectable water or sterile injectable dextrose solution to create one of the three baricities. This, in conjunction with the patient's position following agent

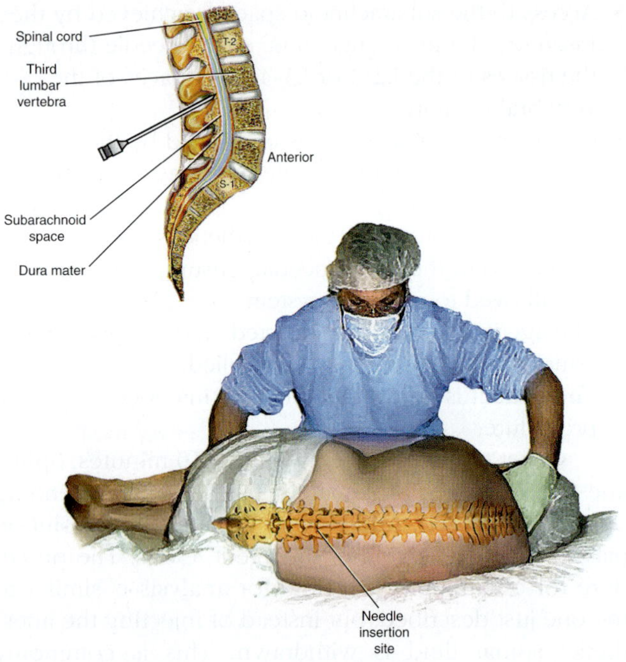

Figure 9-12 Positioning for spinal anesthesia

administration, will be the principal determinant of agent contact and effect.

The most common baricity used is the hyperbaric spinal. The patient is positioned with the operative side in the dependent position. Following agent administration, the patient will remain in this position while the agent settles and affects the nerve roots of the dependent area.

A hypobaric spinal is used for patients undergoing procedures in the prone position. The patient is positioned immediately following agent administration, permitting the agent to settle around the nerve roots of the sacral and caudal areas.

- *Rate of injection:* The rate of agent injection will affect the agent's placement. Rapid injection will promote turbulence as the medication combines with CSF. This may cause the agent to spread over a larger area of nerve roots, resulting in an increased area of effect.
- *Increased CSF pressure:* An increase in CSF pressure may result from the position of the operating table, coughing, straining, or muscle contraction. This can occur in the patient who has a uterine contraction immediately following agent placement, or it may occur during patient self-repositioning following agent placement. An increase in pressure may result in migration of the anesthetic agent and unintended contact with nerve roots controlling major body functions (e.g., respiration). Spinal anesthesia may cause a loss in the sensations associated with breathing or may, in fact, cause loss of sensory and/or motor function of the diaphragm. Should this occur, respiratory assistance is necessary until function is restored.

Spinal Anesthetic Agents and Additives

The most commonly used agent for spinal anesthesia administration is tetracaine hydrochloride. Other agents for use in spinal anesthesia administration include lidocaine hydrochloride and procaine hydrochloride.

Duration of the anesthetic may be enhanced with the addition of epinephrine to the anesthetic solution, preventing rapid redistribution of the agent. Postoperative pain management may also be performed during the same injection by the addition of an intrathecal opioid.

Advantages of Spinal Anesthesia

Spinal anesthesia is advantageous for several reasons. The patient will remain conscious during spinal anesthesia, permitting the patient to remain in control of his airway. Many patients choose not to be fully aware of the surgical environment, and spinal anesthesia is easily supplemented with IV sedation, which induces a lighter, more natural sleep without the systemic effects of a general anesthetic.

Spinal anesthesia is nonirritating to the respiratory tree. Patients do not experience the discomfort of endotracheal intubation or the irritation sometimes caused to mucous membranes of the upper respiratory tract from exposure to inhalation agents.

Spinal anesthesia blockade of the sympathetic and parasympathetic nervous system produces bowel contraction, facilitating exposure within the abdominal cavity during surgical interventions of the abdomen or pelvis.

Spinal anesthesia is also an excellent muscle relaxant, permitting ease of retraction of the abdominal wall without additional pharmacological intervention.

Disadvantages and Complications of Spinal Anesthesia

Some of the disadvantages and complications of spinal anesthesia will be described.

Induced hypotension is a common problem. Following agent administration, blood vessels innervated by the blocked pathways dilate, resulting in pooling of a significant volume of blood. This results in the hypotension commonly seen immediately following injection. It may continue for a period of time until the body's homeostatic mechanisms can adjust. Blood pressure can drop significantly, leading to ischemic-related issues such as angina or myocardial infarction or cerebrovascular accident in patients who are predisposed to these conditions.

Hypotension is treated in several ways. Patients undergoing spinal anesthesia administration are pretreated with a bolus dose of IV fluids during the immediate preoperative period. This provides a readily available source of fluid support to the circulatory system to counteract venous pooling. Higher than normal volume fluid delivery is continued postinjection for those patients able to manage fluid loading.

Following spinal anesthesia agent administration, hypotensive episodes are detected with close monitoring of blood pressure and mean arterial pressure. If a hypotensive crisis is detected, the patient is treated with IV ephedrine administration. Ephedrine is a potent vasoconstrictor, resulting in a rise in blood pressure. When this treatment does not result in significant blood pressure stabilization, the patient may be treated with phenylephrine (Neo-Synephrine).

Nausea or vomiting may be induced by the administration of spinal anesthesia. Hypotensive episodes cause the body to shunt blood away from the gastrointestinal organs. Cerebral ischemia and rapid gastric emptying occur in response to reduced blood flow, resulting in nausea and, commonly, vomiting. Vomiting may also be induced by traction on visceral organs of the abdominal cavity during interventions of the gastrointestinal tract or pelvis.

Dosage control presents another problem. The agent, once delivered to the patient, cannot be titrated or adjusted. The anesthesia provider must use methods other than titration and dose adjustment to manage the side effects and complications of the agent's effects.

Spinal headache is a less frequent complication of spinal anesthesia. Spinal headache results from meningeal layer irritation resulting from a drop in CSF pressure. This commonly occurs as a result of fluid leaking through the dural puncture site. Primary treatment for "spinal headache" includes bedrest, lying in a horizontal position (prone position is the best choice, but impractical), and the administration of increased fluids, either by mouth or parenterally. For persistent fluid leakage, a blood patch may be performed. A blood patch involves the creation of a clot over the dural puncture site by the injection of the patient's blood at the site of leakage.

The potential exists for patients to develop temporary or permanent paraesthesia or paralysis related to spinal anesthesia administration. This may be due to inadvertent patient movement during needle placement, inadvertent injection directly into a nerve, or sepsis related to breaks in sterile technique during administration.

EPIDURAL ANESTHESIA

Epidural anesthesia involves the administration of an anesthetic agent into the tissues directly above the dura mater, through which the agent is then absorbed into the CSF. The epidural can be administered with a single injection to provide anesthesia of short duration. More commonly, a lumbar approach is used to place an indwelling catheter. The catheter is secured and left in place, permitting titration of the agent's effect by permitting readministration of additional agent as the patient's condition warrants. When no longer necessary, the catheter is removed.

The rate and volume of agent delivered at any given time influence the level or area of anesthesia obtained. The more rapidly a bolus of medication is delivered and the larger the volume given in any one injection, the more likely the agent is to spread through the tissue, causing an effect on a larger number of nerve fibers. Patient position and baricity of the anesthetic solution have little to no effect on the level of anesthesia obtained.

CAUDAL ANESTHESIA

Caudal anesthesia is a type of epidural anesthesia that involves the administration of a nerve conduction-blocking agent into the epidural space of the sacral canal. Used primarily in obstetrics for painless childbirth, caudal anesthesia is being replaced by epidural anesthesia.

NONTRADITIONAL ANESTHESIA OPTIONS

Several options for nontraditional therapy are in use today. These may be used alone or to supplement more traditional anesthesia approaches.

Hypnoanesthesia is an adjunctive therapy useful in altering the patient's level of consciousness and awareness of the surgical environment. The patient must be totally compliant and the hypnotherapist must accompany the patient throughout the procedure. On a more practical level, hypnotherapy is particularly useful during the induction stages of general anesthesia for children undergoing mask induction, focusing the child's attention on a familiar or predetermined thought or activity, making her less aware of the induction agent and mask aromas. The anesthesia provider often implements this type of hypnosis.

Acupuncture involves the intense electrical stimulation of specific body sites to alter the perception of pain at the surgical site by the release of endorphins. While a common principal method of intraoperative pain control in Eastern medicine practices, acupuncture is used as an adjunctive therapy in the United States.

TEAM MEMBER ROLES DURING ANESTHESIA ADMINISTRATION

Every surgical team member has a responsibility to the patient during anesthesia administration. Tables 9-9 through 9-13 list those responsibilities with respect to each type of anesthesia. These are typical examples of the chain of events starting in the preoperative waiting (holding) area through admission to the PACU. General

Table 9-9 Preoperative Visit in Waiting Area

ROLE RESPONSIBILITY	CIRCULATOR	ANESTHESIA PROVIDER
1. Introduce self and state reason for visit (assure patient privacy).	X	X
2. Identify patient and verify biographic information (e.g., age, gender, social history).	X	X
3. Review patient chart for completeness (e.g., history and physical, consent[s], reports of diagnostic studies).	X	X
4. Note physical findings (e.g., height, weight, allergies, NPO status, vital signs, medication history, level of consciousness, presence of any physical or sensory defects, presence of pain, existing wounds).	X	X
5. Note mental and emotional status (be certain that the patient has an accurate understanding of events about to occur).	X	X
6. Read surgeon's orders and be sure that all orders have been completed (e.g., bowel preparation, preoperative medications that may include prophylactic antibiotics).	X	X
7. Provide basic orientation information to the patient pertaining to the OR and PACU experiences.	X	X
8. Allow the patient (and family or friends with the patient, if appropriate) an opportunity to express concerns and ask questions.	X	X
9. Provide emotional support as needed and answer any questions asked. Questions may be redirected, to the surgeon, for example, if interviewer is not able to answer.	X	X
10. Order any diagnostic studies and/or consults with other physicians (e.g., cardiologist) regarding patient's condition.		X
11. Order or administer premedication if necessary.		X
12. Assign patient risk status according to ASA guidelines.		X
13. Be sure all preoperative duties have been carried out (e.g., patient appropriately attired, IV inserted and patent, jewelry removed, necessary prosthesis removed).	X	
14. Formulate a plan of care specific to this patient's needs.	X	X
15. Transport patient to OR.	X	Anesthesia provider may assist with transport if available.

and spinal anesthetic situations will be used as illustrative procedures.

PREOPERATIVE VISITS

In most circumstances, the patient is visited in the preoperative waiting area by both the anesthesia provider and the circulator (Table 9-9). This interview may be conducted separately or jointly as much of the same information is obtained or verified by both team members. This is also an opportunity for patient education. The surgeon will often visit to answer any final questions and offer emotional support.

PREOPERATIVE ROUTINE—ALL TYPES OF ANESTHESIA

Each team member contributes to preoperative care in different ways. These roles are summarized in Table 9-10.

TEAM MEMBER DUTIES DURING GENERAL ANESTHESIA

Each team member also contributes during the induction of anesthesia and the anesthetized state. Some common contributions are listed in Table 9-11.

Table 9-10 Routine Preoperative Tasks

ANESTHESIA PROVIDER	CIRCULATOR	STSR	SURGEON
	Transports patient to operating room Has patient transfer to operating table; assists as needed; ensures safety and comfort	Greets patient; introduces self Makes a mental assessment of the patient's size and condition to anticipate items that may be needed for the procedure	
Introduces and applies monitoring devices (e.g., temperature, blood pressure, ECG, pulse oximeter)	Applies monitoring devices as needed; secures arms on armboards; protects ulnar nerves Ensures suction is set up and turned on	Keeps conversation and preparatory noise to a minimum (e.g., do not clank the instruments)	
Induction of anesthesia begins	Resuscitation devices should be readily available if needed		Is available to assist if needed

Table 9-11 Tasks During General Anesthesia Induction and Maintenance

ANESTHESIA PROVIDER	CIRCULATOR	STSR	SURGEON
May preoxygenate patient	Stays at patient's side (usually the right) to provide emotional support for the patient and assistance for the anesthesia provider	Maintains quiet environment while completing preparatory tasks	Is available to assist if needed
Induction begins with IV or inhalation agents	Has suction available	Absolute quiet may be requested at this time; preparatory activities may be halted momentarily	
Provides oxygen support as needed	Observes and monitors patient for any change; reports as necessary		
Intubates patient if planned	Assists with intubation by providing suction, passing instruments and supplies as needed; be prepared to apply cricoid pressure	The possibility of a tracheotomy exists if severe airway problems arise	
Verifies ET tube placement and secures tube	Provides stethoscope	Observes and monitors patient for any change; reports as necessary	

(continues)

Table 9-11 ***(continued)***

ANESTHESIA PROVIDER	CIRCULATOR	STSR	SURGEON
Gives permission for other preoperative activities to begin	Final preparations are achieved (e.g., Foley catheter insertion, application of antiembolic stockings, final positioning, shave, skin prep)	Consults with surgeon as needed; variations specific to the patient may be made in suture or medication routine	Confers with OR team about any specific patient variances in the procedure; assists with patient preparation and positioning if needed; scrubs for procedure
Monitors patient and records necessary information; titrates anesthetic agents as needed; administers IV fluids as needed	Observes patient for any significant changes; reports as necessary; assists sterile team members with gowns	Assists other sterile team members to don sterile attire and assists with draping patient for procedure	Enters OR and prepares for procedure
Maintains optimal homeostatic conditions for the patient and surgeon; reports any significant changes in patient's condition to the surgeon	Receives supplies from the sterile field and attaches as necessary (e.g., electrosurgical cord and suction tubing); turns on operating lights; positions furniture for procedure; provides supplies for patient care as needed to anesthesia provider; helps maintain a sterile field; records operative events on appropriate forms	Passes supplies to circulator to be connected to appropriate devices; positions sterile furniture for use; provides instruments and supplies for surgeon as needed	Initiates incision and performs necessary surgical maneuvers; reports any significant changes in operative plan or patient's condition to anesthesia provider
Allows emergence from anesthetic agents	Performs closing counts; provides dressing material	Provides suture and supplies for closing and accomplishes closing counts	Terminates surgery; surgeon is advised of accuracy of counts
Patient is extubated if planned	Stands by patient; has suction available; notifies PACU staff that patient will be arriving (gives estimated time, if possible) and advises of any special condition or equipment that will be necessary	Applies dressings; removes drapes	Leaves sterile field to write postoperative orders and dictate operative report
Helps transfer patient to gurney or bed and transports to PACU	Assists with transfer and transport	Maintains sterile field until patient is out of operating room; may need to provide assistance with the patient	Assists with transfer and transport as needed

TEAM MEMBER DUTIES DURING SPINAL ANESTHESIA

Spinal anesthesia requires a variation in routines. These are summarized in Table 9-12.

POSTANESTHESIA CARE

Following the surgical procedure, duties change relative to termination of the anesthetized state (usually), transferral of the patient to the PACU, and initiation of postoperative care. These duties are summarized in Table 9-13.

Table 9-12 Duties During Spinal Anesthesia

ANESTHESIA PROVIDER	CIRCULATOR	STSR	SURGEON
Indicates preference for patient position	Prepares necessary positioning supplies	Maintains quiet environment while completing preparatory tasks	Is available to assist as needed
May provide oxygen support and sedation	Assists with oxygen apparatus as needed		
Assists patient with positioning and verifies that position is accurate	Assists with patient positioning and remains at patient's side to provide emotional support and to help the patient maintain the position		
Opens sterile supplies; dons sterile gloves; preps patient's skin	Continues to assist patient in maintenance of the position; informs patient of what to expect (e.g., prep solution may be cold)		
Administers local anesthetic and introduces spinal needle	Encourages patient to remain still	Anesthesia provider may insist on absolute quiet at this time	
Verifies needle placement and introduces anesthetic	Patient must remain still and not strain Observes patient and monitors for any change; reports as necessary	Observes patient and monitors for any change; reports as necessary	
Gives permission for patient to be repositioned	Assists patient to operative position; ensures safety and comfort		Assists with patient positioning if needed
Gives permission for other preoperative activities to begin	Final preparations are, achieved (e.g., Foley catheter insertion, application of antiembolic stockings, shave, skin prep)	Remembers that patient is and will remain awake for the entire procedure; consults with the surgeon as needed; variations specific to the patient may be made in suture or medication routine	Assists with patient preparation as necessary; confers with OR team about any specific patient variations in the procedure; scrubs for procedure

(continues)

Table 9-12 *(continued)*

ANESTHESIA PROVIDER	CIRCULATOR	STSR	SURGEON
Monitors patient and records information; introduces supplementary sedation as needed	Observes patient for any significant changes and reports as needed; assists sterile team members with gowns	Assists other sterile team members to don sterile attire and assists with draping patient for procedure	Enters OR and prepares for procedure
Provides ventilatory support if necessary; administers IV fluids as needed	Receives supplies from the sterile field and attaches as necessary (e.g., electrosurgical cord and suction tubing); turns on operating lights; positions furniture for procedure	Passes supplies to circulator to be connected to appropriate devices; positions sterile furniture for use	
Anesthesia provider may request (or the surgeon may desire) to test the operative site prior to making the incision to be sure that the anesthesia is complete	Quietly stands by patient to provide support if needed, without alarming the patient	Provides device necessary for test; often a needle or tissue forceps with teeth is used	Ensures that the anesthesia is complete; offers assurance to the patient
Maintains optimal conditions for the patient and surgeon; reports any significant changes in the patient's condition to the surgeon	Provides supplies for patient care as needed to anesthesia provider and sterile field; records operative events on appropriate forms	Provides instruments and supplies for surgeon as needed	Caution is used when discussing the patient's condition or requesting instruments so that the patient does not become alarmed (e.g., the surgeon may ask for the Bard Parker, which is a brand of knife blade rather than using the word "knife!"); initiates incision and performs necessary surgical maneuvers; reports any significant changes in operative plan or patient's condition to anesthesia provider
Raises patient's level of consciousness as needed	Performs closing counts; provides dressing material	Provides suture and supplies for closing and accomplishes closing counts	Terminates surgery; surgeon is advised of accuracy of counts

Table 9-12 ***(continued)***

ANESTHESIA PROVIDER	CIRCULATOR	STSR	SURGEON
	Notifies PACU staff that patient will be arriving (give estimated time, if possible) and advises of any special condition or equipment that will be necessary	Applies dressings; removes drapes	Leaves sterile field to write postoperative orders and dictate operative report
Helps transfer the patient to gurney or bed and transports to PACU	Assists with transfer and transport	Maintains sterile field until patient is out of the OR; may need to provide assistance with the patient	Assists with transfer and transport

Table 9-13 Postanesthesia Duties

ANESTHESIA PROVIDER	CIRCULATOR	PACU CAREGIVER	SURGEON
Main responsibility during transport is airway and ventilation	Guides and propels transport device to PACU	Directs OR team with patient to proper cubicle; has suction and monitoring equipment ready	Completes written postoperative orders; accompanies patient to PACU
Gives verbal patient status report to PACU caregiver	Locks transport device in place; assists PACU caregiver with patient care	Provides ventilatory support as needed; applies monitoring devices as needed; listens to verbal report from anesthesia provider	Gives verbal orders as needed; stands by to lend assistance if needed
Ensures patency of airway	Gives verbal patient status report to PACU caregiver	Obtains baseline vital signs and reports to surgeon and anesthesia provider and documents results	Locates patient's family or friends and reports status if appropriate
May leave the immediate area when patient is stable but should remain available for unexpected events and patient discharge	Turns care over to PACU caregiver	Monitors patient, provides ventilatory support as needed; provides ordered medications for pain control as ordered; administers medications and fluids as ordered; maintains dressings as needed; provides emotional support as required	May leave the immediate area when patient is stable, but should remain available for unexpected events

(continues)

Table 9-13 (continued)

ANESTHESIA PROVIDER	CIRCULATOR	PACU CAREGIVER	SURGEON
Discharges patient from PACU when discharge criteria are met		Patient usually remains in PACU for a minimum of 1 hour, longer if necessary; patient is discharged when specific predetermined criteria are met and on the order of a physician	Notifies PACU staff, often by way of written orders, of patient discharge status (e.g., home, hospital ward room, intensive care unit) for which prior arrangements have been made (e.g., hospital room reserved); however, this may be changed according to the patient's condition

CASE STUDY

Tyrone is a healthy 19-year-old athlete at the local college. He has been admitted to the hospital for "outpatient" surgery, an arthroscopic examination of his right knee. Shortly after the administration of the anesthetic agent, the anesthesia provider notices that Tyrone is producing a high amount of carbon dioxide, his muscles appear rigid, and the monitor shows a mild tachycardia and a rapid increase in temperature.

1. What condition is likely affecting Tyrone? Is it dangerous?
2. What are the steps that need to be taken in order to treat this condition?
3. What medication is routinely given for this condition?

QUESTIONS FOR FURTHER STUDY

1. What is cricoid pressure and when is it used?
2. Why might bupivacaine be a better choice of local anesthetic than lidocaine?
3. What is the primary difference between spinal and epidural anesthesia?
4. How are certain medications affected by the hepatic first pass effect?
5. Describe the necessary equipment and procedure used to evoke and evaluate a train-of-four response.
6. Is the placental barrier effective in protecting the fetal environment? Why or why not?

BIBLIOGRAPHY

American Society of Anesthesiologists [Online]. Available from *http://www.asahq.org*

Asperheim, M. K. (1996). *Pharmacology: An introductory text* (8th ed.). Philadelphia: W. B. Saunders.

Bispectral Index™ monitoring [Online]. Available from *http://www.aspectms.com*

Division of Anaesthesiology & Intensive Care of the University of Queensland [Online]. Available from *http://gasbone.herston.uq.edu.au/gasbone.html*

Dripps, R., Eckenhoff, J., & Vandam, L. (1988). *Introduction to anesthesia—The principles of safe practice* (7th ed.). Philadelphia: W. B. Saunders.

Drug Enforcement Agency—Controlled Substances Act [Online]. Available from *http://www.usdoj.gov/dea/pubs/csa.htm*

Egan, T. Remifentanil: An esterase-metabolized opioid [Online]. Available from *http://web2.searchbank.com*

Evans, T. J. The unusual history of "ether" [Online]. Available from *http://www.anesthesia-nursing.com/ether.html*

Fearnley, S. Pulse oximetry. Nuffield Department of Anaesthetics University of Oxford [Online]. Available from *http://www.nda.ox.ac.uk*

Greater Houston Anesthesiology [Online]. Available from *GHAMD@chooseGHA.com*

Hurford, W., Bailin, M., Davison, J., Haspel, K., & Rosow, C. (1998). *Clinical anesthesia procedures of the Massachusetts General Hospital* (5th ed.). Philadelphia: Lippincott-Raven.

Lewis, S., & Collier, I. (1992). *Medical-surgical nursing: Assessment and management of clinical problems* (3rd ed.). St. Louis, MO: Mosby-Year Book.

Malignant Hyperthermia Association of the United States (MHAUS) [Online]. Available from *http://www.mhaus.org/whatismh.html*

McGuiness, A. M., et al. (2002). *Core curriculum for surgical technology* (5th ed.). Centennial, CO: Association of Surgical Technologists.

Miller, R. (1994). *Anesthesia* (4th ed.). New York: Churchill Livingstone.

Pinosky, M. Laryngeal mask airway: Uses in anesthesiology. Southern Medical Association [Online]. Available from *http://www.sma.org*

Salerno, E. (1999). *Pharmacology for health professionals.* St. Louis, MO: Mosby.

Snyder, K., & Keegan, C. (1998). *Pharmacology for the surgical technologist.* Philadelphia: W. B. Saunders.

Spratto, G. R., & Woods, A. L. *Delmar's A–Z NDR—98.* Clifton Park. NY: Delmar Learning.

Wingard, L. B., Brody, T. M., Larner, J., & Schwartz, A. S. (1991). *Human pharmacology: Molecular-to-clinical.* St. Louis, MO: Mosby-Year Book.

Yale Medical School. Managing malignant hyperthermia [Online]. Available from *http://gasnet.med.yale.edu/gta/ mh/clinicalupdate.html*

CHAPTER 10

Instrumentation, Equipment, and Supplies

Paul Price

CASE STUDY

Maria is a surgical technology student working a rotation in the sterile processing department. She has been asked to gather instrumentation and supplies for an emergency procedure involving a gunshot wound to the chest. The patient has just arrived in the emergency department, and the ER nurse has advised the OR team that the patient will be stabilized and on the way to the OR soon.

1. What equipment should be in the room for this procedure?
2. What supplies should be gathered?
3. What instrument sets should be gathered?
4. With limited time, what supplies should be opened first, and what supplies should be opened later?

OBJECTIVES

After studying this chapter, the reader should be able to:

C 1. Discuss the relationship between instrumentation, equipment, and supplies and quality patient care in the OR.

A 2. Identify items that require sterilization prior to use in the sterile field.

R 3. Identify basic instruments by type, function, and name.

4. Demonstrate proper care, handling, and assembly of instruments.
5. Identify types of special equipment utilized in OR practice and demonstrate proper care, handling techniques, and safety precautions.

6. Identify the names and functions of accessory equipment and demonstrate proper care, handling, and assembly.
7. Identify and prepare supplies used in the OR.

E 8. Discuss the relationship between instruments, equipment, and supplies and the OR environment as related to safety.

SELECT KEY TERMS

1. ancillary	8. defibrillator	16. pneumatic	21. stainless steel
2. aperture	9. drain	17. resistance	22. teeth
3. bipolar electrosurgery	10. fenestration	18. retract	23. tube
4. capillary action	11. insufflation	19. scalpel	24. ureteral
5. catheter	12. irrigation	20. serrations	25. urethral
6. cottonoid	13. magnification		
7. cryo-	14. monopolar cautery		
	15. Nd:YAG		

INSTRUMENTATION

Most modern surgical instruments are made of **stainless steel**, which is a combination of carbon, chromium, iron, and a few other metals (alloys). This combination of metals adds strength to the instrument and resistance to corrosion during repeated sterilizations. Instruments with a high percentage of carbon are harder than those with less carbon and are therefore less likely to wear. Chromium increases **resistance** to corrosion.

Manufacturers of surgical instruments add one of three types of finish during fabrication. A highly polished, bright finish increases resistance to corrosion but can be distracting to the surgical team because of its tendency to reflect light. A satin (dull) finish is less reflective and reduces glare. An ebonized (black chromium) finish is nonreflective and virtually eliminates glare. This type of finish is useful for procedures involving a laser because it prevents deflection of the laser beam.

CLASSIFICATIONS

Instruments are classified as cutting/dissecting, grasping/holding, clamping/occluding, retracting/viewing, probing, dilating, suturing, and suctioning. Other instruments that do not fit easily into these classifications are referred to as accessory instruments. These include the ring forceps, used to grasp a folded X-ray-detectable 4-in. × 4-in. sponge for sponging or retraction deep within a wound (with the sponge, it is referred to as a sponge stick); curved ring forceps, which may be used to create tunnels for placement of catheters or arterial grafts; and towel clips, used to hold folded towels together during square-draping and occasionally to grasp, hold, and reduce small fractured bones.

CUTTING/DISSECTING

Instruments with one or more sharp edges that are used for incision, sharp dissection, or excision of tissue are classified as cutting/dissecting instruments. These typically include knives, scalpels, scissors, and bone-cutting instruments (osteotomes, curettes, chisels, gouges, and rongeurs). Saws, drills, biopsy punches, adenotomes, and dermatomes may also be classified as cutting instruments. *Note:* The suffix *-tome* refers to an instrument for cutting. The base word generally describes the type of tissue to be cut. For example, an *osteotome* is an instrument designed to cut bone.

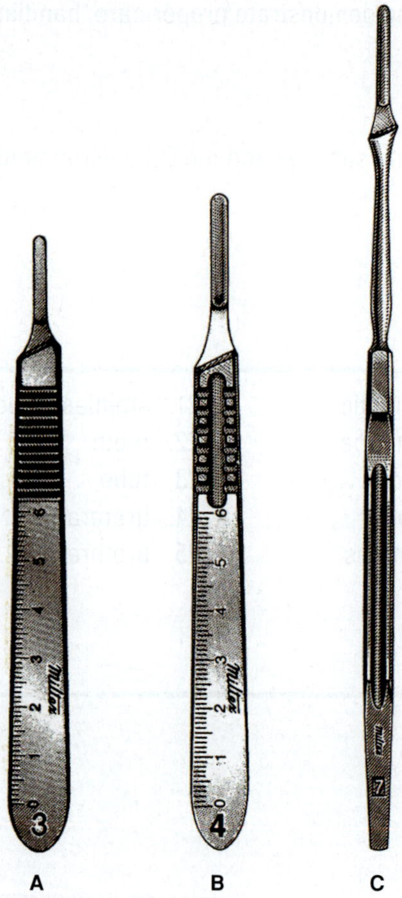

Figure 10-1 Scalpel handles: (A) #3, (B) #4, (C) #7 *(Courtesy of Miltex Instrument Co, Inc.)*

Scalpels

The terms *knife* and **scalpel** are often used interchangeably, although scalpels typically have a detachable disposable blade and nondisposable handle, and, generally, knives refer to a nondisposable handle and blade as a single unit (e.g., amputation knife or cataract knife).

Scalpel handle sizes include #3, #4, #7, and #9. The #3 and #4 handles are 5 in. in length, and the #7 handle is slightly longer (Figure 10-1). The #3 long handles for deeper cuts are 8¾ in. in length and may be angled for access to areas that are difficult to reach. Other knife handles include the miniature blade handle with chuck for eye procedures and other procedures requiring very small incisions. The Beaver blade is designed to fit the miniature blade handle.

Disposable blades are made from carbon steel and slide into a groove on the working end of the scalpel handle, although some scalpel handles have a locking mechanism instead of a groove for easy loading (Figure 10-2). The blades must be loaded onto and removed from the handle with an instrument, typically a needle holder, and never with the fingers. The blades fit specific handles:

- Blades #10, #11, #12, and #15 fit #3, #7, and #9 handles.
- Blades #20–#25 fit a #4 handle.

Any size Beaver blade will fit a miniature blade handle. The most frequently used Beaver blade is a #69.

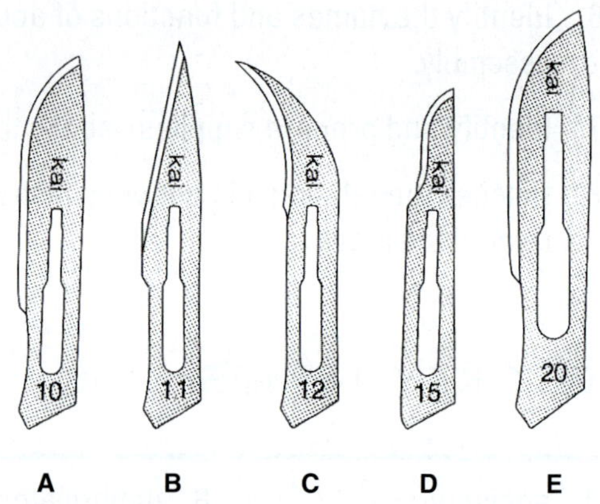

Figure 10-2 Scalpel blades: (A) #10, (B) #11, (C) #12, (D) #15, (E) #20 *(Courtesy of Miltex Instrument Co., Inc.)*

The #10 is the blade most frequently used and is typically loaded onto the #3 handle. The #11, #12, and #15 blades are usually loaded onto the #7 handle, although the #15 blade is frequently used with the #3 handle for superficial procedures requiring a small incision, such as plastic or hand procedures.

Scissors

Scissors used during a surgical procedure may be tissue scissors, suture scissors, wire scissors, or bandage/dressing scissors. In general, tissue scissors should never be used to cut anything other than tissue because it will dull the blades. However, some cardiovascular surgeons prefer to cut polypropylene sutures with Metzenbaum tissue scissors. Wire scissors are only used for cutting wire, but straight Mayo suture scissors are occasionally used for cutting dressings, drapes, drains, and other nonsuture items.

The blades of tissue scissors have sharp cutting edges and are available in varying lengths (in general, the deeper the wound, the longer the scissors needed), degrees of blade curves, and sharpness of tips. In addition to cutting tissue (sharp dissection), scissors can be used to spread and open tissue planes (blunt dissection).

Tissue scissors may be of heavy construction for tough tissue, medium for tissue that is neither tough nor delicate, or light for thin, fragile tissue. Tips may be pointed or blunt, and blades may be straight or curved. Most tissue scissors are curved, however, so that the tips can always be visualized by the surgeon and can reach around other structures. Curved Mayo scissors are often the scissors of choice for heavy tissue, and curved Metzenbaum scissors are used for medium to fine tissue. Delicate tissue is frequently dissected with curved iris, Jamieson, Westcott, or Stephen's tenotomy scissors, Metzenbaum, curved Mayo, and Potts-Smith scissors (Figure 10-3).

Examples of specialized scissors include Potts-Smith scissors for incisions into ducts, veins, or arteries; Jorgenson scissors for hysterectomy; Cushing scissors for dural in-

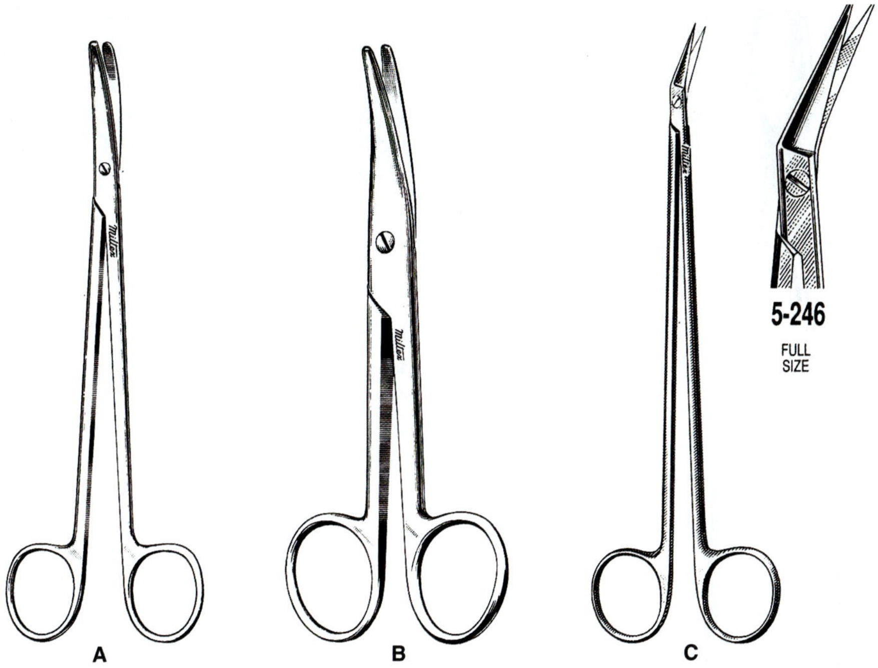

Figure 10-3 Scissors: (A) Metzenbaum, (B) curved Mayo, (C) Potts-Smith ***(Courtesy of Miltex Instrument Co., Inc.)***

cision; and microscissors for microsurgery. Scissors for eye procedures include strabismus, iris, and corneal scissors.

Suture scissors typically have straight blades and blunt tips, although pointed, straight iris scissors are frequently used to cut fine sutures during ophthalmic or plastic procedures, and curved Metzenbaum scissors are occasionally utilized for cutting polypropylene sutures during cardiovascular procedures. Straight Mayo scissors are most frequently used for cutting sutures.

GRASPING/HOLDING

Grasping/holding instruments are designed to manipulate tissue to facilitate dissection or suturing or to reduce and stabilize fractured bone during internal fixation. These instruments may or may not have a ratcheted locking mechanism. *Tissue forceps,* also referred to as *pick-ups* or *thumb forceps,* do not have ratchets and are constructed with a flattened spring handle. Tissue forceps are usually used in the nondominant hand to grasp and hold tissue when suturing or dissecting. Tissue forceps may have **teeth**, **serrations**, or may be smooth and vary greatly in length and type. Common examples include Adson (with and without teeth), Ferris-Smith, DeBakey, Brown, Russian, Gerald (with and without teeth), and Cushing bayonet forceps (with and without teeth) (Figure 10-4). Ratcheted grasping/holding instruments include Allis, Babcock, and Kocher (Ochsner).

Bone-holding clamps are typically ratcheted and are designed to hold a bone in place for eventual pinning or plating. Smaller bone-holding forceps for bones of the hand or foot may resemble the Backhaus towel clamp, but larger bone-holding forceps have working ends that are designed to either encircle a large or medium bone or firmly grasp and hold it with multiple serrated edges. Examples include Lane, Kern, Lowman, and Lewin (Figure 10-5).

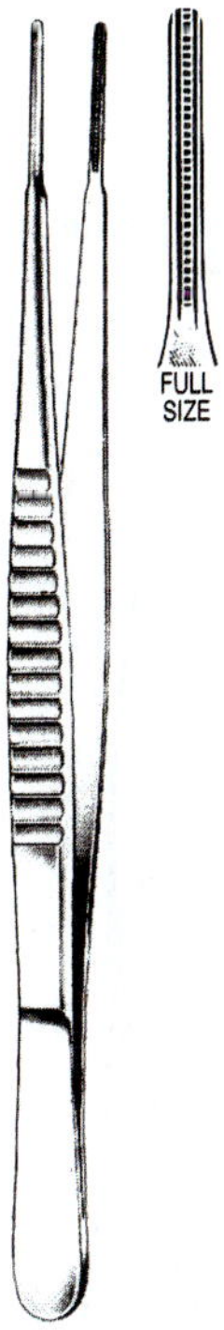

Figure 10-4 DeBakey tissue forceps ***(Courtesy of Miltex Instrument Co., Inc.)***

CLAMPING/OCCLUDING

Clamping/occluding instruments are designed to occlude or constrict tissue and are constructed with opposing ringed

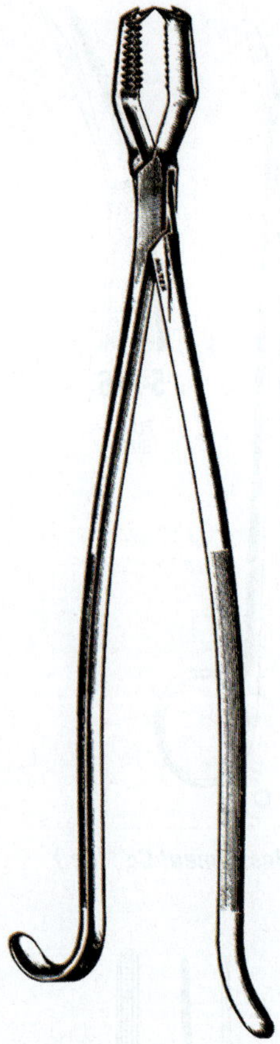

Figure 10-5 **Lane bone-holding forceps** *(Courtesy of Miltex Instrument Co., Inc.)*

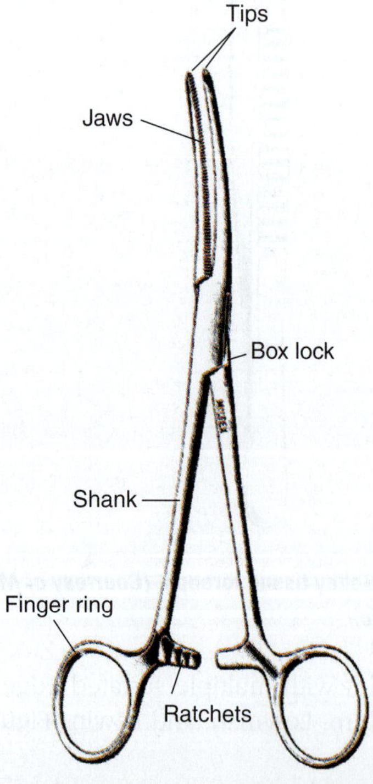

Figure 10-6 **Instrument anatomy** *(Courtesy of Miltex Instrument Co., Inc.)*

handles for fingers, interlocking ratchets located just above the ringed handles to lock the instrument in place, and two shanks that connect the ringed handles to the box lock, or hinge joint of the clamp. The box lock controls the opposing jaws of the instrument. The instrument may be straight or curved in varying degrees, and the tips may be pointed or rounded. Jaw serrations may be horizontal, longitudinal, or cross-hatched for better traction on tissue (Figure 10-6).

Most vascular clamps have atraumatic serrations that run along the length of the jaws and permit the partial or total occlusion of vessels without damage to their delicate tissue. Vascular clamps are also constructed with long, flexible jaws for increased vessel protection during occlusion. Some vascular clamps, such as the Fogarty Hydro-grip, protect the vessel with disposable, protective plastic inserts. Bulldog vascular clamps are small, spring-loaded devices with atraumatic serrations. Bulldog vascular clamps do not have finger rings or ratchets.

Hemostatic clamps are designed to occlude bleeding vessels until they can be ligated, occluded with stainless steel or titanium ligaclips, or coagulated. Hemostats are typically curved, although straight hemostats are frequently utilized for "tagging" sutures.

RETRACTING/VIEWING

Instruments designed for the exposure of the operative site are called *retractors*. Retractors may be handheld or self-retaining and are constructed in a variety of sizes and designs. Many handheld retractors are double ended, with a slight variation of shape on each end, and are frequently used in pairs on opposite sides of the incision. Self-retaining retractors, such as the Balfour retractor, remain in place by mechanical means and often have interchangeable blades for varying depths and tissue types. Self-retaining retractors for abdominal or brain procedures may attach to the OR table for stabilization. Self-retaining retractors are used in virtually all surgical specialties.

Wide-curved retractors with a blunt edge are typically used to **retract** the abdominal wall (Figure 10-7). Retractors for abdominal or thoracic organs are wide and dull and typically have some amount of "give" for protection of delicate tissue. Sharp rake-like retractors are used for retraction of nonvital structures, such as fat or skin. Single-hook or double-hook retractors are utilized for the retraction of skin during plastic procedures. Flat malleable retractors made of low-carbon stainless steel or silastic may be bent into desired positions for various retraction duties. Brain spoons are an example of a malleable retractor that can be hand held or applied to a self-retaining device for retraction of brain tissue.

Viewing instruments may provide retraction; however, their main function is to allow visualization of a structure. For example, a nasal speculum is used to spread the nares, allowing visualization of the internal nose. Specula and endoscopes are examples of viewing instruments.

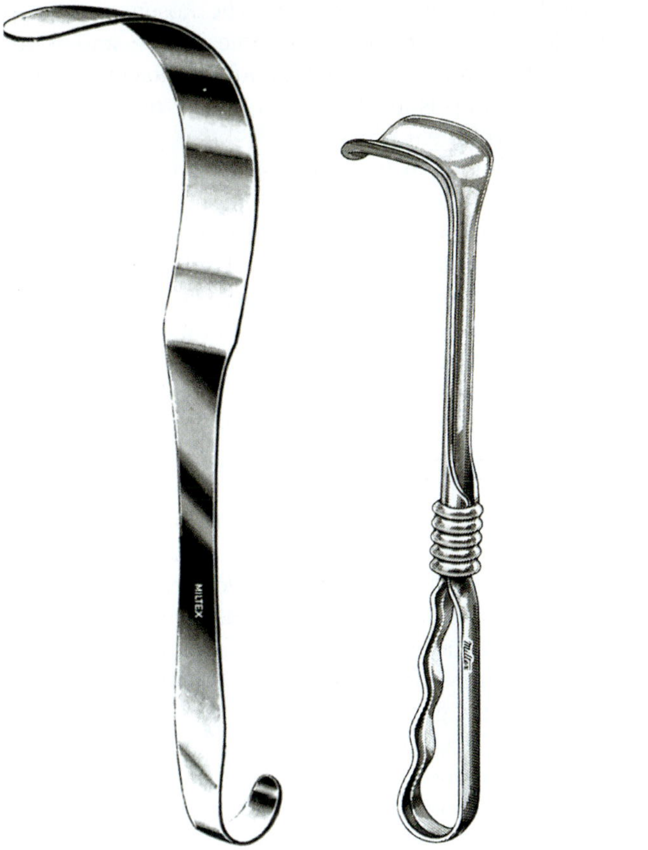

A B

Figure 10-7 Retractors: (A) Deaver, (B) Richardson ***(Courtesy of Miltex Instrument Co., Inc.)***

PROBING

Malleable, wire-like instruments for the exploration of a structure such as a fistula or duct are called *probes*. Probes are typically found in abdominal, gallbladder, or rectal instrument sets and are often used with guides called *grooved directors*. Probes for coronary arteries are small and malleable and can also be used to dilate the coronary artery.

DILATING

Dilators are instruments used to gradually dilate an orifice or duct to allow for introduction of larger instrumentation or to open a stricture. Vessels are sometimes dilated during cardiovascular procedures.

Structures are dilated using the smallest through the largest dilators, so these instruments are usually found in numbered sets. Dilators gradually taper to the distal end from the wider, proximal portion of the working end. Dilators for the cervix are double ended, with the opposite end one size up or down in width. Single-ended female **urethral** dilators are shorter than single-ended urethral dilators for men. Single-ended esophageal dilators are the longest of the dilators, with a long gradual taper to the point of the working end.

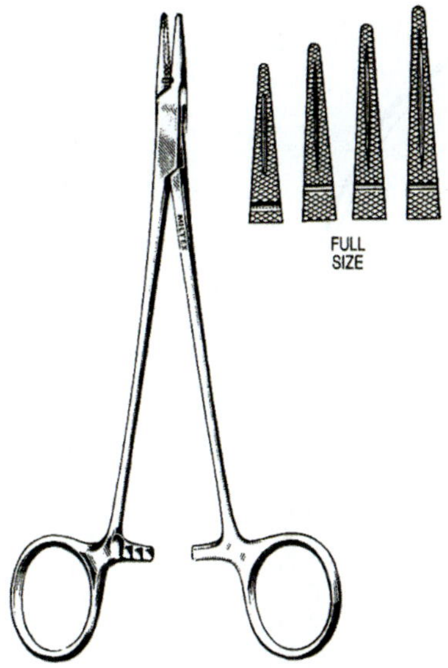

Figure 10-8 Needle holder ***(Courtesy of Miltex Instrument Co., Inc.)***

SUTURING

Instruments used to hold a curved suture needle for suturing are called *needle holders*. Needle holders vary in length and may be fine, regular, or heavy. The choice of needle holder depends on the size of the patient and the size of the needle and suture used. Although most needle holders have straight blades, some are curved for suturing around vital structures. These curved needle holders are used during certain genitourinary and gynecological procedures.

The jaws of a needle holder are designed to prevent the needle from moving during suturing. Jaws with tungsten carbide inserts or cross-hatched serrations are usually effective for needle immobilization.

Most needle holders are constructed as clamps; that is, they are designed with finger holes, ratchets, shanks, box locks, and blades with jaws (Figure 10-8). Needle holders for microsurgical, ophthalmic, and certain vascular procedures, however, have a spring action with a single ratchet that protects the small, delicate suture needle and allows the surgeon to use more subtle maneuvers when suturing.

SUCTIONING

The removal of blood and bodily fluids from an operative site by negative pressure to provide better visualization is accomplished with a hollow suction tip that is connected by plastic tubing to a suction canister. The suction canister is in turn connected to a vacuum device. Suction tips may be nondisposable or disposable and vary in size and design, depending on the procedure and the amount of fluid to be suctioned.

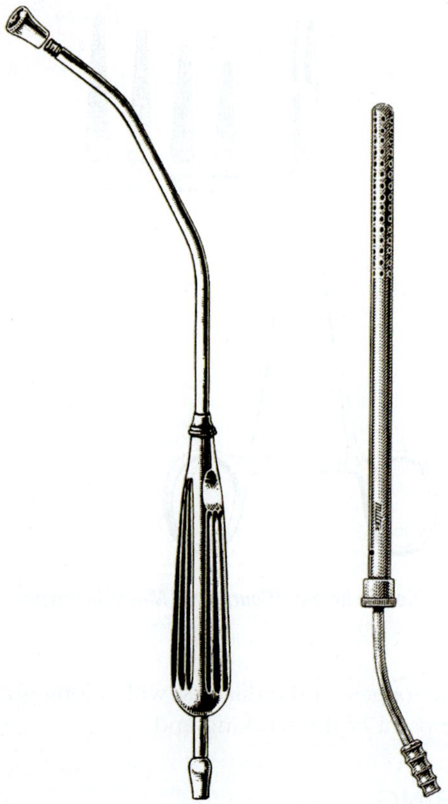

Figure 10-9 **Suction tips: (A) Yankauer, (B) Poole** ***(Courtesy of Miltex Instrument Co., Inc.)***

Neurosurgeons prefer an angled suction tip with a proximal thumbhole that allows for variability in suction strength. This feature prevents neural tissue from being damaged when fluids are aspirated. Because these small-diameter suction tips have a tendency to become obstructed, they are furnished with a flexible stylet that is inserted through the lumen to facilitate cleaning. The Frazier or Baron suction **tube** is an example of this type and is also used by plastic, ORL, and orthopedic surgeons. These suction tips are numbered according to size.

Commonly used for aspiration of abdominal fluids are the Yankauer and Poole suction tips. The Yankauer suction tip was designed for pharyngeal suctioning during tonsillectomy but is frequently used for abdominal procedures. The Poole suction tip has a removable guard with multiple holes that allows the surgeon to rapidly aspirate large amounts of fluid, usually **irrigation**, from the abdominal cavity without interference from abdominal viscera. The guard can be removed for more precise suctioning (Figure 10-9).

Some disposable suction tips have an attached active electrode that allows for simultaneous suctioning and coagulation. These special devices are frequently used by ORL surgeons during tonsillectomy. Other specialty suction tips include the long straight metal devices used during rigid esophagoscopy, laryngoscopy, bronchoscopy, and mediastinoscopy procedures. The Rosen suction tip resembles a large, bent hypodermic needle and is included with an adapter for suction tubing attachment. The Rosen suction tip is available in a variety of sizes and is typically used for ear procedures.

A *trocar* is an instrument with a sharp point and cutting edges that allow for penetration of a body cavity for the drainage of fluid or the introduction of an endoscope. The trocar fits inside a hollow cannula that is left in place after tissue penetration. After removal of the trocar, suction tubing can be attached to the cannula, and the contents of the cavity aspirated. Trocar/cannula assemblies are frequently used to **drain** sinuses or gallbladders.

MICROINSTRUMENTATION

Instruments that are used to perform microsurgery are very small, delicate, and precise devices that, when used in conjunction with an operating microscope, allow the manipulation and repair of very small structures or portions of tissue. These instruments are typically made of titanium or stainless steel, but titanium is preferred because it is stronger yet lighter in weight. The finish is dull so that light from the operating microscope is not reflected into the eyes of the operating team.

Microinstruments are designed to be held with the thumb and forefinger, allowing for more subtle movements than are allowed with finger rings. Scissors and needle holders are typically spring loaded, with a single, delicate ratchet for the locking needle holder. Scalpels for microsurgery are usually of the Beaver type; the arachnoid knife is frequently used for neurosurgery. Microdissectors and nerve hooks are used for blunt dissection, and spring-loaded vascular or aneurysm clips are used to occlude small vessels. Forceps for microsurgery may have fine teeth or may be smooth. Forceps may also be curved or straight. The tips of the forceps must be protected because they are easily bent or thrown out of alignment. Bipolar forceps are frequently used for coagulation of tissue during microsurgery.

INSTRUMENT CARE AND HANDLING

Instruments, as with all tasks related to the surgical procedure, are handled in three phases: preoperative, intraoperative, and postoperative tasks. The combination of these three phases is referred to as the *instrument cycle*.

Preoperatively, the instrument set and other supplies are gathered for the planned surgical procedure according to the surgeon's preference card. The instrument container must be opened, and the instrument set removed from the container. Instruments, and other supplies, are organized and prepared for use on the back table and Mayo stand (refer to Chapter 12).

Intraoperative instrument handling involves a complex set of critical thinking and interactive tasks. The STSR must be able to anticipate, or predict, the needs of the patient and surgical team members. The A POSitive CARE Approach is used to anticipate these needs through knowledge of normal anatomy and physiology, operative pathology, and the planned operative procedure, and an understanding of any variations that may be necessary to accommodate the specific patient (refer to Chapter 12). It is imperative that the STSR observe the progression of the procedure to obtain necessary information.

Postoperative instrument handling involves all of the steps related to preparing the instruments for reuse. These steps include

- Cleaning and decontamination
- Inspection and maintenance
- Reassembly of the instrument set
- Preparation for sterilization
- Sterilization
- Storage

Additional information about the postoperative phase of the instrument cycle is found in Chapters 7 and 12.

All surgical instruments must be handled with great care during all phases of the instrument cycle. This helps to (1) prevent injury to the patient or surgical team members, (2) extend the life of the instrument, and (3) allow the instrument to perform correctly and consistently. Some instruments may be complex and expensive to replace. Delicate instruments, such as microinstrumentation, may require special handling. Instruments are occasionally used for purposes other than intended; this practice is not recommended because damage to the instrument may result.

TYPES OF INSTRUMENT SETS

Instruments are typically assembled into sets, sterilized, and stored for later use. The instruments within each type of set are standardized according to the type of procedure for which they will be used and the needs of the facility. An instrument list or *count sheet* is used to ensure that all necessary instruments are included in the set (Figure 10-10). Generally, some instruments from each category are included in the set. Names for similar instrument sets may vary from one facility to another. For example, the laparotomy set may be alternately referred to as a major or abdominal set.

Some procedures require a smaller, secondary set of specialized instruments in addition to the larger, primary set of instruments. For example, a major (laparotomy) set is necessary to perform a cholecystectomy because it contains all of the basic instrumentation for exposure and closure of the abdomen. A gall bladder set would also be necessary, however, for its common bile duct dilators and scoops, Randall stone forceps, Mixter right angles, and cholangiogram instrumentation. Other specialized instruments that are not included with any set would have to be opened separately.

LAPAROTOMY SETS

General abdominal procedures typically require a major laparotomy or a minor laparotomy set (also called a major or minor procedures set). Refer to Table 10-1 for a suggested list of the instrumentation in a basic laparotomy set. Exploration of the common bile duct or removal of the gallbladder will require a gallbladder tray. The self-retaining Balfour retractor with additional blades for exposure of abdominal contents is occasionally opened separately. Some institutions require a separate bowel resection set for removal of any portion of the bowel. Rectal procedures will require a rectal set in addition to a minor procedures set. Some institutions have assembled a separate hemorrhoid set for hemorrhoidectomy.

Laparoscopic sets, used with increasing frequency for abdominal procedures, are equipped with one set of basic laparoscopic instruments and electrosurgical cords that can be steam sterilized and another set that has the camera, light cord, insufflator hose, and laparoscope that must be sterilized via an alternative method (e.g., Steris) that will not cause damage to the delicate lenses and fiber optics.

OBSTETRIC/GYNECOLOGICAL (OB/GYN) SETS

Obstetric/gynecological procedures require instrument sets specifically for dilatation and curettage (Table 10-2), abdominal hysterectomy, vaginal hysterectomy, laparoscopic procedures (including specific sets for laparoscopic-assisted vaginal hysterectomy, or LAVH), and cesarean section. Specialty instrumentation is discussed in Chapter 15.

OPHTHALMIC SETS

Ophthalmic operations require basic eye procedure sets in addition to conjunctival, muscle, cataract, cornea, globe and orbit, ophthalmoscope, or retinal instrument sets.

OTORHINOLARYNGOLOGY SETS

Otorhinolaryngology procedures require sets for ear procedures, such as myringotomy or tympanoplasty; nasal procedures (Table 10-3), such as nasal septal reconstruction or submucous resection; and sets for removal of the tonsils and/or adenoids. A tracheotomy tray is used for creation of an opening into the trachea. A sinuscope set is also frequently used for endoscopy of the sinuses.

PLASTIC SETS

A basic plastic set is necessary for most cosmetic procedures and generally is equipped with delicate skin instruments, larger soft tissue instruments for breast augmentation, and some small bone instruments for nasal reconstruction. A minor orthopedic, or "hand," set is required for reconstructive hand surgery. A separate set may be required for liposuction.

Instrument List/Count Sheet — Minor Set

Instrument Name	*Quantity*	*Set Assembly*	*Initial Count*	*First Count*	*Final Count*
Halsted mosquito straight 5″	4				
Halsted mosquito curved 5″	8				
Crile curved 5½″	4				
Crile straight 5½″	2				
Rochester-Pean 6¼″	2				
Allis 6″	2				
Babcock 6¼″	2				
Mayo-Hegar needle holder 7″	2				
Crile-Wood needle holder 6″	1				
Mayo scissors straight 5½″	1				
Mayo scissors curved 5½″	1				
Metzenbaum scissors curved 7″	1				
Metzenbaum scissors curved 5½″	1				
Foerster sponge forceps straight 9½″	2				
Backhaus perforating towel clamp 5¼″	4				
Lorna nonperforating towel clamp 5¼″	2				
Senn sharp	2				
Volkman 3 prong sharp	2				
U.S. Army Retractor	2				
Richardson-Eastman medium/large	2				
Yankauer suction tip	1				
Frazier suction tip 9 French with stylet	1				
Probe with eye 5½″	1				
Grooved director 5½″	1				
Tissue forceps without teeth 5½″	1				
Tissue forceps with teeth 5½″	1				
Adson tissue forceps with teeth 4¾″	2				
Knife handle #3	2				

Signature of individual preparing set: ____________________

Figure 10-10 Sample instrument list

Table 10-1 Basic Laparotomy Set

Yankauer suction tip	1 ea.	Mayo-Hegar needle holder, 6 in.	2 ea.
Poole suction tip	1 ea.	Mayo-Hegar needle holder, 7 in.	2 ea.
8-, 10-, and 12-in. DeBakey forceps	1 ea.	Mayo-Hegar needle holder, 8 in.	2 ea.
#3, #4, and #7 knife handles	1 ea.	Mayo-Hegar needle holder, 10½ in.	2 ea.
Mayo scissors straight	1 ea.	Goelet retractor	2 ea.
Mayo scissors curved	1 ea.	U.S. Army retractor	2 ea.
7- and 9-in. Metzenbaum scissors	1 ea.	Ribbon retractor, ¾ in.	1 ea.
Ferris-Smith forceps	2 ea.	Ribbon retractor, 1¼ in.	1 ea.
Adson tissue forceps with teeth	2 ea.	Deaver retractor, 1 in.	1 ea.
Russian tissue forceps	2 ea.	Deaver retractor, 2 in.	2 ea.
Cushing tissue forceps	2 ea.	Richardson retractor, large	1 ea.
Halsted mosquito forceps curved	6 ea.	Kelly retractor, 2½ in.	1 ea.
Crile forceps, 5½ in. curved	12 ea.	Balfour retractor and blades	1 ea.
Rochester-Pean forceps, 8 in.	6 ea.	Lahey gall duct forceps, 7½ in.	2 ea.
Rochester-Ochsner forceps, 6¼ in.	4 ea.	Allis tissue forceps, 6 in.	2 ea.
Mixter forceps, 7¼ in. curved	1 ea.	Allis tissue forceps, 10 in.	2 ea.
Mixter forceps, 9 in.	1 ea.	Babcock tissue forceps, 6¼ in.	2 ea.
Baby Mixter forceps, 5¼ in. curved	1 ea.	Babcock tissue forceps, 9¼ in.	2 ea.
Backhaus towel clamp	8 ea.	Stainless steel ruler	2 ea.
Foerster sponge forceps	2 ea.		

Table 10-2 Dilatation and Curettage Set

#3 and #4 knife handles	1 ea.
Dressing forceps, 8 in.	1 ea.
Heaney tissue forceps, 5 in.	1 ea.
Backhaus towel clamp, 5¼ in.	4 ea.
Foerster sponge forceps	1 ea.
Bozeman dressing forceps, 10½ in.	1 ea.
Heaney needle holder, 8 in.	1 ea.
Graves vaginal speculum, medium	1 ea.
Jackson vaginal retractor	2 ea.
Hegar uterine dilators	8 ea.
Sims uterine sound	1 ea.
Schroeder Braun tenaculum forceps	1 ea.
Jacobs vulsellum forceps	1 ea.
Sims uterine curette, sharp sizes 1, 3, and 5	1 ea.
Sims uterine biopsy curette	1 ea.

GENITOURINARY SETS

Genitourinary procedures typically require the following:

- *Kidney procedures:* A major laparotomy set, basic vascular set, a kidney set, long instrument set, and a chest (thoracotomy) set
- *Prostate procedures (open):* A major set, prostatectomy set (with Judd-Mason, Millin, and/or Denis-Browne retractors), and long instrument set

Some institutions have prepared special sets for pyeloplasty, ureteroplasty, tuboplasty, and vasectomy. These are generally used together with a major or minor procedures set.

ORTHOPEDIC SETS

Orthopedic procedures require a general orthopedic set with soft tissue and basic bone instrumentation. They also require specific sets with instruments for exposure, reduction, and internal fixation of a bone; for replacement of a joint; or for the placement of an intramedullary rod. Procedures for the hand or foot typically require a minor orthopedic, or hand, set.

CARDIAC SETS

Coronary bypass procedures typically require one set with instruments for exposure of the heart and great vessels and cannulization for cardiopulmonary bypass and another set with instruments for saphenous vein harvesting or internal mammary artery dissection and coronary anastomosis. Delicate coronary artery anastomosis instruments (e.g., Diethrich) are generally kept in a separate smaller set. A sternal saw, sternal retractor, and internal mammary artery (IMA) retractor are usually opened separately. Valve retractors and sizers for aortic or mitral valve replacement are also opened separately.

Table 10-3 Basic Nasal Set

Yankauer suction tube	1 ea.	Graefe forceps, 4⅜ in.	1 ea.
#3 and #7 knife handles	1 ea.	Farrell applicator, 6½ in.	1 ea.
Mayo dissecting scissors, 5½ in. curved	1 ea.	Frazier suction tube, 7 French	2 ea.
Metzenbaum scissors, 5½ in. curved	1 ea.	Vienna nasal speculum, medium	1 ea.
Metzenbaum scissors, 7 in. curved	1 ea.	Killian septum speculum, 3 in.	1 ea.
Plastic surgery scissors, 4¾ in. curved	1 ea.	Cottle septum speculum	1 ea.
Adson tissue forceps with teeth	2 ea.	Wilde nasal dressing forceps	1 ea.
Halsted mosquito forceps	6 ea.	Joseph single hook	1 ea.
Backhaus towel clamp, 3¾ in.	4 ea.	Joseph double hook, 2 mm	1 ea.
Halsey needle holder, 5 in.	2 ea.	Joseph double hook, 7 mm	1 ea.
Senn retractor sharp	2 ea.	Aufricht nasal retractor-speculum	1 ea.
U.S. Army retractor	2 ea.	Joseph nasal scissors, 5¾ in. curved	1 ea.
Baby Allis tissue forceps, 5 in.	2 ea.	Joseph nasal scissors, 5¾ in. straight	1 ea.

THORACIC SETS

Instrument sets for thoracic procedures are equipped with instruments needed to remove a rib (e.g., Bethune rib shears, Matson rib stripper/elevator) and expose and repair the organs of the thorax. If exposure requires median sternotomy, a sternal saw and retractor are opened separately. Thoracic sets are also equipped with cardiovascular instrumentation. Thoracic procedures may also require a major set with soft tissue instruments or a general vascular set for additional cardiovascular instruments. Ligaclip applicators of various sizes are sometimes opened separately. Thoracoscopy sets are used frequently.

PERIPHERAL VASCULAR SETS

Peripheral vascular procedures require a vascular set with vascular instruments that are the proper size and fit for the exposure and repair of the vessel to be repaired. A major laparotomy set, with its large abdominal retractors and soft tissue instruments, and a vascular set, with large and medium vascular instruments, will be necessary for abdominal aortic aneurysmectomy or aortofemoral bypass. Some peripheral vascular sets are specific to the procedure; for example, a carotid endarterectomy or creation of arteriovenous (AV) fistula will require a carotid or AV fistula set, respectively. The carotid set can also be used for medium-sized arterial procedures, such as a femoral thrombectomy, and the AV fistula set can be used for repair of small arteries.

Cardiac and vascular surgery have many common instrument requirements (Table 10-4).

NEUROSURGICAL SETS

Neurosurgical procedures require instrumentation for exposure and repair of the brain, spinal cord, and periph-

Table 10-4 Basic Cardiovascular Set

#3 long knife handle	1 ea.	Glover bulldog clamp, 8 cm straight	2 ea.
Metzenbaum scissors, 7 in. curved	1 ea.	DeBakey-Semb ligature carrier, 10¼ in.	1 ea.
Potts-Smith scissors, 7½ in. 25° angle	1 ea.	DeBakey thoracic tissue forceps, 9½ in.	1 ea.
Potts-Smith scissors, 7½ in. 45° angle	1 ea.	DeBakey thoracic tissue forceps, 6 in.	1 ea.
Potts-Smith scissors, 7½ in. 60° angle	1 ea.	Frazier suction tube, 9 French	1 ea.
Potts-Smith tissue forceps, 9¾ in.	1 ea.	Freer elevator, double-ended	1 ea.
DeBakey needle holder, 9 in.	1 ea.	Volkmann retractor, 4 prong sharp	2 ea.
Providence hospital forceps, 5½ in. curved	12 ea.	U.S. Army retractor	2 ea.
Little retractor, 7¾ in.	2 ea.	Harrington retractor, 12 in.	1 ea.
Rummel thoracic forceps, 9 in.	2 ea.	Kelly retractor, 3 in.	1 ea.
DeBakey tangential occlusion clamp, 10¼ in.	1 ea.	Deaver retractor, 3 in.	2 ea.
DeBakey multipurpose clamp, 9½ in.	1 ea.	Ribbon retractor, 1½ in.	1 ea.
DeBakey vascular clamp, 12¼ in.	1 ea.	Cushing vein retractor, 9 in.	1 ea.
Glover bulldog clamp, 8 cm curved	2 ea.		

eral nerves. Craniotomy requires a basic neurosurgical (craniotomy) set and, in some institutions, a minor procedures set for its extra soft tissue instruments. A microsurgical set is often necessary as well.

Laminectomy requires a laminectomy set with bone and neurosurgical instruments and occasionally a minor procedures set for soft tissue instruments. If a fusion is necessary, a basic orthopedic set is required, with osteotomes, curettes, and gouges usually opened separately. A microsurgical set is necessary for laminectomy for tumor removal.

Transphenoidal hypophysectomy requires a transphenoidal, craniotomy, and ORL (nasal) set and, occasioally, a minor procedures set to take a fascial graft. Some institutions combine all of these sets into one transphenoidal set.

A Cloward set is typically used for anterior cervical discectomy and fusion. For ventricular shunts, a minor procedures and craniotomy set are necessary.

Instrument sets for specific procedures are described in the procedures section of the text.

INSTRUMENT LIST/COUNT SHEET

As instrument sets are assembled, an instrument list, or count sheet, with the type and number of instruments is referred to by the assembler to minimize errors (see Figure 10-10). After assembly, this list is signed by the assembler and placed into the instrument pan before wrapping. The signature assures that any mistakes in assembly can be traced to the proper source. During the setup for the surgical procedure, the STSR hands the instrument list to the circulator, who begins a visual and verbal instrument count by referring to the sheet. As each instrument is confirmed by the STSR, the circulator writes the correct number next to the printed instrument name on the count sheet. During closure, the counting process is repeated.

If a count is waived for the procedure, the STSR can confirm that the instrument set is complete by referring to the instrument list afterward.

SPECIALTY EQUIPMENT

Every OR contains a certain amount of standard equipment. Today's OR, however, is increasingly specialized. As technology affects operative practice, an increased amount of specialized equipment is required.

ENDOSCOPES

Endoscopes are used preoperatively, intraoperatively, or postoperatively for diagnosis, biopsy, visualization, and/or repair of a structure within a body cavity or the interior of a hollow organ (Figure 10-11). Because the endoscope is introduced either through a body opening, such as the urethra, or through a small skin incision, hospital stays are shortened and recovery time is less than for a major surgical procedure. Many endoscopic procedures can be done on an out-patient basis.

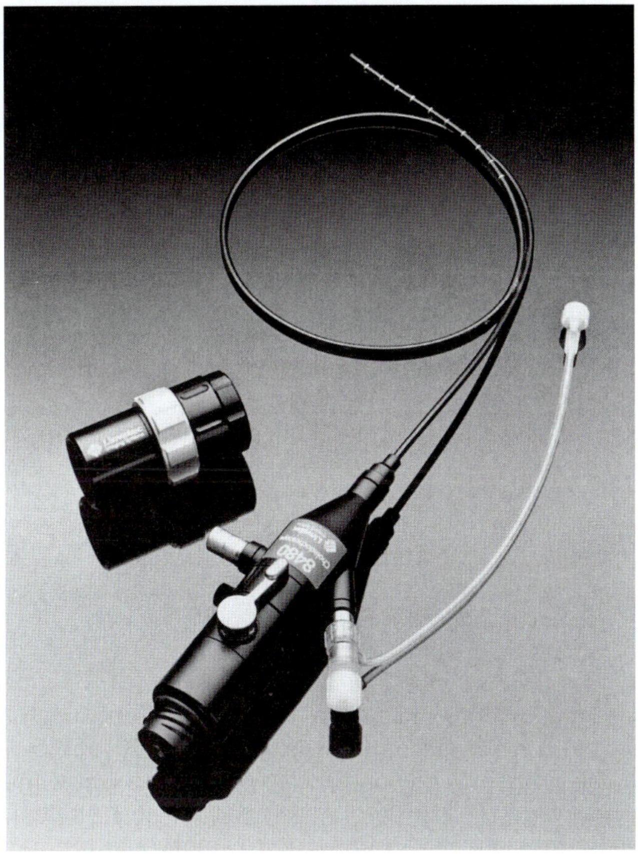

Figure 10-11 Flexible endoscope ***(Courtesy of Linvatec)***

Advances in fiber-optic technology have allowed routine endoscopic access to areas that were once considered beyond reach, such as the ventricles of the brain. Lumbar discectomy can now be performed through an endoscope, as can many abdominal or thoracic procedures.

Scopes with or without cameras can be inserted into body cavities or joint spaces through trocar/cannula assemblies for diagnostic purposes or surgical repair. These include arthroscopes, laparoscopes, and thoracoscopes.

Scopes can also be inserted through body orifices for viewing, repairing, or biopsy of tissue. They may also be used for hemorrhage control or retrieval of a foreign body. These include bronchoscopes, laryngoscopes, colonoscopes, gastroscopes, hysteroscopes, sigmoidoscopes, proctoscopes, sinuscopes, otoscopes, cystoscopes and resectoscopes.

Many modern fiber-optic endoscopes are flexible with a maneuverable tip and channels for the introduction of flexible instruments, suction, and fluid injection. Rigid scopes may be hollow or constructed with a telescopic lens system and eyepiece. Examples of rigid scopes are those typically used for cystoscopy, laparoscopy, thoracoscopy, proctoscopy, sigmoidoscopy, and arthroscopy. Rigid bronchoscopy is preferred for retrieval of a foreign body from a bronchus, but flexible bronchoscopes are most often used for diagnostic purposes.

Lensed endoscopes can be attached to a camera that produces an image on a monitor for viewing by the surgical team. A light cord that has one end attached to the scope and the other attached to an electrical light source produces the illumination necessary for viewing.

Specialty scopes include

- Choledochoscope for exploration of the biliary system
- Mediastinoscope for visualization and biopsy of the structures of the mediastinum
- Ureteroscope for exploration of the ureters
- Angioscopes for visualization of the heart and major vessels, or vascular endoscopes for the interior of smaller vessels
- Ventriculoscopes for exploration of the brain's ventricular system
- Fetoscope for visualization of a fetus *in utero*

Endoscopes can be used with active electrosurgical devices for coagulation or tissue dissection. The resectoscope uses a high monopolar electric current to shave hypertrophied prostate from within the proximal urethra, and instruments with **monopolar cautery** and **bipolar electrosurgery** active electrodes are commonly used during laparoscopy for tissue coagulation and dissection.

Lasers can also be used with endoscopes. For instance, hydrocephalus can be successfully treated in a select group of patients by inserting an endoscope and neodymium-yttrium aluminum garnet (**Nd:YAG**) laser through a ventriculostomy. The laser creates a new pathway for cerebral spinal fluid, bypassing the obstruction that led to hydrocephalus.

POWER TOOLS

Instruments used in the OR that are powered by compressed air or nitrogen, electricity, or battery are called *power tools.* Power tools may be used to drill holes into the skull and then connect the holes to turn a bone flap for access to the brain. They may be used to ream the central shaft of a long bone for rod placement or drill holes for screws to secure a plate on a fractured bone. They may be used to saw the femoral or humeral head for joint replacement or saw through the sternum for access to the heart. Power tools are used to reshape bone for plastic/reconstructive procedures or drive pins to reduce and stabilize fractured bone. Power instruments are also used to cut skin, usually for skin grafting, or grind skin for dermabrasion.

Nitrogen for power instruments is supplied from a tank or is piped in from outside the surgery department. The tank is mobile, allowing for easier hookup for power hoses. Any shaped adapter can be fitted to the tank for the connection of two power hoses. Pressure gauges on the regulator are set by the OR team at the specifications of the manufacturer of the power equipment and should be followed closely to prevent damage to the instrument and its hose or injury to the patient. The internal pressure of the tank is typically 500 psi, while operating pressure is set between 80 and 100 psi.

Larger power equipment is frequently powered by battery or nitrogen, while delicate bone work may require a faster air-powered instrument for greater precision and reduction of heat and vibration. Many older dermatomes for skin grafts are electric powered, but the newer dermatomes and high-speed dermabraders are powered by compressed nitrogen.

Power saws have either a reciprocating (back-and-forth) or oscillating (side-to-side) action for cutting bone, and the blades for these power instruments are available in a variety of sizes and shapes (Figure 10-12). The blade of a craniotome cuts through the cranium with a rotary motion, and the delicate tissue underneath is protected by a dural guard at the foot of the instrument.

Drills utilize a rapid rotary motion for carving bone with burs or drilling holes for wire, pins, or screws. Drivers also utilize a rapid rotary motion for inserting, or "driving," sharp pins to reduce a bone fracture or guide a driven nail. Reamers utilize a slower rotary motion for reaming the shaft of a long bone to insert a nail or rod. Cranial perforators use a rotary motion to drill holes in the cranium and are designed to stop before penetrating the brain.

LASERS

Lasers have been used in the operating room with greater frequency since the first practical model was built in 1960.

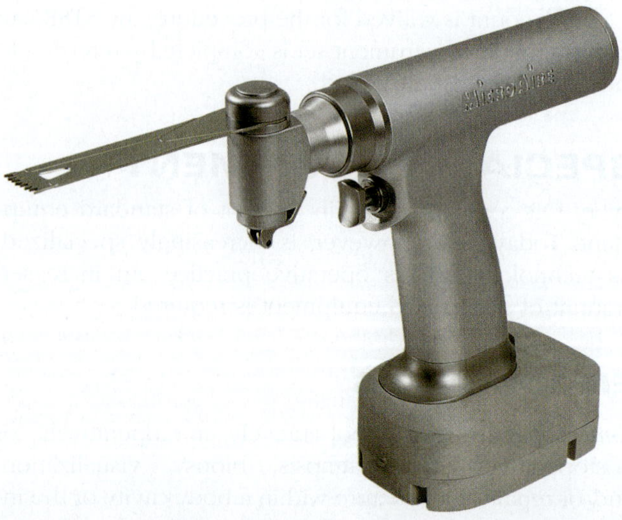

Figure 10-12 Oscillating power saw ***(Courtesy of MicroAire Surgical Instruments)***

Virtually all surgical specialties have incorporated this amazing device into their surgical armamentarium as laser technology has advanced. The acronym "laser" means *light amplification by the stimulated emission of radiation* and refers to the process of converting some form of energy into light energy that extends from the near-ultraviolet portion to the far-infrared portion of the electromagnetic spectrum.

Laser light is different from ordinary light. Laser light is monochromatic, which means that the photons that compose the light are all of the same color or wavelength. Its color will decide how it will react with various tissues; in other words, red laser light is absorbed by red-pigmented tissue. As the laser energy is absorbed by the tissue, heat energy is produced and the tissue is damaged. Laser light is *collimated,* which means that its waves are parallel to each other and do not spread out as they travel away from their source. This property of laser light allows for pinpoint precision for surgical applications. Laser light is *coherent,* meaning that the light waves travel in the same direction and in phase with each other, increasing its amplitude and its power.

The factors that decide the penetration depth of the beam include power, color, wavelength, and duration of exposure to tissue. Tissue consistency also plays an important role.

The parts of a laser system include the excitation source, head, **ancillary** (auxiliary) components, control panel, and delivery system.

The excitation source provides the energy that allows the laser head to produce light. Gas lasers are stimulated by an electrical source, and solid or liquid lasers are stimulated by flash lamps.

The energized active medium that excites the photons of the laser head is what gives the laser its specific name. The classifications of the active media are shown in Table 10-5. Mirrors located on each end of the laser head reflect and amplify the laser energy produced by the active medium.

The ancillary portions of the laser system include the console for protection of internal components; the air or water cooling system, which prevents the laser head from overheating; and the vacuum pump in the CO_2 laser system, which pulls and delivers the active medium to the laser head.

The computerized control panel regulates the modes, duration times, and wattage required for control of the laser sytem. Various safety measures are built into the system and controlled from the panel. These include the stand-by mode, master key for operation, and feedback security measures that monitor the components for proper function of the system.

The delivery system is the laser system component that delivers the laser energy to the tissues from the laser head. Carbon dioxide lasers use a hollow tube with mirrors (articulated arm) that deflect the gas forward. This articulated arm can be attached to a microscope or to a handpiece. The Nd:YAG and argon lasers use laser fibers as a delivery system.

Table 10-5 Active Media

MEDIA	CHARACTERISTIC
Gas	This active medium is energized by electricity to produce the laser light. Examples include carbon dioxide, helium-neon, krypton, argon, and excimer.
Solid	An energy-producing element on a rod is energized by flash lamps to produce the laser light. Examples include ruby and Nd:YAG.
Liquid	An organic dye is energized by a laser beam to produce the laser light in various wavelengths.
Semiconductor crystals	Laser energy is delivered directly to tissue through a filter or slit lamp microscope.

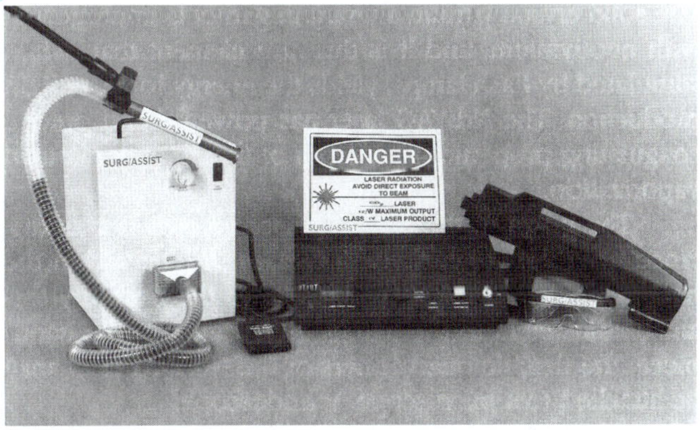

Figure 10-13 Carbon dioxide laser with plume evacuator ***(Courtesy of Surg/Assist, Inc.)***

CARBON DIOXIDE

The carbon dioxide (CO_2) laser is the most frequently utilized laser system in the OR (Figure 10-13). Because its 10,600-nm beam is invisible, a helium-neon beam serves as the aiming device. Its active medium is actually a combination of CO_2, helium, and nitrogen gases.

Unlike the argon or Nd:YAG laser, carbon dioxide laser energy absorption does not depend on the pigment of the tissue affected; therefore, it can be used on light and dark tissues. It is absorbed by water to a depth of 0.5 mm, and its energy is used to heat the intracellular fluid. The increased heat destroys cellular proteins and bursts the cell wall, producing steam from the heated water and cellular debris that proliferates through the air as laser "plume."

ARGON

The argon laser produces a blue light in the approximate range of 488 nm and a green light in the approximate range of 515 nm. The argon laser beam is absorbed by dark and red tissues to a depth of 0.5–2 mm. Because it travels through clear tissues without heating them, it is useful for the treatment of diabetic retinopathy, a condition in which bleeding vessels on the retina impair vision. These posterior bleeding vessels can be coagulated by an argon laser beam that must travel through the clear, anterior portions of the eye without damaging them.

NEODYMIUM:YTTRIUM ALUMINUM GARNET

The Nd:YAG laser has a wavelength of 1064 nm and is located in the near-infrared region of the electromagnetic spectrum. The laser energy is readily absorbed by tissue protein but poorly absorbed by water and hemoglobin. The solid crystal yttrium aluminum garnet is impregnated with neodymium, and it is this rare element that, when stimulated by flash lamps, yields the energy for laser light production. The Nd:YAG laser has powerful and precise coagulating properties to a depth of 6 mm, with minimal vaporization.

The beam of the Nd:YAG laser spreads out as distance from the target tissue increases. A lens within the handpiece delivery system helps focus the beam by distance adjustment to the tissues. In addition to the handpiece, the flexible quartz fibers of the Nd:YAG laser may be attached to a microscope or endoscope.

POTASSIUM TITANYL PHOSPHATE

The potassium titanyl phosphate (KTP) laser produces a green light of 532-nm wavelength with an affinity for red or darker tissues, such as hemoglobin or melanin. The delivery system may be a handpiece or fiber, producing a beam with a smaller diameter than the CO_2 or the Nd:YAG laser for more precise coagulation. The fiber may range from 0.2 to 0.6 mm in diameter.

EXCIMER

The term *excimer* refers to a molecule that loses a photon when energy is lost after initial excitation. The active medium is a halide-oxide dimer or a halide-halide dimer. The excimer's pinpoint ultraviolet laser beam is absorbed by protein with minimal thermal spread, so it is used to reshape the cornea for radial keratoplasty and to destroy plaque within a stenotic artery for angioplasty.

HOLMIUM:YAG

The wavelength of the Ho:YAG laser can be increased to 2100 nm by passing it through a crystal that contains holmium, thulium, and chromium. The result is a precision beam that is absorbed by water. It is used in dentistry and for atherectomy or radial keratoplasty.

LASERS IN ENDOSCOPY

With development of the quartz fiber-optic delivery system in the 1970s, lasers could finally be attached to endoscopes for less invasive repair. The first application for endoscopic laser technology was for gastrointestinal hemorrhage control. An argon laser attached to a gastroscope was used to coagulate bleeding vessels in the stomach for a patient with advanced gastritis, eliminating the need for a major surgical procedure to open the abdomen.

Today, the laser of choice for gastrointestinal endoscopy is the Nd:YAG laser system because its beam penetrates deeply into the tissues for better coagulation and destruction of tumor masses. The argon laser with its shallow beam is still used to treat angiodysplasias within the thin wall of the intestine.

Laser microlaryngoscopy is routinely used for the endoscopic treatment of many benign and malignant tumors of the larynx. Because of the proximity of the laser to the endotracheal tube, precautions must be taken to prevent combustion during anesthesia administration.

Laser bronchoscopy, first described in 1974, has improved access for treatment of certain diseases of the tracheobronchial tree. The CO_2 and Nd:YAG lasers are the instruments of choice for laser bronchoscopy.

Stereotactic laser endoscopy is used for treatment of certain brain tumors to preserve adjacent neural tissue and to reduce postoperative cerebral edema and recovery time.

Arthroscopy is occasionally performed with Nd:YAG, CO_2, or Ho:YAG laser systems to vaporize protein and bond collagen and to cut or smooth cartilage or tissues within joints. Percutaneous disk procedures can also be performed with the Nd:YAG laser.

Endoscopic transurethral prostatectomy is occasionally achieved with an Nd:YAG laser system. Urethral strictures can be released with an Nd:YAG laser attached to a cystoscope. Bladder tumors can be vaporized with an Nd:YAG laser attached to a cystoscope. A fiber-optic ureteroscope introduced through the urethra and bladder can be used to direct a pulsed dye laser beam into the ureters to fragment calculi.

Hysteroscopes can be coupled with an Nd:YAG laser system to excise and vaporize uterine septa, sessile polyps, and smaller fibroids. Menorrhagia can also be treated with this combination. Laparoscopic laser application for other gynecological conditions include endometriosis vaporization with the Nd:YAG/laparoscope combination, neosalpingostomy, uterosacral transection, ovarian cystectomy, and certain instances of ectopic pregnancy.

Laparoscopic laser applications can be used for certain general surgery procedures such as laparoscopic cholecystectomy, performed with an Nd:YAG, KTP, Ho:YAG, or argon laser system.

Colonoscopes combined with argon or Nd:YAG laser systems are used to treat polyps, arteriovenous malformations, bleeding disorders, and the ablation of certain types of tumors.

MICROSCOPES

The compound operating microscope is a binocular apparatus that uses bent light waves for variable **magnification** of tissues during microsurgery. It may be suspended from the ceiling or mounted on a mobile frame with locking casters. Eyepieces and objective lenses are interchangeable according to the needs of the surgeon. The operating microscope consists of the optical lens system, magnification and focus controls, the illumination system, a mounting system for stability, an electrical system, and accessories (Figure 10-14).

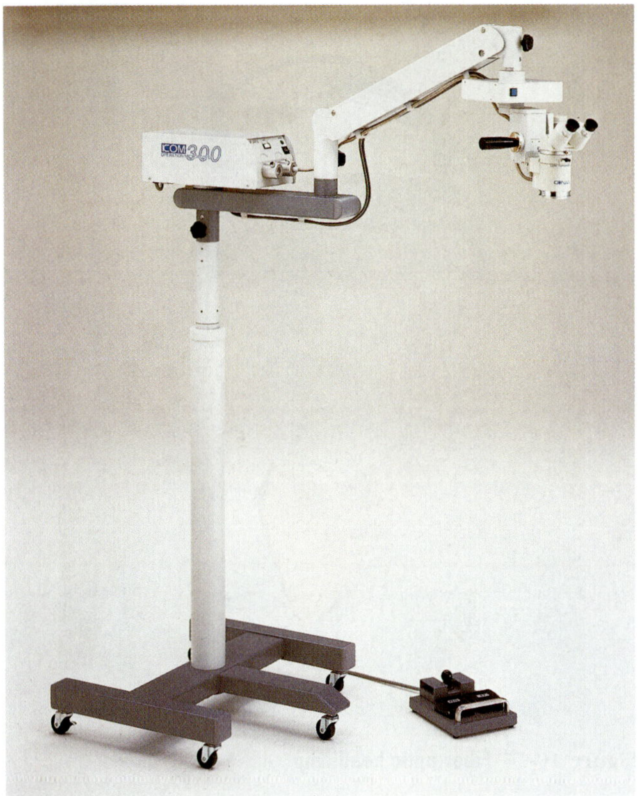

Figure 10-14 **Operating microscope** ***(Courtesy of Konan Medical Corp.)***

MAGNIFICATION

The optical lens system provides the magnification and resolving power necessary to do the surgical work. The *resolving power* of the microscope refers to the ability of the optical system to filter out adjacent images and to clarify detail. The optical system is composed of the objective lens and eyepieces (referred to as *oculars*). The focal length of the objective lens ranges from 100 to 400 mm, signifying the distance of the lens from the target tissue. This distance is referred to as the working distance. The binoculars serve as magnifiers of the actual image provided by the objective lens. Achromatic capabilities of the oculars sharpen the image in the actual colors of the target tissues. A second set of binoculars for an assistant can be attached to the body of the microscope. A beam splitter allows the second set of oculars to match the original set's field of view.

Total magnification is calculated by multiplying the magnifying power of the objective lens with the magnifying power of the oculars. Increases in magnifying power decrease the depth and the width of the field of view. Most operating microscopes are equipped with a zoom lens operated by a foot control that can quickly increase or decrease magnification. Focusing is controlled by a foot pedal and/or hand control.

ILLUMINATION

Light waves for illumination of the operative field are provided by paraxial or coaxial illuminators. Paraxial illuminators contain tungsten or halogen bulbs and focusing lenses mounted to the body of the microscope. This type of illuminator can be angled inward to illuminate the operative site and is equipped with a diaphragm to narrow the beam. Coaxial illuminators use fiber optics to transmit light waves through the microscope's optical system. The light transmitted by this type of illuminator is cool to protect tissues from excessive heat. Light intensity is controlled by a switch on the support arm.

The microscope can be adapted for attachment to a laser or a camera can be attached to the beam splitter for viewing the target tissues on a monitor. The microscope can be covered with a sterile drape by the STSR, or sterile covers can be attached to the focusing knobs by the surgeon for minor procedures.

VIDEO MONITORS, RECORDERS, AND CAMERAS

Video cameras can be attached to microscopes or endoscopes so that the procedure can be viewed on a monitor and recorded for documentation. Still images can be taken with the camera and printed with a microcomputer imaging system for later study. A fiber-optic light cord attached to an electric light source is necessary for illumination of body interiors. Video cameras and light cords should be "cold" sterilized with the peracetic acid system.

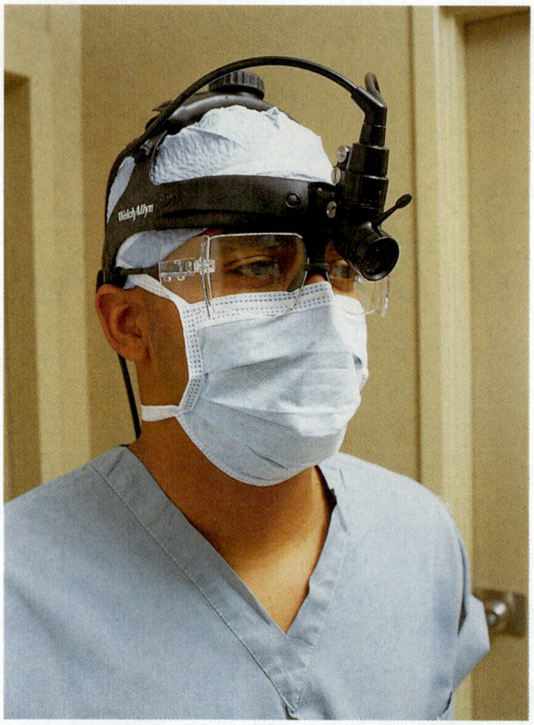

Figure 10-15 Fiber-optic headlamp

FIBER-OPTIC HEADLAMPS AND LIGHT SOURCES

Fiber-optic headlamps are worn by surgeons for additional lighting of the operative site. These devices are worn on the head of the surgeon to focus an intense light beam of small diameter in areas that are poorly illuminated by the overhead operating lights. Light waves are supplied by the electrical light source that is mounted on a mobile cart. Although every specialty makes use of the fiber-optic headlamp, it is most frequently worn by cardiovascular and ORL surgeons (Figure 10-15).

A fiber-optic light cable may be attached to an illuminator mounted on a retractor for illumination of deep pockets or cavities that are not easily reached with the beam of the overhead OR lights. These types of retractors are frequently used for breast augmentation or mastectomy.

IRRIGATION/ASPIRATION UNIT

An *irrigation/aspiration* (IA) device that is powered by nitrogen may be utilized to debride a traumatic or infected wound. The adjustable pulsed saline solution literally pulverizes necrotic tissue or clots, allowing the wound to heal naturally. The surgical team must be protected from the splattered fluids, so a circular shield is often placed on the hand control.

Diseased eye lenses may be fragmented and removed with a Phaco-Emulsifier, a machine that uses ultrasonic energy (cavitation) to fragment the lens, and an irrigator/aspirator to remove the fragments. IA flow is automatically adjusted for pressures within the anterior chamber of the eye. The newer piezoelectric machine uses electric impulses to generate heat and is cooled by air or fluid that flows through the power cord. Aspirant flows through transparent tubes away from the operative site.

CRYOTHERAPY UNITS

A **cryo**therapy unit uses liquid nitrogen, Freon, or carbon dioxide gas to deliver extreme cold through an insulated probe to diseased tissues, creating necrosis without damage to adjacent tissues. The diseased tissue can then be removed under hemostatic conditions. Because cryotherapy preserves neighboring tissue and removes diseased tissue without significant hemorrhage, it is useful for the removal of vascular tumors, brain tumors, and the prostate gland. Cryotherapy is also utilized to repair retinal detachments and extract cataracts.

INSUFFLATORS

Laparoscopic procedures cannot be performed unless carbon dioxide gas is infused into the abdominal cavity through either a Veress **insufflation** needle or a Hasson blunt trocar. Expansion of the abdominal cavity with CO_2 gas, referred to as insufflation, creates a space for viewing with a video camera attached to an endoscope and for work within the cavity through ports inserted at strategic points through the abdominal wall. The machine that infuses the CO_2 gas into the abdominal cavity is called an *insufflator*. The typical intraoperative pressure for laparoscopy is 12–15 mm Hg.

NERVE STIMULATORS

Nerve stimulators produce very small electric currents that, when applied to tissue, help to identify and preserve essential nerves for cranial, facial, neck, or hand reconstructive procedures. The nerve stimulator is especially useful for identification of the seventh cranial (facial) nerve during acoustic neuroma removal and to identify the facial, acoustic, cochlear, and vestibular nerve branches during otological procedures. Anesthesia providers may use the nerve stimulator to assess the actions of neuromuscular blockers administered during anesthesia.

To operate the nerve stimulator, the needle that is attached by wire to the locator probe is inserted into adjacent, nonessential tissue. The structure in question is touched with the probe and the electric current is delivered to the structure. If a nerve is nearby, the surrounding tissue will move slightly, or the tissues that the nerve innervates will respond with movement.

ACCESSORY EQUIPMENT

An assortment of equipment is needed for surgical procedures routinely. This equipment is referred to as accessory equipment.

SUCTION SYSTEMS

Suction apparatus utilize a vacuum to remove fluids from the surgical site and patient's airway. A minimum of two suction units is required in each operating room. One unit must be available at all times to assist with airway maintenance and the other is used within the surgical field. The components of the suction system include:

- *Vacuum source*—May be portable or centralized. The centralized vacuum source is accessed via outlets located in each OR.
- *Vacuum source tubing*—Connects the vacuum source with the collection unit.
- *Collection unit*—May be reusable, disposable, or contain a disposable liner. The collection unit may have incremental markings to allow estimation of the amount of fluid contained within.
- *Tubing*—Connects the collection unit to the fluid source. Is usually disposable and may be sterile or nonsterile according to the situation.
- *Suction tip*—Removes the fluid from the source. May be sterile or nonsterile, disposable or reusable, and one of a variety of styles.

The sterile suction tubing and tip are opened onto the sterile field in preparation for the procedure. The STSR will connect the suction tip to the tubing and set the apparatus aside for placement of the sterile field following drape application. Once the patient has been draped, the suction tubing is secured to the drape with a nonpenetrating device. The end with the suction tip applied remains on the sterile field and the opposite end is passed from the sterile field to the circulator for attachment to the collection device. Once connected, the vacuum is turned on and adjusted by the circulator.

ELECTROSURGICAL UNIT

The electrosurgical unit (ESU) is used to apply electrical current through the patient's tissue to cut and/or coagulate the tissue (Figure 10-16). The electrosurgical unit uses two modes to deliver the electrical current to the tissue: monopolar and bipolar.

The *monopolar* mode, also referred to as *unipolar*, is the most commonly used. Monopolar electrosurgery is most frequently used for coagulation, but may also be used to cut tissue. The generator is capable of blending the coagulation and cutting functions to achieve a combined result.

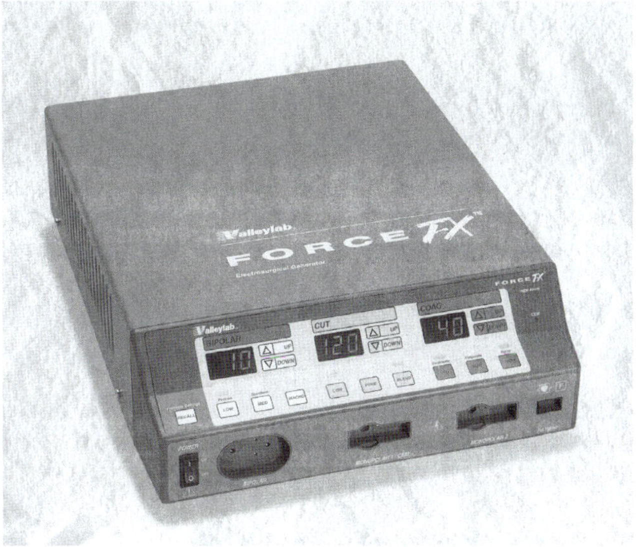

Figure 10-16 Combination bipolar and monopolar ESU ***(Courtesy of Valleylab)***

The *bipolar* mode is used less frequently to protect and preserve delicate nearby tissue. The bipolar mode is only used for coagulation.

HISTORY

In 1891, D'arsonval and Tesla applied high-frequency energy to the human body to generate heat using concepts of electromagnetic waves first discovered by Hertz. In 1908, Von Zeynek applied electromagnetic waves for therapy that he called *diathermy*. Doyen and Czerny used this same equipment, a spark-gap, long-wave diathermy, in the OR to cut tissue, calling it *surgical diathermy*. Attempts were made with these units to generate currents of different qualities by the adjustment of contact gaps. This resulted in a variation of frequency of sparking at the spark gaps, but the results were highly unsatisfactory.

Electrocautery began in earnest 20 years later, when Dr. Harvey Cushing collaborated with William T. Bovie, a physicist, to produce a device that used radio-frequency electric current for coagulation. Later advances in electronics offered the vacuum tube, or valve generator. This new unit allowed a nonmodulated current that was much smoother than the old spark-gap generator. The new tube generators solved many of the problems of the spark-gap generators by ensuring consistent power, freedom from maintenance problems, and silent operation. The high-frequency current generated by the tubes allowed cutting of tissues that was not possible with the spark-gap generators. However, with the high-frequency tube current, it was impossible to use precision cutting electrodes, such as needles or loops.

In the 1970s, solid-state generators were developed as a result of semiconductor technology. These units use transistors, diodes, and rectifiers for electrical current generation. Today's modern electrosurgical units are microprocessor based and are equipped with safety features that reduce the incidence of burns when the path to the inactive electrode is interrupted.

Although the electrosurgical unit of today uses completely different technology than the original device developed by Bovie, the ESU is still referred to as the *Bovie* at many facilities.

COMPONENTS: MONOPOLAR AND BIPOLAR

The monopolar electrosurgical unit consists of three main components: the generator, the active electrode, and the dispersive electrode.

The *generator* provides the source of electrical current (up to 400 W of power) to the active electrode and a pathway for current returning from the dispersive electrode. The generator may be activated by the surgeon with a hand control located on the active electrode or with a foot control device. The generator must be connected via a cord and three-prong hospital-grade plug to a source of electricity that is grounded (the wall outlet).

A power cord is attached to the back of the generator, as are the monopolar and bipolar foot control devices, if needed. Also located on the back of the generator is the volume control. For safety reasons, the volume may be adjusted, but never turned completely off.

The control panel is located on the front of the generator and includes the on/off switch, the receptacles for the active and dispersive electrodes, and the power level and blend adjustments. Some units may be equipped to handle two active electrodes at the same time. This feature is especially useful when multiple procedures are performed on a single patient simultaneously.

Some electrosurgical generators are capable of operating in the monopolar or bipolar mode. If this is the case, a separate area on the control panel is dedicated to the bipolar function. When turned on, the machine performs a self-check prior to entering the "ready" mode.

The *active electrode,* also referred to as the *electrosurgical pencil,* is usually a disposable item packaged in a sterile fashion by the manufacturer and usually includes a protective holster. The pencil is placed on the sterile field along with other sterile supplies when being opened for the procedure.

To prepare the active electrode for use, the STSR will remove any protective devices and packaging material and set the entire unit (pencil with appropriate tip and holster) aside for placement on the sterile field following drape application. Once the patient has been draped, the cord and holster are secured to the drape (according to the manufacturer's instructions or with a nonperforating nonmetallic device). The pencil end remains on the sterile field within the holster, and the opposite end is passed from the sterile field to the circulator for attachment to the generator. Once connected, the power settings are adjusted by the circulator.

The *dispersive electrode,* also called the *grounding pad* or *inactive electrode,* is removed from its protective package, secured to the patient (according to facility policy and the manufacturer's instructions), and connected to the receptacle on the front of the generator.

The dispersive electrode is securely affixed to the patient by the circulator prior to application of the sterile drapes. A burn may occur if the dispersive electrode is improperly placed or is not secure. Refer to the manufacturer's instructions and the facility policy manual for information on proper placement of the dispersive electrode. The dispersive electrode is a disposable item and is available in adult and pediatric sizes.

Note: The dispersive electrode is only necessary when the ESU is operated in the monopolar mode.

Monopolar ESU current ideally utilizes the following pathway:

- Current flows from the generator to the active electrode.
- The active electrode delivers concentrated cutting or coagulating current to the surgical site.
- Electrical current passes through the patient's body.
- Dispersed current exits the patient's body at the site of the inactive electrode.
- Current returns to the generator.

Bipolar electrosurgery utilizes the same three basic components in a slightly different configuration. The active electrode and the inactive electrodes are housed in the tines of a two-prong forceps, eliminating the need for a separate dispersive electrode. Typically, the tip is reusable and the cord may be reusable or disposable. The tip and cord are placed on the sterile field along with other sterile supplies when opening for the procedure. The bipolar unit is prepared by the STSR within the sterile field by removing any protective devices and packaging material and connecting the tip to the cord. The unit is set aside for placement on the sterile field following drape application. Once the patient has been draped, the cord is secured to the drape. The end with the forceps remains on the sterile field (and may be placed within the holster along with the monopolar pencil) and the opposite end is passed from the sterile field to the circulator for attachment to the generator. Once connected, the power settings are adjusted by the circulator.

Bipolar electrosurgical current utilizes the following pathway:

- Current flows from the generator to the active electrode.
- The active electrode delivers concentrated coagulating current to the surgical site.
- Electrical current passes through the tissue between the tines of the bipolar forceps.
- Current returns to the generator.

PRINCIPLES

The principles for the unipolar application of electrosurgical current for tissue coagulation or cutting are relatively straightforward. High-frequency current is generated and conducted through the patient's body via the active electrode from a small surface area and is then dispersed through an inactive electrode with a larger surface area that acts as a ground. The inactive or dispersive electrode channels the low current back to the generator, preventing heat buildup within the patient's tissues.

The heat produced by the high-frequency current is a direct result of the tissues' resistance to the electrical current's path. The amount of heat produced due to this tissue resistance is directly proportional to the square of the current. In addition, the amount of heat produced is equally proportional to the resistance. In other words, tripling the current output is equivalent to a ninefold increase in the amount of heat produced. A tripling of the resistance is equivalent to a threefold increase of heat.

High-frequency currents with frequencies in excess of 500 kHz are necessary to improve the current transfer from the electrodes to the tissues and to prevent damage to nerves and muscles located in the path of the current.

Advantages of electrosurgery include reduced loss of blood and saved time. Hemostasis is brought about either by applying the active electrode directly onto the bleeding tissue or by touching the active electrode to forceps. This reduces blood loss and saves the time needed to apply suture ligatures. Cutting tissue with a high-frequency current eliminates the need to stop and control active bleeding because the cutting current sears the tissue as it is divided. It is possible to seal tissue clefts and lymphatic vessels that would normally ooze fluid postoperatively, reducing resorption of toxic fluids, edema, and postoperative pain.

COAGULATION AND CUTTING FUNCTIONS

A "spray" configuration for coagulation of small bleeding vessels uses a damped waveform to generate intense heat for hemorrhage control. This modulated current generates peak-to-peak voltages of up to 6000V for the solid-state generators, and up to 15,000V for spark-gap generators. The low current and high voltage cause intense sparking between the active electrode and tissue (spray), drawing an arc without direct contact. On the other hand, contact coagulation with blade, ball, loop, forceps, or clamp generates a much lower voltage, around 2000V with a coagulation current, and only 500V is generated when contact coagulating with a cutting current. The blade of the active electrode must be free of charred tissue to work efficiently. Special abrasive cleaners that stick to the drape are available on the market.

Cutting current utilizes a nonmodulated current and is ideal for scalpel-like incisions and simultaneous hemostasis. This undamped waveform generates a constant output at peak voltages of up to 1200V.

A blended current is a modulated current of up to 2000V peak-to-peak. The blend current is a mixture of cutting and spray coagulation (modulated and nonmodulated current) and allows for coagulation that is more precise during electrosurgical cutting.

DISPERSIVE ELECTRODE PLACEMENT

The inactive (dispersive) electrode, also known as the grounding pad, disperses the current and heat generated in tissue. The current flows from the active electrode through the tissues and then traverses back to the grounded generator through the grounding pad, which is attached to the generator by way of a flexible conducting cord.

Most grounding pads are disposable, although metal plates and gel are still occasionally used. The disposable pads are flexible for molding and contain a conductive gel that allows the pad to stick uniformly to the patient without damaging the skin on removal.

A properly placed grounding pad reduces the risk of electrical burns to the patient. After the patient has been positioned, the pad should be positioned over a large fleshy area, preferably a muscle mass, that is clean, dry, and relatively free of scars or hair. The area for pad placement should not be over a metal prosthesis or a bony prominence and should be as close as possible to the operative site so that electrical current through the body is kept to a minimum. After pad placement, the flexible cord of the grounding pad should be firmly secured to the grounding connection on the generator.

GENERAL PATIENT SAFETY MEASURES

In addition to the precautions for grounding pad placement mentioned above, the following safety factors should be considered when electrosurgical units are used:

- Prep solutions that are flammable, such as alcohol, should not be allowed to pool under the patient and should be allowed to dry completely before the procedure begins. These solutions or their fumes can ignite when exposed to a spark from the electrosurgical unit.
- Flammable anesthetics should not be used during electrosurgery. Precautions should be taken to prevent ignition of oxygen or nitrous oxide for procedures around the head.
- Electrocardiogram electrodes have metal tips that can serve as an errant pathway for the current traveling to a ground, burning the patient. Careful placement of electrodes is necessary.

- A pacemaker or internal **defibrillator** can malfunction during electrosurgery. Personnel should monitor the patient for potential interruptions and should be prepared with a defibrillator.
- Jewelry or other metallic objects that belong to the patient should be removed before surgery to prevent possible patient burns from a current that is seeking a ground from the active electrode.

ELECTRICAL SHOCK AND BURN

One of the major dangers with electrosurgery is electrical shock and burn. In addition to the patient, the surgical team members may also be at risk. General patient safety measures and those relating to the placement of the dispersive electrode have been discussed; two other possible causes for shock or burn are radio-frequency (RF) capacitive coupling and high-voltage dielectric breakdown.

RF capacitive coupling occurs when alternating current travels from the active electrode, across intact insulation, causing a burn. For example, a surgeon clamps a hemostat onto a bleeding vessel. The surgeon applies the electrosurgical pencil to the hemostat and activates it to coagulate the vessel. The surgeon's glove normally acts as an insulator protecting the surgeon from the current moving through the metal conductor (hemostat). However, the insulator (glove) is thin (providing little resistance) and the current may travel through the glove (path of least resistance) to the surgeon's skin, causing a burn. In addition to thin insulation, RF capacitive coupling is influenced by the size of the active electrode, duration of activation of the electrode, and the strength of the current.

Dielectric breakdown occurs when high voltage breaks down some insulating material, such as the surgical glove. During electrosurgery, dielectric breakdown may result when the material in the glove is unable to withstand the leakage of current generated by the ESU. High voltage can produce a hole in the glove and consequently the wearer will sustain a burn. Again, the thickness of the insulation, duration of activation of the electrode, and strength of the current influence the outcome.

HAZARDS OF VAPORIZED TISSUE PLUME

Vaporized tissue *plume* (smoke and aerosolized tissue) is formed when tissue is thermally destroyed and vaporized with the use of the ESU, laser, and other surgical devices (e.g., power equipment for cutting bone). Vaporized tissue plume is known to contain harmful chemical and biological by-products and is considered potentially hazardous. Standard Precautions must be used in all patient care situations in which blood, any body fluid, secretions, or excretions (with the exception of sweat), nonintact skin, and mucous membranes may be encountered. Additionally, it is recommended that vaporized tissue plume be collected by an appropriate mechanical evacuation system at all times. The vaporized tissue plume evacuation system should be independent of the fluid aspiration system.

ARGON BEAM COAGULATOR

Argon gas can be used to enhance the effectiveness of the electrosurgical current. Argon gas is inert and incapable of combustion, allowing electric current to pass safely through the gas. Argon gas from a portable tank attached to a specialized electrosurgical unit is emitted from the distal end of a specialized electrosurgical pencil. When the gas is ionized by electric current, it becomes more conductive than air and provides a more efficient pathway along which the current can travel. The energized argon gas appears as a bright beam of light. Because argon gas is heavier than air, the "beam" displaces the air, causing less tissue damage, which in turn produces less vaporized tissue plume than traditional electrosurgery. Remember, the argon-enhanced system uses electrical current that passes through the patient, therefore a dispersive electrode must be utilized.

HARMONIC SCALPEL

The harmonic scalpel uses ultrasonic energy rather than electricity to cut and coagulate tissue at the point of impact. Ultrasonic energy is precise and tissue coagulates at a lower temperature (coagulation occurring at 50–100°C) than electrosurgery (obliterative coagulation occurring at 150–400°C); therefore, the surrounding tissues suffer minimal thermal damage (charring) and less vaporized tissue plume is produced, enhancing visualization especially during endoscopic procedures. Use of a dispersive electrode is not necessary because no electricity passes to or through the patient.

LIGHTS

Obviously, good lighting is necessary for any surgical procedure. White fluorescent overhead lights provide general illumination for the room. Ceiling-mounted overhead operating lights provide the focused lighting necessary for precision illumination during the surgical procedure. Most ORs are equipped with two overhead operating lights, although larger ORs may have more. Rooms equipped for open-heart procedures usually have four, as will some trauma and neurosurgical rooms (Figure 10-17).

Overhead operating lights should be freely adjustable to any angle desired and should make an intense light appropriate for the size of the incision. The diameter and focus of the light pattern can be adjusted with a control mounted on the light fixture. The beam should generally be set at 10–12 in. depth of focus so that the intensity of the beam is relatively equal at the surface and depth of the incision.

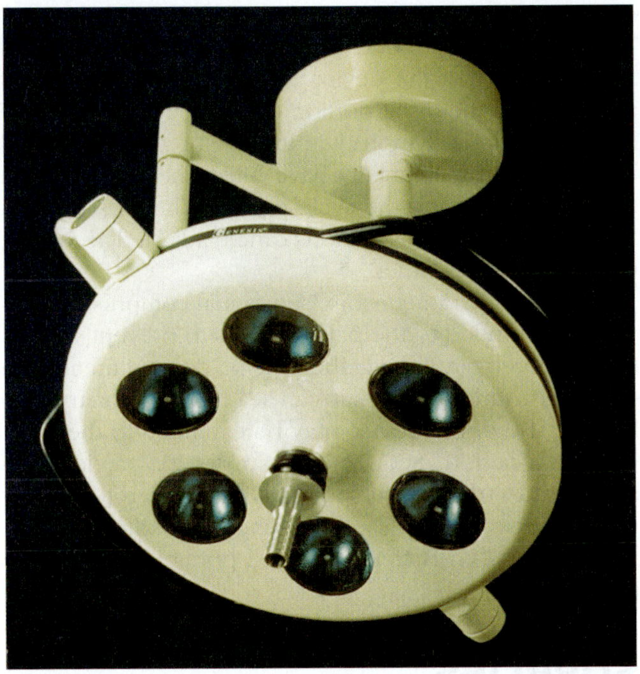

Figure 10-17 **Surgical lights** *(Courtesy of Burton Medical Products)*

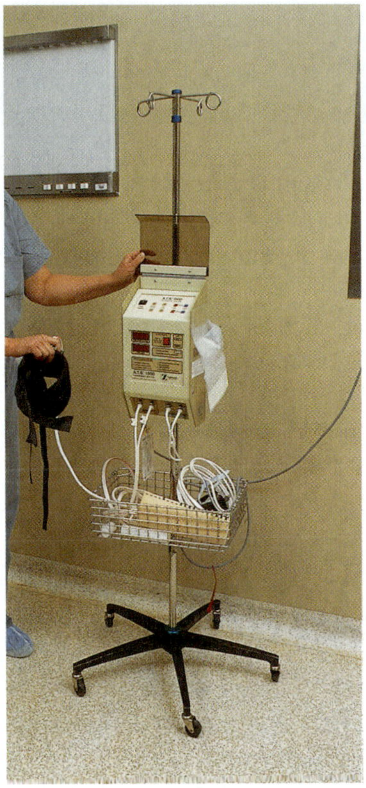

Figure 10-18 **Pneumatic tourniquet system**

The light beam from the overhead OR light should produce no shadows and minimal heat and be near the blue/white color of daylight. The light is typically set within a range of 1800–6500 K. An illumination factor of 5000 K approximates sunlight at noon on a cloudless day. Overhead lights should produce less than 25,000 $\mu W/cm^2$ of radiant energy. The light fixtures and suspension-mounted tracks or central mount should be built so that they are easily cleaned and do not retain dust.

Light fixtures are equipped with a screw or clip device within the center of the fixture for attachment of sterile handles. These autoclavable handles are used by the operative team to manipulate illumination for the operative site. The handles may be left permanently attached to the fixture and covered with disposable sterile plastic covers for each sterile procedure.

Light intensity from overhead operating lights is controlled by a wall-mounted fixture with a rheostat (dimmer) and an on/off switch. The operating room light should never be turned off unless the rheostat has been turned down. This prevents expensive light bulbs from blowing out.

PNEUMATIC TOURNIQUETS

Tourniquet use is necessary during some procedures on the extremities to restrict blood flow to the surgical site. The tourniquet serves two main purposes:

1. The amount of blood lost by the patient is minimized.
2. Visualization of the surgical site for the sterile team members is improved.

The electrically operated **pneumatic** tourniquet consists of the following components (Figure 10-18):

- *Cuff*—Consists of a rubber bladder contained within a fabric or plastic covering, similar to a blood pressure cuff and may house a single or double chamber. The double-chamber tourniquet is used for intravenous regional (Bier) blocks.
- *Tubing*—Connects the cuff to the pressure source.
- *Pressure device*—Consists of an air compressor, pressure controls, pressure gauge, and timer.
- *Power source*—The compressor is run by electricity. The unit is usually plugged in to a wall outlet; however, some units also have a battery that is capable of operating the compressor for a short time. This is useful in case of a power failure and for patient transport from the emergency department to the OR. (Compressed air may also be piped into the OR or may be obtained from a portable tank.)

The technique for tourniquet preparation, application, and use is as follows. *Note:* The surgeon may request a sterile cuff and tubing, requiring a variation of this procedure.

Placement of the cuff is determined by the physician. As a rule, the cuff is placed as far proximally on the extremity as possible. Variations may occur according to the patient's specific situation.

TECHNIQUE

Tourniquet Application

1. All equipment is checked for accuracy, function, integrity, and cleanliness.
2. Preset the pressure according to the physician's order.
3. Padding, such as stockinette or rolled cotton sheeting, is applied circumferentially to the patient's skin.
4. The appropriate size cuff is snugly applied and secured over the padding.
5. The tubing is connected securely to the cuff.
6. If necessary, a protective covering is applied to the cuff.
7. The patient is prepped and draped.
8. The extremity is exsanguinated with the use of gravity and/or an Esmarch bandage.
9. The tourniquet is inflated to the correct pressure and the timer started.
10. The tourniquet is deflated and the time noted.
11. Presence, type, and thickness of padding, size and location of the cuff, inflation pressure, duration of inflation, and condition of the skin prior to and following tourniquet use are documented in the patient's operative record.

Tourniquet pressure is determined by the surgeon and/or anesthesia provider according to the patient's systolic blood pressure and any other related medical conditions(s). Generally, the tourniquet pressure for the lower extremity is higher than the systolic blood pressure by one-half the value. The tourniquet pressure for the upper extremity is approximately 30–70 mm Hg higher than the patient's systolic blood pressure. During a lengthy procedure (duration greater than one hour), it is recommended that the tourniquet be temporarily deflated periodically.

The patient may suffer neurovascular damage from incorrect cuff placement, excessive tourniquet pressure, and/or prolonged inflation.

SEQUENTIAL COMPRESSION DEVICES

The *sequential compression device* consists of a compressor that is electrically operated, connecting tubing, and one or more sleeves that enclose that patient's limb(s). The sleeves house a series of chambers that are filled with fluid or air when the device is activated. Fluid or air is pumped into the distal portion of the sleeve causing any fluid (e.g., blood, lymph) within the limb to move proximally. Once the chambers have filled, they are emptied (decompressed) and the cycle repeats. The pressure and frequency of the compressions can be adjusted according to the physician's order.

In the operating room, sequential compression devices are applied to the patient's legs to prevent venous stasis, thereby reducing the risk of development of a deep vein thrombosis that can lead to pulmonary embolism. Use of the device may be extended to the postoperative period. Sequential compression devices are also used to treat edema and may be applied to the patient's upper extremity following an axillary lymph node dissection. Battery-operated portable devices are available.

SUPPLIES

Supplies refers to a large variety of sterile and nonsterile goods. These include drapes, drains, dressings, casting materials, and so forth.

DRAPES

Surgical drapes are used by the surgical team to isolate and protect the operative site from contaminants that can cause a surgical site infection (SSI). Properly used, drapes serve as a barrier that eliminates the migration of microorganisms from nonsterile areas to the sterile field.

Effective drape materials should be

- Lint free to prevent airborne particles from entering the surgical wound
- Fluid resistant to prevent strike-through contamination
- Antistatic to prevent sparking that could ignite the drapes or flammable gases
- Tear and puncture resistant
- Free of toxic residue
- Porous enough so that body heat is not retained, resulting in hyperthermia
- Finished with a color that does not reflect the operating lights
- Flame retardant so that they do not ignite if exposed to the beam of a laser or spark from an electrosurgical unit

DRAPE MATERIALS

Various materials have been used for surgical draping over the years. Each type has some strengths and weaknesses. Drape materials may be nonwoven textile fabrics, woven textile fabrics, or plastic.

Nonwoven Fabrics

Nonwoven fabric drapes are disposable and are typically made from compressed synthetic fibers, such as nylon or polyester bonded with cellulose. Aluminum-coated materials are preferred during laser procedures for their flame-retardant properties. Nonwoven drapes are light, yet strong, and offer the advantage of disposability. They need not be washed, folded, repaired, or sterilized by OR personnel, and contact with contaminants is minimized.

Disposable drapes have reinforced layers of material surrounding the **fenestration** (opening) of the drape. Some may have a plastic cover with a central slit over a rounded fenestration for snug fits around extremities. They are also equipped with special tags for attachment of suction tubing, electrosurgical cord or other lines or tubing to the drape. A built-in, antimicrobial incise drape across the fenestration is also available for certain specialty drapes.

Woven Textile Fabrics

Reusable drapes are becoming popular with hospitals because they are cheaper to use than disposable drapes. The cotton fibers of the material swell when they become wet, making the material impermeable to liquids. The material is also treated with a fluorochemical finish to further increase its fluid-repellant action.

Reusable drapes have certain disadvantages: They must be laundered, folded, inspected for wear, and sterilized after each use. If a defect is found they must be repaired. Frequent washings cause the fibers of the material to wear down, requiring heat-seal patches. Small holes may be missed, compromising the integrity of the barrier. Because they are reusable, the handlers' risk of exposure to contaminants is increased.

Plastic Adhesive Drapes

A modern classification of drapes is the plastic adhesive drape. These drapes are typically made of a thin, clear, plastic material that has an adhesive backing and can be applied to the skin without blocking vision.

Incise Drapes. *Incise drapes* are made of a thin, clear, plastic material that has an adhesive backing that may be impregnated with an antimicrobial iodine agent that is slowly released after application to destroy bacteria from the patient's skin during the surgical procedure. Incise drapes are typically applied to the patient's skin after four folded towels have been placed around the incision site. The prepped skin should be allowed to sufficiently dry so that the incise drape sticks properly. The incision is made through the drape.

Aperture Drapes. **Aperture** drapes are small, clear plastic drapes with openings that are surrounded by an adhesive backing. They are commonly used to drape eyes. These types of drapes allow the surgeon to view landmarks that would normally be covered.

Isolation aperture drapes are large, clear plastic drapes with an adhesive backing surrounding the fenestration and are frequently utilized as drapes for hip pinning. The isolation drapes are used to drape a patient who has been positioned on a fracture table that maintains traction of the affected extremity. Isolation drapes allow the surgeon to visualize the patient and the C-arm during fluoroscopy.

DRAPE TYPES

Drapes may be fenestrated, meaning that they have openings for exposure of the area to be incised, or they may be nonfenestrated. Each fenestrated drape has openings specific to the area to be exposed. For example, a laparotomy drape has a large, longitudinal fenestration within the center of the sheet because it is used to expose longitudinal incisions of the abdomen. A thyroid sheet has a small, transverse fenestration at the top of the sheet because it is used to expose transverse incisions of the thyroid. The remainder of any drape should always be sufficient to cover the feet and anesthesia screen. For tall patients, a nonfenestrated, reinforced three-quarter sheet may be added to sufficiently cover the feet.

Fenestrated drapes are used for the following procedures:

- Abdomen (laparotomy, or "lap" sheet)
- Pediatric abdomen (pediatric, or "pedi" sheet)
- Thorax and kidney (transverse lap sheet)
- Neck, especially the thyroid (thyroid sheet)
- Extremities (extremity sheet)
- Hip (hip sheet)
- Perineum (single-piece perineal sheet)
- Cranium (craniotomy sheet)

Nonfenestrated sheets may be used to custom "square drape" a surgical site, or to cover unaffected body parts that are not completely covered by the primary drape sheet. "Flat" sheets are square or rectangular sheets that may be placed under an extremity as a base for further draping. They are also used to cover arms on armboards or as a shield for the anesthesia provider. Flat sheets include the minor, medium, and reinforced three-quarter sheets.

Nonfenestrated drapes are also custom designed to cover specific areas. For example, the four-piece perineal sheet is designed to cover a patient in lithotomy position.

The opening for the perineum is created by two leg coverings (leg pockets), an under buttocks drape, and an abdominal drape.

Nonfenestrated split sheets are used to create an opening for a surgical site or to drape an extremity. One end of the split sheet is open down the center, creating a U shape. The free ends of the drape are referred to as the "tails" of the drape. The tails of two split sheets can be overlapped to create a fenestration of desired size, or the tails of one split sheet can be brought around a stockinette-covered extremity.

Stockinettes are designed as stretchable tubes to cover extremities. One end of the tube is closed to encase the distal portion of the extremity. The other is open for the proximal end. The stockinette is packaged in a roll and need only be unrolled over the extremity while the extremity is held aloft. Some stockinettes are covered with plastic to be fluid impermeable. These are frequently used to cover extremities for coronary bypass or hip replacement procedures.

STERILE PACKS

Sterile packs are the first item opened for a surgical procedure and are placed onto the back table to serve as the initial sterile field. Most basic sterile packs contain a Mayo stand cover, two gowns, a suture bag, four sticky paper drapes for square draping, and two paper towels for hand drying. Some sterile packs are packaged and sterilized by the facility with reusable items.

Drapes and specialty supplies are added for specialty packs. For instance, a laparotomy pack contains all of the items within a basic pack, with the addition of a laparotomy drape. A custom pack prepared by the manufacturer at the request of the institution may contain drapes and supplies necessary for specific procedures or specialties. For instance, an open-heart pack will contain supplies necessary to place the patient on cardiopulmonary bypass, in addition to basic draping items.

TYPES

Sterile packs have become highly specialized over the years. Examples of packs for specific specialties include OB/GYN, orthopedic, and ORL packs. Examples of specialized packs for specific procedures include craniotomy, arthroscopy, open-heart, and laparoscopy packs. Each specialized pack contains supplies and drapes that are specific to the specialty or the surgical procedure.

SPONGES AND DRESSINGS

Surgical sponges are used by the operative team to absorb blood and tissue fluids, blunt dissect tissues, and protect important structures during the surgical procedure. Surgical sponges are soft and lint free and contain a radiopaque strip so that they can be located by X-ray if left within a wound. They are counted for most surgical procedures.

Laparotomy sponges are the largest and most absorbant of the surgical sponges and are available in several sizes. These sponges are used on procedures requiring large incisions, such as laparotomy or thoracotomy. They are typically moistened with saline and used as "pads" to protect retracted viscera. Laparotomy sponges are also referred to as *laps, tapes,* or *packs* and are assembled five per package.

Radiopaque four-by-fours are smaller and less absorbent than laparotomy sponges. Typically referred to as *Raytec sponges,* they are used for procedures requiring smaller incisions. Raytec sponges can be folded and clamped onto ring forceps to make sponge sticks for sponging and retracting within an abdominal wound. Loose Raytec sponges are not permitted on the operative field during an open laparotomy procedure because they can be easily lost within the wound. As a rule, Raytec sponges are removed from the operative field and replaced with laparotomy sponges and stick sponges as soon as the peritoneum is entered. Raytec sponges are assembled as 10 sponges per package (Figure 10-19).

Neurosurgical sponges are referred to as *patties* or **cottonoids**. They are used to protect delicate neural tissue when suctioning and to assist with hemostasis during neurosurgical procedures. By placing a moistened neurosurgical sponge onto bleeding neural tissue, suction can be applied without damage to the underlying tissue. Most neurosurgical sponges have a radiopaque string attached to the sponge for easy location within the wound. This type of sponge is moistened with saline before use and is typically arranged

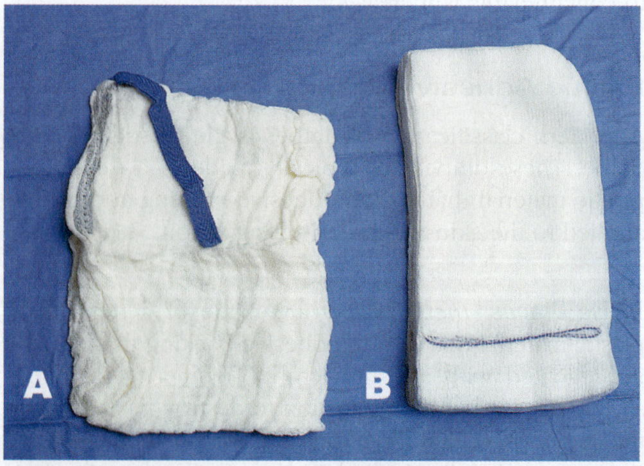

Figure 10-19 Surgical sponges: (A) Laparotomy, (B) X-ray-detectable 4-in. × 4-in.

on a special tray or an upside-down kidney basin on the Mayo stand. These sponges are assembled 10 per package.

Tonsil sponges are cotton-filled gauzes with a string attached. These sponges are used during tonsillectomy to pack the bed after tonsil removal and are typically loaded and passed on an instrument. These sponges are assembled in packages of five.

Kitner dissecting sponges are small rolls of cotton tape that are used to aid the surgeon in blunt dissection of tissues. They are always loaded onto a clamp, such as a Rochester-Pean, for use. These sponges are assembled in packages of five, and the STSR should always have one loaded onto an instrument and four within the carrier (Figure 10-20).

Peanut sponges are small gauze sponges used for blunt dissection or fluid absorption. These sponges are also loaded onto a clamp of some sort before use.

SURGICAL DRESSINGS

A surgical dressing is applied to most wounds (traumatic or surgical) for one or more reasons. Dressings serve the following functions:

- Protect the wound from trauma.
- Protect the wound from microbial contamination.
- Absorb drainage and secretions.
- Support the incision.
- Provide pressure to reduce or eliminate dead space, reduce or prevent edema, assist in maintaining hemostasis, and prevent hematoma formation.
- Maintain an environment that allows for preservation of new epithelial tissue and destruction of microbes.
- Conceal the wound aesthetically.

Prior to application of any type of dressing, the incision and surrounding skin must be clean and dry. A skin preparation material such as tincture of benzoin or Mastisol may be applied prior to application of the dressing. The functional dressing must be of appropriate size and type for the specific wound, secure, and relatively comfortable for the patient.

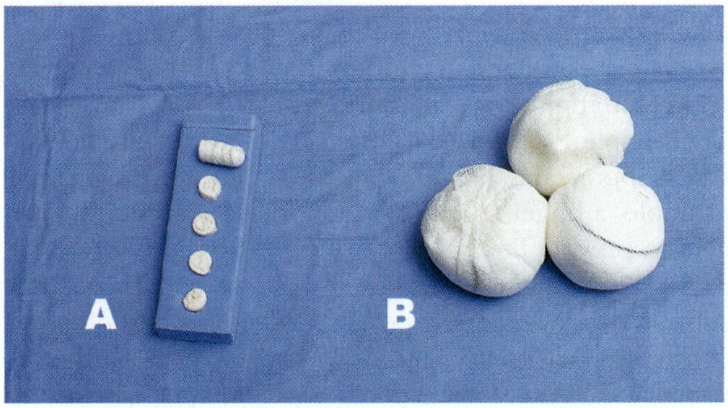

Figure 10-20 Surgical sponges: (A) Kitner, (B) tonsil

In the operating room, dressing application is considered the final step of the surgical procedure and must be carried out under sterile conditions. Dressing changes must also occur under sterile conditions. Dressing changes are occasionally scheduled in the operating room to provide a sterile environment and to allow the patient to be anesthetized if the procedure is expected to be painful or the patient is not cooperative (e.g., infant).

Some dressing materials are referred to as *sponges*. Use caution not to confuse dressing sponges and surgical sponges. Typically, dressing sponges do not contain radiopaque markers, the exception being certain types of packing material that could potentially be inadvertently retained within a body space or cavity (e.g., vaginal pack). To avoid confusion, dressing sponges are not provided to the sterile field until the final count is complete.

Note: Some types of specialty procedure packs may contain the dressings specific to that procedure. In this situation, the dressings are to remain in their original packaging until the final count is complete.

Dressing Types

The type of dressing to be applied is determined by several factors including

- Type, size, and location of the wound
- Amount of drainage expected
- Surgeon preference
- Age and size of the patient
- Underlying medical conditions (including known allergies)
- Condition of the surrounding skin
- Comfort of the patient

Dry sterile dressings are most often applied to closed surgical wounds. The surgeon may desire to place an antiseptic or antibiotic on the wound prior to dressing application.

One-Layer Dressing. A one-layer dressing is used to cover a small incision from which drainage is expected to be minimal (e.g., endoscopic access site). These dressings are also frequently used to cover the site of intravenous access. A one-layer dressing consists of transparent polyurethane film with an adhesive backing. Examples of brand name products used as one-layer dressings include Op-site and Bioclusive. Additionally, liquid *collodion* (a type of liquid chemical dressing) may be applied to the wound and allowed to dry, forming a seal over the incision. Collodion is flammable and may not be permitted in some health care facilities. Other examples of one-layer dressings include aerosol adhesive sprays, foams, gels, hydrocolloids, and skin closure tapes. *Note:* Skin closure tapes are used to maintain approximation of the wound edges and may be used alone or in conjunction with another type of dressing.

Three-Layer Dressing. A three-layer dressing is used to cover any size incision from which drainage (light, moderate, or heavy) is expected. A three-layer dressing consists of the following components: the inner (contact) layer, the intermediate (absorbent) layer, and the outer (securing) layer. The layers of a three-layer dressing may also be referred to as the primary, secondary, and tertiary layers. A three-layer dressing may be as simple as an elastic adhesive bandage (e.g., Band-Aid) or very complex.

The inner contact layer covers the wound completely and remains in direct contact with the wound. The wicking action of the contact layer allows passage of the drainage or secretions away from the healing wound into the intermediate absorbent layer. The contact layer will be one of three types with these purposes:

1. *Nonpermeable (occlusive)*—A nonpermeable dressing is a fine mesh gauze that has been impregnated with an emulsion (e.g., Vaseline Gauze, Xeroform Gauze). The occlusive dressing is used to create an airtight and watertight seal. It is nonadherent and allows passage of drainage to the absorbent layer. A nonpermeable dressing may be placed around an exit wound for a chest tube to prevent air from reentering the pleural space.
2. *Semipermeable (semi-occlusive)*—A semipermeable dressing is a hydrocolloid (e.g., ExuDerm, Tegasorb) or hydrogel (e.g., Nu-Gel, AQUA-GEL). The semi-occlusive dressing is used to create a mechanical surface and allow for passage of air and fluids. A semipermeable dressing may be used to debride a wound. A hydrocolloid dressing may be used on a chronic wound such as a burn or decubitus ulcer.
3. *Permeable (nonocclusive)*—A permeable dressing is a nonadherent material (e.g., Telfa, Adaptic) used to draw secretions from the wound (called *wicking action*) and allow passage of air and fluid. The nonadherent material should allow "painless" removal of the dressing.

The intermediate (absorbent) layer is placed over the contact layer to absorb any drainage or secretions. The thickness of the absorbent layer will vary according to the amount of drainage that is expected. Examples of absorbent dressings include 2-in. × 2-in. gauze sponges, 4-in. × 4-in. gauze sponges (e.g., Toppers, Sof-Wick), fluffed gauze sponges (Kerlix), and abdominal pad (also referred to as an ABD pad or combine pad) dressings (e.g., Surgipad, Tendersorb).

The outer (securing) layer is used to secure the contact and absorbent layers in position. Several options are available for securing the dressing:

- *Tape* (e.g., paper, silk, adhesive)—Used most frequently.
- *Wrap* (e.g., elastic bandage), Ace; *adhesive crinkled gauze,* Coban; *rolled gauze,* Kling; *fluffed rolled gauze,* Kerlix—Used to secure a dressing or a splint to an extremity, provide pressure and support, conform to body contours, or secure a thoracic dressing while allowing for movement of the chest wall during respiration. The wrap may contain a self-adhesive (e.g., Velcro) or may be secured with tape. A wrap (rolled cotton sheeting, Webril) may be applied as padding under a cast. *Note:* Neurovascular damage may result if a wrap is applied too tightly.
- *Stockinette*—Used prior to splint or cast application.
- *Tube gauze*—Used on a digit.
- *Montgomery straps*—Used in situations that may require frequent wound inspections or dressing changes.

Pressure Dressing. A pressure dressing is a type of three-layer dressing to which additional material is added to the intermediate layer or one that is tightly secured to cause compression of the surgical wound. Tissue compression influences wound healing dynamics and may promote wound healing; however, a dressing applied too tightly may cause neurovascular compromise that will negatively influence the wound healing process. The pressure dressing may serve one or more of the following purposes:

- Immobilization of an area
- Support
- Absorption of excessive drainage
- Even pressure distribution
- Elimination of dead space
- Reduced edema
- Reduced hematoma formation

Bulky Dressing. A bulky dressing is a type of three-layer dressing to which additional material is added to the intermediate layer. The bulky dressing is used to immobilize an area, provide additional support to the wound, or absorb excessive drainage.

Rigid Dressings. Casts and splints are examples of rigid dressings applied following a closed traumatic injury (e.g., simple fracture) or surgery to provide support and/or to prevent movement. They are made of plaster or a lightweight synthetic such as fiberglass. Some types of splints may be manufactured of molded plastic or a metal (e.g., aluminum finger splint).

A splint is applied to one side of a structure to provide support and prevent unidirectional movement. For example, a finger splint may be applied after tendon surgery to prevent flexion.

A cast encircles (encases) a body part to provide support or prevent any type of movement. A cast often incorporates the joint(s) proximal and/or distal to the affected area. The most widely used type of cast is the cylindrical cast that is applied to an extremity.

Other common types of cast include these:

- *Body jacket*—Extends from the axillae to the hips to immobilize the lower thoracic and lumbar vertebrae.
- *Walking cast*—Cylindrical cast of the lower extremity that has a polyurethane sole or rubber heel added to allow for ambulation.
- *Spica cast*—Secured to the torso to support the hip or shoulder in the desired position.
- *Minerva jacket*—Extends from the head (incorporating the mandible while exposing the face) to the hips to immobilize the cervical and upper thoracic vertebrae.

Because each cast is custom made, a number of other types of cast may be fashioned to suit the patient's individual situation.

Specialty Dressings. Certain types of dressings have been designed for specific applications or uses. Examples of the specialty dressings include the bolster dressing, the wet-to-dry dressing, the wet-to-wet dressing, the thyroid collar, the ostomy bag, the drain dressing, and the tracheotomy dressing, eye pads and shields, and the perineal pad:

- *Bolster dressing*—Dressing that is sutured into position. The bolster dressing may also be referred to as a "stent dressing" or a tie-over dressing. The bolster dressing is often placed over a skin graft recipient site to apply even pressure and prevent fluid from accumulating under the graft or to secure a dressing to an area that is contoured such as the face, neck, or nose. Long sutures are placed lateral to the wound edges and the suture ends are tied over the dressing to secure it.
- *Wet-to-dry dressing*—Wet gauze (soaked in the liquid of the surgeon's choice; e.g., normal saline, antibiotic solution, Dakin's solution) is applied to the wound and allowed to dry. The dried dressing is removed along with any tissue that has adhered to the dressing. This form of mechanical wound debridement is often performed on burn wounds and may be performed under anesthesia in the OR to provide patient comfort.
- *Wet-to-wet dressing*—Wet gauze is applied to the wound and is changed before it dries. Removal of the dressing while it is still wet provides minimal wound debridement and causes the patient less pain than the wet-to-dry dressing.
- *Thyroid collar (Queen Anne's collar)*—Circumferential neck wrap applied to secure the dressing over a thyroid incision. The thyroid collar may be manufactured or fashioned from a surgical towel. Ensure that the collar is not applied too tightly.
- *Ostomy bag*—Applied over an intestinal stoma to contain excretions. The bag is attached to the patient's skin with an adhesive that is incorporated around the edges of the bag.
- *Drain dressing*—Gauze sponge that is manufactured (e.g., Sof-Wick drain sponge) or fashioned with a scissors (usually a slit or "Y" shape) to accommodate a wound that contains a drain.
- *Tracheotomy dressing*—A drain dressing is placed around a tracheotomy tube, and the tube itself is secured with wide umbilical tape that is tied around the patient's neck. Straps manufactured with Velcro fasteners are also available for this purpose.
- *Eye pad*—Oval-shaped gauze applied over the eyelid to retain medication and keep the lid closed.
- *Eye shield*—Rigid oval shield applied over the eye pad to protect the eye from pressure or trauma.
- *Perineal (peri) pad*—Used to absorb vaginal or perineal drainage (e.g., sanitary napkin). May require the use of a belt or underpants to keep in position.

Packing Material. Packing material is used to assist with hemostasis, provide pressure, support a wound, and/or eliminate dead space. Packing material may be placed in the nose, rectum, vagina, or in an open wound. Packing material is typically a long strip (e.g., 1 yard, 5 feet, 8 feet) of gauze and is available in a variety of widths (e.g., ¼, ½, or 1 in.) The gauze may be plain (e.g., NuGauze Packing Strip-Plain), impregnated with an antiseptic (e.g., NuGauze Packing Strip with Iodoform 5%), or contain a radiopaque marker.

CATHETERS, TUBES, AND DRAINS

A variety of **catheters**, tubes, and drains are available to the health care provider to serve many patient care functions. They are placed within surgical wounds, tubular structures, and hollow organs in order to assist with diagnosis, restore function, promote healing, or prevent complications. Typically, these are hollow, cylindrical-shaped objects that are not easily categorized. For example, a "chest tube" is used to provide drainage of the thoracic cavity; therefore, it can be considered both a tube and a drain. It is imperative that the surgical technologist learn the names and understand the functions of these devices to ensure quality patient care.

CATHETERS

Catheters are used to remove fluid or other objects, such as thrombi and stones, from the body (Figure 10-21). They are also used to monitor body functions and to insert fluids including contrast media and medications. Soft, flexible catheters are manufactured of polyvinyl chloride, Teflon, silicone, latex, polyethylene, and polyurethane among other products. Some nonretaining urethral catheters are made of stainless steel.

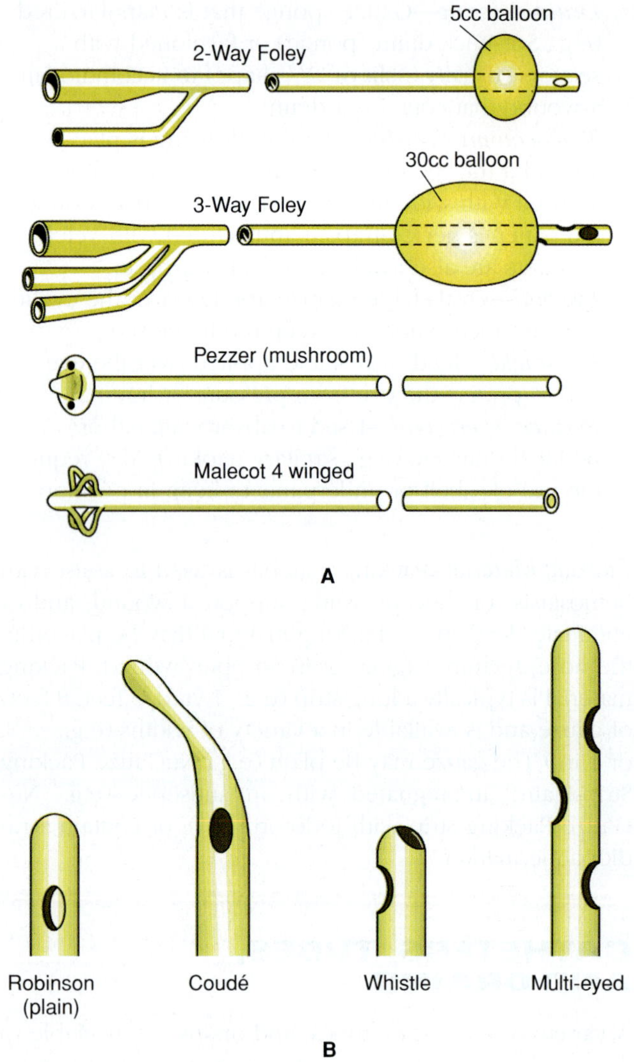

Figure 10-21 Catheter types: (A) Self-retaining, (B) nonretaining

Some of the more common types of catheters are discussed below. Keep in mind that a number of specialty catheters such as the cholangiogram catheter, the Swan-Ganz catheter, and the Tenckhoff catheter are also available. The Tenckhoff catheter is used to infuse dialysis fluid into the peritoneal cavity so that waste can be filtered from the blood.

Urinary Catheters

Urinary catheters are typically used to drain urine, but may have other applications as well. For example, the Robinson catheter may also be used to provide irrigation fluid within a duct. Urinary catheters are classified as urethral, **ureteral**, and suprapubic according to the method for placement, and further classified as nonretaining and self-retaining. Urinary catheters use the French scale for sizing. French (Fr) size is determined by multiplying the diameter of the item in millimeters by three. Most catheter types are available in a variety of sizes. The catheter may possess one or more openings or "eyes" in the tip to allow for drainage. The procedure for insertion of a urethral catheter is described in Chapter 8.

Nonretaining catheters are temporarily inserted through the urethra into the bladder to obtain a urine specimen, decompress the bladder, or maneuver around an obstruction. Examples of the nonretaining urethral catheter include the Robinson, which has a straight, plain tip (may also be referred to as a "red rubber" or "straight cath"), and the Coudé catheter, which has a rigid curved tip. Nonretaining urethral catheters do not require the use of a drainage bag.

Self-retaining or indwelling urethral catheters are called *Foley catheters*. Foley catheters are used to measure urinary output over an extended period or provide bladder decompression. The Foley catheter uses a balloon to retain the catheter within the bladder, allowing for continuous drainage of urine. The balloon may have a 5- or 30-cc capacity. A syringe is used to inflate the balloon with sterile water. Sterile water, rather than normal saline, is used for balloon inflation to prevent erosion of the balloon wall. Typically, 8–10 cc of water is placed within the syringe used to fill a 5cc balloon to compensate for the water that remains in the catheter lumen between the syringe port and the balloon. The two-way Foley has two ports that allow for balloon inflation and drainage of urine. The three-way Foley has an additional port that allows irrigation fluid or medications to enter the bladder. Some Foley catheters contain a thermometer in the tip that is used to measure the patient's core temperature. Self-retaining urinary catheters require the use of a gravity drainage bag (e.g., Urimeter). Various types of drainage bags are available and a specialized adapter (e.g., five-in-one adapter) may be necessary to connect certain types of catheters to the appropriate drainage bag. The gravity drainage bag must be maintained below the level of the bladder to promote drainage and prevent reflux.

The *suprapubic catheter* is placed into the bladder through a surgical opening in the abdominal wall. Examples of catheters that may be placed suprapubically are the Foley, Pezzer (mushroom), and the Malecot (winged tip). The Pezzer and Malecot catheters rely on the shape of their tip for retention, rather than an inflatable balloon. The catheter may be additionally secured to the exterior abdominal wall with heavy nonabsorbable suture. A drainage bag is necessary. The procedure for insertion of a suprapubic catheter is described in Chapter 20.

Ureteral catheters are placed in the ureter(s) with the assistance of a cystoscope. They are used to decompress the kidney, identify and protect the ureter(s) during pelvic procedures, and introduce contrast media during retrograde pyelography. Ureteral catheters are identified by the shape of their tip and typically contain a radiopaque marker. Examples of the ureteral catheter include the whistle tip, the olive tip, and the cone tip. A ureteral drainage bag is needed if the catheter is to be retained.

Intravascular Catheters

Intravascular catheters are used to infuse fluids (including nutrients and medications), obtain a diagnosis, monitor body functions, and remove thrombi. Intravascular catheters may be sized according to gauge or the French method and may contain a single or double lumen. Intravascular access catheters may be inserted percutaneously or via a small incision referred to as a *cut-down*.

Venous access may be achieved peripherally, usually in the upper extremity, or centrally, for example, via the subclavian or jugular vein. The Angio-Cath is an example of a vascular catheter used to provide peripheral access, and the Groshong is one of the more common central vein catheters.

Arterial catheters may be inserted temporarily to draw arterial blood for laboratory study or may be indwelling to provide information about the patient's physiological condition (e.g., arterial blood pressure). Arterial catheters are also used to perform diagnostic studies and various procedures including coronary artery angioplasty.

A Fogarty is a balloon-tipped catheter. The catheter is passed beyond an obstruction within the lumen of a vein, artery, or duct. The balloon is then inflated, and the catheter is withdrawn along with the obstruction (e.g., thrombus or stone). A variation of the Fogarty catheter is used for irrigation of the biliary system.

TUBES

Tubes are used to remove air and fluids from the body for the purpose of decompression. Tubes are also used to maintain the patency of a lumen and for the administration of oxygen, anesthetic gasses, medications, and fluids including nutrition supplements.

Gastrointestinal Tubes

Gastrointestinal tubes are used to aspirate air and fluids from the gastrointestinal tract. The gastrointestinal tube may be passed through the nose or mouth into the stomach or intestine, through the rectum into the intestine, or may be inserted surgically. Gastrostomy (feeding) tubes are also considered gastrointestinal tubes. Many gastrointestinal tubes employ the sump design. The term *sump* refers to a dual-lumen tube in which one lumen is used for evacuation of fluid and the second allows air to enter for equalizing the pressure within the structure, reducing the risk of damage to delicate tissues by preventing constant negative pressure.

Airway Tubes

Airway tubes are used to maintain patency of the upper respiratory tract. Airway tubes include

- *Endotracheal (ET) tube*—Available in adult and pediatric sizes as well as cuffed and uncuffed styles. The ET tube is passed through the nose or mouth, between the vocal cords, and into the trachea of the unconscious patient.
- *Oral airway*—Inserted through the mouth to separate the jaws and depress the tongue.
- *Nasal airway*—Inserted through the nose to prevent obstruction of the airway due to relaxation of the soft palate. Sometimes referred to as a nasal "trumpet" because of its shape.
- *Tracheotomy tube*—Placed directly into the trachea via an incision in the neck. The tracheotomy tube has three components: (1) outer cannula (may be cuffed, uncuffed, or fenestrated), (2) inner cannula, and (3) obturator.

Chest Tubes

Chest tubes are inserted percutaneously to treat pneumothorax and or surgically inserted (through a separate "stab" wound) following cardiothoracic surgical procedures to evacuate air and fluid from the pleural space. If two chest tubes are inserted ipsilaterally, one is placed in the upper portion of the thoracic cavity to allow evacuation of air and the second is placed in the lower portion for evacuation of fluids. The chest tube is secured to the exterior wall of the thorax with heavy nonabsorbable suture. The chest tube is connected to a closed water-seal drainage system (Figure 10-22). Two chest tubes may be connected to the same collection device with the use of a "Y" connector. The water-seal drainage system uses water in the collection unit to prevent air from reentering the pleural space, thereby maintaining the negative pressure necessary for effective respiration. The collection unit must be maintained below the level of the thoracic cavity to promote gravity drainage and prevent reflux. Prior to connecting the water-seal drainage system to the chest tube(s), it must be prepared according to the manufacturer's instructions. It may be necessary to use an adapter to connect the chest tube to the drainage system. Suction may be applied to some types of drainage systems to facilitate evacuation of air and fluid from the thoracic cavity (Figure 10-22).

DRAINS

Drains are used to evacuate air and fluids from a surgical or traumatic wound. Drains function passively or actively.

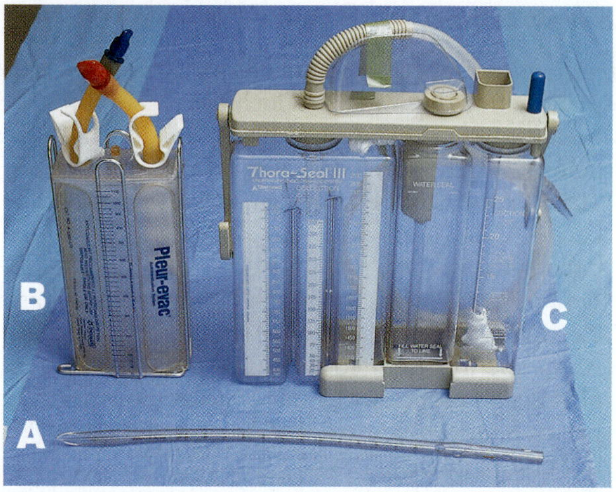

Figure 10-22 Chest drainage systems: (A) Chest tube, (B) Pleur-evac auto transfusion system, (C) Thora-seal (water-seal) system

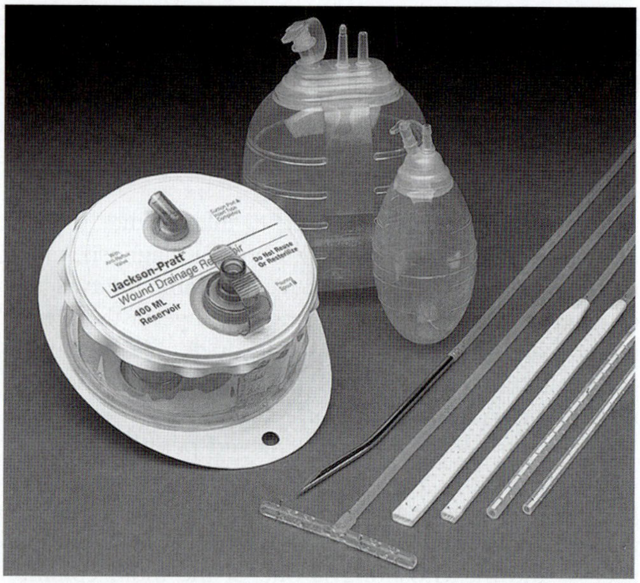

Figure 10-23 Closed-wound drainage systems *(Courtesy of Allegiance Healthcare)*

Passive Drains

Passive drains allow a pathway for fluid or air to move from an area of high pressure to one of lower pressure. A passive drain may be connected to a gravity collection device or the drainage may be contained within an absorbent dressing. Examples of passive drains include

- *Penrose drain*—Latex tubing that is placed partially within the wound, allowing fluid to move out of the wound into the dressing by **capillary action**.
- *Cigarette drain*—Penrose drain with gauze inside to encourage fluid to move out of the wound into the dressing by wicking action.
- *T-tube*—Placed within the biliary system to drain bile via gravity into a specialized collection unit called a *bile bag*.
- *Gastrostomy tube*—Inserted through the abdominal wall into the stomach to remove gastric contents or insert nourishment.
- *Cystostomy tube*—Inserted through the abdominal wall into the urinary bladder to remove urine.
- *Nephrostomy tube*—Inserted percutaneously into the kidney to remove urine.

Active Drains

Active drains make use of negative pressure (Figure 10-23). Negative pressure is created by removing air from the collection device manually or mechanically. An electric or battery-operated pump or the facility's vacuum system may be used to provide mechanical evacuation. Active drains are connected to a collection device. The chest tube and water-seal drainage system is an example of an active drainage system. Additional examples include

- *Hemovac*—Typically used following orthopedic procedures when a moderate amount of drainage is expected.
- *Jackson-Pratt*—Typically used following abdominal procedures when a moderate amount of drainage is expected.
- *Stryker*—Typically used following orthopedic procedures. Effective in reducing dead space due to the strength of the battery-operated evacuation pump.

NONSUTURE NEEDLES

Most needles used in the OR are *suture needles,* employed for passage of suture material through tissue. These needles either are attached (swaged) to the end of a suture or have eyes for threaded suture. However, nonsuture needles, such as hypodermic, arterial, intravenous, biopsy, insufflation, or spinal needles, are commonly utilized during surgical procedures.

Hypodermic needles are used to inject medications into tissues or intravenous tubing. The STSR uses them to withdraw medications into a syringe from a vial held by a circulator. Hypodermic needles may also be used to withdraw fluids from tissues. They are produced in varying sizes and lengths. Needle lengths range in size from ½ to 4 in., and gauge sizes range from 12 to 30, with smaller needles having the larger gauge number.

Spinal needle/cannula assemblies are 3–4 in. long with a sharp, beveled stylet within the metal cannula. These needles are typically employed to introduce anesthetic agents into the epidural or subdural space or to obtain cerebral spinal fluid for diagnostic purposes.

Arterial or *venous/cannula needle* assemblies employ a needle to introduce a plastic indwelling catheter into a vessel. Arterial needle/cannula assemblies are used to obtain arterial blood gases or are attached to a line leading to a transducer to directly monitor arterial blood pressure. Intravenous cannula/needle assemblies, such as the Angio-Cath, are attached to IV lines for the introduction of fluids and/or medications into the patient's system.

Arterial needles, such as the Potts-Cournand needle/cannula assembly, are used to introduce diagnostic or angioplasty guiding catheters over guiding wires into the arterial system. Venous needles with an aspirating syringe are used to puncture large veins for the introduction of monitoring catheters, such as the Swan-Ganz.

Heparin needles attached to syringes are used during open cardiovascular procedures to irrigate open arteries with a saline-heparin solution.

Large percutaneous *biopsy needles* are used to obtain tissue samples from within the body for biopsy. This type of biopsy is sometimes guided with the aid of CT scan or fluoroscopy. Examples of this type of needle include the Dorsey cannulated needle for biopsy of cerebral tissue through a bur hole, the Chiba biopsy needle for biopsy of lung tissue through the chest wall, and the Franklin-Silverman cannulated biopsy needle with a "trap door" tip for biopsy of the liver and other internal organs. Bone marrow trocars introduced through cortical bone may be used to obtain bone marrow.

Biopsy needles attached to syringes may be used to aspirate fluid from a cyst or abscess. Very small biopsy needles can obtain cells from breast lesions, lymph nodes, or other shallow tissues.

IRRIGATORS AND SYRINGES

Syringes may be made of plastic or glass and are used to irrigate wounds, aspirate fluids, or inject medications. Standard syringes are calibrated in milliliters and/or cubic centimeters, while insulin syringes are calculated in units. Tuberculin syringes are calculated in tenths or hundredths of a cubic centimeter.

A syringe consists of a tip that may be plain (Luer-slip) or locking (Luer-Lok). The plain tip accepts needles that simply slip over the syringe tip. This connection is not nearly as secure as the Luer-Lok tip, which locks the needle onto the syringe tip with a twisting motion.

Standard syringes vary in size, containing from 3 to 60 cc of fluid. The 10-cc syringe is the most commonly used standard syringe. Tuberculin syringes contain up to 1 cc of fluid.

Standard 10-cc syringes used for injecting local anesthetics may have finger and thumb holes for better control. These syringes are referred to as *three-ring* or *control* syringes.

Irrigating syringes may be bulb or bulb/barrel syringes or larger standard syringes with a heparin needle attached for intra-arterial irrigation. The standard irrigating bulb/barrel syringe for most procedures is the bulb Asepto syringe, which holds approximately 120 cc. The ear syringe does not have a barrel and is used to irrigate smaller incisions and structures such as the ear and to remove fluids from the nose and mouth of an infant.

CASE STUDY

Chang is a surgical technology student in a clinical rotation. The assignment for the day is to work with the central sterile supply team preparing instruments and instrument sets for sterilization. Chang has been asked to prepare a dilatation and curettage set.

1. How will Chang know what instruments the hospital routinely places in this set?
2. What categories of instruments will be represented in this set?

QUESTIONS FOR FURTHER STUDY

1. What factors determine which type of laser should be used for a specific procedure?
2. What are the strengths and weaknesses of each type of material used for drapes?
3. Why are some instrument finishes dull or black?
4. In what situation(s) is a water-seal drainage system used?
5. What is the purpose of a Tenckhoff catheter?
6. Explain the difference between a scalpel and a knife. List one or more examples of each.

BIBLIOGRAPHY

Ansell Healthcare Products, Inc. (2001). *Understanding the relationship between surgical gloves and electrosurgery* [Brochure]. Massillon, OH: Author.

Atkinson, L. J., & Fortunato, N. (1996). *Berry and Kohn's operating room technique* (8th ed.). St. Louis, MO: Mosby.

Ball, K. A. (1990). *Lasers, the perioperative challenge.* St. Louis, MO: Mosby.

Deitch, E. A. (1997). *Tools of the trade and rules of the road: A surgical guide.* Philadelphia: Lippincott-Raven.

Edgerton, M. T. (1988). *The art of surgical technique.* Baltimore: Williams & Wilkins.

Goldman, M. A. (1988). *Pocket guide to the operating room.* Philadelphia: F. A. Davis.

Hausner, K. (1985). All electrosurgical units are not created equal [Online]. Available from *http://elmed.com/equal/htm*

Hausner, K. (1985). Electrosurgery—Macro vs. micro [Online]. Available from *http://elmed.com/micvsmac.htm*

Hausner, K. (1985). Laser vs. electrosurgery. [Online]. Available from *http://elmed.com/lasvselec.htm*

Hausner, K. (1986). *Electrosurgery.* Addison, IL: Elmed.

McGuiness, A. M., et al. (2002). *Core curriculum for surgical technology* (5th ed.). Centennial, CO: Association of Surgical Technologists.

Meeker, M. H., & Rothrock, J. C. (Eds.). (1995). *Alexander's care of the patient in surgery* (10th ed.). St Louis, MO: Mosby.

Miltex Instrument Co. (1998). *Miltex surgical instruments.* Lake Success, NY: Author.

Valleylab. (2002). *Principles of electrosurgery.* Retrieved October 29, 2002, from *http://www.valleylab.com*

Smith, M. F., & Stehn, J. L. (1993). *Basic surgical instrumentation.* Philadelphia: W. B. Saunders.

CHAPTER 11

Wound Healing, Sutures, Needles, and Stapling Devices

Paul Price

CASE STUDY

Frances, a 63-year-old woman, has been suffering from right upper quadrant pain. Diagnostic tests have confirmed the presence of gallstones. Her physician has scheduled her for an open cholecystectomy with a common bile duct exploration. Frances also has diabetes and is obese.

1. What is the surgical wound classification expected to be?
2. What considerations should be made during closure because of Frances' underlying conditions?
3. By what method is Frances' wound expected to heal?

OBJECTIVES

After studying this chapter, the reader should be able to:

C 1. Define terms relevant to wound healing.

2. List the possible complications of wound healing.

A 3. Explain the classifications of surgical wounds.

4. Define and give examples of types of traumatic wounds.

5. List the factors that influence healing and describe the manner in which they affect the healing process.

R 6. Describe the characteristics of inflammation.

7. List and define common suture terms.
8. Identify suture materials and stapling devices and their usage.
9. Describe the types, characteristics, and uses of natural and synthetic absorbable suture materials.
10. List and describe the common natural and synthetic nonabsorbable sutures, stating their sources, common trade names, and uses.
11. Discuss preparation and handling techniques for suturing and stapling devices, and list the factors relating to the choice of each.
12. List and define common suture techniques.
13. Discuss the basic uses and advantages of stapling instruments.
14. Identify, describe the use of, and demonstrate proper handling of the various types of surgical needles.
15. **E** List the types of injury that cause damage to tissues.
16. List the characteristics of the types of healing.
17. Describe the stages/phases of wound healing.

SELECT KEY TERMS

1. adhesion
2. anastomosis
3. approximated
4. chromic gut
5. chronic wound
6. cicatrix
7. dead space
8. debridement
9. dehiscence
10. devitalized
11. evisceration
12. first intention
13. fray
14. French-eyed needle
15. friable
16. herniation
17. immuno-suppressed patient
18. inflammation
19. laceration
20. ligated
21. monofilament
22. packing
23. primary suture line
24. PTFE
25. second intention
26. secondary suture line
27. swaged
28. tensile strength
29. third intention
30. vessel loop

INTRODUCTION

The surgical technologist must have an understanding of the various types of wounds—surgical (intentional) and traumatic (accidental)—and the processes involved in tissue repair and wound healing. Incision choice, tissue-handling techniques, wound closure options, and possible complications all influence wound healing. Ideal wound healing involves restoration of continuity, strength, and appearance to the tissue.

TYPES OF WOUNDS

The word *wound* is described as any tissue that has been damaged by either intentional (surgical) or accidental (traumatic) means.

SURGICAL WOUND

Surgical wounds are either incisional or excisional. An *incision* is an intentional cut through intact tissue for the purpose of exposing or excising underlying structures. *Excision* is removal of tissue.

CLASSIFICATION OF SURGICAL WOUNDS

Surgical wounds are further classified into four categories according the degree of microbial contamination and are often referred to in the patient record by roman numeral (Table 11-1). The categories are as follows:

Class I: Clean (Infection Rate 1–5%)

- Incision made under ideal surgical conditions
- No break in sterile technique during procedure
- Primary closure
- No wound drain
- No entry to aerodigestive or genitourinary tract

Class II: Clean Contaminated (Infection Rate 8–11%)

- Primary closure
- Wound drained
- Minor break in sterile technique occurred
- Controlled entry to aerodigestive (includes biliary tract) or genitourinary tract

Class III: Contaminated (Infection Rate 15–20%)

- Open traumatic wound (less than 4 hours old)
- Major break in sterile technique occurred
- Acute **inflammation** present
- Entry to aerodigestive (includes biliary tract) or genitourinary tract with spillage

Class IV: Dirty/Infected (Infection Rate 27–40%)

- Open traumatic wound (more than 4 hours old)
- Microbial contamination prior to procedure
- Perforated viscus

Surgical wound classification is subject to change during the procedure according to the situation. The final wound classification is assigned at the end of the procedure and is included in the permanent documentation.

TRAUMATIC WOUND

Traumatic wounds are classified in several different ways, according to severity. A single wound may fall into more that one category. The classifications are:

- *Closed wound:* The skin remains intact, but underlying tissues suffer damage.
- *Open wound:* The integrity of the skin is destroyed.
- *Simple wound:* The integrity of the skin is destroyed. There is no loss or destruction of tissue and there is no foreign body in the wound.
- *Complicated wound:* Tissue is lost or destroyed, or a foreign body remains in the wound.
- *Clean wound:* Wound edges can be **approximated** and secured. A clean wound is expected to heal by **first intention**.

Table 11-1 Wound Classification

CLASSIFICATION	DEFINITION	EXAMPLES
Clean (Class I)	Uninfected, uninflamed operative wound in which the respiratory, alimentary, genital, or uninfected urinary tracts are not entered	Coronary artery bypass graft, craniotomy
Clean contaminated (Class II)	Uninfected operative wound; respiratory, alimentary, genital, or urinary tract is entered under controlled circumstances without unusual contamination	Appendectomy, cholecystectomy
Contaminated (Class III)	Acute, nonpurulent, inflamed operative wound or open, fresh wound, or any surgical procedure with major breaks in sterile technique or gross spillage from the gastrointestinal (GI) tract	Open fracture, colon resection with gross spillage of GI contents
Dirty (Class IV)	Clinically infected operative wound or perforated viscera or old, traumatic wounds with retained necrotic tissue	Resection of ruptured appendix

- *Contaminated wound:* Contamination occurs when a dirty object damages the integrity of the skin. Contamination can become infection within a short period of time (4–6 hours). **Debridement** is necessary. Debridement involves wound irrigation to wash out contaminants and removal of **devitalized** tissue.

Another method of classifying traumatic wounds is by the mechanism of injury. Some examples are

- *Abrasion:* Scrape
- *Contusion:* Bruise
- ***Laceration***: Cut or tear
- *Puncture:* Penetrating wound
- *Thermal:* Heat or cold (can be chemical)

CHRONIC WOUND

Chronic wounds are those that persist for an extended period of time. A chronic wound may develop because of an underlying physical condition that the patient suffers from or it may be due to infection.

INFLAMMATORY PROCESS

Inflammation is the body's protective response to injury or tissue destruction. The inflammatory process serves to destroy, dilute, or wall off the injured tissue. The classic local signs of inflammation are

- Pain (dolor)
- Heat (calor)
- Redness (rubor)
- Swelling (tumor)
- Loss of function (functio laesa)

An inflammatory reaction occurs when injured tissues release histamine from the damaged cells. The histamine causes the small blood vessels in the area to dilate, increasing the blood flow to the area, resulting in the heat, redness, and swelling.

TYPES OF WOUND HEALING

Three types of wound healing are identified. They are listed as first intention (primary union), **second intention** (granulation), and **third intention** (delayed primary closure). The type of wound healing will be determined by the type and condition of the tissue.

FIRST INTENTION (PRIMARY UNION)

First intention healing occurs with a primary union that is typical of an incision opened under ideal conditions. Healing occurs from side to side in a sterile wound in which **dead space** has been eliminated and the wound edges have been accurately approximated. Wounds heal rapidly with no separation of the edges and minimal scarring. Wound **tensile strength** plateaus at the third month at 70–80% of original strength. Healing by first intention occurs in three distinct phases (Figure 11-1).

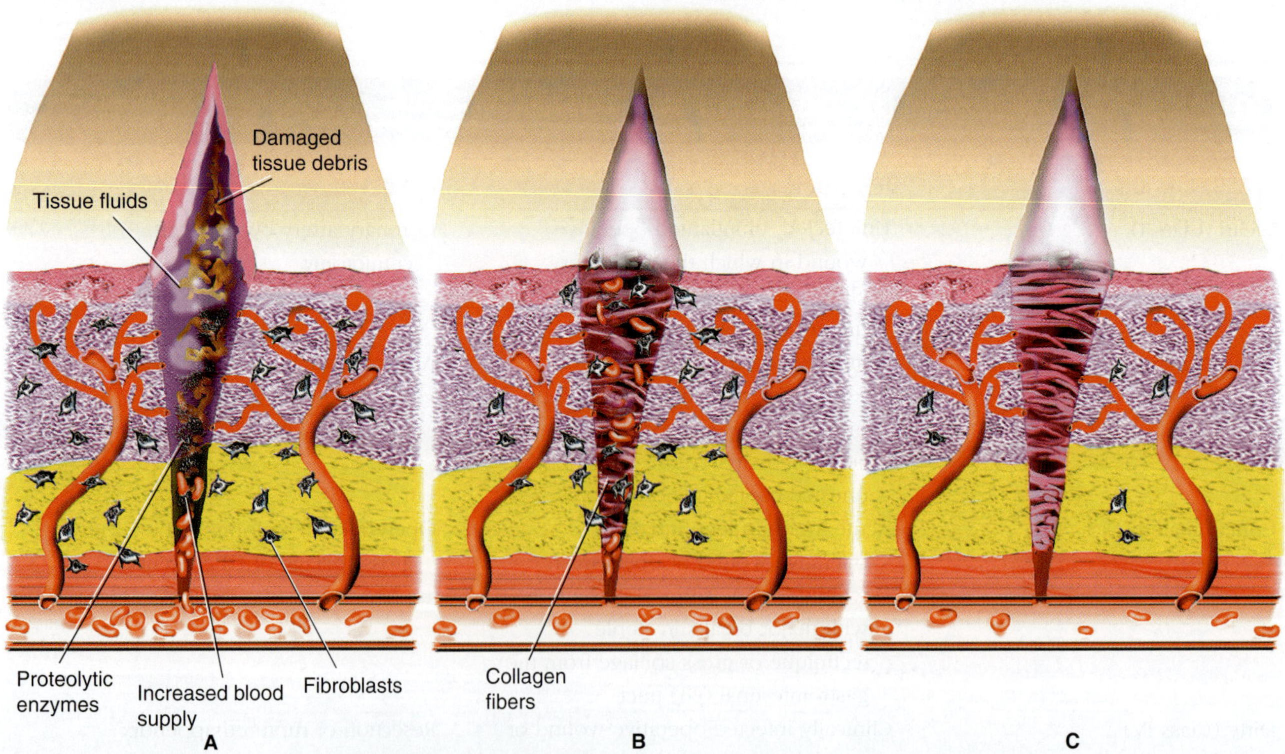

Figure 11-1 Tissue response to injury: (A) Phase 1, inflammatory response and debridement process; (B) phase 2, collagen formation (scar tissue), (C) phase 3, sufficient collagen laid down ***(Reproduced with permission from Ethicon, Inc., Somerville, NJ, 2002)***

PHASES OF WOUND HEALING BY FIRST INTENTION

PHASE 1: LAG PHASE OR INFLAMMATORY RESPONSE PHASE

This stage begins within minutes of injury and lasts approximately 3–5 days. It is defined by the physiological changes associated with inflammation manifested as heat, redness, swelling, pain, and loss of function. The warmth and redness associated with inflammation are a result of the arterial dilatation that increases blood flow to the area. This stage of reparation controls bleeding through platelet aggregation, delivers blood to the injured site through vessel dilation, and forms epithelial cells for repair. A scab forms on the surface to seal the wound, preventing serous leakage and microbial invasion. Increased capillary permeability triggered by chemicals released by injured cells permits leakage of protein-rich fluid into the extravascular fluid compartment, and results in edema and localized pain.

Leukocytes move to the endothelial lining of the small vessels within hours after the injury, eventually moving through the endothelial spaces outside of the vessels. Once in the extravascular space, they are drawn to the site of the injury. The neutrophils and macrophages begin to neutralize foreign particles by phagocytosis.

Basal cells migrate across the skin edges, closing the surface of the wound. Fibroblasts in the deeper tissue begin the reconstruction of the nonepithelial tissue. The wound does not gain tensile strength during this phase.

PHASE 2: PROLIFERATION PHASE

This stage begins on approximately the third postoperative day and continues for up to 20 days. Fibroblasts multiply and bridge the wound edges. The fibroblasts secrete collagen that forms into fibers that give the wound approximately 25–30% of its original tensile strength. New networks from existing capillaries are established by the 5th to 8th day, and lymphatic networks are reformed by the 10th day, many of which diminish during the final phase of wound healing.

PHASE 3: MATURATION OR DIFFERENTIATION PHASE

This stage begins on the 14th postoperative day and lasts until the wound is completely healed (up to 12 months). During this phase, the wound undergoes a slow, sustained increase in tissue tensile strength with an interweaving of the collagen fibers. Wound contraction resulting from the work of dermal and subcutaneous myofibroblasts is completed in approximately 21 days. Collagen density increases and formation of new blood vessels decreases, causing the scar tissue to pale. A small, white, mature surface scar, called a **cicatrix**, appears during the maturation phase.

Key words to remember include

Cicatrix: Normal scar formation (expected)

Keloid: Raised, thickened scar due to excessive collagen formation

"Proud flesh": Excessive granulation issue

Tensile strength: Ability to resist rupture

SECOND INTENTION (GRANULATION)

Second intention healing occurs when a wound fails to heal by primary union. It generally occurs in large wounds that cannot be directly approximated or in which infection has caused breakdown of a sutured wound. It also occurs in a wound in which the risk of infection is so great that primary wound closure would result in infection. Second intention healing may be allowed following the removal of necrotic tissue or after a wide debridement. The wound is left open and allowed to heal from the inner layer to the outside surface. This is a more complicated and prolonged process than healing by primary union. Granulation tissue that contains myofibroblasts forms in the wound, causing closure by contraction.

As the wound heals, large gaps in tissue fill, from the bottom upward, with granulation tissue, leaving a weak union and a wide, irregular scar that may result in **herniation**. Excessive granulation tissue, sometimes referred to as "proud flesh," may protrude above the defect margins and block re-epithelialization.

THIRD INTENTION (DELAYED PRIMARY CLOSURE)

Third intention healing, or delayed primary closure, occurs when two granulated surfaces are approximated. The traumatic (Class III or Class IV) surgical wound is debrided and purposely left open to heal by second intention (granulation) for approximately 4 to 6 days. The patient may be treated with systemic antibiotics and special wound care techniques may be used to treat or prevent infection. The infection-free wound is then closed and allowed to finish the healing process through first intention (primary closure). The result is a wound that heals by contraction, granulation, and connective tissue repair, with intermediate tensile strength and scarring. This method of repair works well for contaminated or dirty wounds that result from trauma and tissue loss.

FACTORS INFLUENCING WOUND HEALING

Three main factors influence the rate at which wound healing occurs, the strength of the healed wound, and the risk of infection.

The first consideration is the physical condition of the patient, which includes

- *Age:* Pediatric and geriatric patients may have decreased vascularity or poor muscle tone.
- *Nutritional status:* Dietary deficiencies can alter the healing process.
- *Disease (chronic or acute):* Metabolic disease, cardiovascular or respiratory insufficiency, obesity, malignancy, and the presence of infection all negatively impact wound healing.
- *Smoking:* Smoking causes vasoconstriction, diminishes oxygenation, and causes coughing that can put stress on a healing wound.
- *Radiation exposure:* Patients undergoing radiation treatment in large doses may experience a decrease in blood supply to the irradiated tissue.
- *Immunocompromised or* ***immunosuppressed patients***: The patient's immune system may be deficient due to congenital or acquired conditions.

The second consideration is intraoperative tissue handling, which includes

- Length and direction of the incision
- Dissection technique (sharp or blunt)
- Duration of surgery (surgical time should be minimized)
- Amount of tissue handling (tissue should be handled as little and as gently as possible)
- Achievement of hemostasis
- Precise tissue approximation
- Elimination of dead space
- Secure wound closure

The third consideration is the application of the principles of asepsis through the use of sterile technique:

- Any microbial contamination of the wound could lead to an infection, causing an increase in morbidity or mortality.

COMPLICATIONS OF THE HEALING WOUND

Tissue disruption, whether intentional or accidental, leaves the patient vulnerable to infection and other complications. Meticulous application of sterile technique alone will not ensure that the patient will remain complication free. Many factors influence wound healing:

- ***Dehiscence***: Dehiscence is the partial or total separation of a layer or layers of tissue after closure. Dehiscence frequently occurs between the 5th and 10th postoperative day and is seen most often in debilitated patients with **friable** (easily torn) tissue. However, dehiscence can also be caused by abdominal distention, too much tension on the wound, inappropriate type or strength of suture material, or improper suturing technique. The patient often reports a "popping" or tearing sensation associated with coughing, vomiting, or straining. Dehiscence can result in retrograde infection, peritonitis, or evisceration if an abdominal incision is involved. Surgery may be required to correct the defect, depending on the severity of the separation.
- ***Evisceration***: Evisceration is exposure (protrusion) of the viscera through the edges of a totally separated wound. Evisceration is an emergency situation that requires immediate surgical intervention to replace the viscera and close the wound.
- *Hemorrhage:* Hemorrhage may be concealed or evident and occurs most frequently in the first few postoperative hours. Hemorrhage can result in postoperative shock. Surgery is frequently required to achieve hemostasis.
- *Infection:* Infection of a wound occurs when microbial contamination overrides the resistance of the host. It results in increased morbidity and mortality. In addition to antibiotic therapy, additional surgery may be required as part of the treatment regimen.
- ***Adhesion***: An adhesion is an abnormal attachment of two surfaces or structures that are normally separate. Fibrous tissue can develop within the peritoneal cavity because of previous surgery, infection, improper tissue handling, or the presence of a foreign body (lint or powder granule). The fibrous tissue that develops can cause abnormal attachments of the abdominal viscera that may cause pain and/or bowel obstruction.
- *Herniation:* Herniation is a result of wound dehiscence and occurs most often in lower abdominal incisions. A hernia is usually discovered 2–3 months postoperatively, and could result in bowel incarceration. Surgery may be required to correct this condition.
- *Fistula:* A fistula is a tract between two epithelium-lined surfaces that is open at both ends. It occurs most often after bladder, bowel, and pelvic procedures. Abnormal drainage is a prevalent sign. Surgery is required for correction.
- *Sinus tract:* A sinus is a tract between two epithelium-lined surfaces that is open at one end. Its occurrence is highest in bladder, bowel, and pelvic procedures. Abnormal drainage is a common sign. Surgery is often required to correct this condition.
- *Suture complications:* Suture complications occur because of either a failure to properly absorb the suture material or an irritation caused by the suture that results in inflammation. It occurs most frequently with silk or cotton materials, and is characterized by a "spitting" of the suture material from the wound or sinus tract formation.
- *Keloid scar:* Keloid formation is a hypertrophic scar formation and occurs most frequently in dark-skinned individuals. Corticoid injections and use of pressure

dressings can help reduce the size of the scar, but surgery may be required for correction.

INTRAOPERATIVE WOUND CARE

Intraoperative wound care involves local (at the wound site) and systemic features such as use of sterile technique, tissue perfusion, and antibiotic therapy. The surgical team is most directly involved with the factors that will decrease the chance of dehiscence or infection. Table 11-2 lists factors in preventing dehiscence and Table 11-3 lists factors in preventing infection.

Dead space is a separation of wound edges that have not been closely approximated, or air that has become trapped between tissue layers (Figure 11-2). The

Table 11-2 Factors in Preventing Dehiscence

FACTOR	RESPONSE
Long paramedian incisions	Avoid when possible. Provide careful closure.
Adequacy of closure	Provide careful closure. Use interrupted, nonabsorbable suture on fascia.
Intra-abdominal pressure	Use special closing techniques. Use interrupted, nonabsorbable suture on fascia. Use retention suture; secondary suture line.
Deficient wound healing	Provide for local tissue perfusion. Treat systemic problems. Use interrupted, nonabsorbable suture on fascia. Use retention suture.
Infection (already present)	Use scrupulous sterile technique. Irrigate wound (antibiotic solution may be used). Close dead spaces. Leave wound open to heal by second intention when necessary.

Table 11-3 Factors in Preventing Infection

FACTOR	RESPONSE
Degree of contamination	Use scrupulous sterile technique. Irrigate wound. Close dead spaces. Leave wound open to heal by second intention if necessary.
Virulence of organism	Respond proactively to probable infective agents.
Amount of nonviable tissue	Debride nonviable tissue. Handle tissue carefully.
Adequacy of local blood supply	Use hemostatic agents cautiously. Autonomic awareness.
Presence of dead space	Close all dead spaces or leave open for healing by second intention or delayed primary closure. Drain wound appropriately.
Presence of coagulated blood	Irrigate wound. Drain wound appropriately.
Presence of excessive suture	Use proper suturing technique.
Presence of undrained serum	Drain wound appropriately. Leave wound open.
Presence of foreign material	Remove gross material. Irrigate wound.

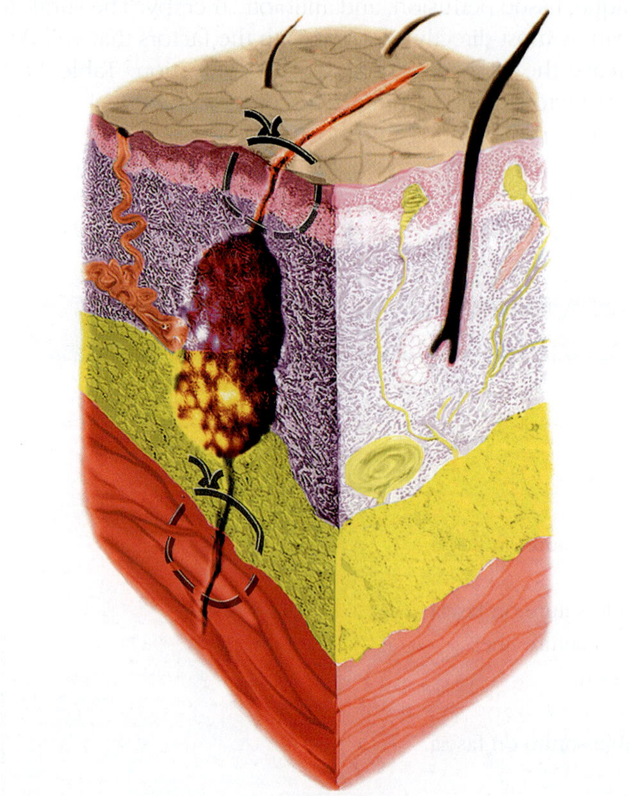

Figure 11-2 Dead space in a wound ***(Reproduced with permission from Ethicon, Inc., Somerville, NJ, 2002)***

space may allow for serum or blood to collect and provide a medium for microbial growth that may result in a wound infection. Dead space can be reduced or eliminated with the use of proper suturing techniques, wound drains, or pressure dressings.

POSTOPERATIVE WOUND CARE

The goal of postoperative wound care is prevention of infection and other complications. Postoperative wound care may include the use of drains and protection of the wound with different types of dressings.

WOUND DRAINS

Drains are devices that have been designed to remove unwanted fluids or gases from the body. Drainage can occur preoperatively, intraoperatively, and postoperatively. Not every drain is necessarily a "wound" drain. A single patient may need more than one type of drainage system as part of the postoperative care. Refer to Chapter 10 for a complete description of the types of drains and how they work.

DRESSINGS

Dressings are an important part of postoperative wound care and the STSR should be familiar with the types of dressings (refer to Chapter 10) and the uses for each. This knowledge should include proper application technique and awareness of potential complications. The types of dressing applied varies with the type of procedure, specialty, surgeon preference, and patient status.

Dressings are applied using sterile technique in the OR as the final step of the procedure. The purpose of the dressing is to provide an optimal physiological environment to promote wound healing. If a dressing must be changed within 48 hours of initial application, or if the wound is open, sterile technique and Standard Precautions must be employed. Dressings are removed or changed if they become wet or soiled or if the patient shows signs of infection. They are generally removed after 48 hours for closed nonchronic wounds. Stomas or areas affected by incontinence may require the use of special products to provide safe drainage.

For a contaminated wound, the skin and subcutaneous tissues are generally left open and packed loosely with fine mesh gauze, such as Iodoform. **Packing** is removed after 4–5 days and, if no infection is present, the wound may be closed at that time. If the wound is still infected, it is allowed to heal by second intention. For this type of healing, the wound should be repacked twice daily with wet-to-dry dressings.

SUTURE

The surgical technologist is, by nature of the role, knowledgeable about sutures and basic suturing techniques. The STSR should be aware of the factors that directly affect suture choice and technique. The surgeon selects the best suture for the particular task and patient and uses the technique that provides optimal patient recovery. The STSR should learn to think about suture in the same way the surgeon thinks about suture.

HISTORY

Since the beginning of recorded history, healing arts practitioners have searched for ways to control hemorrhage and bring wound edges together for healing. As far back as 3000 B.C.E., healers were using linen strips and animal sinews to close wounds. Later, around 600 B.C.E., cotton, leather, horsehair, and bark tree fiber were used in India with some success. During the first century, a Roman physician named Celsus and a Greek physician named Galenus began ligating bleeding vessels.

Until the development of sterile technique during the 19th century by Lister and Pasteur, patients generally succumbed to tetanus, gangrene, or septicemia. Pasteur believed that living organisms outside the body might be responsible for disease and suggested that surgeons sterilize anything introduced into the body during surgery by "passing it through boiling water or, better still, through a flame."

Lister, an English surgeon, accepted Pasteur's theory of living organisms. He believed that infection was a result of "disease dust" in the air that made its way into an open wound during surgery. This fundamental basis of asepsis, that microbes must be kept out of an open wound and that those already present must be destroyed, is still practiced today.

By 1867, Lister was using carbolic acid as a bacteriocide, and he began soaking his sutures in carbolized oil. Suture ends that were typically left dangling from the wound were cut short by Lister because he recognized that the dangling strands were an entry portal for bacteria into a wound. Lister succeeded in significantly lowering the infection rate of his patients, but most surgeons of the late 19th century still opposed antiseptic concepts.

By the early 20th century, most suture materials used for surgical procedures were made from the intestinal walls of sheep (catgut), although some preferred silk, linen, or kangaroo tendon. The surgical gut was sold in a dehydrated state and sterilized in open glass tubings. After the surgical gut was heat sterilized, preservative solution was added and the tube was sealed. In 1909, the Davis & Geck Company perfected a method for sterilizing the surgical gut after the tubes were sealed. By 1930, the company had introduced suture materials for specific specialties that included surgical gut, silk, linen, cotton, and celluloid-linen.

Suture tubes were eventually replaced by a plastic packet containing the sterile suture strand surrounded by a peel-away plastic wrapper that could be transferred onto a sterile field, alleviating the need for sterile transfer forceps. By the late 1950s, surgical silk was improved by braiding and waxing it for easier passage through tissues and improved handling. The first synthetic absorbable suture material was fabricated from polyglycolic acid in the early 1960s, resulting in a suture material with high tensile strength and minimal tissue reaction.

Today, the surgeon can choose from a variety of suture materials, each designed for specific tissues and purposes. Although the perfect suture does not exist, if it did, it would exhibit the following characteristics:

- It would be pliable and flexible with good handling characteristics.
- It would be easy to tie, and would hold knots securely.
- It would not **fray** as it was tied.
- It would slide through tissues effortlessly.
- The smallest diameter would never break.
- It would not cause tissue reaction of any sort.
- The tensile strength of the absorbable suture would be maintained only as long as the wound required support.
- The absorbable suture would disappear completely the second the wound could support itself.
- Absorption would be predictable in every patient.
- It could be used in infected wounds.
- It could be used in every surgical situation.
- It would be inert, nonallergenic, and economical to use.
- It would be inexpensive and easily sterilized.

TYPES OF SUTURE MATERIAL

Suture material may be classified as *absorbable,* meaning it is capable of being absorbed by tissue within a given period of time, or *nonabsorbable,* meaning that it resists enzymatic digestion or absorption by tissue. Suture material can also be classified as **monofilament**, made of a single thread-like structure, or *multifilament,* consisting of multiple thread-like structures braided or twisted into a single strand.

Absorbable sutures are designed to hold tissue edges together until they heal and can withstand normal stress. Sutures are treated as foreign material by the body, and the longer they dwell within tissues, the more likely the tissues will react negatively and impair the healing process. Ideally, the absorbable sutures should be completely absorbed at the very moment that the tissue no longer requires them for stability. Therefore, suture absorption time should closely coincide with the time that it takes the tissue to heal.

Monofilament sutures are relatively inert and do not readily harbor bacteria. They glide through tissues more easily than multifilament sutures, resulting in minimal tissue damage because they encounter little resistance within the tissue. Monofilament sutures, however, do not hold knots as well as multifilament sutures and are relatively difficult to handle.

Multiple-strand sutures exhibit a characteristic called *capillarity,* which is the capability to harbor bacteria and retain tissue fluids that can be communicated along the length of the strand. For this reason, multifilament sutures should not be used in the presence of infection. Multifilament sutures handle well and hold knots securely. Their multistrand configuration affords them greater tensile strength, pliability, and flexibility. Many brands are coated for enhanced handling capability and easier passage through tissues.

Suture material may be natural, meaning that it is made from naturally occurring substances, such as cellulose, an animal product, or animal tissue; or synthetic, consisting of polymers from petroleum-based products. Synthetic absorbable sutures are hydrolyzed by the body. Water within the tissue penetrates the strand and breaks down the synthetic fiber's polymer chain, resulting in minimal tissue reaction. Natural absorbable sutures are digested by body enzymes that attack the suture strand, eventually destroying it.

Suture provides support for healing tissues in the early phases of wound healing and should have a certain amount of elasticity to accommodate tissue swelling and the strains placed on the wound by coughing or vomiting.

SUTURE SIZES

Suture sizes are selected to correspond to the size of the tissue to be sewn. Heavy tissue requires a heavy-gauged suture; fragile tissue requires a small-gauged suture.

The sizing method for sutures is derived from a time when sewing thread was used as suture material. The suture diameter is referred to as the *gauge* of the suture. The United States Pharmacopeia (USP) specifies diameter range for suture materials. The diameter of stainless steel sutures is identified by the Brown & Sharpe (B&S) commercial wire gauge numbers. The largest available suture for use in surgery is #5; it is approximately the size of commercial string. The progression downward in size is listed in Table 11-4.

USP suture sizes #1 through 4–0 are the most commonly used. Sizes #1 and #0 are used frequently for closure of orthopedic wounds and abdominal fascia. Suture sizes 4–0 and 5–0 are typically used for aortic **anastomosis**, whereas suture sizes 6–0 through 7–0 are used for smaller vessel anastomoses, such as those on the coronary or carotid arteries. Size 8–0 through 11–0 sutures are used for microvascular and eye procedures. Size 4–0 sutures are used to close dural incisions; size 3–0 and 4–0 sutures are used for most subcuticular skin closures. Suture lengths range from 13 to 150 cm.

GENERAL FACTORS AFFECTING CHOICE OF SUTURE

Factors that must be considered when choosing suture material are the type of procedure, the condition of the patient's tissue, the nature of the disease process, the surgeon's preference, suture availability, and cost. The choice of suture is often a matter of opinion. The surgeon typically sticks to what he or she learned during surgical training.

Table 11-4 Comparison of Suture Gauges

USP	B&S	METRIC
#5 (largest)	20 g	7
#4	22 g	6
#3	23 g	6
#2	24 g	5
#1	25 g	4
0	26 g	3.5
2–0	28 g	3
3–0	30 g	2
4–0	32 g	1.5
5–0	35 g	1
6–0	40 g	0.7
7–0		
8–0		
9–0		
10–0		
11–0 (smallest)		

The surgeon must decide what size suture to use for each particular type of tissue encountered, and if the suture should be multifilament or monofilament, absorbable or nonabsorbable.

Absorbable sutures are often the first choice for tissue that does not need continued support. Nonabsorbable sutures are used where continued strength is necessary, for instance, to close abnormal openings in the heart. They are typically used to close the dura over the brain or spinal cord, and for fascia and skin closure. Silk sutures are commonly used for ligating vessels. Absorbable sutures are used for subcutaneous tissue and the mucosal layer of the intestine.

The condition of the patient's tissue is an important factor in suture choice. Not all tissues are alike. Some tissues are stronger than others, and some heal faster. Fascia and skin are strong but heal slowly. Gastrointestinal tissue is relatively weak but heals quickly. The normal strength and healing characteristics of a tissue are modified by the condition of that tissue in each patient. Some factors modifying the normal condition of tissue are as follows:

- Age of the patient
- Weight of the patient
- Metabolic factors
- Carbohydrates
- Proteins
- Vitamins
- Dehydration
- Vascularization
- Thickness of tissue at a given time
- Edema or induration
- Incision relative to fiber direction
- Amount of devitalized tissue within wound

The nature of the disease process is also important to consider in suture choice because disease affects the patient's metabolic processes, which in turn modify the condition of the tissues as noted above. Wound healing and suture selection are affected by these factors. Some individual disease processes affecting suture choice that the STSR should be aware of are

- Diabetes mellitus
- Immune system diseases
- Pituitary gland dysfunction
- Localized infection
- Systemic infection

CHARACTERISTICS OF COMMON SUTURES

Suture materials have distinguishing characteristics that can be compared. Physical characteristics include configuration, capillarity, ability to absorb fluid, size (diameter), tensile strength, knot strength, elasticity, and memory. Sutures may vary in pliability, how easily they pass through tissue, how easily they tie, and how secure the knots are. Each suture has a certain predictable effect on the tissue in which it is used.

MONOFILAMENT ABSORBABLE SUTURES

Monofilament absorbable sutures have the following characteristics:

Plain Gut

- *Type:* collagen (submucosa of sheep intestine or serosa of beef intestine)
- *Absorption rate:* enzymatic digestion in 70 days; absorbed faster in the presence of infection
- *Tensile strength:* significant decrease in 7–10 days; 0% in 2–3 weeks
- *Tissue reaction:* marked inflammatory reaction
- *Common usage:* superficial hemostasis; tissue with rapid healing time
- *Package color:* yellow
- *Other:* stored in alcohol solution; strength varies along suture strand; sinus tract formation common

Chromic Gut

- *Type:* collagen (submucosa of sheep intestine or serosa of beef intestine) treated with chromium salts to delay rate of absorption
- *Absorption rate:* significant enzymatic digestion in 14–21 days; absorbed faster in the presence of infection
- *Tensile strength:* significant decrease in 21 days
- *Tissue reaction:* moderately high, but delayed inflammatory reaction
- *Common usage:* internal ligation; may be used on peritoneum and fascia and infected or contaminated areas
- *Package color:* beige
- *Other:* stored in alcohol solution; strength varies along suture strand; sinus tract formation common

Polydioxanone (PDS II, Ethicon)

- *Type:* synthetic fiber from petroleum by-products
- *Absorption rate:* hydrolyzed in 180–240 days
- *Tensile strength:* 50% retained in 28 days; 25% retained in 40–45 days
- *Tissue reaction:* minimal
- *Common usage:* tissue that requires long-term tensile strength
- *Package color:* silver
- *Other:* may be dyed or clear

Polyglecaprone (Monocryl, Ethicon)

- *Type:* copolymer of glycolide and epsilon-caprolactone
- *Absorption rate:* complete at 91–119 days by hydrolysis
- *Tensile strength:* 50–60% remains at 1 week; 20–30% remains at 2 weeks
- *Tissue reaction:* slight
- *Common usage:* general soft tissue approximation and/or ligation; subcuticular closure
- *Package color:* coral
- *Other:* undyed

MONOFILAMENT NONABSORBABLE SUTURES

Monofilament nonabsorbable sutures have the following characteristics:

Polypropylene (Prolene, Ethicon; Surgilene, Davis & Geck)

- *Type:* synthetic fiber from polymerized propylene
- *Absorption rate:* nonabsorbable
- *Tensile strength:* excellent
- *Tissue reaction:* least reactive of all synthetic materials
- *Common usage:* tissue that requires long-term tensile strength; general, cardiovascular, and plastic procedures; low coefficient of friction
- *Package color:* deep blue
- *Other:* one of the most inert suture materials, especially useful in the presence of infection; suture of choice for vascular anastomosis; commonly used as mesh for tissue reinforcement, especially for hernioplasty

Nylon (Ethilon, Ethicon; Dermalon, Davis & Geck)

- *Type:* synthetic fiber polyamide polymer of coal, air, and water
- *Absorption rate:* nonabsorbable
- *Tensile strength:* degrades at a rate of 15–20% per year
- *Tissue reaction:* minimal
- *Common usage:* skin closure; retention sutures
- *Package color:* mint green
- *Other:* one of the most inert suture materials; useful in ophthalmic, microsurgery, and tendon repair; somewhat more difficult to handle and tie, and the knot holds poorly

Stainless Steel

- *Type:* 316L stainless steel (chromium and nickel alloys)
- *Absorption rate:* nonabsorbable
- *Tensile strength:* indefinite
- *Tissue reaction:* minimal
- *Common usage:* abdominal wound closure; hernia repair; sternal closure (#5 most common); cerclage; tendon repair; bone repair; retention sutures
- *Package color:* yellow-ochre

- *Other:* considered the most inert of the suture materials; can be used in infected wounds; requires special handling techniques; must not be used in the presence of other types of metal prostheses or implants; may be braided

Polybutester (Novafil, Davis & Geck)

- *Type:* monofilament strand of copolymers glycol and butylene
- *Absorption rate:* nonabsorbable
- *Tensile strength:* high
- *Tissue reaction:* low
- *Common usage:* tissue that requires long-term tensile strength
- *Package color:* seafoam green
- *Other:* has the greatest ability to stretch in response to a given load

MULTIFILAMENT ABSORBABLE SUTURES

Multifilament absorbable sutures have the following characteristics:

Polyglactin 910 (Vicryl, Ethicon)

- *Type:* synthetic fiber from a copolymer of glycolide and lactide; absorbable material is braided
- *Absorption rate:* minimal for 40 days; complete in 60–90 days for coated form
- *Tensile strength:* 50% retained at 21 days
- *Tissue reaction:* minimal
- *Common usage:* tissue that requires long-term tensile strength and absorbable suture is desired; general soft tissue approximation and/or ligation
- *Package color:* violet
- *Other:* one of the most popular sutures used today; uncoated monofilament also available; knot security fair, but ties easily

Polyglycolic acid (Dexon, Davis & Geck)

- *Type:* synthetic fiber from a homopolymer of glycolic acid; absorbable material is braided
- *Absorption rate:* significant absorption at 30 days
- *Tensile strength:* 50% of original remaining at 21 days
- *Tissue reaction:* minimal
- *Common usage:* tissues that require long-term tensile strength but absorbable suture desired
- *Package color:* gold
- *Other:* coated and uncoated forms available; little memory; ties easily with good knot security

MULTIFILAMENT NONABSORBABLE SUTURES

Multifilament nonabsorbable sutures have the following characteristics:

Surgical Silk

- *Type:* natural fiber from silkworm cocoons
- *Absorption rate:* nonabsorbable (disappears in about 2 years)
- *Tensile strength:* high; most lost in 1 year
- *Tissue reaction:* less than gut; more than synthetics
- *Common usage:* serosa of gastrointestinal tract and fascia in absence of infection; frequently used for suture ligatures
- *Package color:* baby blue
- *Other:* virgin and dermal forms available; excellent knot security and handling characteristics; no memory

Surgical Cotton

- *Type:* natural cellulose fiber
- *Absorption rate:* nonabsorbable
- *Tensile strength:* weak nonabsorbable; stronger when wet
- *Tissue reaction:* moderate
- *Common usage:* not commonly used today
- *Package color:* pink
- *Other:* used primarily as umbilical tape; used in the OR for vessel or duct isolation; easy, secure knots with excellent handling characteristics; no memory

Braided nylon (Nurolon, Ethicon; Surgilon, Davis & Geck)

- *Type:* long-chain aliphatic polymer nylon 6 or nylon 6,6
- *Absorption rate:* nonabsorbable with gradual encapsulation by fibrous connective tissue
- *Tensile strength:* very high, though progressive hydrolysis may result in gradual loss of tensile strength
- *Tissue reaction:* minimal
- *Common usage:* general soft tissue approximation where continual strength is necessary; commonly used for neurosurgical closures
- *Package color:* mint green
- *Other:* polybutilate, polytetrafluoroethylene, and silicone coatings used to reduce tissue drag; knot security and handling characteristics excellent (similar to silk but much stronger)

Polyethylene terephthalate (Mersilene, Ethicon)

- *Type:* braided polyester fiber
- *Absorption rate:* nonabsorbable with encapsulation by fibrous connective tissue
- *Tensile strength:* very high; no significant change known to occur
- *Tissue reaction:* minimal
- *Common usage:* general soft tissue approximation where continual strength is necessary
- *Package color:* turquoise
- *Other:* 10–0 and 11–0 available as monofilament for ophthalmic procedures; knot security and handling characteristics excellent

Polyethylene Terephthalate Coated with Polybutilate (Ethibond, Ethicon; Dacron, Davis & Geck)

- *Type:* braided, coated polyester fiber
- *Absorption rate:* nonabsorbable with encapsulation by fibrous connective tissue
- *Tensile strength:* very high
- *Tissue reaction:* minimal
- *Common usage:* general soft tissue approximation where continual strength is necessary; commonly used to close incisions of the heart
- *Package color:* orange
- *Other:* available for use as ligature ties; knot security and handling characteristics excellent

Tantalum

- *Type:* alloy
- *Absorption rate:* nonabsorbable
- *Tensile strength:* excellent
- *Tissue reaction:* minimal
- *Common usage:* hernioplasty
- *Other:* must not be used in the presence of other types of metal prostheses or implants; memory is straight but can be kinked; knot security good

PACKAGING OF SUTURE

Suture dispenser boxes contain one to three dozen suture packets and provide clear product identification through color coding, bold graphics, and descriptive symbols. The most important information that the STSR should learn to look for on the box are suture size and material and the type and size of needle. Other important information displayed on the suture box includes

- Surgical application
- Product code number
- Suture length and color
- Metric diameter equivalent of suture size and length
- Shape and quantity of needles (shown in silhouette)
- Needle point geometry
- Lot number
- Expiration date, if necessary

The primary suture packet is color coded and identifies the product code, number, material, size (USP and metric), and needle type and number. A suture strand with only one needle is represented by a single, actual-sized needle silhouette on the packet. A double-armed (two-needle) suture is represented by two needle silhouettes. Any needle number greater than 2 is represented by a single needle silhouette and the number of needles is written in red. Rapid release needles are designed to "pop off" the suture strand after a single suture has been placed.

The primary suture packet is sterile and contained within an outer wrapper similar to a peel pack. The contents of the wrap are sterile; however, the outside of the package is not.

LIGATURES

Ligatures, also referred to as *ties,* are used to occlude vessels for hemorrhage control or for organ or extremity removal. For example, the occlusion of the femoral artery is necessary to prevent hemorrhage when amputating the leg. Typically, vessels that are not coagulated or occluded with stainless steel clips are **ligated** with suture. Ties are available as full-length or precut suture strands in a package, or wound onto radiopaque reels for superficial bleeders.

Standard lengths for non-needled suture material are 54 in. for absorbable material and 60 in. for nonabsorbable material. These strands may be cut in half-, third-, or quarter-lengths by the STSR. Single strand ligating material is available in precut lengths of 18-, 24-, and 30-in. strands. Superficial bleeders will usually require ligatures no more than 18 in. in length. Deeper bleeders require a suture length of between 18 and 30 in.

Ligatures are placed around a hemostatic clamp that has been affixed to a bleeding vessel. After the first knot is thrown, the surgical assistant removes the clamp and the ligature is secured with a surgeon's knot. The assistant then cuts the excess suture. Monofilament sutures, because the knots can slide, are typically cut leaving ¼ in. ends. Multifilament sutures can be cut closer to the knot (⅛ in.) because they do not slide as readily as monofilament sutures.

LIGATING METHODS

Ligating methods include the free-tie, the suture ligature, the reel tie, and the instrument tie (tie-on-a-pass).

FREE-TIE

Ligating material may be used as either single-strand ties or as continuous ties from a reel or other device. Precut ties that are removed as single strands from the package and placed into the opened hand of the surgeon for use as ligatures are referred to as *free-ties.* This type of tie is not on a reel and is not loaded onto an instrument (Figure 11-3).

SUTURE LIGATURE (STICK TIE)

Large vessels are typically occluded with *suture ligatures,* or *stick ties,* to prevent suture slippage that can lead to uncontrolled hemorrhage. Stick ties are sutures with a **swaged** atraumatic needle loaded onto a needle holder for placement through the center of a large vessel after a hemostat clamp has been applied. The ends of the suture are brought around the clamp so that the vessel is doubly ligated (Figure 11-4). For superficial bleeders, 18-in. stick ties are used, and 27-in. stick ties are used for deeper vessels. Sizes 2–0 and 3–0 are the most commonly used stick-tie sizes, and silk is the preferred suture material. In

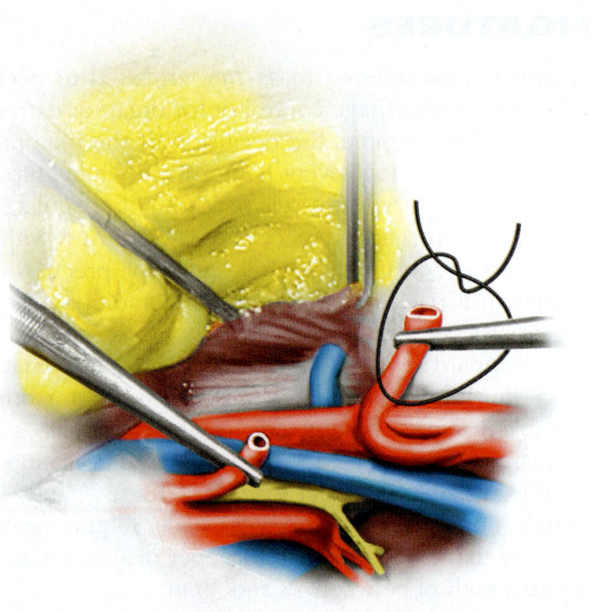

Figure 11-3 Free-tie ligature ***(Reproduced with permission from Ethicon, Inc., Somerville, NJ, 2002)***

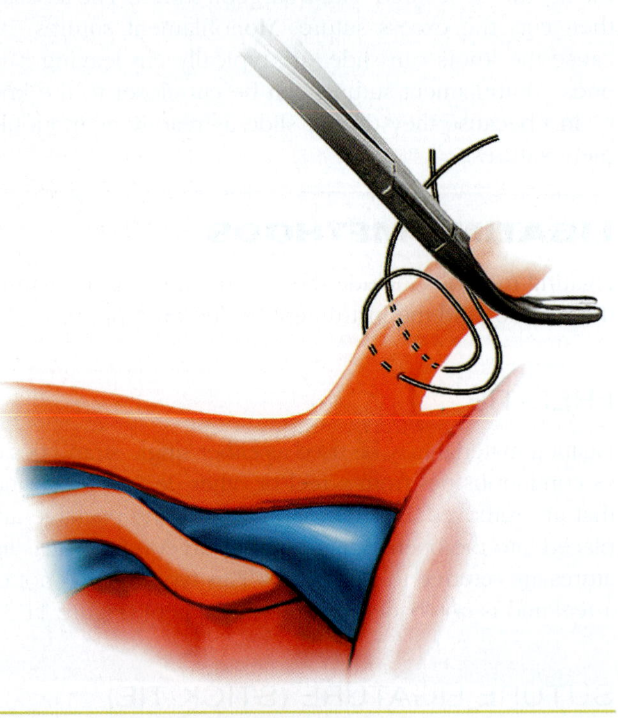

Figure 11-4 Stick-tie ligature ***(Reproduced with permission from Ethicon, Inc., Somerville, NJ, 2002)***

theory, however, any suture material can be used as a stick-tie ligature; it depends on the tissue to be sutured.

LIGATURE REEL

Ligature reels may be wound with absorbable or nonabsorbable sutures and are typically used to occlude superficial bleeders. Reels with absorbable suture material are frequently used on superficial bleeders of subcutaneous tissue just after the incision is made. The most commonly used ligature reels are chromic, plain, or polyglactin 910 sutures. Silk ligature reels are still available for use, as well.

Ligature reels are radiopaque and are included in the count in many institutions because they can easily be lost within a wound. The most commonly used sizes are 2–0, 3–0, and 4–0. The size of the material is indicated by the number of holes visible on the side of the reel. The STSR should prepare the reel by unhooking the end of the suture strand and pulling it 1 in. away from the reel so that the surgeon can grasp the suture without struggling to find the end.

INSTRUMENT TIE

Deep bleeding vessels that have been occluded with a hemostat clamp may be inaccessible for a free-hand ligature. Therefore, a suture is loaded onto an instrument (*tie-on-a-pass*), usually a Crile hemostat, Schnidt tonsil clamp, Adson clamp, or Sarot clamp, for easier placement around the tip of the occluding hemostatic clamp.

SUTURE FOR THE PROCEDURE

To determine what sutures will be necessary for a particular surgical procedure, the STSR should consult the surgeon's preference card and gather the sutures accordingly. Preference cards contain the surgeon's suture "routine," suture sizes, needles, and product code numbers for specific procedures. The STSR should consult with the surgeon to find out if any sutures from the preference card can be excluded or if any need to be added, or if the patient's size or condition requires modification of the suture routine.

The STSR should open only as many suture packets as are necessary because leftover sutures cannot be resterilized and must be discarded. Inexperienced surgical technologists tend to overcompensate for lack of suture knowledge by opening too many packets. However, if too few packets are opened, the surgical procedure may be prolonged unnecessarily while the circulator retrieves the additional sutures. Good communication between the STSR and the surgeon, in addition to regularly updated preference cards, can minimize waste and keep supply costs down.

After the suture packets have been opened onto the sterile field (sutures are often opened into the sterile basin set), the STSR can arrange the sutures in the order in which, they will be used during the procedure. Ligature reels should be removed from their packets and placed onto the Mayo stand with the strand end extended slightly. Free-ties should be opened at the end of the packet and placed on the Mayo stand with the suture strands protruding for easy access. Longer free-ties can be removed from their packets completely and placed into a rolled or folded towel. If hemorrhage is anticipated, stick ties should be loaded onto needle holders in advance of need and placed within reach, and ties-on-passes should also be loaded and ready. For routine procedures, such as coronary bypass, sutures can be loaded onto needle holders and arranged in the order in which they will be used. Otherwise, the suture packets are left unopened on the sterile field until they are needed.

Suture needs can be anticipated by the STSR by paying close attention to the course of the procedure and listening to the comments of the surgeon and assistants. The STSR should have a clear understanding of the anatomy encountered and the sequence of the procedure.

PLACEMENT ON FIELD

The sterile suture package is transferred to the sterile field using one of the two techniques used for opening any type of peel-packed item (refer to Chapter 12). It may be placed onto the sterile field or secured by the STSR (Figure 11-5).

LOADING THE SUTURE

Suture with a needle attached is prepared for use in the following manner (Figure 11-6). The STSR chooses an appropriate needle holder based on the size of the suture needle to be used, the surgeon's preference, and the depth of tissue to be sutured. The needle holder is clamped approximately one-third of the distance from the swaged end of the needle to the needle point. Tougher tissue may require the needle holder to be moved to the half-point of the needle. The swaged area of the needle (that part of the needle in which the suture enters the needle) should never be clamped. Modern suture packets allow the STSR to load the needle without touching it.

After loading the suture onto the needle holder, the STSR should straighten the suture with a gentle pull. Other handling tips include:

- Do not attempt to pull or stretch surgical gut or collagen. Excessive handling with rubber gloves can weaken and fray these sutures. Nylon sutures should be drawn between gloved fingers to remove memory.
- Do not place any tension on the needle suture attachment (swage).
- Avoid crushing or crimping sutures with instruments.
- Keep surgical gut away from heat.
- Never soak surgical gut.
- Do not wet rapidly absorbing sutures.
- Keep silk dry, and cotton wet.
- Do not bend stainless steel wire.

The surgeon should receive the needle holder and suture with the needle pointed toward the surgeon's thumb. The STSR should control the trailing end of the suture to prevent snagging. After use, the surgeon should place the needle holder onto a safety zone between the Mayo stand and the operative site. The STSR should not attempt to remove the armed needle holder from the surgeon's hands. Facility policy may require the use of a "safe transfer" method, rather than hand-to-hand transfer.

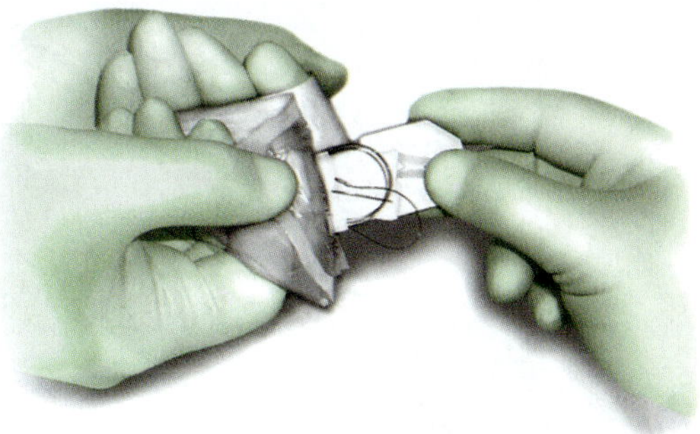

Figure 11-5 **Sterile suture transfer to the STSR** ***(Reproduced with permission from Ethicon, Inc., Somerville, NJ, 2002)***

LAYER CLOSURE

Abdominal wounds are closed in layers. From inner to outer, these layers include the peritoneum, fascia, muscle, subcutaneous, subcuticular, and skin layers (Figure 11-7).

PERITONEUM

The peritoneum, a fast-healing, thin membrane lining the abdominal cavity, lying beneath the posterior fascia, may not require suturing if the posterior fascia is closed properly. If the surgeon chooses to close the peritoneum, a continuous 3–0 absorbable suture is frequently utilized.

FASCIA

The fascia is a layer of tough connective tissue covering the body's muscles. It is the primary supportive soft tissue structure of the body, and great care must be taken to close the abdominal fascia layer securely. This layer heals slowly and must endure the brunt of wound stress; therefore, interrupted, heavy-gauge, nonabsorbable sutures with multifilament strands are preferred for added strength. If an absorbable suture material is used, it should be slow absorbing and have high-tensile strength. If the fascial layer is weak, surgical synthetic polypropylene mesh may be sutured in with polypropylene sutures for structural support.

MUSCLE

Muscles are typically not closed with suture because they do not tolerate suture material well. Muscles are usually separated or retracted and, therefore, do not need to be closed (Figure 11-8). If they are incised, however, they should be loosely approximated with interrupted absorbable sutures.

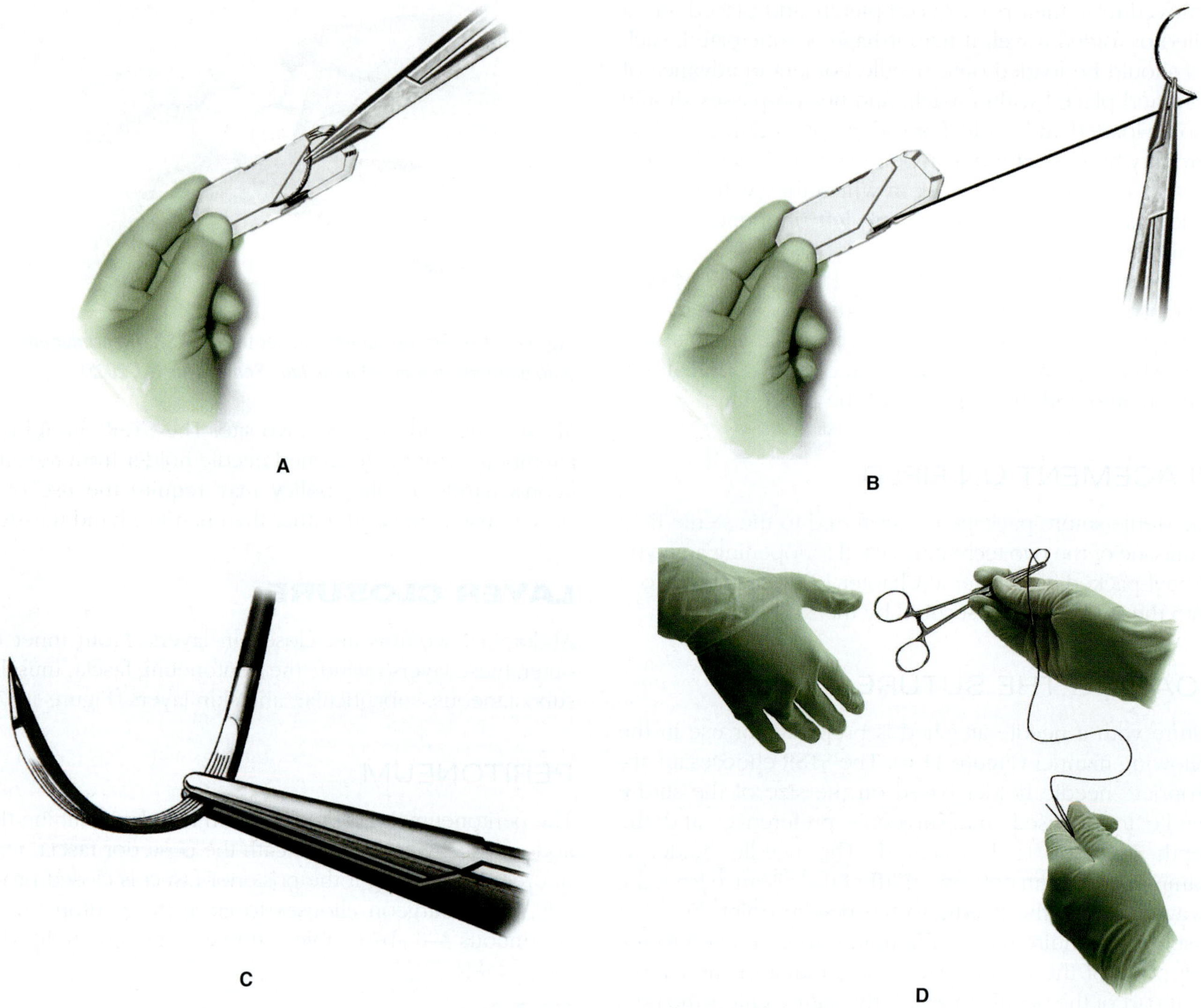

Figure 11-6 Loading the suture: (A) Needle holder is clamped onto the needle approximately one-third the distance from the swage. (B) Suture is removed from the package without placing tension on the swage. (C) Close-up of needle correctly armed on needle holder. (D) Placement of the armed needle holder in the surgeon's hand ***(Reproduced with permission from Ethicon, Inc., Somerville, NJ, 2002)***

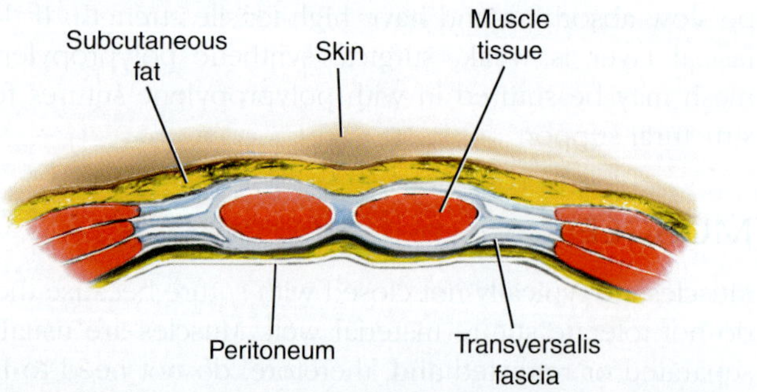

Figure 11-7 The abdominal wall ***(Reproduced with permission from Ethicon, Inc., Somerville, NJ, 2002)***

SUBCUTANEOUS

Like muscle, subcutaneous tissue does not tolerate sutures well. Many surgeons prefer to place a few interrupted sutures into this layer to prevent dead space, especially for obese patients. Plain gut is often the preferred suture material for subcutaneous closure.

SUBCUTICULAR

The subcuticular layer is an area of tough connective tissue just beneath the skin and just above the subcutaneous layer. A subcuticular closure is often utilized to minimize

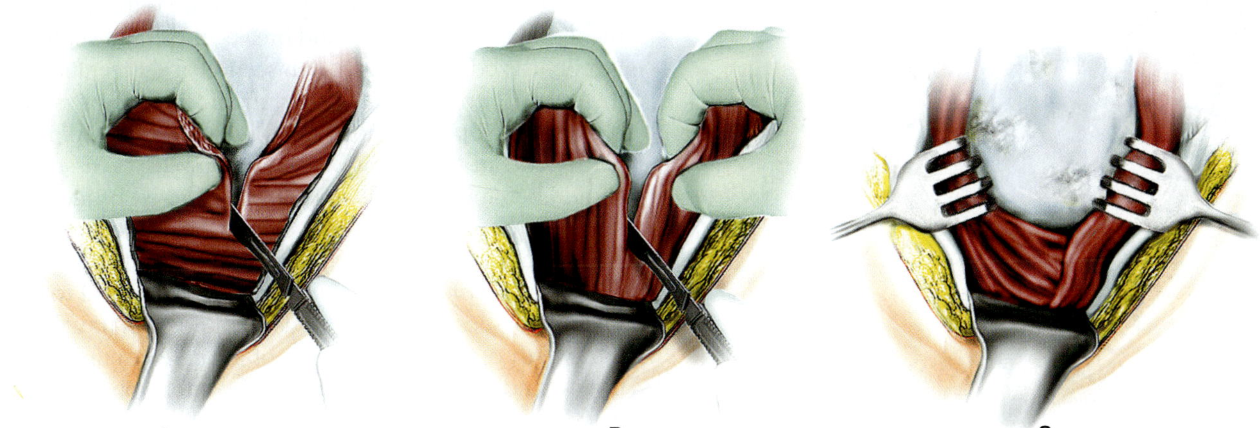

Figure 11-8 **Muscle separation: (A) Cutting, (B) splitting, (C) retracting** ***(Reproduced with permission from Ethicon, Inc., Somerville, NJ, 2002)***

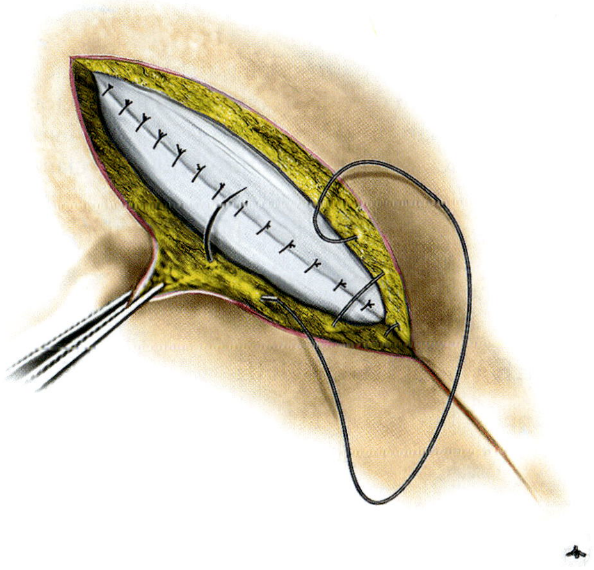

Figure 11-9 **Subcutaneous sutures** ***(Reproduced with permission from Ethicon, Inc., Somerville, NJ, 2002)***

scarring. Short lateral stitches are placed in a continuous fashion just under the epithelial layer of the skin, in a line parallel to the wound (Figure 11-9). Absorbable sutures preferred and are used more frequently than nonabsorbable sutures because the surgeon need not remove them. Nylon is preferred but must be removed after the wound can support itself. Small-gauge sutures can be utilized for these types of closures because the fascia endures the brunt of tension for the healing wound. Skin closure tapes are often used in conjunction with subcuticular closures to further minimize scarring.

SKIN

Skin may be closed with interrupted or continuous monofilament, nonabsorbable sutures on a cutting needle, or with stainless steel staples. Polypropylene or nylon are the preferred suture materials; however, stainless steel staples result in less tissue reaction. The drawback to skin closure is that the wound scars more than with a subcuticular closure, and sutures must eventually be removed.

ENDOSCOPIC SUTURE

Use of a suture ligature through a trocar cannula during endoscopy requires that the ligatures be preknotted into loops before insertion. Plastic delivery devices with the sutures loaded into them facilitate delivery. For suturing, the suture and swaged needle are introduced through a suture introducer that is inserted through a cannula.

SUTURING TECHNIQUES

Suturing techniques include the various methods for proper closure of wounds under any conditions. All wounds are not the same, and one technique for closure may not be applicable in all situations.

PRIMARY SUTURE LINE

The **primary suture line** refers to the sutures that approximate wound edges for first intention healing. These sutures are placed in either an interrupted or continuous fashion.

The *continuous,* or *running, suture* is a primary suture line consisting of a single strand of suture placed as a series of stitches. The strand is tied after the first stitch is placed at one end, and then tied again after the last stitch is placed at the other end. Evenly distributed tension along the suture line is a hallmark of the continuous suture closure (Figure 11-10). The surgical assistant "follows" or "runs" the suture by holding the lower quarter of the suture taut and away from the area of closure. This process keeps the proper amount of tension on the suture line and keeps the suture strand out of the surgeon's line of view.

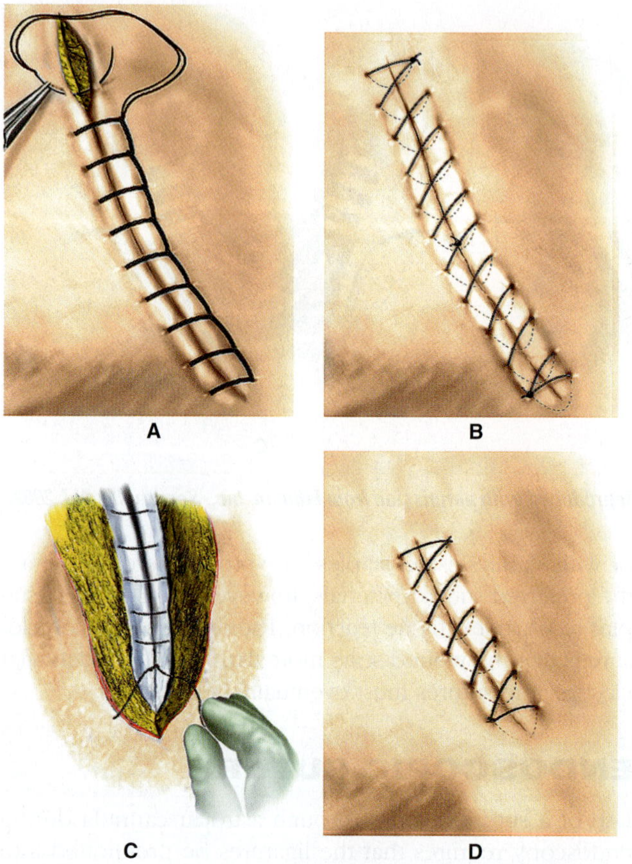

Figure 11-10 Continuous suturing techniques: (A) Interlocking stitch, knotted at each end, (B) two strands, knotted at each end and in the middle, (C) looped suture, tied to itself, (D) over-and-over running stitch ***(Reproduced with permission from Ethicon, Inc., Somerville, NJ, 2002)***

The drawback to this type of closure is that if any segment of the continuous strand breaks, the entire suture line is jeopardized, resulting in dehiscence or evisceration. For this reason, continuous sutures should be not be used to close tissues that are under a lot of tension. Abdominal fascia and heart wall incisions are examples of tissue that should be closed with a series of interrupted or individual sutures, rather than a single, continuous suture strand.

In addition to the closure of choice for tissues under tension, the *interrupted suture line* is also useful to close infected tissues. Bacteria and tissue fluids can travel along the length of a wound by way of a single continuous suture strand. The interrupted suture "interrupts" the pathway of the bacteria, localizing the area of infection to a smaller area of the wound (Figure 11-11). For these and other reasons, Halsted condoned the use of small-gauge, interrupted sutures for wound closure.

TRACTION SUTURES

Traction sutures are used to retract a structure that may not be easily retracted with a conventional retractor instrument. A nonabsorbable suture is placed into or around the structure and the suture ends are clamped with a hemostatic clamp. The structure is then pulled to the side of the operative site. Examples of traction sutures are those placed into the sclera of the eye, the myocardium of the heart, or the tongue.

PURSESTRING SUTURE

A drawstring suture placed in a circular fashion around a structure in such a way that pulling on the suture ends

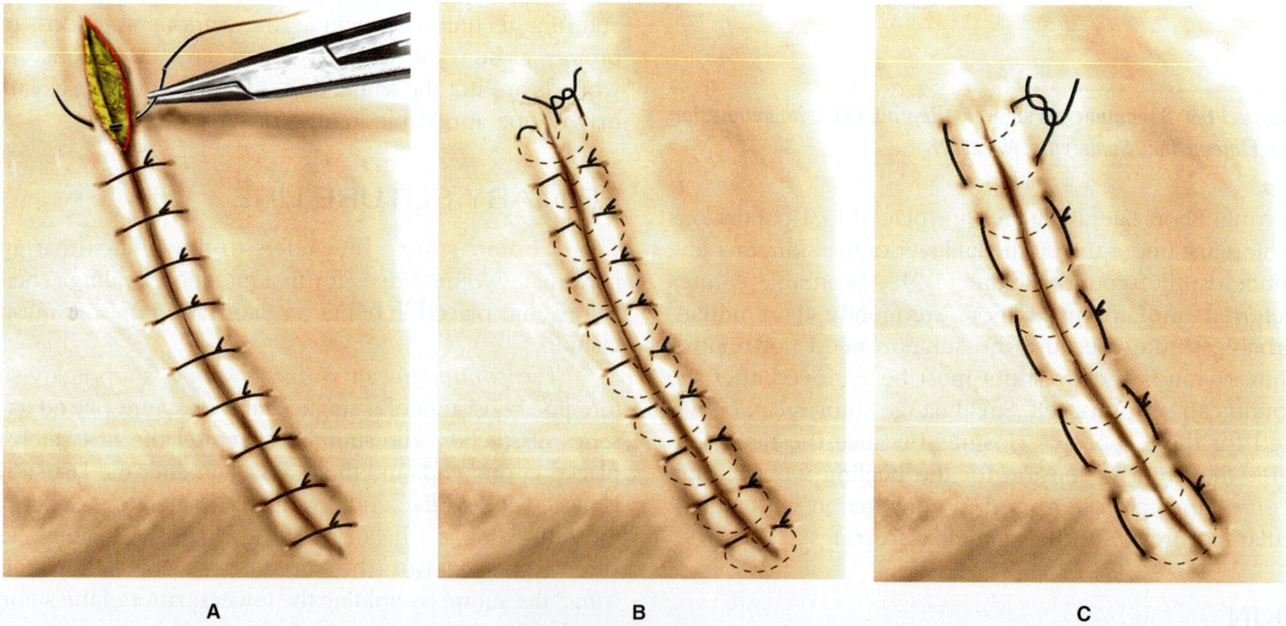

Figure 11-11 Interrupted suturing techniques: (A) Simple interrupted, (B) interrupted vertical mattress, (C) interrupted horizontal mattress ***(Reproduced with permission from Ethicon, Inc., Somerville, NJ, 2002)***

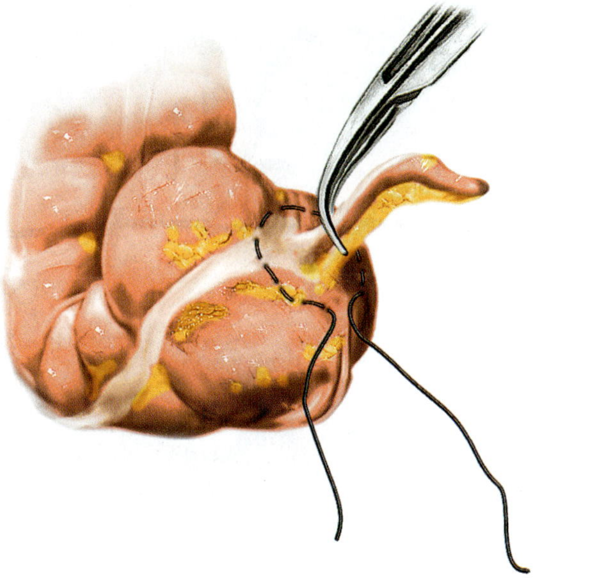

Figure 11-12 Pursestring suture ***(Reproduced with permission from Ethicon, Inc., Somerville, NJ, 2002)***

tightens and closes an opening is called a *pursestring suture* (Figure 11-12). Pursestring sutures are placed into the cecum around the proximal portion of the appendix so that once the appendix is removed, the suture ends can be tightened and tied, closing the opening into the cecum. Pursestring sutures are also placed into the right atrium and ascending aorta for introduction of cannulae for cardiopulmonary bypass.

SECONDARY SUTURE LINE

A **secondary suture line** is useful for support of the primary suture line. It helps to ease tension on the primary suture line, thus reinforcing the wound closure and obliterating any dead spaces. Retention sutures are an example of a secondary suture line.

RETENTION

Retention sutures are large-gauge, interrupted, nonabsorbable sutures placed lateral to a primary suture line for wound reinforcement. These sutures may be placed through all layers of the tissue. They are used when the surgeon suspects that the wound will not heal properly or will heal slowly due to immunosuppression, obesity, diabetes, or other compromising factors. Retention sutures can also prevent wound disruption that may result from sudden increases in abdominal pressure created by postoperative vomiting or coughing (Figure 11-13).

ACCESSORY DEVICES

Accessory devices for wound closure include bolsters and bridges, buttons, lead shots, and adhesive skin closure

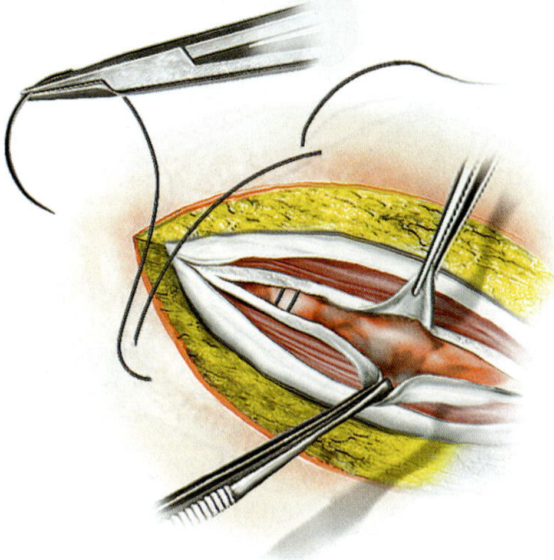

Figure 11-13 Retention suture

tapes. Although **vessel loops** and umbilical tapes are not used for closure of a wound, they are described here.

BRIDGES AND BOLSTERS

Various devices are employed to keep retention sutures from cutting into the skin. *Bridges* are plastic devices that "bridge" the closed incision. Retention suture ends are brought up through holes on each end of the bridge and tied at the middle. A circular tightening device on the bridge allows tension to be adjusted on the retention sutures (Figure 11-14).

Bolsters are pieces of plastic or rubber tubing threaded over the retention suture ends before the ends are tied. Once tied, the bolsters cover the retention sutures and prevent them from cutting into the skin.

BUTTONS AND LEAD SHOTS

Tendon sutures may be pulled through *buttonholes* and tied over a button to prevent tissue damage. *Lead shots* may be placed onto the ends of subcuticular sutures after skin closure.

UMBILICAL TAPE

Cotton *umbilical tape* was once used to ligate the severed ends of the umbilical cord after childbirth. It is used in the OR as a retraction and isolation device for bowel, nerves, vessels, or ducts. Umbilical tape is usually packaged with two strands in a pink packet, and is best used moistened with saline and loaded onto a hemostat.

VESSEL LOOPS

Silicone *vessel loops* have, for the most part, replaced umbilical tape as isolation/retraction devices for vessels,

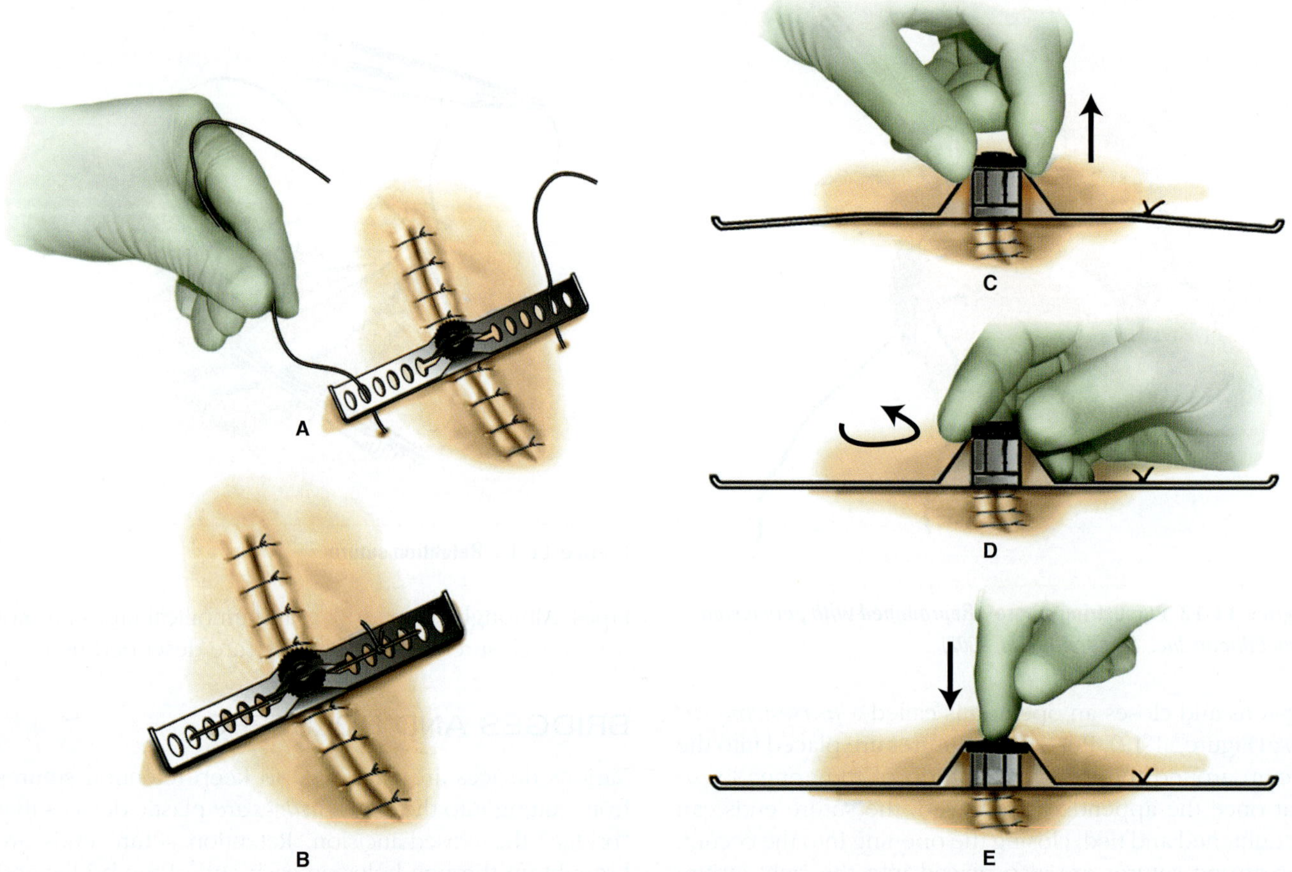

Figure 11-14 Adjustment of retention suture bridge: (A) Pass the retention suture through the appropriate holes in the bridge. (B) Place the suture with tension over the slit in the capstan and tie. (C) To adjust tension, lift capstan. (D) Rotate capstan until desired tension is attained. (E) To lock, press capstan down into bridge ***(Reproduced with permission from Ethicon, Inc., Somerville, NJ, 2002)***

nerves, or ducts. The elasticity of the vessel loops makes them ideal for retraction of delicate structures or for temporary occlusion of a vessel. Vessel loops are colored for easy identification of different adjacent structures. Typically, white and yellow loops are for nerves or ducts, red loops are for arteries, and blue loops are for veins. They are packaged in pairs.

ADHESIVE SKIN CLOSURE TAPES

Skin closure tapes are adhesive-backed strips of nylon or polypropylene tapes used to reinforce a subcuticular skin closure, or to approximate wound edges of small incisions or superficial lacerations when sutures may not be necessary (Figure 11-15). They should be applied to dry skin or skin that has been prepared with tincture of benzoin so that they stick properly. Skin closure tapes are available in ⅛-, ¼-, and ½-in. widths.

Skin Adhesive

Skin adhesive is a sterile liquid that is applied topically (Figure 11-16). It is used on the surface of a wound that will not be under tension in place of adhesive skin closure tapes, staples, or suture. The adhesive is applied after the area has been cleaned and dried. The wound edges are approximated and the adhesive is applied in layers to seal the skin edges, creating a microbial barrier. Application of the adhesive is faster than suture insertion and may provide a better cosmetic result. The adhesive remains intact for 5–10 days and is sloughed off naturally, eliminating the need for removal.

STAPLING DEVICES

Stainless steel, titanium, and absorbable *staples* are frequently used during a surgical procedure to anastomose or approximate tissue edges. Staples are also used to ligate tissues. The staples are designed to form a noncrushing B shape when inserted into tissue. This shape allows blood to pass through the line of staples, preventing tissue necrosis and promoting healing.

Staplers may be disposable or nondisposable with disposable color-coded staple cartridges. Nondisposable staplers are not always as reliable as the disposable staplers and must be assembled by the STSR during case setup.

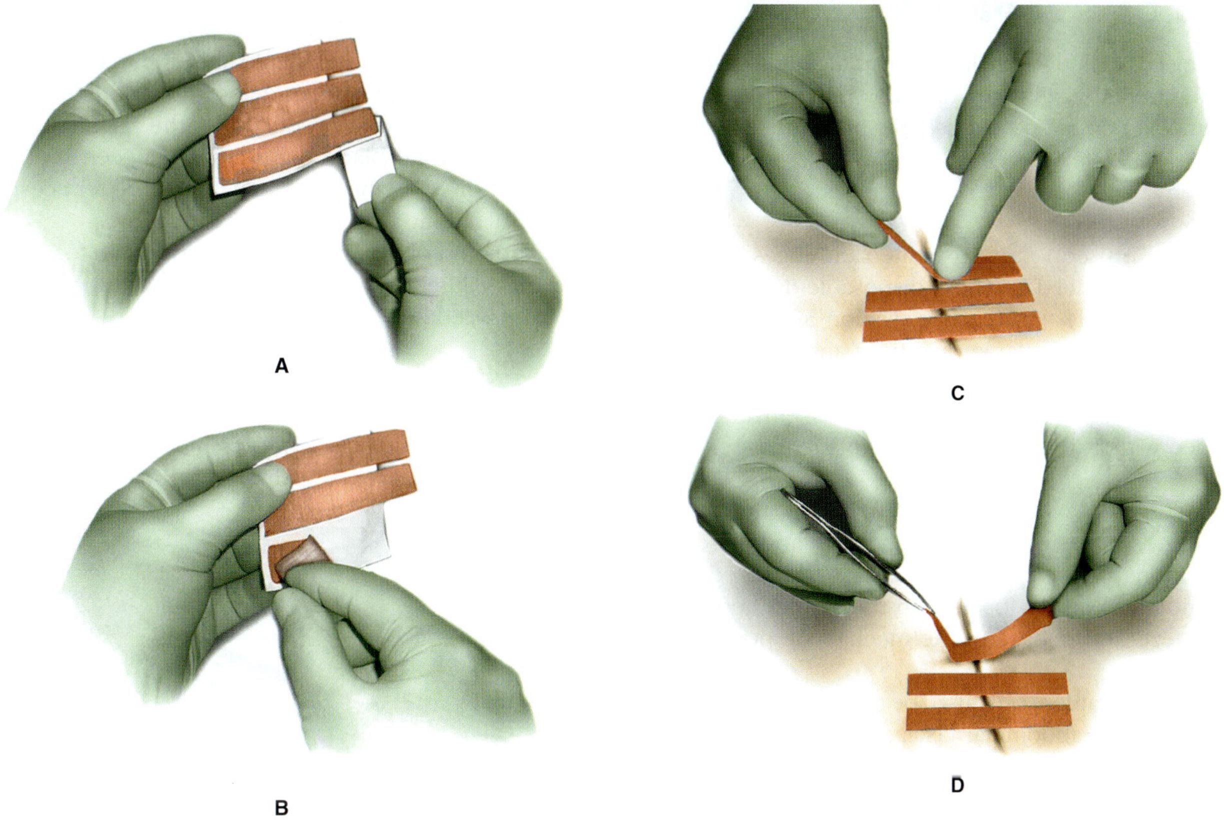

Figure 11-15 **Application of skin closure tapes: (A) Using sterile technique, remove card from sleeve and tear off tab. (B) Peel off tapes as needed in a diagonal direction. (C) Apply tapes at 1/8-in. intervals as needed to complete apposition (*make sure the skin surface is dry before applying each tape*). (D) When healing is judged to be adequate, remove each tape by peeling off each half from the outside toward the wound margin. Then, gently lift the tape away from the wound surface** ***(Reproduced with permission from Ethicon, Inc., Somerville, NJ, 2002)***

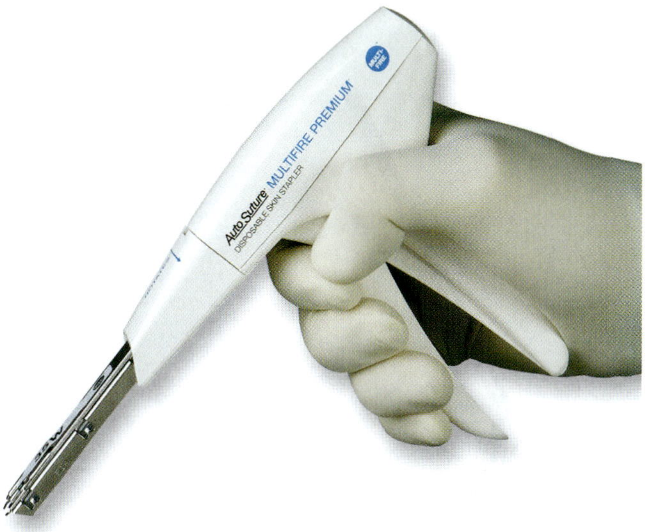

Figure 11-16 **Skin stapler** ***(Copyright ©2003 United States Surgical. All rights reserved. Reprinted with the Permission of United States Surgical, a division of Tyco Healthcare Group LP.)***

Disposable staplers are preassembled, packaged, and sterilized by the manufacturer and need only be discarded after use. Disposable staplers also have removable, disposable cartridges so that a new stapler is not required each time the stapler is fired.

Stapling offers the following advantages over suturing:

- *Less tissue reaction:* Stainless steel is the least reactive of all wound closure materials.
- *Accelerated wound healing:* Tissues are not handled as much as they would be with suturing, increasing the odds that the wound will heal without incidence. The B shape of the staples allows nutrients to pass through the staple line to the tissue edges.
- *Less operating and anesthesia time:* Stapling takes less time to perform than suturing, resulting in less blood loss during the procedure.
- *Efficiency:* Staples create an airtight and leak-proof anastomosis or closure.

The disadvantages of staple use include:

- Increased cost.
- Staples must be precisely placed. Errors in technique for linear or circular stapling are much more difficult to correct than suturing errors.

TYPES OF STAPLERS

Stapling devices include skin, linear (stapling and cutting), ligating, and intraluminal types. Stapler styles are available to accommodate open and endoscopic procedures.

SKIN

Skin staplers are used to approximate skin edges during skin closure (Figure 11-17). These disposable devices dispense a single staple with each activation and they are supplied in a variety of staple quantities and widths. For example, staplers loaded with 35 wide or regular width staples are used to close most long incisions. Smaller staplers loaded with 5–10 staples are available to close small incisions.

The surgeon everts and approximates the skin edges with Adson tissue forceps with teeth, and the operator positions the stapler at the approximated edges with the aid of an arrow located on the stapler head. A single squeeze and release of the mechanism positions the staple.

Individual staples can also be used to close the tough tissue of the abdominal fascia. This layer is thick, and heals slowly. The nonreactive nature of metallic staples makes them an ideal choice for fascia.

LINEAR STAPLERS

Linear staplers are used to insert two straight, staggered, evenly spaced, parallel rows of staples into tissue (Figure 11-18). Linear staplers are typically used to staple tissue to be transected within the alimentary tract or thoracic cavity, although they have many other surgical applications as well. The linear stapler is available in various lengths.

To operate the linear stapler, the tissue is placed within the jaws of the stapler at the level of transection. The stapler is closed, compressing the tissue. The safety mechanism is removed and the stapler is activated. A scalpel is used to sever the tissue distal to the staple line.

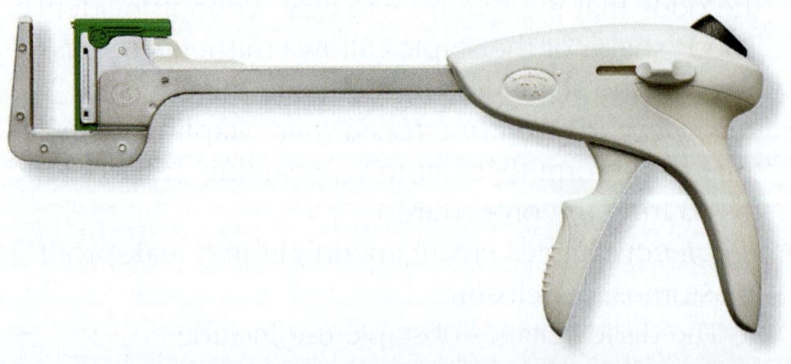

Figure 11-17 **Linear stapler** ***(Copyright ©2003 United States Surgical. All rights reserved. Reprinted with the Permission of United States Surgical, a division of Tyco Healthcare Group LP.)***

Linear Cutters

The *linear cutter* is used to staple and transect the tissue (Figure 11-19). Linear cutters deliver *two* double staple lines (similar to the one produced by the linear stapler) and contain a knife blade that passes between the two staple lines, dividing the tissue. The linear cutter is especially useful during gastrointestinal procedures.

A variation of the linear cutter is available for endoscopic procedures and is especially useful during gynecological procedures (Figure 11-20).

Ligating Clips

A *ligating clip* is used to occlude a single small structure, such as a blood vessel or a duct. A structure to be di-

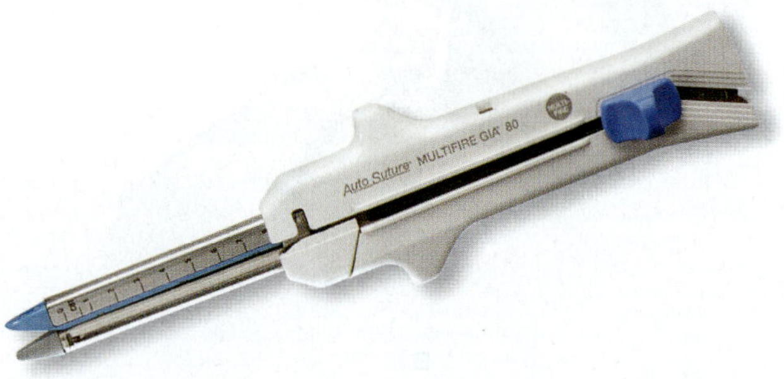

Figure 11-18 **Linear cutter** ***(Copyright ©2003 United States Surgical. All rights reserved. Reprinted with the Permission of United States Surgical, a division of Tyco Healthcare Group LP.)***

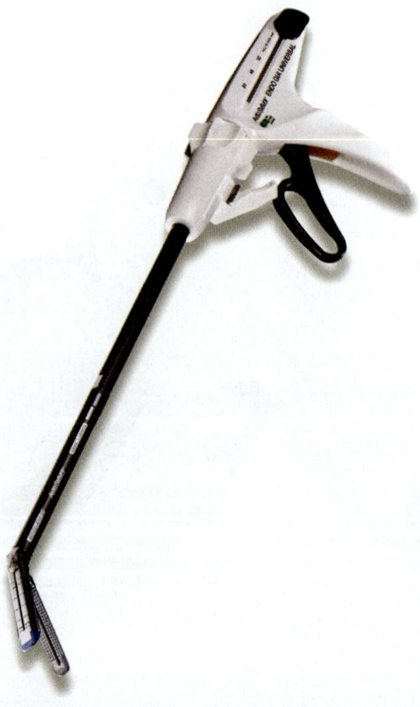

Figure 11-19 **Endoscopic linear cutter** ***(Copyright ©2003 United States Surgical. All rights reserved. Reprinted with the Permission of United States Surgical, a division of Tyco Healthcare Group LP.)***

vided must have at least two individual clips placed (one or more proximally and one or more distally). The structure is then divided with a scissors or a scalpel. The stainless steel, titanium, or absorbable clips are available in an automated disposable applier (Figure 11-21) or may be manually loaded onto a reusable device. A variation of the automated disposable applier is available for endoscopic procedures and is especially useful during cholecystectomy.

Ligating Cutters

The *ligating cutter* ejects two ligating clips side by side and then divides the tissue between the clips with a single activation. It is especially useful during gastrointestinal procedures for division of the greater omentum.

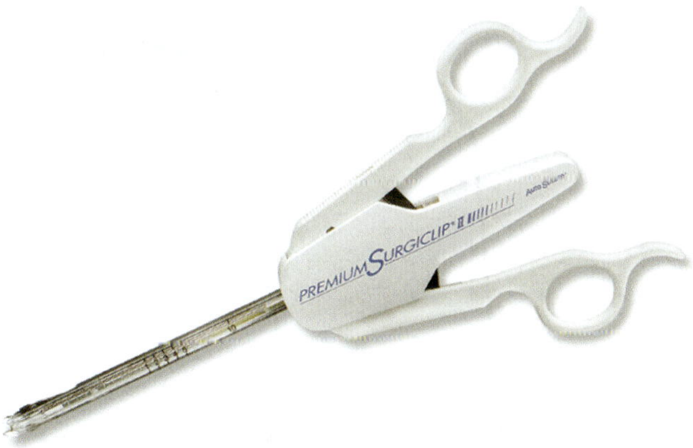

Figure 11-20 Automated ligating clip applier *(Copyright ©2003 United States Surgical. All rights reserved. Reprinted with the Permission of United States Surgical, a division of Tyco Healthcare Group LP.)*

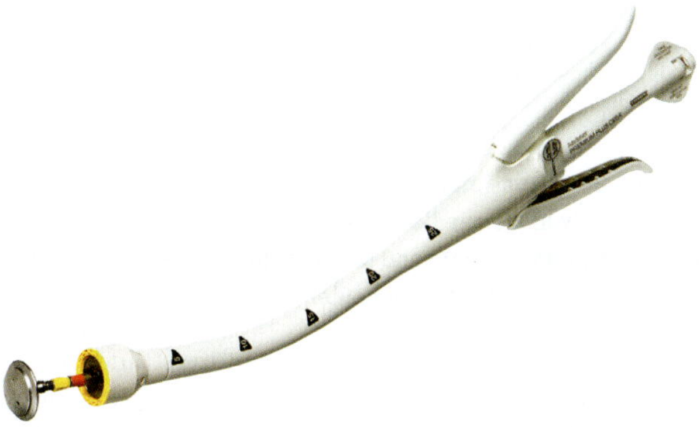

Figure 11-21 Open intraluminal stapler *(Copyright ©2003 United States Surgical. All rights reserved. Reprinted with the Permission of United States Surgical, a division of Tyco Healthcare Group LP.)*

INTRALUMINAL STAPLERS

Intraluminal (circular) staples are used to anastomose tubular structures within the gastrointestinal tract (Figure 11-22). This stapler fires a double row of circular staples and then trims the lumen with a knife located within the head of the stapler. These staplers are commonly used during resection and reanastomosis of the distal colon or rectum.

MESHES OR FABRICS

Synthetic materials can be used as a bridge for tissues that cannot be brought together without placing a great deal of tension on the tissues. They may also be used as a reinforcement for fascia defects. The lattice-like structure of the material allows connective tissue to proliferate within the mesh, creating a strong bridge for native tissues. Surgeons often make use of meshes to shore up fascia during hernia repair. Examples of synthetic meshes include:

- *Polypropylene mesh:* This is a relatively inert material that can be used in the presence of infection. It has excellent elasticity and high tensile strength.
- *Polyglactin 910 mesh:* This is an absorbable material that provides temporary support during healing.
- *Polytetrafluoroethylene* (**PTFE**) *mesh:* This is a soft, flexible material that is not absorbable and should not be used in the presence of infection.
- *Stainless steel mesh:* This material is rigid and hard to apply, resulting in discomfort for the patient. It is, however, the most inert of the mesh materials, and can be used in the presence of infection or during second-intention healing.
- *Polyester fiber mesh:* The least inert of the synthetic meshes, it should never be used in the presence of infection because its multifilament fiber construction can harbor bacteria.

Biological materials for tissue repair include fascia lata from the muscle of cattle or from the patient's own thigh.

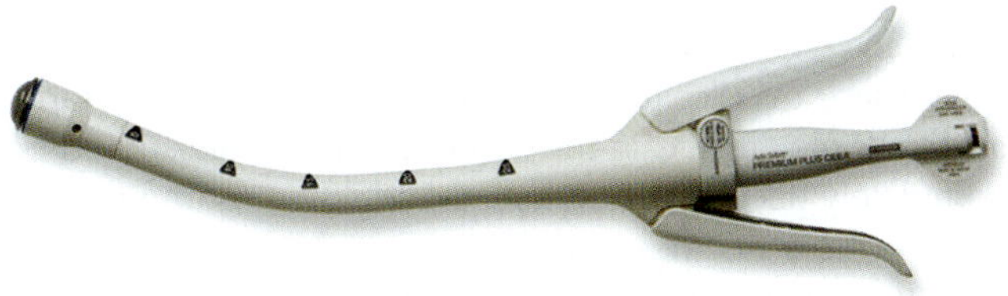

Figure 11-22 Closed intraluminal stapler *(Copyright ©2003 United States Surgical. All rights reserved. Reprinted with the Permission of United States Surgical, a division of Tyco Healthcare Group LP.)*

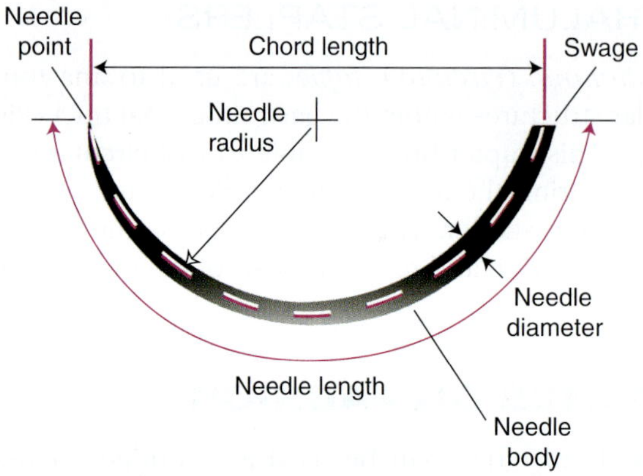

Figure 11-23 Needle anatomy ***(Reproduced with permission from Ethicon, Inc., Somerville, NJ, 2002)***

NEEDLES

Surgical needles are used to insert suture material into tissue and are available in a wide variety of sizes and shapes. Only a few types are used consistently, however. They are made of steel and should be strong enough so that they do not bend or break during suturing.

Needles can be described in terms of the following characteristics: eye, point, body, and shape (Figure 11-23).

NEEDLE EYE

The *eye* is the portion of the needle where the suture strand is attached. Surgical needles may be closed-eyed, French-eyed, or eyeless (swaged) (Figure 11-24).

Closed-eyed needles may have round or square holes and are loaded by inserting the end of the suture material through the hole. The eyed needle allows the use of a wide variety of sutures with a wide variety of needles. Loading the eyed needle with the suture strand can be a cumbersome process when wearing gloves or if the needle is small. The eyed needle causes more tissue damage than the eyeless (swaged) needle because the suture strand is not continuous with the needle.

The **French-eyed needle** is loaded by pulling the taut strand into a V-shaped area just above the eye. This type of needle is loaded more quickly than a closed-eyed needle, but still results in more tissue damage than the eyeless needle.

Needles that are manufactured with suture strands inserted into one end are referred to as *eyeless* or *swaged needles*. These needles are continuous with the suture strand, and the hole created in the tissue by the needle should be completely filled by the suture strand when suturing.

Eyeless needles may have a single-arm attachment or a double-arm attachment. The single-arm attachment is a single needle swaged to the suture strand. These may by used for interrupted or continuous suturing.

The double-arm attachment involves a needle swaged to each end of the suture strand. These are commonly used for anastomosis of vessels.

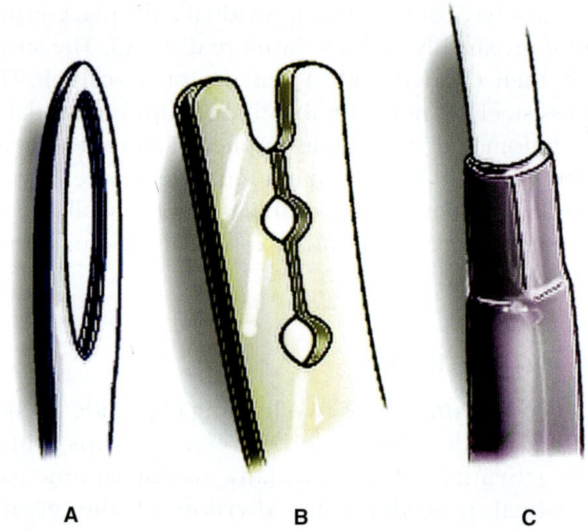

Figure 11-24 Types of needle eyes: (A) Closed, (B) French, (C) swaged ***(Reproduced with permission from Ethicon, Inc., Somerville, NJ, 2002)***

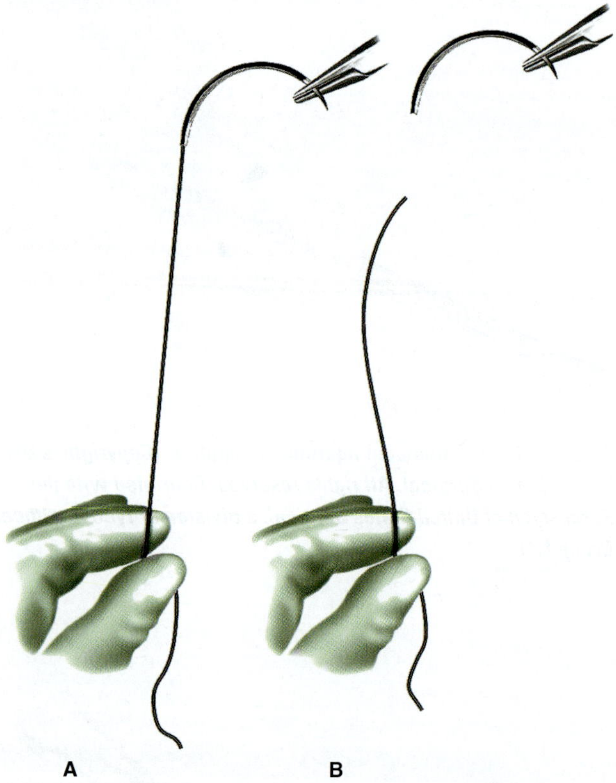

Figure 11-25 Rapid-release needle technique: (A) Hold the needle securely in the needle holder. The suture should be grasped securely and pulled straight and taut. (B) The needle is released with a straight tug of the needle holder

Eyeless needles may have the suture strand permanently attached, or the needle may be detached from the suture strand with a quick pull. This detachable needle is referred to as a *control-release needle* and is typically used for rapid, efficient placement of interrupted sutures (Figure 11-25).

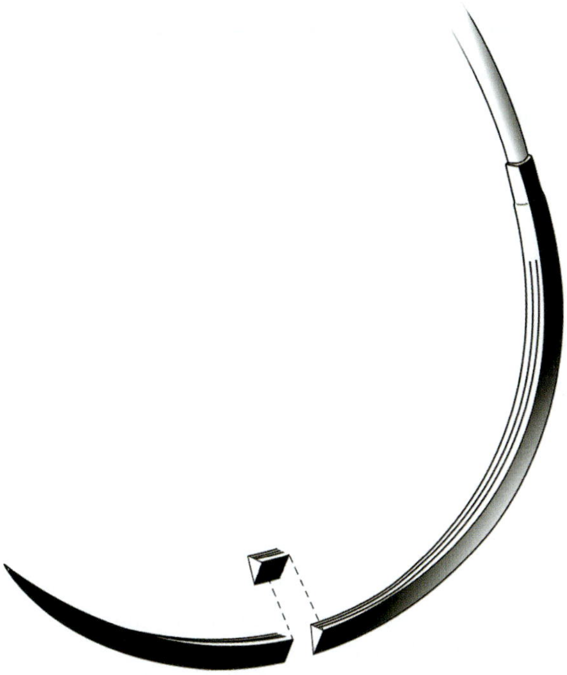

Figure 11-26 **Reverse cutting needle** ***(Reproduced with permission from Ethicon, Inc., Somerville, NJ, 2002)***

NEEDLE POINT

Needle points may be cutting, tapered, or blunt. Cutting needles are used for tough tissue that is difficult to penetrate. The sharp edges of this type of point actually cut the tissue as they penetrate it. Cutting needles are typically used for the sclera of the eye, tendons, or skin, and may be either curved or straight.

Conventional cutting needles consist of three cutting edges that are directed along the inner curve of the needle. These needles place a small cut in the direction of the pull of the suture.

Reverse cutting needles consist of opposing cutting edges in a triangular configuration that extend into the full length of the shaft (Figure 11-26). They are used for the skin because they have a flat edge in the direction of the pull. This results in less tearing of tissue.

Side cutting needles are used primarily for ophthalmic procedures because they will not penetrate into deeper tissues.

Trocar points have three sharp cutting edges that end in a sharp cutting tip. These points are used to penetrate tissue for the delivery of endoscopes into body cavities or joint spaces. They are also used to insert postoperative drains.

Tapered point needles have a round shaft without a cutting edge, so they penetrate tissue without cutting it. These points are used for delicate tissues, such as the tissue of the gastrointestinal tract.

Blunt points have a round shaft that ends in a blunt tip. These points are used primarily for the kidney or liver.

Prosthetic grafts sewn onto vessels require the use of a needle that is sharp enough to penetrate the graft but delicate enough to prevent damage to the vessel. The *ground point wire needle* has a point with sharp edges, but the round body of a tapered needle that permits easy passage through the graft without damage to the vessel.

NEEDLE BODIES

The shaft, or body, of the needle is located between the suture strand and the point. Its size and shape are variable, and choice depends on the type of tissue it is to be used for. Typically, the heavier the tissue, the heavier the body. Length is determined by the depth of the "bite" of the tissue to be sutured.

The point of the needle determines the shape of the body. Body shapes are typically round, triangular, or flattened. Tapered and blunt needles have round bodies, while cutting needles have triangular configurations.

The shape of the body may be straight, ¼ circle, ⅜ circle, ½ circle, ⅝ circle, or ½ curve. The shape is determined by how it is to be used. The ½ circle is the most commonly used body shape. Microsurgical needles and retention suture needles are usually ⅜ circle, as are needles for skin closure.

CASE STUDY

A surgeon working deep within the abdomen suddenly asks the STSR for a stick tie.

1. Describe what should be passed to the surgeon, and include the length of the needle holder, the length of the suture, the type of needle that should be used, and the type and gauge of the suture material.

QUESTIONS FOR FURTHER STUDY

1. During what situations would a control-release needle be used?
2. What type and gauge of suture would be used to anastomose a synthetic aortic graft onto an aorta during an abdominal aortic aneurysmectomy?
3. Under what conditions are retention sutures used?
4. What are the classic signs of systemic inflammation?
5. How does phagocytosis contribute to wound healing?
6. What tissue layers are encountered during closure of a McBurney's incision?

BIBLIOGRAPHY

Atkinson, L. J., & Fortunato, N. (1996). *Berry and Kohn's operating room technique* (8th ed.). St. Louis, MO: Mosby.

Bell, J., et al. (2002). *Core curriculum for surgical assisting*. Centennial, CO: Association of Surgical Technologists.

Buerk, C. A., & Van Way, C. W., III. (1986). *Pocket manual of basic surgical skills*. St. Louis, MO: Mosby.

Caruthers, B. L., May, M., & Ward-English, L. (1995). *The surgical wound*. Englewood, CO: Association of Surgical Technologists.

Ellis, H., & Lamont, P. M. (1989). *Problems in general surgery—wound healing*. Philadelphia: J. B. Lippincott.

Ethicon, Inc. (1999). *Wound closure manual*. New Brunswick, NJ: Author.

McGuiness, A. M., et al. (2002). *Core curriculum for surgical technology* (5th ed.). Centennial, CO: Association of Surgical Technologists.

Meeker, M. H., & Rothrock, J. C. (Eds.). (1995). *Alexander's care of the patient in surgery* (10th ed.). St Louis, MO: Mosby.

O'Toole, M. (Ed.). (1992). *Miller-Keane encyclopedia & dictionary of medicine, nursing, & allied health* (5th ed.). Philadelphia: W. B. Saunders.

Ravitch, M. M., Steichen, F. M., & Welter, R. (1991). *Current practice of surgical stapling*. Philadelphia: Lea & Febiger.

Stroumtsos, O. (1978). *Perspectives on sutures*. St. Louis, MO: Davis & Geck (American Cyanamid Company).

United States Surgical Corporation. (1974). *Stapling techniques in general surgery*. Norwalk, CT: Author.

CHAPTER

12

Surgical Case Management

Bob Caruthers
Teri Junge
Ben D. Price

CASE STUDY

During a lumbar discectomy procedure, the STSR removed a specimen from the jaws of a pituitary rongeur. She looked at the specimen and said to the neurosurgeon, "I think you should stop and look at this specimen. It does not look like disk material to me." "How so?" the surgeon asked. "It has a lumen," she said. The surgeon looked at the tissue, had the circulator call a genitourinary specialist, completed the procedure, and assisted on the repair of the ureter.

1. What did the STSR have to know in order to make this important observation?
2. What is the relationship between anatomical and physiological knowledge and practical application in the OR?
3. Did the STSR handle the situation well? Explain your response.

OBJECTIVES

After studying this chapter, the reader should be able to:

C 1. Describe the role of the STSR in caring for the surgical patient.

A 2. Demonstrate techniques of opening and preparing supplies and instruments needed for any operative procedure with the maintenance of sterile technique at all times.

3. Demonstrate the proper techniques for the surgical hand scrub, gowning, gloving, and assisting team members.

4. Demonstrate the proper technique for preparing supplies and instruments on a sterile field.

R 5. Demonstrate and explain in detail the procedure for counting instruments, sponges, needles, and other items on the sterile field.

6. Demonstrate the initial steps for starting a procedure.
7. Demonstrate intraoperative handling of sterile equipment and supplies.
E 8. Explain and demonstrate postoperative routines.

SELECT KEY TERMS

1. adhesive
2. anticipate
3. antimicrobial
4. biohazard
5. circumferentially
6. count
7. craniotomy
8. cylindrical
9. donning
10. foreign body
11. handwash
12. indicator
13. lap sponge
14. mask
15. neutral zone
16. pathology
17. PPE
18. resident organisms
19. scrub (sterile) attire
20. sterile team member
21. stockinette
22. surgeon's preference card
23. surgical scrub
24. transient organisms
25. wraparound-style gown

INTRODUCTION

The surgical technologist is responsible for the three phases of surgical patient care, or surgical case management, with minimal direction or supervision from other surgical team members. The three phases of case management are the preoperative, intraoperative, and postoperative phases. The surgical technologist normally functions in a sterile capacity during the surgical procedure, but also performs many nonsterile duties (known as *circulating duties*) throughout the course of the workday.

1. The preoperative case management phase occurs prior to initiation of the surgical procedure (creation of the incision or insertion of an endoscope). Some of the duties of the surgical technologist during the preoperative case management phase include
   - **Donning** operating room attire and personal protective equipment (**PPE**)
   - Preparing the OR
   - Gathering the necessary instrumentation, equipment, and supplies for the planned procedure
   - Creating and maintaining the sterile field
   - Scrubbing and donning sterile attire
   - Organizing the sterile field for use
   - Counting necessary items
   - Assisting team members during entry to the sterile field
   - Exposing the operative site with sterile drapes
2. The intraoperative case management phase occurs while the surgical procedure is being performed (time frame between initiation and termination of the procedure). Some of the duties of the surgical technologist during the intraoperative case management phase include
   - Maintaining of the sterile field
   - Passing instrumentation, equipment, and supplies to the surgeon and surgical assistant(s) as needed
   - Assessing and predicting (anticipating) the needs of the patient and surgeon and providing the necessary items in order of need
   - Preparing and handling medication
   - Counting necessary items
   - Caring for the specimen(s)
   - Applying dressings
3. The postoperative case management phase begins when the surgical procedure is terminated (application

of the dressing or extraction of the endoscope). Some of the duties of the surgical technologist during the postoperative case management phase include

- Maintaining of the sterile field until the patient is transported to the postanesthesia care unit or critical (intensive) care unit
- Removing used instrumentation, equipment, and supplies from the OR
- Caring for and maintaining instrumentation, equipment, and supplies following use
- Preparing the OR for the next patient

APPLIED THEORY

Several theoretical concepts must be applied by the surgical technologist in order to provide optimal care to the surgical patient during all three phases of surgical case management. Many of these topics have been introduced in previous chapters; however, their importance merits review and further discussion.

PRINCIPLES OF ASEPSIS

The principles of asepsis are designed to achieve a specific goal, which is to keep the microbial count within the sterile field to an irreducible minimum, thereby protecting against the transmission of disease (refer to Chapter 7).

The three principles of asepsis are as follows:

1. A sterile field is created for each surgical procedure.
2. **Sterile team members** must be appropriately attired prior to entering the sterile field.
3. Movement in and around the sterile field must not compromise the sterile field.

Once the principles of asepsis are understood, the need for applying them becomes obvious. The principles of asepsis have many applications, and they are collectively referred to as the *practice of sterile technique*.

Several concepts, or rules, are key to the implementation of sterile technique. Each concept is related to one or more of the principles of asepsis and must be followed when performing the basic skills. These rules are applied in all patient care situations that involve an invasive procedure, while keeping in mind the goal of reduction of the microbial count within the sterile field to an absolute minimum. Strict adherence to sterile technique is a necessity that is governed by an individual's surgical conscience.

Irreducible Minimum

The term *irreducible minimum* is used in relation to the microbial count when sterility is discussed for three main reasons:

1. Living tissue cannot be sterilized.
   - The skin of the patient and surgical team members harbors microbes that cannot be removed via the skin prep, hand washing, or **surgical scrub**.
   - Adequate preparation of some surgical sites is impossible due to the presence of a large number of microbes (e.g., nose, intestinal tract).
   - The wound may already have been exposed to contaminants (e.g., compound fracture).
   - Infection may already be present (e.g., ruptured appendix).
2. Environmental hazards are present.
   - Environmental decontamination may be ineffective.
   - Airborne contaminants may come in contact with the sterile field.
   - Destruction of microbial barriers results in contamination (e.g., tears, exposure to moisture).
   - Movement in and around the sterile field may cause contamination.
3. Sterility is not absolute and cannot be effectively proven all the time.
   - Chemical indicators (external and internal) only verify exposure to the sterilization process. They are not proof of sterility.
   - All types of packaging materials for sterilization have disadvantages.
   - Human error can affect the outcome of the sterilization cycle.
   - Handling and storage conditions may compromise sterility.
   - Microbes that have not yet been identified may be a threat.

The term *sterile* is relative and is used descriptively, even though sterility may not be absolute 100% of the time due to one or more of the factors listed above.

SURGICAL CONSCIENCE

All surgical team members must strictly adhere to the principles of asepsis and the practice of sterile technique. The honesty and moral integrity necessary to uphold these standards, as discussed in an earlier chapter, is called *surgical conscience*. Each individual must be conscientious enough to recognize and correct breaks in sterile technique, whether committed alone or in the presence of others. Each surgical team member is accountable for his or her actions. The surgical team member who hesitates or refuses to admit a break in sterile technique has no place in the operating room.

There is no compromise of sterile technique. Sterility cannot be taken for granted; it must constantly be checked and maintained. Surgical team members constantly monitor their own technique, as well as that of the other team members. Breaks in sterile technique are identified and corrective measures are taken. Each team member must be expecting and able to accept critique from others. The safety and well-being of the patient must come first. Any lapse in sterile technique may put the patient at risk for surgical site infection (SSI) that could potentially lead to death.

Breach of the Sterile Field

What happens when one or more of the principles of asepsis are violated and the goal of keeping the microbial count within the sterile field to an irreducible minimum is not met? Three options are available to the surgical team if break in technique occurs:

1. *Disregard the contamination.* This is a real option, but has only one temporary application. The contamination may only be disregarded when the patient's life is immediately at risk. Once the patient is stabilized, the contamination must be reported and appropriate corrective measures taken (e.g., the surgeon may want to place the patient on prophylactic antibiotics).
2. *Remove the contaminated item from the sterile field.* This is the most common action chosen and is appropriate in most situations. The contaminated item is removed from the sterile field and replaced with a sterile one. Any items subsequently contaminated must also be removed (e.g., gloves) or covered. Typically, the circulator (wearing appropriate PPE) will assist with removal of the contaminated item(s) from the sterile field.
3. *Cover the contaminated item or area.* Some contaminated items cannot be removed from the sterile field due to the timing or other circumstances of the contamination. An impervious drape may be placed over the contaminated area, thereby reestablishing the sterile field.

Keep in mind, not every SSI is the result of human error or a problem with the surgical environment. Patient factors such as age, nutritional status, presence of disease (acute or chronic), and smoking influence the risk of acquiring an infection.

Considered Contaminated

An item is *considered* contaminated in a situation where a violation of one or more of the principles of asepsis *may* have occurred. The term *considered* means that the situation has been thought about carefully and a decision has been made to "deem" or "regard" the situation in the same manner as a blatant contamination. Whenever any question about sterility arises, the item is considered contaminated and corrective action must be taken. The catch phrase "When in doubt—throw it out!" is often used in reference to a situation in which sterility is questionable. For example, a slight watermark is noticed on the exterior of a wrapper of a package that contains towels. The towel pack is considered contaminated and the towels are not placed onto the sterile field. Instead, the package is opened and the contents are discarded or set aside for reprocessing.

REVIEW OF STANDARD PRECAUTIONS

According to the guidelines defined by the Centers for Disease Control and Prevention (CDC) in 1996, Standard Precautions are implemented to prevent the transmission of disease (refer to Chapter 5). *All* individuals are considered potentially infectious, whether they show signs of disease or not. Blood, all body fluids, secretions, excretions (with the exception of sweat), nonintact skin, and mucous membranes are considered potentially infectious. Exposure control policies have been developed to reduce the risk of exposure using PPE to prevent parenteral, mucous membrane, and nonintact skin exposures. The surgical technologist must be familiar with the policy at her facility and know the procedure to follow if an exposure incident occurs.

Standard Precautions recognize the following modes (routes) of transmission for disease transfer:

- *Airborne*—droplet contamination is considered an airborne mode
- *Contact*—direct and indirect
- *Common vehicle*—infection carried in blood
- *Vector*—microbes transmitted from one host to another via an animal (e.g., fly)

In the OR, the two sources for exogenous microbial contamination are the environment and the personnel. The patient presents the third source of contamination (endogenous).

1. Environmental sources of contamination are
   a. *Fomites*—Many microbes are capable of survival on inanimate objects.
      - Fomites must be thoroughly cleaned, disinfected, and/or sterilized prior to use.

   b. *Air*—Dust, lint, skin squamae, and moisture droplets must be filtered out of the air.
      - Air is introduced at the ceiling and exhausted near the floor.
      - High-efficiency particulate air (HEPA) filters are used.
      - A minimum of 15 filtered air exchanges must occur per hour, 3 of which must be fresh (outdoor) air.
      - Positive air pressure is maintained in the OR with respect to adjacent areas and corridors to allow air movement from "clean" to "less clean" areas.

   - Recommended air temperature and humidity must be maintained.
   c. *Vectors.*
   - Must be eliminated
2. Surgical team members present microbial hazards from several sources including
   a. *Hair*—A source of staphylococcus and a gross contaminant.
      - Must be clean and covered to reduce the microbial population and contain shed particles.
   b. *Skin and subungual areas*—An individual sheds several thousand skin particles per minute that may also contain staph. Resident flora below the skin surface (glands and hair follicles) also present a hazard.
      - The highest level of personal hygiene must be carried out by all personnel.
      - OR attire is worn to cover as much skin as possible to limit particle shedding.
      - Hand washing and the surgical scrub are used to remove **transient organisms** and reduce the number of **resident organisms** on the hands and arms by chemical and mechanical action.
   c. *Blood and body fluids*—Surgical personnel may be carriers of diseases (e.g., HIV, TB, or other infection) that can be transmitted to the patient. Additionally, the nasopharynx acts as a microbial reservoir expelling contaminants during breathing, talking, coughing, and sneezing.
      - PPE provides some protection, but may not be completely effective.
   d. *Human error*—Any breach in technique may put the patient at risk of contracting a nosocomial infection that could prove deadly.
3. The surgical patient presents many of the same hazards as the surgical personnel including
   a. *Hair*
   b. *Skin*
   c. *Blood and body fluids*

Personal protection, within and outside the workplace, includes:

1. Washing hands frequently (The basic hand washing technique is found in Chapter 7.)
2. Getting a HBV vaccine
3. Abstaining from sexual activity or practicing "safe sex"
4. Not sharing personal items (e.g., razor, toothbrush, eating utensils)
5. Using PPE according to the situation (e.g., OR attire, protective attire, scrub attire)
6. Using environmental controls
   - Positive/negative pressure ventilation
   - Surface decontamination
   - Handling of soiled patient care items (e.g., linen, diapers, bedpans)
   - Handling of sharps (e.g., needles, scalpel blades, sharp instruments and devices)
     - Do not recap needles by hand.
     - Do not remove used needles from syringes by hand.
     - Do not bend, break, or manipulate used needles by hand.
     - Place sharp items in puncture-resistant containers for disposal.
     - Use caution when handling sharps (e.g., effective communication, use of a safe transfer method).

CRITICAL THINKING

Critical thinking is a systematic method of organizing one's thoughts and activities, enabling one to make appropriate case management decisions. The A POSitive CARE Approach is designed to prompt critical thinking abilities.

The critical thinking process involves the following five basic steps:

1. Identifying the goal or problem
2. Gathering and evaluating as much information as possible, using the A POSitive CARE Approach
3. Generating one or more responses and considering the implications (a response may be a series of actions)
4. Implementing the best response
5. Assessing the results of the action(s) taken and making adjustments, if necessary

The critical thinking process is an ongoing cycle that does not end with the fifth step. As the results are assessed, a new goal or problem may emerge and the cycle is repeated.

ANTICIPATION

The ability to implement critical thinking activities provides the STSR with the ability to **anticipate**, or predict, the needs of the patient and surgical team members. Information gathered during the preoperative phase of case management (e.g., **surgeon's preference card**, communication with surgical team members) is integrated into the procedure as needed. Additional information is obtained during the intraoperative case management phase by observing the progression of the procedure, processing the information, and making available any necessary items, in advance of their need.

For example, the STSR who is participating in an appendectomy, using the traditional approach on an adult patient, will be expecting the surgeon to initiate a McBurney's incision. To make the incision, the surgeon will require a #10 scalpel blade loaded onto a #3 scalpel handle. Immediately after the incision is made, the wound will most likely bleed. The STSR will be prepared to assist in achieving hemostasis by offering the surgeon the electrosurgical pencil or hemostats, such as curved Criles. It will then be necessary to separate the wound edges for the dissection to continue. Due to the small size of the McBurney's incision and its location in the abdominal wall, the STSR predicts that the surgical assistant will want to use a pair of U.S. Army or small Richardson retractors. Alternatively, if a surgical assistant is unavailable, the surgeon may prefer to use a small self-retaining retractor such as a Weitlaner.

Notice that the sequence of events described above applies not only to the appendectomy procedure, but also to virtually any surgical procedure. The STSR can predict, or anticipate, that for most procedures an incision will be made, hemostasis achieved, exposure provided, and so on. Rather than memorizing the steps of a specific surgical procedure, the STSR should focus on organizing his thoughts and activities to enable application of learned information to manage successfully virtually any surgical procedure.

THE A POSITIVE CARE APPROACH

The A POSitive CARE Approach uses acronyms designed to serve as memory tools to provide the surgical technologist with a systematic method for surgical problem solving. The A POSitive CARE Approach has two divisions.

The CARE division establishes a broad context in which the surgical technologist places the introductory and foundational information that dominates the profession. The CARE acronym is intended to serve as a conceptual reminder, rather than as a one-to-one correlation, to the surgical technologist that all activities affect the care given to the patient.

- **C**aring Attitude—care directed toward the patient and surgical team members
- **A**pplication—application of the principles of asepsis to the practice of sterile technique
- **R**ole—individual role
- **E**nvironmental concern—a general awareness and concern for the patient care environment

The A POSitive division relates directly to surgical procedures with the CARE concept as the underlying theme. The A POSitive acronym does allow the one-to-one correlation and should be used to conduct a review before each surgical procedure.

- **A**natomy—the normal anatomy
- **P**athology—the related pathological condition
- **O**perative procedure—the planned operative procedure
- **S**pecific variations—any variations that may be necessary to accommodate this specific surgeon or patient

COMMUNICATION

Technical skills are critical to surgical patient care. However, they are only part of the skills required of an efficient and effective STSR. Verbal and nonverbal communication skills are very important. The modern surgical environment is clinically and technologically complicated and surgery is inherently dangerous. Even though the surgeon bears primary responsibility for the patient, the surgeon can neither see nor do everything required for safe patient care alone. Many important facts must be shared with various surgical team members. Some examples of necessary communication are shown in Table 12-1.

Some basic communication principles can make the workplace environment more pleasant and protect the patient more effectively. Some of these principles are

- Always speak respectfully and professionally.
- Keep communication focused on the patient and the procedure.
- Express needs clearly (e.g., "May I have a cord gas tube, please?").
- Always repeat complicated orders, names of medications or solutions, and count information (e.g., "The syringe contains 1% lidocaine with epinephrine.").
- If unsure, ask (e.g., "Are you ready to switch from irrigation solution to contrast medium?").

Table 12-1 Examples of Communication of Important Information

INFORMATION NEEDED BY	INFORMATION NEEDED FROM STSR
Anesthesia provider: checking blood loss	"500 cc of irrigation has been used."
Anesthesia provider: beginning of craniotomy	"We have 25 cc of 1% lidocaine with epinephrine in the scalp."
Surgeon: as cholangiocath is passed	"Cholangiocath has been irrigated with normal saline. Syringe contains normal saline."
Surgeon: as peritoneum is being closed	"First closing count is correct."
Circulator: change in expected procedure	"We are going to need the GI suture after all. 3–0 chromic and 3–0 silk please."

- If concerned about an action that another individual is about to take, state the concern in the form of a question (e.g., "Should we switch from the monopolar to the bipolar electrosurgical unit at this point?").
- Always tell the truth. The patient's well-being may depend on it (e.g., "I did not verify what medication is in that syringe during the relief report. It must be discarded.").

TEAMWORK

All members of the surgical team know their individual roles and typically do not have to be told what to do or when to do it by another team member. Every team member has the best interest of the patient in mind and all must work together to ensure patient safety. Everyone must be observant of the events occurring around them and use effective verbal and nonverbal skills to communicate with one another. Effective use of communication skills is essential to teamwork.

PREOPERATIVE CASE MANAGEMENT

The preoperative case management phase typically begins at the start of the workday and may be repeated several times throughout the day according to the caseload. A basic preoperative routine and the related concepts and technical activities (skills) are presented later in this chapter. The situation described is "ideal"; keep in mind that the variations to this routine can occur for a variety of reasons (e.g., product differences, facility policy).

ATTIRE

The STSR reports to the facility in street clothes at the designated time (or is "called in" to participate in an emergent procedure); signs in, if necessary; and enters the department. Authorized personnel in street clothes may pass through the nonrestricted area and proceed to the locker room to change into OR attire.

Three types of attire are required to enter the operating room (semirestricted and restricted areas; refer to Chapters 5 and 7) and perform various case management functions: OR attire, protective attire (PPE), and **scrub (sterile) attire**. Certain types of attire may be listed in more than one category. For example, the hair cover is a component of OR attire, but is also considered protective attire.

Each facility should have a written policy specifying the type of attire to be worn in each area.

OR ATTIRE

OR attire is worn in the semirestricted and restricted areas of the operating room to protect both the patient and the staff by keeping microbial counts to a minimum and limiting microbial spread (Figure 12-1). OR attire consists of the scrub suit and hair cover. A **mask** and shoe covers may also be required. The use of cosmetics (e.g., makeup, fragrance, nail polish, and false nails or tips) and wearing of jewelry (of any type, including a wedding band) may be restricted according to facility policy.

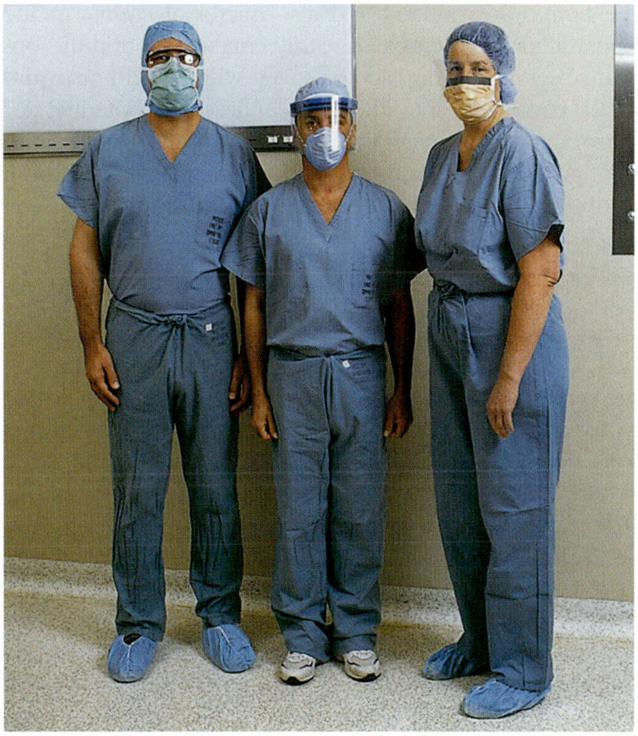

Figure 12-1 OR attire

Scrub Suit

Each surgical team member must don a scrub suit ("scrubs") prior to entering any restricted or semirestricted area. Scrub suits come in a variety of sizes and styles. Usually one style is chosen by the facility based on cost and comfort. Some facilities provide scrub suits on a "check out" basis: A scrub suit is checked out and another is not provided until the first suit is returned. The intent of this system is to contain costs and maintain a clean environment.

The scrub suit has been shown to reduce particle shedding into the environment from the body, which helps maintain the clean operative environment. Scrub suits should therefore be close fitting and shirts and drawstrings should be tucked into the pants.

After each daily use, or if the scrubs become wet or soiled, they should be removed and placed in the appropriate receptacle to be laundered by the approved laundry facility. Some facilities are beginning to use a system in which scrubs are checked out and laundered at home. Further studies are warranted to learn how this practice affects the home environment and also microbial counts in the operating room. Scrubs are easily contaminated in the operative setting. Taking scrubs soiled with blood-borne and other pathogens into the home raises the potential for spreading pathogens in the home and to other members of the household. If scrubs become soiled or wet with blood, body fluids, sweat, or food, they should be changed immediately. This helps prevent cross-contamination and generally adds to the comfort of OR personnel.

Some facility policies require that individuals wear a clean cover gown or laboratory ("lab") coat, buttoned or tied, over their scrubs when they leave the surgical services area for other areas of the facility, either for meals or for patient transport. The rationale for this practice has long been the reduction of bacterial contamination of the scrubs from outside sources, although some have argued that exogenous bacteria from the individual wearing the scrub is the major source of contamination. The use of cover gowns or lab coats to cover scrub suits certainly provides a more professional appearance and prevents soiling of the scrubs with food or drink, but this practice has not been shown to reduce the rate of surgical site infection. In addition, some facility policies require that scrubs be changed each time a team member leaves the surgical services area. While this certainly ensures that clean scrubs are always worn in the OR, time and cost constraints sometimes prevent this practice. Scrubs worn outside the facility should not be worn in the OR; they should instead be exchanged for a clean set.

Hair Cover

While in the semirestricted and restricted areas of the surgery department, a cap or hood is worn to cover all hair of the head and face. Hoods that cover both the head and the sides of the face are provided for individuals with beards. Hair has been shown to be a heavy source of contamination; therefore, no hair should be left exposed while in the surgical environment. Hair covers are donned prior to the scrub suit to decrease the possibility of hair or dandruff being shed onto the scrub suit or into the surgical wound. Hair covers also decrease microbial dispersal. Head coverings include hats, caps, hoods, and even "space helmets" that completely enclose the head and provide their own ventilation system. "Space helmet" systems are usually used in high-infection-risk environments, such as open-joint orthopedic surgery. Skullcap-type hair covers should not be used unless the individual has very short hair that can be completely covered by this type of cap. Personnel with longer hair should wear bouffant-type caps or hoods. Most caps are disposable, single-use items, although some hospitals allow reusable head covers if they are laundered daily by a hospital-approved facility. If reusable head covers are used, they should be made of a densely woven, lint-free material. Disposable head covers are made of lint-free nonwoven material. After use, disposable hair covers should be immediately placed in a designated receptacle. Hair covers should be changed if they become wet or soiled.

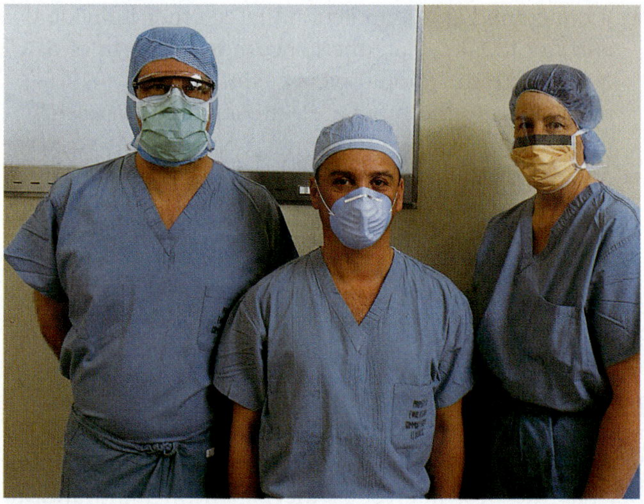

Figure 12-2 Examples of mask types

Mask

A mask must be worn at all times in any restricted area where sterile supplies are open and while surgery is in progress (Figure 12-2). The mask should be tied to fit snugly over the mouth and nose. Most disposable masks have a metal or plastic noseband that can be contoured to fit over the bridge of the nose. To prevent fogging of protective eyewear, tape may be used to cover this portion of the mask, but care should be taken to use a nonirritating type of tape, because the skin under the eyes is very sensitive and prone to irritation.

The mask is secured to the head with either an elastic band or two pairs of strings. To ensure a snug comfortable fit, the strings of the mask should not be crisscrossed when tied. Some mask styles incorporate protective eyewear. High-filtration masks are available for use with known tuberculosis patients; however, the CDC and the National Institute for Occupational Safety and Health recommend the use of a mask/respirator.

Masks are worn to contain and filter moisture droplets expelled from the mouth and nasopharynx during talking and normal breathing, as well as from sneezing and coughing. The mask also filters inhaled air and serves to protect the user from fluid splashes to the mucous membranes of the face.

Masks should be either on or off. They should never be untied and allowed to hang down around the neck, because they harbor many microorganisms and will further contaminate the scrub suit. In addition, masks should be handled by the strings and only minimally. If a mask is not in use, it should be removed and discarded in the proper container. Masks should also be changed between cases.

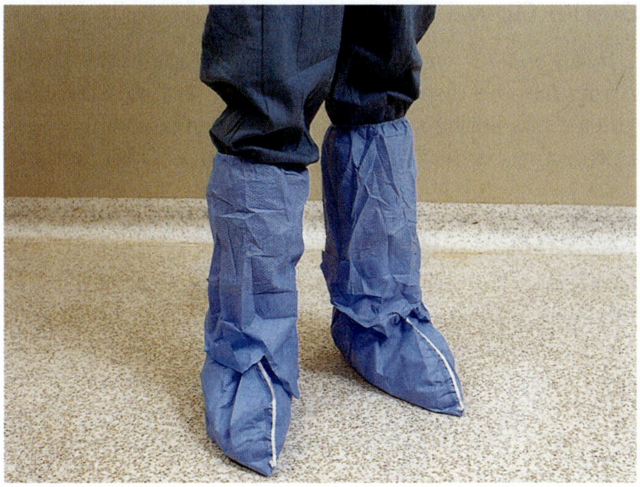

Figure 12-3 Impervious boots

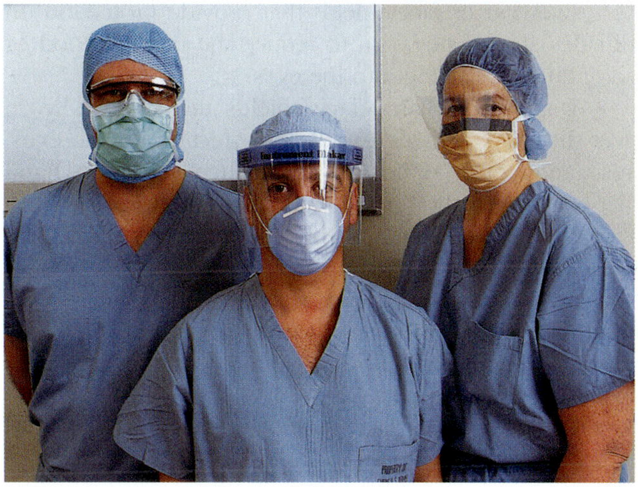

Figure 12-4 Examples of protective eyewear

Shoe Covers

Protective shoe covers are worn in the semirestricted and restricted areas of the surgery department, primarily as personal protective equipment to shield the shoes and feet from gross fluid contamination. When a procedure will require large amounts of irrigation fluid or large spills may occur, some individuals prefer to wear the larger impervious boot style shoe covers (Figure 12-3).

Some facilities allow specifically designated shoes to be worn within the surgical suite without shoe covers. These shoes must not, however, be worn outside the surgical suite to prevent cross-contamination to and from the outside areas of the facility. If shoe covers are used, they must be removed whenever they become soiled or wet and must always be removed when leaving the surgical suite.

Even if shoe covers are not required at a certain facility, their use may still be indicated for personal protection according to the situation.

TECHNIQUE

OR Attire

1. Apply hair cover prior to donning scrub suit.
2. Don scrub suit.
3. Remove body adornments and excess cosmetics, as needed.
4. Apply identification badge and radiation monitoring device, if necessary.
5. Change into shoes appropriate to the OR; apply shoe covers, if necessary.
6. Apply mask and eyewear, as needed.

PROTECTIVE ATTIRE

Personal protective equipment is worn to protect the health care provider and the patient not only from microbial contact, but also from environmental hazards (e.g., radiation, lasers). The scrub suit, mask, hair cover, and shoe covers have already been discussed as part of the OR attire. Additional PPE includes nonsterile gloves, protective eyewear, and radiation protection.

Note: Sterile team members must don some types of protective attire (e.g., eyewear, sternal/thyroid shield) prior to performing the surgical scrub. In some situations, the sterile attire is worn over the PPE (e.g., lead apron).

Nonsterile Gloves

As part of standard precautions, *gloves* must be worn any time contact with broken skin or body fluids is expected. When this contact is to occur outside the sterile field, nonsterile latex or vinyl gloves are available. Some individuals have a sensitivity or allergy to latex. If either the patient or staff person is latex sensitive, vinyl or other synthetic gloves must be used. Clean items should not be handled with soiled gloves, and gloves should be removed immediately after use and discarded in the appropriate receptacle. A **handwash** should be performed immediately following glove removal.

Protective Eyewear

Protective eyewear should be worn any time an environmental hazard exists or exposure to blood or body fluids may occur (Figure 12-4). In a study of occupational blood exposures in the operating room at six different facilities, the most vulnerable location for serious blood exposure was identified to be the eye, and individuals in the circulating role were found to have the same number of exposures as those in the scrub role.

Eyewear or face shields that provide protection on all sides should be worn to reduce the risk of blood or body fluids splashing into the eyes.

Disposable plastic face shields that can be worn over the mask provide excellent protection for the eyes, nose, and mouth. Many have an attached foam brow band that offers protection from fluid falling into the eyes from above. Experimentation with different types of face shields may be necessary to find one that offers protection, comfort, and maximum visibility. Mask-shield combinations without the upper foam band should be worn with caution, because they afford little protection from splashes from above.

Regular eyeglasses with side and top shields applied or goggles are other options for eye protection. Prescription goggles are available.

Specialized eyewear is also available to offer protection from radiation and laser injury. Use caution when selecting laser eyewear to ensure that the optical density of the lens is compatible for protection from the specific type of laser in use.

Radiation Protection

Radiation is routinely encountered in the OR in the form of X-rays; however, various other radioactive elements may also be used. Lead shielding devices are available to protect the staff and the patient from unnecessary exposure:

- *Portable lead screen*—Brought into the OR to shield team members who cannot leave the room.
- *Lead apron*—Shields the torso. Aprons are worn over OR attire and are available in a variety of sizes and styles.
- *Lead sternal/thyroid shield*—Wrapped around the neck and secured with Velcro.
- *Leaded glasses*—Protect the eyes from radiation as well as body fluids.
- *Lead-impregnated gloves*—May be sterile or nonsterile.

Other Protective Attire

According to the situation, additional protective attire may also be required. A fluid-proof apron may be worn by environmental services personnel and individuals working in the decontamination area of the sterile processing department. Sterile gowns are also available with fluid-proof panels in the front of the gown and around the sleeves.

SCRUB (STERILE) ATTIRE

Scrub attire is worn by the sterile surgical team members and is donned after performing the surgical scrub. Scrub attire is necessary for entry into the sterile field and consists of the sterile gown and gloves.

Sterile Gown

A *sterile gown* is worn by all sterile team members. Sterile gowns may be disposable or reusable and must be constructed of a lint-free woven or nonwoven fabric that offers a protective barrier. The front of the gown from the midchest level to the waist and the sleeves **circumferentially** to 2 in. proximal to the elbows is considered sterile. The woven fabric cuff of the gown is the weak link. The cuff acts as a wick if fluid seeps under the top of the glove, and it likewise wicks perspiration to the outer layer of the cuff. For this reason, *the cuffs of the gown must be considered nonsterile and must always be covered by the cuff of the glove.* The industry is currently working on ways to address this problem, including the use of reinforcements and extended length gloves.

Various types of gowns are available to provide protection from the expected degree of fluid (body fluid or irrigation solution) exposure. Fluid-resistant gowns are cost effective, but provide a low level of fluid-protection. Impervious gowns contain fluid-proof reinforcements in the front and in the sleeves. Full-coverage systems, sometimes referred to as space suits, are available for orthopedic and other high-risk procedures. The gown portion envelops the wearer's body to below the knees and has a hooded face shield or helmet that covers the head, neck, and shoulders. The full-coverage gown contains a ventilation system and many also contain communication systems because the noise generated by the ventilation system makes it extremely difficult to hear other surgical members.

Sterile Gloves

Sterile gloves are worn by all sterile team members. The sterile gloves are applied immediately after donning the sterile gown. Sterile gloves are available in a variety of styles and sizes and have been developed for specific surgical specialties (e.g., ophthalmology, orthopedics). Lead gloves are available when the use of X-rays is expected. Extra protection from puncture or seepage of fluid through the gloves may be afforded by wearing glove liners (e.g., steel, Kevlar) or double gloving (Figure 12-5). Studies have shown that the incidence of disease contracted from puncture injuries drops sharply when the injury occurs to a double-gloved hand. As a sharp item passes through the layers of the gloves, fluid and debris are removed and less biological material (bioburden) is present on the item if a skin puncture occurs.

Additionally, double gloving is recommended for the following reasons:

- Fat is known to degrade latex.
- The barrier efficiency of latex decreases over time.
- The structure of latex is lattice-like, containing many spaces that fill with fluid during the surgical procedure. As the gloves become saturated with fluid,

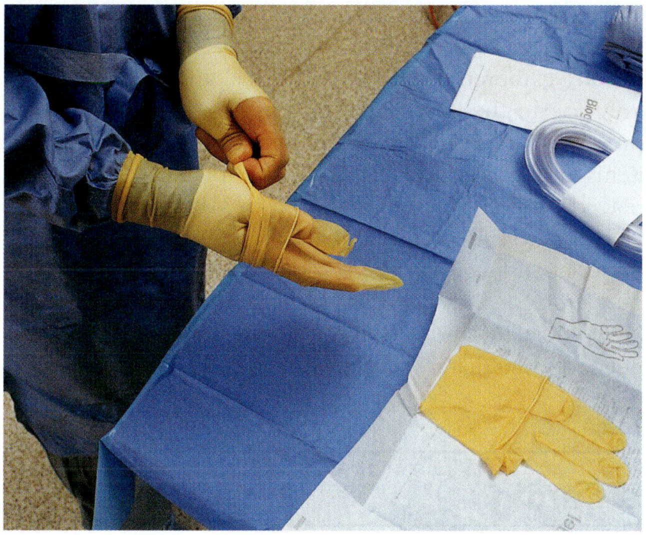

Figure 12-5 Double gloving

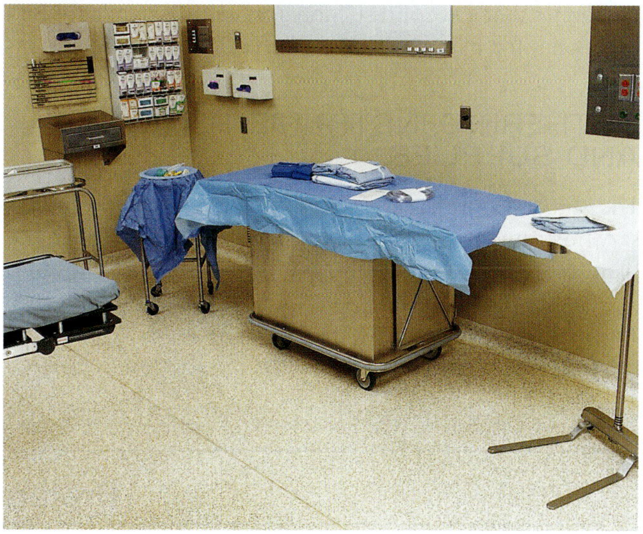

Figure 12-6 Furniture placement in the OR

pathways may be created through the latex, allowing the passage of fluid to the wearer's skin.

Numerous studies have shown double gloving to reduce significantly the amount of blood contamination of the hands. One such study showed that during 45 surgical procedures, visible contamination of the hands occurred in 38% of the cases with single gloving. This number was reduced to 2% when double gloves were worn.

When double gloving, extra comfort may be achieved by wearing the under glove one-half to one full size larger than the wearer's normal glove size, and the outer glove of normal size. While this method may seem backward, it often does provide a greater level of comfort than two pairs of gloves of the same size. Experimentation with different glove types and sizes will allow the wearer to achieve the desired level of comfort and tactile awareness.

Note: Sterile gloves may be utilized without a sterile gown to allow a nonsterile team member to perform a sterile activity, such as urinary catheterization. However, in that situation they are not considered "scrub attire."

PREPARING THE OR

Once properly attired, the STSR reports to the control desk to obtain necessary information about her assignment. Preparation for the first surgical case of the day is slightly different from preparation for subsequent cases because some of the activities need only be performed once per day or are included in the postoperative case management activities and do not have to be repeated. At many facilities, ancillary personnel may perform some of the tasks listed.

On entering the restricted area, a basic handwash is performed. According to facility policy, application of the mask may be necessary at this time. All equipment and horizontal surfaces are wiped down with disinfectant solution and another handwash is performed.

OR SETUP

Verify that all necessary furniture (e.g., IV stands, anesthesia provider's cart) and equipment (e.g., electrosurgical unit, microscope) is present in the OR and remove any unnecessary items. Furniture and equipment are arranged for ease of use, efficiency, and the best possible sterile technique. Whenever possible, the back table, Mayo stand, and ring stands should be positioned so that the sterile field is established in the area furthest from the door. When the OR doors open and close, air movement is at its highest; therefore, it is advantageous to establish the sterile field as far as possible from the movement of the doors and from human traffic into and out of the room. All tables to be set up as part of the sterile field should be placed at least 12–18 in. away from walls and all furniture should be placed side by side and away from any major traffic paths (Figure 12-6).

The OR table is positioned under the operating lights in whatever orientation is required for the procedure, with the anesthesia machine typically placed at the head of the table. The operating lights are checked at this time for functionality and positioned close to where they will be focused for the procedure. All other equipment (e.g., patient monitors, electrosurgical unit, tourniquet) is tested for functionality.

Bags for laundry, clean waste, and biohazardous waste should be in the hamper frames, and these are positioned so that waste can be easily disposed of during initial setup, but at a safe distance from the sterile field. Kick buckets are lined with impervious **biohazard** liners. Suction canisters should have new suction liners, and the suction tubing should be attached to the wall vacuum outlet.

Be certain that a second suction apparatus is available and functional for management of the patient's airway.

GATHERING INSTRUMENTATION AND SUPPLIES

The surgeon's preference card is obtained and the necessary instrumentation and supplies are gathered for the planned surgical procedure and placed on a case cart. The preference card may be computer generated (Figure 12-7) or handwritten. Additional information concerning the procedure may be obtained from other sources such as the patient, the patient's chart, or other surgical team members. At some facilities, ancillary personnel may have already gathered the necessary items, and the STSR must only locate the case cart and ensure that everything is present. The case cart is brought into the OR and the items are positioned for use. The back table pack is placed on the back table, the basin set is placed on the appropriate ring stand, and the instrument set is placed on a flat surface near the back table. If instruments must be sterilized, they are placed in the sterilizer (steam or peracetic acid) and processed at this time. Any items not needed immediately (e.g., dressing materials) are placed

Preference Card

Surgeon:	**Dr. Mitchell**	
Procedure:	**Appendectomy - Adult (Traditional Approach)**	
Position:	**Supine**	
Glove Size/Style:	**8 white with 7½ ortho over**	Dominant Hand: **Right**
Equipment:	**Electrosurgical unit with dispersive electrode** **Standard setting: 40/40 Blend 1** **Suction Apparatus** **Headlamp (available)**	
Supplies:	**Basic pack (customized)** **Laparotomy sheet (vertical fenestration)** **Double basin set** **Gloves for all sterile team members** **Poole suction tip—disposable** **Electrosurgical pencil** **Aerobic and anaerobic culture tubes (available)**	
Instrumentation:	**Minor instrumentation set** **Medium Richardson retractor**	
Suture and Usage:	**Ties:**	**2-0 Vicryl Reel**
	Pursestring:	**3-0 Vicryl SH**
	Peritoneum:	**2-0 Vicryl CT-1**
	Fascia:	**2-0 Vicryl CT-1 x 3**
	Sub-Q:	**None or 3-0 Vicryl CT-1 (obese patient)**
	Skin:	**Staples or 3-0 Nylon (if ruptured)**
Dressings:	**Bacitracin ointment** **Telfa** **4x4 gauze** **2″ Paper tape**	
Skin Prep:	**Shave, if necessary** **Betadine—5 minute**	
Medications:	**Bupivacaine 0.5% (available for postoperative pain control)** **Control syringe (if needed)** **25 gauge 1½″ Needle (if needed)**	

Figure 12-7 **Sample surgeon preference card**

in a location that will be convenient for the circulator to retrieve and open during the procedure, if/when needed.

CREATING AND MAINTAINING THE STERILE FIELD

The mask must be applied prior to creation of the sterile field and is worn by all individuals in the presence of the sterile field. The door of the OR is closed prior to creation of the sterile field and although it is necessary to use the door, it remains closed as much as possible, as long as the sterile field needs to be maintained. The key concepts (rules) that relate to the three principles of asepsis must be applied for sterile technique to be implemented.

1. The concepts that relate to the first principle of asepsis (a sterile field is created for each surgical procedure) are as follows:
   - Only sterile items are used within the sterile field. If the sterility of an item is in doubt, the item should not be used. Evidence of moisture on an item renders the item nonsterile.
   - Destruction of the integrity of a microbial barrier results in contamination. Moisture that seeps through a barrier renders the item nonsterile.
   - The sterile field is located within the operating room as far away as possible from doors and high-traffic areas.
   - The sterile field is created as close as possible to the time of use. Sterile items may not be covered with a sterile drape for later use. Facility policy may dictate a specific time frame for use of opened sterile items.
   - The sterile field is kept in constant view; team members (sterile and nonsterile) may not turn their backs on the sterile field.
   - Edges of a wrapper are initially considered contaminated around a 2-in. perimeter.
   - Wrapper or drape edges that are placed below table level are considered contaminated and must not be brought back up to table level.
   - Table edges will ultimately define the sterile area. Any item that extends beyond or below the table edge is considered nonsterile.
   - Once positioned, a sterile wrapper or drape may not be relocated.
   - Sealed edges of a peel pack are considered nonsterile.
   - A sterile package is opened away from the nonsterile individual.
   - Nonsterile individuals must remain at least 12–18 in. away from the sterile field.
   - The sterile field must remain at least 12 in. from nonsterile items (e.g., wall, furniture).
   - Nonsterile individuals or items may not touch, reach across, or pass over the sterile field.
   - Nonsterile individuals or items may not pass between or be placed between two sterile fields.
2. The concepts that relate to the second principle of asepsis (sterile team members must be appropriately attired prior to entering the sterile field) are as follows:
   - Sterile individuals must be appropriately attired, including PPE and scrub attire.
   - Self-gowning is performed from a separate sterile surface to prevent contamination of the back table when entering the sterile field.
   - The closed glove method is recommended when gowning and gloving oneself.
   - The knit cuff of the gown is completely enclosed within the cuff of the glove.
   - The sterile gown is considered sterile from the waist or table level to the mid-chest line in the front of the gown. The hands and arms are considered sterile to 2 in. proximal to the elbow. This is considered the sterile "zone."
   - The back of a **wraparound-style gown** is not considered sterile.
   - Sterile individuals must keep their hands in sight at all times and within the sterile zone. Elbows are kept close to the sides, and hands are never placed in the underarm area.
3. The concepts that relate to the third principle of asepsis (movement in and around the sterile field must not compromise the sterile field) are as follows:
   - Talking and movement within and around the sterile field are kept to a minimum.
   - Sterile individuals must remain well within the sterile area.
   - Sterile individuals pass each other face to face or back to back by rotating 360°.
   - Sterile individuals keep their backs to a nonsterile individual or area and allow at least 12–18 in. of space.
   - Sterile individuals always face the sterile field.
   - Sterile individuals are allowed to sit down only when the entire procedure will be performed in the sitting position.
   - Tubing and cords are secured to the sterile field with nonperforating devices to prevent slippage and destruction of the sterile barrier.
   - Sterile individuals or items may touch only sterile items and reach or pass over the sterile field.
   - Addition of sterile items to the sterile field is accomplished by a nonsterile team member. The item may be placed directly onto the sterile field or be secured by the STSR.
   - When transferring sterile solutions to the sterile field, only the lip of the nonsterile bottle is positioned over the sterile container. The STSR will position the container at the edge of the sterile field

to facilitate the transfer of the sterile fluid. The bottle is held at least 12–18 in. above the container.

- Sterile team members must avoid leaning over the sterile field, if possible.
- When assisting a team member entering the sterile field, a safe distance is maintained, and the gloved hands are protected by "cuffing" the towel, gown, and gloves over the hands to prevent contact with the nonsterile individual.
- Nonsterile surfaces that will have sterile drapes applied are draped first toward the sterile individual to prevent contamination of the gown and to avoid reaching over the nonsterile area. The gloved hands are protected by "cuffing" the drape over the hands to prevent contact with the nonsterile area. Until the sterile drape is applied, the sterile individual must maintain a safe distance.

Opening Sterile Supplies

Before opening any sterile item:

- Verify that the item has been exposed to a sterilization process by inspecting the chemical **indicator** for the appropriate color change.
- Examine the integrity of the packaging material to be sure that it is dry and does not have any tears, perforations, or watermarks.
- Ensure that the expiration date, if present, has not passed.

Any item that does not meet these criteria is not used.

Because of its central location, it is recommended that the back table pack be opened first. This allows freedom of movement around the back table. As the pack is opened it covers the back table, creating a sterile field and exposing the sterile supplies within. If an item is double wrapped, it will be necessary to open both wrappers at this time. If disposable packaging material is sealed with tape, the tape should be broken at the seal rather than removed because removal can damage the integrity of the packaging material.

As additional items are opened, the sterile field is expanded. Typically, the larger items such as the basin set and the instrument set are opened next and then smaller remaining wrapped and peel-packed items are placed onto the existing sterile field. To reduce the risk of contamination of the sterile field, it is recommended that the STSR's gown and gloves be opened on a separate surface, such as the Mayo stand, rather than the back table.

TECHNIQUE: Opening the Back Table Pack

Refer to Figure 12-8A–C.

1. Check the integrity of the outer packaging material.
2. Remove the outer packaging material.
3. Check the integrity of the inner packaging material.
4. Orient the pack correctly on the back table.
5. Break or remove the seal.
6. Unfold the first flap away from you.
7. Unfold the second flap toward you.
8. Remove any accessory items, if included.
9. Reposition yourself as necessary to open the third flap.
10. Insert your hands under the cuff, grasp, and extend the drape to cover the table.
11. Move to the opposite side of the table and open the fourth flap.

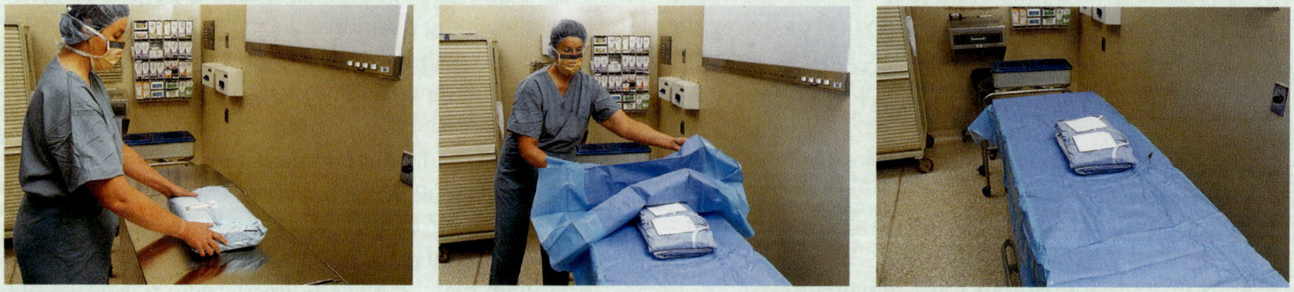

A B C

Figure 12-8 Opening the back table pack: (A) Position pack on back table. (B) Place hands under the cuff and unfold. (C) Pack opened

TECHNIQUE Opening the Basin Set

Refer to Figure 12-9.

1. Check the integrity of the outer packaging material.
2. Remove the outer packaging material.
3. Check the integrity of the inner packaging material.
4. Orient the basin set on the appropriate size ring stand.
5. Break or remove the seal.
6. Unfold the first flap away from you.
7. Unfold the second flap toward you.
8. Reposition yourself or the ring stand to facilitate opening the third flap.
9. Insert your hands under the cuff, grasp, and extend the drape to cover the ring stand.
10. Move to the opposite side or rotate the ring stand; open the fourth flap.
11. Place the ring stand in proximity to the back table.

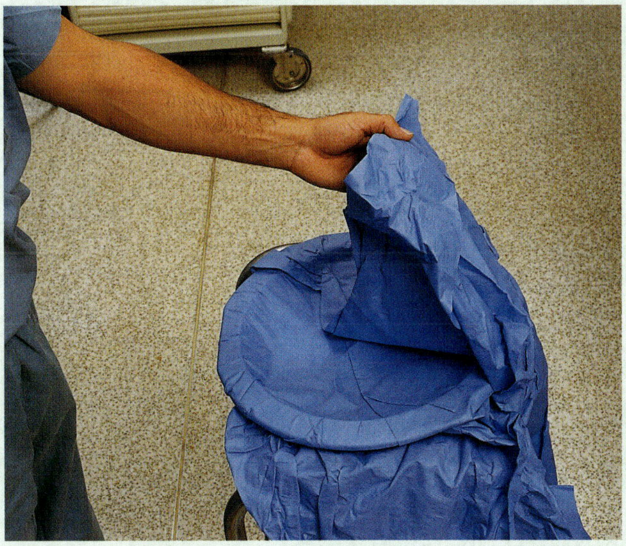

Figure 12-9 Opening the basin set

TECHNIQUE Opening a Small Wrapped Package, (Such as Initial Gown) onto a Clean Surface

1. Check the integrity of the packaging material.
2. Orient the gown package on the Mayo stand.
3. Break or remove the seal, if present.
4. Grasp the tab and open the first flap away from you.
5. Grasp the tab and open the second and third flaps in the appropriate directions.
6. Grasp the tab and open the fourth flap toward you.
7. Open the appropriate size gloves.

TECHNIQUE Opening a Small Wrapped Package onto the Sterile Field

Refer to Figure 12-10.

1. Check the integrity of the packaging material.
2. Orient the package in one hand so that the first flap will be opened away from you.
3. Break or remove the seal.
4. Grasp the tab and open the first fold away from you with your opposite hand.

(continues)

(continued)

5. Secure the flap in the hand that is holding the sterile package.
6. Open the second fold and secure the flap without reaching over the exposed sterile item.
7. Open the third fold and secure the flap.
8. Open the fourth fold toward you and secure the flap.
9. Transfer the item onto the sterile field by tossing gently without crossing the boundary for the sterile field.
10. Retract your hands as soon as the item is airborne.
11. Discard the wrapper.

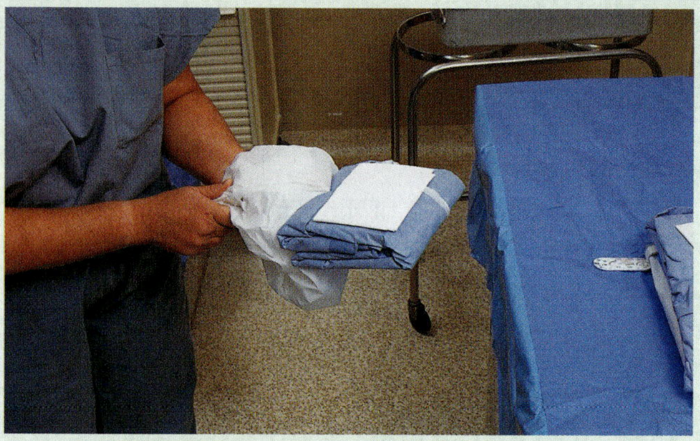

Figure 12-10 Opening a small wrapped package

TECHNIQUE Opening a Peel Pack

Refer to Figure 12-11.

1. Check the integrity of the packaging material.
2. Orient package in both hands by grasping one edge of the peel pack in each hand.
3. Slowly separate the sides of the peel pack.
4. Balance the item within the package to prevent contamination.
5. Maintain a safe distance from the sterile field while continuing to open the package.
6. Transfer the item onto the sterile filed by tossing gently without crossing the boundary for the sterile field.
7. Retract your hands as soon as the item is airborne.
8. Discard the wrapper.

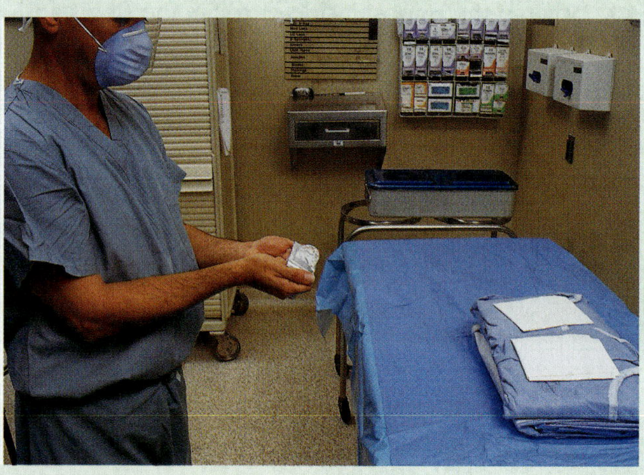

Figure 12-11 Opening a peel pack

TECHNIQUE Opening the Instrument Set (Container System)

1. Place the instrument container on a suitable surface.
2. Verify the presence of filters and color change of external chemical indicator(s).
3. Break or remove the seals, ensuring that fragments of the seal do not become airborne.
4. Release the mechanism securing the lid.
5. Lift the lid vertically 12–18 in. above the container, then step back.
6. Invert the lid and inspect; verify that the inner surface of the lid is dry and that the filter is dry and intact.
7. Place the lid in a convenient location.

SCRUBBING AND DONNING STERILE ATTIRE

Once the sterile field is established, the STSR performs the surgical scrub and dons the sterile attire in preparation for entry to the sterile field (principle of asepsis #2). Be sure that all personal needs are taken care of and that all necessary PPE (e.g., protective eyewear, radiation shield) has been donned prior to initiating the surgical scrub.

TECHNIQUE

The Surgical Scrub

Counted Brush Stroke Method

Refer to Figure 12-12A–J.

1. Don all PPE.
2. Inspect the integrity of the hands and arms to rule out the presence of wounds or infection.
3. Inspect nails and cuticles.
4. Open the brush package and place in a convenient location.
5. Turn on the water and adjust the temperature.
6. Wet hands and arms, apply antiseptic, and lather to 2 in. above the elbows (basic handwash).

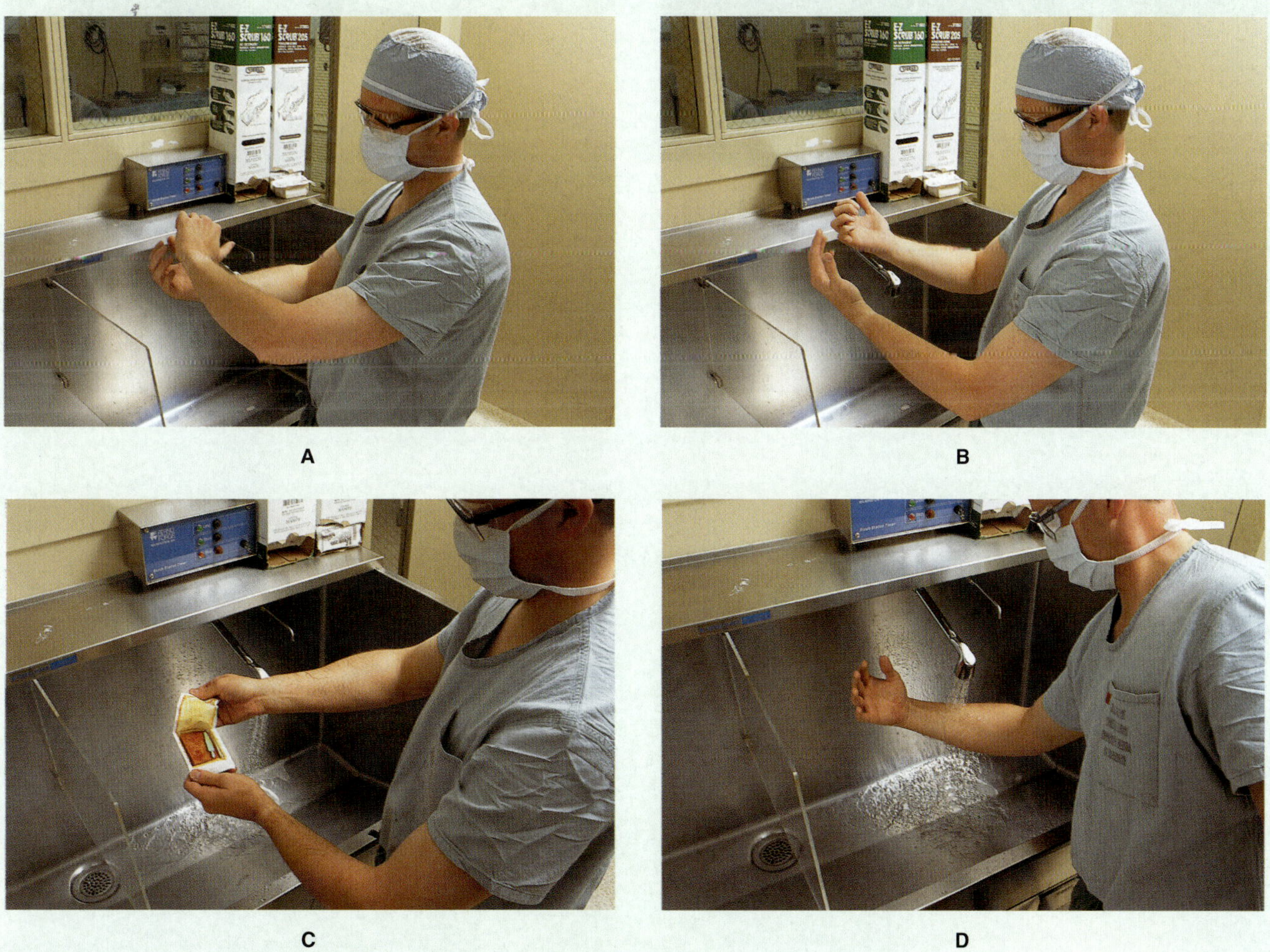

Figure 12-12 The surgical scrub (counted brush stroke method): (A) Inspect hands and arms. (B) Inspect nails and cuticles. (C) Open brush package. (D) Apply water.

(continues)

(continued)

7. Obtain the nail cleaner.
8. Clean each subungual space and around the cuticles (if necessary) under running water.
9. Discard the nail cleaner.
10. Rinse hands and arms.
11. Keep the hands above the elbows and keep elbows bent to allow water to run off the elbows.
12. Obtain the scrub brush; wet and lather.
13. Begin scrubbing the first hand by placing the fingertips together and scrubbing all of the nails and cuticles 30 brush strokes (one stroke is the combined back and forth motion).
14. Use 10 brush strokes for all subsequent planes.
15. Scrub each finger by dividing it into four planes.
16. Scrub each web space as a separate plane.
17. Progress in an orderly fashion to ensure that all surfaces receive adequate chemical exposure and mechanical action.
18. Conserve water, if possible.
19. Add antiseptic, as needed.
20. Scrub the hand by dividing it into four planes; use circular motions.
21. Divide the arm into three sections.
22. Further divide each section into four planes and scrub each individually using circular motions.
23. Continue the scrub to 2 in. proximal to the elbow.
24. Transfer the brush to the scrubbed hand and repeat the process on the opposite extremity.

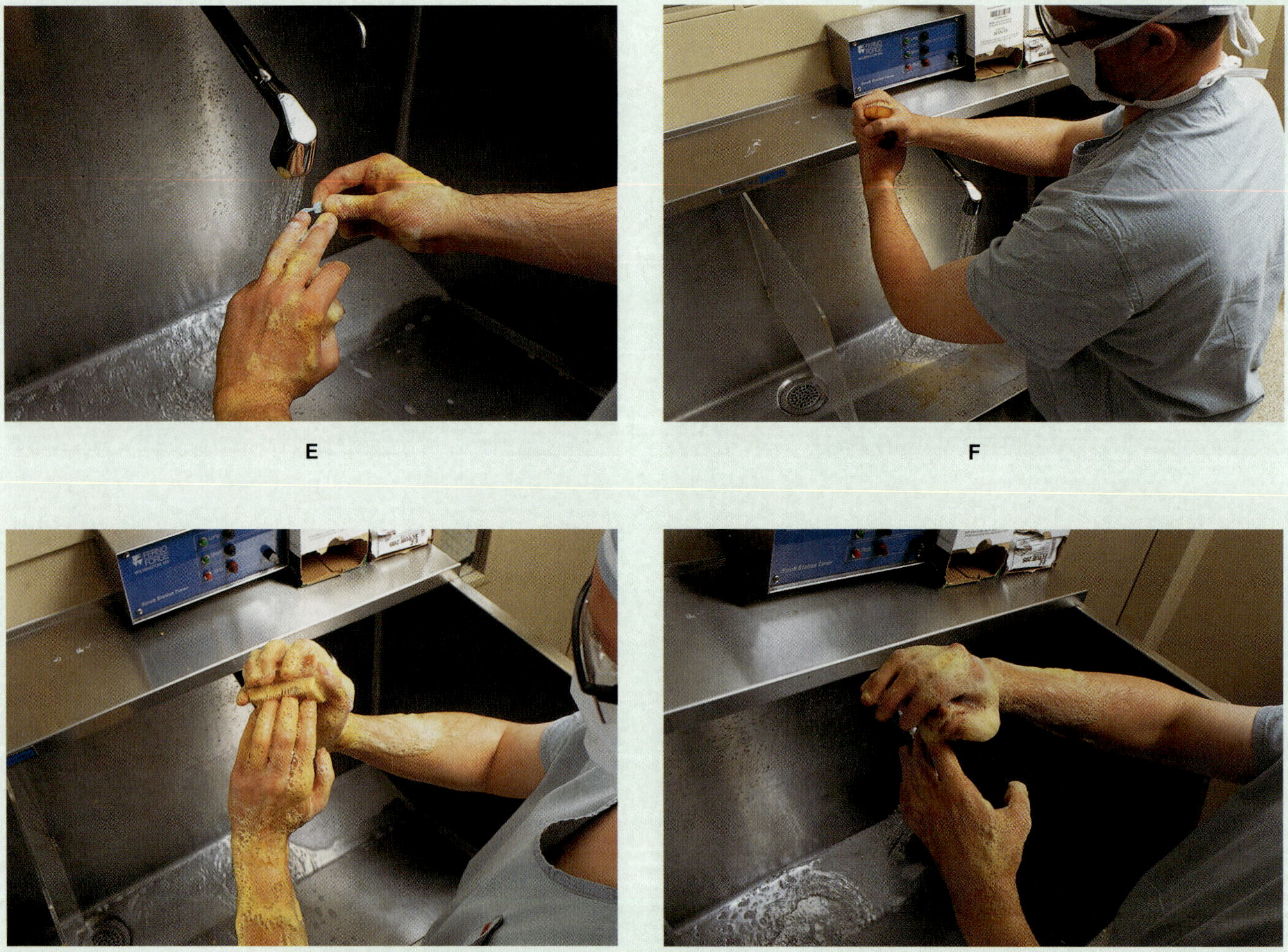

E F G H

Figure 12-12 ***(continued)*** **(E) Clean under each nail. (F) Apply antiseptic. (G) Scrub nails (30 strokes). (H) Scrub all planes of all fingers (10 strokes per plane).**

25. Discard the brush.
26. Rinse one extremity from the fingertips to the elbows while keeping the elbows bent. Note and avoid all environmental hazards (e.g., faucet, edges of sink).
27. Repeat rinse on the opposite extremity.
28. Turn off the water.
29. Allow the excess water to drip into the sink.
30. Proceed to the OR with elbows bent and hands between the mid-chest and waist level. Do not touch anything.
31. Open the OR door with your hip and proceed to the table where the gown and gloves are open.

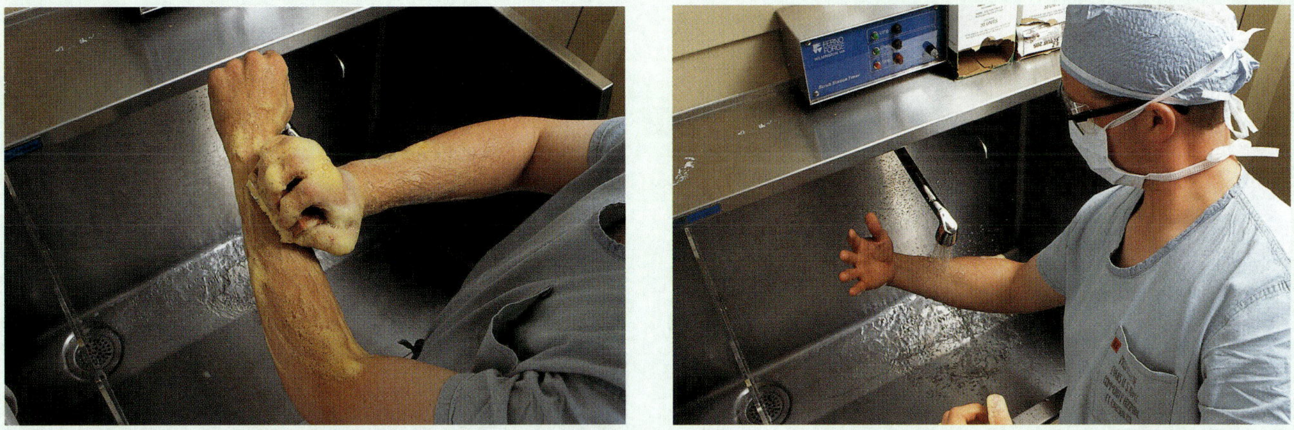

I J

Figure 12-12 ***(continued)*** **(counted brush stroke method): (I) Scrub hands and arms (10 strokes per plane). (J) Rinse thoroughly**

The Surgical Scrub

Any individual who will enter the sterile surgical field, touch sterile instruments, or an incisional wound, must scrub their hands and arms to 2″ above the elbows with an **antimicrobial** scrub solution (refer to Chapter 7) prior to each surgical procedure. This surgical scrub is intended to remove as many microorganisms as possible from the hands and arms, and to render them surgically clean prior to donning the sterile gown and gloves.

Two types of organisms live on and in the skin. Transient organisms are organisms that have been acquired by touching other objects (fomites) contaminated with these organisms. These organisms are on the surface of the skin and are easily removed by handwashing or scrubbing. Resident organisms (flora) thrive deeper below the surface of the skin and are therefore more difficult to remove. The flora cannot be totally removed by scrubbing, although mechanical action does bring some of them to the surface. Over time, these microorganisms work their way to the surface of the skin, contaminating the skin. For this reason, it is preferable to use a surgical scrub solution that provides a film of protection lasting for several hours. This film will continue to kill any resident microbes that may reach the surface of the skin in the several hours following the surgical scrub.

Equipment for the Surgical Scrub. Each facility provides a variety of disposable scrub brushes impregnated with antiseptic solution. When a plain brush is used, containers of various antiseptic solutions (refer to Chapter 7) are provided. These are operated with a foot pump so that the antiseptic can be dispensed without the use of the hands.

One of two methods for the surgical scrub may be used: the timed method or the counted brush stroke method. In the timed method, the hands and arms are scrubbed for a prescribed length of time. The counted brush stroke method requires a measured number of brush strokes for each anatomical area to be scrubbed. Although either method is effective when performed properly, the counted brush stroke method is more likely to produce a thorough surgical scrub for individuals just learning to scrub.

Self-Drying and Gowning

As soon as the scrub is complete, the surgical team member proceeds directly to the OR, enters by pushing the door open with the hip, keeps hands between the waist and the mid-chest, and avoids touching anything with the hands or arms. The gown and gloves for the STSR are opened onto a Mayo stand or other small table during the establishment of a sterile field. The STSR approaches this table immediately upon entering the room. The STSR will dry, gown, and glove himself and then assist the other team members. Once the hands and arms are dried, the STSR is prepared to don the gown.

Donning a surgical gown requires some big movements. These should be minimized. *The STSR must have a heightened awareness of the total environment in order to avoid contamination.*

After the gown has been donned, the fasteners at the shoulders and waist must be secured. The circulator will assist in this process by pulling the gown all the way onto the shoulders and around the body. Care must be taken not to turn your back on the sterile field at any time. The final step of gowning, called *turning,* is accomplished after the gloves have been donned, using the closed glove technique. The back of a wraparound-style gown is not considered sterile.

TECHNIQUE: Drying the Hands and Arms

Refer to Figure 12-13.

1. Approach the sterile field with caution.
2. Keep the elbows bent; stoop down to secure the towel.
3. Pinch and lift the towel from the sterile field without dripping on or touching the gown, gloves, or wrapper.
4. Step away from the sterile field with the arms extended.
5. Unfold the towel without allowing the edges to fall below the waist.
6. Bend slightly at the waist so that the towel does not come in contact with the scrubs.
7. Hold the towel in the palm of one hand while drying the opposite hand and arm using a patting motion.
8. Transfer the towel to the opposite hand without crossing the hands or passing the towel over the scrubbed hands.
9. Dry the opposite hand and arm.
10. Discard the towel.

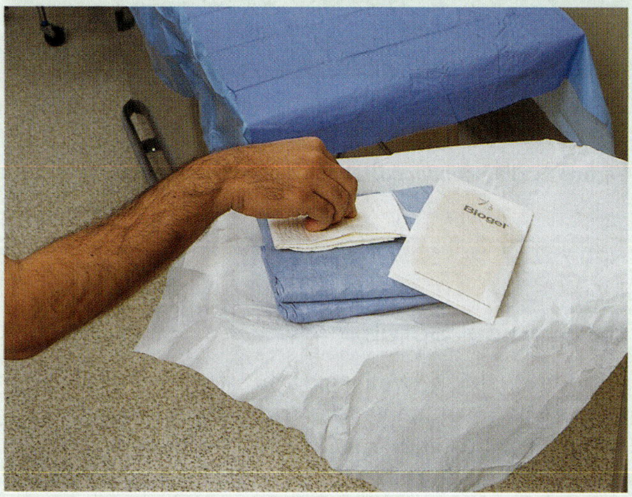

Figure 12-13 Drying the hands and arms

TECHNIQUE: Self-Gowning

Refer to Figure 12-14A–F.

1. Approach the sterile field with caution.
2. Grasp the gown at the center near the neck without touching the gloves or the wrapper.
3. Lift the gown from the wrapper and step back with the gown still folded.
4. Hold the inside of the gown near the shoulders and allow the gown to unfold.
5. Begin donning the gown by slipping the hands and arms into the sleeves.
6. Slide the gown over the arms using a "swimming" motion.

7. Keep the hands within the cuff of the gown.
8. Flex the elbows to hold the gown in place.
9. Allow the circulator to assist with the final gown adjustments and secure the neck and back of the gown.

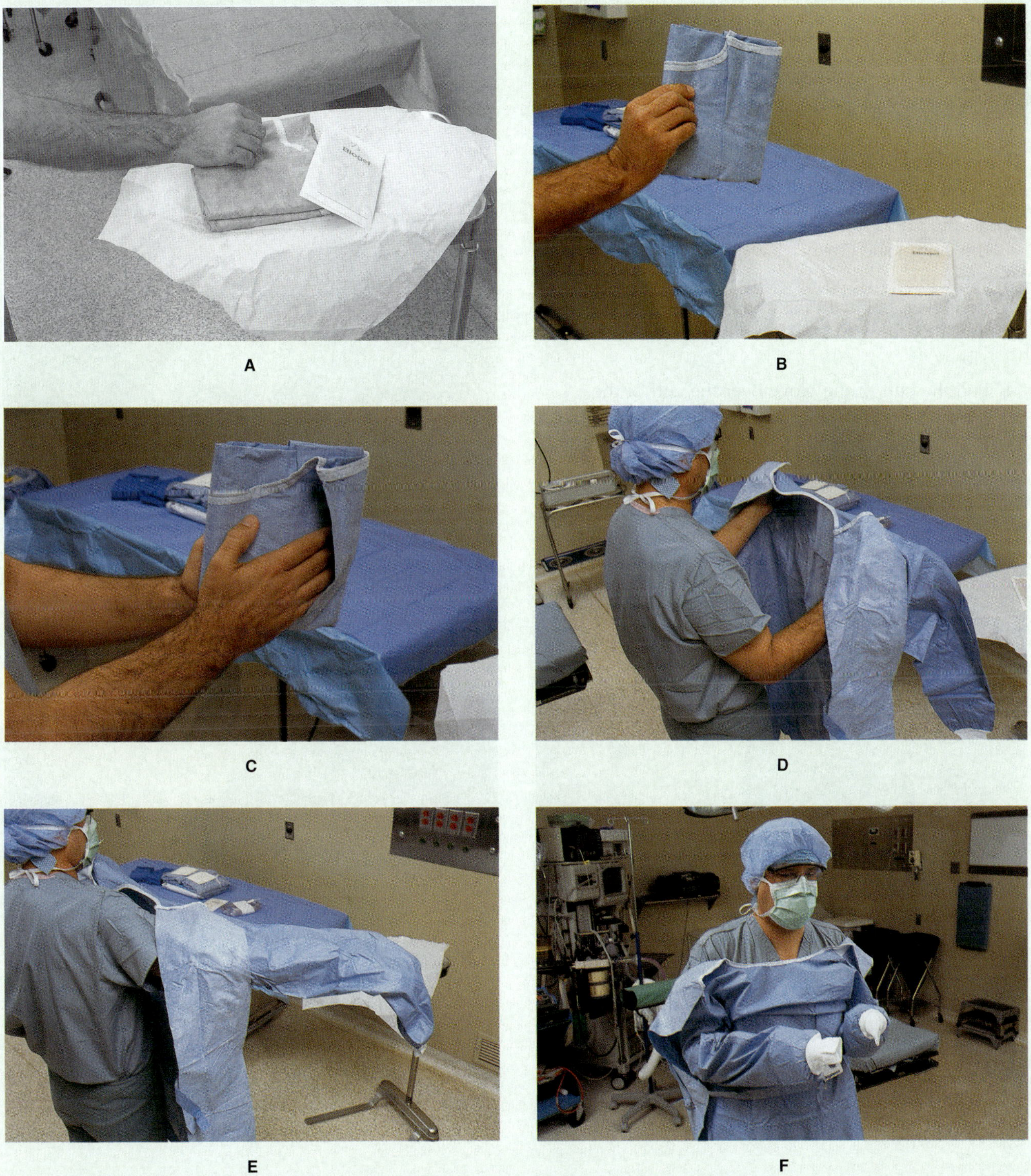

Figure 12-14 **Self-gowning: (A) Pick up gown after drying hands and arms. (B) Lift gown while keeping body away from Mayo stand. (C) Identify collar and orient gown. (D) Release lower portion and identify arm openings. (E) Enter sleeves. (F) Flex arms to hold gown in place**

Closed Gloving

The closed glove technique is used for donning the gloves following the surgical scrub and after the sterile gown has been donned. The individual gloving should always work from a separate table, never the back table, to prevent contamination. Only the STSR who scrubs first should use this technique. All other team members should be assisted by the STSR.

TECHNIQUE Closed Gloving

Refer to Figure 12-15A–C.

1. Approach the sterile field with caution.
2. Secure the first glove, keeping the fingers within the cuff of the gown.
3. Align the glove on the palm of the hand that will be gloved first with the thumb side of the glove toward your palm and the fingertips toward the elbow.
4. Pull the cuff of the glove over the cuff of the gown.
5. Unfold the cuff of the glove to completely cover the cuff of the gown.
6. Grasp the glove and the gown at the wrist level.
7. Work the fingers into the glove as the glove is pulled into position.
8. Secure the second glove and apply using the same technique.
9. Double glove.

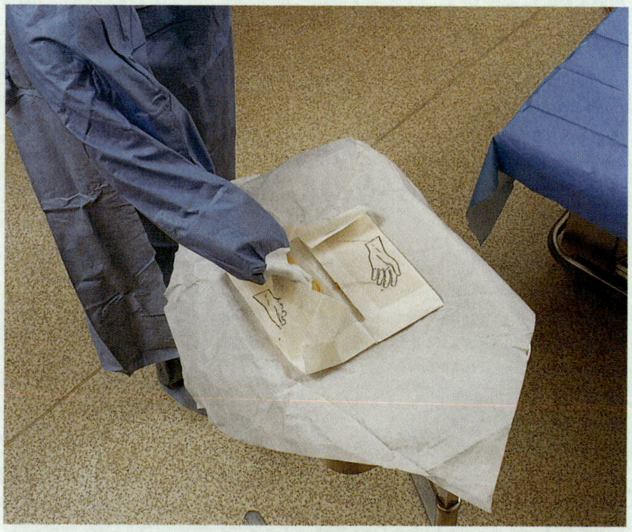

A

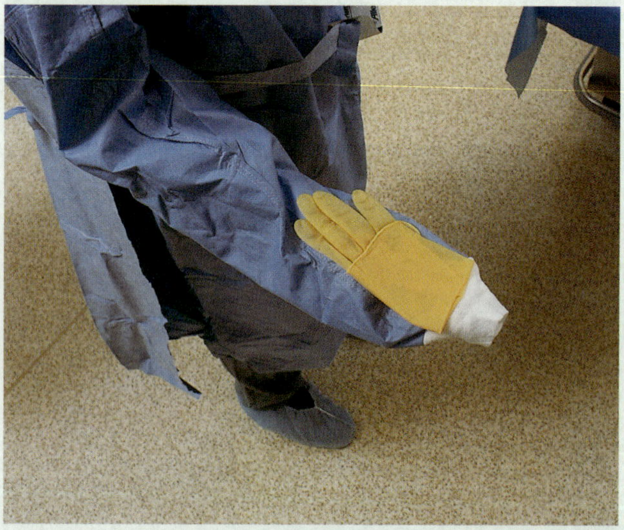

B

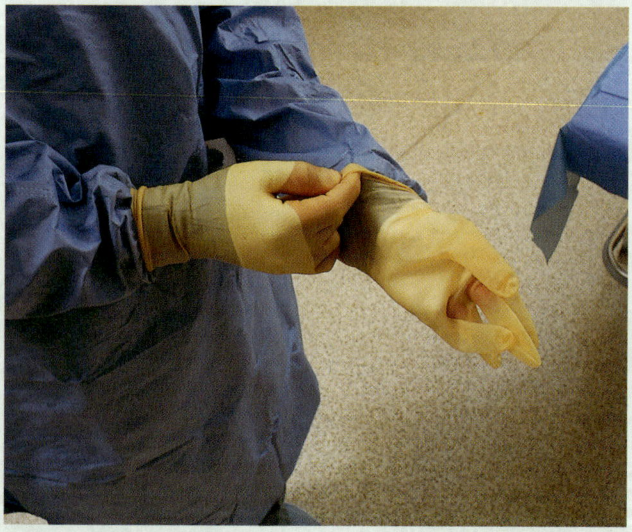

C

Figure 12-15 Closed gloving: (A) Keep hands in cuffs; remove glove from wrapper. (B) Position first glove palm to palm, thumb to thumb. (C) Pull on and adjust glove

Turning the Gown

The circulator assists in turning the wraparound-style gown. Because one sterile and one nonsterile team member and large movements are involved, extreme vigilance is required during this maneuver. The gowned individual maintains an appropriate distance from the other sterile areas until the gown has been completely secured, and should continue to face the sterile field at all times, never turning the back on a sterile area. Once the back of the gown has been turned, it is considered nonsterile. This technique is used not only for the STSR but also for subsequent sterile team members as well.

TECHNIQUE

Turning the Gown

Refer to Figure 12-16A–C.

1. Remain facing the sterile field.
2. Secure the tag in the right hand and the gown tie in the left hand and separate.
3. Hold the tag in such a way that the circulator has space to grasp the tag.
4. Pass the tag to the circulator at the right side.
5. The circulator will move around to the left side.
6. Transfer the gown tie from the left to the right hand.
7. Receive the gown tie from the circulator at the left side.
8. The circulator retains and discards the tab.
9. Secure both gown ties.

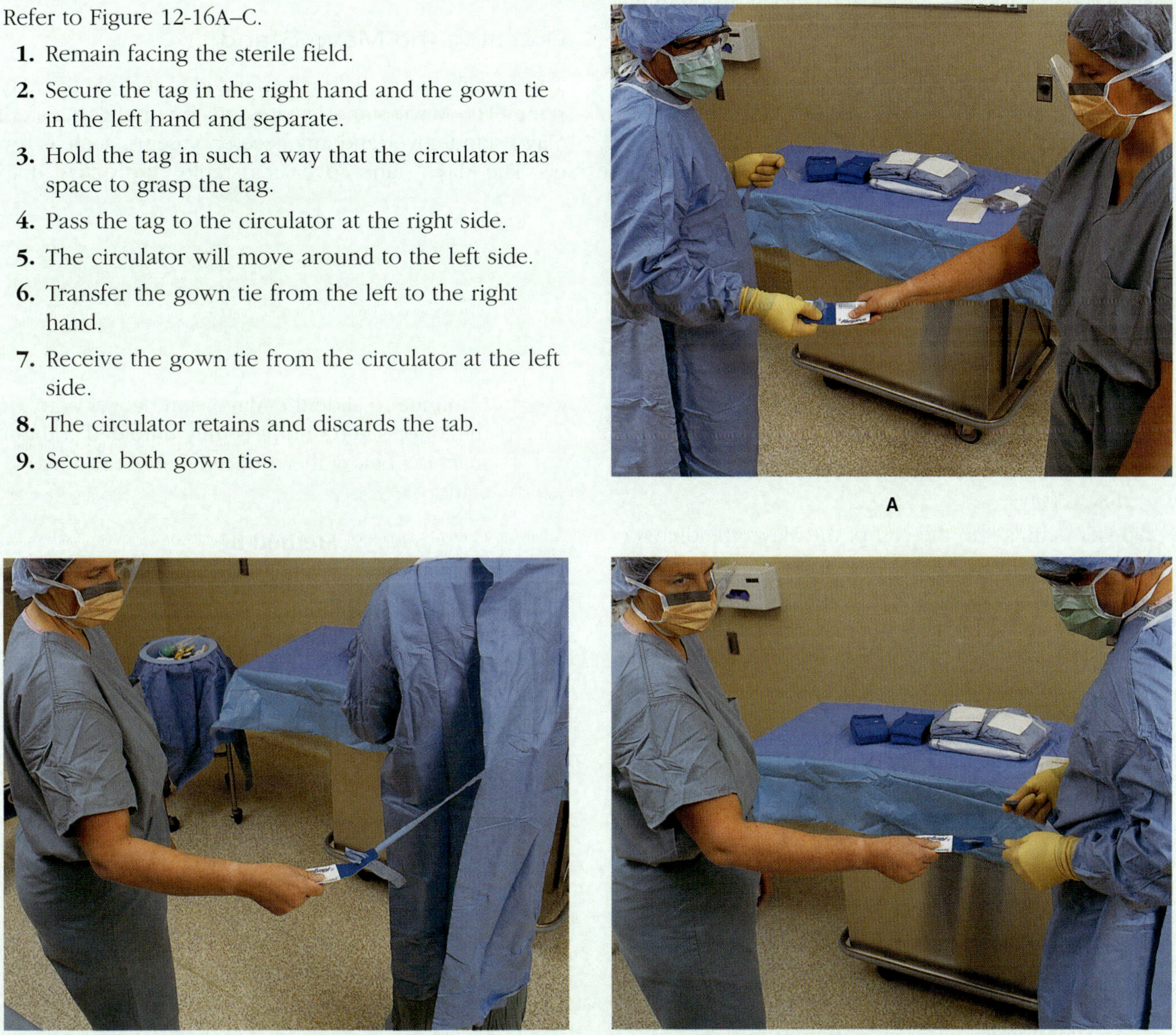

A

B

C

Figure 12-16 Turning the gown: (A) Disengage the tab and hand it to the circulator. (B) Circulator moves behind the STSR. (C) STSR rotates shoulders to receive the tie with the left hand

Open Gloving

This method is used to don gloves for skin prep, for catheterization, or for any procedure to be performed in a sterile fashion but without the surgical hand scrub or use of a sterile gown. Hands should always be washed and dried before gloves are donned and as soon as feasible following removal. The open gloving technique is not recommended when wearing a sterile gown. The technique for open gloving is found in Chapter 8.

PREPARATION OF THE STERILE FIELD

Once the STSR has entered the sterile field, a number of tasks must be performed quickly and efficiently prior to initiation of the surgical procedure. Keep in mind that practical realities conflict with the practice of strict sterile technique. For example, one of the concepts that relates to the second principle of asepsis states: "Sterile individuals must keep their hands in sight at all times, and within the sterile zone." This becomes impossible when the sterile individual is required to reach above his or her head to place sterile covers on the light handles. As long as direct contamination does not occur, the hand and arm of the individual applying the light handle covers is *considered* sterile.

A logical and efficient pattern (routine) must be established and repeated during preparation for all types of surgical procedures. The following is a sample organizational routine for a laparotomy in which everything runs smoothly and according to plan. Be aware that variations (such as contamination, product differences, surgeon's preference, the patient's situation, and school or facility policy) can occur. Plan in advance the steps that will be taken when a variation does occur.

Dressing the Mayo Stand

The existing sterile field is expanded to include the Mayo stand. The Mayo stand is "dressed" by applying a sterile Mayo stand cover and any accessory items, such as towels. The Mayo stand cover is a sterile **cylindrical** drape

TECHNIQUE: Dressing the Mayo Stand

Refer to Figure 12-17A–C.

1. Partially open and orient the Mayo stand cover on the back table according to the manufacturer's instructions.
2. Insert hands into the cuff of the Mayo stand cover as directed.
3. Grasp all layers contained within the cuff of the cover with both hands to prevent slippage.
4. Open the pocket in the folded Mayo stand cover that will eventually present to the bare Mayo stand.
5. Approach the Mayo stand, ensuring that items that are to remain sterile do not touch the bare Mayo stand.
6. Secure the Mayo stand by placing one foot on the base of the stand.
7. Use the method that best suits your situation to apply the Mayo stand cover.

Method A

- Stand directly in front of the Mayo stand.
- Begin to slide the Mayo stand cover onto the Mayo stand. Do not let the folded portion of the Mayo stand cover unfold and slip below the level of the Mayo stand.
- Continue to slide the Mayo stand cover onto the Mayo stand until it is fully unfolded without reaching below the surface level of the Mayo stand.

Method B

- Stand slightly to the side of the Mayo stand.
- Begin to slide the Mayo stand cover onto the Mayo stand. Do not let the folded portion of the Mayo stand cover unfold and slip below the level of the Mayo stand.
- Keep one hand within the cuffed portion of the Mayo stand cover and begin to push the cover toward the back of the Mayo stand.
- Extend the cover one fold at a time with your opposite hand.
- Continue to slide the cover onto the Mayo stand until it is fully unfolded without reaching below the surface level of the Mayo stand.

8. Make any final adjustments.
9. Fold or tuck any excess material.
10. Place towels on the Mayo stand, if needed.
11. Continue with preoperative case management duties.

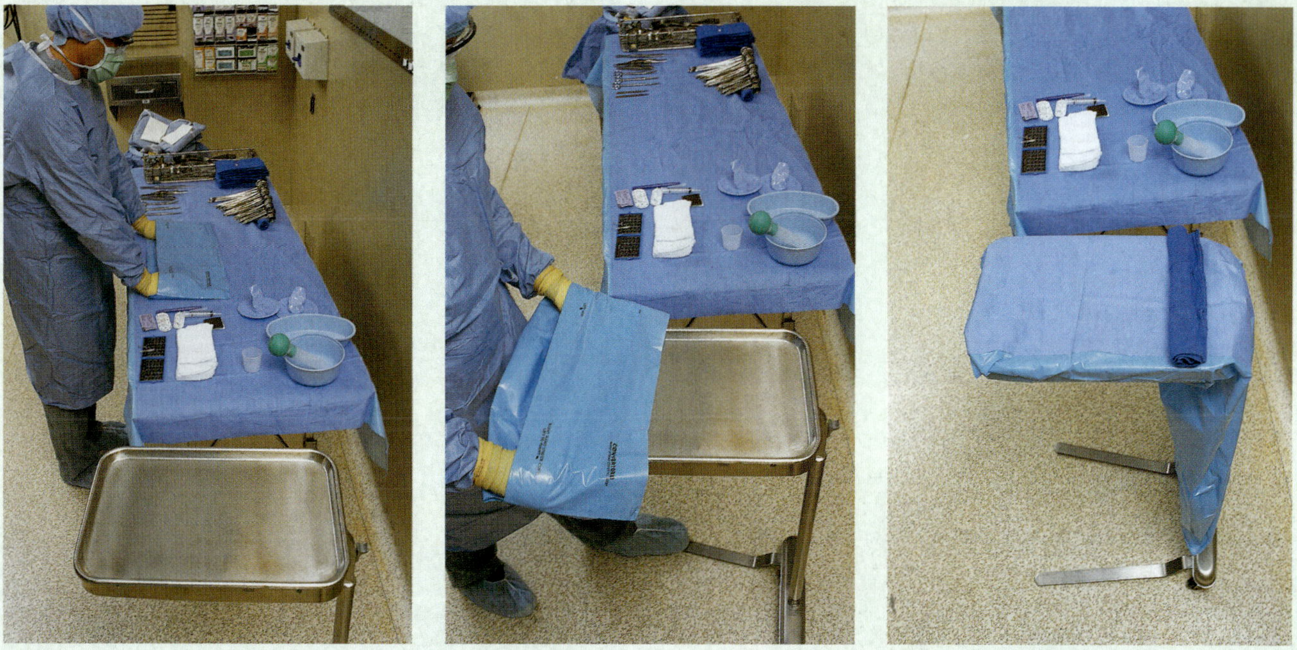

Figure 12-17 **Dressing the Mayo stand: (A) Orient the Mayo stand cover on the back table. (B) Initial placement of the Mayo stand cover. (C) Mayo stand dressed**

that is closed at one end and encircles the upper portion of the Mayo stand.

ORGANIZING THE BACK TABLE

The back table provides a large sterile area for preparation and storage of sterile items. Instruments less likely to be used, redundant instruments, or instruments of specific and often one-time use are left on the back table. The back table is typically the first sterile area prepared by the STSR (Figure 12-18A–C).

Several principles of practice are applied while organizing the back table:

- Move about as little as possible.
- Keep the body centered in a "box" and move just the shoulders and hands.
- Work in sections at the table.
- Handle each item only once.
- Learn a logical and efficient pattern for back table organization and repeat it case after case.
- Be aware of the total environment, especially the movement of others.

Organization of the back table requires that drapes and supplies included in the back table pack itself be rearranged. This may be a relatively small number of items or quite complex. Small basins must be moved from the basin set and placed to receive sterile solutions. Instrument sets must be moved from a container system or wrapper to the back table. Sharps and medications must be arranged. Items must be organized in such a way as to allow for safe and efficient **count** procedures. Ultimately some items will be transferred to the Mayo stand and the patient. A good piece of advice is "Think fast but move carefully." The STSR should have a basic plan in mind before beginning back table organization. A good time to begin this activity is at the scrub sink using the A POSitive CARE Approach. For the student, the time at the scrub sink is well spent reviewing the first five or six steps that should be taken once the scrub attire is donned. As experience is gained, the time at the sink is best spent reviewing the needs of the surgeon and the steps of the procedure. The STSR with considerable experience will typically think of variations in anatomy, **pathology**, and operative procedures and develop a mental game plan for responding to specific variations.

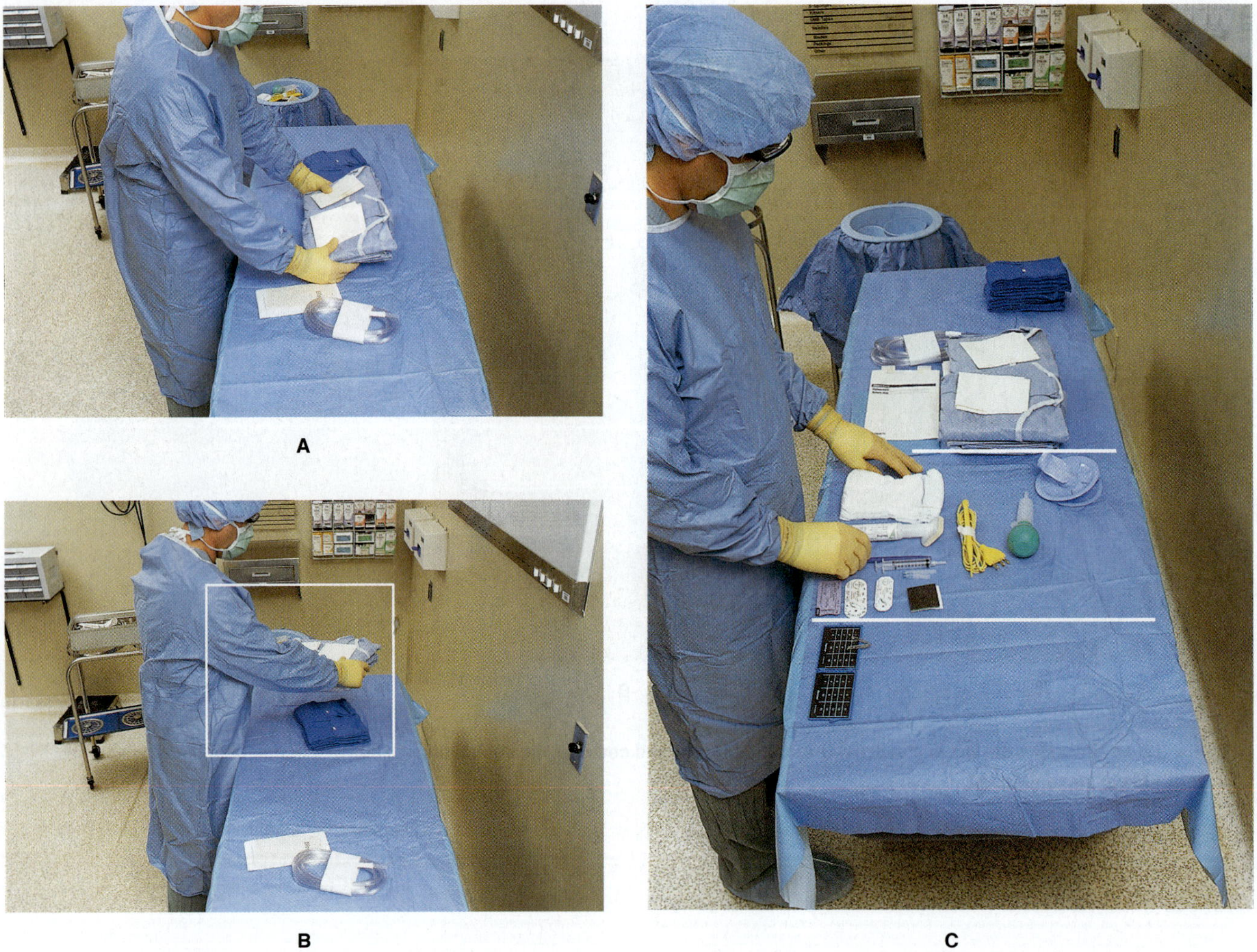

Figure 12-18 **Principles of back table setup: (A) Move as little as possible. (B) Keep body within an imaginary box. (C) Work in sections at the back table**

TECHNIQUE

Organizing the Back Table

Refer to Figure 12-19A–D.

1. Arrange all items that were placed into or packaged within the basin set (and all items that were opened onto or contained within the back table pack) by placing them in their final location on the back table. Handle each item only once.
    - Secure the sterile suture/trash bag in a convenient location.
    - Place small basins and medicine cups near the edge of the table to allow the circulator access for placement of solutions or medications. (Refer to the Pouring Sterile Fluid technique. Medication handling techniques are presented in Chapter 9.)
    - Place all sharps in a common location.
    - Organize the suture material in the predicted order of need according to the surgeon's preference card.
2. Organize all drapes and accessory items related to the draping procedure in an empty basin in the

order in which they will be needed. Complete each task prior to moving to the next item in the organizational routine.

- Connect the Yankauer suction tip to the suction tubing and place in the basin.
- Prepare the electrosurgical pencil by removing and discarding any packaging material and place in the basin.
- Place the light handles or covers in the basin.
- Place the laparotomy sheet over the items already in the basin. Be sure that it does not extend beyond the sterile field.
- Four drape towels are prepared and placed on top of the laparotomy sheet.
- If a lower body sheet will be used, place it on top of the towels.
- Place the surgeon's and assistant's gloves, gowns, and towels on the top of the stack.

3. Space is now available on the back table for the instrument set, which must be removed from its container. (Refer to the Removal of the Instrument Set from the Container System technique.)
4. The instruments are organized by category. For example, all retracting instruments are placed in one area, all cutting instruments are placed in another, and so on. Instrument structure, classification, and usage information is found in Chapter 10.
5. The initial count is performed at a mutually convenient time by the circulator and the STSR.
   - Items are counted in the same order for every procedure (e.g., sponges first, sharps second, and instruments last) according to facility policy.
   - The name of the item is stated prior to counting (e.g., "Lap sponges—1, 2, 3, 4, 5.").
   - Each item is separated by the STSR and visualized by both team members.

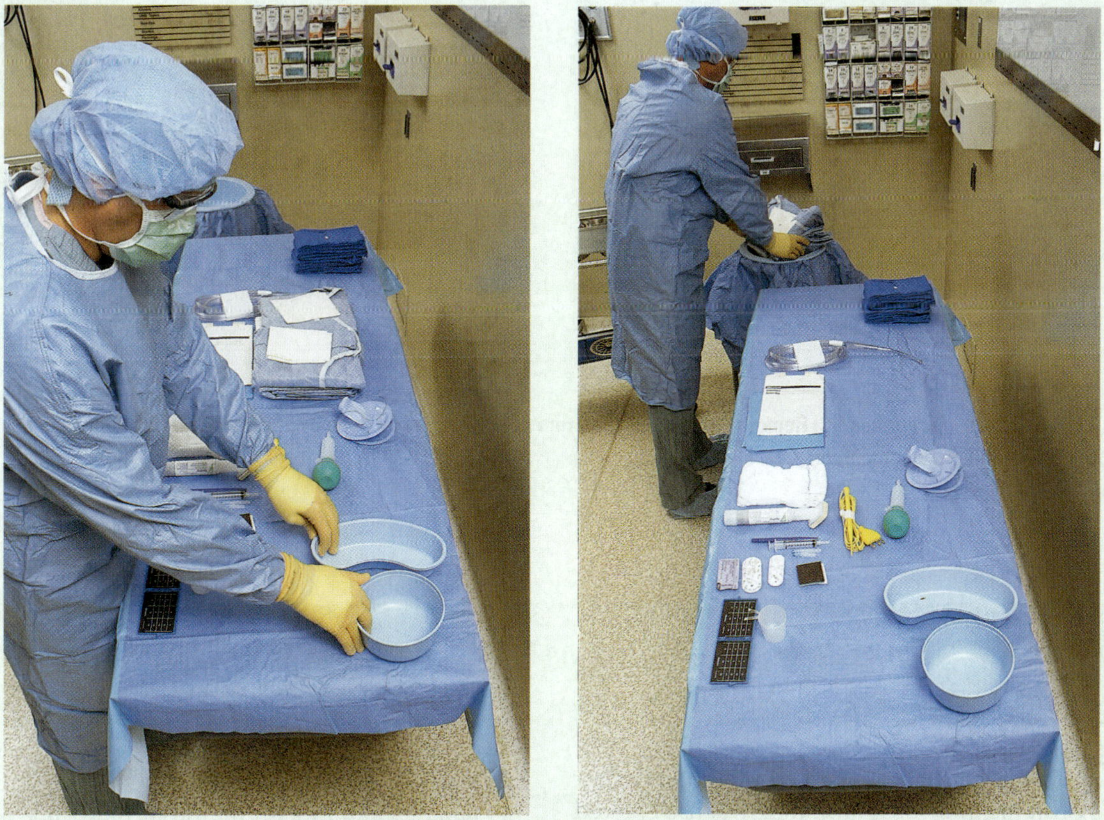

A B

Figure 12-19 Organizing the back table: (A) Place the small basins near, but not over, the edge of the table. (B) Move drapes, gowns, and gloves to the large basin area.

(continues)

(continued)

- Each item is verbally counted by both team members. This may be accomplished in unison or by repeating the count according to facility policy.
- Each item, or group of items, is recorded by the circulator.

6. Continue with preoperative case management duties.

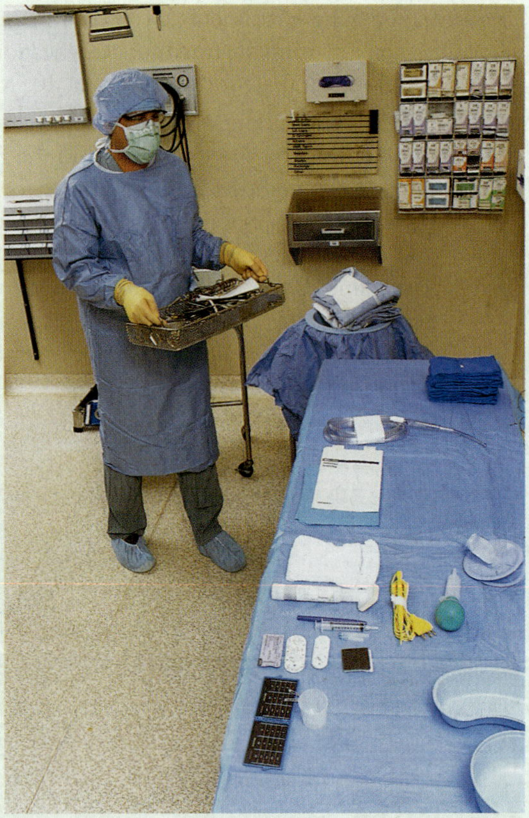

C

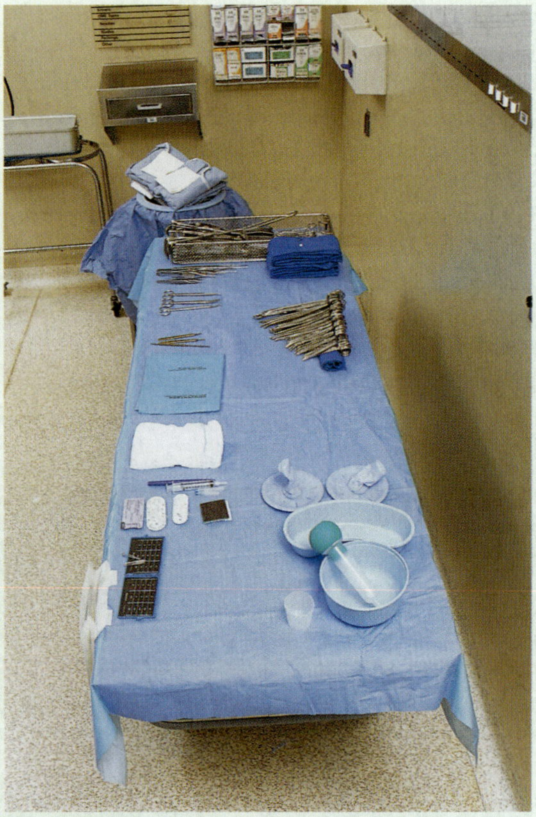

D

Figure 12-19 ***(continued)*** **(C) Remove instrument tray from container; verify exposure to sterilization process. (D) Back table setup complete**

TECHNIQUE

Pouring Sterile Fluid

(*Note:* this skill is typically performed by the circulator or other nonsterile individual once the STSR has entered the sterile field.)

1. Obtain sterile fluid (sterile water and saline are routinely used) according to the surgeon's preference card (first verification).
2. Verify that the "five rights" are met (refer to Chapter 9).
3. Verify the patient's allergy status.
4. Remove and discard the protective outer seal from the fluid container.
5. Remove the inner seal using sterile technique.
6. Approach the sterile field while maintaining a 12-in. minimum distance.

7. Ensure that the fluid does not spill, drip, or run down the outer surface of the container.
8. The circulator and STSR visually and verbally verify the name, strength, and expiration date of the fluid (second verification).
9. Hold the lip of the container approximately 12 in. above the basin and pour without splashing or dripping. It is not necessary to completely empty the solution container.
10. Once the fluid is on the sterile field, another visual/verbal verification of the fluid label is performed (third verification).
11. The fluid container may be saved for future reference or discarded according to facility policy.
12. The fluid container may *NOT* be recapped for later use of the remaining solution. However, it may be recapped for disposal.
13. The fluid is labeled by the STSR according to facility policy.
14. Fluid is prepared for use (Refer to next technique, Filling a Bulb Syringe).
15. Continue with preoperative case management duties.

TECHNIQUE Filling a Bulb Syringe

1. Assemble the components of the bulb syringe, if necessary.
2. Expel the air from the bulb.
3. Maintain pressure on the bulb.
4. Insert the tip of the syringe into the basin containing the sterile fluid.
5. Release the pressure on the bulb and allow the syringe to fill.
6. Tip the syringe upward allowing the sterile fluid to enter the bulb. If the syringe is not completely filled, repeat steps 2–5. Be sure that the sterile fluid within the syringe is not accidentally expelled while continuing to fill the syringe.
7. Label the bulb syringe (if necessary) according to facility policy.
8. Place the bulb syringe in a safe location until needed.
9. Continue with preoperative case management duties.
10. Remember to state the contents of the syringe when passing it to the surgeon or surgical assistant, when needed.
11. Remember to keep track of the amount of fluid used and report usage to the anesthesia provider and/or circulator, as necessary.

TECHNIQUE Removal of the Instrument Set from the Container System

1. Request the circulator's assistance at a mutually convenient time.
2. Verify exposure to the sterilization process by observing the chemical indicator for the appropriate color change.
3. Approach the container cautiously, ensuring that the gown front/sleeves do not contact the exterior of the container.
4. Reach carefully into the container and grasp the tray/basket containing the instrumentation.
5. Lift the tray/basket vertically and step away from the container.
6. Hold the tray/basket (without allowing it to touch the sterile gown) while the circulator verifies that the container interior is dry and that the filter is intact.
7. Place the tray/basket gently in the prepared location on the back table.
8. Continue with preoperative case management duties.

ORGANIZING THE MAYO STAND

The Mayo stand is prepared to receive the instruments and supplies that will be used most frequently and commonly during the surgical procedure. Items placed on the Mayo stand vary greatly. The instrumentation on the Mayo stand for a laparoscopic procedure varies greatly from a laparotomy setup, even if the intent is the same, for example, removal of the gallbladder. Instrumentation for orthopedics is radically different from ophthalmic surgery. Each facility may require basic setups. There is no way for a student to learn "the" setup because it does not exist. However, it is important for students to learn the setup(s) for the institutions in which they practice. Like the back table, a logical and sequential routine should be established and followed consistently.

Mayo setups vary too much for a single description. However, some key principles of practice apply without regard to the particulars of instrument location:

- Place only those items (instruments and supplies such as sponges) most likely to be used on the Mayo stand.
- Instruments from each category are inspected for damage and functionality then conveniently arranged on the Mayo stand.
- Typically, instruments are placed on the Mayo stand in pairs (or even numbers if more than two like items are required).
- Ratcheted instruments are closed to the first ratchet as they are moved from the back table to the Mayo stand.
- Handles of ringed instruments may be placed over a rolled towel to facilitate order.
- Use caution when placing sharp items.

Perhaps the most important tip is to habituate an efficient procedure for Mayo setup. The less time the STSR spends worrying about the mechanics of the setup, the more time can be spent making mental plans for variations in the procedure.

ASSISTING A TEAM MEMBER

The STSR (or another team member) who has already scrubbed and donned sterile attire assists other team members who have performed their surgical scrub and are ready to enter the sterile field. Typically, the surgeon and surgical assistant begin their surgical scrub when the circulator begins the patient's skin prep and enter the OR just about the time the prep is finished.

DRAPING THE SURGICAL PATIENT

Drapes are applied to the surgical patient as an extension of the sterile field that has already been created in prepa-

TECHNIQUE
Assisting a Team Member

Drying, Gowning, and Gloving

Refer to Figure 12-20A–D.

1. Lift the towel from the sterile field and step away from the field without turning your back on the sterile field.
2. Unfold the towel without allowing the ends of the towel to fall below waist level.
3. Protect your gloved hands by rolling the towel over the gloved fingers.
4. Present the towel to the team member by holding it taut and placing the edge of the towel on the team member's extended palm without making contact.
5. Lift the folded gown from the sterile field while the team member is drying her hands and arms.
6. Step away from the sterile field without turning your back on the sterile field and unfold the gown so that the outside of the sterile gown is toward you.
7. Place your hands near the shoulder area of the gown, allowing the neck/shoulder area of the gown to fold back over your hands protecting them from contact with the individual you are assisting.
8. Present the gown to the team member by extending your arms.
9. Remain still while your team member places her arms into the gown sleeves.
10. Drop the gown onto the team member's upper arms.
11. Expose the team member's hands, if necessary.
12. Secure the right glove from the wrapper.
13. Step back from the sterile field and prepare the glove by unfolding and orienting it with the thumb of the glove facing the team member.
14. Roll the glove cuff over your fingertips to create a circular opening.

15. Extend the glove toward the team member and hold securely while she inserts her right hand.
16. Ensure that the cuff of the glove completely covers the cuff of the gown.
17. Repeat the procedure for the left glove.
18. The circulator will assist with the final gown adjustments, secure the neck and back of the gown, and assist with turning the back of a wraparound-style gown.

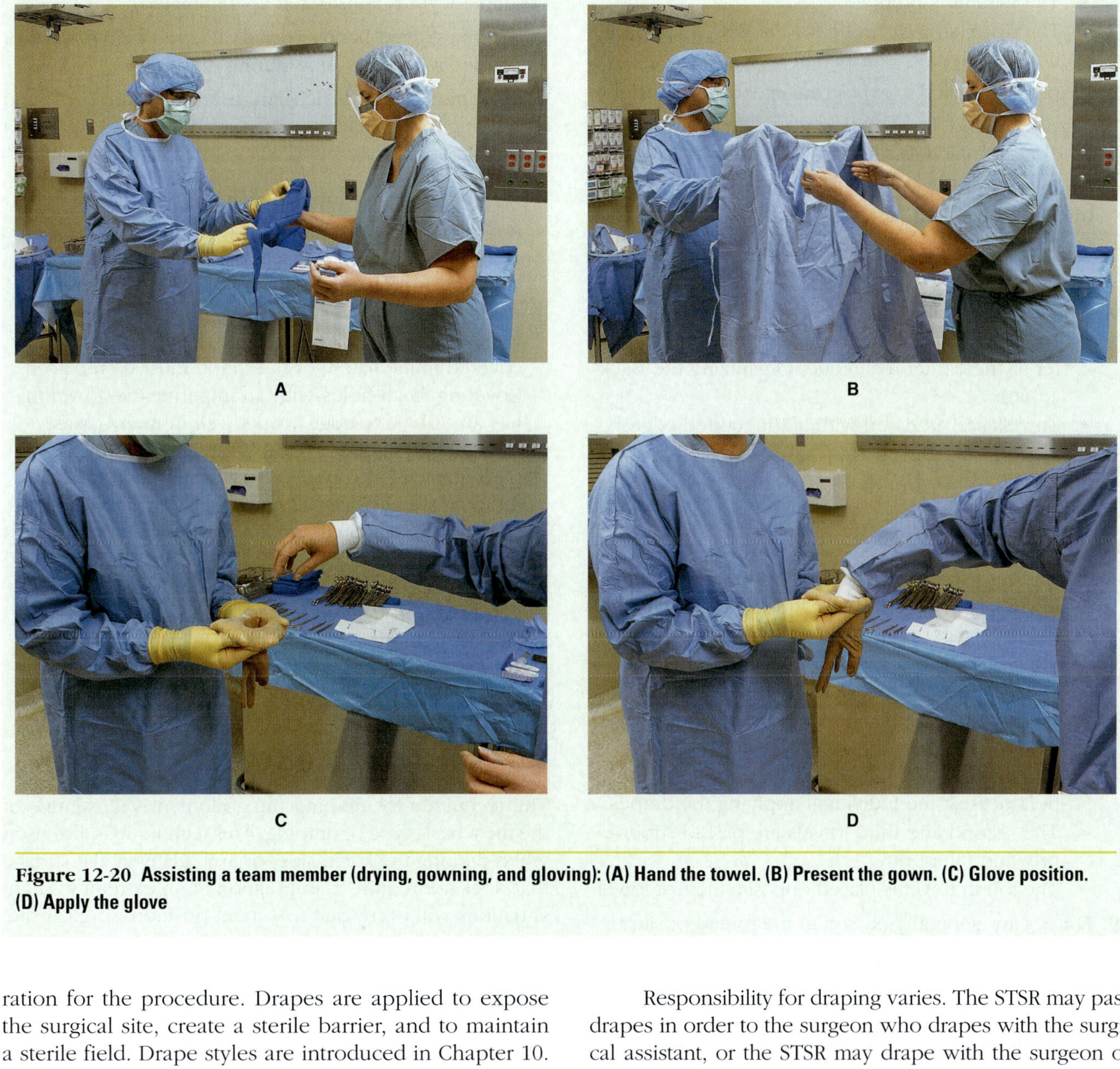

Figure 12-20 **Assisting a team member (drying, gowning, and gloving): (A) Hand the towel. (B) Present the gown. (C) Glove position. (D) Apply the glove**

ration for the procedure. Drapes are applied to expose the surgical site, create a sterile barrier, and to maintain a sterile field. Drape styles are introduced in Chapter 10.

Draping is another variable procedure. Draping for most abdominal procedures is common to several specialty areas; however, many specialty areas require specific kinds of drapes and draping techniques. In this section, several key concepts (principles) that apply to all draping activities and four types of draping procedures—abdomen, perineum, extremity, and **craniotomy**—are presented in some detail.

Responsibility for draping varies. The STSR may pass drapes in order to the surgeon who drapes with the surgical assistant, or the STSR may drape with the surgeon or with the surgical assistant. All parties involved are expected to know proper draping procedures. The STSR must know the draping procedures, details about the drapes themselves, folding patterns, and potential difficulties associated with specific drape types. Because some drapes are large and because the possibility of contamination is increased during draping, the circulator should participate as a careful observer of the procedure.

The principles (rules) that relate to draping, without regard to the type of surgical procedure or the type of draping, are as follows:

1. Typically, the following is accomplished prior to drape application:
   - The patient is anesthetized.
   - A Foley catheter is inserted, if necessary.
   - The patient is positioned.
   - The patient is prepped.
   - The dispersive electrode for the ESU is applied, if necessary.
2. Drapes are applied to expose the intended surgical site.
3. Drapes should be constructed of fluid-resistant or fluid-proof materials.
4. Drapes should have a high tensile strength, be lint free, antistatic, and flame resistant.
5. Drapes should be flexible enough to contour to the shape of the patient or item.
6. Organize the drapes in advance of need.
   - Drapes are stacked in order of intended use (Refer to the earlier technique, Organizing the Back Table).
   - Towels are prepared with a 2-in. cuffed edge.
7. Drapes are not passed over nonsterile areas. It may be necessary to carry the drape to the opposite side of the operating table.
8. Towel placement.
   - All four towels and the four towel clips, if needed, are carried to the individual applying the drapes at one time.
   - Towels are presented one at a time to the individual applying the drapes.
   - Towels are placed with the folded edge down and the gloved hands protected from contamination.
   - The first towel is placed on the side of the patient nearest the individual applying the drapes.
   - The second and third towels are placed superiorly and inferiorly.
   - The fourth towel is placed opposite the first towel.
9. Drapes are generally passed in the folded position.
10. The protective covering is removed from a self-adherent drape prior to use.
11. A folded towel may be useful in applying and smoothing the self-adherent impervious drape.
12. Place the folded drape on the patient and unfold using sterile technique.
13. The sterile gown and gloves may not contact nonsterile personnel or items.
14. Maintain a safe distance from the operating table until the drapes have been applied.
15. Drapes are not relocated after initial placement.
16. Sterile gloved hands are covered by a cuff of the drape when extending the drape to the periphery of the sterile field.
17. Misplaced drapes may be covered with another drape, if necessary.
18. A contaminated drape is removed by the circulator and discarded; it may be necessary to re-prep the area.
19. Any portion of the drape that falls below waist or table level is considered contaminated.
20. Sterile gloved hands are not allowed below waist or table level at any time during draping.
21. Nonperforating devices are used to secure cords and tubing to the drapes.

Problem Solving

- Any contamination offers three possible responses: ignore, discard and replace, or cover. (Ignoring a contamination is only allowed in the most extreme emergencies!)
- Holes discovered or made after draping must be covered immediately or the drape must be replaced. Covering small holes with an impermeable towel that has an **adhesive** edge works well in many cases.
- Perforating towel clips, if unfastened after initial placement, should be removed from the field and replaced if necessary with another sterile towel clip. (*Note:* The individual handling the towel clip may need to change gloves.)
- Small **foreign bodies** (e.g., hair) are grasped with a hemostat and handed to the gloved hand of the circulator and the area covered. (The hemostat should be placed in a convenient place off the sterile field for inclusion in closing counts.)

DRAPING THE ABDOMEN

The technique for draping the abdomen is illustrative of the most basic type of draping. This technique is also used when draping the back, side, or any relatively flat surface that does not require manipulation of an extremity. Slight variations will occur due to patient position, surgical site, size of the area to be draped, and surgeon's preference.

DRAPING THE PERINEUM

One-piece lithotomy drapes that will both cover the legs while in stirrups and provide access to the perineum are available. However, a series of special drapes, including an under-the-buttocks sheet, special drapes for each leg and stirrup (leggings), and a fenestrated sheet, are more typically used. The technique described presumes an isolated vaginal procedure and not a laparoscopic combination. This type of draping runs an unusually high risk of glove contamination; therefore, double gloving is recommended.

TECHNIQUE

Draping the Abdomen

Refer to Figure 12-21A–C.

1. A sheet may be used to cover the patient's lower body.
   - Present the edge of the sheet to the individual assisting with application of the sheet.
   - Unfold the sheet as both individuals approach the patient.
   - Protect the gloved hands by cuffing the sheet.
   - Do not reach below the surface of the operating table.
2. Four towels are used to outline the intended surgical site.
3. Provide towel clips, if necessary.
4. If desired, a self-adherent impervious drape may be placed.
5. Prepare (e.g., remove protective covering from adherent portion of drape) and orient the laparotomy sheet.
6. It may be necessary to move to the opposite side of the operating table to facilitate application of the laparotomy sheet.
7. Place the fenestration over the intended surgical site.
8. Slowly unfold the sheet bilaterally.
9. Do not let the head end of the sheet fall below table level.
10. Stabilize the sheet.
11. Extend the head end of the sheet.
    - Be sure the arm boards are adequately covered.
    - Protect the gloved hands from contamination.
    - If necessary, hold the sheet until a nonsterile team member is able to take it from you and secure it.
12. Reposition hands and continue to stabilize the sheet.
13. Extend the foot end of the sheet.
    - Protect the gloved hands from contamination.
    - Do not reach below the surface of the operating table.
14. Proceed with other preoperative activities such as placement of the electrosurgical cord, suction tubing, and light handles.

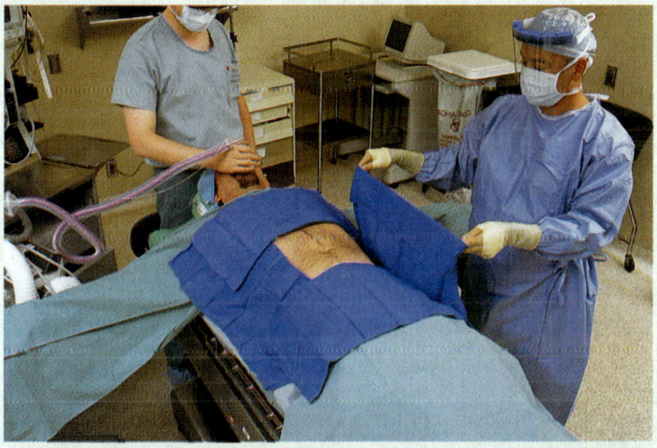

A

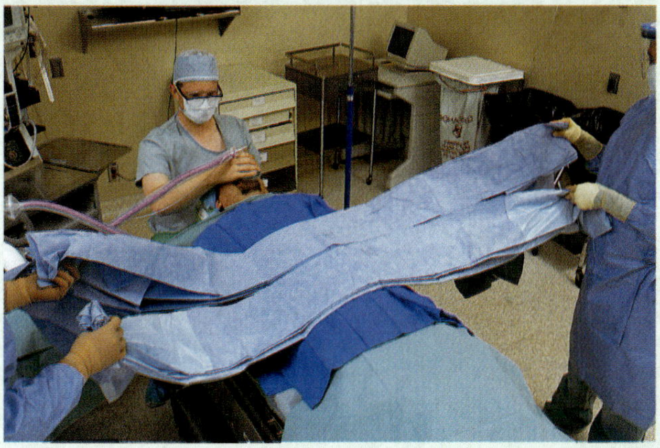

B

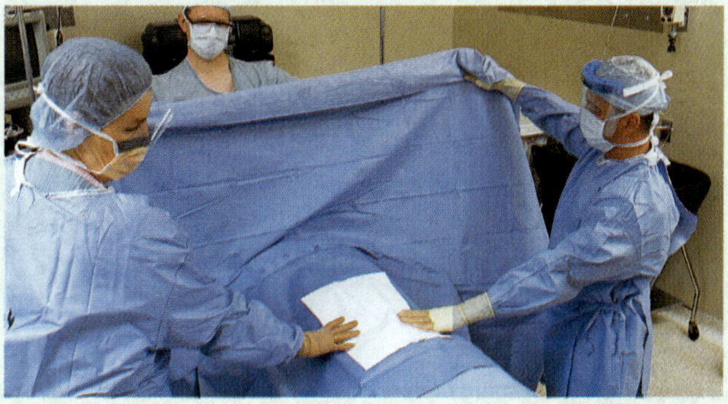

C

Figure 12-21 Draping the abdomen: (A) Towels are used to define the planned incision site. (B) Unfold laparotomy sheet. (C) Protect hands as laparotomy sheet is unfolded

TECHNIQUE

Draping the Perineum

Refer to Figure 12-22A–C.

1. Present the under-the-buttocks drape to the team member applying the drapes so that the hands may be inserted into the cuff of the drape.
2. Let the drape unfold toward the floor.
3. The drape is tucked under the patient's buttocks with the hands protected within the cuff of the drape and an awareness of environmental hazards (e.g., the patient's legs).
4. Two or three towels may be applied to outline the intended surgical site.
   - Present the first two towels that have been folded diagonally, one at a time to the team member applying the drapes.
   - If necessary, a third towel is placed horizontally to isolate the anal area.
5. Provide towel clips, if necessary.
6. Present the first legging to the team member applying the drapes so that the hands may be inserted into the cuff of the drape.
7. The legging is unfolded as it is applied to the leg suspended in the stirrup.
8. Present the second legging to the team member applying the drapes so that the hands may be inserted into the cuff of the drape.
9. The legging is unfolded as it is applied to the leg suspended in the stirrup.
10. The fenestrated sheet is applied to expose the perineum. Alternatively, a drape sheet or towel may be applied across the abdomen.
11. Proceed with other preoperative activities such as placement of the electrosurgical cord, suction tubing, and light handles.

Note: A common variation to this draping technique is to apply the leggings prior to placement of the under-the-buttocks drape.

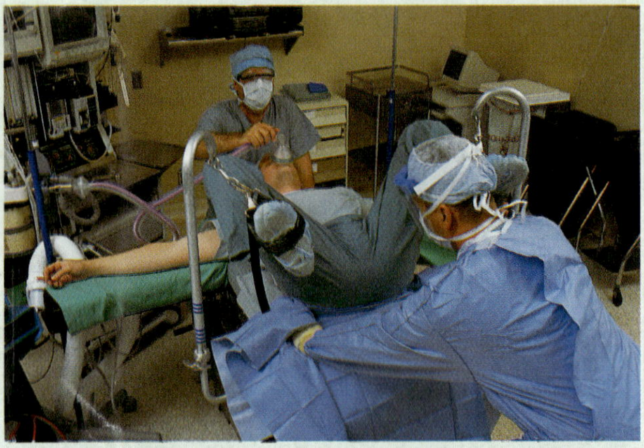

A

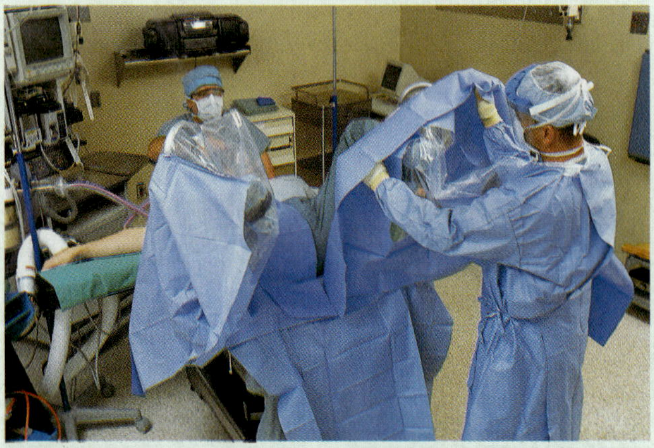

B

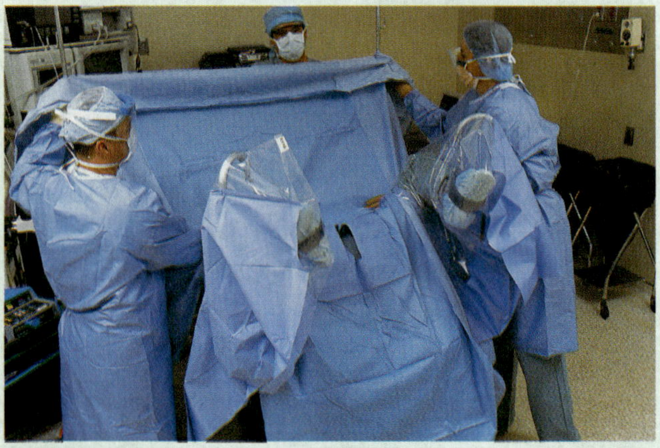

C

Figure 12-22 Draping the perineum: (A) Place the under-the-buttocks sheet. (B) Place the leggings. (C) Place the fenestrated sheet

DRAPING AN EXTREMITY

Draping an extremity provides three unique problems not faced in the first two draping scenarios:

- The body part to be draped for surgery is cylindrical in shape.
- Because the cylindrical shape requires a nonsterile team member to hold the extremity while the skin is being prepped, the extremity must be received from the nonsterile team member. Typically, the nonsterile team member wearing sterile gloves will be holding the extremity in an elevated position at approximately a 45° angle. If the patient's condition allows, the extremity may also be abducted.
- The body part will most likely be manipulated through some range of motion during the procedure.

TECHNIQUE: Draping the Extremity

Refer to Figure 12-23A and B.

1. The circulator maintains elevation of the extremity following the prep.
2. A sheet or towels may be placed superiorly.
3. A sheet is placed inferiorly (under the extremity).
   - Present the edge of the sheet to the individual assisting with application of the sheet.
   - Unfold the sheet as both individuals approach the patient.
   - Be aware of the position of the circulator to avoid contamination.
   - Protect the gloved hands by cuffing the sheet.
   - Do not reach below the surface of the operating table.
4. Adherent split ("U") sheets may be placed superiorly and/or inferiorly.
5. Present the prepared **stockinette** to the team member assisting with draping.
   - As the stockinette is applied, the responsibility for elevating the extremity is transferred from the circulator to the sterile team member as the extremity is accepted into the sterile field.
   - The STSR may be required to hold the extremity while the stockinette is unrolled to the proper level.
   - If necessary, the stockinette is secured by wrapping it with an elastic or adherent bandage.
6. Prepare and orient the extremity sheet.
7. It may be necessary to move to the opposite side of the operating table to facilitate placement of the extremity sheet.

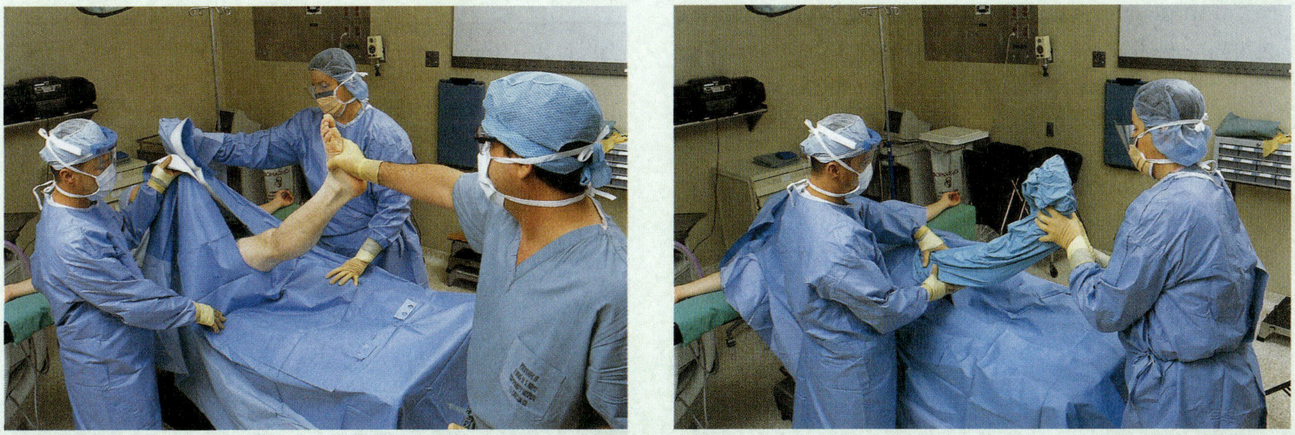

A B

Figure 12-23 Draping an extremity: (A) Place the split sheet under the extremity. (B) Place the cylindrical covering (stockinette)

(continues)

(continued)

8. Prepare the fenestration for insertion of the extremity.
9. Place the fenestration at the proper level for the planned procedure.
10. Slowly unfold the sheet bilaterally.
11. Do not let the head end of the sheet fall below table level.
12. Extend the head end of the sheet as far as possible.
    - Protect the gloved hands from contamination.
13. Extend the foot end of the sheet.
    - Protect the gloved hands from contamination.
    - Do not reach below the surface of the operating table.
14. The extremity is placed on the sterile surface. Alternatively, the surgeon may prefer that the extremity remain elevated to facilitate tourniquet usage.
15. The stockinette is cut to expose the surgical site.
16. Proceed with other preoperative activities such as placement of the electrosurgical cord, suction tubing, and light handles.

DRAPING FOR CRANIOTOMY

Draping for a craniotomy illustrates another type of draping with unique specifications. It also presents three rather unique problems:

- The patient and the operating table may be in a variety of positions (e.g., sitting, lateral, supine).
- A relatively small access area is required but it is on a rounded surface.
- One end of the craniotomy drape may be placed over or on the Mayo stand or Mayfield table containing the instruments.

TECHNIQUE Draping for a Craniotomy

Refer to Figure 12-24.

1. The intended surgical site is outlined with three to four sterile towels.
    - If cloth towels are used, they may be sutured in position or secured with towel clips.
2. The craniotomy drape is applied.
    - If necessary, remove the protective covering from the adhesive portion of the drape.
    - Hand one end of the craniotomy drape to the surgeon.
    - Unfold the drape bilaterally.
    - The fenestration is positioned to expose the surgical site.
    - The superior end of the drape (with fluid collection pouch) is allowed to fall toward the floor.
    - The inferior end of the drape is extended over the patient.
    - The drape may be allowed to rest on the patient's body or may be placed on the Mayo stand or Mayfield table and secured by the weight of the instruments and supplies or with adhesive or clamps.
3. Additional sheets may be used as necessary.
4. Proceed with other preoperative activities such as placement of the electrosurgical cord, suction tubing, and light handles.

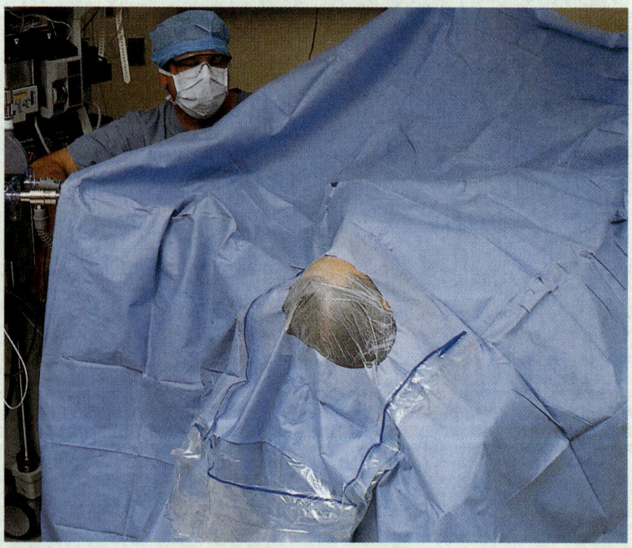

Figure 12-24 Patient draped for a craniotomy

There is little room for error in craniotomy draping. Since the critical steps of the surgical intervention take place inside the skull, the opening must be in precisely the correct place or access to the corresponding brain area is difficult or denied. Many times, *the preoperative skin prep routine will include the surgeon marking the skin incision with a scalpel or sterile marking pen prior to draping*.

The craniotomy drape is normally a large fenestrated sheet with a round opening that can be adjusted in circumference. Some surgical units use Mayfield tables for neurosurgical instrumentation and some use Mayo stands. In either case the instrument stand is positioned over the patient's body. The craniotomy drape may be placed over the Mayo stand or on the front of the Mayfield table. This prevents gravity from pulling the drapes toward the floor.

POSITIONING OF THE STERILE TEAM MEMBERS AND THE FURNITURE

Following drape application, the sterile team members take their places around the operating table and the furniture is moved into position. Positioning of the sterile team members and the furniture is affected by a number of factors. Variations are often necessary to accommodate a specific situation. Factors affecting positioning of sterile individuals and items include

- Planned surgical procedure
- Planned patient position
- Size of the patient
- Preference of the sterile team members (e.g., a right-handed surgeon may prefer the STSR to consistently be to his right)
- Height of the sterile team members
- Dominant hand of the sterile team members
- Configuration of the OR
- Placement of nonsterile personnel or items (e.g., anesthesia provider or X-ray machine)

Following drape application the surgeon and surgical assistant may be provided with the light handles or covers, suction apparatus, and the electrosurgical pencil for placement on the sterile field while the STSR moves the furniture into position.

The Mayo stand is typically the first sterile item that is moved into position. To move the Mayo stand, the STSR lifts the front of the Mayo stand slightly, without disturbing the items that have been placed thereon, and slowly rolls it into position. The Mayo stand is constructed to allow the tray portion to be placed over the draped patient. This allows the STSR to stand behind the Mayo stand (with access to the foot control, should height adjustment be necessary) facing the instruments and supplies on the Mayo stand while observing the procedure, and allows efficient passage of instruments and supplies to other sterile surgical team members. Once positioned over the patient, the underside of the Mayo stand is considered nonsterile even though the sterile drape is in place, because the area cannot be readily observed.

The ring stand containing the basin(s) may be positioned next followed by the back table or vice versa, according to the situation. The STSR maneuvers the sterile item into position by placing her hands on the surface of the item and rolling the item into position. The circulator may independently move or assist the STSR with movement of the ring stand or back table by squatting down, grasping the item below the level of the sterile drape, and then maneuvering the item into position.

The back table should be positioned to allow the STSR to retrieve items without turning her back to the remainder of the sterile field. Since this may be a practical impossibility, the back table must be distant enough from the STSR to allow safe movement between the sterile areas.

While the circulator connects and activates the electrosurgical unit, suction apparatus, and any other necessary items, the STSR places two surgical sponges near the operative site, ensures that everything is ready, and prepares to pass the scalpel to the surgeon. The preoperative case management phase ends just prior to initiation of the incision.

INTRAOPERATIVE CASE MANAGEMENT

The intraoperative phase of case management begins when the incision is made. The intraoperative responsibilities of the STSR extend far beyond "passing" the instrumentation and supplies to the surgeon and other sterile team members. An awareness of the total surgical environment is necessary to allow the STSR to anticipate, or predict, the needs of the patient, the surgeon, and other surgical team members.

GENERAL PRINCIPLES

The information in this section is not intended to allow the STSR to memorize the steps related to a particular surgical procedure. Rather, it is to provide focus on organization of thoughts and activities (using the A POSitive CARE Approach) to enable application of the information to management of virtually any surgical procedure. (Specific *technical considerations* are presented in Chapters 14 through 24.)

It is the intraoperative activity of the STSR that is most illustrative of the classic role of the STSR. This is the period of time in which the A POSitive CARE Approach becomes critical to efficient and effective case management. Throughout this period, the STSR should constantly compare the anatomy and pathology being seen to what should be expected and the progress and success of the procedure to the norm. The specific variations observed should lead to predictions about procedural sequence and needs of the surgeon. The efficient and effective STSR always

- Observes the details of anatomy, pathology, and procedure.
- Handles the specific skills of instrument care and passing proficiently.
- Works to predict actions and needs two to three steps in advance.
- Pays attention to the entire OR environment: physical, mental, and emotional.
- Communicates effectively with all members of the surgical team, particularly the surgeon and the circulator.

The STSR is constantly observing the operative field and comparing what is seen to what is expected. The typical variations that must be accounted for are

- Differences between normal and variant anatomy
- The nature of the pathology causing the intervention and its variations, plus surprises from unknown or unpredictable pathology
- Differences in surgeons' approaches to the procedure
- The knowledge, skill level, and confidence of the individuals making up the surgical team
- Problems with equipment, instruments, and technology

Some brief examples of each variation are presented below.

So-called "normal" anatomy is a statistical term. For practical purposes there are three general anatomical conditions:

1. *Normal anatomy:* anatomy that approximates the statistical norm
2. *Normal variation:* variations that occur relatively frequently and are not pathological
3. *Abnormal anatomy:* variations that are pathological or problematic

The STSR should be familiar with the basic normal anatomy of all bodily systems and well versed in those specialty areas in which he works frequently. The first question is always something like this: Does the basic gross anatomy appear normal? Normal variations are found frequently and include:

- The arterial branches to the liver and gallbladder have several well-documented patterns.
- The course of the recurrent laryngeal nerve has several well-documented patterns.
- Female pelvic structure has several defined types.

Each of these is a variation of the norm. However, each may affect the decisions made in patient intervention. It is important to ligate and cut the cystic artery and not the hepatic artery or any of its branches during a cholecystectomy. The course of the recurrent laryngeal nerve must be identified and preserved during a thyroidectomy to avoid postoperative speech complications. Pelvic structure is a significant contributor to the decision to perform a cesarean section. In each case, the anatomy determines changes from the routine. The STSR must prepare for these changes in advance. In the first two examples, the changes may be subtle. The STSR may verify that there are enough ligating clips remaining or recognize that the pattern of dissection will follow a different sequence. In the third instance, the variation may cause a change in procedure from normal delivery to cesarean section or may affect visibility during a hysterectomy resulting in the use of different retractors. Sometimes the STSR cannot actually see the variation but can identify it from the surgeon's comments. In every instance, the STSR should use the information to predict the sequence of events to follow.

Pathological or problematic variations in anatomy also affect the procedure. At times the abnormality may be the reason the procedure is being done (e.g., aortic aneurysm, bowel obstruction, or congenital anomaly). At other times the abnormality may be discovered as part of the procedure (e.g., adhesions, bicornuate uterus, or retrocecal appendix). Each condition affects the procedural sequence and presents unique technical problems. The STSR should immediately ask herself: What are the possible solutions to this problem and how will it affect the procedure?

Several examples of pathological conditions and some of the problems presented by each condition are described briefly below:

- Meningiomas usually have a rich vascular supply from their meningeal origin. Excessive bleeding may begin with the perforation of the bone and may be problematic throughout the procedure.
- A severely infected and friable gallbladder may need decompressing prior to any attempt to remove it.
- A bowel obstruction resulting in leakage of intestinal contents may lead to the use of retention sutures.
- Abnormal placental position may cause a change from a low cervical to a classical incision into the uterus during a cesarean section.

Each problem of pathology usually has several different solutions. Some of the responses are determined more by the anatomical and pathological variables combined than any other factor. Some are more affected by the training and preference of the surgeon. Some are affected by current research studies. All responses are ultimately affected by a combination of these variables. The effective STSR must be conscious of the variables and use them to predict the future path of the procedure.

Probable changes or special needs should be communicated as early as possible to the circulator. For instance, if there is a bowel obstruction with spillage and the STSR knows that the specific surgeon always uses retention sutures in this circumstance, this information should be communicated as early as possible. This allows for efficient and effective case management in the circulator's role. For instance, one might state, "There is spillage of bowel contents. We may anticipate copious irrigation and the use of retention sutures. Dr. Doe usually uses #1 nylon, double armed." This allows the circulator to plan an efficient course of action. The circulator will be thinking: When will these be needed? Are there other items (such as bolsters) that will be needed? When is it best for me to leave the room in order to obtain the supplies?

Anatomy and pathology are the primary determinants of the procedure and its variations. However, the STSR can only make predictions about the future course of action if the operative procedure is known and understood. *Two items the STSR should never be in doubt about: the instrumentation and the normal operative steps of a procedure.* It is not sufficient to memorize the steps of a procedure, although that is a necessary starting point. Textbooks present an idealized situation and not the actual procedure involving the specific anatomy, pathology, surgeon, and team involved in the procedure being performed at a given time in the OR. Procedures must be understood in order to make the best predictions about future events. Understanding procedures begins with a solid foundation in anatomy, physiology, and pathology. Only then do the procedural steps and the actual surgical techniques make sense. The procedure and the problems presented are logical when set into the context of anatomy and physiology.

It is often difficult for students to grasp the subtleties of the point being made. An illustration may help. Consider a cholecystectomy. The gallbladder lies in a bed underneath the liver. It is attached to the common bile duct by its own bile duct, the cystic duct. Knowing that, it is easy to see that (1) the cystic duct must be ligated and divided in order to remove the gallbladder and (2) the common duct must remain functional after the operation. It is important, then, to identify, ligate, and divide the cystic duct. Normally, this is done before the gallbladder is dissected from the liver bed. However, the cystic duct is not always easy to identify. If there is any doubt as to the anatomy, what can be done? There are three technical options:

- Continue careful dissection of the structures of the lesser omentum.
- Place a clamp on Hartmann's pouch and retract the gallbladder inferiorly.
- Dissect the gallbladder from the liver bed until the cystic duct is identifiable at the distal end.

Sometimes identification of the cystic duct is simply a matter of continuing dissection until the structures can be visualized well enough for certain identification. Knowing that the cystic duct and the common duct generally form a Y at their connective site, tension on Hartmann's pouch, directed inferiorly, causes the arms of the Y to separate, making identification easier. Finally, in difficult cases, the one sure way to find the cystic duct is to free the gallbladder first. The duct arising from the gallbladder is the cystic duct. Here we see three solutions to a common surgical problem. Understanding the anatomy allows one to understand the procedure and its variants. The STSR can make predictions about instrumentation based on this understanding.

The task of predicting presumes variability. If there were only one way to perform a procedure, there would be no need for predictions. To a great extent, the most challenging work of the STSR is predicting specific variations and their probability of occurrence. The STSR does this by

- Knowing normal anatomy and comparing that knowledge to what is seen in the actual patient
- Understanding basic physiology and pathology and comparing that knowledge to the structural and physiological effects seen in the actual patient
- Understanding operative procedures, their sequence of steps, instrumentation, and general techniques and the variations required based on anatomy, pathology, and surgeon's preference

These three components interplay with each other. As knowledge and experience grow, the STSR becomes more adept at seeing subtle changes and predicting the effects of the changes on the procedure.

SAFETY

Standard Precautions must be used at all times. Additionally, a number of intraoperative safety measures must be employed to protect the patient and the surgical team members. Some examples include

- Placement of the electrosurgical pencil in the holster when not in use
- Use of safe transfer techniques
- Cautious handling of sharps
- Double gloving
- Appropriate protection from environmental hazards (e.g., lasers, X-rays)

INTRAOPERATIVE COMMUNICATION

Along with the ability of the STSR to anticipate the needs of the patient and surgical team members, verbal and nonverbal methods of communication are also used to facilitate the surgical procedure.

Verbal Communication

Verbal communication occurs between all members of the surgical team. However, the majority of the intraoperative verbal communication takes place within the sterile field. The surgeon or surgical assistant typically calls out the name of the desired item and the STSR responds by providing it directly to the individual requesting the item. For example, if the surgeon asks for a scalpel, the STSR responds by placing the scalpel in the surgeon's dominant hand or by placing it in the preestablished "**neutral zone**" (according to facility policy). If the requested item is readily available, a verbal response from the STSR may not be necessary. However, if a requested item is not readily available, the STSR should acknowledge the request and inform the team member(s) when the item is expected. For example, if the surgeon calls for culture tubes that were not opened onto the sterile field, the STSR may respond with, "I'm getting them now" and provides them to the surgeon as soon as they become available.

Nonverbal Communication

Hand signals are used to keep talking, and its resultant microbial contamination, to a minimum (Figure 12-25A–D). Additionally, hand signals often replace verbal requests if the patient is not under general anesthesia. The STSR must be vigilant of the activities at the surgical site to receive and accurately respond to nonverbal requests.

PASSING THE INSTRUMENTS (AND OTHER SUPPLIES)

Specific techniques are used for handling each of the types of instruments used in surgery. This section considers general techniques for passing instruments and the specific problem of handling sharps. The reader is also referred to the sections on the neutral zone and sharps safety in Chapter 5. The basic principle of instrument passing is simple: Pass the instrument so that it is received in a position ready for use.

The discussion on instrument passing presumes a laparotomy procedure. The Mayo stand is placed in the area of the patient's lower thighs. Surgeon and assistant are positioned on each side of the patient at the level of the abdomen. The STSR should be directly behind the Mayo stand. The surgeon may be positioned on the same or opposite side of the operating table as the STSR. The relationship between the surgeon and the STSR will determine the technique used to pass the instruments. The STSR must be aware of the visual fields of the surgeon and assistant. The surgeon's field of vision should not be obstructed when passing instruments to the assistant. Passing techniques are described in Table 12-2.

The scalpel represents one of the more dangerous instruments used. Several practices have been defined and practiced in recent years, including:

1. Handing the scalpel to the surgeon and receiving the scalpel back from the surgeon
2. Handing the scalpel to the surgeon but having the surgeon place it in a designated safe area on the Mayo stand where it is retrieved by the STSR (Chapter 5)
3. No-hand technique where the scalpel is placed in the neutral zone by the STSR, retrieved and used by the surgeon, returned to the neutral zone by the surgeon, and retrieved by the STSR
4. No-hand technique using a basin as the safe area (beware danger of reaching into basin with sharps; refer to Chapter 5)

It is not clear if any of these techniques are any safer than the others in the long run. Practical experience suggests that the most dangerous component is the return exchange from surgeon to STSR. The surgeon is solely focused on the procedure and there is no clear, habituated technique for this pass. Given the realities versus theoretical concerns, option 2 seems to provide the best and

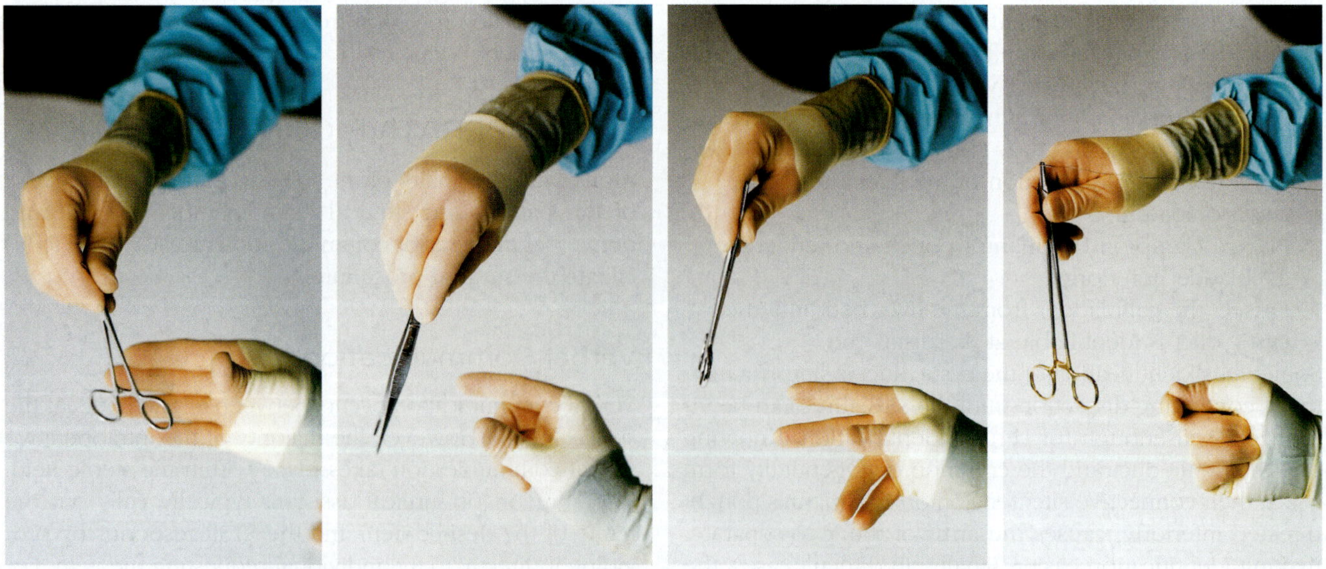

A B C D

Figure 12-25 Hand signals: (A) Request for a hemostat, (B) request for a tissue forceps, (C) request for a scissors, (D) request for a suture

Table 12-2 Techniques for Passing Instruments: Which Hand to Use

RECEIVER'S POSITION	STSR'S PASSING HAND	SPECIAL TECHNIQUE
Surgeon on same side of table as STSR and to STSR's left		
Pass to surgeon's right hand	STSR uses right hand	
Pass to surgeon's left hand	STSR uses right hand	Arm must be bent to avoid surgeon's right hand
Pass to assistant's right hand	STSR uses right hand	Avoid surgeon's visual field
Pass to assistant's left hand	STSR uses right hand	Avoid surgeon's visual field
	These passes must be made without hitting Mayo with side or back	
	May use left hand if the pass does not interfere with surgeon's right hand	
Surgeon on same side of table as STSR and to STSR's right		
Pass to surgeon's left hand	STSR uses left hand	
Pass to surgeon's right hand	STSR uses left hand	Arm must be bent to avoid surgeon's right hand
Pass to assistant's left hand	STSR uses left hand	Avoid surgeon's visual field
Pass to assistant's right hand	STSR uses left hand	Avoid surgeon's visual field
	These passes must be made without hitting Mayo with side or back	
	May use right hand if the pass does not interfere with surgeon's right hand	
Surgeon across table from STSR	See technique for passing to assistant	

safest compromise. The STSR is focused on the exchange, the surgeon is habituated to presenting the receiving hand a certain way, and the exchange can be made confidently. The return is not confidently made; therefore the surgeon should set the scalpel down in a designated place. The STSR may then secure the scalpel and return it to its designated storage location on the Mayo stand. It is probably best to remove both the skin and deep "knives" to a secure sharps area on the back table as soon as they are no longer needed.

If handed, the scalpel is placed into the surgeon's hand "pencil" style. The STSR should use the fingers of the passing hand to protect the others from the blade. This is accomplished by holding the scalpel handle with the index and middle finger near the blade. With the palm of the passing hand facing the OR table, the blade rests in the open area formed by the cupped hand. The knife handle is placed firmly in the surgeon's hand. When the surgeon has securely grasped the knife, the STSR moves the passing hand up and away from the blade (Figure 12-26).

Ringed instruments are passed by holding the shaft of the instrument and placing the rings in the palm of the surgeon's open receiving hand. The instrument should be placed firmly into the surgeon's hand. Remember the surgeon's eyes and thoughts are on the anatomy and next step of the procedure. A quick snap of the wrist will place the rings into the surgeon's palm with a slight "snap." This is the proper pressure. (The student should note that microsurgical instruments are not passed with the same speed or pressure at which general laparotomy instruments are passed.) The surgeon will know the instrument

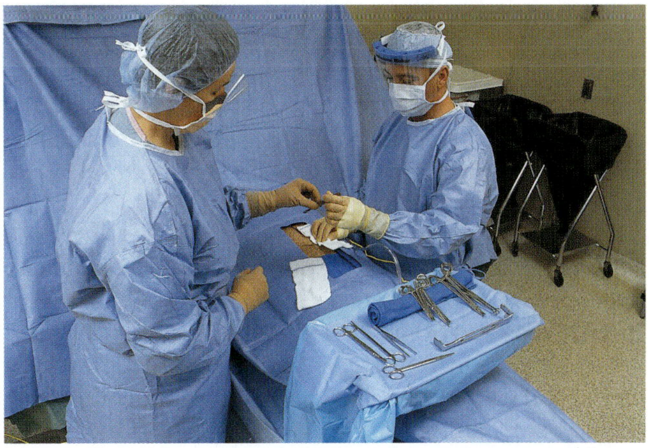

Figure 12-26 Passing the scalpel to the surgeon

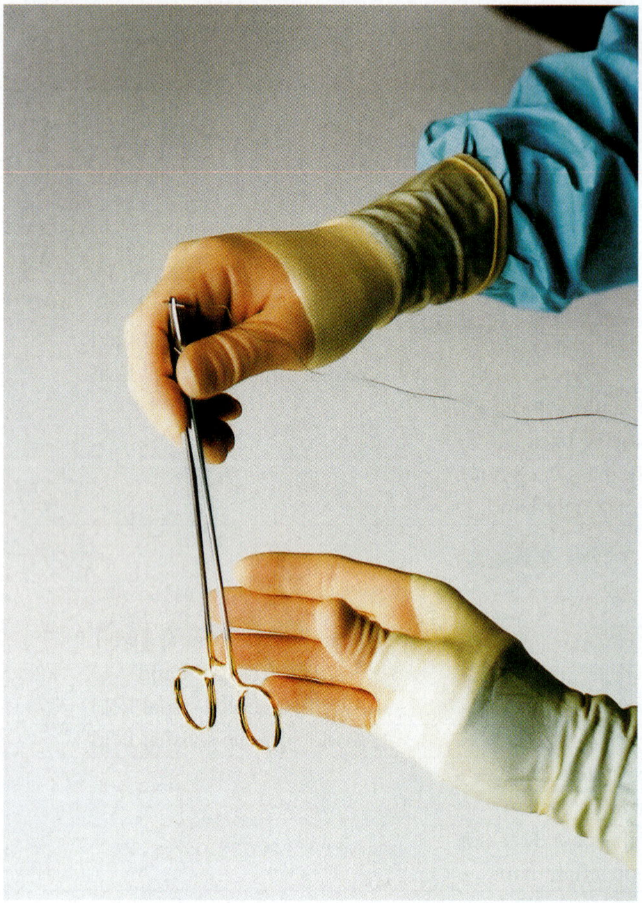

Figure 12-27 Passing the suture to the surgeon

is there and close the receiving hand around the rings. Curved instruments should be placed in the hand with the point curving in the same direction as the surgeon's fingers. Ringed instruments are passed closed. During the procedure, all instruments are returned to a designated area by the surgeon where they are retrieved, cleaned, and replaced on the Mayo stand by the STSR.

Needle holders are ringed instruments with the added complexity of having a sharp needle held at the end (Figure 12-27). As mentioned above, the instrument should be passed from the STSR to the surgeon but placed in the safe area by the surgeon after use to be retrieved by the STSR. Typically, needles are placed near the tip of the needle holder and set at 90° to the long line of the needle holder. Other needle positions are used for specific purposes, but the surgeon will ask for these variations when needed. Suture should be draped over the back of the hand so the STSR's delivering hand prohibits the suture from entering the surgeon's hand with the instrument. Long sutures should be controlled by the STSR until the surgeon has full control of the suture. The use of a neutral zone is recommended to minimize the incidence of sharps injury; other passing methods should only be employed when the neutral zone cannot be safely utilized.

Retractors come in a variety of shapes, weights, and types. They should be passed carefully. The handles of handheld retractors are placed in the palm of the surgeon's or surgical assistant's hand with gentle pressure. Self-retaining retractors are presented according to the type of retractor. Those with rings are held along the shaft with the rings presented. Some retractors (e.g., Gelpi) must be handled according to sharps rules. Some retractors are large and require the addition of multiple pieces. These must be passed with extra care because of their weight.

Lap sponges are passed unfolded. The sponges may be used moistened or dry. If moistened, they are soaked in body temperature saline and squeezed out before use. The solution in which sponges are soaked should not be used as irrigation; fiber particles may contribute to the formation of adhesions. 4-in. × 4-in. sponges are usually opened one fold, converting them to 4 in. × 8 in. Use of these sponges is generally restricted to the skin and subcutaneous tissues unless the sponge is folded and held in the jaws of a sponge forceps. Laparotomy sponges are sometimes "packed" into the abdominal cavity to hold some portion of the contents away from the operative site. The best practice is to count the sponges as they are packed into the abdomen, report it to the circulator and record it on a count board. Keep an ongoing count of these sponges. If you are preparing to close and you notice that four sponges were packed into the abdomen but only three are marked as removed, you should notify the surgeon. It is easier to retrieve the sponge before closure has started than after.

The volume of laparoscopic procedures performed today dictates changes in handling and passing of instrumentation. The often rapid-fire exchange of the classic laparotomy has been replaced with slow and methodical passing of long and somewhat cumbersome laparoscopic instruments. Because of their length and thin shafts, these instruments are especially fragile. Once received by the surgeon, the tips must be guided into a port for passage into the abdomen. Speed is less important than precision.

Specialties such as orthopedics and neurosurgery involve many specialized instruments and power equipment. Specialties such as ophthalmic surgery not only have many specialized instruments but most of them are microsurgical instruments. The specific requirements for safe and efficient handling of these instruments will be discussed when appropriate within the procedural chapters.

MAINTAINING ORDER WITHIN THE STERILE FIELD

The STSR must not only keep up with the needs of the sterile team members, but must also maintain the sterile field in a safe and orderly fashion to facilitate the surgical procedure and counting.

All instruments and supplies are arranged on the Mayo stand so that each one is picked up and passed us-

Table 12-3 Responsibility for Counts

	INSTRUMENTS	SPONGES	SHARPS/NEEDLES
Prior to opening	Sterile processing	Manufacturer	Manufacturer
Opening/closing	STSR/circulator	STSR/circulator	STSR/circulator
Intraoperative additions	STSR/circulator	STSR/circulator	STSR/circulator
Circulator change	(Usually not possible)	STSR/incoming circulator	STSR/incoming circulator
STSR change	(Usually not possible)	Incoming STSR/circulator	Incoming STSR/circulator
Team change	STSR/circulator	STSR/circulator	STSR/circulator

ing one smooth movement, ensuring a safe transfer and conserving time and movement within the sterile field.

Each time the electrosurgical pencil is used, the tip should be checked for cleanliness (and cleaned if necessary), the cord may need to be untangled, and the pencil must be returned to the holster for storage.

Clean sponges are added to the field as needed, and then the used ones are removed and placed in the kick bucket.

With the exception of the scalpel, most instruments are placed on the drapes when no longer needed by the surgeon or surgical assistant. Typically, the scalpel is placed on the Mayo stand or in a designated neutral zone when no longer needed. Loose instruments are picked up as soon as feasible, cleaned if necessary, and returned to their storage location on the Mayo stand or back table.

Blades, suture needles, and other sharps not in use are typically placed on the back table in (or near) the sharps container and organized in an orderly fashion to facilitate counting. Excess suture material is removed from the needle and discarded to prevent entanglement.

Additional instruments and supplies may be added to the field during the procedure and must be placed in position and accounted for.

ADDITIONAL SUPPLIES

Often, it is necessary to add instruments and supplies to the sterile field. The STSR typically verbally requests the additional item(s); however, the circulator may anticipate a specific need and provide the item(s) without being asked. The circulator obtains the item, inspects and opens the package, and either places the item in a convenient location on the sterile field or allows the STSR to retrieve the item from the packaging material. Any additional packaging material is removed and discarded by the STSR and the item either used immediately or placed in its storage location for future use. Countable items (e.g., sponges) are counted and added to the count as soon as feasible. Addition of items to the sterile field should not disrupt the progression of the surgical procedure.

Table 12-4 When to Count

Opening 1	All items open on back table; prior to Mayo stand setup
Additional items	As added
Team changes	Before exiting team member leaves room
Closing 1	As soon as closure of peritoneum initiated or any first layer of a cavity (Example: Start closing count 1 while uterus is being closed on a cesarean section. Have an extra count on such procedures.)
Closing 2	As soon as closure of fascia initiated or layer before subcutaneous
Final	As soon as skin closure initiated

COUNTING

Instrument, sponge, and sharps counts are very important. They are important for both patient safety and legal reasons (Table 12-3). Counts should be performed according to facility policy and should be done with precision.

Instruments are counted in the sterile processing area and the initial instrument count sheet is signed by the individual preparing the instrument set. The count sheet is removed from the instrument set by the STSR and handed to the circulator during the preoperative phase. The proper time to complete the first count is when all items are on the back table but before preparation of the Mayo stand has begun (Table 12-4). While it is not always possible to meet this recommended practice, it should serve as the expected norm. Counting requires that both the STSR and circulator visualize each individual item. Items should be counted as listed on the count sheet. Any disagreement with the initial count from sterile processing should result in a recount. If

Table 12-5 Problems with Counts

PRIOR TO INCISION	ACTION
Instruments	Change count sheet to match the actual count; initial change
Sponges	Count twice; still incorrect, remove entire package from room; document problem; open new package and count again
Sharps/needles	Count twice; still incorrect, remove entire package from room; document problem; open new package and count again
CLOSING COUNT	**ACTION**
Instruments	Inform surgeon immediately; recount; still incorrect, inform surgeon again; check cavity; document all actions and findings
Sponges	Inform surgeon immediately; recount; still incorrect, inform surgeon again; check cavity; document all actions and findings
Sharps/needles	Inform surgeon immediately; recount; still incorrect, inform surgeon again; check cavity; document all actions and findings
Diagnostic imaging may be used to demonstrate the presence or absence of the item in a body cavity or wound. However, every effort should be made to find the missing item.	

the count remains at variance, the actual number should be written and initialed. If the facility has a policy and procedure for reporting this type of error, that procedure should be initiated (Table 12-5). Extra instruments should be listed and counted. When both the STSR and circulator agree on the instrument count, they move to sponges.

Sponges are prepackaged by the manufacturer, typically in groups of 5 or 10. All sponges on the back table must be counted. Dressing sponges should not be opened onto the back table until after the final closing count. For laparotomy sponges, the count verifies the number of sponges, that each sponge has a radiologically detectable strip attached, and that the strip is firmly attached to the sponge. The 4-in. × 4-in. sponges are also completely

TECHNIQUE Counting

1. State the name of the item to be counted (e.g., "4 × 4s").
2. Verify that the circulator can see the item.
3. Separate the items as they are counted.
4. Verbalize the numbers.
5. Repeat at the end of the cycle (e.g., "4 × 4s: 1, 2, 3, . . . , 10. Ten 4 × 4s").
6. Circulator repeats the count (e.g., "Ten 4 × 4s").
7. Circulator writes the number on count sheet or board.
8. At the end of sponge and sharps counts, repeat the totals (e.g., "Five laps, ten 4 × 4s, 2 knife blades, 4 needles").

Counts would not be performed if real problems did not exist. Most problems with counts result in the team correcting the problem immediately (Table 12-5). The failure to recognize or solve a problem can result in severe consequences for a patient later.

separated and counted one at a time. Radiologically detectable indicators are identified. All other sponges are counted using similar procedures.

Sharps are counted. The STSR should point to each item during the count. Since needle packets are not commonly opened until the time of use, needles must be recounted as opened. The initial count can be accomplished by showing the circulator the needle picture on the suture packet. One must take care with multiple needle packets. When opened, the circulator must be in a position to see each needle.

MEDICATION HANDLING

The STSR should be familiar with anesthetic agents, medications, and solutions used during surgical intervention. Procedures and practices concerned with the handling of medications are covered in Chapter 9. No amount of vigilance can prevent some patients from reacting negatively to a medication, but vigilance can reduce medication errors to an absolute minimum.

SPECIMEN CARE

According to the situation, specimen care may occur during the intraoperative or postoperative phases of case management. For example, a specimen obtained for frozen section (e.g., lymph node) is generally removed from the sterile field intraoperatively, prepared and identified according to facility policy, and sent to the lab as soon as possible. However, a specimen obtained for permanent section (e.g., appendix) may remain on the sterile field until the procedure is completed and will be cared for postoperatively. A general discussion of specimen care is found in Chapter 13 and details that are more specific to each surgical specialty are available in each of the procedural chapters as needed.

DRESSING APPLICATION

There are too many types of postoperative wound dressings to list the technique for application of each. However, it is important to recognize that the last skin suture or staple does not end the team's responsibility for wound care. Given our presumed laparotomy, it is to be expected that the area around the incision is both bloody and covered with prep solution. It is also true that for comfort reasons the best time to clean the patient is immediately following the completion of the procedure.

The intraoperative phase of case management ends with application of the dressing.

TECHNIQUE: Dressing Application

1. All necessary items are prepared in advance.
   - Moist and dry sponges are prepared.
   - Dressing materials are obtained (following wound closure and completion of the final count) and arranged in the order in which they will be applied.
2. The area around the wound is cleaned and dried using caution not to disrupt the wound edges.
3. The dressing is applied. Use of a temporary dressing is not recommended because the risk of contamination of the wound is increased when replacing it with the permanent dressing.

PROGRESSION OF THE SURGICAL PROCEDURE

Although each patient and procedure differs in detail, most open procedures follow the same sequence of events. During each event within the sequence, the STSR must anticipate the needs of the patient and the surgical team members. The surgeon and surgical assistant should not have to ask for each item; the STSR must be able to predict the sequence of the needed items. A sample sequence of events for an open operative procedure and the technical considerations (expected actions) for the STSR are found in Table 12-6.

Table 12-6 Sample Sequence of Events for an Open Procedure

STEPS OF THE OPERATIVE PROCEDURE	TECHNICAL CONSIDERATIONS FOR THE STSR
1. An incision is made.	• Pass the scalpel or "skin knife" to the surgeon's dominant hand (or use a safe transfer method). • Prepare the electrosurgical pencil for use. • Expect the surgeon to return the scalpel to the Mayo stand (or neutral zone) and keep hands out of the way.
2. Hemostasis is achieved.	• Place the electrosurgical pencil in the surgeon's dominant hand. • The surgical assistant may use the suction apparatus to remove excess blood and electrosurgical plume, as needed—the surgical assistant will likely be able to retrieve the suction apparatus without the assistance of the STSR due to its location on the sterile field. • Anticipate the use of hemostats if the electrosurgical pencil is not effective in achieving hemostasis. • Retrieve the skin knife and place it in its storage location on the back table—reuse of the skin knife is not anticipated. • Clean surgical sponges are added to the field as needed, and then the used ones are removed and placed in the kick bucket—it may be necessary to switch from small sponges to larger ones as the wound size/depth increases.

(continues)

Table 12-6 *(continued)*

STEPS OF THE OPERATIVE PROCEDURE	TECHNICAL CONSIDERATIONS FOR THE STSR
3. Dissection continues through the necessary tissue layers.	• Sharp dissection may be carried out with the "deep knife" (provided to the surgeon's dominant hand) or with a scissors (provided to the surgeon's dominant hand) and a tissue forceps (provided to the surgeon's nondominant hand). • Blunt dissection may be carried out with the use of a dissecting sponge (e.g., peanut) or with the surgeon's fingers. • Retrieve the electrosurgical pencil, clean the tip if necessary, and place the pencil in the holster—reuse of the electrosurgical pencil is anticipated. • Anticipate the continuing need for hemostasis and provide the electrosurgical pencil or hemostats as needed—if hemostats are used, anticipate the use of the electrosurgical pencil or suture material and the suture scissors. • As the wound deepens, anticipate the need for longer instruments. • Any instrument not in use is secured, cleaned as needed, and replaced in its storage location for possible reuse—contaminated items are isolated as needed (e.g., bowel technique).
4. The wound edges are retracted to provide exposure.	• Expect the surgical assistant to retract the wound edges and provide the appropriate size retractor or pair of retractors when needed—as the incision deepens larger/deeper retractors will be used. • Exposure and isolation of structures may also be achieved with the use of surgical sponges (e.g., moistened laparotomy sponges).
5. The procedure is performed.	• Provide specialty instrumentation and suture material for the specific procedure. • Anticipate the continuing need for hemostasis. • Retrieve and care for sharps and other items as needed. • Care for the specimen as needed.
6. Hemostasis is maintained.	• Prior to closure, a final wound inspection is made to ensure that there is no active bleeding. • If necessary, hemostasis may be achieved mechanically (e.g., ligating clips), thermally (e.g., electrosurgically), or pharmaceutically (e.g., topical thrombin)—provide necessary items.
7. Wound is irrigated.	• Prior to wound closure, the surgeon may irrigate the wound with body temperature normal saline (or antibiotic solution according to the situation). • Pass the container (e.g., bulb syringe or pitcher) containing the irrigation fluid and be sure to state the name of the contents (e.g., normal saline). • Provide the Poole suction tip if necessary. • A small basin (e.g., kidney basin) placed near the dependent wound edge may be useful for collection of excess irrigation fluid. • Make a mental note of the amount of irrigation fluid used. • Retrieve and refill the fluid container if necessary. • Remove and replace the Poole suction tip as needed.
8. Wound is closed.	• Provide appropriate retractors to the surgical assistant. • Hemostats may be needed to secure the wound edges prior to closure.

Table 12-6 *(continued)*

STEPS OF THE OPERATIVE PROCEDURE	TECHNICAL CONSIDERATIONS FOR THE STSR
	• Provide necessary wound closure material to the surgeon's dominant hand and a tissue forceps to the nondominant hand. • Provide the suture scissors to the surgical assistant. • Perform necessary counts as needed and report the results. • Provide additional wound closure material as needed. • Retrieve and care for sharps and other items as needed. • As closure of the wound progresses, smaller/shallower retractors may be needed.
9. Dressing is applied.	• Dressing materials are provided after the wound is closed and the final count is performed. • The dressing materials are organized in the order in which they will be applied. • The skin around the wound is cleaned and dried using caution not to disrupt the wound edges. • The dressing is applied.

POSTOPERATIVE CASE MANAGEMENT

The postoperative phase of case management begins once the dressing is applied. Students should take careful note that it is relatively easy to become lax about the postoperative case management routine. The tension and excitement of the case are over. The STSR may be fatigued; however, the OR and all instruments, equipment, and supplies must be returned to their original state of readiness and cleanliness for the next patient and this must occur without cross-contamination.

PRESERVATION OF THE STERILE FIELD

Following dressing application, the STSR ensures that all sharps and nondisposable items are removed from the drapes. The sterile back table, Mayo stand, and basin set are moved away from the operating table. This portion of the sterile field is maintained until the patient is transported to the postanesthesia care unit (PACU). Preservation of the sterile field until the patient is transported is considered "best practice." However, not all facilities require it for all types of procedures.

DRAPE REMOVAL

As soon as the items that must remain sterile are moved away from the operating table, the STSR removes his or her outer pair of gloves (if double gloved) and returns to the operating table to assist with drape removal. In some situations, the STSR may be required to remain sterile while other surgical team members remove the drapes.

TECHNIQUE Drape Removal

1. The STSR stabilizes the dressing while a nonsterile team member (e.g., anesthesia provider) releases the suspended portion of the drape.
2. The drape is rolled as it is removed, containing any biohazardous material or disposable items.
3. It will be necessary for the STSR to switch the hand stabilizing the dressing as the drape is rolled over that area to facilitate removal of the remainder of the drape.
4. The drape is placed in the linen or waste receptacle as needed.
5. The wound towels and towel clips (if used) are removed.
6. The towels are placed in the linen or waste receptacle and the towel clips are set aside for later placement with the other used instruments.

   Note: The following steps are not part of the drape removal process, but are carried out immediately following drape removal.
7. If necessary, the patient's skin adjacent to the dressing is cleaned and dried.
8. The dressing is secured.

GOWN AND GLOVE REMOVAL

Following removal of the drapes, the STSR removes his or her soiled gown and gloves, disposes of them in the appropriate receptacle(s), and dons a pair of nonsterile gloves in order to assist with the immediate postoperative care of the patient.

Note: The technique for removal of the gown and gloves during a sterile procedure (for replacement due to a contamination) is slightly different from the technique used at the end of the procedure.

TECHNIQUE: Gown and Glove Removal at End of Procedure

1. If necessary, the circulator unfastens the back of a reusable gown. The back of a disposable gown may be torn by the STSR.
2. Grasp the gown near the shoulders and roll the gown away from you.
3. Touch only the gown with the gloved hands.
4. Place the gown in the proper receptacle.
5. Grasp the palm of the glove to be removed first with your opposite hand without touching your bare skin.
6. Remove the glove by inverting it.
7. Retain the removed glove in the hand that remains gloved.
8. Initiate removal of the remaining glove by sliding the degloved hand between the skin of the wrist and the glove.
9. Invert the second glove as it is removed to contain both gloves.
10. Dispose of the gloves in the proper receptacle.
11. Wash your hands as soon as feasible.

IMMEDIATE POSTOPERATIVE PATIENT CARE

Several tasks must be performed before the patient is ready to be transferred onto the gurney and transported to the PACU. Some of these tasks include:

- Any excess prep solution is removed from the patient's skin.
- If used, the dispersive electrode is removed and the condition of the patient's skin is noted.
- The patient may be extubated.
- Monitoring devices are removed.
- A warm blanket may be provided if necessary.

PATIENT TRANSFER AND TRANSPORTATION

In preparation for transfer to the gurney, the gurney is brought into the OR, positioned adjacent to the operating table, and the wheel locks applied. A transfer device, such as a roller, is obtained and positioned for use. The IV bag is moved onto the IV pole that is attached to the gurney and the tubing is freed.

Typically, four individuals are needed to transfer an anesthetized patient from the operating table to the gurney. The anesthesia provider remains at the patient's head and coordinates the transfer. Additional team members position themselves at the patient's sides and feet. When the anesthesia provider gives the signal, the patient's head and feet are supported and the patient is rolled away from the gurney using the draw sheet. The transfer device is placed under the patient's torso and the patient is gently rolled back onto the transfer device. Be sure that the individuals at the patient's sides brace their bodies against the operating table and the gurney to prevent slippage and verify that no tension will be placed on the IV tubing (or any other tubing

TECHNIQUE: Gown and Glove Removal for Replacement During a Procedure

1. Step away from the sterile field and request a new gown and gloves as soon as the contamination is recognized.
2. Remain still with your back toward the circulator so that the gown can be unfastened.
3. Face the circulator once the gown is unfastened.
4. Remain still and maintain an appropriate distance from the circulator while he removes the gown.
5. Extend both arms with the palms upward to allow the circulator to grasp the glove exteriors and remove them.
6. Rescrub, if necessary.
7. Don the new gown and gloves using the appropriate method.
8. Return to the sterile field and continue with the necessary tasks.

such as a Foley catheter or chest tube) during the transfer. The anesthesia provider will again signal when she is ready to complete the transfer. The patient's head and feet are supported while the patient is gently moved onto the gurney. Following transfer, the transfer device is removed, the side rails raised, and the wheel locks released.

When the anesthesia provider determines that the patient is ready, he is transported to the PACU. Typically, the anesthesia provider and the circulator transport the patient; however, in certain situations (e.g., additional equipment must be moved with the patient), the STSR may be required to assist with the transport.

BREAKDOWN OF THE SETUP

Once the patient leaves the OR, the STSR may begin breakdown of the setup. If needed, additional PPE (e.g., nonsterile gloves) is donned. A sample routine for breakdown of the setup follows:

- The specimen is cared for as needed.
- All sharps are placed in the sharps container on the back table.
- The sharps container is closed and placed in a puncture-proof biohazardous waste container (Figure 12-28).
- Instruments are removed from the Mayo stand, opened or disassembled as needed, and placed in a basin of water.
- The basin containing the soiled instruments is placed in/on the case cart.
- Instruments on the back table that were not used for the procedure may be replaced into the instrument tray.
- The instrument tray is placed in/on the case cart.
- All linen items are placed in the hamper.
- All disposable items are placed in the waste receptacle.
- Suction canisters and tubing are discarded.
- The OR furniture is positioned.
- The case cart is taken to the decontamination area.
- PPE is removed and discarded.
- A handwash is performed.

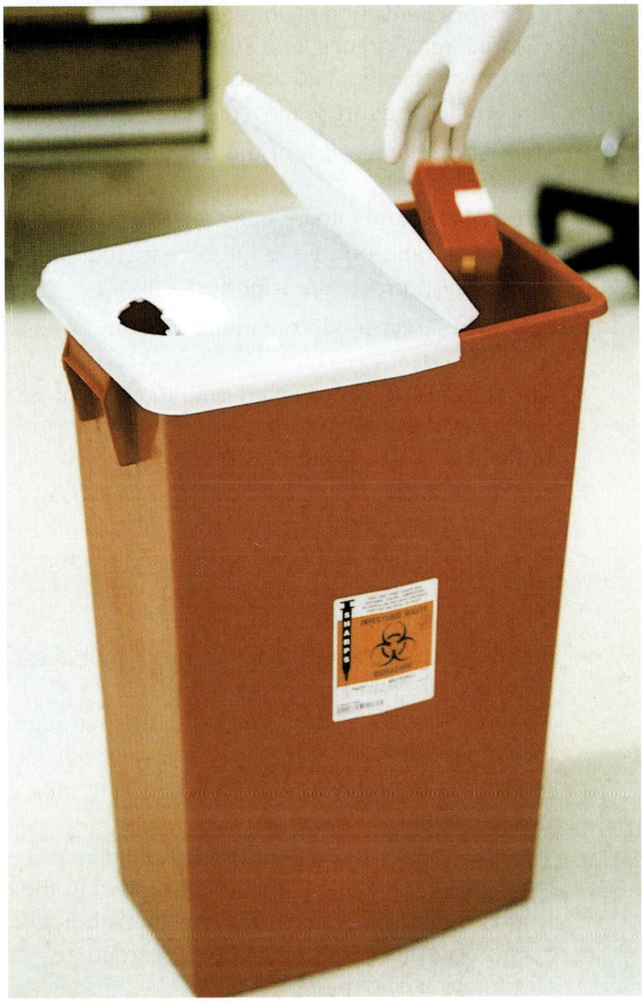

Figure 12 28 Disposal of the sharps container

THE OPERATING ROOM CYCLE

The basic steps of the OR cycle correlate with the three phases of surgical case management. Typically, additional personnel such as the anesthesia technologist and environmental services personnel are available to assist with completion of the OR cycle. However, in some situations (e.g., "on call") the STSR and the circulator may be responsible for some or all of the following duties:

1. *Preoperative phase*—preparation of the OR for a specific surgical procedure
    - Prior to the first case of the day, all surfaces are cleaned with a damp cloth; facility policy will determine the type of disinfectant used. This step is eliminated for subsequent cases.
    - Necessary furniture and equipment are brought into the OR and any extraneous items are removed, according to the type of procedure planned and the surgeon's preference.
    - Function of all equipment is verified.
    - The case cart is brought into the OR and the items to be opened are positioned for use. The remaining items are kept available for possible later use. They are placed in a location that will be convenient for the circulator to retrieve and open during the procedure, if needed.
    - The sterile field is established and prepared for the intraoperative phase of the OR cycle.
    - The patient and all surgical team members (nonsterile and sterile) are present in the OR.
    - The patient is anesthetized, positioned, prepped, and draped.

- Accessory items (e.g., light handles or covers, electrosurgical pencil, and suction apparatus) are placed, connected, and activated.
- The sterile furniture is moved into position.

2. *Intraoperative phase*—use of the OR during the surgical procedure
   - The doors to the OR are kept closed.
   - Traffic into and out of the OR is restricted.
   - The surgical procedure is performed.
3. *Postoperative phase*—decontamination and basic setup of the OR
   - The sterile field is preserved until the patient is transported to the PACU.
   - Immediate postoperative patient care is provided; then the patient is transferred to the gurney and transported to the PACU.
   - The setup is broken down and reusable items are placed in/on the case cart and taken to the decontamination area.
   - Sharps are placed in a puncture-proof biohazardous waste container.
   - All unused supplies are returned to their storage locations.
   - Anesthesia equipment is cared for and any disposable items are discarded.
   - The specimen is taken to the collection area where it will be picked up and transported to the laboratory for later examination by the pathologist.
   - Suction canisters and tubing are discarded according to facility policy.
   - Any remaining linen and waste (biohazardous materials are kept separate) are placed in the appropriate receptacles.
   - Bags are removed from the receptacles, sealed, and processed according to facility policy.
   - The OR is decontaminated according to facility policy (additional personal protective equipment may be needed).
     - All surfaces are cleaned with a disinfectant.
     - The floor is cleaned with a disinfectant using a wet vac or a mop.
     - Cleaning supplies are returned to their storage location.
     - PPE is removed and discarded.
     - Hands are washed.
   - The OR is set up for reuse.
     - Bags are replaced in the waste and linen receptacles.
     - Sheets are placed on the operating table.
     - Anesthesia cart and machine are restocked.
     - Suction canisters and tubing are replaced.
     - All furniture and accessories are placed in their storage locations.
     - Any items used during the procedure are replaced (restocked).

THE INSTRUMENT CYCLE

The basic steps of the instrument cycle also correlate with the three phases of surgical case management. Typically, additional personnel are available in the sterile processing department to assist with completion of the instrument cycle. However, in some situations (e.g., "on call") the STSR and the circulator may be responsible for some or all of the following duties.

1. *Preoperative phase*—preparation of the instrumentation for a specific surgical procedure
   - Instrumentation needed for the specific surgical procedure is obtained (according to the surgeon's preference card) from the storage area, placed in/on the case cart, and brought to the OR.
   - The instrument container is positioned and opened.
   - The instrument set is removed from the container.
   - Any additional instruments are opened, as needed.
   - Instruments are organized, counted, and prepared within the sterile field for use during the surgical procedure.
2. *Intraoperative phase*—use of the instrumentation during the surgical procedure
   - The STSR provides the necessary instruments to the surgeon and surgical assistant, as needed.
   - Instruments are retrieved, cared for, and prepared for reuse by the STSR.
   - Instruments are counted, according to facility policy, during the surgical procedure.
3. *Postoperative phase*—care of the instrumentation following the surgical procedure
   - Decontamination of the instruments begins in the OR as the instruments are opened or disassembled and placed into the basin of water. An enzyme may be added to the water to begin the breakdown of organic matter on the instruments. The process continues once the instruments are delivered to the decontamination area. Ideally, they undergo terminalization in an instrument washer-sterilizer. Typically, lubrication and drying are part of the washer-sterilizer process (refer to Chapter 7).
   - Instruments that have been processed in a washer-sterilizer are rendered safe to handle, once they have cooled. The instruments are taken to the preparation area and are inspected to ensure cleanliness and proper function. The set is reassembled according to the instrument list or count sheet and the sheet is signed by the individual preparing the instrument set. The instrument set or individual instruments

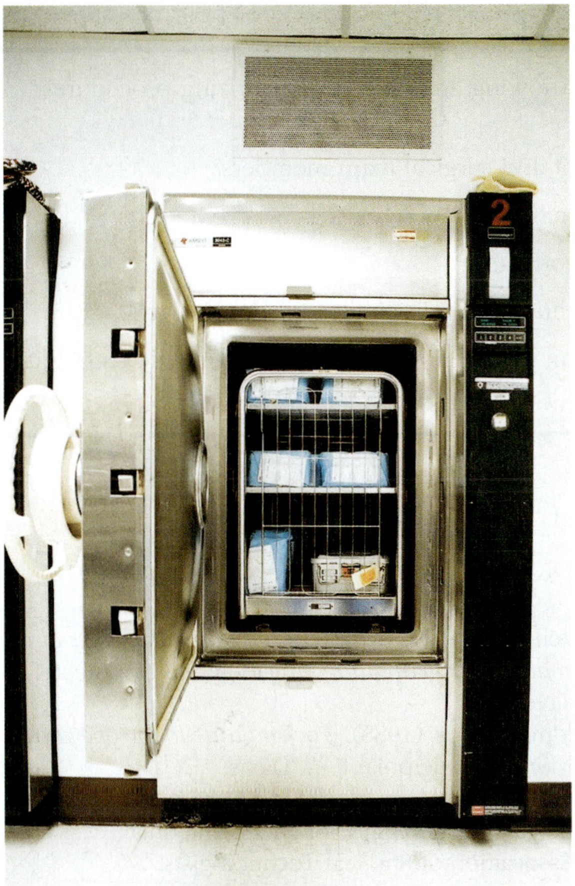

Figure 12-29 Instrument sterilization

are packaged for sterilization. An instrument set in its tray may be wrapped; however, a container system is more typically used. The signed count sheet is included with the instrument set. A chemical indicator is placed in a visible location before the container system, wrapper, or peel pack is sealed (refer to Chapters 7 and 10).

- The instruments are sterilized (Figure 12-29).
- Exposure to the sterilization process is verified.
- The set is stored for future use (Figure 12-30) (refer to Chapter 7).

The postoperative phase of case management ends when the operating room and the instrumentation are ready for reuse.

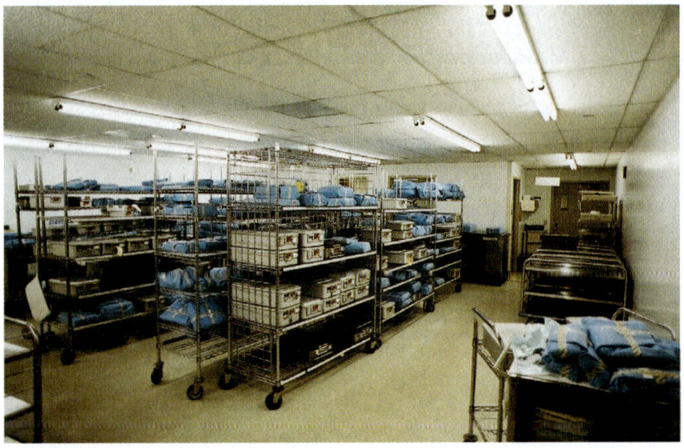

Figure 12-30 Instrument storage

CASE STUDY

During the repair of a midline episiotomy, the family practice resident closing the episiotomy said, "Something's wrong but I can't identify it." The STSR said, "I'm worried too. Do you think this patient may have DIC (disseminated intravascular coagulopathy)?" "Why do you ask?" the resident asked. "I've seen this before and the blood doesn't look right. I placed some of the patient's blood in a plain test tube. It's been seven minutes, and there is no clot forming." The resident asked the circulator to call the obstetric faculty to the room and alerted the anesthesia provider. The patient's blood pressure dropped for a while, but the quick response of the team held off any severe complications and the patient was dismissed several days later without further complications.

1. What observation did the STSR make that helped the patient?
2. How did applying the A POSitive CARE Approach help the STSR?
3. Was the STSR's response appropriate? Discuss your opinion.

QUESTIONS FOR FURTHER STUDY

1. Which is more important for the STSR in the long run, knowing anatomy or memorizing procedures? Why?
2. Why is it important to anticipate the needs of the patient and surgical team members?
3. What are the procedures for correct counting of instruments and sponges?
4. What steps must be taken if any part of the count is incorrect?
5. Describe the OR cycle and explain how the surgical technologist participates in the OR cycle.
6. What corrective options are available to the surgical team members when a breach in sterile technique occurs?

BIBLIOGRAPHY

Atkinson, L. J., & Fortunato, N. (1996). *Berry and Kohn's operating room technique* (8th ed.). St. Louis, MO: Mosby.

Ball, K. A. (1990). *Lasers, the perioperative challenge*. St. Louis, MO: Mosby.

Caruthers, B. L., Price, J. P., Price, B., & Junge, T. (1999). *Asepsis and sterile technique* [CD-ROM]. Centennial, CO: Association of Surgical Technologists.

Deitch, E. A. (1997). *Tools of the trade and rules of the road: A surgical guide*. Philadelphia: Lippincott-Raven.

Goldman, M. A. (1988). *Pocket guide to the operating room*. Philadelphia: F. A. Davis.

McGuiness, A. M., et al. (2002). *Core curriculum for surgical technology* (5th ed.). Centennial, CO: Association of Surgical Technologists.

SECTION 3

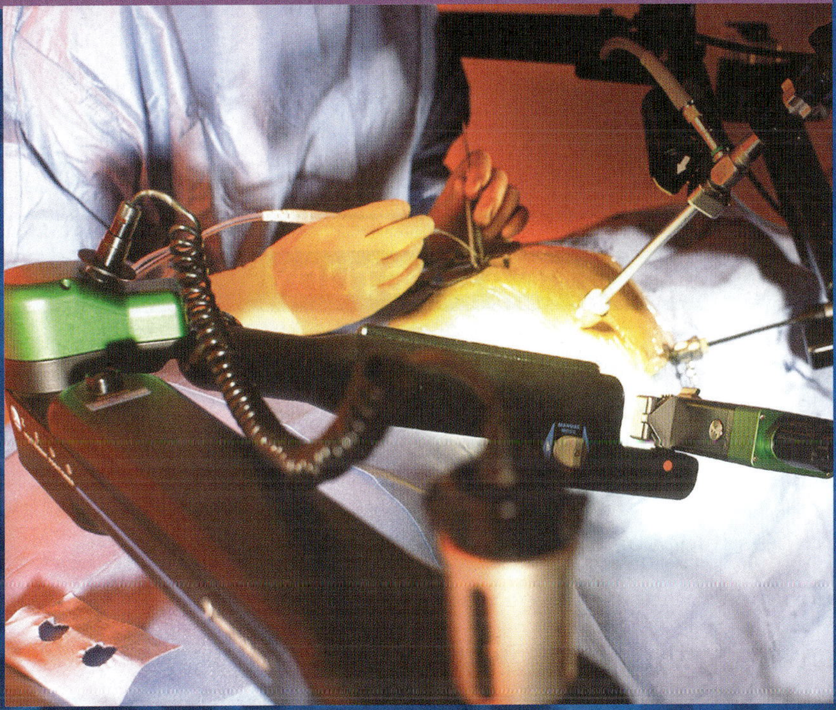

Surgical Procedures

CHAPTER 13

Diagnostic Procedures

Paul Price

CASE STUDY

Dathan, an 8-year-old male, was brought to the emergency department by his parent. He complained of generalized periumbilical pain that has now localized to the right lower quadrant. His mother states that his appetite has been poor and that he is now experiencing nausea, vomiting, and a fever.

1. What structures might be involved in the right lower quadrant?
2. What diagnostic studies might be performed?
3. What diagnostic study will indicate the presence of infection?

OBJECTIVES

After studying this chapter, the reader should be able to:

A 1. Apply knowledge of anatomy and physiology to determine which diagnostic examinations will be useful.

P 2. List the sources of patient data.

3. List and discuss techniques used to establish the diagnosis.

O 4. Determine which diagnostic procedures will require surgical intervention.

5. Identify the major indications for surgical intervention.

S 6. Understand the surgical technologist's role in caring for each specific type of specimen.

SELECT KEY TERMS

1. angina	8. CSF	15. -graph	21. Roentgenography
2. auscultation	9. cystoscopy	16. indwelling	22. sign
3. biopsy	10. ECG	17. isotope scanning	23. symptom
4. capnography	11. EEG	18. obstruction	24. urinalysis (UA)
5. C-arm	12. frozen section	19. palpation	25. ultrasonography
6. cholangiography	13. -gram	20. prosthesis	
7. contrast media	14. Gram stain		

SOURCES OF PATIENT DATA

Information about a patient's condition can be obtained in several ways from many sources, including

- History and physical examination
- Diagnostic imaging
- Laboratory findings
- Electrodiagnostic studies
- Endoscopic studies
- Pulmonary diagnosis
- Plethysmography and phleborheography

HISTORY AND PHYSICAL EXAMINATION

The first step in determining the etiology of a patient's condition is gathering medical, social (including any ethnic and/or religious information that may impact the course of treatment), and psychological information about the patient and, if applicable, the patient's family. This is generally achieved in a personal interview with the patient or some other responsible party (parent, spouse, paramedic) if the patient is unable to respond as a result of age or condition. The examination may be routine, or the individual may have one or more **symptoms** that have caused her to seek medical attention.

A physical examination should be performed. The physician performing the examination will verify the symptoms that the patient is experiencing and may discover other **signs** that will indicate the presence of a pathological condition. The physical exam should not focus on just the area of complaint, but should be inclusive of all body systems. The patient's height, weight, temperature, pulse, respiration, and blood pressure (BP) information should be assembled and recorded.

Several tools and methods are available to the physician to facilitate the physical exam, including

- Direct visualization
- Enhanced visualization (otoscope/ophthalmoscope)
- Indirect visualization (pharyngeal mirror)
- **Palpation** external (abdominal or thyroid) and/or internal (pelvic exam or digital rectal exam)
- **Auscultation** (stethoscope)

In addition to the physical exam, the physician may request that the patient undergo one or more imaging or laboratory tests. Once the results of the physical examination and the ordered tests have been assimilated, treatment may begin or more advanced diagnostic procedures may be advised.

The same tools used for preliminary diagnosis continue to be available during treatment (surgical or otherwise) for reevaluation of the condition; they may also have therapeutic applications.

DIAGNOSTIC IMAGING

Diagnostic imaging is a term that refers to the various techniques now available for producing images of the human body. Historically, the radio**graph** or X-ray was the predominant, if not the only, imaging technique available. *Radiography,* or **Roentgenography**, remains a viable source of diagnostic information. Large surgical departments typically have diagnostic imaging personnel assigned solely to the OR.

RADIOGRAPHY (ROENTGENOGRAPHY)

X-rays used to view internal structures for diagnostic purposes are high-energy electromagnetic radiation produced by the collision of a beam of electrons with a metal target within an X-ray tube. Penetrability of the X-ray beam is related to the unit of energy called a joule measured in rads (radiation absorbed dosage), the standard unit of an absorbed dose of ionizing radiation.

Preoperative plain radiographic films of the chest are frequently ordered by the anesthesia provider for identification of lung abnormalities that may interfere with the exchange of gases during anesthesia.

Thoracic surgeons can discover a good deal about the status of the ribs, sternum, and internal thoracic organs from a plain chest film. Fractures of the bones of the thorax may be revealed, as well as primary or metastatic tumors. Examination of the lung fields may reveal diffuse lung disease patterns or a collapsed lung, and examination of the pleural space may reveal effusion or tumor. Examination of the vessels in the lung field can reveal pulmonary arterial or venous hypertension. Interstitial edema appears as a diffuse haziness, and alveolar edema will produce a lung opacification. Structures within the mediastinum may also be examined for lesions.

In the OR, plain radiographic films from a fixed X-ray tube (typically included in **cystoscopy** rooms for retrograde urography or cystography) or portable X-ray machines are used for these purposes:

- Identify the location of abnormalities and foreign bodies (such as bullets, ingested items, or calculi).
- Locate retained sponges, sharps, or instruments.
- Discover fluid or air within body cavities.
- Verify the correct location for an operative procedure (such as the level of a cervical disk to be removed).
- Aid in bone realignment and **prosthesis** placement.
- Verify placement of **indwelling** catheters, tubes, and drains.

A portable X-ray machine must be moved into the OR in order to make radiographs (Figure 13-1). The making of a radiograph requires that a cassette, containing unexposed X-ray film, be positioned opposite the tube. Anterior/posterior (AP) radiographic views require that the film be placed underneath the patient, lateral views demand placement next to the body. In the radiology department, film placement is not difficult; in the operating room, however, specially developed assistive devices may be required. The primary goal of the STSR during intraoperative radiography is to protect the sterile field from contamination. The STSR may accomplish the dual goals of keeping the field sterile and allowing for the radiographic study using several methods. The X-ray cassette can be covered by the STSR with a sterile cassette cover to allow the cassette to be placed within the sterile field. If the X-ray tube is to be positioned over the operative field, the tube itself may be covered with a sterile drape or the wound may be protected with a sterile towel. Lateral films require the use of a portable cassette holder that can be positioned opposite the tube. This portable holder should be covered with a sterile drape before it is positioned near the OR table.

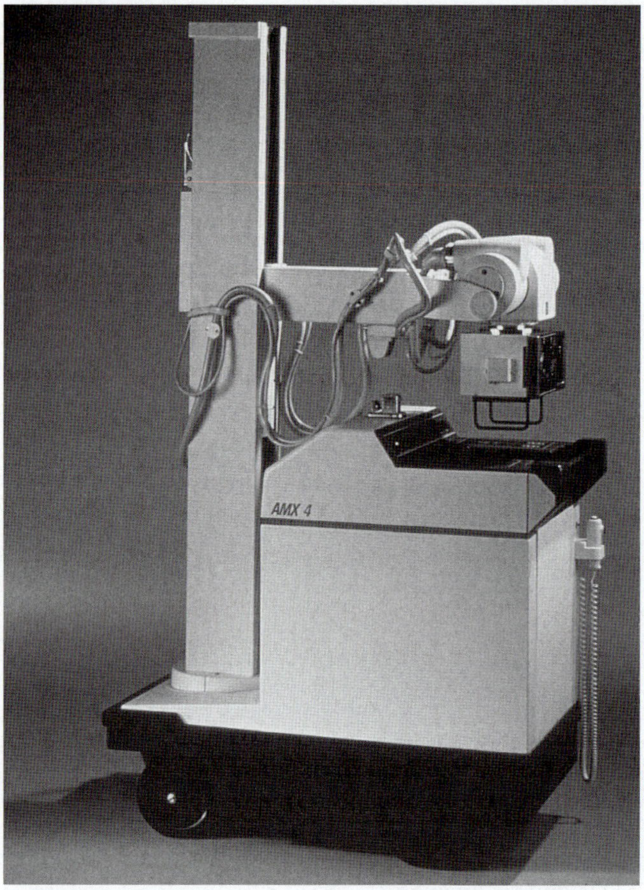

Figure 13-1 Portable X-ray machine *(Courtesy of GE Medical Systems)*

Once the film has been exposed to the radiation, it must be processed prior to viewing. The film is removed from the cassette in a darkroom and passed through a developing machine. Many operating rooms are equipped for this procedure; otherwise the film must be taken to the radiology department for processing, which can be time consuming. Often the surgeon will "read" the film intraoperatively; in some situations the expertise of the radiologist may be requested (Figure 13-2).

Mammography

Mammography utilizes X-rays to locate tumors of the breast in their early stages (Figure 13-3). The breast is tightly held in a device intended to decrease the density of the tissue for better visualization. Mammography

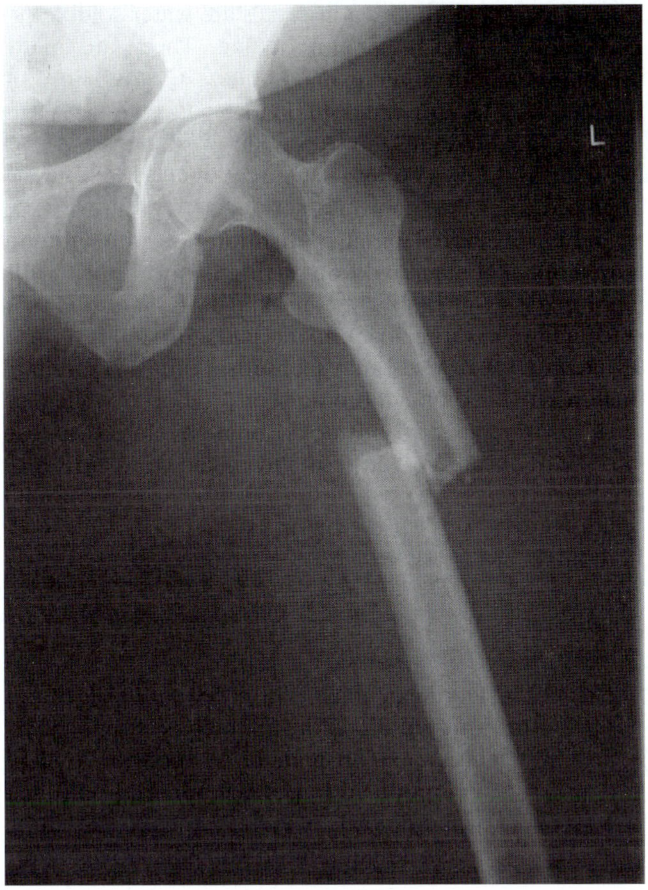

Figure 13-2 **X-ray depicting a femur fracture**

should not be painful, but the positioning of the breast can be uncomfortable for the patient.

Mammography can be performed in conjunction with a needle aspiration biopsy during which a very fine, long needle may be used to **biopsy** a tumor after it is localized on the X-ray film.

A mammo**gram** may be sent with the patient to the OR for breast biopsy and local excision of breast masses.

Myelography

Myelography is used to evaluate the spine for patients with neck, back, or leg pain. Magnetic resonance imaging (MRI) has largely replaced this technique, but it may still be used in some cases. MRI is useful in imaging the spinal cord, nerve roots, and disks, but myelography has the added benefit of clearly outlining bone tissue. Myelography is also useful for patients who are unable to undergo MRI because of metallic implants or allergy to **contrast media**.

For myelographic studies, contrast medium is injected into the cerebrospinal fluid at the lower lumbar level. This contrast medium outlines the spinal cord and nerve roots on X-ray film studies. Computed axial tomography studies may also be performed along with plain radiography to identify osteophytes (bony spurs) or disk extrusions.

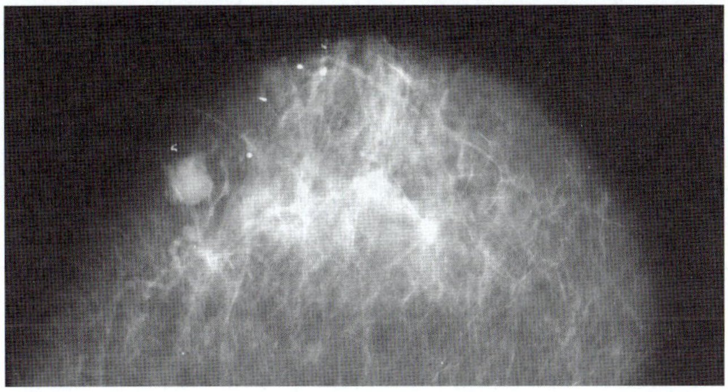

Figure 13-3 **Mammogram depicting a sarcoma**

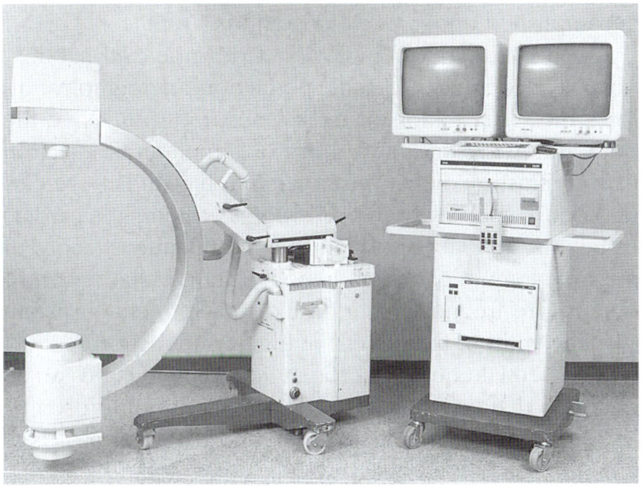

Figure 13-4 **C-arm with monitor**

FLUOROSCOPY

A fluoroscope utilizes X-rays to project images of body structures onto a monitor. Amplification is achieved with the use of an image intensifier. The images may be viewed during movement and projected in "real time," allowing the action of joints and organs to be viewed directly. Fluoroscopic images taken during angiography can be digitalized with background images subtracted for enhanced visualization of the structures.

The portable image intensifier is referred to as the **C-arm** because of its configuration (Figure 13-4). It is designed so that the image intensifier and tube are always in opposition. The C-arm is frequently used in conjunction with a special radiographic table that allows X-rays to pass through the tabletop.

Fluoroscopy has many intraoperative applications:

- Angiography (including cardiac catheterization)
- **Cholangiography**

- Retrograde urography
- Aid in bone realignment and prosthesis placement
- Verification of catheter placement (epidural/central venous pressure) and lead (pacemaker) introduction
- To direct instrumentation (neurosurgery/orthopedics)

Angiography

Angiography remains the reference standard for assessing the cause and severity of peripheral vascular disease. It is the preliminary diagnostic technique necessary for acute planning of many therapeutic procedures, including endarterectomy, angioplasty, bypass grafting, and embolectomy. Angiography is an invasive procedure that must be accomplished under sterile conditions.

The technique, employing videotape and subtraction of background (digital subtraction angiography) allows the visualization of most veins and arteries of the body following the intravenous or intra-arterial injection of a contrast medium. Most angiographic studies are carried out in specially equipped rooms, such as the cardiac catheterization laboratory, or the special studies room of the radiology department, although intraoperative arteriograms are frequently performed in the operating room (usually without the benefit of digital subtraction).

Essential equipment for angiography includes an X-ray unit that is capable of making both fluoroscopic (recorded on videotape) and still pictures, film changers for the still shots, pressure injectors, contrast media, catheters, guidewires, and needle/cannula assemblies.

The film changer allows tracking of the course of the injected contrast medium as it travels through the portion of the arterial or venous system being studied. It exchanges film rapidly after each exposure so that the area under study is completely outlined. Rapid serial film changers capable of at least two films per second are essential for areas of high-velocity blood flow (e.g., thoracic and abdominal aorta or cerebral vessels).

Single-plane units (utilizing only one film) are sufficient for angiographic studies done in the operating room during the surgical procedure, but generally biplane studies are necessary to truly evaluate the anatomy of a vessel, particularly the posterior wall.

A pressure injector is useful for areas of nonselective angiography where large amounts of contrast solution must be injected quickly. It is universally used for angiography of the aorta and left ventricle.

Contrast, as defined in radiology, is the difference in optical density in a radiograph that results from a difference in radiolucency or penetrability of an object. Contrast materials are solutions that are injected into the arteries or veins during angiography that are not penetrable by X-rays (that is, they are radiopaque) and therefore stand out in contrast to the surrounding tissues during angiographic study.

The modern contrast materials are water-soluble organic molecules with bound iodine. There are many brand names, such as Hypaque, Cystografin, or Renografin, each with varying iodine concentration. It is the iodine content that determines the radiodensity of the material. The exact concentration of iodine is listed on the label. Often the brand name reflects the area of intended use (e.g., the brand name Renografin implies that the intended target area is the kidney).

The trade names and numbers of the various agents can be confusing to the surgical technologist. For example, the iodine contents of Renografin 60 (meglumine diatrizoate) and Hypaque 50 (sodium diatrizoate) are almost identical. Most contrast media are hypertonic, viscid solutions, some with high sodium as well as iodine content. In proper dosage, they are quite safe, but they are toxic in overdosage and when allowed to remain in tissues for extended periods of time due to low cardiac output or dehydration.

The amount and the site of the injection of contrast media cannot be rigidly applied to every patient. Nonselective aortography may require from 30–50 mL of the more concentrated solutions at a rate of 10–25 mL/sec. Selective arterial injections—for example, carotid studies—require 10–12 mL at 7–8 mL/sec. Less concentrated solution is recommended for the selective studies. The volume and the flow rate of the contrast material into the vessel are the determining factors in the quality of the angiogram. In the demonstration of peripheral arteriosclerosis, relatively slow rates and large volumes of contrast solution make the best combination for successful study.

Catheters (needle/cannula combinations that may include a stylet or guidewire) are tubular, flexible instruments for intra-arterial or intravenous injection of contrast solutions. New catheter materials are continually appearing on the market. Selective catheterization of vessels often requires specially designed, preformed catheters. The smaller the radius of the catheter, the safer the procedure. Thin-wall catheters of sizes 5–7 French (Fr) are sufficient for most applications. Catheters with multiple side holes are necessary for nonselective aortograms. All catheters should be frequently irrigated (flushed) with a normal saline/heparin mixture (1000–2000 u/500 mL) to prevent clots from forming within the catheter.

Many different needle/cannula assemblies are available for angiography. Most consist of an innermost obturator within a sharp, pointed needle and an external cannula with a blunt, tapered end. The most common size is 18 Fr. The Potts-Cournand arterial needle/cannula assembly is frequently used for angiography.

Flexible, atraumatic guidewires protect the intima of the vessel from the catheter tip and "guide" the catheter to the proper location within the cardiovascular system. The guidewires also serve as mechanisms for catheter exchange. The guidewires come in various diameters, lengths, and tip styles. The guidewire length and diameter must correspond with the internal diameter and length of the catheter being used. The typical guidewire is called a *J-wire* because the flexible tip at the end is shaped like the letter J. The floppy curve at the end of the guidewire is useful for negotiation of tortuous, sclerotic vessels.

The percutaneous intra-arterial catheter placement described by Seldinger and called the *Seldinger technique* allows easy entrance into most vessels of the body. The femoral route is the method of choice for study of the entire aorta and its branches, including the cerebral vessels and those of the lower limbs.

With the Seldinger technique, the skin and subcutaneous tissues in the femoral region are injected with Xylocaine 1%, and a small incision is made with a #11 knife blade. The subcutaneous tissues are spread with a hemostat for free passage of the catheter and guidewire. The needle/cannula is then inserted into the femoral artery at an angle of 45–60 degrees, and the stylet is gently and slowly withdrawn until blood spurts forcefully from the proximal end of the cannula. The guidewire is then inserted through the cannula and into the artery. The cannula is removed over the guidewire and, while pressure is applied to the puncture site, the catheter is threaded over the guidewire and into the artery. With the tip of the guidewire protruding from the distal end, the catheter is positioned at the proper level under fluoroscopy, and the guidewire is removed. The catheter is then flushed with heparinized saline. Contrast material is injected and X-rays are taken.

Cardiac Catheterization

Cardiac catheterization permits the evaluation of heart function, visualization of coronary arteries and cardiac chambers (especially the left ventricle), and the measurement of pressures within the cardiac chambers. It is used to diagnose coronary artery, valvular, pulmonary, and congenital heart disease (Figure 13-5).

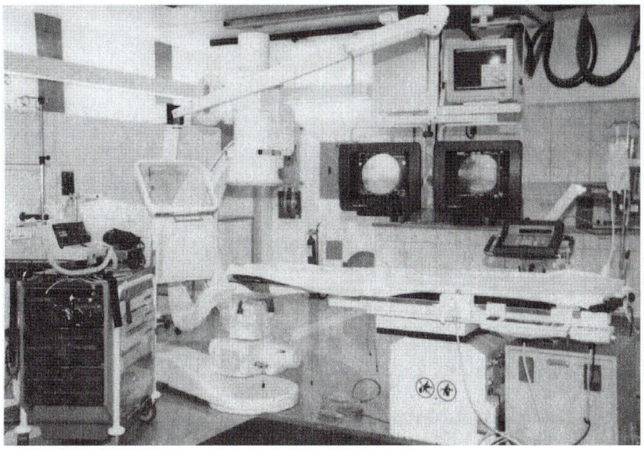

Figure 13-5 Cardiac catheterization laboratory *(Courtesy of GE Medical Systems)*

Studies may be made of the left and right heart with catheters introduced into the femoral artery and femoral vein, or the brachial artery and brachial vein, right subclavian, or internal jugular vein. Because the introduction of a catheter into the brachial artery involves an incision and "cut-down" of the vessel, the percutaneous femoral route is by far the most popular.

Left heart studies include left ventriculogram, coronary artery arteriogram, and measurement of left ventricular pressures. The ejection fraction, which is calculated from planimetric measurements from the ventriculogram during diastole and systole, is a good indicator of general cardiac function.

Utilizing the Seldinger technique described previously for peripheral vessel angiography, a catheter is introduced into the femoral artery and positioned into the ostia of the left coronary system under fluoroscopy. Contrast medium is injected, and, with the aid of computerized digital subtraction, cinefluorograms are taken. Any lesions of the left coronary system are clearly outlined. Catheters are exchanged, and the technique is repeated for the right coronary system.

After coronary angiograms are completed, coronary catheters are exchanged for a multiple-hole pigtail catheter that is positioned across the aortic valve and into the left ventricle. Chamber pressures are measured and recorded, and the catheter is hooked up to a pressure injector capable of injecting a large volume of contrast material into the left ventricle. A ventriculogram is made outlining the left ventricular wall. Wall movement is examined for any deficiencies related to myocardial infarction, and the ejection fraction is calculated from the ventriculogram.

Right heart studies are accomplished with the aid of a balloon-tipped, Swan-Ganz pulmonary artery catheter attached to a transducer and monitor. Pressures are taken in the right atrium to rule out right or left ventricular failure, hypovolemia, or embolism. Pressures are also taken in the right ventricle to rule out mitral valve insufficiency, left ventricular failure, or congestive heart failure; and in the pulmonary artery to rule out changes in pulmonary vascular resistance that may occur in hypoxemia, respiratory insufficiency, pulmonary edema, or pulmonary embolism.

The catheter is inserted into the femoral vein (or, occasionally, the subclavian or internal jugular vein), advanced through the inferior or superior vena cava, and positioned into the right atrium for chamber pressure measurements. When an RA (right atrial) waveform appears on the oscilloscope, the balloon is inflated with air to facilitate catheter advancement with blood flow across the tricuspid valve and into the right ventricle, where a typical RV (right ventricular) waveform appears on the oscilloscope. After recording, the catheter is advanced across the pulmonary semilunar valve and into the pulmonary artery, where a PA (pulmonary artery) waveform is noted and recorded. The flow of blood through the pulmonary artery carries the catheter balloon into one of the smaller pulmonary artery branches, where it wedges and occludes the vessel. This wedge has a distinct waveform, and is referred to as the pulmonary capillary wedge pressure (PCWP). PCWP reflects end-diastolic pressures, and so is an important determinant in the functioning of the left side of the heart. After recording of the PCWP, the balloon is deflated and the catheter slips back into the pulmonary artery, where a PAP (pulmonary artery pressure) is measured and recorded.

Cholangiography

As a diagnostic tool preoperatively, and intraoperatively during cholecystectomy or common bile duct exploration, a catheter can be inserted and contrast medium injected into the biliary system to outline calculi or other **obstructions** under fluoroscopy. Accomplished either with plain films or fluoroscopy, cholangiography may be done during open or laparoscopic cholecystectomy (Figure 13-6).

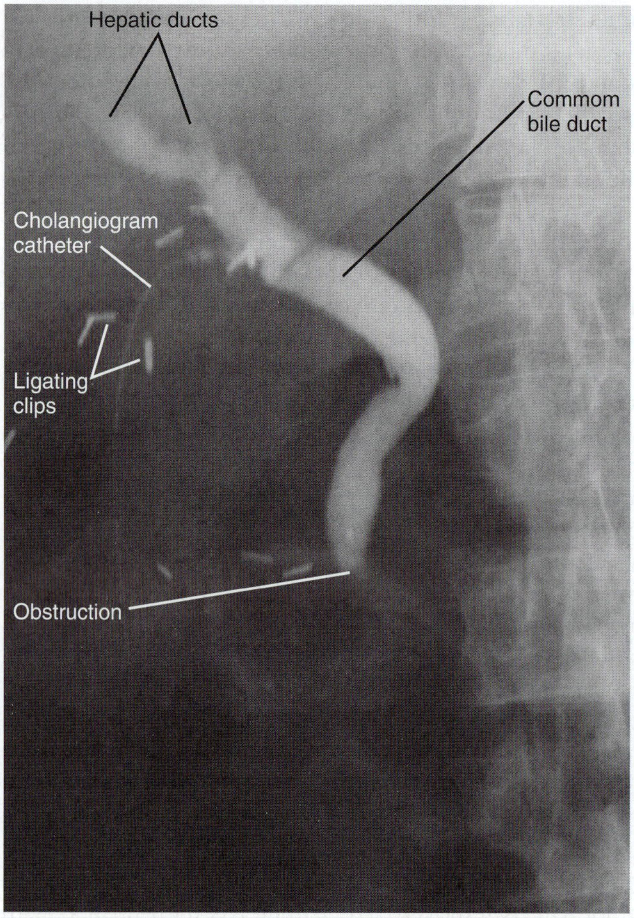

Figure 13-6 Intraoperative cholangiogram depicting gallstones

COMPUTED AXIAL TOMOGRAPHY (CAT SCAN)

Computed axial tomography (CT or CAT scan) is the use of a specialized X-ray machine that produces pictures of a body part in "slices" for evaluation by a radiologist (Figure 13-7). The CT scanner is adjustable to make the slices as thick or thin as desired. Most slices are 2–10 mm thick. The CT scan uses electromagnetic radiation to create an image from approximately 4,000 different tissue densities that are sorted into 16 different groups. Each group is assigned a shade of gray. The detailed cross sections of the CT scan are useful for detection and examination of masses within the body. The CT image can sometimes be enhanced with the use of an iodine-based contrast medium, which is given to the patient intravenously. The contrast medium cannot be used in individuals who are allergic to iodine.

As a neurological diagnostic tool, CT scanning is better than MRI for emergencies related to the brain because it is faster and better able to detect fresh bleeding. The CT scan is also useful for the detection of cerebral infarction and can be used with contrast for the detection of tumors and infection. This iodinated solution tends to leak into brain tissues that have suffered damage from tumor or infection, causing them to be seen as bright spots on the CT scan.

To undergo a CT scan, the patient must enter the scanning device, which is tubular in shape. The exam can be lengthy and the patient is expected to remain still for the duration of the scan. This is difficult for young children who may become frightened, or for an adult patient who may experience a feeling of claustrophobia. Either of these situations may require the patient to be sedated or placed under general anesthesia.

POSITRON EMISSION TOMOGRAPHY

Positron emission tomography (PET scanning) combines CT and radioisotope brain scanning. PET scanning helps to identify how different areas of the brain function by highlighting chemical or metabolic activity.

MAGNETIC RESONANCE IMAGING

Magnetic resonance imaging uses two different forms of energy to create an image. A spinning hydrogen atom is placed into a magnetic field, forcing the atoms to line up and "spin" at a particular frequency. Applied radio waves force the hydrogen atoms to cycle in phase. As the radio waves shut down, the atoms release a radio wave of the characteristic frequency that is measured and transformed into an image. MRI uses these radio waves in a strong

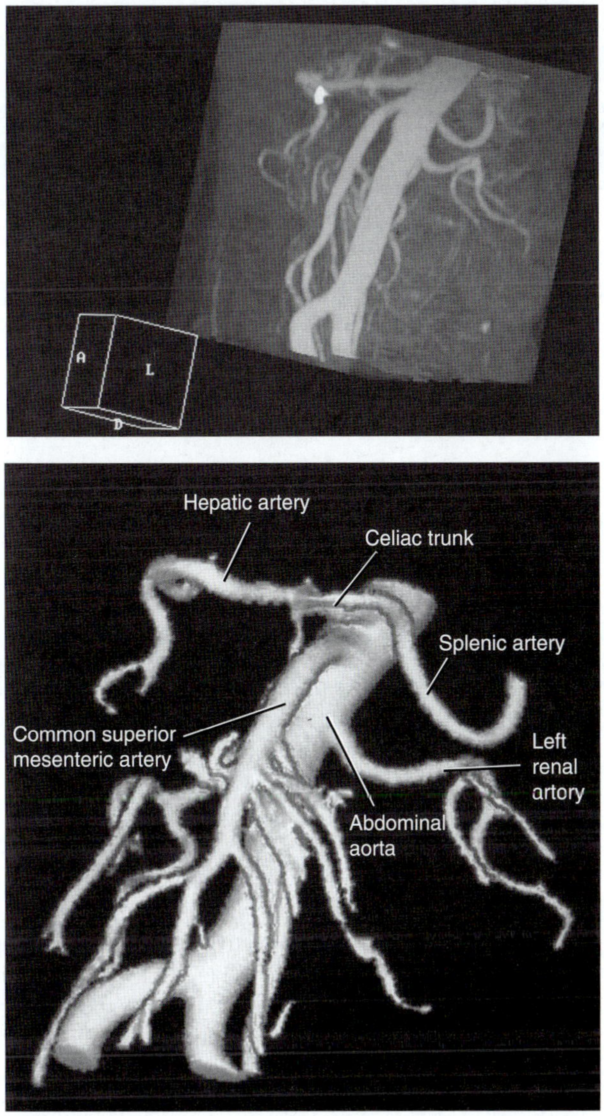

A

B

Figure 13-7 Computed tomography angiography: (A) Demonstration of the abdominal aorta with its main branches, (B) 3D reconstruction

magnetic field to form pictures of parts of the body in slices, much like a CT scan. However, MRI slices may be taken from any direction, a feature that CT scanners are unable to provide. In addition, MRI scanning uses no X-ray radiation.

MRI is especially good for imaging soft tissue, so it is often used for the evaluation of brain disorders and for providing images of a herniated disk and its relationship to the spinal cord (Figure 13-8).

As with CT scanning, contrast media may be injected intravenously to help spotlight tumors and infections. For detection of brain or spine tumors and infections, MRI images are taken before and after injection of contrast. The contrast medium used for MRI is not iodine based, so that patients with iodine allergy are not adversely affected.

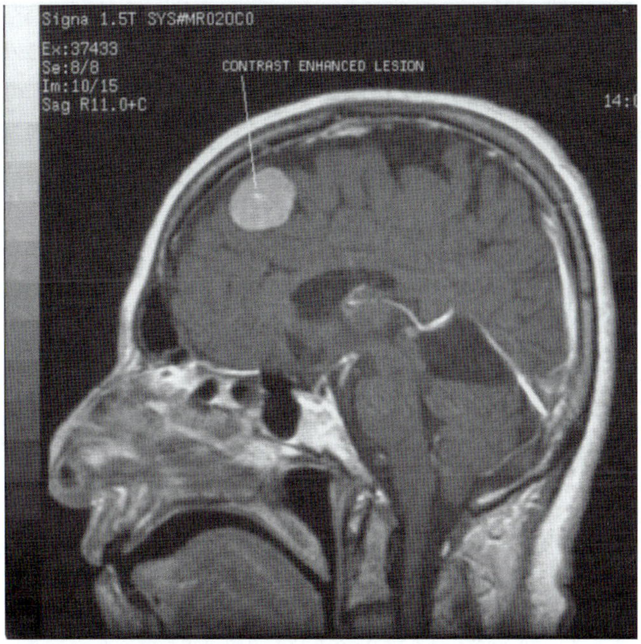

Figure 13-8 MRI depicting a brain tumor

Like the CT scan, the MRI exam is lengthy and the unit is tubular in shape, potentially causing fear and anxiety in the patient. In addition, the MRI device makes repeated loud noises that can complicate the patient's ability to remain calm and still. Again, sedation or an anesthetic may be used.

ULTRASONOGRAPHY

During an ultrasound examination, high-frequency sound waves are directed into the body and reflected from the tissues to a recording device for diagnostic purposes. Frequencies of 1–10 million Hz are necessary for diagnostic studies. The lower the frequency, the greater the depth of sound wave penetration into the body.

Ultrasonic waves are produced when a crystal (transducer) is stimulated electrically. The beam that is produced is directed into the body and variances in tissue density are reflected back to the transducer as echoes. These echoes are then converted into electrical impulses that can be viewed as images.

Ultrasound is a useful diagnostic tool for examination of the heart and abdominopelvic cavity. It is also useful for identifying carotid artery stenosis. Because ultrasound waves cannot pass through structures that contain air, **ultrasonography** is not used to examine the lungs. Ultrasonography is ideal for examination of the fetus because it does not use ionizing radiation.

Echocardiography

Echocardiography is a noninvasive study that provides a two-dimensional image of the heart by directing beams of

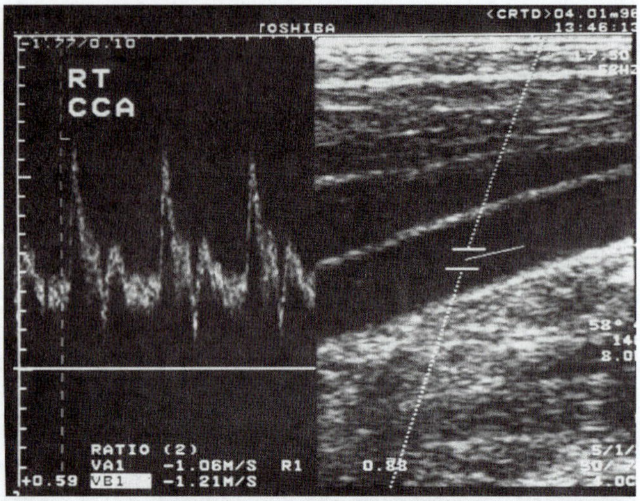

Figure 13-9 Doppler ultrasound, venous system

ultrasonic waves from a sonar-like device through the chest wall. These sound waves echo from the heart and surrounding structures to provide information about cardiac structural abnormalities. Color Doppler techniques of echocardiography are useful for mapping blood flow through the heart.

Transesophageal echocardiography, a slightly more invasive procedure, involves the introduction of a transducer attached to the end of a gastroscope into the esophagus, bringing the probe into closer approximation with the heart. It is useful for the assessment of valvular function and intraventricular blood volume during cardiac surgery and for the detection of cardiac chamber enlargement and septal defects.

Doppler Ultrasonography

A measurement can be taken of the shift in frequency of a continuous ultrasonic wave proportional to the velocity of blood flow in vessels (Figure 13-9). The Doppler monitor measures blood flow that transmits the sound of moving red blood cells to the transducer. The difference in pitch between the transmitted and reflected sounds produces a tone that can be amplified by the machine. *Doppler ultrasonography* is used in the OR to determine the patency of arterial anastomosis. The Doppler probe is covered with a sterile drape for use within the sterile field.

The measurement of segmental limb pressures is easily achieved with the Doppler probe. Pressure in the thigh can be determined by applying a tourniquet and determining the pressure at which flow is extinguished in the popliteal or tibial artery using the Doppler probe. By placing the cuff around the calf, pressure measurements of the calf can be obtained as the examiner determines which pressure is associated with the loss of pedal flow.

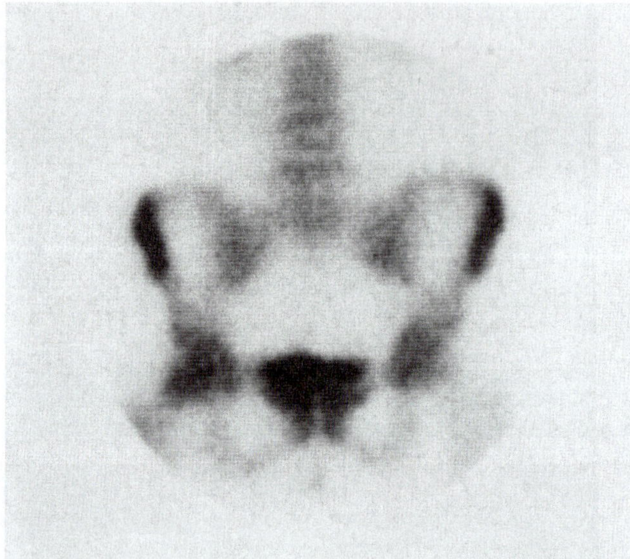

Figure 13-10 Radionuclide scan, lumbar

Calf and thigh pressures are compared with each other and with the brachial artery pressure to provide an objective assessment of the degree of arterial disease.

ISOTOPE SCANNING

Isotope scanning, sometimes referred to as a nuclear medicine study or radionuclide imaging, involves the intravenous injection of a radioactive isotope into the patient prior to the imaging study (Figure 13-10). A variety of isotopes are available that are taken up metabolically by specific types of tissue. The metaiodobenzylguanidine (MIBG) scan will be specifically discussed in Chapter 20 as it relates to the adrenal gland. Collections of isotopes in a certain area are referred to as a "hot spot" and may indicate the presence of a pathologic condition. A bone scan is an example of an isotope scan.

RADIATION THERAPY

Radiation kills cells by interfering with their metabolic activity. *Radiation therapy* is used in predetermined doses to treat specific types of neoplasms that are susceptible to radiation by exposure to the radiation source. Radiation can be administered to the patient with a beam that passes through the tissue or by direct tissue contact with an implantable radiation source.

LABORATORY REPORTS

The laboratory or pathology department is responsible for countless types of examinations on every type of body fluid and tissue that exists. Findings from these studies are extremely valuable in sorting out what may be normal for one patient and abnormal for another. Every type of exam cannot possibly be listed here simply because they are too numerous; only the basics will be covered in this text. A blood test, for example, may be run to provide the practitioner with some broad general information, or may be ordered to obtain one specific value. Only normal values are listed here. Abnormalities as they pertain to a patient's pathological condition will be discussed in the procedural chapters.

The surgical technologist plays an important role in specimen care and handling. This is more thoroughly discussed in the procedural chapters. As always, whenever handling any body substances, Standard Precautions are used.

HEMATOLOGIC STUDIES

Venous or arterial blood is drawn from the patient for visual or computerized examination in the laboratory setting. Many methods for collection are available. Normal laboratory findings are illustrated in Table 13-1, and normal blood gas findings are listed in Table 13-2.

Table 13-1 Hematology Values

Red blood cell (RBC) count	
Male: 4.3–5.9 × $10^6/mm^3$, 4.3–5.9 × $10^{12}/L$ (SI units)	
Female: 3.5–5 × $10^6/mm^3$, 3.5–5.0 × $10^{12}/L$ (SI units)	
RBC indices	
Mean corpuscular hemoglobin (MCH), 27–33 pg (standard and SI)	
Mean corpuscular hemoglobin concentration (MCHC), 33–37 g/dL, 330–370 g/L (SI units)	
Mean corpuscular volume (MCV) 76–100 μm^3, 76–100 fL	
Hemoglobin	
Male: 13.5–18 g/dL, 135–180 g/L (SI units)	
Female: 11.5–15.5 g/dL, 115–155 g/L (SI units)	
Glycosylated (HbA1-C), <7.5%, 5–6% (desired)	
Hematocrit	
Male: 40–52% (0.40–0.52)	
Female: 35–46% (0.35–0.46)	
Platelets	130–400 × $10^3/mm^3$
White blood cells (leukocytes)	5,000–10,000/mm^3
Neutrophils	50–70%
Segments	50–65%
Bands	0–5%
Basophils	0.25–0.5%
Eosinophils	1–3%
Monocytes	2–6%
Lymphocytes	25–40%
T-lymphocytes	60–80% of lymphocytes
B-lymphocytes	10–20% of lymphocytes
Bleeding time	1–3 min (Duke)
	1–5 min (Ivy)
Coagulation time (Lee White)	5–15 min
Prothrombin time	10–15 sec (same as control)
Partial thromboplastin time (PTT)	60–70 sec
Thrombin time	Within 5 sec of control
INR recommended range	
Standard therapy	2.0–3.0
High-dose therapy	2.5–3.5
Activated partial thromboplastin time (APTT)	30–45 sec

Table 13-2 Blood Gas Values

Whole blood oxygen, capacity	17–24 vol %
Arterial	
Saturation	96–100% of capacity
pCO_2	35–45 mm Hg
pO_2	75–100 mm Hg
pH	7.38–7.44
Bicarbonate, normal range	24–28 mEq/L
Base excess (BE)	+2 to −2 (±2 mEq/L)
Venous	
Saturation	60–85% capacity
pCO_2	40–54 mm Hg
pO_2	20–50 mm Hg
pH	7.36–7.41
Bicarbonate, normal range	22–28 mEq/L

Table 13-3 Urinalysis Values

Reference Values (Adult)	
Color	Light straw to dark amber
Appearance	Clear
Odor	Aromatic
Foam	White (small amount)
pH	4.5–8.0 (average is 6)
Specific gravity (SG)	1.005–1.030 (1.015–1.024, normal fluid intake)
Protein	2–8 mg/dL (negative reagent strip test)
Glucose	Negative
Ketones	Negative
Microscopic examination	
RBC	1–2 per low-power field
WBC	3–4
Casts	Occasional hyaline

URINALYSIS

Urine collection methods vary according to the type of test to be performed. A simple voided specimen is collected as the patient urinates into a clean container. A clean-catch sample involves cleaning the urinary meatus prior to voiding and "catching" the sample midstream into a sterile collection device. Catheterized specimens are obtained under sterile conditions and placed in a sterile specimen container. Normal **urinalysis** (**UA**) values are shown in Table 13-3, and urine chemistry values are listed in Table 13-4.

Urine may be collected over a 24-hour period and the entire sample tested for electrolytes and nitrogenous wastes.

TISSUE SPECIMENS

Fluid and tissue samples are removed from the body to determine the exact nature of a disease or for treatment of a condition. Several methods exist for removing fluid and tissue from the body:

- *Needle aspiration:* A fine needle and syringe are used to withdraw the sample.
- *Incisional biopsy:* The lesion is incised and a portion is removed for study.
- *Excisional biopsy:* The entire tumor is removed and examined.

During biopsy, small amounts of suspect tissue or fluid may be aspirated by needle or excised through a surgical incision and sent to the laboratory to determine the type of infection or neoplasm, or the degree of tumor metastasis (staging).

Intraoperatively, if an immediate diagnosis is necessary for a decision to remove more tissue, the biopsy sample is sent directly to the pathologist for a **frozen section**, which involves freezing the tissue sample, slicing it into thin sections, staining, and microscopic viewing. The pathologist is then able to give an opinion about the nature of the sample. This method is not 100% accurate and the final diagnosis may be deferred to the results of the "permanent section."

If a frozen section is not indicated, the tissue is placed into a container of sufficient size with a fixative solution, such as formalin, before being sent to the laboratory. Some very large specimens, such as amputated limbs, may require improvised techniques for transport to the laboratory.

The STSR should be aware of the identity and origin location of the specimen when receiving it from the surgeon, and should communicate this information to the circulator when passing it off the sterile field. Orientation of the specimen becomes important when the margins of the wound must be proven to be free of tumor. The tumor edges may be marked (with suture or another method); the STSR should accurately communicate the significance of the markers to the circulator or pathologist.

If the specimen must be removed from the sterile field intraoperatively, this must be done in a sterile manner. The specimen should be placed in or on a sterile specimen container, Telfa pad, towel, or basin. A counted surgical sponge should never be used for transport of a specimen. If the specimen is to remain on the back table for any reason, precautions should be taken to prevent it from drying.

Table 13-4 Urine Chemistry Values

Aldosterone	2–26 μ/24 hr, 5.6–73 nmol/ 24 hr (SI units)
Amylase	4–37 U/L/2 hr
Bilirubin and bile	Negative to 0.02 mg/dL
Electrolytes	
Calcium	7.4 mEq/24 hr
Chloride	70–250 mEq/24 hr
Magnesium	15–300 mg/24 hr
Phosphorus, inorganic	0.9–1.3 g/24 hr
Potassium	25–120 mEq/24 hr
Sodium	40–220 mEq/24 hr
Glucose	0
5-Hydroxyindoleacetic acid (HIAA)	2–10 mg/24 hr
Ketones	0
Nitrogenous constituents	
Ammonia	30–50 mEq/24 hr
Creatinine clearance	100–200 mL/min
Creatinine	Males: 20–26 mg/kg/ 24 hr Females: 14–22 mg/kg/ 24 hr
Protein	0–5 mg/dL/24 hr
Urea	6–17 g/24 hr
Uric acid	0.25–0.75 g/24 hr
Osmolality	200–1,200 mOsm/L
Porphobilinogen	0.2 mg/24 hr
Steroids	
17-Hydroxycorticosteroids	Males: 5–15 mg/24 hr Females: 3–13 mg/24 hr
17-Ketosteroids	Males: 8–25 mg/24 hr Females: 5–15 mg/24 hr
Urobilinogen	0–4 mg/24 hr
Vanillylmandelic acid (VMA)	1.5–7.5 mg/24 hr

BACTERIOLOGIC TESTS

Tissue or fluid that is suspected of being infected may be cultured so that the pathogen can be identified and treated. This is called *culture and sensitivity*. The culture is performed to determine the exact organism; once the organism is identified, a determination is made as to which form of treatment it will be sensitive to. Sterile cotton-tipped swabs are exposed to the tissue or fluid to be cultured, and then placed into the transport container. Aerobic and anaerobic studies may be ordered, each requiring its own specialized transport container. Anaerobic bacteria die quickly if exposed to air; therefore the swab should be placed quickly into the growth medium or vacuum transport tube for eventual incubation in the laboratory.

Table 13-5 Cerebrospinal Fluid Values

Cell count	0–8/mm^3
Chloride	118–132 mEq/L
Culture	No organisms
Glucose	40–80 mg/dL
Pressure	75–175 cm water
Protein	15–45 mg/dL
Sodium	145–150 mg/dL

Gram Stain

The **Gram stain**, developed in 1844, remains a valuable tool in identifying bacteria. Bacteria to be cultured are collected in the sterile transport tube and taken to the laboratory for analysis. There the bacterium is exposed to stains of crystal violet and iodine, then exposed to alcohol and stained again. Bacteria that retain the blue are called *gram positive* and those that fade to pink are *gram negative*. This quick method of identification helps the physician determine an initial course of treatment, which may be altered when the culture and sensitivity results are available.

Many other staining techniques for specific organisms have been developed following Gram's principles.

Spinal Tap

Cerebrospinal fluid (**CSF**) is withdrawn ("tapped") from the lumbar area of the spinal column for analysis. The fluid is normally clear. The physician can make a preliminary diagnosis by observing if the fluid is bloody or cloudy, allowing initial treatment to begin. Final diagnosis is reserved until the CSF has undergone laboratory analysis (Table 13-5).

Thoracentesis

Thoracentesis involves the placement of a needle into a posterior portion of the pleural space for the analysis of pleural effusion. The procedure is generally performed as an aid in the diagnosis of inflammatory or neoplastic diseases of the pleura or the lung. Therapeutic applications for thoracentesis include the removal of fluid accumulations from within the thoracic cavity. CT scan or ultrasonography may accompany thoracentesis to ensure accurate needle placement.

ELECTRODIAGNOSTIC STUDIES

The body consists of cells that contain polarized molecules. The communication systems of the body are bioelectrical or biochemical. Microelectrical impulses can be measured and provide useful diagnostic information.

ELECTROCARDIOGRAPHY

The *electrocardiogram* (**ECG**) is a valuable tool for the detection and evaluation of all forms of heart disease, especially myocardial infarction (Figure 13-11). However, the ECG should not be the only diagnostic tool used because, in certain instances, it may appear normal in patients with cardiac conditions. It may also appear abnormal in patients in good cardiac health; therefore, the ECG is best utilized in the detection and evaluation of cardiac dysrhythmias and conduction disturbances. Cardiac dysrhythmias are discussed in Chapter 22.

Electrocardiography is performed by placing a number of electrodes in predetermined locations on the skin of the arms, legs, and torso to record the electrical activity of the heart. The number of electrodes (also referred to as *leads*) varies according to the patient situation and the type of information desired. Typically, a five-lead configuration is utilized in the operating room.

The Holter monitor allows 24-hour monitoring for asymptomatic and symptomatic dysrhythmias. The system is composed of a portable tape recorder, one or two electrocardiographic leads, and a computer system capable of quantifying rhythm disturbances. The patient wears the monitor while attending to daily activities.

ECG is also useful for graded exercise testing. The patient walks on a treadmill at an increasing rate while heart rate, blood pressure, and ECG are closely monitored for significant changes. Exercise testing evaluates the delivery of oxygen via coronary circulation in response to increased demands. It also indicates the presence of myocardial ischemia for patients with **angina**.

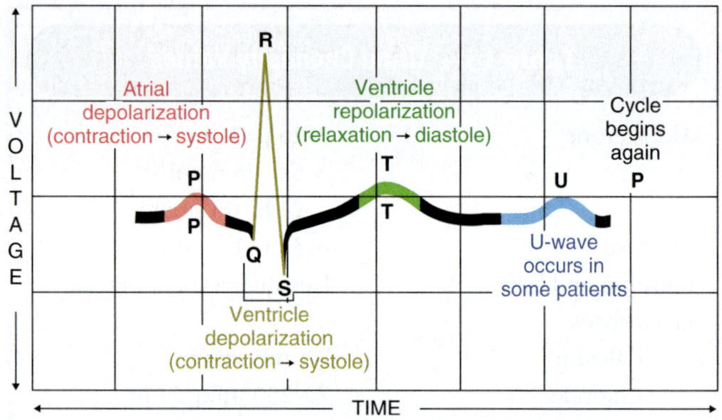

Figure 13-11 ECG and cardiac cycle

ELECTROENCEPHALOGRAPHY

Electroencephalography (**EEG**) is a display and recording of the electrical activity of the brain by measurement of changes in electric potentials. Electrodes may be placed on the scalp or on the brain's surface intraoperatively. The signals picked up by these electrodes are sent to an amplifier, which compares the signals from the two electrodes involved. A wave pattern based on the difference in the electrical activity picked up by the two electrodes is then printed for review. A baseline measurement is usually recorded with the patient lying down and with the eyes closed.

EEG is used to help diagnose seizure disorder, brain tumor, epilepsy, and other diseases and injury to the brain. In addition, EEG is used intraoperatively during certain cranial, spinal, and vascular procedures for monitoring of neurological function.

When used in the diagnosis of seizures, EEG measurements are taken during a seizure and during a period of normal brain activity. This helps to localize the origin of the seizure within the brain and to confirm seizure activity. EEG patterns are also analyzed to help determine the area of the brain affected by a tumor or other abnormality.

EEG brain topography uses computers to simultaneously record a large number of digitized EEG channels. This information is analyzed and plotted on a screen or printer using different colors to depict EEG activity. This method gives a more accurate view of the location of alterations in brain wave activity in relation to the surface of the skull.

ELECTROMYOGRAPHY

Electromyography (EMG) is the study and recording of the electrical activity of skeletal muscle. Electric stimulation is applied to the muscle via a probe that is inserted through the skin into the muscle. Information about muscle contractility and innervation can be assembled.

PULMONARY DIAGNOSIS

Respiratory status and the severity of several pulmonary conditions is evaluated in several ways. One of them, blood gas analysis, has already been mentioned.

PULSE OXIMETRY

Arterial saturation of hemoglobin with oxygen is measured by passing a light through the tissues to determine the optical density of the blood. The lighted noninvasive device is most often placed on the finger, toe, or earlobe. The pulse oximeter measures the oxygen saturation in percentages. The normal value is 95–97%. Oxygen administration should increase the percentage.

CAPNOGRAPHY

Capnography was designed to estimate arterial levels of carbon dioxide noninvasively for surgical patients requiring mechanical ventilation. Measurment of the amount of carbon dioxide that is exhaled makes the estimation. This is referred to as the *end-tidal* CO_2. The sensor is located within the anesthesia circuit or ventilation tubing and sends the information to a monitor, which displays the information in graph (wave) form. This is helpful in detecting dislocated endotracheal tubes and acidosis.

SPIROMETRY

Spirometry is another noninvasive technique used for evaluating the patient's respiratory status. Information about the lung capacity, resistance, and ventilatory pressure is obtained and displayed in numerical and graph form on a monitor. This technique is useful in detecting leaks in the ventilatory system and patient conditions such as chronic obstructive pulmonary disease (COPD) and adult respiratory distress syndrome (ARDS).

ENDOSCOPY

Endoscopes can be used preoperatively or intraoperatively to directly visualize internal structures for diagnostic purposes. Chapter 10 provides a detailed description of the various types of endoscopes and their uses for diagnosis and therapy and individual procedural chapters for specific endoscopic procedures.

PLETHYSMOGRAPHY AND PHLEBORHEOGRAPHY

Plethysmography is useful in patients with diffuse small vessel arterial disease, especially diabetics. A plethysmograph is an instrument for determining and registering variations in the volume of an extremity and in the amount of blood present in the extremity or passing through it. Common plethysmographic techniques include a mercury strain gauge and air plethysmography (pulse volume recorder). With the use of a mercury strain gauge, changes in leg volume that accompany arterial pulsation are sensed by the strain gauge and translated as a waveform on a strip chart recorder. A pulse volume recorder detects changes in the volume of an inflated air bladder that is expressed on a strip chart recorder. In each case, changes in the volume of the examined part are measured, rather than changes in blood velocity of a particular artery, as in Doppler studies. Thus, while their waveforms are similar, plethysmography and Doppler ultrasonography are measuring two related but separate parameters and provide different information. Although plethysmography measures blood flow quite well, it does not measure the flow of a particular artery in the way that Doppler studies can.

Diagnosis of deep-vein thrombosis can be made by *phleborheography,* a plethysmographic technique in which rhythmic changes in venous volume in the legs associated with respiration are recorded.

INDICATIONS FOR SURGERY

Surgical intervention can occur for many reasons. The patient's condition will dictate if the imminent procedure should be classified as emergent, urgent, elective, or optional. Some of the reasons for an individual to undergo surgery are listed below:

- Diagnostic procedures
- Trauma
- Metabolic disease
- Infection
- Repair congenital defect
- Treat a neoplasm
- Relieve obstruction
- Reconstruction
- Aesthetics

CASE STUDY

Fredrick is scheduled as the STSR on a laparoscopic cholecystectomy for a patient diagnosed with cholecystitis and cholelithiasis. He is assembling supplies and preparing the operating room for the case.

1. What laboratory studies do you expect to find on the patient's chart?
2. Are diagnostic image studies likely to be part of the patient's preoperative workup? If so, what kind? How will they be viewed in the OR?
3. Is it likely that any studies will be performed during the procedure? What kind? How might this affect the room preparation?

QUESTIONS FOR FURTHER STUDY

1. What type(s) of specimen(s) should the STSR be prepared to handle intraoperatively?
2. Would a CT scan or X-ray best demonstrate a soft tissue tumor? Why?
3. What is the first priority of the STSR when an intraoperative X-ray is being taken?
4. What is a cholangiogram?
5. Contrast media and isotopes are both used to enhance diagnostic imaging studies. How do they differ?
6. Describe a patient situation in which a frozen section may be requested intraoperatively.

BIBLIOGRAPHY

Atkinson, L. J., & Fortunato, N. M. (1996). *Berry and Kohn's operating room technique* (8th ed.). St. Louis, MO: Mosby.

Carter, D. C., & Dudley, H. (Eds.). (1985). *Rob & Smith's operative surgery* (4th ed.). St. Louis, MO: C. V. Mosby.

Delmar Publishers. (1998). *Delmar's radiographic positioning and procedures: Image library* [CD-ROM]. Clifton Park, NY: Author.

Estes, M. E. Z. (1998). *Health assessment and physical examination.* Clifton Park, NY: Delmar Publishers.

Gazes, P. C. (1990). *Clinical cardiology* (3rd ed.). Philadelphia: Lea and Febiger.

Harvey, A. M., Johns, R. J., McKusick, V. A., Owens, A. H., & Ross, R. S. (Eds.). (1988). *The principles and practices of medicine* (22nd ed.). East Norwalk, CT: Appleton & Lange.

McGuiness, A. M., et al. (2002). *Core curriculum for surgical technology* (5th ed.). Centennial, CO: Association of Surgical Technologists.

O'Toole, M. (Ed.). (1997). *Miller-Keane encyclopedia & dictionary of medicine, nursing, and allied health* (5th ed.). Philadelphia: W. B. Saunders.

Sabiston, D. C., Jr. (1997). *Textbook of surgery. The biological basis of modern surgical practice* (15th ed.). Philadelphia: W. B. Saunders.

Spratto, G. R., & Woods, A. L. (1998). *Nurse's drug reference.* Clifton Park, NY: Delmar Publishers.

CHAPTER 14

General Surgery

Bob Caruthers
Gary Allen

CASE STUDY

Laura is a 45-year-old woman who is somewhat overweight, eats a typical American diet, and is generally healthy. She has been developing severe colicky pain in her right upper quadrant about 2 hours after meals. After a history and physical, she was diagnosed with cholelithiasis.

1. What does cholelithiasis mean?
2. What causes the condition?
3. Name three possible treatments for cholelithiasis.

OBJECTIVES

After studying this chapter, the reader should be able to:

A 1. Discuss the relevant anatomy and physiology of the abdominal wall, digestive system, hepatic and biliary system, pancreas, spleen, thyroid, and breast.

P 2. Describe the pathology and related terminology of each system or organ that prompts surgical intervention.

3. Discuss any preoperative diagnostic procedures and tests.

4. Discuss any special preoperative preparation procedures related to general surgery procedures.

O 5. Identify the names and uses of general surgery instruments, supplies, and drugs.

6. Identify the names and uses of special equipment related to general surgery.

7. Discuss the intraoperative preparation of the patient undergoing general surgical procedures.

8. Define and give an overview of illustrative general surgery procedures.

9. Discuss the purpose and expected outcomes of the illustrative procedures.

10. Discuss the immediate postoperative care and possible complications of the illustrative procedures.

S 11. Discuss any specific variations related to the preoperative, intraoperative, and postoperative care of the general surgery patient.

SELECT KEY TERMS

1. absorption	8. -cysto-	15. -oma	21. portal venous system
2. anastomosis	9. -docho-	16. -ostomy	22. -stasis
3. ascites	10. -ectomy	17. -otomy	23. stenosis
4. bile	11. excision	18. parietal	24. ulcer
5. chole-	12. incision	19. peristalsis	25. viscera
6. chyle	13. lysis	20. peritoneum	
7. chyme	14. necrosis		

ANATOMY

General surgery involves most of the organ systems in the human body at some time or another. Most commonly, general surgery involves the abdominal wall, abdominal cavity, and the contents of the abdominal cavity. This area will receive the most attention in this chapter. A separate anatomy section in the latter portion of the chapter discusses the anatomy of the breast and thyroid gland.

ABDOMINAL CAVITY: GENERAL DIMENSIONS

The abdominal cavity, containing the abdomen proper and lesser pelvis, extends from the diaphragm to the base of the pelvis and is enclosed by musculature that maintains the position of the abdominal and pelvic structures. The abdomen is also bounded by bony structures: the ribs superiorly as well as superoanteriorly and superoposteriorly, the iliac crests inferolaterally, the pelvic girdle inferiorly and inferoposteriorly, and the vertebrae posteriorly. Bony landmarks of significance in abdominal surgery are the xiphoid process (the distal portion of the sternum), the subcostal margin (the plane along each angle of the rib cage), the anterior iliac crests (or spines), and the symphysis pubis (the most distal point of the anterior abdomen). These landmarks serve as reference points for muscular attachments and **incisions** into the abdomen to access the internal organs.

The abdomen proper contains a large portion of the digestive tract (alimentary canal), the liver, gallbladder, pancreas, spleen, kidneys, and suprarenal glands, as well as numerous blood and lymph vessels, lymph nodes, and nerves. The funnel-shaped lesser pelvis contains coils of the digestive tract and its most distal portions, blood and lymph vessels, lymph nodes, and nerves. The lesser pelvis also contains most of the structures of concern in urology and gynecology (refer to Plate 1 in Appendix A).

The abdomen may be divided into nine regions: the epigastric, right and left hypochondriac, the umbilical, the right and left lumbar, the hypogastric or pubic region, and the right and left inguinal (or iliac) regions (Figure 14-1A). The abdomen is also spoken of in terms of quadrants: the right and left upper quadrants and the right and left lower quadrants (Figure 14-1B).

SURFACE FEATURES

Surface features other than bony structures may be used to identify regions of the abdomen and serve as reference

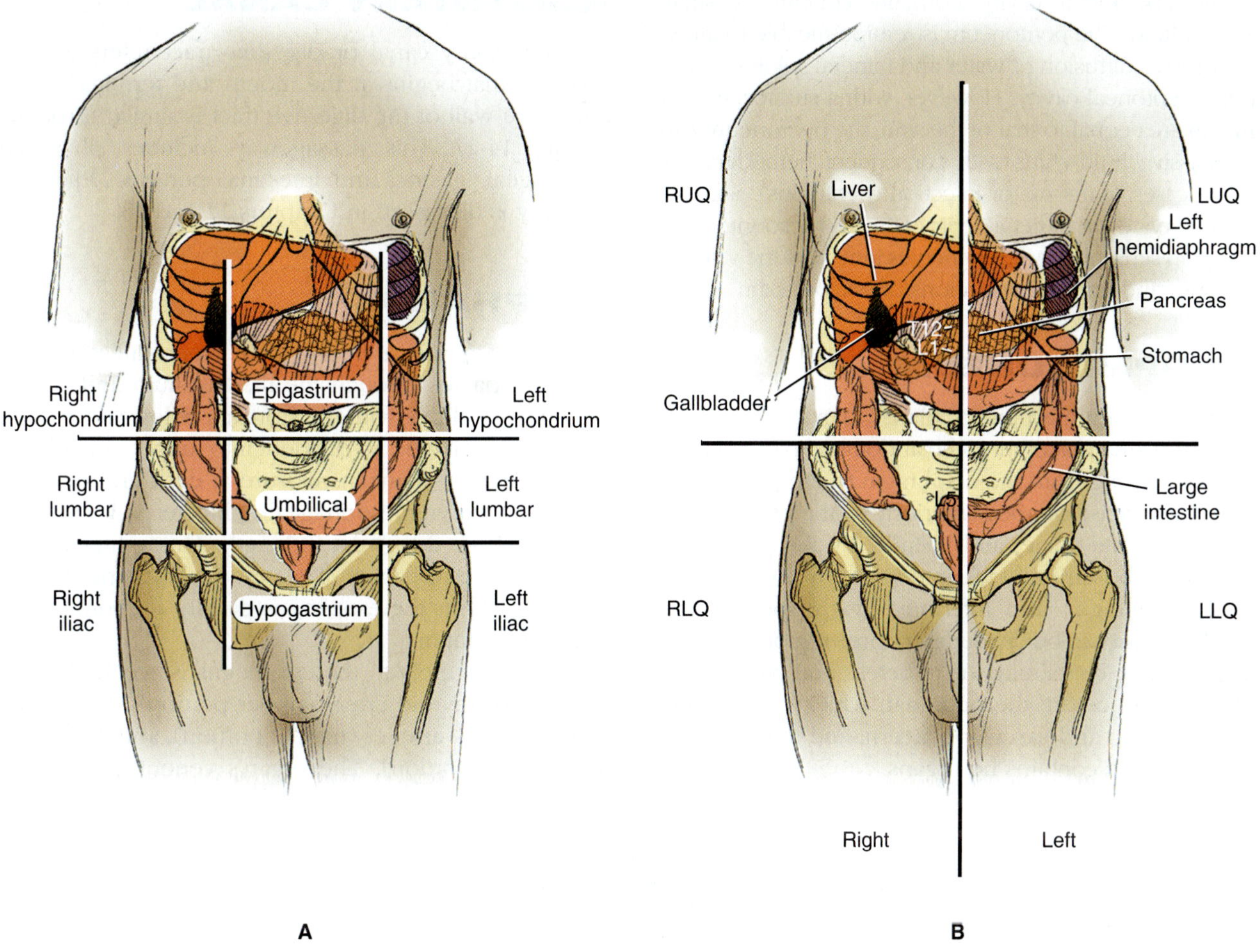

Figure 14-1 Abdominopelvic divisions: (A) Regions, (B) quadrants

points for the underlying musculature and internal organs. These features include the

- Umbilicus (generally at the level of the disk between the third and fourth lumbar vertebrae)
- Linea alba (a median groove created by the joining of the abdominal aponeuroses)
- Semilunar lines of Spieghel (demarcating the lateral margins of the rectus abdominis muscles)
- Bilateral abdominocrural creases (between the thigh and abdomen)

ABDOMINAL MUSCULATURE

Commonly encountered muscles in abdominal surgery are those on its anterior surface: the external and internal oblique, the transverse abdominis, and the rectus abdominis. The oblique groups and the transverse abdominis, the three "flat" muscles, attach at varying levels to the lower ribs and the iliac crests. The rectus abdominis, a long strap-like muscle, arises from the costal margin and the sides of the xiphoid process and extends to the symphysis pubis (refer to Plates 12A and B in Appendix A).

The abdominal muscles are wrapped in fibrous fascia varying both in thickness and intrinsic strength. The transverse abdominis and the obliques each have a dense white tendon of insertion, the aponeurosis. These aponeuroses come together in the midline to form the "sheath" around the rectus abdominis and the midline linea alba.

PERITONEUM

The abdominal cavity, as well as the organs contained within it, is lined with a continuous band of fibrous to flimsy tissue called the **peritoneum**. The **parietal** peritoneum lines the anterior, lateral, and posterior abdominal walls, the pelvis, and the inferior surface of the diaphragm. It is loosely attached and can be easily stripped from most surfaces. The visceral peritoneum covers all organs of the peritoneal cavity and is intimate with them in that it is essentially continuous with the matrix of the visceral wall. The primary function of the peritoneum is to provide a slippery surface over which the **viscera** can freely glide.

The abdominal cavity normally contains a small amount of fluid. The peritoneum is semipermeable to allow for the passive diffusion of water and mineral solutes to and from the peritoneal cavity. However, with a surface area of 1.7 m^2, an area equal to that of the skin, the peritoneum can cause massive fluid shifts with consequent hemodynamic effects in cases of trauma or infection (peritonitis). Somatic nerves innervate the parietal peritoneum and account for localized pain sensation. Afferent nerves innervate the visceral peritoneum and transmit sensations of "vague" pain.

RETROPERITONEUM

The retroperitoneum is more a "plane" than a "space" and occupies the area posterior to the abdominal parietal peritoneum extending from the diaphragm to the pelvis. The retroperitoneum is bounded anteriorly by the peritoneum, posteriorly by the spine, and laterally by the psoas and quadratus lumborum muscles, superiorly by the 12th ribs and the diaphragm, and inferiorly by the pelvis. The retroperitoneum can be divided into three regions: the anterior pararenal, containing the pancreas and parts of the duodenum and colon; the perirenal, which holds structures of urologic and vascular concern; and the posterior pararenal, which contains no organs.

ALIMENTARY CANAL

The alimentary canal or digestive tract refers to a passageway that begins at the mouth and terminates at the anus. The wall of the digestive tract is similar throughout (Figure 14-2). This passageway includes pharyngeal, esophageal, gastric, and intestinal portions. Pharyngeal anatomy is discussed in Chapters 17 and 18.

ESOPHAGUS

The esophagus is a hollow tube approximately 24 cm long that passes through the mediastinum and connects the pharynx above with the stomach below (refer to Plate 1). The esophagus is divided into upper, middle, and lower thirds. It maintains closure at each end by sphincters. The pharyngoesophageal sphincter is a clearly defined structure 2 to 3 cm in length. This sphincter closes the upper esophagus. The esophagogastric (cardiac) sphincter closes the esophagus distally at about the level of the diaphragm.

Blood supply to the esophagus is accomplished by the inferior thyroid artery (upper portion), the bronchial and intercostal arteries (middle portion), and the celiac artery (lower portion). The organ's venous drainage, im-

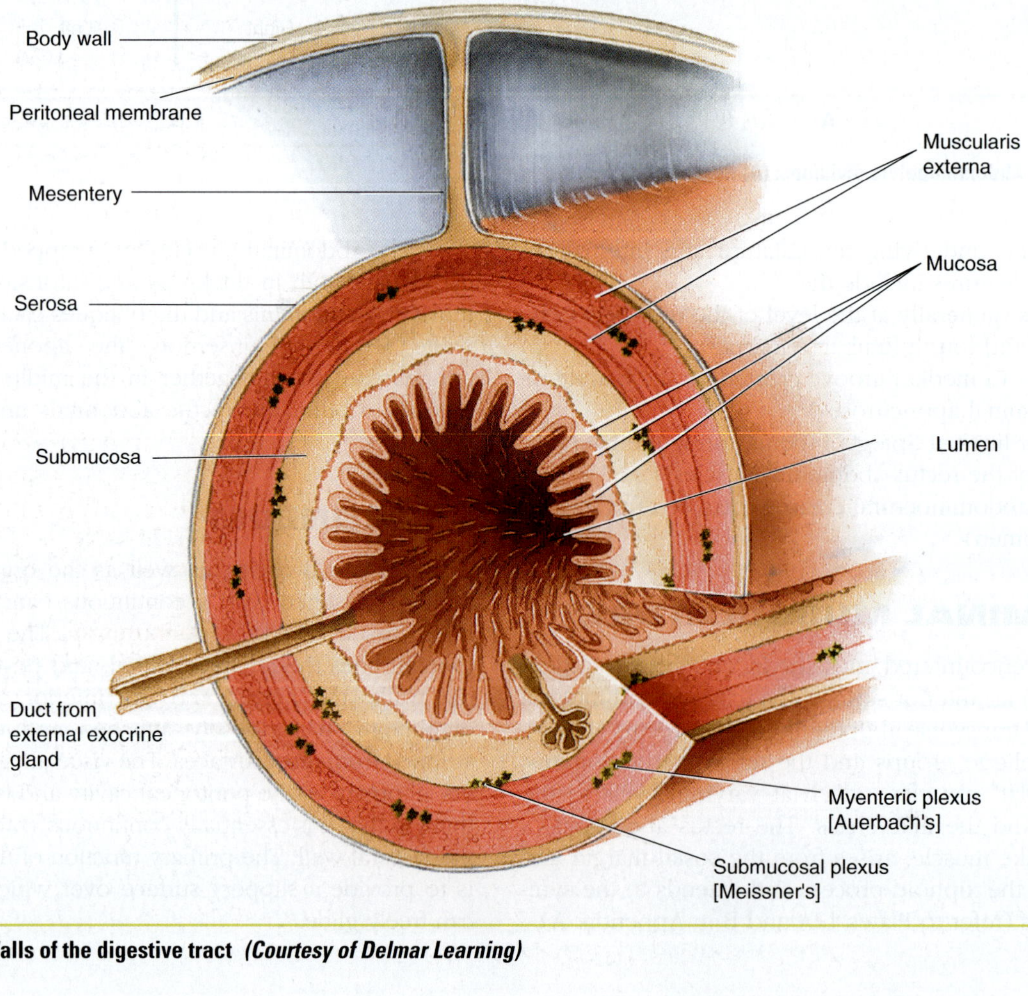

Figure 14-2 Walls of the digestive tract *(Courtesy of Delmar Learning)*

portant in the discussion of esophageal varices, is via the right and left gastrics, and lymphatic drainage is associated with the internal jugular, tracheal, intercostal, diaphragmatic, and gastric nodes. Both parasympathetic fibers from the vagus nerve and sympathetic nerves from the cervical and thoracic ganglia innervate the esophagus.

STOMACH

The sac-like stomach is the most dilated portion of the alimentary canal and lies in the epigastric, umbilical, and left hypochondriac regions of the abdomen. The sections of the stomach are the cardia, fundus, corpus, antrum, and pylorus. The cardia is a small area at the esophagogastric junction. It opens into the largest region, the corpus (body) of the stomach. Above this area is the fundus and below it is the antrum, which extends to the pylorus, the distal region of the stomach at the duodenal junction. The shape of the stomach presents two anatomical curves. The lesser curvature is the superior surface and the greater curvature is the inferior border (Figure 14-3).

The musculature of the stomach consists of three layers. The inner layer, which at the esophageal junction is continuous with the circular layer of the esophagus, is said to be "incomplete," thicker in the fundus than it is in the antrum. The middle layer is the only "complete" muscle layer and is composed of circular fibers that increase in number from the fundus to the pylorus, running from the lesser to the greater curvature. This layer plays a dominant role in gastric emptying as part of the antral "pump" mechanism. Distally the pyloric sphincter, a thick band of muscle, separates the pylorus from the duodenum. The outer layer of muscle is continuous with the longitudinal fibers of the esophageal musculature and runs along the lesser and greater curvatures, converging at the pylorus and becoming continuous with the longitudinal muscle of the duodenum.

Blood supply to the stomach is via the left gastric artery, the first and smallest branch of the celiac artery, and the left gastroepiploic and short gastric branches of the splenic artery. The gastroduodenal artery, the first branch of the left gastric artery, contributes as well. Five veins drain the stomach. The left gastric (coronary) vein serves the cardia, fundus, and lesser curvature. The right gastric drains the pylorus. The short gastrics, left and right gastroepiploics, drain the greater curvature (Figure 14-4A).

Parasympathetic innervation of the stomach is by the left (anterior) and right (posterior) vagal nerve trunks. Sympathetic innervation comes from thoracic roots 7 to 9. Vagal innervation is an important factor to consider in the resolution of many gastric conditions because it affects both gastric motility and pepsin production. The sympathetic nerves supply vasomotor control to the gastric vessels and provide the main pathway for gastric pain (Figure 14-4B).

The digestive function of the stomach begins with the mucous secretions of the cardia, easing passage of foodstuffs to the gastric regions. The fundus produces hydrochloric acid. The corpus produces acid as well, but also secretes pepsinogen and mucus. The antrum is a nonacid-producing region of the stomach that secretes both mucous and gastrin from its cellular lining. The pylorus is essentially a storage area before the lysed foodstuffs (**chyme**) pass into the duodenum.

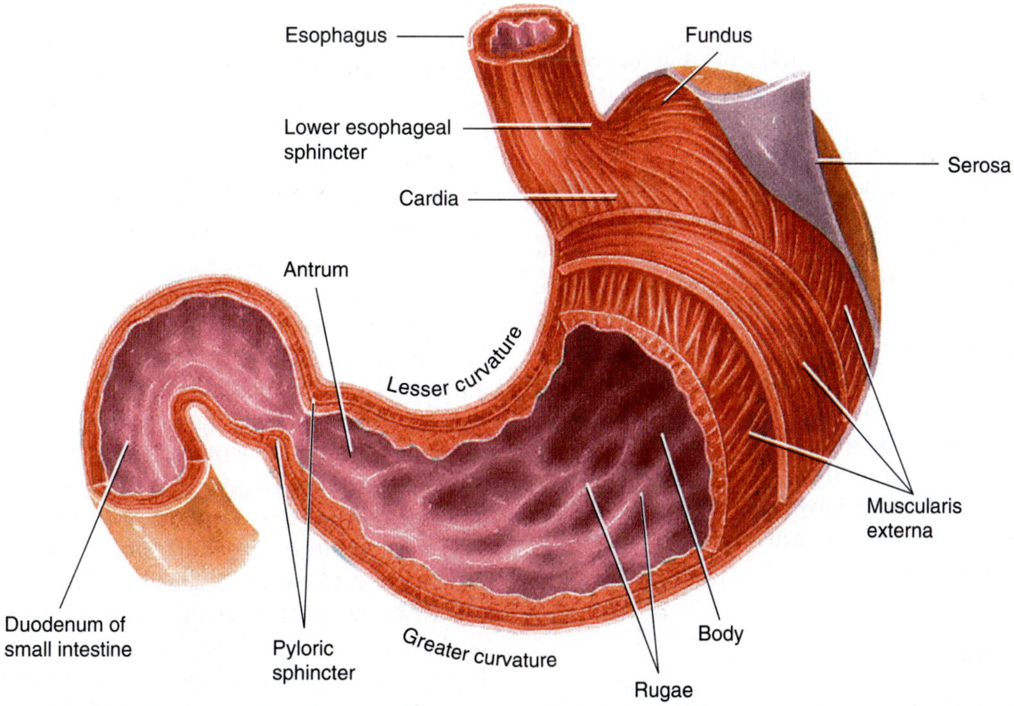

Figure 14-3 Stomach anatomy ***(Courtesy of Delmar Learning)***

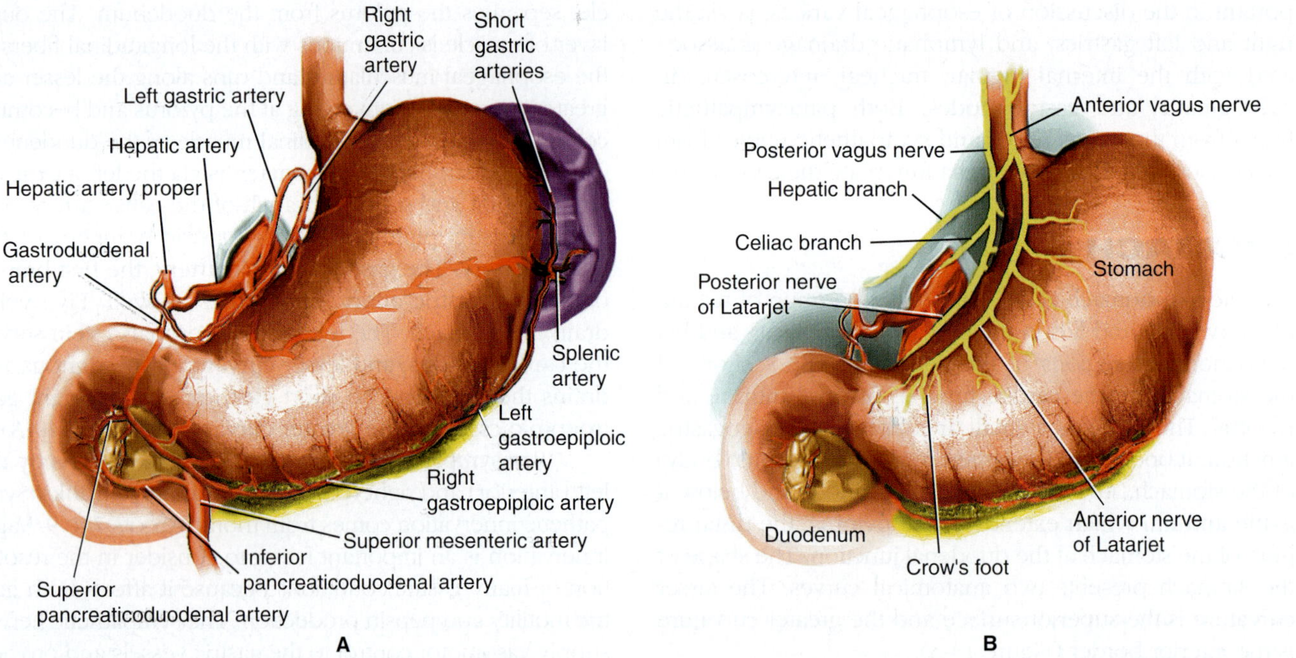

Figure 14-4 Stomach: (A) Arterial supply, (B) neural supply

SMALL INTESTINE

The small intestine begins at the pyloric sphincter and is composed of three contiguous sections: proximally, the duodenum, then the jejunum, and distally, the ileum. The latter two segments are termed the "mesenteric" small intestine. Overall the small intestine is approximately 6 to 7 m in length and varies in luminal diameter from 3 to 5 cm. The small intestine, which is the longest portion of the alimentary canal, digests foodstuffs, absorbs nutrients, and produces the various acids and enzymes necessary for these functions.

Blood supply to the duodenum arises from the right gastric, supraduodenal, right gastroepiploic, and the superior and inferior pancreaticoduodenal arteries. The duodenum also receives blood from branches of the hepatic and gastroduodenal arteries. The adjoining venous system ends in the splenic, superior mesenteric, and portal veins. The superior mesenteric artery, via the jejunal and ileal branches, supplies blood to the mesenteric small intestine. Venous drainage is to the superior mesenteric vein.

Innervation to the small intestine is via the celiac plexus, vagus, and thoracic splanchnic nerves, and serves to either initiate or inhibit both **peristalsis** and sphincter activity, as well as stimulate intestinal secretions. Lymph drainage originates at two levels, mucosal and muscularis, and drains to the mesentery.

DUODENUM

The duodenum is the first of three segments of the small intestine. The duodenum is horseshoe shaped. Its name comes from the Greek word for "12 fingers." The duodenum is about 12 finger breadths (30 cm) in length and averages 3 to 5 cm in width. This portion of intestine is subdivided into four portions. The first portion, the duodenal "cap," is a cone approximately 5 cm long with a base continuous with the pylorus and an apex joining with the second portion. Unlike the remainder of the duodenum, longitudinal mucosal folds line the duodenal cap. This portion of the small intestine is the most mobile segment. It is enclosed in peritoneum, which forms the hepatoduodenal ligament from its anterior and posterior planes. This ligament carries the portal vein, hepatic artery, and common **bile** duct (CBD). The free edge of hepatoduodenal ligament constitutes the anterior border of the foramen of Winslow. The duodenal cap is also the most frequent site of peptic **ulcers**.

The second portion of the duodenum is approximately 10 to 12 cm long. Entirely retroperitoneal, this portion descends to the right of midline from the first to third lumbar vertebrae and is intimately associated with the pancreas along it medial border. The second portion of duodenum exhibits the transverse mucosal folds common to the rest of the alimentary canal. The hepatopancreatic ampulla of Vater, where the CBD joins the pancreatic ducts of Wirsung and Santorini, is located at the midpoint. The third portion runs horizontally right to left for approximately 15 cm at the level of the third lumbar vertebra. Also retroperitoneal, this portion lies directly over the descending aorta and the inferior vena cava (IVC). The fourth portion of the duodenum is 8 cm long and passes upward, forward, and to the left of the aorta staying below the level of the body of the pancreas. Ultimately, the fourth portion terminates at the ligament of Treitz, which delineates the beginning of the mesenteric small intestine.

JEJUNUM AND ILEUM

The mesenteric small intestine is longer in men than in women. This section of intestine averages 5 m in length. Although no clear distinction exists, the proximal two-fifths of the mesenteric small intestine is referred to as the jejunum (Latin for "empty"). The distal three-fifths is called the ileum (Greek for "roll" or "twist"). The jejunum occupies the left upper abdominal cavity and the ileum lays in the right abdomen and pelvis. The jejunum has a thicker wall and wider lumen than the ileum, yet the ileum displays more vascularity and fat in its mesentery. The mesenteric small intestine exhibits a gradual narrowing of its lumen from its junction with the duodenum to the distal ileum.

The walls of the mesenteric small intestine are composed of five layers: the innermost mucosa, the submucosa, the muscle layer (muscularis propria), the subserosa, and the outermost serosa. Villi, which in the jejunum are longer and appear more "frondlike," line the lumen. Villi aid in the transport of nutrients and secrete digestive enzymes produced mainly by their epithelial cells but also by their associated crypt (goblet and Paneth) cell structures. Epithelial cells produce disaccharides and amino peptidases. Goblet cells secrete acid mucopolysaccharides and glycoproteins (mucus), and Paneth cells, which are most numerous in the ileum, produce lysosomal enzymes and a carbohydrate-protein complex. Villi also contain columnar absorption cells over their entire surfaces.

The submucosa, a network of loose connective tissue rich in blood vessels, nerves, and lymphatics, is separated from the mucosa by the muscularis mucosae. The muscularis propria of the entire small intestine is composed of an inner circular and outer longitudinal layer of nonstriated muscle and is thickest in the duodenum. The serosa is the visceral peritoneum, an extension of the mesentery.

MESENTERY

The mesenteries are peritoneal folds and include the mesentery of the small intestine, the mesoappendix, the transverse mesocolon, and the sigmoid mesocolon. These mesenteries contain the blood vessels, nerves, and lymph vessels that serve the adjoining organs. The root of the small intestine's mesentery, the point at which it is attached to the posterior wall of the abdominal cavity, begins at a level left of the second lumbar vertebra and extends diagonally downward 15 cm to the fourth or fifth lumbar vertebrae. From this point the mesentery fans out to meet the entire length of the small intestine, changing in length from 20 cm at the proximal jejunum to 5 cm at the distal ileum.

The arterial structure of the mesenteric small intestine increases in complexity from the duodenum to the terminal (distal) ileum and demonstrates both "end arteries" and looping vascular "arcades." Vascular supply to the small intestine requires more than 12 branches of the superior mesenteric artery (SMA).

The mesoappendix is a triangular fold that attaches the whole length of the appendix to the ileal mesentery, and carries the appendicular vessels within. The transverse mesocolon, carrying the middle colic vessels, spreads across the posterior aspect of the transverse colon and attaches to the posterior abdominal wall, passing around the head and body of the pancreas. The sigmoid mesocolon secures the sigmoid to the pelvis at the level of the sacrum. It carries the sigmoid and superior rectal vessels and the left ureter.

COLON

The length of the colon averages 90 to 125 cm and its lumen ranges from 8.5 cm at its most proximal point to 2.5 cm at the distal sigmoid section. The colon can be referred to by right and left segments but is more commonly divided into specific anatomical sections: the proximal cecum, the ascending colon, the transverse colon, the descending colon, the sigmoid colon, and the rectum (Figure 14-5).

The wall of the colon consists of four layers: mucosa, submucosa, muscularis, and serosa. The colon's mucosal epithelium is similar in structure to that of the small intestine, but contains more mucus-producing goblet cells and is relatively "flat," lacking the villi common in the small intestine. A thin, indistinct muscularis separates the mucosa from the submucosa, which contains a vast network of arteries, veins, lymph vessels, and the nerve plexus of Meissner. The inner muscularis layer, which can be differentiated into two layers by cellular configurations, is well developed and is arranged in a series of strictly circular rings. It is peculiar to the colon that the outer longitudinal muscularis propria is arranged in three separate taenia (coli) rather than as a continuous enveloping layer, allowing for greater distensibility.

Overall, the colon is responsible for the **absorption** of water and electrolytes, the compaction of fecal waste, and the production of vitamin K by its intestinal flora. The left colon is primarily a storage unit and as such plays almost no role in digestion and absorption. In its water absorption role, the colon is subject to about 2 L of the more than 8 L of water and endogenous secretions that enter the alimentary canal daily, and reclaims all but 150 to 200 mL.

The cecum, ascending colon, and right portion of the transverse colon are supplied with blood from the ileocolic, right colic, and middle colic branches of the SMA. The left transverse colon, descending colon, sigmoid, and rectum derive their blood supply from the

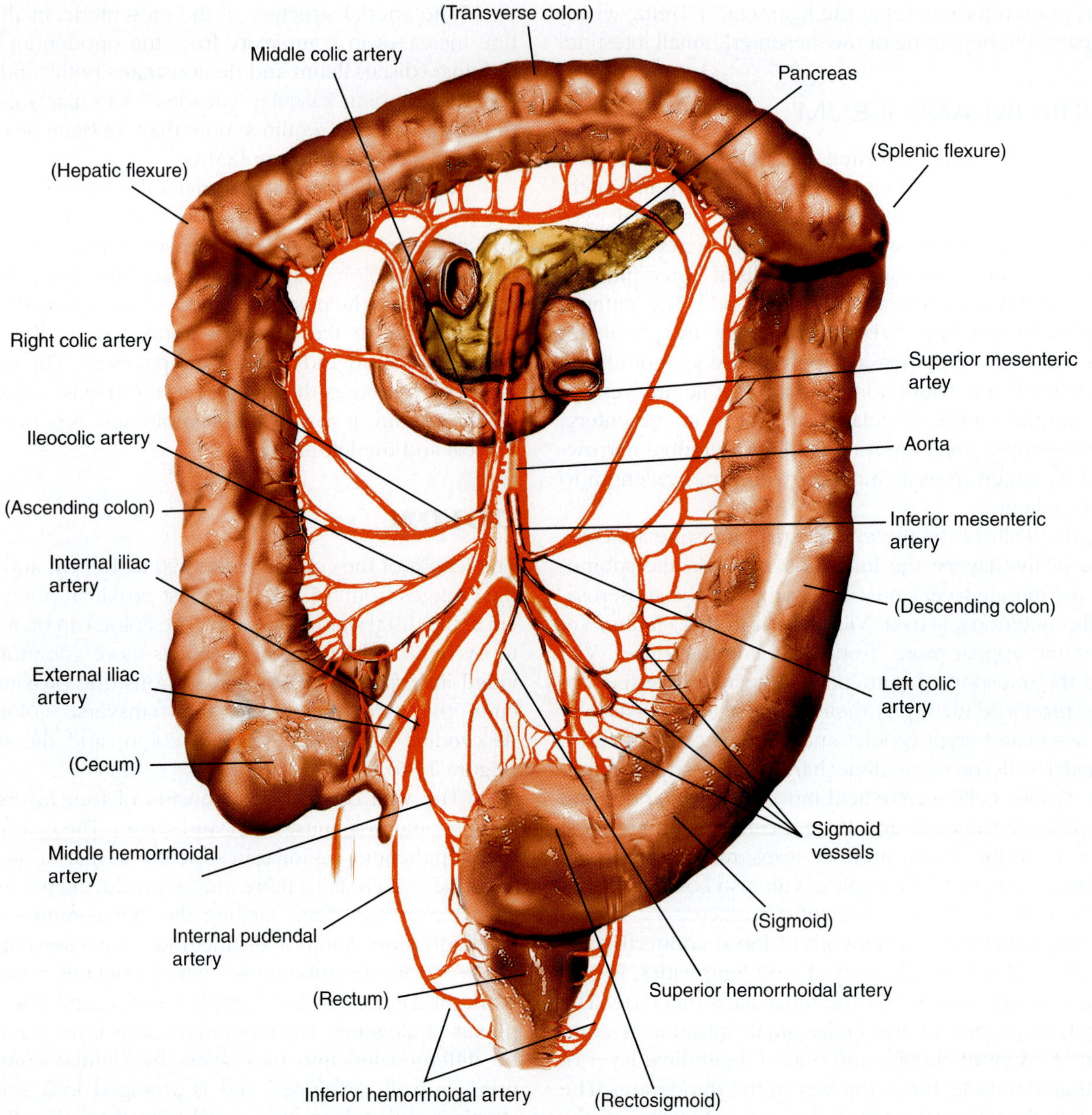

Figure 14-5 Anatomy/blood supply of the colon and rectum

superior left colic, sigmoid, and superior rectal (hemorrhoidal) branches of the inferior mesenteric artery (IMA). Venous return is by accompanying veins bearing the same names as the arteries. Lymphatic drainage courses alongside the arterial supply, and the mesentery is full of bean-shaped lymph nodes. The chain-like paracolic, intermediate, and central nodes drain the visceral lymph fluid (**chyle**) to the cisterna chyli, a 5-cm sac in the region of the aorta.

Innervation of the colon is primarily autonomic, involving both sympathetic and parasympathetic support. This innervation is from the celiac, superior mesenteric, intermesenteric, and superior and inferior hypogastric plexuses, as well as fibers from the splanchnic and tenth cranial (vagus) nerves, and the third and fourth sacral segments.

CECUM

The cecum (Latin for "blind") is a mobile pouch with no mesenteric attachment, situated in the right lower abdominal cavity, that is wider (8.5 cm) than it is long (6.5 cm). It is at the superior aspect of the cecum that the ileum terminates at the ileocecal junction. Located 15 cm diagonal to the ligament of Treitz, this area contains a semilunar valve, the competency of which is of clinical importance in assessing colon obstruction.

APPENDIX

Attached to the cecum is the vermiform appendix, an embryonic extension of the apex (inferior aspect) of the cecum. The appendix is a worm-like blind tube, 0.8 cm wide and averaging 8.5 to 22.5 cm in length. The base is usually retrocecal and the distal tip can be found in almost any position. The appendix derives its blood supply from the mesoappendix.

ASCENDING COLON

The ascending colon is approximately 20 cm in length and begins at a point level to the ileocecal junction, extends upward along the right side of the abdominal cavity to the level of the lower pole of the right kidney, and ends in a hepatic flexure at the inferior surface of the liver. The ascending colon is fixed retroperitoneally to the posterior abdominal wall and its anterior surface is in contact with the ileum, greater omentum, and anterior abdominal wall. A peritoneal fold extending down from the hepatorenal ligament also provides support for the hepatic flexure.

TRANSVERSE COLON

The transverse colon begins at the hepatic flexure and traverses the anterior abdomen in a gentle upward curve, finally attaching to the undersurface of the diaphragm in the left hypochondriac region at the level of the 10th and 11th ribs. It is connected to the diaphragm by the phrenocolic ligament, which also supports the spleen, and is thus pulled upward creating the splenic flexure. The transverse colon is the longest section of the colon at 40 to 50 cm, and is also the most mobile segment.

Haustra (Latin for "that which draws water, as a bucket") are normal outpouchings of the colon wall that are demarcated by strands of circular muscle. In the transverse colon, haustra are more readily noticeable than in other segments and their absence in the transverse colon is abnormal. The splenic flexure is so acute that the end of the transverse colon usually overlaps the front of the descending colon, making radiographic examination difficult.

DESCENDING COLON

The descending colon begins at the acutely angled splenic flexure and routes inferiorly along the lateral border of the left kidney, toward the pelvis. The descending colon is 30 cm long, has the heaviest muscle layer and thinnest lumen of the organ, and is covered with peritoneum on only the anterior two-thirds of its surface. The posterior aspect of the descending colon is intimately associated with the posterior abdominal wall.

SIGMOID COLON

The sigmoid colon is the primary site of colon cancer and is the section of colon most susceptible to volvulus (twisting). It can vary in length from 15 to 50 cm and is attached to generous mesentery, allowing for substantial mobility during resection. The sigmoid is named for its redundant shape that resembles the Greek letter sigma and results in a corrugated pattern of mucosal loops that command careful inspection during diagnostic endoscopy. The sigmoid colon is readily identified by its regularly spaced, fat-laden epiploic appendices on its serosal layer.

RECTUM

Latin for "straight," the rectum is a 10 to 12 cm long curved tube that displays a "zig-zagged" lumen and three prominent interior folds, two on the left wall and one on the right wall, that are referred to as the superior, middle, and inferior valves of Houston. The rectum is continuous with the sigmoid and descends along the sacrococcygeal concavity, exhibiting an anteroposterior curve, the sacral flexure, as it passes through the funnel-shaped pelvic diaphragm to join the anus below. It is at the rectum that the taenia arrangement of the outer longitudinal coat, common to the rest of the colon, changes to a continuous enveloping layer of muscle.

ANUS

The anal canal is only 3 cm long but is surrounded by a complex musculature of involuntary and striated tissues that form the anal sphincters. The internal sphincter is a continuation of the circular smooth muscle layer of the rectum, and extends distally to within 1 cm of the anal orifice. The muscle fibers of the external sphincter form a collar around the anus and intermingle with those of the levator ani. They are separated from the internal sphincter by a thin layer of longitudinal muscle continuous with the outer longitudinal coat of the rectum. This separation can sometimes be visually distinguished in the anus as the "white line of Hilton" and is usually palpable. The upper half (about 15 mm) of the anus is lined with mucosa, which is plum red in color due to the proximity of the rectal venous plexus. Within the lining of the anus there is also a transition from the mucus-secreting columnar epithelium of the intestines to the stratified squamous epithelium of the skin. This change can occur anywhere within the length of the anus but generally occurs at a level of the anal papillae, the terminal portions of the longitudinal folds of the rectal lining. Membranes connecting the papillae form the anal valves, above which are recesses, termed the anal sinuses (crypts), that can clog with fecal matter and develop abscesses.

Except in the lower anus, innervation is both sympathetic and parasympathetic. The sympathetic innervation to the upper anus is derived from the lumbar part of the trunk and the superior hypogastric plexus. The parasympathetic supply is via the pelvic splanchnic nerve and inhibitory to the internal anal sphincter. The external sphincter is controlled by the inferior rectal branch of the pudendal nerve. The external sphincter is also innervated by motor fibers from the fourth sacral segment of the spinal cord.

OMENTA

The omenta are comprised of the lesser and greater omentum. The lesser omentum is continuous with the peritoneum covering the anterosuperior and posteroinferior surfaces of the stomach and the first 2 cm of the duodenum. From its attachment at the lesser curvature of the stomach and the duodenum, the lesser omentum ascends as a double fold to the porta hepatis. These layers enclose the hepatic artery, portal vein, and bile duct, as well as lymph vessels, lymph nodes, and nerves, as the lesser omentum connects the duodenum to the liver, forming the hepatoduodenal ligament. Posterior to this ligament is the foramen of Winslow, a communication between the lesser omentum (sac) and the peritoneal cavity.

The greater omentum is the largest of the peritoneal folds and is a double sheet folded on itself to form four layers. The greater omentum is usually thin, but it is a major site of fat disposition in the abdomen, and in obese individuals the greater omentum may be massive. The greater omentum stores fat and limits peritoneal infection, but it is less absorptive than other peritoneal folds. The greater omentum descends from the greater curvature of the stomach and the cap of the duodenum. It may be congenitally absent, and can be excised without any apparent ill effect to the patient.

PANCREAS

The pancreas is an elongated, flattened, gray to tan organ that weighs between 70 and 120 g and is divided into regions designated as head, neck, body, and tail. The head lies within the duodenal curve and can be imbedded into the wall of the second portion of the duodenum. The boundary between the head and neck is a groove that accommodates the gastroduodenal artery (Figure 14-6).

The neck of the pancreas, about 2 cm long, adjoins the pylorus and merges into the body of the pancreas, which is a prism-like section with anterior, posterior, and inferior surfaces. It extends obliquely upward and to the left about 10 cm to the tail of the pancreas. The tail is narrow and usually reaches the gastric surface of the spleen. It is contained between two layers of the splenorenal ligament along with the splenic vessels.

The pancreas lacks a definitive capsule and is instead surrounded by fine connective tissue. Approximately 80% of the parenchyma (structural framework) of the pancreas

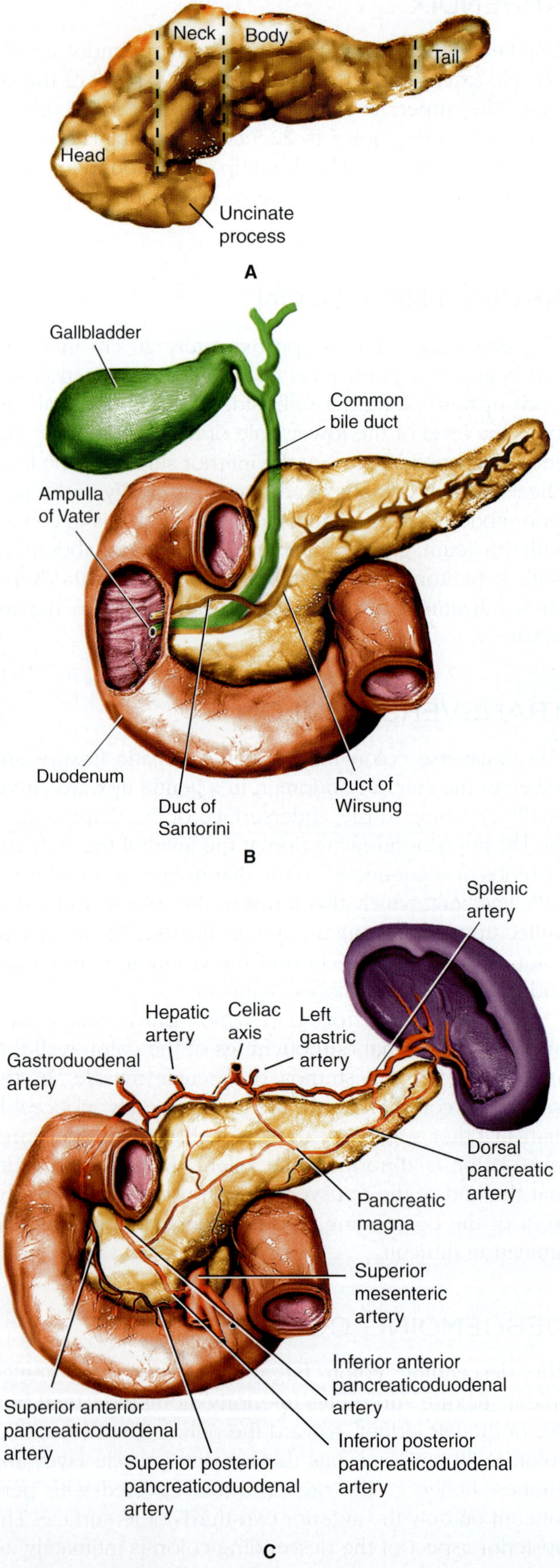

Figure 14-6 Pancreas: (A) Segments, (B) ducts, (C) blood supply

is divided into lobules consisting of acini (exocrine secreting glands). Acini are spherical or curved structures and are composed of tall pyramid cells containing eosinophilic zymogen granules that relate to functional secretion. Acini surrounding islets of Langerhans appear to be larger and contain more granules than other acini.

The acinar secretions serve two primary functions. First, the hydrolytic enzymes break down fats, proteins, carbohydrates, nucleic acids, the digestive secretions of other organs, and sloughed epithelial cells. Second, bicarbonate secretion helps maintain a neutral intraluminal pH, which is important if the duodenal mucosa is to survive the onslaught of gastric acid and pepsins. These secretions reach the alimentary canal by the main pancreatic duct, and occasionally a second accessory duct.

The islets of Langerhans are endocrine secreting glands that number 1,000,000 and account for only 1% of the pancreatic mass. With this fact in mind, it is interesting to note that the islets receive 25% of the pancreatic blood supply. The islets are composed of glucagon-secreting alpha cells, insulin-secreting beta cells, somatostatin-secreting delta cells, and PP, or pancreatic peptide-secreting cells. The relative concentration of these cells within the islets varies considerably depending on their location within the pancreas. The primary function of these structures is to maintain blood sugar levels.

The pancreas has a rich arterial supply from branches of the celiac artery and superior mesenteric arteries as well as the great pancreatic branch of the splenic artery. The pancreatic and pancreaticoduodenal veins drain the pancreas into the splenic, portal, and superior mesenteric veins. The lymphatic system follows the vascular routes, draining into the pancreaticosplenic lymph nodes.

Innervation of the pancreas is supplied by the vagus and splanchnic nerves by way of the hepatic and celiac plexuses. The parasympathetic vagus innervates the acini, ducts, and islets, and also mediates visceral pain. The sympathetic nerves influence the pancreatic blood vessels.

SPLEEN

The spleen is the single largest mass of lymphatic tissue in the body. It lies in the left upper quadrant of the abdomen, between the fundus of the stomach and the diaphragm, and is largely shaped by nearby structures (stomach, left kidney, splenic flexure of the colon, and tail of the pancreas). The spleen varies in size and weight with age, but it is generally 12 cm long, 7 cm thick, and 3 to 4 cm wide, and weighs about 150 to 200 g. It is suspended by several ligaments, most notably the gastrosplenic, splenorenal, splenophrenic, and pancreaticosplenic. The spleen is made up of "red pulp," which is predominantly vascular (75% of its volume), and "white pulp," which is primarily lymph tissue.

The spleen is essentially a filtration mechanism and its function is directly related to its structure. The spleen's red pulp serves as a red blood cell (erythrocyte) storage area in youth and holds 35–80% of the adult body's platelets. The white pulp contains lymphocytes, involved with immune responses related to T-cell and B-cell activities, and macrophages that clear the blood of cellular debris. The spleen is not absolutely necessary for life, as its function can be carried by the liver and other lymph tissue, but its **excision** can lead to an impairment of immunologic response that can become life threatening.

Blood supply to the spleen is usually via the splenic artery from the celiac trunk of the aorta, but in about 15% of individuals the splenic artery is a separate aortic branch. The splenic artery generally divides into two branches that in turn divide into 3 to 40 subsequent branches. The splenic vein arises from the hilum of the spleen and is eventually joined by the superior and inferior mesenteric veins to form the portal vein. Innervation of the spleen is from the medial and anterior parts of the celiac plexus and may also arise from the vagus nerve. Lymphatic drainage arises from the splenic capsule and hilum and follows the blood vessels to empty into the pancreaticosplenic and celiac nodes.

LIVER

The liver, the largest organ in the abdomen, weighs between 1,200 and 1,500 g and accounts for 2% of the adult body weight. It lies in the right upper quadrant of the abdomen, under the protection of the thorax (refer to Plate 1 in Appendix A). The liver is divided anatomically into right and left sides by the falciform ligament, which connects the liver to the diaphragm and anterior abdominal wall, and the fissures through which the ligamentum venosum and ligamentum teres pass. It is further divided into four lobes: right, left, quadrate, and caudate. The right side of the liver, which is six times larger than the left, contains the caudate and quadrate lobes. The liver is covered by a thin connective tissue of type I and type II collagen called Glisson's capsule.

The liver has a double blood supply. The hepatic artery, which provides all the oxygen the organ requires, carries 25% of the blood into the liver, and the portal vein, from the viscera and pancreas, provides the nutrients the liver needs while carrying 75% of the blood to the liver. The point at which the hepatic artery and portal vein enter, and the bile duct exits, is termed the porta hepatis. It is at this point that the hepatic artery and portal vein divide into right and left branches. The right and left hepatic ducts meet at the porta hepatis to form the common hepatic duct. This triad of artery, vein, and duct continues to divide and eventually communicates with every functional unit (lobule) of the liver.

Lobules are typically polyhedral units roughly 0.7 by 2.0 mm in size that contain a variety of cells. Lobules provide metabolism of lipids, proteins, carbohydrates, and hormones; store vitamins; produce cytotoxins; degrade microorganisms, drugs, and endotoxins; harbor immunoglobulin-producing cells; and secrete bile. The triads run along the outside of the lobule while the terminal venule of the hepatic vein, which drains the liver, lies within its core.

The cellular structure of the liver includes a variety of cell types due to the multiple functions of the organ. The most prominent of these cell types are the hepatocytes, the Kupffer cells, the pit cells, and the lipocytes. Hepatocytes occupy 80% of the liver's volume, carry out the major metabolic activities of the liver, and are arranged in a pattern radiating from the central vein to the lobule's periphery. Kupffer cells are large fixed macrophages that take up bacteria, endotoxins, and cellular debris, are thought to clear the blood of circulating tumor cells, and play a role in iron metabolism. Pit cells possess natural killer activity and play a dominant role as a cytotoxin of tumor cells. Lipocytes are usually in close contact with Kupffer cells and produce fibronectin, laminin, chondroitin sulfate, hyaluronic acid, and, in response to injury, large quantities of collagen. The cells of the liver perform a variety of functions:

- Produce bile
- Metabolize carbohydrates, fats, and proteins
- Store sugar as glycogen
- Store fat-soluble vitamins A, D, E, and K plus iron and copper
- Detoxify many harmful substances by phagocytic action
- Synthesize prothrombin and fibrinogen

The liver is drained by the right and left hepatic veins emptying into the inferior vena cava at a level below the diaphragm. The liver bile collects in ductules (canals of Hering) adjacent to the lobules and eventually drains into the right and left hepatic ducts which merge to form the common hepatic duct (CHD). As it exits the porta hepatis, the CHD lies anterior to the portal vein and to the right of the hepatic artery.

Hepatic innervation arises from the hepatic plexus and contains both sympathetic and parasympathetic fibers that run alongside the vascular and ductile components of the triad. Primary lymph drainage is into the portal system, but there is some drainage into the internal mammary nodes transdiaphragmatically.

BILIARY TRACT

The biliary tract communicates between the liver and the duodenum and consists of the gallbladder, the cystic duct, the CHD, and the CBD, which terminates at the sphincter of Oddi. The function of the biliary tract is to transport, store, and release bile to aid the digestion and absorption of fat.

The gallbladder is a bluish, pear-shaped bag that lies partly in a fossa on the inferior surface of the right hepatic lobe above the transverse colon and next to the duodenal cap (Figure 14-7). It is generally 9 cm long and has a bile storage capacity of approximately 50 mL. The gallbladder is divided into four regions: fundus, body, infundibulum, and neck. The fundus is the rounded end lying directly anterior to, and extending about 1 cm past, the free edge of the liver. It is the palpable portion of the gallbladder during physical examination. The body, which is not clearly separated from the fundus and infundibulum, is the largest portion of the gallbladder and is closely attached to the inferior surface of the liver. It lies near the cap and upper portions of the duodenum. The infundibulum is a transitional area between the body and the neck and is firmly attached to the cap of the duodenum by an avascular portion of the hepatoduodenal ligament. It is less wide than the body and narrows to the neck. The neck of the gallbladder is attached to the liver by loose connective tissue, which houses the cystic artery. The neck is the tapering portion of the infundibulum. It is approximately 5 to 7 cm long and follows a tortuous S-shaped path curving upward and forward, then abruptly downward to its junction with the cystic duct. It is in this area that a small bulge can form that extends down onto the duodenum. Called Hartman's pouch, this is a common area for cystic calculi (gallstones) to gather and clog the passage of bile into the cystic duct. When this condition is present the cystic duct will appear to leave the gallbladder at a point on the left side rather than at the apex.

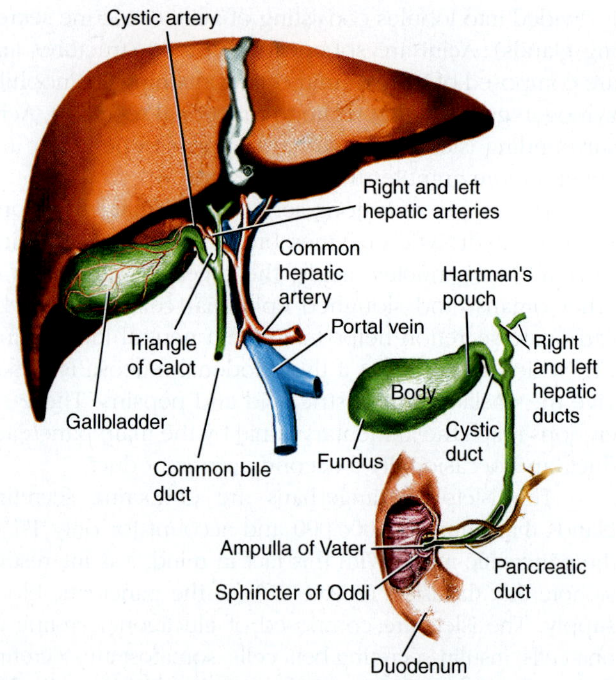

Figure 14-7 Gallbladder, bile ducts, and porta hepatis

The gallbladder has four tissue layers. The outer serosa covers all of the fundus but only the inferior surface of the remainder of the gallbladder. The perimuscular (subserosal) layer is connective tissue and adipose peritoneal tissue. The fibromuscular layer of the gallbladder contains smooth muscle arranged in longitudinal, circular, and oblique bundles. The innermost mucosa is generally a yellowish-brown color with a corrugated honeycomb appearance. Mucosal folds are evident only when the gallbladder walls are relaxed and disappear with distention. The mucosa actively absorbs water and solutes from the bile it collects from the liver and concentrates it. In the neck of the gallbladder these mucosal folds convolute obliquely into a spiral pattern.

The cystic duct is a tubular structure that connects the neck of the gallbladder to the CBD. The cystic duct can vary considerably in length (0.5 to 8 cm) and circumference (3 to 12 mm) but ultimately connects with the hepatic duct to form the CBD. The mucosa of the cystic duct has 10 to 14 successively crescentic folds that appear as a spiral valve (valves of Heister), which respond to changes in intraductal pressure and thereby control the flow of bile in either direction.

The CBD is formed by a junction of the cystic and hepatic ducts and varies in length from 5 to 17 cm on its path to the duodenum. It is between 3 and 15 mm wide and has a lumen 9 to 11 mm in diameter. The mucosa of the CBD is continuous with that of the cystic and hepatic ducts but it has no distinct muscle layer. The distal CBD courses behind the upper border of the pancreatic head, passing through its parenchyma to join with the pancreatic duct to form the ampulla of Vater in the duodenum. Although the singular ampulla of Vater usually enters the duodenum at a point 8 to 10 cm distal to the pylorus, in about 10–15% of the population the pancreatic ducts and CBD open into the duodenum independently along various points of the duodenal length. The sphincter of Oddi, which has a thick coat of longitudinal and circular smooth muscle, controls flow of bile into the duodenum.

Blood supply to the gallbladder is through the cystic artery, right hepatic artery, and the posterior superior pancreaticoduodenal artery. Veins draining the upper ductile system and the gallbladder course into the liver while those draining the lower ductile system flow into the portal vein. The lymphatic pathways follow the venous system collecting first at the nodes around the cystic duct and then anastomose with the lymphatics of the pancreas and eventually go to the nodes at the porta hepatis.

The gallbladder receives its parasympathetic vagal innervation from the submucosal and myenteric plexuses common to the alimentary canal. Sympathetic innervation reaches the gallbladder and bile ducts via the splanchnic nerve and hepatic plexus. The nerves have motor and sensory function and communicate with fibers of the right phrenic nerve, which is thought to explain "referred" shoulder pain with gallbladder disease.

GENERAL SURGERY INSTRUMENTATION

Instrumentation varies widely with geographic region, hospital availability, and surgeon's preference. Many factors influence the selection of instrumentation both for the facility and the surgeon. For this reason, the instrumentation lists that follow are basic and relatively standard. This is intended to provide the student with a starting point from which to learn the instrumentation of general surgery.

MAJOR SET

The foundation set for many surgical procedures is the *major laparotomy set* (Table 14-1).

Many types and sizes of retractors are used in general surgery. An illustrative sample is shown in Figure 14-8.

MINOR SET

The intent of the major laparotomy set is to provide instrumentation for almost any procedure that can be performed in the abdominal cavity. In fact, most thoracic,

Table 14-1 Major Laparotomy Set

Yankauer suction tip	1 ea.
Poole suction tip	1 ea.
8″, 10″, and 12″ DeBakey forceps	2 ea.
#3, #4, and #7 knife handles	1 ea.
Mayo scissors straight	1 ea.
Mayo scissors curved	1 ea.
7″ and 9″ Metzenbaum scissors	1 ea.
Ferris-Smith forceps	2 ea.
Adson tissue forceps with teeth	2 ea.
Russian tissue forceps	2 ea.
Cushing tissue forceps	2 ea.
Halsted mosquito forceps curved	6 ea.
Crile forceps 5½″ curved	12 ea.
Rochester-Pean forceps 8″	6 ea.
Rochester-Ochsner forceps 6¼″	4 ea.
Mixter forceps 7¼″ curved	1 ea.
Mixter forceps 9″	1 ea.
Baby Mixter forceps 5¼″ curved	1 ea.
Backhaus towel clamp	8 ea.
Foerster sponge forceps	2 ea.
Mayo-Hegar needle holder 6″	2 ea.
Mayo-Hegar needle holder 7″	2 ea.
Mayo-Hegar needle holder 8″	2 ea.
Mayo-Hegar needle holder 10½″	2 ea.
Goelet retractor	2 ea.
U.S. Army retractor	2 ea.
Ribbon retractor ¾″	1 ea.
Ribbon retractor 1¼″	1 ea.
Deaver retractor 1″	1 ea.
Deaver retractor 2″	1 ea.
Richardson retractor, small	2 ea.
Richardson retractor, large	1 ea.
Kelly retractor, 2½″	1 ea.
Balfour retractor and blades	1 ea.
Lahey gall duct forceps 7½″	2 ea.
Allis tissue forceps 6″	2 ea.
Allis tissue forceps 10″	2 ea.
Babcock tissue forceps 6¼″	2 ea.
Babcock tissue forceps 9¼″	2 ea.
Stainless steel ruler	1 ea.
Schnidt tonsil forceps 7½″	2 ea.

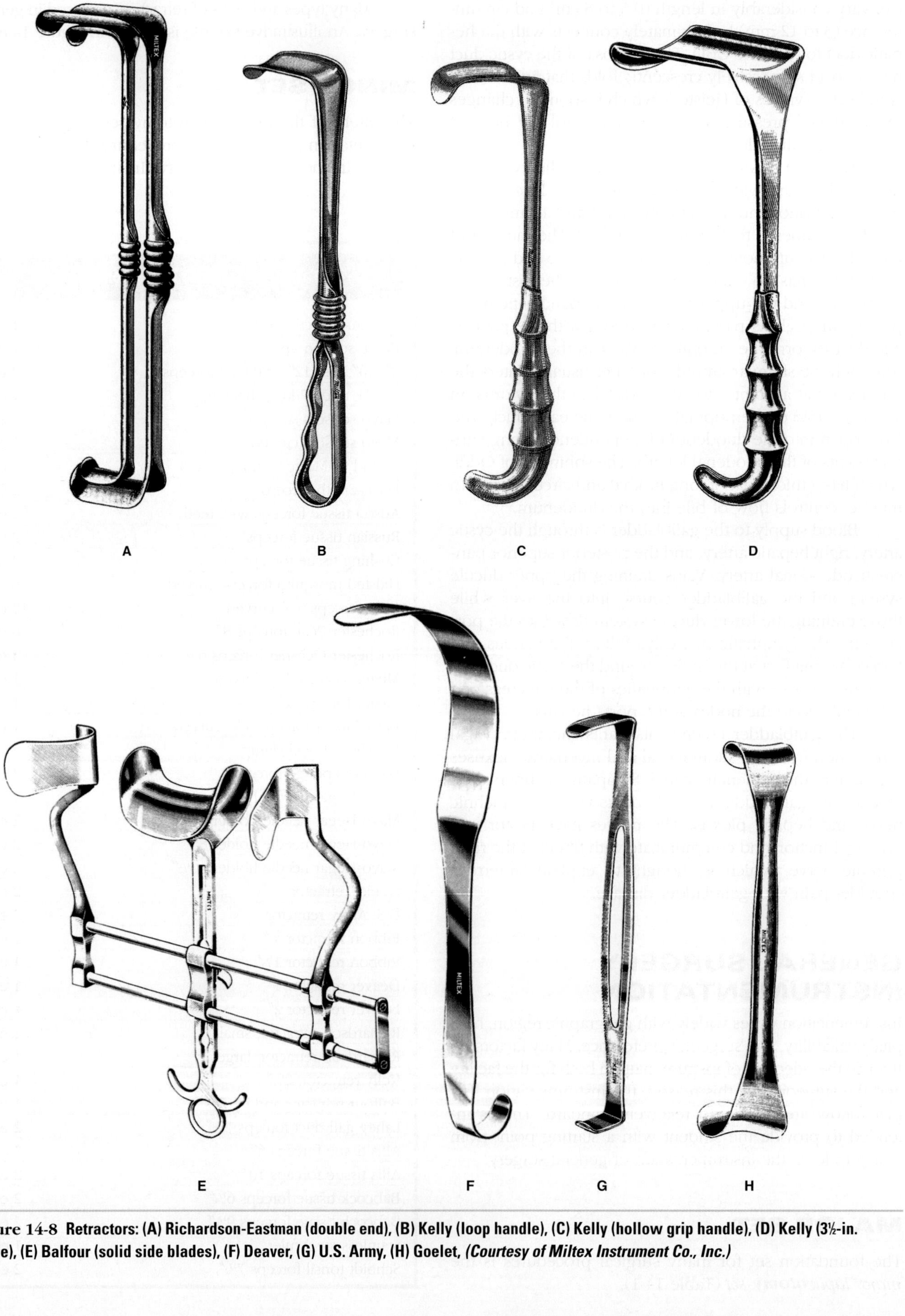

Figure 14-8 **Retractors: (A) Richardson-Eastman (double end), (B) Kelly (loop handle), (C) Kelly (hollow grip handle), (D) Kelly (3½-in. blade), (E) Balfour (solid side blades), (F) Deaver, (G) U.S. Army, (H) Goelet,** ***(Courtesy of Miltex Instrument Co., Inc.)***

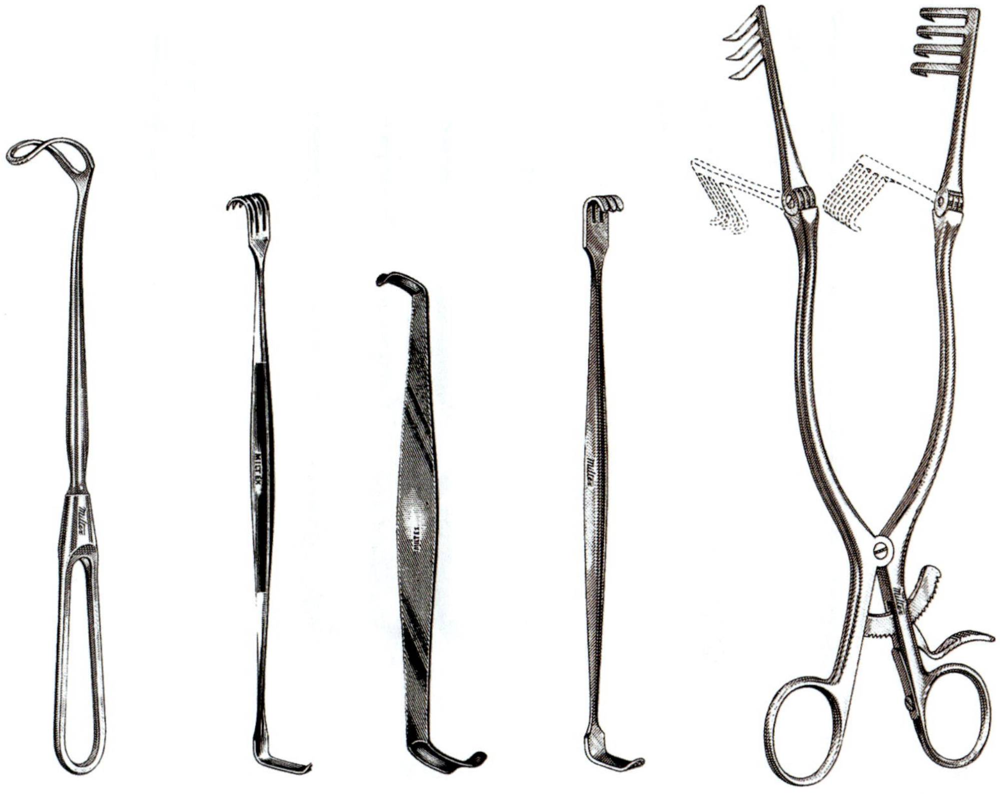

Figure 14-8 *(continued)* **(I) Green, (J) Senn, (K) Crile, (L) Mathieu, (M) Beckman-Weitlaner** *(Courtesy of Miltex Instrument Co., Inc.)*

vascular, gynecologic, and genitourinary surgery can be performed with the basic major laparotomy set. Many common procedures do not require the same amount of instrumentation. Most hospitals will have a less extensive instrument set called a *minor set* (Table 14-2).

Table 14-2 General Surgery – Minor Set

Yankauer suction tip	1 ea.
#3 knife handles	2 ea.
Mayo scissors straight	1 ea.
Mayo scissors curved	1 ea.
7″ Metzenbaum scissors	1 ea.
Adson tissue forceps with teeth	2 ea.
Halsted mosquito forceps curved	6 ea.
Crile forceps 5½″ curved	6 ea.
Backhaus towel clamp	6 ea.
Foerster sponge forceps	2 ea.
Mayo-Hegar needle holder 6″	2 ea.
Mayo-Hegar needle holder 7″	2 ea.
U.S. Army retractor	2 ea.
Allis tissue forceps 6″	2 ea.
Babcock tissue forceps 6¼″	2 ea.
Probe with eye 5½″	1 ea.
Grooved director with probe tip 5½″	1 ea.
Senn retractor, double ended, sharp	2 ea.
Volkman retractor 3 prong	2 ea.
Frazier Ferguson suction tip	1 ea.
Schnidt hemostatic forceps	2 ea.

LOCAL EXCISION INSTRUMENTS

Small instrument sets may be used for local excision. These instrument sets consist of most of the instruments in the minor set with the addition of some "plastic surgery" instruments.

BILIARY INSTRUMENTS

For exploring the common bile duct a variety of ductal (Randall stone) forceps and stone "scoops" (Mayo, Moynihan, or Moore) are available. The surgeon may also request Potts scissors for opening the duct, a Lahey duct forceps to clamp the duct, and a set of sequentially sized ductal dilators (Bakes #3–#10). To decompress the gallbladder, an Ochsner gallbladder trocar is used. A sample of biliary instruments is shown in Figure 14-9.

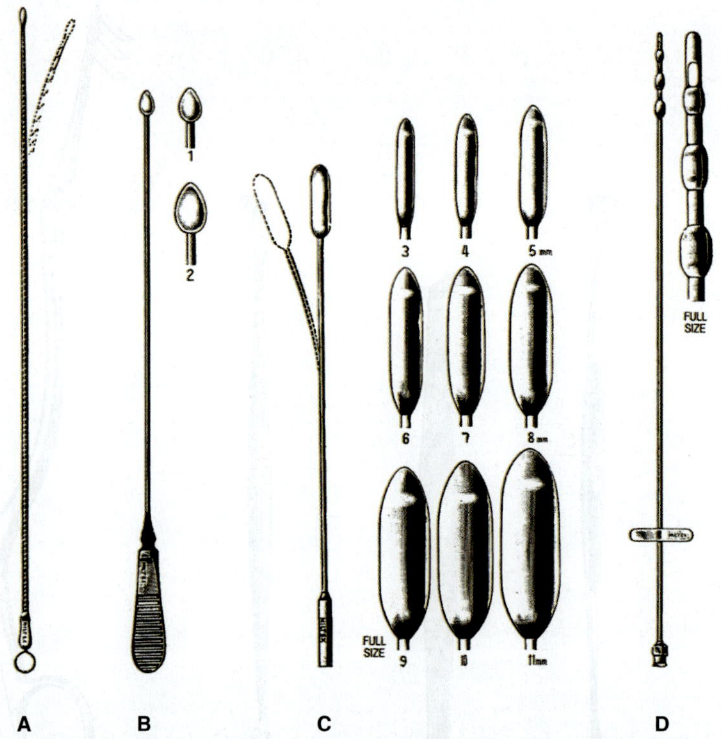

Figure 14-9 **Gallbladder instruments: (A) Ochsner (Fenger) gall duct probe, (B) Mayo common duct probe, (C) Bakes common duct dilator set, (D) Mixter irrigating dilaprobe** ***(Courtesy of Miltex Instrument Co., Inc.)***

INTESTINAL INSTRUMENTS

Intestinal instruments include a variety of bowel clamps, such as Payr, Allen, Doyen, or Best, as well as stapling devices such as the linear stapler, linear cutter, and the circular stapler with accompanying sizers and circular suturing devices (refer to Chapter 11). An intestinal set may also include extra forceps and an extra Poole-type suction tip for intraluminal work. A sample of intestinal instruments is shown in Figure 14-10.

OTHER GENERAL INSTRUMENTS

Some procedures require specific and unique instrumentation. These include items such as triple tenaculums for grasping large breast masses, ligature carriers to pass sutures in tight spaces (as in low sigmoid resections), esophageal (Maloney) dilators (bougie), liver retractors, and clamps. Skin staplers are commonly used.

ROOM SETUP

For most general surgery procedures, a standard OR table with Trendelenburg capability is suitable. Anesthesia personnel are invariably positioned at the head of the table.

POSITIONING

Supine is the position of choice for most surgery of the abdominal cavity or the breast. Arms are usually placed on armboards at less than a 90° angle to the body. The patient restraint (safety strap) is applied over the anterior thighs and secured to each side of the OR table. Because access to the operative site is mandatory, cases such as excision of a lip**oma** on the back or flank may require lateral or "rolled" positioning. Anal surgery can be performed in lithotomy, lateral, or jackknife position. Positioning devices, such as kidney rests, sandbags, or rolls may be necessary for cases in which a corkscrew position is required. This aligns the upper body at a 45° tilt and the rest of the trunk in lateral, and is used for thoracoabdominal approaches for extensive esophageal surgery.

DRAPING

The majority of draping requirements for general surgery are for laparotomy draping. Some procedures require lithotomy, and some, extremity draping. Draping procedures are covered in detail in Chapter 12. Minor procedures require the use of towels to square drape an operative area and covering the area with the appropriately sized fenestrated sheet.

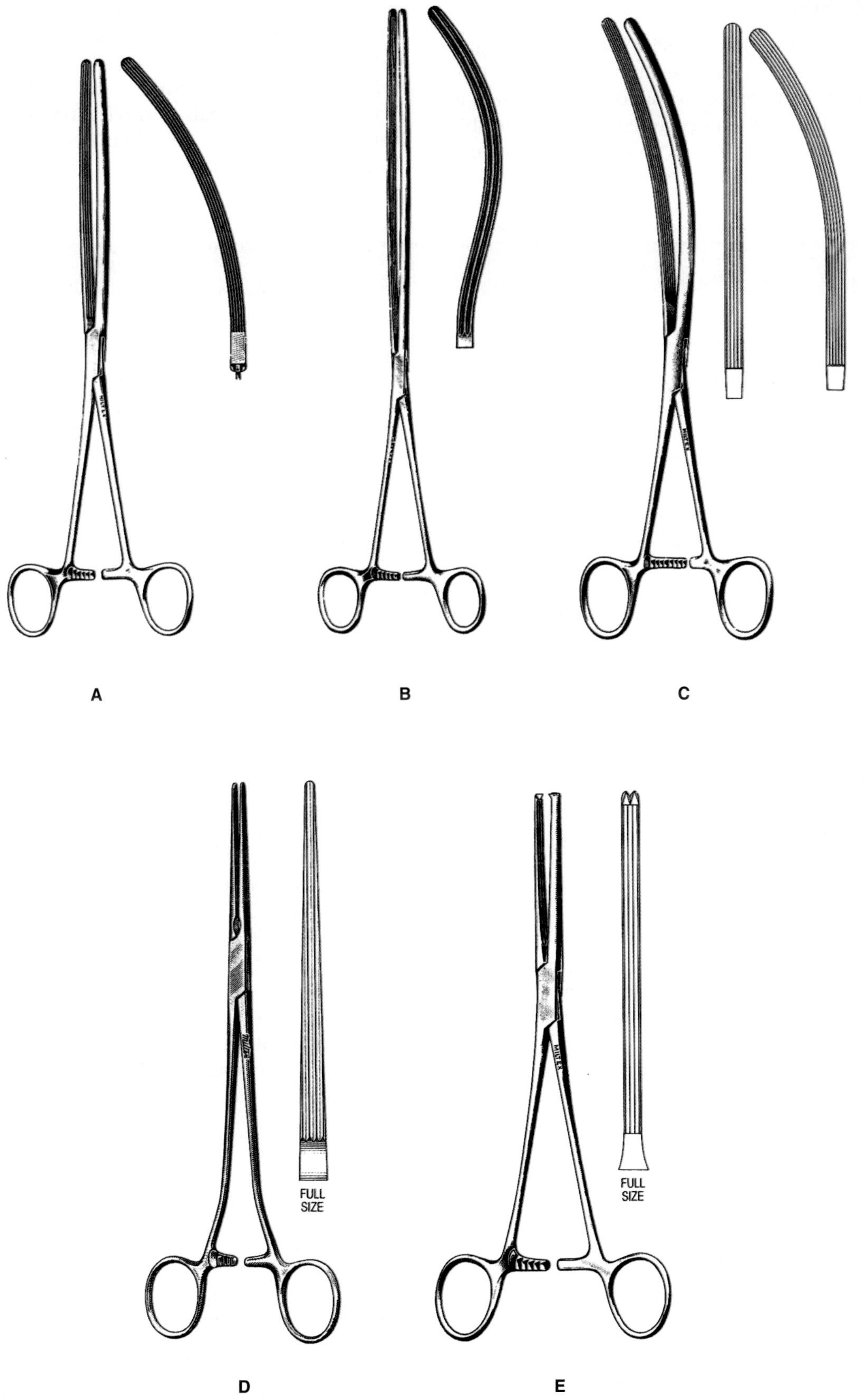

Figure 14-10 **Intestinal instruments: (A) Doyen forceps, (B) Kocher forceps, (C) Mayo-Robson forceps, (D) Dennis clamp, (E) Allen clamp** ***(Courtesy of Miltex Instrument Co., Inc.)***

INCISIONS

In general surgery a variety of incisions are used to gain access to the abdominal contents (Table 14-3). The type chosen depends on the access desired, the procedure to be performed, the surgeon's preference, the extensibility, and wound security. Other considerations include the patient's physical condition, speed of entry required, and sites of previous surgery. The types of incisions are vertical (median or midline, paramedian, supraumbilical, and infraumbilical), transverse, oblique (oblique lateral, McBurney "muscle-splitting," and Kocher subcostal), and thoracoabdominal. Complications of wounds and their closure include infection, herniation, disruption, pain, and nerve damage.

Table 14-3 Abdominal Incisions

VERTICAL INCISION—MEDIAN

Use
- Access to any organ in the abdominal cavity
- Ventral herniorrhaphy
- Trauma

Advantages
- Provide good access
- Can be extended caudad or cephalad
- Provide rapid entry into the abdomen
- Least hemorrhagic

Disadvantages
- Wide scar formation
- Highest incidence of wound disruption (dehiscence) and postoperative herniation

Types
- Epigastric (supraumbilical)
- Subumbilical
- Full midline—a combination of the two, curving around the umbilicus and extending from a point below the xiphoid to a point above the symphysis pubis

Opening Technique
- Skin and subcutaneous tissue incised in a line over the linea alba
- Small bleeding vessels "bleeders" are coagulated
- Linea alba and extraperitoneal fat incised to the peritoneum
- Peritoneum entered at a point closest to the umbilicus to avoid injury to the bladder below or the falciform ligament above

Closing Technique
- Closed in layers
- Peritoneum closed separately with a continuous 2–0 absorbable suture or incorporated with other layers
- Fascia closed #0 or #1 braided nonabsorbable sutures placed 1 cm apart
- Skin closed with 4–0 nylon, 4–0 subcuticular absorbable sutures, or skin staples

Variations
- Trauma: the entire thickness of the wound, from peritoneum to skin, may be closed in one layer, called "through-and-through"
- Tissue layers up to the skin are incorporated as one layer, using running #2 polypropylene sutures
- Subcutaneous tissue and skin may be left open to heal by granulation, or for "delayed" closure 3 to 5 days later

VERTICAL INCISION-PARAMEDIAN

Use
- Same as median except for trauma
- Lower left excellent for sigmoid surgery

Advantages
- Better wound strength than median
- Better cosmesis
- Lower incidence of incisional herniation

Disadvantages
- Increased intraoperative bleeding
- Increased infection rates
- Greater postoperative pain
- Nerve damage
- Atrophy of the rectus abdominus muscle

Types
- Upper (may require an oblique extension toward the xiphoid)
- Lower
- Lateral (junction of the middle and outer thirds of the rectus sheath)

Opening Technique
- Skin and subcutaneous tissue incised to the anterior rectus sheath
- Anterior rectus dissected away from the muscle
- Rectus muscle retracted laterally
- Posterior rectus sheath and peritoneum are incised in the same plane as the anterior sheath

Closing Technique
- Peritoneum and posterior rectus sheath are closed as one layer, 2–0 or 0 absorbable suture
- Anterior sheath closed, 0 absorbable or nonabsorbable
- Subcutaneous tissue may be approximated with interrupted 3–0 catgut or similar suture
- Skin closed as in median incision

OBLIQUE INCISION—GENERAL FEATURES

Use
- Access to specific structures, especially those located laterally in the abdominal cavity

Advantages
- Access to specific organ(s)
- Strong closure

Table 14-3 *(continued)*

Disadvantages
Hemorrhagic
Muscle splitting
May endanger nerves

Types
Subcostal (Kocher)
McBurney's
Lateral

OBLIQUE INCISION—MCBURNEY'S

Use
Access to the appendix and extraperitoneal drainage of an abscess

Opening Technique
Obliquely downward and inward over "McBurney's point," the junction of the middle and outer third of the line that joins the umbilicus and the anterior superior iliac spine
External oblique muscle is divided in the direction of its fibers
Small incision is made in the underlying internal oblique adjacent to the rectus sheath
The opening is then spread with the tips of scissors until it is big enough to allow two fingers to be placed within
Small retractors (e.g., U.S. Army or small Richardson) are then placed to retract the muscle and expose the peritoneum
Peritoneum is grasped with forceps, incised, and the resultant hole is spread with the index finger, creating a circular opening
Note: A variation of this incision is the Rocky-Davis incision, which encounters the same abdominal structures, but runs more transversely.
Note: If further surgery (e.g., colon resection) is needed, the entire incision can be extended in either a medial or lateral direction.

Closing Technique
Begins with a "pursestring" closure of the peritoneum, or by incorporating the peritoneum with the transversalis fascia in a running closure with 2–0 absorbable suture
Transverse abdominis and internal oblique may be approximated with two or three interrupted 2–0 absorbable sutures
External oblique approximated with 2–0 absorbable or polypropylene sutures
Subcutaneous tissues may be closed with interrupted 3–0 or 4–0 absorbable sutures
Skin is closed with a subcuticular 4–0 suture or skin staples

OBLIQUE INCISION—KOCHER SUBCOSTAL

Use
Biliary tract (right) and spleen (left)

Opening Technique
Incision begins at the midline 2.5 to 5 cm below the xiphoid and extends obliquely lateral about 12 cm, staying 2.5 cm below the costal margin
Rectus sheath and muscle are divided electrosurgically
Underlying lateral musculature is incised in an outward direction for a short distance and retracted to expose the peritoneum
The small eighth dorsal nerve may be divided; however, the ninth dorsal nerve must be preserved to prevent subsequent weakening of the abdominal musculature
Peritoneum is incised the length of the incision

Closing Technique
Peritoneum and fascia closed with 0 synthetic absorbable or nonabsorbable suture
Subcutaneous tissue may be approximated with 2–0 absorbable suture
Skin is closed with interrupted 4–0 nylon subcuticularly, or with staples

TRANSVERSE INCISION

Use
Curved transverse upper abdominal incision is used for access to the pancreas and abdominal exploration in cases of blunt trauma
Lower transverse incision used for access to pelvic viscera

Advantages
Access to specific organ(s)
Strong closure

Disadvantages
Hemorrhagic
Muscle splitting
May endanger nerves

Types
Upper transverse (a bilateral subcostal incision that is joined through the midline)
Lower transverse (Pfannenstiel, Maylard, and Cherney; see Chapter 15)

Opening Technique
Upper transverse: incised bilaterally as described in the subcostal incision, and joined at the midline
Lower transverse: see Chapter 15

(continues)

Table 14-3 *(continued)*

Closing Technique
Peritoneum and fascia closed with 0 absorbable or nonabsorbable suture
Subcutaneous tissue may be approximated with a 2–0 absorbable suture
Skin closed with interrupted or running 4–0 nylon suture, subcuticularly or with staples

THORACOABDOMINAL

Use
Converts the pleural and peritoneal spaces into one cavity, and is used when particular access is required for extensive esophagogastric surgery (left) or emergency hepatic resection (right)

Advantages
Access to specific organ(s)
Access to both pleural and peritoneal spaces

Disadvantages
Difficult patient positioning
Hemorrhagic
Same as median
Same as thoracic (requires chest tube)
Difficult for patient postoperatively

Opening Technique
Incision begins as a standard midline or left upper paramedian incision
Extended obliquely over the thorax along the eighth costal interspace
Diaphragm is divided radially toward the esophageal hiatus for as far as necessary

Closing Technique
Begins with repair of the diaphragm with #1 silk
A chest tube is placed through a stab wound in the ninth intercostal space along the posterior axillary line
Standard closure of the chest
Standard median or paramedian closure

Incisions are illustrated in Figure 14-11.

SURGERY OF THE ABDOMINAL WALL: HERNIAS

A hernia (Latin for "rupture"; Greek for "bud") is defined as a protrusion of a viscus through an opening in the wall of the cavity in which it is contained. The hernial orifice is the defect in the abdominal wall and the hernia sac is the outpouching of the peritoneum. A hernia is termed external if it protrudes through the abdominal wall, interparietal if the sac is contained within the abdominal wall, and internal if the hernia is within the visceral cavity. A hernia may be congenital, acquired, or a combination thereof.

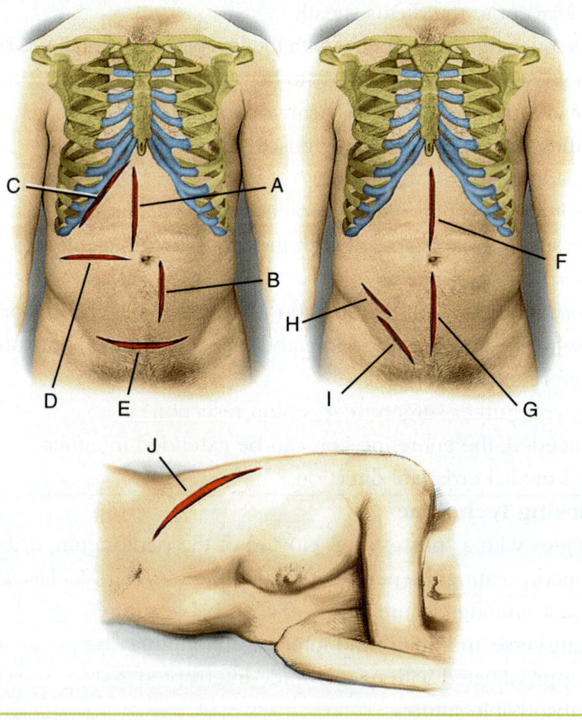

Figure 14-11 Abdominal incision options: (A) Right upper paramedian, (B) left lower paramedian, (C) right subcostal, (D) right midline transverse, (E) Pfannenstiel, (F) upper longitudinal midline, (G) lower longitudinal midline, (H) McBurney's, (I) right inguinal oblique, (J) right thoracoabdominal

SPECIFIC ANATOMICAL FEATURES OF THE GROIN AREA

The tissue layers encountered in groin herniation repair are, in order of descent, skin and subcutaneous tissues, Scarpa's fascia, innominate fascia, external oblique muscle, inguinal ligament, interparietal fascia, internal oblique muscle, transverse abdominis muscle, transversalis fascia, Cooper's ligament, rectus abdominis muscle, and peritoneum. Within these tissue layers are other structures such as the superficial and inferior epigastric vessels, the iliofemoral vessels, the spermatic cord and its blood supply, and the ilioinguinal nerve. Other pertinent structures include the lacunar ligament, the inguinal (Poupart) ligament, the conjoined ligament (falx inguinalis), the cremaster muscle and fascia, Hesselbach's triangle, the femoral canal, and the iliopubic tract.

Scarpa's fascia is a homogenous membranous sheet attached to the iliac crest, linea alba, and pubis that is intimate with the subcutaneous tissues. The innominate fascia separates the aponeurosis of the external oblique muscle from the overlying tissues and contains the intercrural fibers. The fasciae situated between the external and internal obliques and between the internal and transverse abdominis muscles are termed interparietal and are the zones for interparietal (interstitial) herniation.

Transversalis fascia is the main focus of groin herniation and separates the abdominal musculature from the preperitoneal fat. This structure is a continuation of the fascia completely containing the abdominal cavity and is inherently weak in the area of Cooper's ligament and the iliopubic tract, lending to inguinal herniation. Cooper's ligament is reinforced periosteum of the pubis and is important in the repair of both femoral and direct inguinal hernias.

The inguinal canal is made up of the superficial (internal) and deep (external) inguinal rings. At the level of the skin, the internal inguinal ring is located superolateral to the pubic tubercle, and the deep inguinal ring is located halfway between the symphysis pubis and the iliac spine along the abdominocrural crease. The inguinal canal passes obliquely medial from the internal ring to the external ring, serving as passage for the spermatic cord.

Femoral hernias are more common in females than males due to anatomical differences in the femoral area. A muscular vascular outlet (fossa ovalis) of the pelvis into the thigh permits passage of the iliopsoas muscle, blood vessels, nerves, and lymphatics supplying the lower extremity. This outlet is bounded posteriorly by the ilium, anteriorly by the pubis, and medially by the rectus muscle. Anteriorly, the iliopubic tract, running beneath the deep inguinal ring, overlies this triangle (femoral canal).

The femoral sheath is divided into three compartments. The smallest is the medial compartment, which constitutes the femoral canal. The iliopubic tract, which is connected to the transversalis fascia, defines the medial border of the femoral canal. Cooper's ligament and the femoral vein demarcate the other boundaries.

HERNIAS

The anatomical features of the abdomen and the various types of pathology result in several different but recognizable types of hernia. These are summarized in Table 14-4.

Indirect, direct, and femoral distinctions are illustrated in Figure 14-12.

HERNIA REPAIR

All hernia repairs have some common goals and the procedures have some common features, also. These are listed in Table 14-5.

INGUINAL HERNIORRHAPHY

The classic procedures that remain in current use are

- *Marcy repair:* Simple closure of the inguinal ring
- *Bassini or Bassini-Shouldice repair:* A new inguinal canal is made by uniting the edge of the internal oblique muscle to the inguinal ligament
- *McVay/Lotheissen:* The transversus abdominis muscle and its associated fasciae (transversus layer) are sutured to the pectineal ligament (Cooper's ligament repair)

The repairs have the same intentions and differ only to the extent to which the myopectineal orifice is repaired (Table 14-6). Endoscopic approaches are increasingly common today. These approaches typically place a synthetic mesh over the defect. The mesh may or may not be sutured or stapled in place. Figure 14-13 illustrates this technique with a mesh repair of the defect.

OTHER HERNIA REPAIRS

Other repairs follow the same principles as the inguinal hernia: Identify the structures, reduce the hernia, and repair the defect. They vary only in location and the unique problems created by the size of the defect and the contents of the sac.

PEARL OF WISDOM

A Penrose drain is often used to retract the spermatic cord. Wet the drain in normal saline immediately prior to use.

Table 14-4 Hernia Types

TYPE	FEATURES: ANATOMICAL LOCATION
Groin	Hernias of the inguinal and femoral areas
	Inguinal: above the abdominocrural crease (>95% male)
	Femoral: below the abdominocrural crease (97% female)
Ventral	Present on the anterior abdominal wall at any point other than the groin
	May present along the linea alba (epigastric, umbilical, and hypogastric) or at the semilunar lines (Spigelian hernia)
Incisional	Hernias at sites of previous surgery and at stomal sites
Diaphragmatic	Hernias in the diaphragm, usually at the esophageal hiatus

TYPE	FEATURES: CONDITION
Reducible	Manual manipulation (taxis) can return the hernia contents to the abdominal cavity
Irreducible or incarcerated	Manual manipulation (taxis) cannot return the hernia contents to the abdominal cavity
Strangulated	Hernia with luminal viscera entrapment that compromises the vascularity of the viscera
Richter's	Incarcerated or strangulated bowel spontaneously reduces and the subsequent gangrenous portion of bowel may be overlooked during hernia repair
Sliding	The abdominal viscera forms part of the hernia sac
Direct	Inguinal hernia
	Acquired type
	Presents through Hesselbach's triangle (bounded by the inguinal ligament, the inferior epigastric vessels, and the lateral border of the rectus abdominis)
Indirect	Inguinal hernia
	Congenital type
	Follows congenital defects that dilate the internal inguinal ring and pass through the deep inguinal ring to the scrotum
	Hernia sac is generally confined to the spermatic cord and the posterior inguinal wall remains intact
Pantaloon	Indirect inguinal hernia
	Peritoneum protrudes on either or both side(s) of the inferior epigastric vessels
Femoral	Sacs originate from the femoral canal through a defect in the medial femoral sheath and emerge through the fossa ovalis into the subcutaneous tissues of the thigh, inferior to the inguinal ligament
	Lymph nodes in this area are commonly caught in the hernia sac forming a palpable mass
	Prone to incarceration and strangulation
Epigastric	Midline hernias above the umbilicus
Hypogastric	Midline hernias below the umbilicus
Umbilical	In children: usually congenital; often spontaneously close
	In adults: usually acquired
	Occur in women at a rate three times that of men and are associated with recurrent pregnancy and obesity
	Hernia consists of a peritoneal sac (or sacs) and its contents (omentum or abdominal viscera) protruding through the umbilical ring

CATEGORY	INCIDENCE
Hernias by region	75% inguinal
Hernias by type	50% indirect, inguinal
	24% direct, inguinal
	10% incisional & ventral
	3% femoral
	5–10% other/unusual
Hernias by gender	Vast majority are male
	25% of males develop an inguinal hernia
	2% of females develop an inguinal hernia
Hernias by side	More frequent on right than left

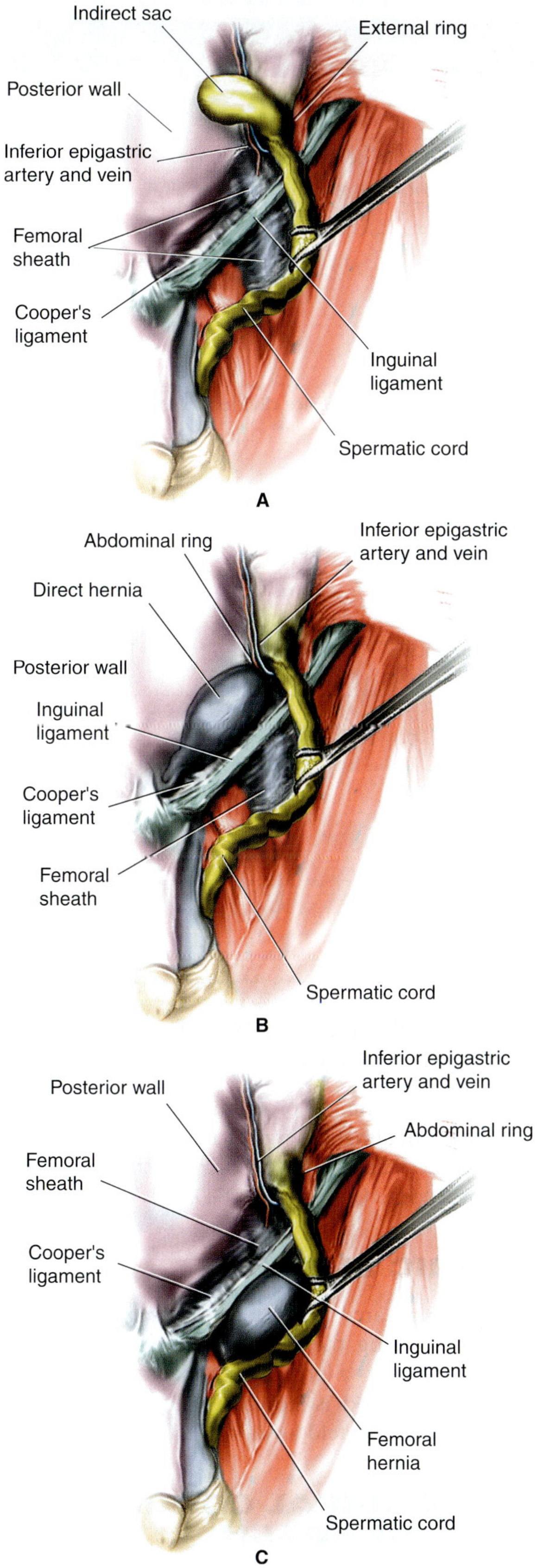

Figure 14-12 Hernia types: (A) Indirect inguinal, (B) direct inguinal, (C) femoral

Table 14-5 Common Features of Hernia Repairs

Instrumentation	Minor instrumentation set
Position	Supine
Prep	Varies with position of hernia
Drape	• Varies with position of hernia • Fenestrated laparotomy sheet or minor sheet over incision site
Anesthesia	• Local • Local with mild sedation—monitored anesthesia care (MAC) • General
Principles	• Identify structures • Protect neural and vascular structures • Free herniated structures and return them to normal anatomical position • Close defect
Postoperative	• Normal wound care • Patient directed not to strain (increases intra-abdominal pressure)
Complications	• Recurrence • Nerve injury • Ischemic orchitis and testicular atrophy • Loss of bowel function • Infection • Complications associated with all open procedures (e.g., hemorrhage, infection)

SURGERY OF THE ALIMENTARY CANAL

The digestive tract is susceptible to internal and external influences. The digestive system constitutes the major portion of surgery performed by the general surgeon. The alimentary canal shares a common structural feature throughout its course, namely, it is tubular in shape. Surgical procedures on the digestive tract must consider this tubular structure. Many of the procedures appear to be variations on a common theme because of the anatomical nature of the digestive tract. This section will look at surgery of the alimentary canal moving from cephalad to caudad.

Table 14-6 Classic Inguinal Hernia Repairs

FEATURE	COMMONALITIES AND DETAILS
Intent	• Preserve the shutter mechanism of the deep inguinal ring • Maintain the oblique orientation of the inguinal canal
Incision	• All use an anterior groin incision
Classic techniques: three stages	• Dissection • Repair • Closure
Procedural steps: open repair	• Inguinal canal is opened • Ilioinguinal nerve is preserved • Cremaster muscle and neurovascular bundle are divided to expose the inguinal ring • Spermatic cord is mobilized • Exposure of the parietal defect in the innermost aponeurotic fascial layer • Elimination of the hernia sac • Cord lipoma removed • Relaxing incision made if needed • Reconstruction of inguinal ring • Replacement of anatomical structures • Closure
Procedural steps: endoscopic approach	• Normal endoscopic approach • Identification of structures and defect • Reduction of hernia contents • Placement of prosthetic mesh • Suturing or stapling of mesh (optional) • Removal of instrumentation and closure
Outcome factors	• Quality of surgery • Integrity of tissues • Tension on suture line

SURGERY OF THE ESOPHAGUS

The esophagus provides a muscular conduit for the passage of material from the mouth to the stomach and vice versa. The esophagus is a muscular tube originating at the level of the cricoid cartilage and terminating with the fundus of the stomach. The esophagus has no serosal layer. This fact has a direct bearing on pathology and surgical intervention. The esophagus is easily perforated and difficult to reconstruct.

ESOPHAGEAL PATHOLOGY

Pathological conditions of the esophagus fall into four major categories: hiatal hernia and reflux esophagitis, esophageal motility disorders, neoplasms, and trauma (Table 14-7).

SURGICAL INTERVENTION ON THE ESOPHAGUS

The anatomy and pathological conditions of the esophagus determine the type and means of surgical treatment available (Table 14-8).

LAPAROSCOPIC NISSEN FUNDOPLICATION

Acid reflux is a common problem. When uncontrolled by conservative treatment, surgical intervention is possible. The laparoscopic approach has become the preferred operative procedure (Procedure 14-1).

GASTRIC SURGERY

The alimentary canal continues its passage caudally with the stomach being the next anatomical structure. The stomach represents a large pouch-like structure in which the passage of food is slowed. The stomach also produces hydrochloric acid as part of the digestive process.

PATHOLOGICAL CONDITIONS OF THE STOMACH

The stomach is a common area for a number of complaints and conditions that eventually lead to surgery (Table 14-9).

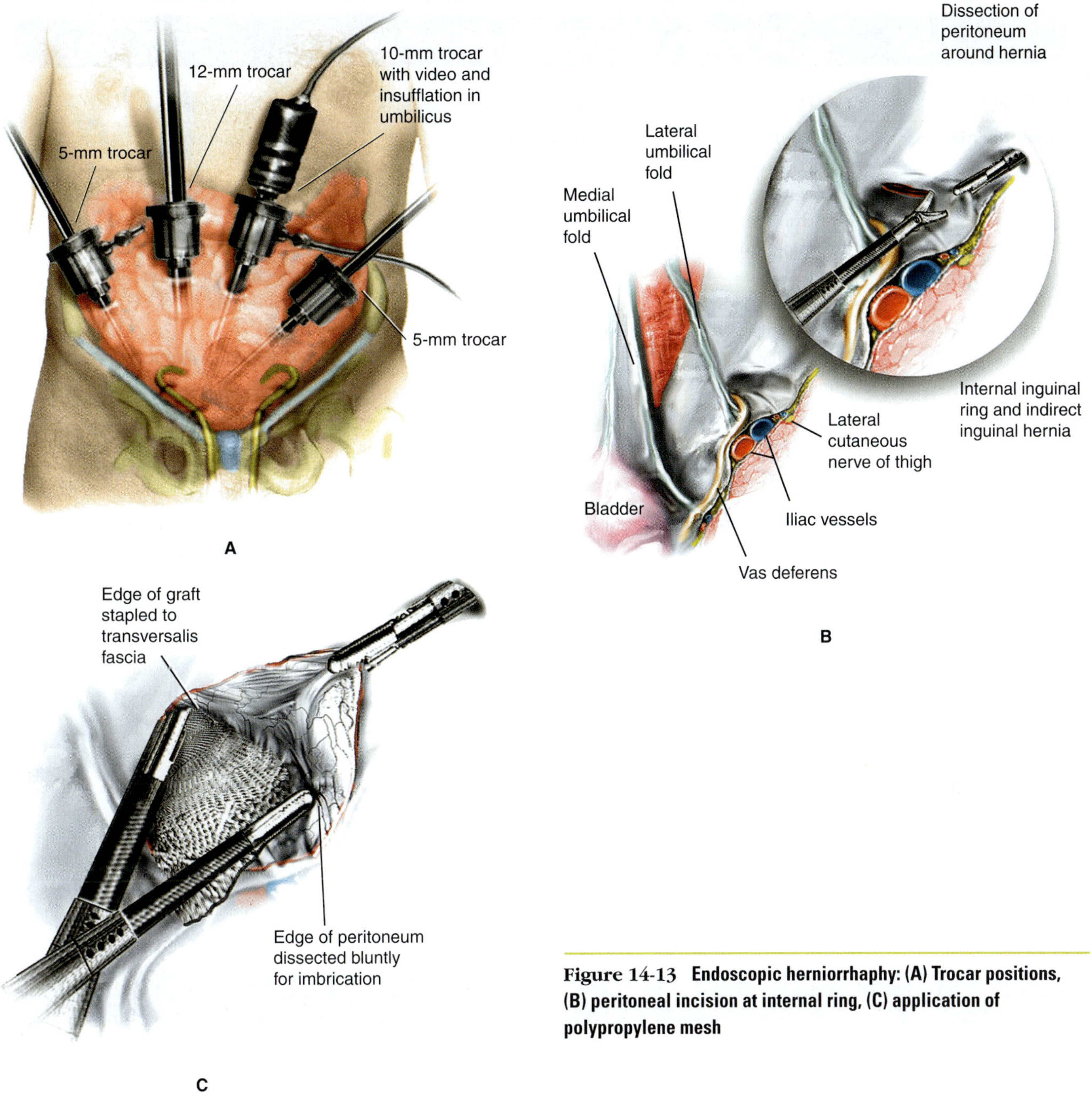

Figure 14-13 Endoscopic herniorrhaphy: (A) Trocar positions, (B) peritoneal incision at internal ring, (C) application of polypropylene mesh

PEARL OF WISDOM

Maloney dilators cannot be inserted from the sterile field. They are passed down the esophagus by the anesthesia provider. Be sure everyone knows where the Maloney dilators are and remind team members when you are nearing the time of use.

GASTROSTOMY

A gastr**ostomy** is the surgical creation of an opening (fistula tract) from the gastric mucosa to the skin and is performed to provide nutrition "feeding" to the patient or to decompress and drain the stomach. A gastrostomy may be lined with mucosa for long-term or permanent usage, or serosa for temporary measures, depending on technique. Often tumors of the larynx, pharynx, esophagus, and proximal

(Text continues on page 413)

Table 14-7 Pathology of the Esophagus

CONDITION	SYMPTOMS/SIGNS	DIAGNOSTICS	TREATMENTS
Hiatal hernia	• Acid reflux • Mucosal erosion, ulceration, scarring, stricture • Burning, non-radiating pain • Pain is positional	• History • Fluoroscopy during barium swallow • Endoscopy • Manometry	Medical treatment Surgical • Correction of anatomical defect • Reconstruction of valve mechanism in lower esophagus
Motility disorders	• Dysphagia • Regurgitation of undigested food	• X-ray with contrast medium • Cineradiography	Medical • Usually unhelpful
Achalasia	• Weight loss • Pain is uncommon • Aspiration pneumonia	• Manometry	Surgical • Invasive endoscopic procedure • Transection of the muscle
Diverticula	• Regurgitation of recently swallowed material • Choking • Foul breath odor	• X-ray with contrast medium	Surgical • Excision of diverticula • Correction of cause
Neoplasm (benign tumors are rare)	• Asymptomatic early • Dysphagia • Weight loss • Pain	• Barium contrast studies • CT scan	• May be limited to palliation • Radiotherapy • Tracheostomy • Extirpation of the esophagus • Reconstruction
Trauma	• Perforation (usually the result of instrumentation) • Ingestion of caustic substances	• Varies with type	Surgical • Immediate intervention

Table 14-8 Esophageal Surgery

PROCEDURE	PURPOSE
Endoscopic visualization and biopsy	Diagnostic procedure
Esophageal dilation	To correct esophageal stricture
Esophagomyotomy	Severance of the muscles at the esophagogastric junction to correct obstruction secondary to cardiospasm
Hiatal herniorrhaphy	Correction of defect and restoration of the cardioesophageal junction
Diverticulectomy	Removal of esophageal diverticulum
Esophagectomy	Removal of the esophagus (en bloc)
Esophagogastrostomy	Distal esophagectomy, removal of diseased lower esophagus and reconstruction of the union of esophagus and stomach

PROCEDURE 14-1 Laparoscopic Nissen Fundoplication

Equipment

- Video tower (typically includes monitor, processing unit for video camera, light source, VCR, printer for still photography)
- Insufflator
- Irrigation system
- Suction apparatus
- Electrosurgical unit with dispersive electrode

Instruments

- Laparoscopy instrumentation set (may include basic instrumentation, e.g., scalpel handle, tissue forceps, needle holders, hemostatic clamps), camera, variety of scopes (e.g., 0°, 30°), electrosurgical cord, insufflation tubing, connectors, and reusable laparoscopic instruments)
- Major instrumentation set (available)

Supplies

- Prep set
- Basic pack
- Basin set
- Gloves
- Laparotomy drapes (leggings, if needed)
- Blades: #11 or #15
- Electrosurgical pencil
- Disposable trocars (typically, 10 mm × 3, 5 mm × 2)
- Disposable laparoscopic instruments (may include liver retractor, coagulation hook, grasping forceps × 2, ligating clip applier with clips of various sizes)
- Pharmaceuticals according to surgeon's preference
- Suture according to surgeon's preference (will likely include 2–0 silk for fundoplication)
- Dressing material according to surgeon's preference (typically elastic bandages)
- Lubricant
- Maloney dilators

Operative Preparation

Anesthesia

- General
- Lubricate and protect patient's eyes
- Local anesthetic may be used in conjunction with general anesthesia to minimize bleeding and postoperative pain

Position

- Supine with thighs abducted and slightly flexed (may require stirrups)
- 20° reverse Trendelenburg

Prep

- Insert Foley catheter, if ordered
- Shave may be necessary, especially for the male patient
- Prep from mid-chest to thighs and laterally as far as possible

Draping

- Apply leggings, if necessary
- Anticipated surgical area is outlined with towels secured with adhesive or towel clips
- Laparotomy sheet

(continues)

PROCEDURE 14-1 Laparoscopic Nissen Fundoplication *(continued)*

Practical Considerations

- X-rays and barium studies in room
- Check insufflator and video equipment prior to patient's arrival
- It may be necessary to sterilize delicate items (e.g., camera) just prior to the procedure
- Surgeon typically stands between the patient's legs, the surgical assistant on the patient's left, and the STSR on the patient's right
- Be prepared for rapid conversion to laparotomy, if complications arise

Operative Procedure	Technical Considerations
1. Five trocars are typically used in the following locations • Above umbilicus in midline • Right subcostal • Left subcostal • Between the umbilical and left subcostal • Under the xiphoid process • A 30° angled laparoscope is used in the periumbilical port	**1.** The probable order of trocar use is • 10 mm • 5 mm • 5 mm • 10 mm • 10 mm
2. Surgical assistant retracts left lobe of liver exposing esophageal hiatus.	**2.** Have liver retractor ready.
3. The lesser omentum is opened. Extra gastric vagal branches may be sacrificed. The right pillar of the hiatus is identified.	**3.** Have ready: • Laparoscopic scissors • Coagulation hook • Ligating clips
4. An incision is made into the peritoneum covering the phrenoesophageal ligament and the phrenogastric ligament is severed.	**4.** Have grasper and dissector of choice ready.
5. The right pillar of the crus is dissected until lower left pillar is reached.	**5.** Prepare grasping forceps of choice.
6. Grasping forceps are placed on the stomach and the stomach is retracted caudally and laterally.	**6.** Grasping forceps are placed through the uppermost port.
7. The left pillar is localized and the posterior vagus nerve identified. The retroesophageal areas are dissected.	**7.** Have ready: • Laparoscopic scissors • Coagulation hook • Ligating clips

PROCEDURE 14-1 Laparoscopic Nissen Fundoplication *(continued)*

Operative Procedure	Technical Considerations
8. The left pillar is dissected cephalad.	**8.** Prepare needle holder with 2–0 silk and have ready: • A second grasping forceps • Coagulation hook • Ligating clips
9. Grasping forceps are applied to stomach and counter traction is applied to expose gastrosplenic ligament. Vessels are isolated with coagulation hook and clipped.	**9.** Check with anesthesia provider to verify that Maloney dilators are ready.
10. The fundus is grasped and passed behind the esophagus and regrasped from other side. Maloney dilator introduced to prevent torsion or stricture.	**10.** Sutures are interrupted. Have scissors available.
11. Interrupted 2–0 silk sutures are placed through stomach and the anterior wall of the esophagus, creating the gastric "wrap." Maloney dilator is removed and replaced with nasogastric tube.	**11.** Anticipate use of 4 to 6 stitches. • Count
12. Hemo**stasis** is achieved; instruments removed; and the incisions are closed in normal laparoscopic manner.	**12.** Have dressing supplies ready.

Postoperative Considerations

Immediate Postoperative Care

- Transport to PACU

Prognosis

- Return to normal activities within 2–4 weeks

Complications

- Esophageal or gastric perforation
- Pleural perforation
- Conversion to laparotomy
- Dysphagia
- Necrosis of wrap
- Pulmonary infection
- Incisional hernia
- Wound infection
- Hemorrhage
- Failure to gain relief from preoperative complaint

stomach, as well as esophageal stricture, dictate this need. There are a variety of ways in which this fistula tract can be created, including placement of synthetic tubes (Stamm or Witzel procedures), rolling the gastric tissues into a tube (Spivak-Watsuji gastrostomy), raising a flap of gastric tissue (Janeway gastrostomy), and utilizing a transected portion of jejunum. A gastrostomy can be created by open, percutaneous, endoscopic, and laparoscopic means. The Stamm and Spivak-Watsuji methods are described here.

The Stamm gastrostomy is a temporary measure that can often be performed under local anesthesia. It is quick, has the widest application, and is technically easy to perform, providing sufficient venting of the stomach (Procedure 14-2).

One variation on the gastrostomy procedure that is used is the Spivak-Watsuji gastrostomy. The steps in this procedure are as follows:

1. An upper midline incision is made.
2. A "flap" of gastric wall full thickness is raised with its base toward the lesser curvature.
3. The flap is then "rolled" and sutured to form a tube.
4. The defect in the gastric wall is closed in layers around the tube.
5. Enfolded gastric mucosa forms a "valve" at the base of the tube to prevent gastric "reflux" through the gastrostomy tube.

Table 14-9 Pathologic Conditions of the Stomach

CONDITION	SYMPTOMS/SIGNS	DIAGNOSTICS	TREATMENTS
Gastric ulcer disease	• Epigastric pain radiating to the back • Pain on ingestion of food • Weight loss	• Upper GI series • Endoscopy • Biopsy to rule out malignancy	Medical • Dietary control • Medication control • Antacids Surgical • Vagotomy • Excision of ulcer
Gastritis	• Diffuse erythema • Mucosal disruption • Nausea • Vomiting • Bleeding	• History • Upper GI series • Endoscopy	• Withdrawal of noxious agents • Decompression of stomach • Antacids • H_2 blockers
Gastric polyp (rare)	• Typically asymptomatic	• Endoscopy	• Biopsy • Conservative treatment related to histological findings
Bezoar (mass of indigestible vegetable fiber)	• Pain • Indigestion	• History • Endoscopy	• Endoscopic removal • Surgical removal
Carcinoma	• Asymptomatic early • Weight loss • Epigastric pain • Dysphagia • Hematemesis • Melena	• Laboratory studies • Upper GI • Endoscopy • Biopsy	• Surgical resection
Lymphoma, leiomyoma, leiomyosarcoma	• Same as above	• Same as above	• Same as above • Benign have good results • Malignant, very poor results

6. The free end of the tubular stoma is secured to the abdominal wall at the skin.
7. A catheter can then be threaded through the stoma into the stomach as needed.

Endoscopic developments allow for another variation on the traditional gastrostomy, the percutaneous endoscopic gastrostomy (PEG). The procedure uses an industry prepared kit and the procedural steps are as follows:

1. Skin site exit point is one-third of the way between the midclavicular line at the rib margin and the umbilicus.
2. Placement site for gastrostomy incision is midstomach.
3. Pediatric gastroscope is introduced and the stomach is insufflated with air.
4. A finger is pressed into the abdominal wall and indentation of the stomach is observed through the endoscope.
5. Local anesthesia is injected at the incision site and a trocar needle is passed into the stomach.
6. Placement of the needle is confirmed visually and the trocar is removed.
7. A wire or nylon loop is passed through the needle and snared by a loop from the gastroscope.
8. The gastroscope is removed, pulling the snare out the patient's mouth where it is attached to the percutaneous gastrostomy tube.
9. The procedure is reversed, pulling the gastrostomy tube down the esophagus into the stomach with the proximal end being drawn through the stab incision and secured.

PROCEDURES RELATED TO GASTRIC SECRETION, ULCERS, AND NEOPLASM

Humans secrete gastric hydrochloric acid even in a fasting state. Hydrochloric acid secretion has three phases: cephalic, gastric, and intestinal. Although hypersecretion

PROCEDURE

14-2 Gastrostomy

Equipment

- Suction apparatus
- Electrosurgical unit with dispersive electrode
- Headlamp available

Instruments

- Minor instrumentation set
- Ligating clip appliers and clips

Supplies

- Prep set
- Basic pack
- Basin set
- Laparotomy drapes
- Electrosurgical pencil
- Gloves
- #10 blades × 2
- Suture according to surgeon's preference
- Dressing material according to surgeon's preference
- Gastrostomy tube of choice (e.g., Foley or Pezzer)
- Sterile catheter plug
- Gastrostomy drainage bag of choice

Operative Preparation

Anesthesia

- General (preferred)
- Lubricate and protect patient's eyes
- Local or MAC (possible)

Position

- Supine

Prep

- Shave may be necessary, especially for the male patient
- Prep from mid-chest to thighs and laterally as far as possible

Draping

- Anticipated surgical area is outlined with towels secured with adhesive or towel clips
- Laparotomy sheet

Practical Considerations

- Have a variety of gastrostomy tubes available

Operative Procedure	Technical Considerations
1. An upper midline incision is made.	**1.** Verify gastrostomy tube type prior to incision if possible.
2. The stomach is identified, and a site on the middle anterior wall of the stomach is selected for tube placement.	**2.** Have ready: small abdominal wall retractors (U.S. Army or small Richardson).
3. The gastric site is grasped with a Babcock and elevated, and a small puncture wound is made through the layers of the gastric wall.	**3.** Have ready: • Babcock clamps • Deep knife (do not reuse) • Verify size of catheter desired and prepare the pursestring suture

(continues)

PROCEDURE

14-2 Gastrostomy *(continued)*

4. #20 to #26 French Foley, Malecot, or Pezzer catheter is inserted 3 to 5 cm into the stomach and secured with two concentrically placed pursestring sutures in the gastric wall.	4. Hand first pursestring and prepare second.
5. The exit site at the skin level in the left hypochondriac region is identified and a stab wound is made in the abdominal wall and the catheter is passed through the opening to the skin.	5. Be sure to use the skin knife. A hemostat is usually passed through incision to receive the catheter.
6. The stomach is secured to the anterior abdominal wall with several heavy sutures placed through the gastric serosa and parietal peritoneum.	6. Prepare sutures. Closure happens quickly, so be prepared to initiate count.
7. The tube is then secured to the skin and the midline incision is closed.	7. Place a sterile plug in the catheter or connect to drainage bag. Prepare dressings.

Postoperative Considerations

Immediate Postoperative Care

- Transport to PACU

Prognosis

- Depends on response to primary condition

Complications

- Hemorrhage
- Exit wound infection
- Erosion of the skin
- Leakage

PEARL OF WISDOM

The stomach may have considerable gastric material inside. Have the suction ready for use as soon as the incision is made into the stomach.

PEARL OF WISDOM

Patients routinely have nasogastric tubes in place. Be sure the position of the nasogastric tube is identified before the linear cutter is placed and activated.

of hydrochloric acid may not result in ulcers, it is thought to be a contributor. Several surgical approaches used alone or in combination are related to gastric secretion and gastric ulcers (Table 14-10).

TOTAL GASTRECTOMY

Total gastr**ectomy** involves removal of the stomach and reconstitution of the alimentary tract (Procedure 14-3). The most common reasons for total gastrectomy are malignancy or bleeding which is uncontrolled by conservative means.

PROCEDURES FOR MORBID OBESITY

Several gastric procedures have been developed over the years to help patients suffering from morbid obesity. These approaches include open gastric stapling, laparoscopic gastric stapling, and laparoscopic banding. A number of special considerations may be involved with anesthesia, safe positioning, and preoperative and postoperative care. However, intraoperatively, these procedures present no significantly different problems than other gastric procedures. They commonly require the use of extra long instruments.

SURGERY OF THE SMALL BOWEL

Small bowel resection can occur anywhere along its considerable length from the ligament of Treitz to the ileocecal junction. Indications for bowel resection include trauma,

Table 14-10 Procedures Related to Gastric Secretion, Ulcers and Neoplasm

PROCEDURE	VARIATION	DEFINITION/PURPOSE	NOTES
Vagotomy	Truncal	Interruption of the vagal trunks at or above the esophageal hiatus of the diaphragm denervates: • Parietal cell mass • Antral pump • Pyloric sphincter • Majority of abdominal viscera	Must be combined with a gastric drainage procedure: • Pyloroplasty • Antrectomy and Billroth I • Antrectomy and Billroth II
	Selective	Total denervation of the stomach from above the crus of the diaphragm to and including the pylorus Spares parasympathetic innervation of the abdominal viscera	Must be combined with a gastric drainage procedure: • Pyloroplasty • Antrectomy and Billroth I • Antrectomy and Billroth II
	Proximal (parietal)	Interruption of branches of the vagus nerve along the lesser curvature Denervates parietal cell mass only so antral pump and pyloric sphincter continue to function	Does not require gastric drainage procedure Contraindicated by gastric outlet obstruction secondary to peptic ulcers
Pyloroplasty		Reconstruction of the pyloric sphincter accomplished by incising the pyloric muscle longitudinally and closing with staples or suture transversely, thereby increasing gastric drainage	Most common type is the Heineke-Mikulicz pyloroplasty
Gastroduodenostomy Billroth I		Antrectomy removes the distal portion of the stomach and the pylorus Reanastomosis is to the duodenum	Preferred approach
Gastrojejunostomy Billroth II		Antrectomy removes the distal portion of the stomach and the pylorus Reanastomosis is to the jejunum	Preferred when the duodenum is scarred End of duodenum must be closed
Gastrectomy		Removal of the stomach Partial or total gastrectomy may be performed for other conditions	More difficult technically Requires a Roux-en-Y antecolic esophagojejunostomy or end to side antecolic esophagojejunostomy

diverticula, lesions, Crohn's disease, strangulation and subsequent **necrosis**, and preparation for stoma creation.

SMALL BOWEL PATHOLOGY

The pathological conditions that affect the small bowel are summarized in Table 14-11.

PRINCIPLES OF BOWEL RESECTION AND ANASTOMOSIS

There are numerous variations in pathology and anatomy that result in variations in procedures of the small bowel; however, most procedures are more alike than different. This is true for most surgical specialties, and it is true for the alimentary tract. Surgically the overriding characteristic of the alimentary tract is that it is a flexible tube that must allow for the movement of various contents. No matter what area is resected or anastomosed some common principles apply. These are summarized as follows:

- The affected bowel must be mobilized.
- Pathological tissue is removed with a margin of healthy tissue.
- An adequate blood supply to the remaining bowel must exist.
- Relatively equal diameter segments of bowel should be sewn together.

PROCEDURE 14-3 Total Gastrectomy

Equipment

- Suction apparatus
- Electrosurgical unit with dispersive electrode
- Headlamp available

Instruments

- Major instrumentation set
- May require extra long instruments
- Gastric and/or bowel resection set
- Ligating clip appliers and clips
- Staplers of choice

Supplies

- Prep set
- Basic pack
- Basin set
- Gloves
- Laparotomy drapes
- Electrosurgical pencil
- Blades #10
- Suture according to surgeon's preference
- Dressing material according to surgeon's preference
- Chest tubes and drainage unit if thoracoabdominal approach

Operative Preparation

Anesthesia

- General
- Lubricate and protect patient's eyes

Position

- Supine

Prep

- Insert Foley catheter, if ordered
- Shave may be necessary, especially for the male patient
- Prep from mid-chest to thighs and laterally as far as possible

Draping

- Anticipated surgical area is outlined with towels secured with adhesive or towel clips
- Laparotomy sheet

Practical Considerations

- Have X-rays in room
- Check that blood has been ordered
- Prepare to monitor blood loss carefully
- Thoracoabdominal approach is possible
- Notify pathology department if frozen sections will be performed
- Be prepared to use clean closure technique

Operative Procedure

1. A generous upper midline incision, bilateral subcostal incisions (chevron), or thoracoabdominal incision is made.
2. The lesser sac is entered and the greater and lesser curvatures mobilized. Any adhesions or peritoneal attachments to the pancreas and posterior peritoneum are divided to mobilize the entire stomach.

Technical Considerations

1. Be prepared for incision of choice and have self-retaining retractor of choice ready.
2. Have prepared:
   - Short and long Metzenbaum scissors
   - Short and long hemostatic clamps
   - Ligating clips
   - Wet lap sponges

PROCEDURE 14-3 Total Gastrectomy *(continued)*

3. The vessels of the greater curvature of the gastroepiploic and inferior short gastrics are ligated and divided. The right and left gastric vessels are ligated and divided. The dissection moves toward the duodenum and extends to include at least one centimeter of the duodenum.	**3.** Prepare stapler of choice.
4. The duodenum is divided with a linear cutter. Devascularization of the stomach is completed. The duodenum and stomach are left attached while the posterior row of anastomosis sutures are placed.	**4.** Prepare for "bowel" technique procedures used at your facility.
5. The dissection is completed and the esophagus is transected.	**5.** Prepare stapler for reuse.
6. The reconstruction of choice is a Roux-en-Y esophagojejunostomy. Eighteen inches of jejunum is needed for a tension-free loop that prevents reflux. Transection is made as far proximal as possible with a linear cutter. Anastomosis can be antecolic or retrocolic as needed. Reconstruction requires two anastomoses: esophagojejunal and an end-to-end jejunojejunal anastomoses.	**6.** Sutures: commonly 3–0 absorbable and 3–0 nonabsorbable on a gastrointestinal needle.
7. Abdomen is closed in the usual manner.	**7.** Prepare closure suture. Initiate count.

Postoperative Considerations

Immediate Postoperative Care
- Transport to PACU or ICU

Prognosis
- Depends on response to primary condition
- Somewhat restricted lifestyle

Complications
- Hemorrhage
- Wound infection
- Failure of anastomosis

- The **anastomosis** should be tension-free and leak-proof.
- The mesenteric defect is closed.
- Functional and anatomical continuity is maintained.

COMMON FEATURES OF RESECTION AND ANASTOMOSIS

While there are several options for the type of anastomosis to be used (Table 14-12), all small bowel resection and anastomosis procedures have some common features:

- Supine position, general anesthesia.
- Abdomen is prepped and draped for midline exposure.
- Adequate retraction is secured.
- Site of injury or pathology is identified and the margins of resection are selected.
- Mesentery is inspected to ensure good blood flow to the remaining segments of bowel.
- A window is bluntly created in the mesentery close to the bowel.
- The proximal and distal mesentery is divided to the apex.
- Lap pads are placed to isolate the operative area from the rest of the abdominal contents.
- Bowel clamps are placed and the small intestine is then transected with a linear cutter, at points distal and proximal to the pathology, and the specimen is removed.

Table 14-11 Pathological Conditions of the Small Bowel

CONDITION	SYMPTOMS/SIGNS	DIAGNOSTICS	TREATMENTS
Meckel's diverticulum	• Peptic ulceration • Inflammation of the ileal mucosa • Congenital umbilical fistula, iron deficiency anemia, malabsorption • Neoplastic formation • Impacted foreign body • Fistula • Incarcerated hernia	• History • Sudden profuse and painless hemorrhage in a child • Radionuclide scans • GI series	Simple diverticulum • Diverticulectomy broad-based diverticulum • Bowel resection
Benign neoplasm	• Obstruction • Volvulus • Bleeding • Pain	• GI series • CT scan	Resection
Malignant neoplasms	• Obstruction • Bleeding • Pain	• GI series • CT scan	Wide resection
Obstruction	• Various complaints • Fluid and electrolyte imbalance • Sepsis • Colic • Distension • Nausea and vomiting • Constipation	• GI series • Barium studies • CT scan	• Treat the cause (e.g., **lysis** of adhesions) • Resection
Crohn's disease	• Decreased body weight • Chronically ill • Hypoproteinemia • Edema • Muscle weakness • Increased basal metabolic rate • Vitamin deficiencies	• GI series • Barium studies	Medical • Treat symptoms • Manage complications Surgical • Treat obstruction, perforation, abscess formation, bleeding fistulas • Resection if necessary

- Anastomosis can be with a two-layer closure by hand, or with staples.

FEEDING JEJUNOSTOMY

Feeding jejunostomy is performed to provide prolonged nutritional support to a patient following gastrointestinal surgery or trauma, especially that involving the duodenum. It can be done at the time of other surgery or as a separate procedure. There are two types of feeding jejunostomy: needle and Witzel techniques. The patient is positioned supinely, general anesthesia is administered, and the skin is prepped. Draping exposes the left flank. The techniques are compared in Table 14-13.

Postoperatively, within 24 hours the patient is started on a dietary formula that is enriched over the course of the next few days until full nutritional support is provided. Complications of feeding jejunostomy include leakage at the site of enterotomy, sepsis, catheter dislodgement, catheter obstruction, and perforation.

APPENDECTOMY

Appendectomy is performed for acute appendicitis or incidentally during other surgery as a prophylactic measure (Procedure 14-4). Acute appendicitis is usually caused by obstruction of the appendiceal lumen, which manifests as inflammation that can affect other nearby organs. Perforation of the appendix or gangrene can result. Pylephlebitis, septic thrombosis of the **portal venous system**, can also occur. Symptoms of acute appendicitis include pain, which can be diffuse, central, or localized in the right lower quadrant, nausea and vomiting, and constipation or diarrhea. An elevated white blood cell count and fever are also common. Physical examination reveals tenderness especially on rebound or a palpable abdominal mass in the area of the appendix.

(Text continues on page 425)

Table 14-12 Small Bowel Anastomosis Options

TYPE	FEATURE	NOTES
End-to-end	Attachment of two ends of approximately the same sized structures	• Best accomplished by a two-layer closure technique • Continuous 3–0 absorbable for mucosa-to-mucosa anastomosis • 3–0 silk interrupted sutures for seromuscular closure • Entire staple line from transection is excised electrosurgically on the distal and proximal ends prior to anastomosis • Open ends of bowel may be suctioned to remove any residual fecal material prior to anastomosis
End-to-side	Attachment of the end of one section of bowel into the side of another section (T-like)	• Best accomplished by a two-layer closure technique • Continuous 3–0 absorbable for mucosa-to-mucosa anastomosis • 3–0 silk interrupted sutures for seromuscular closure • Staple line from transection is removed electrosurgically on the "end" section prior to anastomosis • Open ends of bowel may be suctioned to remove any residual fecal material prior to anastomosis • End-to-side positioning has one oriented at right angle to other to maintain opening
Side-to-side	Creation of parallel opening in two sections of bowel with anastomosis	• Especially good technique between lumens of unequal dimensions • Best realized with staplers • Technique requires opening the bowel minimally to allow passage of the "halves" of the linear cutter into each lumen, followed by activation of the device to divide the bowel, thereby creating a terminal tube pouch twice the diameter of the bowel • End of the "tube" is closed with a linear stapler
Roux-en-Y	Roux-en-Y is a specific technique of anastomosis that allows for a variety of applications in gastric, intestinal, biliary, and pancreatic surgery. Roux-en-Y is used in partial or total gastrectomy, with pancreatic resection, and in surgery of the bile duct, and is an integral part of the Whipple pancreaticoduodenectomy	The jejunum is divided with a linear cutter at a point about 20 cm distal to the ligament of Treitz. The distal portion of the jejunum is mobilized to the point of anastomosis. This anastomosis may be to the common bile duct (choledochojejunostomy), the stomach (gastrojejunostomy), the pancreas (pancreatojejunostomy), the duodenum (duodenojejunostomy), or another structure such as the gallbladder (chole**cysto**jejunostomy). The proximal portion is reanastomosed to the jejunum (jejunojejunostomy) in an end-to-side fashion. The result is a continuous alimentary tract with an available side branch for anastomosis to another organ.

Table 14-13 Jejunostomy Techniques

NEEDLE TECHNIQUE	WITZEL TECHNIQUE
• A short midline incision is made.	• A short midline incision is made.
• A loop of proximal jejunum is delivered through the wound.	• A loop of proximal jejunum is delivered through the wound.
• The ligament of Treitz is identified and an area 25 cm distal to that point is selected for the placement of the jejunostomy tube.	• The ligament of Treitz is identified and an area 25 cm distal to that point is selected for the placement of the jejunostomy tube.
• A 14–16 gauge needle is inserted into the jejunum at an angle that creates a tunnel in the subserosa prior to entering the jejunal lumen.	• A pursestring of 3–0 absorbable suture is placed in the proposed site of jejunostomy on the antimesenteric border.
• A 7 Fr catheter is introduced through the needle and advanced 30 to 40 cm into the lumen, and the needle is withdrawn.	• A small opening is made in the jejunum electrosurgically and a soft rubber catheter is introduced into the jejunal lumen and advanced distally. • The pursestring is tightened and secured around the catheter.
• The jejunum is anchored to the abdominal wall. The catheter is brought out through a separate stab wound and secured to the skin with 4–0 nylon.	• The catheter is brought through a separate stab wound and secured at the skin level with 4–0 nylon, and the jejunum is secured to the parietal peritoneum of the anterior abdominal wall.
• The midline incision is closed.	• The midline incision is closed.

PROCEDURE 14-4 Appendectomy

Equipment

- Suction apparatus
- Electrosurgical unit with dispersive electrode
- Head lamp available

Instruments

- Minor instrumentation set

Supplies

- Prep set
- Basic pack
- Basin set
- Gloves
- Blades (#10 × 2)
- Suture according to surgeon's preference
- Laparotomy drapes
- Electrosurgical pencil
- Dressing material according to surgeon's preference
- Culture tubes (aerobic and anaerobic) available
- Penrose drain available
- Irrigation solution (antibiotic may be used)

PROCEDURE 14-4 Appendectomy *(continued)*

Operative Preparation

Anesthesia
- General
- Lubricate and protect patient's eyes

Position
- Supine

Prep
- Shave may be necessary, especially for the male patient
- Prep from mid-chest to thighs and laterally as far as possible

Draping
- Anticipated surgical area (right lower quadrant) is outlined with towels secured with adhesive or towel clips
- Laparotomy sheet

Practical Considerations

- Have a major instrumentation set available
- Procedure can be performed via laparoscopic approach

Operative Procedure

1. The McBurney's incision is typically used.
2. The appendix is identified by following the cecal taenia to the appendiceal base. This may require the gentle mobilization of the cecum into the wound (see Figure 14-14A).

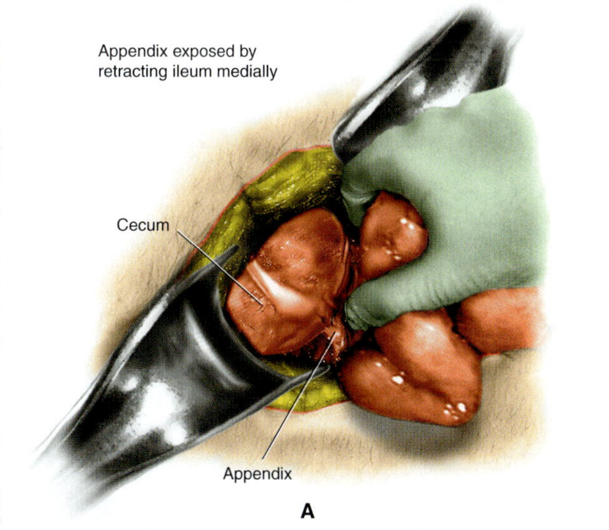

Figure 14-14 Appendectomy: (A) Cecum and appendix identified

3. The mesoappendix is transected from the free end tip of the appendix toward the base, by a series of double clamping, cutting, and ligation with 3–0 absorbable ties (Figure 14-14B).

Technical Considerations

1. Small retractors are placed and may be redirected several times as the incision proceeds through the muscle layers.
2. Be prepared to culture free fluid, if present, as soon as the peritoneum is entered.
3. This procedure may be reversed if the appendix is severely adhered or retrocecal or if anatomy is otherwise distorted.

(continues)

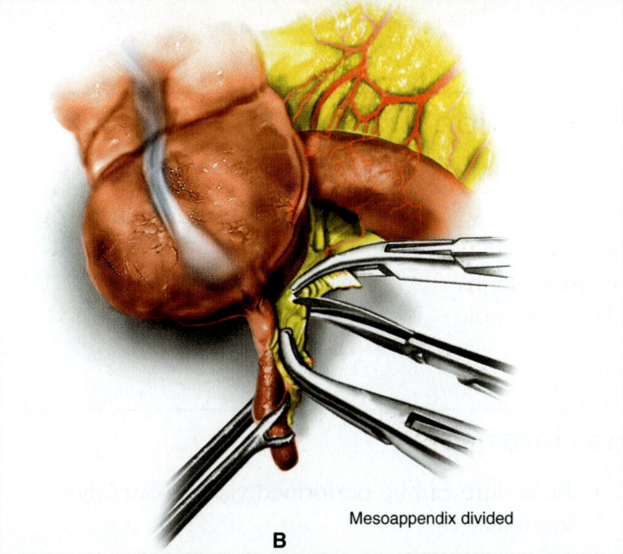

Figure 14-14 Appendectomy: (B) Appendiceal artery ligated

4. A clamp is placed across the appendix near the base, crushing the appendix, and is then removed and reapplied slightly distally.

4. Prepare pursestring suture if surgeon uses that technique.

5. A 3–0 absorbable suture on a small taper needle may be passed through the cecum, around the base of the appendix, in a pursestring manner (see Figure 14-14C).

5. Be sure to treat suture and needle as contaminated.

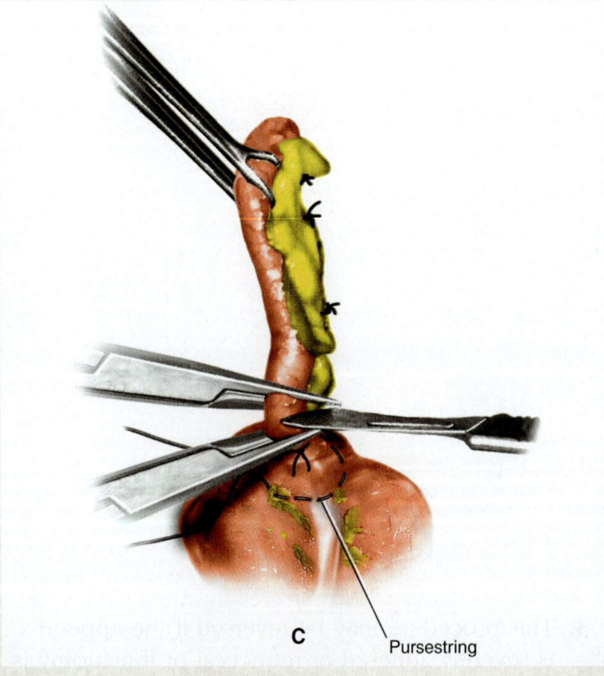

Figure 14-14 Appendectomy: (C) Excision of appendix

PROCEDURE 14-4 Appendectomy *(continued)*

6. The crushed base is then ligated with an 0 absorbable tie and the appendix is amputated electrosurgically or with scissors or a scalpel.	**6.** Have a basin on the field to contain the appendix and contaminated instruments. A Penrose drain may be placed.
7. The incision is closed in layers.	**7.** Small incision. Be prepared to perform counts quickly.

Postoperative Considerations

Immediate Postoperative Care

- Transport to PACU

Prognosis

- Return to normal activities within 4–6 weeks

Complications

- Hemorrhage
- Wound infection
- Intestinal obstruction due to resultant adhesions
- Stump rupture
- Sepsis

COLON SURGERY

The pathology of the colon and the techniques of colon resection are very similar to those for the small bowel (Table 14-14). The same principles of resection and anastomosis apply.

COLON RESECTION

There are several reasons for performing a colon resection:

- Ileocecal disease
- Strangulated bowel
- Colorectal cancer

Table 14-14 Pathological Conditions of the Colon

CONDITION	SYMPTOMS/SIGNS	DIAGNOSTICS	TREATMENTS
Diverticular disease (diverticulosis, diverticulitis)	• Subacute onset of left lower quadrant pain • Alteration in bowel habits • Palpable mass • Fever	• History • Physical examination • Abdominal X-rays • Barium studies • Fiberoptic endoscopy	Medical • Treat complications Surgical • Colectomy
Neoplasm (polyps and carcinoma)	• Determined by anatomical location	• History • Physical examination • Abdominal X-rays • Barium studies • Fiberoptic endoscopy	Surgical • Adequate local incision • Hemicolectomy or colectomy
Ulcerative colitis and Crohn's disease	• See small bowel pathology • Watery diarrhea • Cramping • Abdominal pain	• History • Physical examination • Abdominal X-rays • Barium studies • Fiberoptic endoscopy	Medical • Treat symptoms Surgical • Colectomy with ileostomy • Continent ileostomy
Obstruction, volvulus, intussusception, impaction	• Abdominal distension • Cramping abdominal pain • Nausea • Vomiting	• History • Physical examination • Abdominal X-rays • Barium studies • Fiberoptic endoscopy	Surgical • Relieve condition • Resection if necessary

- Perforation
- Ulcerative colitis
- Polyp and diverticular disease
- Mesenteric disease
- Obstruction
- Fistula excision
- Stoma formation

Prior to the procedure the patient has often undergone colonoscopy, barium enema studies, and CT or ultrasound to identify and locate pathology. Often, a bowel prep is done prior to surgery to cleanse the bowel of fecal matter and bacteria. Because the colon has the largest population of intestinal flora, it is most susceptible to postoperative infection, and therefore the use of prophylactic antibiotics is routine.

Colon resection for cancer is commonly undertaken as a hemicolectomy, which may be a right from the ileocecal junction, cecum, appendix, and ascending colon past the hepatic flexure or a left from just proximal to the splenic flexure to the sigmoid colon. Colon resection commonly requires a subsequent anastomosis between lumens of unequal diameter such as is the case with anastomosis to the ileum. To overcome this disparity, the smaller lumen is cut at a slant to provide a wider aperture for anastomosis, or a side-to-side technique is used. Anastomosis can be by a two-layer hand closure technique or with staples.

Colon resection requires mobilization of the segment to be excised, which can dictate division of colic ligaments, (e.g., splenocolic and/or the omentum). It also may involve creation of a permanent or temporary stoma. Resection of cancer requires a distal margin 5 cm from pathology, and a proximal margin determined by colonic blood supply. Because of the larger vessels, the mesenteric division usually requires larger hemostats in place of the smaller ones used in small bowel resection. Heavier ties are often required. Vessels encountered during colon resection include the right, middle, and left colic arteries, the inferior and superior mesenteric arteries, the intercolic and sigmoid arteries, and the superior rectal artery. Sigmoid resection involves only that portion of the large intestine. The options for colon resection are illustrated in Figure 14-15.

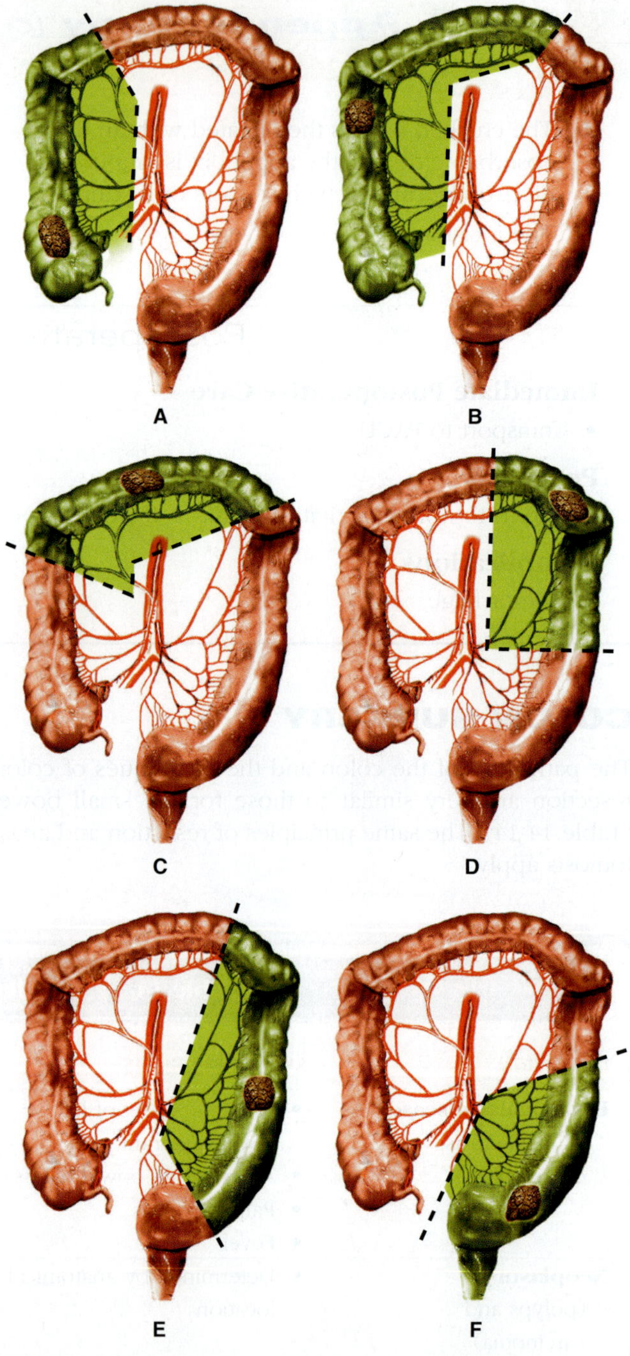

Figure 14-15 Colon resection options: (A) Right colectomy, (B) right hemicolectomy, (C) transverse colectomy, (D) left colectomy, (E) left hemicolectomy, (F) abdominoperineal resection

PEARL OF WISDOM

The appendix and all instruments and needles associated with its removal are contaminated. They are placed in a basin and removed from the immediate field. The basin is placed in a predefined area on the back table and left there until the case is completed. Instruments and needles are counted by pointing, not by touching.

Complications of colon resection are identical to those for small bowel resection and also include ureteral injury, thromboembolism, a greater chance of sepsis and obstruction, and the complications associated with stoma construction and maintenance.

STOMAS

A stoma ("ostomy") is a communication of a section of bowel with the outside of the abdominal cavity created to divert the fecal stream. This "diversion" is done temporarily to protect a recent intestinal anastomosis, to avoid potential abdominal "spillage" postoperatively, or as an end (permanent) result of bowel resection. In this section of the chapter, a stoma is in reference to an ileostomy or colostomy.

Stomas are created from either an end section or loop of the ileum (ileostomy) or colon (colostomy). The sigmoid colon is also used as an "end" colostomy following abdominoperineal (A/P) resection. Stomas created as "end" stomas have a single aperture at the skin surface, and those created from "loops" generally have two apertures in the same wound. Loop-type stomas have an afferent functioning aperture and an efferent nonfunctioning aperture, and may be created with the bowel in continuity or separated.

There are numerous potential complications common to all stomas. They include ischemia, **stenosis**, stomal prolapse, stomal retraction, parastomal hernia, fistula formation, bleeding from varices around the stoma, leakage from the "appliance," offensive odors, contact dermatitis, laceration, urinary tract calculi, gallstones, infection, hyperplasia, and bowel obstruction secondary to stomal creation.

In stoma creation, a site is selected at a point below the costal margin, above the belt line, and usually at the appropriate lateral edge of the rectus abdominis muscle. Site selection is preferably accomplished prior to surgery, with the site marked on the patient after review of the area in both the standing and sitting positions. This provides maximum comfort for the patient. In some cases, of course, stoma creation is a result of intraoperative decision making, and therefore preoperative site selection is a moot point. However, selection of the site will still follow the basic guidelines just described. Stoma types are listed in Table 14-15.

Table 14-15 Stoma Types

STOMA TYPE	DESCRIPTION
End ileostomy	• Constructed from a terminal portion of ileum • Temporary or permanent
Loop ileostomy	• Primarily a temporary stoma for fecal diversion
End-loop ileostomy	• A modification of the loop method in which the loop is divided with a linear cutter and both ends are brought out through the skin incision
End colostomy	• Created from the descending colon and sigmoid
Loop colostomy	• Utilizes the transverse colon • Not generally used as a permanent colostomy as it discharges a semiliquid stool • The most frequently used method of stoma creation for temporary fecal diversion
End-loop colostomy	• A modification of the loop method in which the loop is divided with a linear cutter and both ends are brought out through the skin incision
Sigmoid colostomy	• Most common type of permanent colostomy • Created at the time of A/P resection • Created as an end colostomy in the lower left quadrant

ANORECTAL SURGERY

The rectal area must be taken into consideration during interventions in the pelvic area. These interventions include general surgery, genitourinary surgery, obstetric and gynecologic surgery, and radical cancer procedures. The associated procedures are discussed in the relevant sections of this book. Anorectal surgery itself is most often concerned with four rather common conditions.

ANORECTAL PATHOLOGY

Pathological conditions of the anorectal area are summarized in Table 14-16.

Anorectal pathology presents with a variety of signs and symptoms (Table 14-17). For most conditions, a conservative approach to treatment is followed before surgical options are exercised.

FISTULOTOMY/FISTULECTOMY FOR FISTULA-IN-ANO

Fistulotomy or fistulectomy is performed in the jackknife or lithotomy position under spinal or general anesthetic. The steps of the procedure are as follows:

1. An anal speculum is inserted and the internal opening is identified.
2. A grooved director is inserted in the tract (provides surface against which to make incision).

Table 14-16 Anorectal Pathology

CONDITION	DEFINITION/TYPES
Fistula-in-ano	A chronic form of perianal abscess that fails to heal after draining and becomes an inflammatory tract characterized by primary internal and secondary external openings Categorized into four groups based upon their relation to the sphincter muscles: • Intersphincteric • Transsphincteric • Suprasphincteric • Extrasphincteric Causes: infectious diseases, malignancy, and trauma; associated with active pulmonary tuberculosis and Crohn's disease
Anal fissure	• Tears in the epidermis of the anal canal extending from the dentate line to the margin of the anus • Primary fissures: trauma, childbirth, or the passage of hard stools • Secondary fissures: associated with other systemic conditions, such as Crohn's disease, leukemia, aplastic anemia, superinfection in HIV patients, and agranulocytosis
Pilonidal disease	• An acute abscess in the sacrococcygeal area, exclusively in the midline, that ruptures spontaneously, resulting in an unhealed sinus tract with chronic drainage • Sinus tract is generally 2 to 5 cm and can be mistaken for a fistula-in-ano • Lesions are often secondarily invaded by hair
Hemorrhoids	• Congestion and dilatation of the submucosal and subcutaneous venous plexuses that line the anal canal caused by persistent or repeated intra-abdominal pressure, heavy physical exertion, constipation, heredity, age, and diet • Most common anal lesions • Classified as external or internal and by location

3. The fistula is incised with a scalpel from the skin surface to the lumen of the tract.
4. Granulation tissue is curetted and the edges of the wound are "marsupialized."
5. The wound is left open.
6. A loose dressing is applied, and a T-binder or underpants are used to hold the dressing in place.
7. The wound heals by second intention (granulation).

Even in this relatively simple procedure there are variations. Fistulectomy is excision of the tract with a margin of normal tissue around it. Excision of the tract is performed by "coring" or by incising the tissues around it. This creates substantial tissue loss and results in a larger separation of the ends of the sphincter muscles, leading to longer healing time and a greater chance of fecal incontinence. Another option involves the use of a seton. A seton is a suture, usually silk, that is drawn through the fistula and tightened around the muscles covering the fistula. This serves to internally cut the external sphincter with minimal tissue disruption. This action is progressive. The seton will delineate the amount of muscle beneath the fistula tract and also acts as a drain while the tract and muscles heal by fibrosis. Seton placement is usually followed by fistulotomy 6 to 8 weeks later.

Complications include damage to the pudendal nerve, urinary retention, hemorrhage, hemorrhoid thrombosis, fecal impaction, pain, recurrence, anal stricture, rectovaginal fistula formation, and most commonly fecal incontinence secondary to division of the internal and external sphincters.

ANAL FISSURES

Treatment of anal fissure is a relatively common procedure. These procedures are performed in the jackknife position with local, spinal, or general anesthesia. The basic procedural steps are as follows:

1. A bivalve Pratt anal speculum is inserted into the anal canal and the fissure is identified.
2. A longitudinal incision is made in the left or right lateral aspect of the anal canal, separating the anoderm and intersphincteric plane from the internal sphincter muscle.
3. An Allis clamp is used to encircle and elevate the internal sphincter and the muscle is divided electrosurgically through its full thickness.
4. Large sentinel piles or skin tags are also excised in an elliptical fashion.

Table 14-17 Anorectal Pathology—Diagnosis and Treatment

CONDITION	SYMPTOMS/SIGNS	DIAGNOSTICS/TREATMENT
Fistula-in-ano	• Purulent or serosanguinous drainage • Palpable fistula tract may be evident • External opening at skin level • Internal opening	Diagnosis • Anoscopy • Hydrogen peroxide injection study • Fistulography • Examination under anesthesia • Probing of the fistula tract • MRI (complex fistulas) • Ultrasonography (complex fistulas) Treatment • Fistulotomy • Fistulectomy • Placement of a "seton"
Anal fissure	• Pain in the anus during and after defecation • Bleeding, over 70% of patients • Swelling that can form a "sentinel pile" • Fibrosis which may lead to skin tag formation • Constipation • Spasm • Pain may be severe and incapacitating	Diagnosis • Visualization • Anoscopy under anesthesia • Digital examination Treatment • Acute fissures usually heal spontaneously in 6 weeks • Chronic fissures generally require surgical intervention • Conservative treatment includes application of topical anesthetics or hydrocortisone ointments, warm baths, and bulk-forming agents, such as bran or psyllium seed, to relieve constipation, and anal hygiene • Surgical treatment: lateral internal sphincterotomy
Pilonidal disease	• More frequent in obese males in their twenties or thirties • Acute abscess, pain can be severe • Chronic sinus formation, pain is minimal, but a seropurulent drainage is present • A pit is evident in the midline approximately 5 cm above the anus	Diagnosis • Visual examination Treatment • Incision and drainage • Various techniques used for the sinus path
Hemorrhoids	• Generally asymptomatic • Painful protrusions that bleed and itch • Mucoid discharge • Inspection of the anal orifice reveals thickening of the columns of Morgagni that appear as bluish lumps beneath the skin or as distinct, prolapsed purplish bodies	Diagnosis • Anoscopy Treatment • Nonoperative treatments: sitz baths, dietary supplements, topical medications, and injections • Hemorrhoidectomy for severe prolapse or other complications • Rubber-band ligation is a conservative intervention that is usually done in the office setting

5. The wound may be closed with 3–0 running chromic suture or left open to heal by second intention.

Sphincterotomy may also be approached in a "closed" fashion, in which a small stab incision is made with a #11 blade in the lateral aspect of the anal canal, the scalpel is advanced to the level of the internal sphincter and rotated 90°, dividing the internal sphincter.

Fissurectomy may be performed and involves excision of the torn tissues followed by closure with a "V-Y" triangular skin flap, the base of which is at the perianal skin level and the apex is at the deepest level of the fissure.

Complications include bleeding, abscess formation, anal stenosis and stricture, failure to heal, recurrence rate up to 25%, temporary paralysis, and fecal incontinence. Biopsy should be performed on any fissure that does not heal after surgical treatment.

INCISION AND DRAINAGE OF A PILONIDAL FISTULA

Incision and drainage of a pilonidal fistula is also a relatively common procedure. These procedures are performed in the jackknife position with local, spinal, or general anesthesia. The basic procedural steps are as follows:

1. A longitudinal midline skin incision is made that is deepened until the abscess cavity is entered.
2. Copious irrigation and curettage of the abscess cavity is performed.
3. Any hair that is present must be removed.
4. Skin edges are trimmed to make the abscess cavity an open wound.
5. The wound is lightly packed with fine mesh gauze and left to heal by second intention.

Complications of incision and drainage include delayed wound healing, wound dehiscence, recurrence, and scarring.

HEMORRHOID LIGATION AND EXCISION

Hemorrhoids are quite common in the population. Successful treatment is usually conservative including dietary restrictions and medications. An intermediate but conservative procedure, rubber band ligation, may be performed at the physician's office. This procedure is done with the patient in the knee chest position. The rectal vault is thoroughly cleansed and local anesthesia 2% lidocaine jelly is applied. An anoscope is introduced and its obturator is withdrawn. The anus is examined and the hemorrhoid is located and grasped. The band is loaded onto the applicator. Several bands may be required. The applicator is passed over the tissue to the base of the hemorrhoid and the band is applied. The hemorrhoid is released from the grasper.

The pressure from the band strangulates the hemorrhoid and it sloughs away in 48 to 72 hours. Only one or two groups of hemorrhoids are ligated in a session, and this routine is repeated on groups of hemorrhoids at 3-week intervals. Complications include pain, bleeding, external thrombosis, stenosis, and sepsis.

HEMORRHOIDECTOMY

Hemorrhoidectomy is undertaken in the OR setting and is indicated in cases of third and fourth degree hemorrhoids (Procedure 14-5). Inflammatory bowel disease and irritable bowel syndrome are both contraindications to this procedure, as is immunosuppression and coagulopathy.

SURGERY OF THE LIVER AND BILIARY TRACT

The anatomical complexities, rich blood supply, physiological importance, and frequent incidence of pathology make the liver and biliary tract a frequent site of general surgery.

SELECT PATHOLOGY OF THE LIVER AND BILIARY TRACT

Liver pathology and surgical conditions are diagnosed via patient history, physical examination, changes in laboratory data, sonography, liver scan, CT scan, and biopsy. Arteriograms may be required to diagnose suspected vascular lesions. The biliary tract is subject to the same diagnostic examinations (Table 14-18). Some biliary stones will show on routine X-ray.

LIVER BIOPSY

Liver biopsy is a diagnostic procedure that plays a central role in the evaluation of suspected liver disease or in diagnosing liver graft (transplant) rejection. It is a low-risk procedure (serious complications below 0.5%) that has a consistently high rate of success (95–98%). Liver biopsy is used when hepatic disorders cannot be diagnosed by histologic, physical, or noninvasive methods. Indications for the procedure include abnormal liver function tests, staging of chronic hepatitis, identification of alcoholic liver disease, fever of unknown origin, determination of the nature of intrahepatic masses, evaluation of cirrhosis, and screening for familial disease. The most common indication is to confirm a suspected hepatic neoplasm prior to surgery. Under current techniques, lesions as small as 0.5 cm can be targeted for biopsy. Liver biopsy can be

PROCEDURE 14-5 Hemorrhoidectomy

Equipment

- Electrosurgical unit with dispersive electrode
- Suction apparatus
- CO_2 laser may be used for vaporization and coagulation of hemorrhoidal tissue
- Headlamp available

Instruments

- Rectal set
- Anoscope
- Rectal speculum
- Rectal dilators
- Buie pile forceps
- Crypt hook

Supplies

- Prep set
- Basic pack
- Basin set
- Electrosurgical pencil
- Gloves
- Blades (#10 × 2)
- Suture according to surgeon's preference
- Drapes according to planned position
- Surgicel or Gelfoam
- Local anesthesia 0.5% lidocaine with 1:100,000 epinephrine may be administered as a hemostatic agent
- Lubricant

Operative Preparation

Anesthesia

- Spinal
- General
- Local

Position

- Jackknife
- Lithotomy
- Modified lateral

Prep

- Enema 1–2 hours preoperatively
- Shave may be required, especially for the male patient
- Benzoin applied to buttocks
- Tape used for retraction of buttocks
- Formal prep may not be required
- Rectal area

Draping

- Small fenestrated sheet

Practical Considerations

- Benzoin under tape protects skin; do not overuse

Operative Procedure	Technical Considerations
1. A Fansler speculum is inserted to expose the anal canal past the anorectal ring dentate line.	**1.** Lubricate speculum for ease of insertion.

(continues)

PROCEDURE 14-5 Hemorrhoidectomy *(continued)*

2. Hemostats are placed on the protruding components.
3. The area around the hemorrhoid group is incised in an elliptical manner with care taken not to cross the dentate line.
4. External hemorrhoids are dissected from the external and internal sphincters.
5. A hemorrhoid clamp is then applied to the internal hemorrhoids, and all tissue above the clamp is removed.
6. The resultant pedicle is suture ligated with 3–0 chromic, released, and oversewn.
7. The mucosa is then approximated with interrupted 3–0 chromic.
8. The excision procedure is repeated on the other group(s) of hemorrhoids.
9. Gelfoam 100 sheet may be flattened, rolled, and inserted into the anal canal to provide hemostasis, and a dry dressing is applied over it.

2. The largest, most redundant group is approached first.
3. Pass scalpel.
4. Have hemorrhoidal clamp ready.
5. Specimens are labeled and sent to pathology for microscopic examination. Have suture ready.
6. Assist with suture as needed.
7. Prepare to repeat process.
8. Have suture ready. Count.
9. Surgicel may be preferred.

Postoperative Considerations

Immediate Postoperative Care

- Transport to PACU

Prognosis

- Return to normal activities

Complications

- Pain
- Infection
- Hemorrhage
- Recurrence
- Constipation

PEARL OF WISDOM

If the width of the elliptical excision surpasses 1.5 cm, the wound may be left open to heal by second intention.

performed via percutaneous, laparoscopic, transvenous, or open means. Specimens are collected by hollow-bore needles, core biopsy needles, or wedge resection. Several conditions eliminate liver biopsy as an option:

- Coagulopathy: a prothrombin time greater than 3 or 4 seconds, and a platelet count below 50,000
- **Ascites**
- Hepatic hemangioma

Prior to biopsy, blood transfusion services and a surgeon should be available. Percutaneous and transvenous biopsies are both done in conjunction with imaging guidance (ultrasound or CT). Ultrasound is less expensive, faster, avoids radiation, and provides "real time" surveillance, allowing for subtle adjustments in needle placement. CT ensures more precise needle placement but requires greater breathing control from the patient. Percutaneous biopsy is performed with a 20- or 22-gauge needle, or a 1.2- to 1.9-mm core biopsy (Tru-Cut) needle that is guided into the liver capsule via a subcostal or intercostal route. The specimen is ob-

Table 14-18 Select Pathology and Treatment of Liver Disorders

PATHOLOGY	SYMPTOMS/SIGNS	TREATMENT
Primary malignancy	• Abdominal pain and weight loss • Palpable mass, arterial bruit, friction rub, ascites	• Partial hepatectomy • Arterial ligation • Chemotherapy
Secondary malignancy (metastasis)	• Same as primary	• Chemotherapy for the primary neoplasm
Hepatic adenoma	• Right upper quadrant pain in females taking birth control pills • Right upper quadrant mass • Massive intra-abdominal hemorrhage	• Discontinue birth control pills and observe • Enucleation • Partial hepatectomy when symptomatic
Nodular hyperplasia	• Usually asymptomatic • Right upper quadrant discomfort not associated with birth control pills	• Surgical removal only if symptomatic
Hemangioma	• Occasional pain or discomfort • Palpable mass • May rupture	• Excision if symptomatic • Radiotherapy • Arterial ligation
Hepatic cysts	• Occasional right upper quadrant discomfort • Occasional mass	• Usually none • Percutaneous or open drainage if symptomatic
Hepatic abscess	• High fever • Right upper quadrant pain • Jaundice • Enlarged and tender liver	• Percutaneous or open drainage • Antibiotics
Trauma/laceration	• Intra-abdominal bleeding • Hypovolemic shock	• Surgical repair of laceration • Partial resection • Arterial ligation

tained and the needle withdrawn. The specimen obtained is extracted from the needle and fixed on a glass slide and immediately sent for cytologic analysis. It may also be placed in 10% buffered formalin. The needle tract in the liver may be plugged with Gelfoam; this technique has proved to be beneficial in preventing postoperative bleeding.

In transvenous liver biopsy, a catheter is placed through the jugular vein and into the hepatic vein, and a biopsy needle is introduced. Several passes are required to obtain an adequate amount of tissue. Laparoscopic liver biopsy can incorporate either needle biopsy or wedge resection of a larger specimen and, obviously, requires the techniques and instrumentation of laparoscopy (see Chapter 15 for laparoscopic procedure). Because of the success rates of these methods, the open approach to liver biopsy is only performed "incidentally" during the course of other surgery when a suspicious lesion is noted. In this procedure two 2–0 chromic sutures on large blunt needles are passed through the liver edge and a wedge of tissue is taken between them. The sutures are then tied together to approximate the liver edges.

Postoperatively, the patient remains hospitalized for observation for 6 to 8 hours and is encouraged to lie on the right side, putting pressure on the operative site. The incidence of admission to the hospital following liver biopsy is about 5%; the patient should remain near the hospital for 24 hours following biopsy. Complications of liver biopsy include pain at the biopsy site, hemorrhage, intrahepatic hematoma formation, pneumothorax, infection, malignant "seeding," and death (rare). Referred pain to the shoulder and bile leakage are also seen following liver biopsy.

REPAIR OF LIVER LACERATION

The liver is the most commonly injured organ in both blunt and penetrating abdominal trauma, including motor vehicle accidents, gunshot wounds, and stab wounds (Procedure 14-6). In patients who have suffered trauma and require laparotomy, 40–45% will have injury to the liver. Repair of a liver laceration is primarily indicated in cases of penetrating wounds and the most critical factor is the control of bleeding.

(Text continues on page 436)

PROCEDURE

14-6 Repair of Liver Laceration

Equipment

- Electrosurgical unit with dispersive electrode
- Suction apparatus
- Sternal saw and thoracic instruments in or near room
- Cell-Saver available
- Laser or argon beam coagulator available
- Headlamp available

Instruments

- Major instrumentation set
- Vascular instruments
- Ligating clip appliers and clips
- Long instruments
- Gallbladder instruments available
- Thoracotomy set available

Supplies

- Prep set
- Basic pack
- Basin set
- Gloves
- Blades (#10 × 2)
- Laparotomy drapes
- Electrosurgical pencil
- Suture according to surgeon's preference
- Dressing material according to surgeon's preference
- Extra laparotomy sponges
- Gelfoam or Surgicel
- Liver suture: chromic with blunt needle
- Passive and positive pressure drains
- Chest tubes and drainage system available

Operative Preparation

Anesthesia

- General
- Lubricate and protect patient's eyes

Position

- Supine

Prep

- Insert Foley catheter, if ordered
- Shave may be necessary, especially for the male patient
- Prep from shoulders to thighs and laterally as far as possible

Draping

- Anticipated surgical area is outlined with towels secured with adhesive or towel clips
- Laparotomy sheet

Practical Considerations

- Patient may be in shock
- Notify blood bank of probable need
- Fluid pumps and solution warmers prepared

Operative Procedure	Technical Considerations
1. Initially opened with long midline incision that may be extended to a thoracoabdominal incision.	**1.** Have scalpel and retractors ready. Have at least ten lap sponges opened and counted on the back table prior to incision.

PROCEDURE

14-6 **Repair of Liver Laceration** *(continued)*

2. Gross blood or intestinal contents are evacuated from the abdomen using lap sponges and suction.
3. Secure adequate exposure and evaluate the liver for severity of injury.
4. *Note:* Treatment choice depends on severity of injury. Severe lacerations require some degree of liver mobilization.
5. Mobilization is achieved by dividing the falciform and round ligaments, which attach the liver to the anterior abdominal wall, and releasing the triangular ligament (diaphragm attachment) on the affected side.
6. Large bleeders within the liver parenchyma may require suture ligation prior to closure of the surface laceration.
7. Once hemostasis is achieved, and the need for hepatic resection is ruled out, the laceration is closed with a 2–0 chromic suture swaged onto a large, blunt (liver) needle.
8. The omentum, with its vascularity intact, may be laid over the laceration and incorporated in the suturing of the laceration.
9. The abdomen is irrigated with warm saline; the liver is inspected for persistent bleeding (which may be controlled by direct pressure).
10. The abdomen is explored for other injuries and then closed.

2. Be sure suction is operational and Cell-Saver, if requested, is ready. The laps will initially be used dry. A basin for clots is useful.
3. Initial exposure may be with handheld retractors such as Richardson, Deaver, or Harrington. Prepare to switch quickly to a self-retaining retractor.
4. Try to anticipate the items that will be necessary for the repair or resection.
5. Cholecystectomy may also be necessary to gain access to the laceration. Be sure gallbladder instruments are available. Long scissors and tissue forceps will be necessary for the dissection.
6. Have at least two sutures loaded and ready to pass if needed. Hemostatic agents may be used.
7. Prepare suture in advance.
8. Pass suture of choice and tissue forceps. The surgical assistant will need the suture scissors.
9. Check temperature of irrigation fluid and keep mental note of amount used. Valsalva's maneuver may be performed to evaluate diaphragmatic patency. Antibiotics may be requested.
10. Handheld retractors may again be necessary. If other injuries are discovered, attempt to anticipate additional items that will be needed. Pass closing suture and tissue forceps to surgeon and scissors to assistant. Initiate closing count.

Postoperative Considerations

Immediate Postoperative Care

- Transport to PACU or ICU

Prognosis

- Depends on initial systemic shock and systemic response

Complications

- Hemorrhage
- Wound infection
- Intrahepatic hematoma
- Perihepatic abscess
- Biliary fistula
- Hepatic artery pseudoaneurysm

PEARL OF WISDOM

Prioritize! This is the key concept to preparing for trauma surgery. What must be ready first in order to save a life? What must be ready to correct the condition? Then, what must be ready to create a better outcome? Organize your mind and instruments accordingly.

Lacerations less than 1 cm may be treated with local pressure, electrosurgery, or application of a hemostatic agent. Lacerations of 1 to 3 cm deep are suitable for suture repair or application of fibrin glue. For deeper lacerations hepatic resection should be considered. In the case of severe bleeding, the Pringle maneuver, clamping the hepatic inflow contained within the hepatoduodenal ligament, or hilum, may be necessary.

LIVER RESECTION

Liver resection is most commonly performed to excise pathology (hepatocellular carcinoma) (Procedure 14-7). It may also be performed as part of the course of treatment for carcinoma of the gallbladder, to resolve uncontrollable

PROCEDURE 14-7 Liver Resection

Equipment

- Electrosurgical unit with dispersive electrode
- Suction apparatus
- Hypo/hyperthermia unit
- Manometer
- Cell-Saver available
- Cavitron or plasma knife available
- Headlamp available

Instruments

- Major instrumentation set
- Vascular instruments
- Gallbladder instruments available
- Thoracotomy set in OR
- Ligating clip appliers and clips
- Long instruments

Supplies

- Prep set
- Basic pack
- Basin set
- Gloves
- Blades (#10 × 2)
- Laparotomy drapes
- Electrosurgical pencil
- Suture according to surgeon's preference
- Dressing material according to surgeon's preference
- Gelfoam or Surgicel
- Vessel loops available

Operative Preparation

Anesthesia
- General
- Lubricate and protect patient's eyes

Position
- Supine
- Modified lateral

Prep
- Insert Foley catheter, if ordered
- Shave may be necessary, especially for the male patient
- Prep from shoulders to thighs and laterally as far as possible

Draping
- Anticipated surgical area is outlined with towels secured with adhesive or towel clips
- Laparotomy sheet

PROCEDURE

14-7 Liver Resection *(continued)*

Practical Considerations

- Confirm availability of blood
- Procedures for monitoring blood loss in place

Operative Procedure	Technical Considerations
1. Incision choice varies but most common is an ipsilateral subcostal (Kocher) incision.	**1.** All items prepared and counted for use.
2. After entering the abdomen, the liver is appropriately mobilized and inspected for extent and possibility of resection.	**2.** Handheld retractors may be used for initial evaluation. Present long instruments for mobilization. Procedure may be terminated at this point.
3. Prior to beginning liver resection the Pringle maneuver is often performed to control blood flow (allows up to 60 minutes before tissue damage occurs). Control of blood supply may also be performed by balloon occlusion or clamping of the infrahepatic and suprahepatic inferior vena cava.	**3.** Prepare vascular clamp for Pringle maneuver or necessary items for other methods to control blood supply. Be sure suction is readily available. Cell-Saver may not be used if tumor is present.
4. Division of the parenchyma is undertaken in a "segmental" or "lobular" fashion, utilizing a scalpel and/or electrosurgery, and ligation of the artery/vein/duct triad is performed, addressing each structure individually, as they are encountered.	**4.** An extension for the electrosurgical pencil is useful. Ligating clips loaded and ready to pass. Right angle clamps will be used for separation of structures. Long length suture on passers ready.
5. Resection continues until the desired amount of liver is excised, preserving as much of the functional liver parenchyma as possible.	**5.** Observe progress of procedure and anticipate moves of other team members. Many steps will be repeated several times.
6. After resection, occlusive devices are released, and hemostasis is achieved. Hemostatic agents may be applied to the parenchyma, and the abdomen is closed.	**6.** Hemostatic agents should be readily available. Anticipate closure. Secure warm irrigation fluid. Prepare closing suture. Organize items and initiate count.

Postoperative Considerations

Immediate Postoperative Care

- Transport to PACU or ICU

Prognosis

- Depends on response to primary condition

Complications

- Hemorrhage
- Wound infection
- Liver resection among select candidates carries a 5% mortality rate
- Infection
- Bile leak
- Liver failure
- Tumor recurrence

PEARL OF WISDOM

Monitoring blood loss is always important. In procedures such as liver trauma and resection it is essential. Keep a sterile marker and a sterile piece of paper to write notes on. Log how much irrigation has been used. Place a scale in the room so the circulator can weigh sponges. Listen for the anesthesia provider to ask questions about blood loss. Be prepared to communicate how many sponges and how much irrigation have been used.

bleeding or parenchymal maceration following abdominal trauma, or for transplant. Liver cancer is one of the most common solid organ cancers worldwide; the liver is a common site for metastatic disease from other organs as well. Although resection is an effective intervention, many patients are not good candidates. Factors such as associated liver disease, extrahepatic metastases, large tumor size, or major hepatic vascular involvement may make resection untenable. The ideal setting for liver resection is a small (2 to 5 cm) tumor in a noncirrhotic liver, but this is uncommon. Cirrhosis of the liver is associated with hepatocellular carcinoma as a result of viral hepatitis or alcohol abuse.

As important as the liver is to life, loss of significant portions of the liver can be survived. The liver is divided into eight segments, each with its own arterial supply, venous drainage, and ductal system (Figure 14-16). For this reason liver resection of up to 80–90% of the organ can be safely performed. Compensatory hypertrophy and hyperplasia, occurring within 3 to 6 weeks after resection (partial hepatectomy), can result in regeneration of the liver to almost normal size.

SURGICAL TREATMENT OF GALLSTONES AND GALLBLADDER DISEASE

Gallbladder disease and associated conditions are seen daily in the operating room. In this section, a logical sequence will be presented so the student can appreciate the pathology, conservative interventions, and a progres-

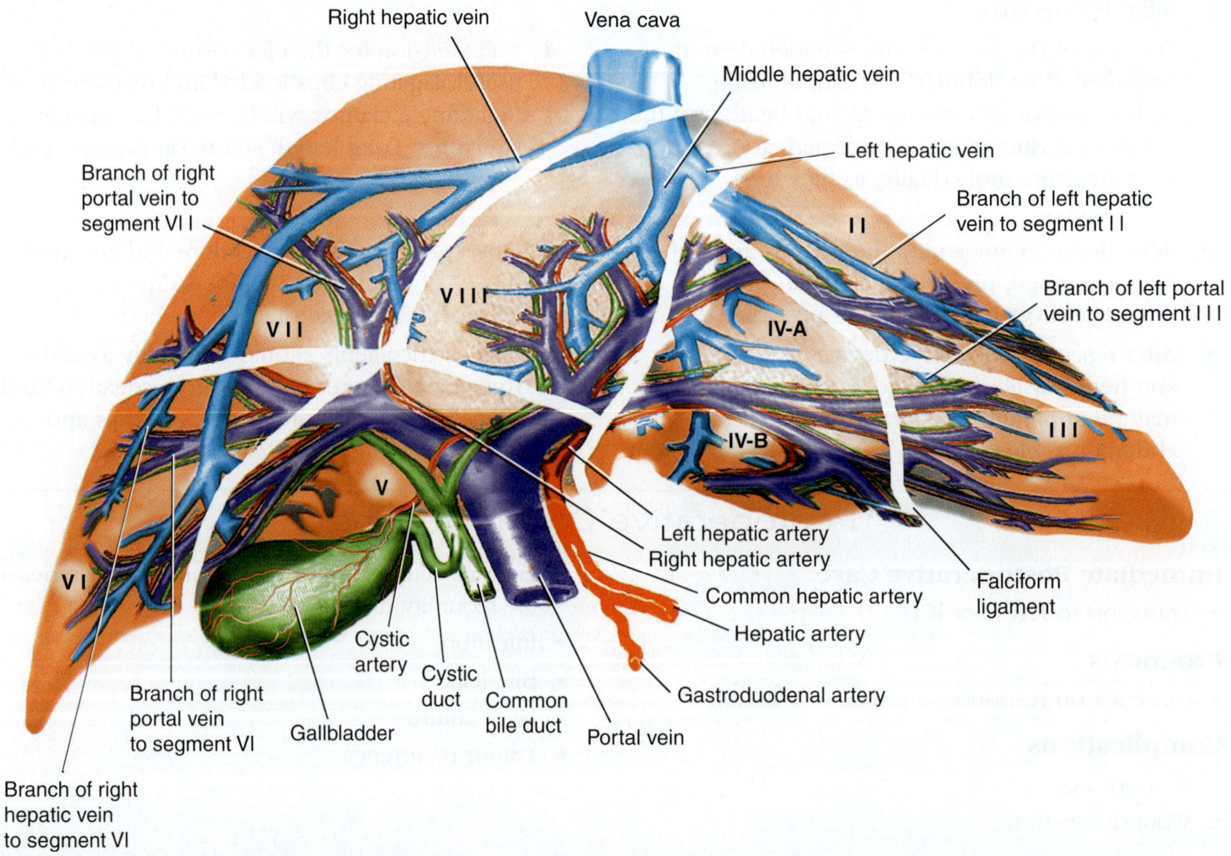

Figure 14-16 Segmental blood supply and ductal system of the liver

sively complicated series of surgical interventions. The sequence is as follows:

- Conservative, noninvasive treatment
- Invasive exploration of the common bile duct
- Open **chole**cystectomy (the procedural steps are essentially the same for the laparoscopic approach with the variations of laparoscopy)
- Cholecystotomy with intraoperative cholangiogram, a procedure performed when cholecystectomy is too risky
- Chole**docho**jejunostomy, the creation of a new drainage pathway

Gallstones (cholelithiasis) represent a significant health problem in the United States. Gallstones (calculi) are classified as being either cholesterol or pigmented. Cholesterol gallstones are a by-product of liver bile that is supersaturated with cholesterol, which then precipitates from the bile to form crystals that grow to macroscopic stones (cholelithiasis). Pigment gallstones are composed of calcium bilirubinate, bilirubin polymers, bile acids, iron, and phosphorus, and may be black, dark brown, yellow, or green.

Conservative Treatment for Cholelithiasis

Gallstones (cholelithiasis) can be treated with medications designed to dissolve them or by extracorporeal shock-wave lithotripsy (ESWL). The electro-generated shock waves pass through soft tissue without harm, but the solid gallstones absorb them and become fragmented. ESWL fragments the gallstones into pieces that are small enough to pass down the cystic duct and common bile duct (CBD) into the alimentary system, where they can be expelled with fecal material. Ultrasound is used to compute the exact location of the target gallstones. The ideal patient for ESWL will have a solitary gallstone less than 2 cm in diameter.

Medications for treatment of cholelithiasis include ursodiol, which reduces cholesterol saturation, and oral bile acids. These medications attack only calcium free gallstones; about 15% of patients with gallstones are candidates for pharmaceutic treatment. This form of therapy may follow ESWL to dissolve the fragments created by that procedure. Although dissolution is usually achieved (50% success rate) within 2 years, half of all patients will develop more gallstones within 5 years of treatment. Methyl tert-butyl ether (MTBE) may also be used to dissolve gallstones by direct injection into the gallbladder through a 7 Fr catheter introduced via the percutaneous transhepatic method. Liver hemorrhage may occur; packing the tract with Gelfoam lowers this risk.

COMMON BILE DUCT EXPLORATION

Common bile duct (CBD) exploration is performed to investigate and resolve obstruction (Procedure 14-8). The procedure requires incision into the CBD (choledochotomy),

PROCEDURE 14-8 Common Bile Duct Exploration

Equipment

- Suction apparatus
- Electrosurgical unit with dispersive electrode
- OR table must accept X-ray cassette or be C-arm compatible

Instruments

- Major instrumentation set
- Common bile duct exploration instrumentation tray
- Fogarty balloon and irrigation catheters and related supplies (e.g., syringe)
- Ligating clip appliers and clips
- Long instruments
- Dorman stone basket
- Choledochoscope and related supplies
- Supplies for intraoperative cholangiogram
- Gallbladder instruments

(continues)

PROCEDURE 14-8 Common Bile Duct Exploration *(continued)*

Supplies

- Prep set
- Basic pack
- Basin set
- Gloves
- Blades (#10 × 2, #11 × 1)
- Laparotomy drapes
- Electrosurgical pencil
- Suture according to surgeon's preference
- Dressing material according to surgeon's preference
- Catheter of choice for cholangiogram
- T-tubes and bile collection device
- Closed wound drainage system available

Operative Preparation

Anesthesia
- General
- Lubricate and protect patient's eyes

Position
- Supine
- May use roll to elevate right side

Prep
- Shave may be necessary, especially for the male patient
- Prep from mid-chest to thighs and laterally as far as possible

Draping
- Anticipated surgical area is outlined with towels secured with adhesive or towel clips
- Laparotomy sheet

Practical Considerations

- Have X-rays or other diagnostic films in room
- Plan for intraoperative cholangiogram

Operative Procedure	Technical Considerations
1. May be accomplished laparoscopically. Right subcostal incision preferred for open approach.	**1.** Prepare for routine laparotomy and normal incisional sequence.
2. Structures of the right upper quadrant of the abdomen are identified and moist packs are used to protect those not involved in the procedure.	**2.** Warm moist packs ready for insertion. Keep count of the number of packs inserted.
3. The lesser omentum is opened and the CBD is identified.	**3.** Anticipate the use of long instruments for dissection.
4. A longitudinal incision about 1.5 to 2 cm is made in the CBD just distal to the junction of the cystic duct. Traction sutures of 4–0 chromic are placed in each edge of the incision.	**4.** CBD incision will require use of #11 blade, Potts scissors, and small suction tip (Frazier) to extract bile. Have traction sutures and "tags" ready.
5. The incision is then "spread" bluntly with a right angle clamp, and any palpable gallstones are "milked" to the choledochotomy site by hand.	**5.** Have ready: fine right angle clamp and blunt tissue forceps for assistant to retrieve stones. Have a specimen container for stones.
6. The CBD is explored with stone forceps (Randall) from the point of incision toward the liver and down to the ampulla of Vater.	**6.** Dilation of duct may be necessary prior to insertion of stone forceps. Have dilators sequentially organized. Present surgeon with a variety of stone forceps so that the correct angle and length for the specific patient may be chosen.

PROCEDURE

14-8 Common Bile Duct Exploration *(continued)*

7. A Fogarty style balloon-tipped catheter or a Dorman stone basket may also be passed to extract any stones. This method requires that the balloon or basket be passed beyond the suspect stone, then inflated/opened, and withdrawn.

7. There are many options available to the surgeon for exploring the duct. Effective communication will help you anticipate the need for baskets, ballooned or irrigation catheters, stone baskets, or choledochoscope. Prepare items as needed. Several methods may be attempted.

8. A T-tube drainage catheter is placed in the CBD with one arm of the "T" running distally and the other proximally. The choledochotomy is closed around the T-tube.

8. Secure requested size T-tube. Surgeon may wish to alter tube to suit patient's anatomy. Have heavy scissors available. Remove any debris from the field.

   T-tube will be sutured into place. The existing traction sutures may be used or new ones placed.

9. A cholangiogram is then performed to demonstrate "free flow" of the contrast medium into the duodenum.

9. Have cholangiogram supplies ready. Drape X-ray equipment if necessary.

10. The projecting end of the T-tube is then brought out through the skin using a separate stab incision that lies in as straight a line as possible to the duct.

10. Skin knife for stab wound and clamp to make tract to exteriorize T-tube and wound drain if used. Connect T-tube and wound drain to closed drainage system components. Drain may be sutured to the skin. Prepare for routine closure and counts.

Postoperative Considerations

Immediate Postoperative Care

- Transport to PACU

Prognosis

- Return to normal activities

Complications

- Hemorrhage
- Wound infection
- Direct injury to the CBD or adjacent structures
- Retained stones
- Pancreatitis
- Stricture of the CBD
- Bile leakage
- Dislodgment of the T-tube
- Development of carcinoma of the gallbladder

PEARL OF WISDOM

Ensure that all air has been expelled from cholangiography system—air bubbles can resemble stones on an X-ray. Hold syringe with plunger up so microscopic bubbles do not get injected.

and can incorporate endoscopic measures (choledochoscopy). Obstruction of the CBD is commonly caused by gallstone migration from the gallbladder. Gallstones in the CBD constitute a condition known as choledocholithiasis. Indications for the procedure include acute or chronic cholecystitis, hyperbilirubinemia, CBD stricture, or presence of a gallstone demonstrated by ultrasound or radiologic examination, jaundice, and the palpation of gallstones within the duct intraoperatively. The procedure may be performed in conjunction with a cholecystectomy.

CHOLECYSTECTOMY AND CHOLANGIOGRAPHY

Cholecystectomy is excision of the gallbladder (Procedure 14-9). Approximately 450,000 are performed annually in the United States. This procedure is primarily performed for acute cholecystitis. Cholecystitis most commonly results from obstruction of the cystic duct by gallstones trapped in Hartman's pouch. Other indications include chronic cholecystitis, calcified gallbladder, tumor of the gallbladder, the presence of asymptomatic gallstones larger than 2 cm, biliary peritonitis, and traumatic rupture of the gallbladder. Contraindications for the procedure include cirrhosis of the liver, advanced age, and the presence of small asymptomatic gallstones.

Acute cholecystitis manifests as moderate to severe pain in the right upper quadrant, fever, nausea and vomiting, and tenderness along the right costal margin. The pain may be referred to the right scapular area. Jaundice is also common. Laboratory findings usually reveal an increased white cell count, and elevated serum bilirubin. Acute cholecystitis is also associated with bacterial inflammation. *Escherichia coli,* salmonella, streptococci, and clostridia have all been implicated. Acute cholecystitis is a serious condition that, if left untreated, can lead to empyema, perforation of the gallbladder or adjacent structures, abscess formation, cholecystenteric fistula, ischemia, impairment of venous return, and necrosis. For this reason most surgeons favor early surgical intervention (within 24 to 48 hours). Symptoms present most commonly in females who are over 40 years of age, premenopausal, and obese.

Cholecystectomy is performed through laparoscopic means in up to 90% of all cases, and this route is successful

PROCEDURE 14-9 Cholecystectomy

Equipment

- Suction apparatus
- Electrosurgical unit with dispersive electrode
- OR table must accept X-ray cassette or be C-arm compatible

Instruments

- Major instrumentation set
- Long instruments
- Ligating clip appliers and clips
- Gallbladder instruments
- CBD exploration supplies (refer to Procedure 14-8)

Supplies

- Prep set
- Basic pack
- Basin set
- Gloves
- Blades (#10 × 2, #11 × 1)
- Laparotomy drapes
- Electrosurgical pencil
- Suture according to surgeon's preference
- Dressing material according to surgeon's preference
- Cholangiogram (refer to Procedure 14-8)
- Closed wound drainage system available

Operative Preparation

Anesthesia

- General
- Lubricate and protect patient's eyes

Position

- Supine
- May use roll to elevate right side

PROCEDURE 14-9 Cholecystectomy *(continued)*

Prep

- Shave may be necessary, especially for the male patient
- Prep from mid-chest to thighs and laterally as far as possible

Draping

- Anticipated surgical area is outlined with towels secured with adhesive or towel clips
- Laparotomy sheet

Practical Considerations

- X-rays or other diagnostic films in room
- Anticipate intraoperative cholangiogram

Operative Procedure	Technical Considerations
1. Several incisional options exist; right subcostal (Kocher) is preferred.	**1.** Prepare for routine laparotomy. Normal incision and exposure procedures will be followed. Kocher incisions are muscle-cutting incisions. The electrosurgical pencil will be used heavily and a vaporized tissue plume evacuation system should be employed.
2. The gallbladder is explored and any apparent adhesions are first released by blunt or sharp dissection. Packs are placed to protect adjacent visceral structures and to further isolate the gallbladder, and retractors are placed.	**2.** Prepare warm, moist lap pads for packing and retractors according to patient size and surgeon preference. Peanut sponges on a long instrument may be used for blunt dissection.
3. The lesser omentum is opened and the associated ducts and vasculature are identified.	**3.** Long scissors, tissue forceps, and right angle clamps will be used. Have ligating clips loaded and ready for use.
4. Once the gallbladder is exposed, a Kelly clamp is placed near the ampulla and traction is applied inferiorly and medially to place the peritoneum overlying the cystic duct and artery under tension.	**4.** Traction clamps will be applied. Electrosurgery may be used to free gallbladder from liver bed. A long angled tip may be useful.
5. The peritoneum is incised with Metzenbaum scissors. Using a right angle and blunt dissection, the cystic artery is identified and followed toward the gallbladder until it is certain that the structure is not the right hepatic artery.	**5.** Scissors, tissue forceps, and a right angle will be used repeatedly. Keep available for immediate reuse.
6. The cystic artery is then double ligated with 2–0 silk or ligating clips are placed across it near the gallbladder, and the artery is transected between the ties or clips.	**6.** Ties will likely be used on passers; have them loaded in advance.
7. The cystic duct, which lies inferior and lateral to the cystic artery, is then isolated by blunt dissection, and its junction with the CBD is identified.	**7.** Anticipate the same procedure for securing and transecting the cystic duct as was carried out on the cystic artery.

(continues)

PROCEDURE

14-9 Cholecystectomy *(continued)*

8. If necessary, an intraoperative cholangiogram is performed at this point. A stab incision is made in the cystic duct, about 2 cm from the CBD, and 4–0 chromic stay sutures are placed on either side of the wound.	**8.** Have cholangiogram supplies ready in advance. Drape radiologic equipment as necessary. A #11 blade followed by Potts scissors will be used for choledochotomy. Two stay sutures and tags are needed.
9. The duct is gently probed for patency and usually bile will ooze out. A cholangiogram catheter is introduced into the duct and secured with a ligating clip across the duct.	**9.** Surgeon may request culture of bile; have supplies available. Suction will be needed to remove bile.
10. The duct is aspirated until bile is drawn into the saline syringe and the duct is flushed with the saline. The dilute contrast medium is then instilled into the duct and an X-ray is taken.	**10.** Be sure all team members are protected from radiation.
11. The X-ray should reveal the structure of the CBD and hepatic duct, as well as demonstrate spillage into the duodenum without any sign of ductal gallstones. (Percutaneous cholangiography requires the same basic steps.)	**11.** Anticipate CBD exploration if stones are visible on X-ray.
12. Traction is then reapplied to the gallbladder in changing directions as needed. With blunt and sharp dissection, the gallbladder is excised from the liver bed. Small bleeders in this area are controlled electrosurgically.	**12.** Prepare for removal of gallbladder. Have electrosurgical pencil or hemostatic agent of choice available.
13. Excision of the gallbladder is usually performed from the cystic duct to the fundus. However, if these structures are difficult to discern, dissection may begin at the fundus and proceed to the duct.	**13.** Receive specimen in a container. Gallbladder bed may be cultured. Anticipate drain placement.
14. The specimen is removed from the wound, the area is irrigated and checked for hemostasis, and the abdomen is closed.	**14.** Warm irrigation on field. Anticipate routine closure and counts.

Postoperative Considerations

Immediate Postoperative Care

- Transport to PACU

Prognosis

- Return to normal activities

Complications

- Hemorrhage
- Wound infection
- Atelectasis (a collapsed or airless condition of the lung)
- Ileus (small bowel obstruction)
- Hepatic artery or bile duct injury
- Damage to structures of the porta hepatis
- Persistent bile drainage
- Retention of duct stones

PEARL OF WISDOM

Cholecystectomy with cholangiogram is one of those procedures that illustrates a routine problem: significant movement by nonsterile team members around the sterile field. Observe carefully the movement of the radiology technologist and the protect the sterile field from potential contamination.

95% of the time. However, conversion to the open procedure does occur and some patients are best treated in this manner. Open cholecystectomy is presented in Procedure 14-9.

For comparison purposes, Figure 14-17A and B illustrate the laparoscopic approach. The actual steps in removal of the gallbladder are the same. The variance occurs with the use of trocars to enter the abdomen and the method of extracting the gallbladder through a port.

CHOLECYSTOSTOMY

Cholecystostomy may be performed when cholecystectomy is deemed unsafe because of local or systemic conditions. It is an infrequently seen procedure, but is also a life-saving one.

Indications for cholecystostomy include acute cholecystitis with gallstones, chronic calculous cholecystitis, acute pancreatitis with obstructive jaundice, and some instances of carcinoma of the pancreas. Cholecystostomy is performed by an open technique as described on page 447, or

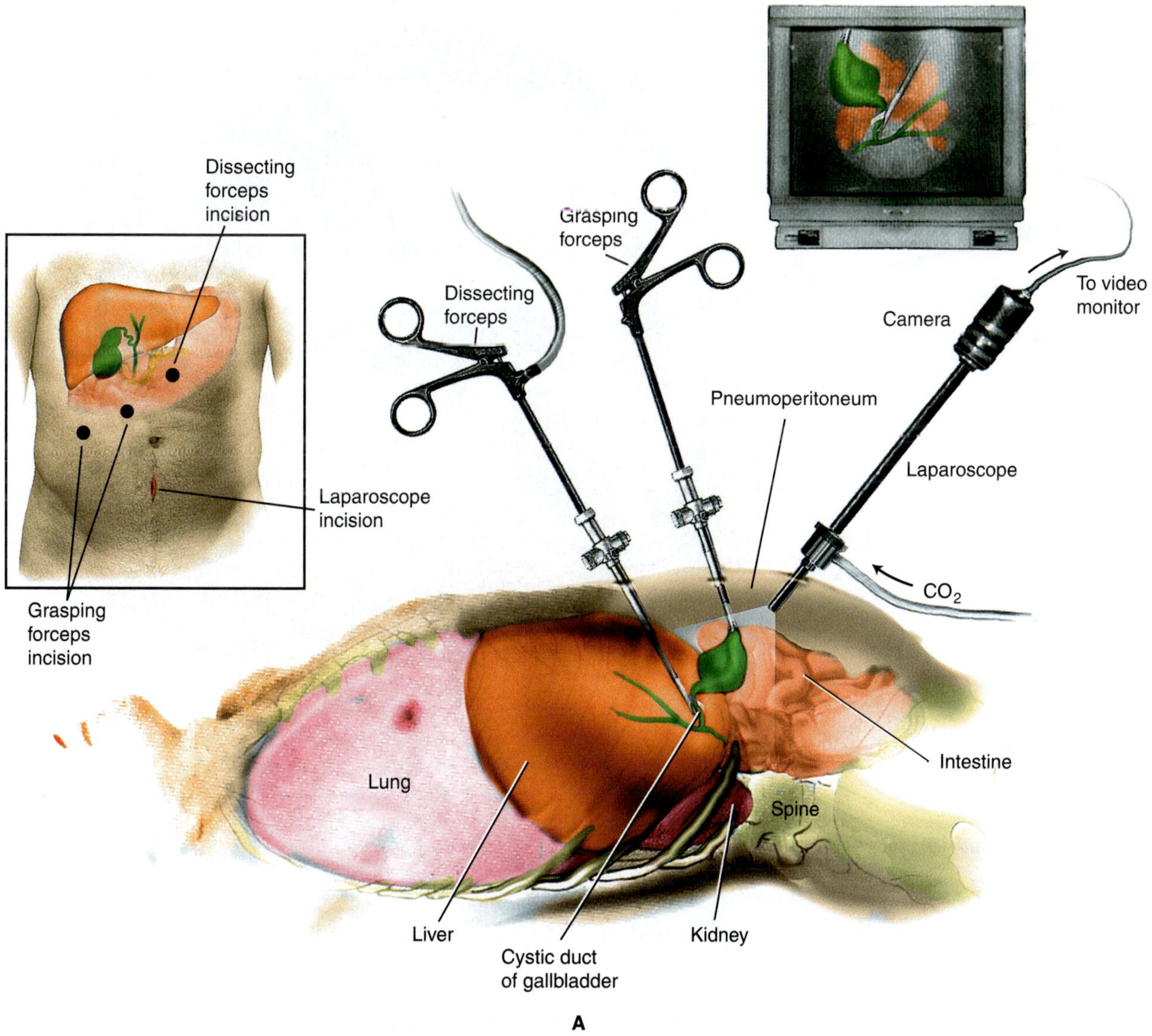

Figure 14-17 Laparoscopic cholecystectomy: (A) Lateral view *(continues)*

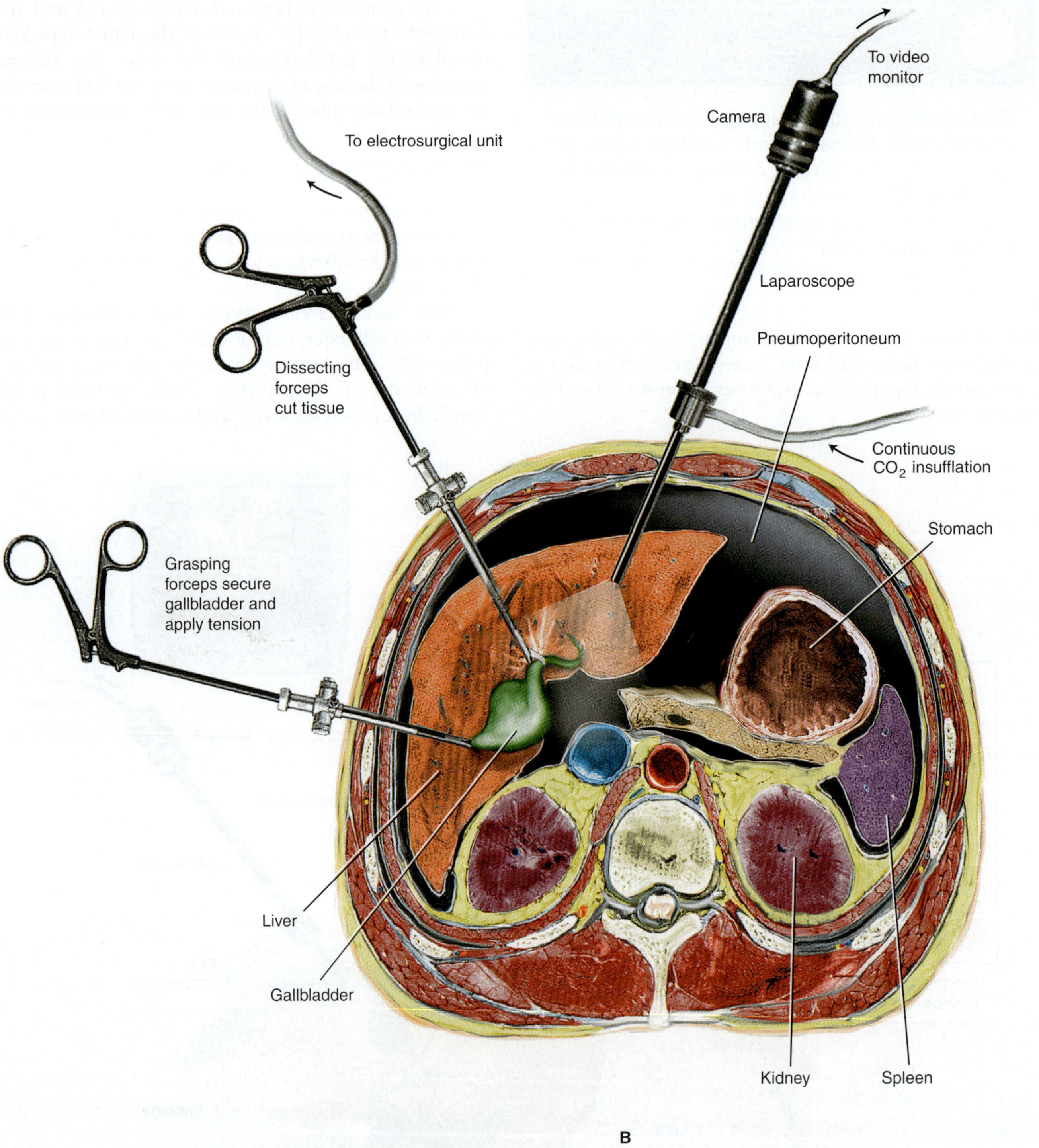

Figure 14-17 ***(continued)*** **(B) cross-section view**

through a percutaneous method guided by ultrasound or fluoroscopy, in which case a drain may be left in place. Complications can be significant for this procedure because of the patient's initial condition. Complications include

- Infection
- Residual stones in the gallbladder and CBD
- Fistula formation
- Recurrent cholecystitis
- Carcinoma
- Subsequent cholecystectomy

Cholecystostomy also carries higher morbidity and mortality rates than cholecystectomy.

Cholecystostomy involves the following actions after a routine opening:

- Once access to the gallbladder is achieved, a 3–0 chromic traction suture is placed in the fundus to elevate the organ into the wound.
- A 3–0 chromic pursestring suture is then placed in the fundus around the area of proposed catheter placement, and a stab incision is made through the serosa.
- A gallbladder trocar is introduced through the incision to decompress the organ.
- Once the gallbladder is decompressed, the trocar is withdrawn and any gallstones present are removed.
- A Pezzer or Malecot catheter is inserted in the incision and the pursestring suture is tightened around it.
- The catheter is brought out through a separate stab wound in the abdomen.
- Routine abdominal closure is carried out.

Choledochojejunostomy

A choledochojejunostomy is undertaken during biliary surgery when pathology or injury makes an easy anastomosis between the bile duct and the duodenum (because of their proximity to each other) impossible. This communication may be made to a simple loop of jejunum, but is more often anastomosed to the side branch of a Roux-en-Y. In this instance, the Roux-en-Y branch is about 50 to 60 cm long and is brought into place through a defect created in the transverse mesocolon.

Anastomosis is commonly made as a one-layer closure in an end- (of the duct) to-side (of the jejunum) fashion and a transhepatic stent or a T-tube may be passed through the jejunum to ensure ductal patency. An opening, similar in diameter to that of the bile duct, is made electrosurgically in the antimesenteric border of the jejunal loop or the terminal branch of a jejunal Roux-en-Y. The bile duct is anastomosed to the jejunum using several interrupted 4–0 or 5–0 absorbable sutures. The Roux-en-Y branch is secured to the hepatic capsule and the abdomen is irrigated, checked for hemostasis, and closed.

Postoperatively, the transhepatic catheter remains in place for 4 to 8 weeks. Diet progresses from liquid to normal over the course of several weeks, and when bowel function has returned to normal a cholangiogram is performed. Complications of this procedure are those common to anastomosis (stricture, leakage, etc.) as well as jaundice, catheter obstruction, and hemorrhage.

SURGERY OF THE PANCREAS AND SPLEEN

Throughout much of history the pancreas was essentially unapproachable. Modern surgical methods and a better understanding have made pancreatic surgery possible and effective. The spleen is commonly traumatized and removed during emergency surgery. Much like the liver and biliary structures, the complex anatomy and physiology provide a challenge to the general surgeon.

SELECT PATHOLOGY OF THE PANCREAS

Pathological conditions of the pancreas are listed in Table 14-19.

Table 14-19 Pancreatic Pathology, Symptoms, and Diagnosis

PATHOLOGY	SYMPTOMS AND DIAGNOSTICS
• Pancreatitis is associated with both primary pancreatic tumors and metastases, primarily from gastric cancer. • Although the inflammatory process of chronic pancreatitis can involve the whole organ, in 20% to 30% of cases it is limited to the pancreatic head. • Carcinoma of the pancreas is the fourth most common malignancy in the United States. • The incidence of pancreatic cancer is the highest in the pancreatic head and ampulla of Vater, and lesions in these areas tend to grow to a large size and metastasize prior to the onset of symptoms. • The majority of patients (over 80%) with pancreatic cancer never undergo curative surgical intervention, while the remainder are treated by the Whipple pancreatoduodenectomy.	• The most common symptom (95% of patients) is intractable upper abdominal (epigastric) pain that is constant and dull. • Other signs and symptoms include malabsorption of nutrients leading to diarrhea and weight loss, nausea, vomiting, low-grade fever, respiratory problems, absence of normal bowel sounds, jaundice secondary to CBD compression, and diabetes. • Diagnosis is commonly made through physical examination that reveals a large palpable mass, low serum bilirubin levels, abnormal radiographs of the abdomen, needle biopsy, CT scan, ERCP, and ultrasonography. • Laparoscopy may also be performed prior to submitting the patient to a laparotomy.

DRAINING PANCREATIC CYSTS

Cystic (fluid-filled) lesions of the pancreas are far less common than solid tumors, and are grouped as simple (true) cysts, neoplasms, and inflammatory pseudocysts. The most common cystic lesion of the pancreas, seen in 10% of all patients with pancreatic disease, is the pseudocyst, which lacks the epithelium-lined structure of a true cyst. True cysts are rare in the pancreas and include congenital and acquired varieties such as solitary or multiple cysts, enterogenous cysts, serous cystadenoma, cystic teratoma (dermoid), papillary cystic tumor, and cystic islet cell tumor. Cysts may become malignant if left untreated. Pancreatic cysts may be drained by one of several techniques.

As laboratory evaluation is generally inconclusive in pancreatic cystic disease, diagnosis is best accomplished through imaging techniques such as CT, endoscopic ultrasonography (EUS), and endoscopic retrograde cholangiopancreatography (ERCP). Ultrasound-guided needle aspiration and needle biopsy are also employed for diagnosis and therapy of pancreatic pathology. The usual approach to treating pancreatic cysts is through drainage or resection techniques and depends upon the size, location, and symptoms of the cystic lesions.

Indications for drainage include infection, gastrointestinal obstruction, hemorrhage, spontaneous cyst rupture, and failure to resolve spontaneously over time. Techniques for drainage are found in Table 14-20.

Postoperative care includes monitoring the drainage, removal of external drains in 7 to 10 days (or longer), and follow-up imaging to confirm cystic atrophy. Complications of treatment include hemorrhage, infection, fistula formation, pseudocyst recurrence, obstruction, and rupture. External drainage is associated with higher mortality rates.

PANCREATIC RESECTION

Pancreatic resection is performed in cases of cysts that cannot be drained, resectable tumors, chronic pancreatitis, and with an inflammatory pancreatic mass in which the duodenum is uninvolved and can therefore be preserved. Resection is also performed for trauma or severe pain and is the only potential cure for pancreatic cancer. Diagnosis of these conditions is usually made through CT scan and needle biopsy. Other procedures undertaken prior to pancreatic resection include thorough physical examination, endoscopic retrograde cholangiopancreatography to determine ductal involvement and anatomy, resolution of pathology of other organs, and establishing metabolic baselines.

PANCREATECTOMY

Pancreatectomy is the surgical removal of the pancreas (Procedure 14-10). It is most often performed as part of a combination procedure, the pancreaticoduodenectomy (Whipple).

WHIPPLE PANCREATICODUODENECTOMY

The Whipple procedure requires both resection and reconstruction. Resection is an en bloc excision of the head of the pancreas, the distal one-third (antrum and pylorus) of the stomach, all of the duodenum, the proximal 10 cm of the jejunum, the gallbladder, the cystic and common bile ducts, and peripancreatic and hepatoduodenal lymph nodes. Re-

Table 14-20 Drainage of a Pancreatic Cyst

APPROACH/TYPE	DEFINITION AND TECHNICAL NOTES
Endoscopic	Endoscopic placement of a stent or catheter directly into the cyst allowing it to drain into the pancreatic ductal system, other organ (e.g., the duodenum), or to the outside.
Percutaneous	Percutaneous placement of a stent or catheters directly into the cyst allowing it to drain into the pancreatic ductal system, other organ (e.g., the duodenum), or to the outside. A transduodenal drainage approach is used in which a needle is guided by imagery into the duodenal lumen, and a catheter is passed through the needle and into the pancreatic duct via the papilla of Vater, to ultimately communicate with the cyst.
Laparotomy	Laparotomy approach and placement of a stent or catheters directly into the cyst allowing it to drain into the pancreatic ductal system, other organ (e.g., the duodenum), or to the outside. Internal drainage is accomplished by constructing an ostomy between the pancreatic cyst and the nearest organ. Cystogastrostomy: cyst anastomosed to the stomach Cystoduodenostomy: cyst in the pancreatic head anastomosed to the duodenum Cystojejunostomy: cyst in the pancreatic body or tail, if extremely large, or if not adherent to the stomach (requires mobilizing a loop of jejunum to allow a "tension-free" anastomosis with the pancreatic cyst) anastomosed to the jejunum

section is performed in eight steps (Figure 14-18A), and reconstruction in three steps (Figure 14-18B), with variable methods employed for each.

RESECTION

1. A wide subcostal or upper midline approach
2. Exploration of the abdomen and assessment of the extent and resectability of the tumor
3. Cholecystectomy
4. Partial gastrectomy
5. Vagotomy
6. Division of the pancreas
7. Dissection of the retropancreatic vessels
8. Division of the jejunum

RECONSTRUCTION

1. Pancreaticojejunostomy
2. Hepaticojejunostomy (choledochojejunostomy)
3. End-to-side gastrojejunostomy

Prior to closure of the abdomen, a standard Braun jejunostomy is performed to keep the jejunum decompressed during the postoperative period. A nasogastric tube is also inserted to keep that organ decompressed. A closed wound drainage system is placed behind the pancreatic and biliary anastomoses. The Volker tube (in the choledochojejunostomy) is brought out through a stab wound in the right flank, and the wound drain exits through a similar wound located 5 cm from the Volker tube. These are secured at the skin level with 3–0 silk. The jejunostomy tube is also brought out through the lateral abdominal wall. The abdomen is then closed.

Postoperative care is crucial and complex. Complications following the Whipple pancreaticoduodenectomy are serious and include abdominal sepsis, pancreatic fistula formation, diabetes, hemorrhage, possibility of reoperation, peptic ulcer formation, disrupted nutrient absorption, delayed gastric emptying, and death. Some degree of complications are experienced by 20–40% of all patients. Hospital mortality following Whipple has traditionally been around 20%, but in the past decade this has been reduced to under 5%.

PROCEDURE 14-10 Pancreatectomy

Equipment

- Suction apparatus
- Electrosurgical unit with dispersive electrode
- Headlamp available

Instruments

- Major instrumentation set
- Vascular instruments
- Biliary instruments in room
- Long instruments
- Bowel resection set
- Harrington retractors
- Ligating clip appliers and clips

Supplies

- Prep set
- Basic pack
- Basin set
- Gloves
- Blades (#10 × 3, #11 × 1)
- Laparotomy drapes
- Electrosurgical pencil
- Suture according to surgeon's preference
- Dressing material according to surgeon's preference
- Hemostatic agents
- Active and passive drains available
- Staplers

(continues)

PROCEDURE 14-10 Pancreatectomy *(continued)*

Operative Preparation

Anesthesia
- General
- Lubricate and protect patient's eyes

Position
- Supine

Prep
- Insert Foley catheter, if ordered
- Shave may be necessary, especially for the male patient
- Prep from mid-chest to thighs and laterally as far as possible

Draping
- Anticipated surgical area is outlined with towels secured with adhesive or towel clips
- Laparotomy sheet

Practical Considerations

- Verify availability of blood
- Monitor blood loss carefully

Operative Procedure	Technical Considerations
1. A left subcostal or upper midline incision is made and retractors are placed for exposure.	**1.** All considerations for cholecystectomy, choledochojejunostomy, and small bowel resection may apply in these procedures.
2. The entire anterior surface of the pancreas is exposed by opening the lesser sac of the omentum and mobilizing the hepatic flexure of the colon.	**2.** Have warm, moist packs and self-retaining retractor ready for placement.
3. The pathology is palpated and the extent of the required resection is determined. Intraoperative ultrasound may be used to outline the structure of the pancreatic duct prior to resection and anastomosis.	**3.** Have available throughout: suture ligatures, ligature on a passer, and ligating clips.
4. A Satinsky type vascular clamp is placed across the pancreas distal to the point of resection. The pancreatic parenchyma is divided sharply with a scalpel.	**4.** Long scissors, long tissue forceps, long right angles, and tonsil hemostats may be needed.
5. The posterior vessels are divided. The pancreas is dissected from the spleen, including division of the splenic artery and vein. The tail and body of the pancreas are removed and any retained pancreatic stump is closed.	**5.** Prepare to receive specimen. Anticipate suture use for stump closure.
6. Hemostasis of the proximal pancreas is achieved with fine mosquito clamps, electrosurgery, and 3–0 silk ties or suture ligatures. The pancreatic duct is prepared for anastomosis to the jejunum.	**6.** Bowel clamps and suture or staplers for bowel closure should be available. Prepare for and maintain bowel technique per facility policy.

PROCEDURE

14-10 Pancreatectomy *(continued)*

7. Reconstruction (pancreaticojejunostomy) is carried out by use of a jejunal loop that is defunctionalized by a Roux-en-Y anastomosis.
8. The pancreatic duct is anastomosed end-to-side to the jejunal loop with a mucosa to mucosa closure. The parenchyma of the pancreas is then secured to the jejunal serosa.

7. Plan for copious irrigation, use of Poole suction, and placement of drains.
8. Prepare suture for closure. Initiate count.

Postoperative Considerations

Immediate Postoperative Care

- Transport to PACU

Prognosis

- Depends on response to primary condition

Complications

- Hemorrhage
- Wound infection
- Fistula formation
- Recurrence of pathology
- Leakage of anastomosis
- Nutritional/digestive concerns
- Ileus

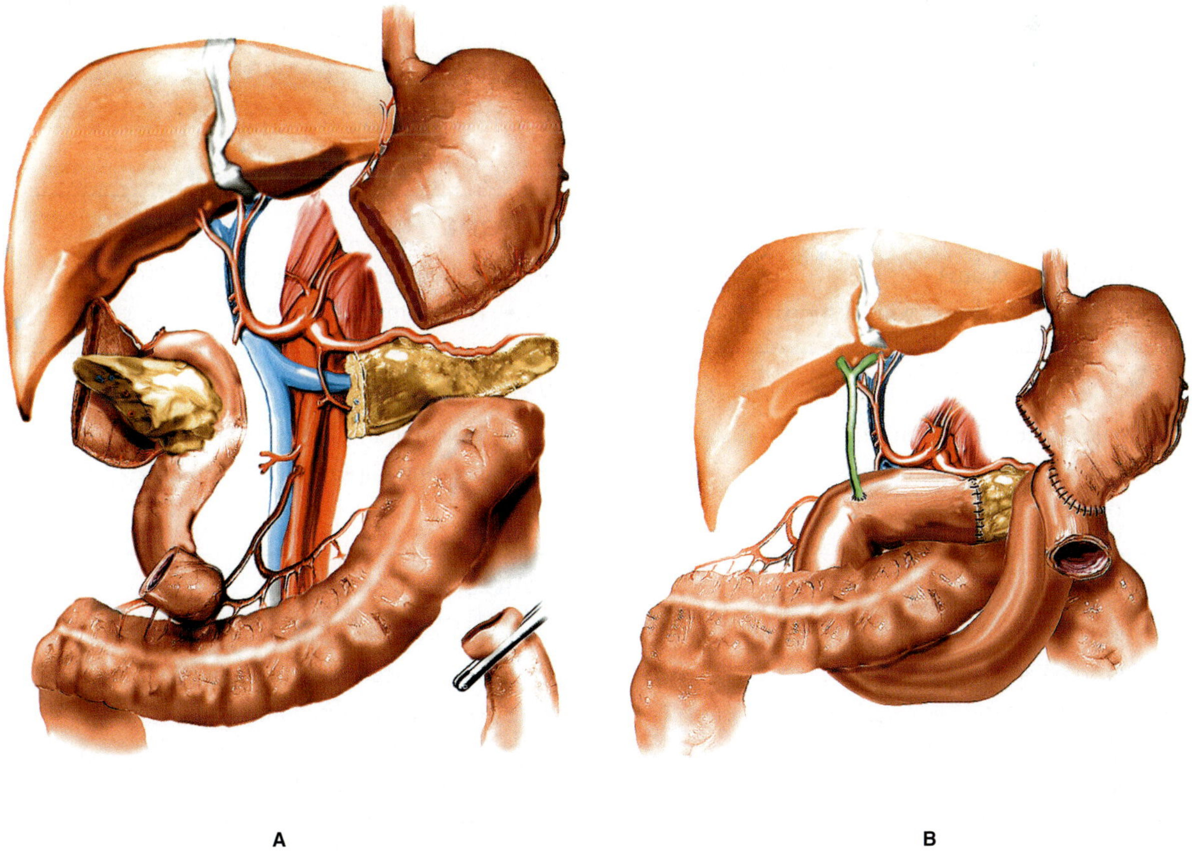

A B

Figure 14-18 **Whipple procedure: (A) Resection, (B) reconstruction**

PEARL OF WISDOM

Listen carefully to the conversation between the surgeon and surgical assistant. It will help you determine which options and procedures will be required. These are very complex procedures but they are made up of a series of smaller procedures. Organize for one basic procedure at a time.

SURGERY OF THE SPLEEN

Trauma, with subsequent intraperitoneal bleeding, is the primary indication for splenectomy. Other disorders that may warrant splenectomy include intraoperative injury, thrombocytopenia (an acquired autoimmune phenomenon that results in the destruction of platelets), splenomegaly, splenic abscess, parasitic cysts of the spleen, and spontaneous rupture resulting from disease.

Signs and symptoms of rupture include hypovolemia, hypotension, bradycardia, and pain. Thrombocytopenia manifests as acute bleeding with low platelet counts. Abscesses and splenic parasitic cysts generally trigger infection and left upper quadrant tenderness. Diagnosis of splenic maladies is commonly confirmed by CT scan. Preoperative care includes platelet infusion, administration of a pneumococcal vaccine, and low-dose heparin therapy.

SPLENECTOMY

Splenectomy is performed for hematologic disorders, splenic anemia, neutropenia, tumors, cysts, and splenomegaly, but the most frequent reason is laceration secondary to trauma (Procedure 14-11).

SPLENIC SALVAGE

Splenic salvage includes repair of lacerations or partial splenectomy. Either option is considered when preservation of the spleen is desired such as in cases involving individuals who may refuse blood transfusions, if existing pathology is limited (such as a small cyst), or when the patient is hemodynamically stable and has no other injuries. Lacerations can be caused by blunt or penetrating trauma,

PROCEDURE 14-11 Splenectomy

Equipment

- Suction apparatus
- Electrosurgical unit with dispersive electrode
- Cell-Saver available
- Headlamp available

Instruments

- Major instrumentation set
- Sarot or other large clamps
- Long instruments
- Vascular and bowel sets available
- Ligating clip appliers and clips

Supplies

- Prep set
- Basic pack
- Basin set
- Gloves
- Blades (#10 × 2)
- Laparotomy drape
- Electrosurgical unit
- Suture according to surgeon's preference
- Dressing material according to surgeon's preference
- Hemostatic agents
- Staplers

PROCEDURE 14-11 Splenectomy *(continued)*

Operative Preparation

Anesthesia
- General
- Lubricate and protect patient's eyes

Position
- Supine

Prep
- Insert Foley catheter, if ordered
- Shave may be necessary, especially for the male patient
- Prep from mid-chest to thighs and laterally as far as possible

Draping
- Anticipated surgical area is outlined with towels secured with adhesive or towel clips
- Laparotomy sheet

Practical Considerations

- Verify availability of blood
- Monitor blood loss carefully

Operative Procedure

1. An upper midline or left subcostal incision is used. Appropriate retractors are placed.
2. Left upper quadrant is explored. Suspensory splenic ligaments are identified and ligaments are then divided by blunt dissection or scissors as required (Figure 14-19).

Technical Considerations

1. Prioritize if patient is hemorrhaging. Dry laps will be used initially.
2. When hemostasis obtained, sponges may be removed and replaced with clean ones. These should be warm and moist to protect the bowel and other structures.

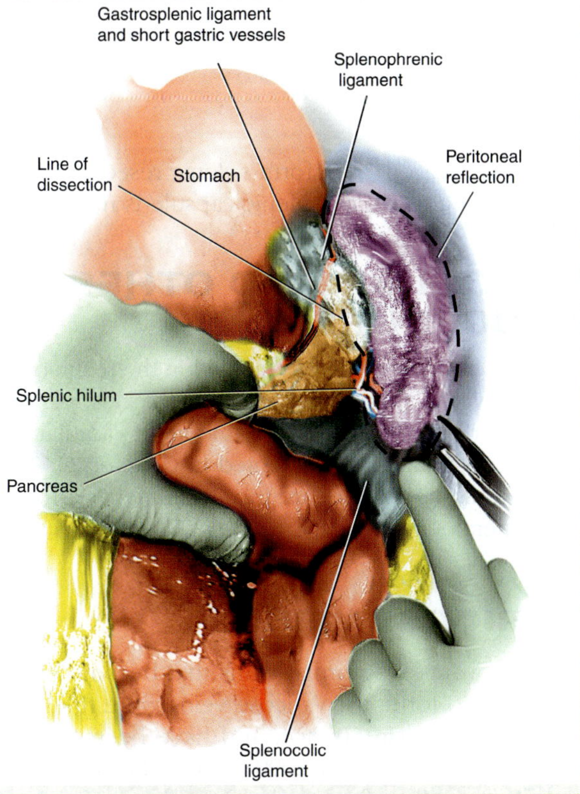

Figure 14-19 Splenectomy

(continues)

PROCEDURE 14-11 Splenectomy *(continued)*

3. The short gastric veins that run to the stomach are identified, ligated, and cut. The spleen is "mobilized" into the wound.
4. Dissection is carried out at the splenic hilum to identify splenic vessels. The splenic artery is double ligated, suture ligated, and divided. The splenic vein is double ligated and divided.
5. The spleen can now be removed and hemostasis is achieved.
6. A drain may be placed and the wound is closed.

3. Have both suture ligatures and ligatures on a right angle passer available, usually 0 silk. Have ligating clips available (medium and large).
4. Provide suction as needed. A small basin for clots may be useful.
5. In trauma, the entire abdomen will be explored following hemostatic control. Damage to the pancreas, stomach, and bowel are common.
6. Drain prepared. Closing sutures ready. Initiate count.

Postoperative Considerations

Immediate Postoperative Care
- Transport to PACU

Prognosis
- Return to normal activities
- Immunologic response may be impaired

Complications
- Hemorrhage
- Wound infection
- Dehiscence

PEARL OF WISDOM

Splenectomy for trauma usually involves a large amount of bleeding. The procedure is relatively straightforward but visualization may be a problem. Large clamps such as Sarot clamps and many lap sponges may be needed (this is not the case with elective splenectomy).

as well as during other surgery, and partial splenectomy is warranted in cases of irreparable damage to a portion of the spleen or to one of its arteries.

Repair of a splenic laceration can entail the application of topical hemostatic agents (e.g., Avitene, Gelfoam), suturing, or wrapping of the spleen with mesh or the omentum, whereas dissection, electrosurgery, CUSA (Cavitron Ultrasonic Aspirator), or lasers, is utilized when partial splenectomy is preferred. In either event, mobilization of the spleen is necessary to enable access to the lacerated area or to perform splenic resection. Maintaining the integrity of the splenic capsule is mandatory.

VASCULAR AND OTHER PROCEDURES

Most vascular interventions fall within the realm of the peripheral vascular specialist. In some locales, general surgeons perform a considerable amount of vascular surgery. These procedures are presented in Chapter 23. The procedures discussed here are those routinely performed by the general surgeon.

VARICOSE VEINS

Varicose veins are normal veins that become elongated, dilated, and tortuous. Varicose veins were first observed by Hippocrates in 500 B.C. and have been treated with surgery for more than 2000 years. The term "varicose veins" generally refers to the affected superficial veins of the lower extremity, but can also be applied to varices of the lower esophagus, spermatic cord (varicocele), and in the anorectal region (hemorrhoids). Those of the lower extremity are addressed in this section.

Varicose veins, a disease that is progressive and incurable, occur in half of the male population and three-quarters of all women. Varicose veins are categorized as primary or secondary, and causes of this condition include heredity, female sex hormones (especially progesterone), constricted clothing, long periods of standing, obesity, incompetent venous valves, pregnancy, gravitational hydrostatic forces, physical inactivity, smoking, hypertension, and hydrodynamic muscular compartment forces. Primary varicose veins consist of protuberant superficial veins, and secondary varicose veins are a complication of deep venous disease.

Symptoms of varicose veins include nonspecific aching and heaviness of the lower extremity which worsen during the day, associated leg cramping at night, mild edema, fatigue, visible protrusions, pigmentation, ulceration, eczema, tenderness, and internal and external bleeding. Indications for therapy include pain, easy fatigability, recurrent thrombophlebitis, external bleeding, appearance, and complications of varicose veins, such as dermal atrophy, hemorrhage, and cellulitis. Contraindications to treatment include pregnancy during the first and second trimester, significant leg edema, arterial occlusive disease, and immobility. Varicose veins may be treated with conservative measures (walking, leg elevation, and elastic stockings), with sclerotherapy (injections), or by surgery (ligation and stripping) (Table 14-21).

VASCULAR ACCESS PROCEDURES

Vascular access refers to the cannulation of arteries and veins. This section focuses on venous access, which is performed to monitor central venous pressure (CVP), to infuse blood products, to provide parenteral nutritional support, and to deliver chemotherapeutic medications and antibiotics. The cut down procedure of the cephalic vein and the percutaneous approach to the subclavian vein (Table 14-22) are described in this section.

Venous access for these purposes is accomplished by the introduction of intravenous access devices (IVADs). The resultant cannulation in this regard can be "transcutaneous" (e.g., Hickman, Broviac, or Groshong catheter) or totally implantable port-catheter systems (e.g., Port-a-Cath). Transcutaneous catheters are available in various diameters, and can have one to three lumens that are accessed through externalized, attachable Luer "hubs." These catheters also have a Dacron "cuff" at a point along their length that is buried subcutaneously and serves as both an anchoring device and a barrier to infection. The Groshong catheter is unique in that it has attached hubs and a two-way valve within. The Port-a-Cath also has a catheter that is placed intravenously; however, access to it is through a "port" of stainless steel, plastic, or titanium that is implanted below the skin and accessed by a noncoring (Huber) needle. These ports can be infiltrated 1,500 to 2,000 times.

Indications for IVAD are

- Intravenous chemotherapy, nutrition, or blood products
- Patients with difficult or exhausted peripheral veins
- Needle phobia
- Central venous pressure must be monitored
- Patient age (pediatric)

Complications of vascular access surgery are vein thrombosis, vascular "steal," catheter thrombosis, venous hypertension, infection, pneumothorax, disruption of vascular surfaces, and luminal dissection. Postoperatively, the wounds require simple dressings, the patient receives antibiotics for 24 hours, the catheters must be flushed with heparinized saline periodically, and the implanted catheters can be used for various lengths of time from months to years.

Table 14-21 Treatment of Varicose Veins

TREATMENT	DEFINITION AND PROCEDURAL NOTES
Sclerotherapy	• Injection into small varicosities (usually less than 3 mm in diameter) that cannot be approached surgically. • Permanently obliterates the lumen of the varicosity by causing a fibrotic reaction within it. • Agents most commonly used for this therapy are sodium chloride 23.4% and 3% sodium tetradecyl sulfate, 40% dextrose, and 25% saline solution.
Vein ligation and stripping	• Involves ligation of the saphenous vein and its tributaries at its junction with the common femoral vein in the groin. • Removal of the saphenous vein from its "bed" in the lower extremity by use of an intraluminal vein stripper.

Table 14-22 Vascular Access Procedures

TREATMENT	DEFINITION AND PROCEDURAL NOTES
Cut-down procedure	• Safest approach for realizing venous access. • Anatomical position of vein identified, local anesthesia administered, incision over the vein carried to the vein. • A 2-cm segment of the vein is isolated from the surrounding tissues and 2–0 silk ties are placed at the proximal and distal points. • A catheter exit, or implantable port, site is identified and developed. • The catheter is then tunneled from the exit/pocket site through the subcutaneous tissue to the cephalic vein until the Dacron cuff is buried a few cm into the tunnel. Catheters are flushed with heparinized saline prior to insertion into the vein.
Percutaneous procedure	• Performed under fluoroscopy and requires an "introduction" kit. • The kit contains a 2¾-in., 18-gauge needle, a 12-mL syringe, a 50-cm 0.38- or 0.32-in. flexible-tipped (J-shaped) guidewire, a guidewire tip "straightener," and a cannulated dilator within a peel-away sheath. • The subclavian vein is located and the exit site (or port pocket site) for the catheter is selected. • Local anesthesia is administered and a 1-cm incision is made in both of these areas. • The catheter is then tunneled from the exit/port site to the venipuncture site and flushed with heparinized saline prior to insertion into the vein. • Catheter position is confirmed with fluoroscopy.

MUSCLE AND NERVE BIOPSIES

Biopsy of skeletal muscle or peripheral nerve is performed in patients with neuromuscular disorders, such as myopathy or neuropathy. Commonly the vastus lateralis, biceps, or deltoid muscles are biopsied in proximal limb disorders, and the gastrocnemius or tibialis anterior muscles are approached for lower extremity pathology. The sural nerve, located near the ankle, is the most common site of nerve biopsy, followed by the radial nerve in the wrist and the superficial peroneal nerve in the calf. Determination for the need for muscle or nerve biopsy is done in conjunction with electromyogram (EMG) and nerve conduction studies.

The patient is appropriately positioned, prepped, and draped to allow access to the biopsy site. Local anesthesia is commonly used. The 3- to 5-cm skin incision follows the Langer lines and is usually superficial, requiring minimal dissection of subcutaneous tissues prior to exposing the target nerve or muscle. A section of the nerve or muscle is isolated, ligated, and divided without disruption of the integrity of the biopsied tissue. The specimen is immediately sent for laboratory examination. The wound is closed with a running subcuticular 4–0 absorbable suture or interrupted 4–0 nylon stitches. A light dressing is applied. Complications following these procedures are few.

INCISION AND DRAINAGE

Simple incision and drainage (I&D) is exactly what it sounds like, an incision with subsequent drainage, and is indicated when there is a need to open an abscess to allow it to drain. This often relieves the pain associated with inflammation as well as reducing the risk of spreading of the infection. It is performed under local, general, or spinal anesthesia, and patient positioning, skin prep, and draping depend on the site of the I&D. A small incision is made directly over, and into, the abscess with a #11 or #15 blade, and a blunt clamp is introduced to "spread" any nerves and vessels out of the way. Aerobic and anaerobic cultures may be obtained. Copious irrigation is applied into the wound, and in most cases the incision is left open, packed with gauze, and secondary closure is performed 3 to 5 days later. Dressings are changed 24 hours after I&D and then every other day thereafter. Further surgical debridement of the necrotic tissue that can develop may be necessary, leading to possible skin graft or tissue flap procedures.

EXCISION OF LESION

Excisions of lesions (lymph nodes and lipomas) are performed for several reasons, primarily to obtain tissue for biopsy, often as curative treatment, and infrequently for cosmesis. The site of pathology can be anywhere on the body, but often lipomas appear on the arm, back, and anterior abdomen. Lymph nodes become enlarged in the femoral and axillary regions, and lesions develop on the arms, legs, and back. These lesions, lymph nodes, and lipomas usually present as painless, sometimes mobile, superficial masses.

Excisional surgery involves incising the skin (along the Langer lines) directly over the pathology, dissection of the subcutaneous tissues, shelling out the dense encapsulated tissue without having to excise any of the normal tissue around it. This approach is generally reserved for lesions 3 to 5 cm. Closure is usually simple, requiring a subcutaneous layer of interrupted 3–0 or 4–0 absorbable and a 5–0 absorbable running subcuticular stitch.

ENDOSCOPY

Endoscopy refers to the use of an endoscope to visualize an anatomical area. Most endoscopes used today are flexible, fiberoptic scopes; however, rigid scopes are useful in specific situations. Procedures include direct visualization, biopsy, and surgical intervention. Common procedures include esophagoscopy, gastroscopy, choledochoscopy, sigmoidoscopy, and colonoscopy. Endoscopy may be performed as a stand-alone procedure or in combination with other surgical interventions.

BREAST SURGERY

In some locales, breast surgery is performed by the gynecologist. Throughout most of the country, however, it remains within the domain of the general surgeon. While the vast majority of breast cancer cases are female, breast cancer is not limited to the female breast. Today, treatment of breast cancer is multidisciplinary.

BREAST ANATOMY

The breasts or mammary glands are modified sweat glands located anterior to the pectoralis major muscle between the second and sixth ribs (refer to Plate 12A). The breasts rest lateral to the sternum and extend to the axilla. The nipples lie at the level of the fifth rib. The mammary glands are accessory to the reproductive function in the female, secreting milk for the nourishment of the infant. Breasts are rudimentary and functionless in the male.

The mammary gland is a flattened circular mass of glandular tissue. It is white or reddish-white in color. The breast is thicker underneath the nipple and thinner at the periphery. The gland is composed of some fifteen to twenty lobes. Each lobe is somewhat pyramidal in shape with its apex oriented toward the nipple and its base toward the periphery. Each lobe contains a lactiferous duct. The ducts are divergent at the base but parallel at the nipple. Each lobe and its lobules are surrounded by loose connective tissue, and the entire gland is surrounded by connective tissue. The connective tissue is not organized well enough to form a true capsule, however. The nipple is conical in shape with a rounded and fissured tip. The nipple receives the openings of the lactiferous ducts. The darkly pigmented skin around the nipple that covers smooth muscle is called the areola.

The mammary glands receive a rich blood supply. The arteries are mostly branches of the subcutaneous vessels of the anterior thorax. These branches include the internal thoracic, lateral mammary, and intercostal arteries. The main vessels enter the breast at its superomedial or superolateral border. Relatively few vessels are found inferiorly. Venous drainage follows the arterial course. Lymphatic drainage is of particular importance because of the frequency of breast cancer in the population. The anterolateral thoracic wall contains a cutaneous lymphatic network that is continuous with the abdomen below and the neck above. The mammary cutaneous lymphatics are part of this lymphatic network.

The nerves of the breast are cutaneous nerves from the anterior thorax. Most anterior and medial mammary branches arise from anterior branches of the lateral cutaneous divisions of the second through sixth intercostal nerves. The upper skin covering the breasts is further innervated by terminal branches of the supraclavicular nerves. The nerves of the breast are both sympathetic and sensory. The skin, smooth muscle of the areola and nipple, blood vessels, and glandular tissue have nerve supply.

BREAST AND AXILLA: PATHOLOGY AND DIAGNOSIS

Like most conditions involving malignancy, breast cancer has been staged. One system is presented in Table 14-23.

Diagnosis of breast cancer clinical Stages I to IV or ductal carcinoma *in situ* usually begins with initial detection through breast examination or mammography. Follow-up endeavors include chest X-ray and bone scanning.

Some general facts about breast cancer that affect surgical intervention are

- Tumor size directly related to the presence of regional metastases and progressive deterioration after treatment
- Breast-conserving surgery possible in 90% of cases
- Men suffer from breast disorders such as breast enlargement (gynecomastia) and less commonly cancer

BREAST SURGERY (NONCOSMETIC)

Breast biopsy should be performed if any of the following conditions exist:

- Clinically suspicious mass persisting through a menstrual cycle
- Cystic mass that fails to collapse completely when aspirated
- Spontaneous serous or serosanguineous discharge from the nipple
- Suspicious mammographic findings

The trend in breast surgery is an evolution from the total removal of all breast tissue to the conservation of as much breast tissue as possible while excising the entire tumor (Figure 14-20). This approach is often combined with dissection of lymph nodes for cancer staging, and postoperative chemotherapy and/or irradiation therapy. Staging refers to the classification of breast cancer by anatomical extent.

Table 14-23 Breast Cancer Staging

CANCER IN SITU	
Stage I	• Tumor 2 cm or less in greatest diameter • No evidence of regional or distal spread
Stage II	• Tumor greater than 2 cm but not more than 5 cm in greatest diameter • With or without movable axillary nodes • Without distal spread
Stage IIIa	• Tumor up to 5 cm in diameter • May or may not be fixed • Homolateral clinically suspicious regional spread or • Tumor greater than 5 cm diameter • May or may not be fixed • With or without clinically suspicious homolateral regional spread • No evidence of distant metastases
Stage IIIb	• Tumor of any dimension • Unequivocal homolateral metastatic supraclavicular or interclavicular nodes or • Edema of the arm, but without distant metastases
Stage IV	• Tumor of any size • With or without regional spread • Evidence of distant metastases

Adapted from *Essentials of Obstetrics and Gynecology,* 3rd ed., by N. F. Hacker and J. G. Moore. Copyright 1998 by W. B. Saunders.

Surgical considerations for all procedures include supine positioning, a wide prep and adequate draping of the incision site, access to the underarm for axillary dissection, and anesthesia as required, local with sedation to general.

BIOPSY/LUMPECTOMY

Breast biopsy may be accomplished with a needle or by surgical removal. Lumpectomy is a common term that also refers to the removal of a breast mass without removal of surrounding tissue. Biopsy is used for diagnostic purposes. Lumpectomy is of diagnostic value but is also part of a treatment regimen. Radiation or chemotherapy may be added to the treatment regimen.

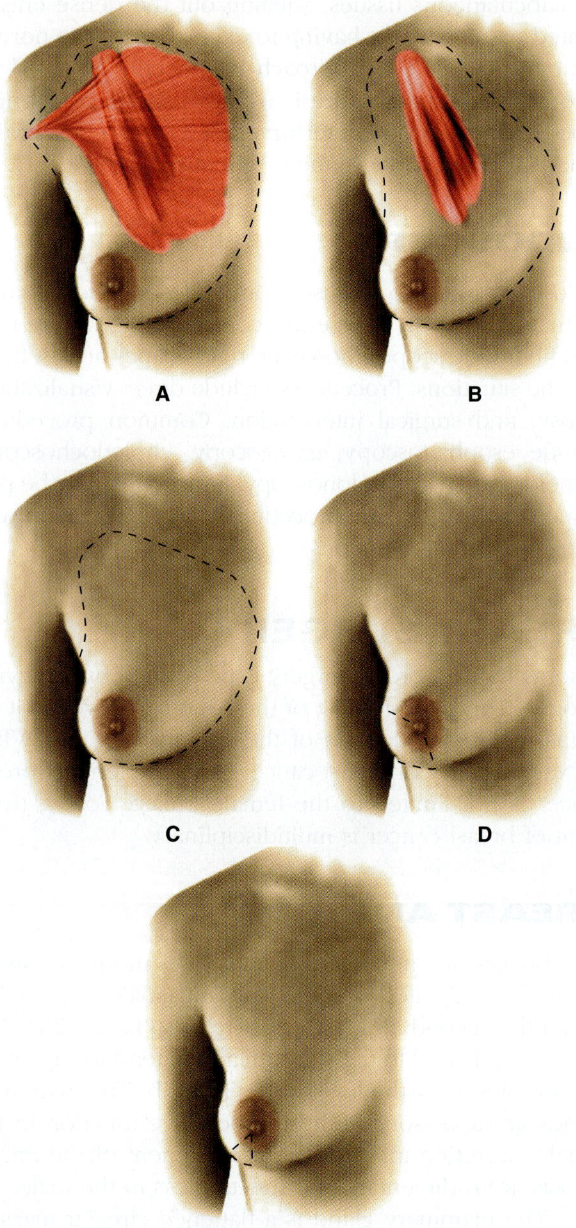

Figure 14-20 Breast surgery options: (A) Radical mastectomy, (B) modified radical mastectomy, (C) simple mastectomy, (D) segmental resection, (E) lumpectomy

SEGMENTAL RESECTION AND AXILLARY DISSECTION

Segmental resection is part of a trend in breast-conserving surgery and has shown survival rates equal to those of radical mastectomy when combined with axillary dissection and subsequent irradiation and/or chemotherapy. Segmental resection removes only the tumor and a reasonable margin of healthy tissue. Incisions are made based on tumor location. Preservation of the subcutaneous tissue is important for cosmesis. Wound closure involves 3–0 absorbable subcutaneous closure, and a 5–0 absorbable subcuticular suture and application of wound closure strips. A light dressing is applied. The most common complications of segmental resection are hematoma formation, infection, and poor cosmetic results, but reexcision is also encountered.

Axillary dissection follows closure of the breast and provides for lymph node sampling and subsequent staging of the disease. A transverse incision extending from the lateral border of the pectoralis major muscle to the anterior border of the latissimus dorsi muscle is made in a skin crease two finger breadths below the axillary crease. Skin flaps are developed by scalpel or electrosurgically. The axillary vein, the lateral edges of the pectoralis muscles, the latissimus dorsi, and the tail of the breast are exposed. Pectoralis fascia is incised to allow mobilization and retraction of the muscles and enables identification of the medial pectoral neurovascular bundle, which is preserved. Dissection proceeds along the course of the axillary vessels, within the boundaries of the axilla, and all fat and lymph tissue is sampled. The specimen is removed, the wound is irrigated, and hemostasis achieved. A closed wound drainage system is placed in the axilla, the wound is closed, and a light, fluffy dressing is applied.

RADICAL AND MODIFIED RADICAL MASTECTOMIES

Mastectomy is the removal of the entire mammary gland breast (Procedure 14-12). This approach is used in Stage I and II breast cancer or in conjunction with chemotherapy and radiation treatments for Stage III and IV breast cancer. Radical mastectomy is not performed as often as it was only a few years ago because

PROCEDURE 14-12 Mastectomy

Equipment

- Suction apparatus
- Electrosurgical unit with dispersive electrode
- May need extra armboard or special armrest

Instruments

- Minor instrumentation tray
- Extra hemostats
- Plastic set may be needed for reconstruction
- Ligating clip appliers and clip

Supplies

- Prep set
- Basic pack
- Basin set
- Chest/breast drapes
- Electrosurgical pencil
- Gloves
- Blades (#10, several)
- Suture according to surgeon's preference
- Dressing material according to surgeon's preference
- Closed wound drainage system × 2

Operative Preparation

Anesthesia

- General
- Lubricate and protect the patient's eyes

Position

- Supine
- Arm on affected side may be on armrest

Prep

- Chest
- Neck
- Axilla
- Arm (circumferential)

(continues)

PROCEDURE 14-12 Mastectomy *(continued)*

Draping

- Anticipated surgical area is outlined with towels secured with adhesive or towel clips
- Chest/breast sheet
- Draping of the arm includes placement of a sheet on the armboard and application of a stockinette over the entire arm

Practical Considerations

- Have mammograms in room
- Notify pathology if frozen sections will be required

Operative Procedure	Technical Considerations
1. The extent of the skin flaps is marked and an elliptical transverse incision is made along these markings allowing for a 4-cm margin around any lesion.	1. Have marking pen available.
2. Tapering skin flaps are developed. Dissection continues down to the chest muscles and laterally to the border of the pectoralis minor muscle. Breast tissue and underlying pectoralis fascia are removed en bloc. The tail of Spence is included in the specimen.	2. *Note:* Most of the procedure is soft tissue dissection so have scalpel, scissors, and/or electrosurgical pencil and/or hemostats available at all times. May ligate large vessels.
3. The pectoralis minor may be divided, stripped, or excised. Excision is used when a lesion is present on the muscle, causing compromise of pectoral innervation.	3. Large clamps may be required for the muscle excision.
4. Two wound drains are usually placed, one in the anterior chest and the other in the axilla. Excess skin is excised and the wound is closed.	4. Have drains of choice available. Prepare suture and initiate count.

Postoperative Considerations

Immediate Postoperative Care

- Transport to PACU

Prognosis

- Return to normal activities (depends on response to treatment)

Complications

- Hemorrhage
- Wound infection
- Anesthesia of the skin and anterior chest wall
- Impaired arm motion "frozen shoulder"
- Skin flap necrosis
- Seromas
- Lymphedema
- Phantom breast syndrome
- Cellulitis
- Hematoma formation

PEARL OF WISDOM

Two setups may be required if reconstruction is being done immediately following the mastectomy to prevent seeding.

of the emphasis on breast-conserving techniques. This technique involves removal of the breast and pectoralis minor muscle, and division of the medial and lateral pectoral nerves. Radical mastectomy is indicated in cases of breast sarcomas, multicentric ductal carcinoma, lobular carcinoma *in situ,* as prophylaxis against future breast cancer, and when breast-conserving techniques are contraindicated.

Modified radical mastectomy proceeds exactly like radical mastectomy but the pectoralis muscles and fascia are preserved and axillary dissection proceeds as previously described. There is no apparent difference in survival or recurrence rates among patients undergoing either radical or modified radical mastectomy.

SURGERY OF THE THYROID AND PARATHYROID

The thyroid gland may fall within the realm of other specialties in some locales; however, the general surgeon commonly operates on the thyroid and parathyroid glands.

ANATOMY OF THE THYROID AND PARATHYROID

The thyroid gland consists of two separate groups of cells that produce hormones (refer to Plate 5). Follicular cells produce, store, and release thyroxine and triiodothyronine, hormones that play a major role in the regulation of the basal metabolic rate. Parafollicular cells secrete calcitonin. Calcitonin helps maintain calcium homeostasis. Adult thyroid glands weigh between 12 and 25 g and consist of two lobes residing anterior to the larynx. The lobes are connected by the thyroid isthmus about the level of the second tracheal ring. The overall structure has an "H" shape. A pyramidal lobe may extend cephalad from the isthmus or its junction with one of the lobes. A fibrous capsule invests the thyroid. The infrahyoid muscles and their associated fasciae overlie the thyroid. The thyroid crosses both the trachea and esophagus. The superior portions of the lateral lobes mold to the cricoid and thyroid cartilages. The carotid sheaths are positioned posterolateral to the gland.

The blood supply is rich and predominantly from the superior and inferior thyroid arteries. The superior thyroid artery is usually the first branch of the external carotid artery. The superior thyroid artery courses downward and forward to the apex of the lateral lobe. The arteriol branches provide blood supply to other structures in the area. The inferior thyroid artery is the largest branch of the thyrocervical trunk of the subclavian artery. The inferior thyroid artery ascends along the medial margin of the anterior scalene muscle and ultimately lies behind the lateral lobe of the thyroid. There it descends to the inferior pole of the thyroid gland where it turns cephalad again and branches to supply the lobe. It provides branches to the pharynx, trachea, and esophagus. The superior thyroid vein crosses the common carotid and empties into the internal jugular vein just superior to the thyroid cartilage. The middle thyroid vein also crosses the carotid and empties into the lower portion of the jugular vein. The inferior thyroid vein descends on the surface of the trachea and behind the manubrium of the sternum to empty into the left and right brachiocephalic veins.

The nerves supplying the thyroid serve some vasomotor functions but primarily innervate the epithelial cells of the follicles of the thyroid gland. The nerves consist of unmyelinated postganglionic fibers traveling with the cardiac, superior laryngeal, and inferior laryngeal nerves following the course of the arteries. One must be aware of the bilateral existence of a recurrent laryngeal nerve during dissection.

The parathyroid glands number from two to six and are small, flat, oval structures lying on the dorsal side of the thyroid gland. The parathyroid glands are covered by the thyroid sheath but have their own capsule also. They produce parathormone which maintains the normal relationship between blood and skeletal calcium. Removal of all parathyroid glands results in tetany and death. The parathyroids are supplied by branches of the inferior or superior thyroid arteries and venous drainage is via the thyroid plexus. The nerve supply is rich, vasomotor in function, and arises from the thyroid branches of the cervical sympathetic ganglia.

PATHOLOGICAL CONDITIONS OF THE THYROID AND PARATHYROID GLANDS

Pathological conditions affecting the thyroid and parathyroid glands are summarized in Tables 14-24 and 14-25.

THYROIDECTOMY

Thyroidectomy is the surgical removal of the thyroid gland (Procedure 14-13). It remains a common procedure. The parathyroid glands, intimately related to the thyroid glands, must be spared.

TRACHEOTOMY

Tracheotomy is a procedure performed by surgeons in many specialties. It may be performed for several reasons including extreme emergencies. Tracheal anatomy is covered in Chapter 17.

INDICATIONS FOR TRACHEOTOMY

Indications for tracheotomy are presented in Table 14-26.

(Text continues on page 467)

Table 14-24 Pathological Conditions of the Thyroid

CONDITION	SYMPTOMS/SIGNS	DIAGNOSTICS	TREATMENTS
Hyperthyroidism	• Nervousness • Restlessness • Emotional lability • Fast speech • Tachycardia • Palpitations • Arrhythmias • Dyspnea • Heat intolerance • Sweating • Fatigue • Weakness • Tremor • Hair loss • Nail separating from nail bed	• History • Physical examination • Serum levels of TSH	• Medical blocking of the hormone and its effects • Radioiodide ablation of active thyroid tissue • Surgical resection
Thyroid carcinoma	• May be asymptomatic • May show signs of hyper- or hypothyroidism according to tumor type • Hoarseness • Signs of tracheal or esophageal compression	• History • Physical examination • Serum levels of TSH • Ultrasound • Laryngoscopy • Scans • Biopsy	• Surgical resection for localized carcinoma (unless anaplastic carcinoma or lymphoma)

Table 14-25 Pathological Conditions of the Parathyroid

CONDITION	SYMPTOMS/SIGNS	DIAGNOSTICS	TREATMENTS
• Hyperparathyroidism	• Asymptomatic early on • Skeletal damage	• Laboratory studies • Ultrasound • Biopsy • CT/MRI scan	• Varies with cause • Surgical resection of affected gland

PROCEDURE 14-13 Thyroidectomy

Equipment

- Suction apparatus
- Electrosurgical unit with dispersive electrode
- Roll or thyroid rest for extending the neck

PROCEDURE 14-13 Thyroidectomy *(continued)*

Instruments

- Thyroidectomy set
- Bipolar forceps with cord
- Ligating clip appliers and clips

Supplies

- Prep set
- Basic pack
- Basin set
- Thyroid drapes
- Electrosurgical pencil
- Gloves
- Blades (#10, #15)
- Suture according to surgeon's preference
- Dressing material according to surgeon's preference
- ¼-in. Penrose drain

Operative Preparation

Anesthesia

- General
- Lubricate and protect patient's eyes

Position

- Supine with neck extension

Prep

- Point of chin to mid-chest and laterally as far as possible

Draping

- Wadded absorptive towels may be placed bilaterally
- Anticipated surgical area is outlined with towels secured with adhesive or towel clips; surgeon may prefer to staple or suture the towels
- Thyroid sheet

Practical Considerations

- A Queen Anne's dressing or thyroid collar may be used
- A tracheotomy tray may be transported with the patient postoperatively

Operative Procedure

1. A symmetrical, transverse incision following the Langer lines is made over the thyroid. Size varies to provide optimal access. Typically two fingerbreadths above the clavicular head.

Technical Considerations

1. Hemostasis
    - Hemostasis will be secured as the procedure progresses
    - Usually via electrosurgical pencil or bipolar forceps
    - May clamp and tie some vessels
    - May use ligating clips

(continues)

PROCEDURE

14-13 Thyroidectomy *(continued)*

2. The incision is extended through the subcutaneous tissues and the platysma muscle is divided. Superior and inferior flaps are mobilized and retractors placed (Figure 14-21A).

2. Prepare self-retaining retractor of choice.

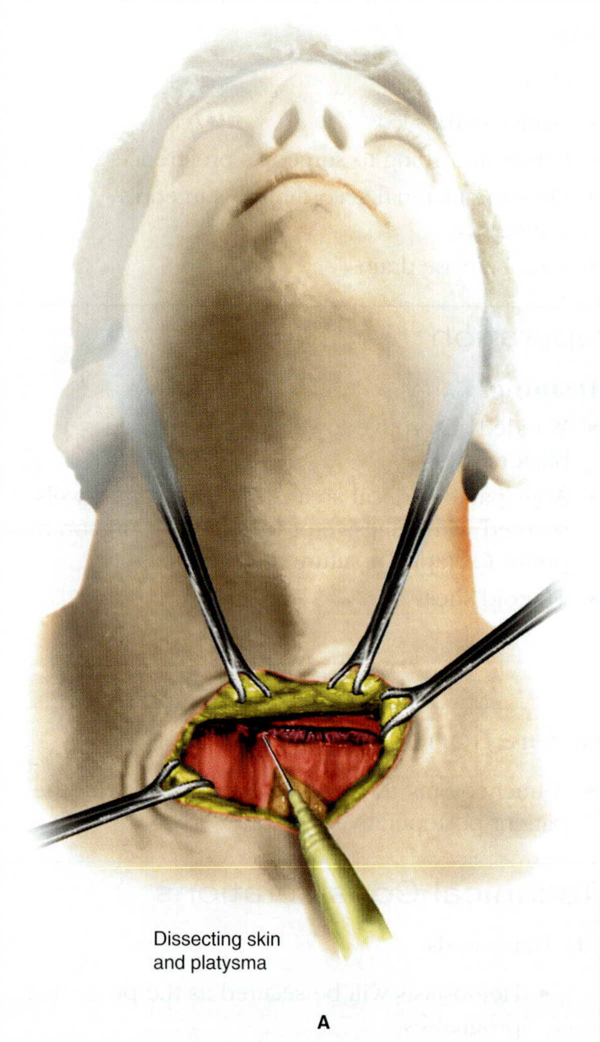

Figure 14-21 Thyroidectomy: (A) Incision

3. The strap muscles are separated and the thyroid lobe is exposed. The middle thyroid vein is exposed, divided, and ligated.

3. *Note:* Most thyroidectomy procedures will move carefully and methodically. Keep fresh dry sponges available. Mosquito hemostats may be used.

PROCEDURE 14-13 Thyroidectomy *(continued)*

4. The superior poles are retracted caudally and the superior vessels are identified. The laryngeal nerves must be identified at this point. The vessels are divided and ligated (Figure 14-21B).

4. This may require the use of small right angle clamps. May require ligature on a passer.

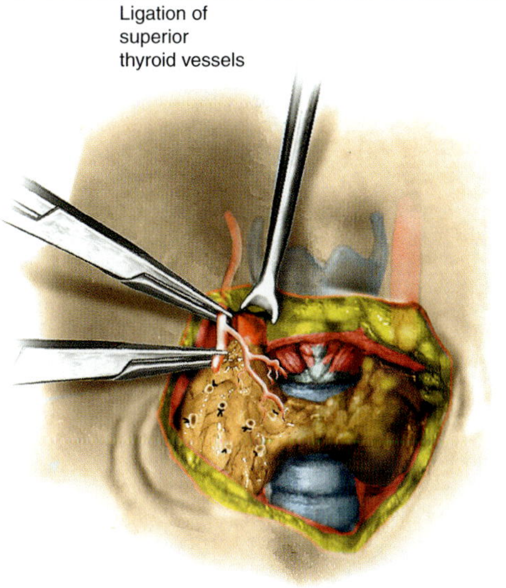

B

Figure 14-21 Thyroidectomy: (B) Ligation of superior thyroid vessels

5. The parathyroid glands, inferior thyroid artery, and recurrent laryngeal nerve are identified. The parathyroid glands are mobilized and vascular supply is preserved (Figure 14-21C).

5. Many procedural steps are repeated. Keep two clamps, scissors, and ties ready.

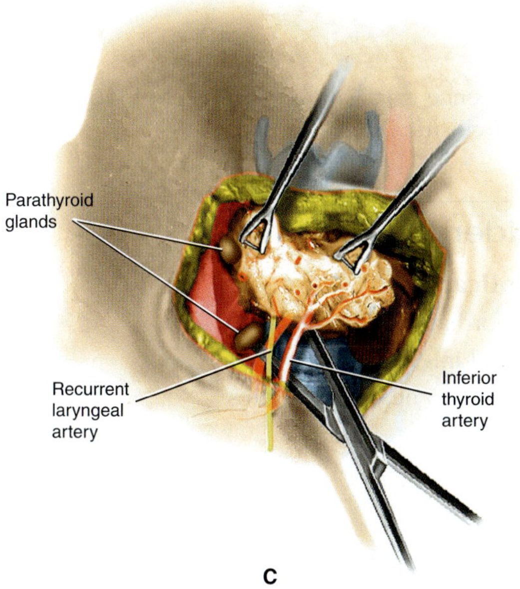

C

Figure 14-21 Thyroidectomy: (C) Identification of parathyroid glands and recurrent laryngeal nerve

(continues)

PROCEDURE 14-13 Thyroidectomy *(continued)*

6. Branches of the inferior thyroid artery are divided and ligated. The superior connective tissue is divided. Hemostasis is achieved with electrosurgical unit (ESU). *Note:* Recurrent nerve must be spared.

6. May alternate between sharp dissection, blunt dissection, and ESU.

7. The thyroid is dissected from the trachea (Figure 14-21D).

7. *Note:* If only one lobe is taken, the isthmus is divided so that it is removed with resected lobe as is the pyramidal lobe.

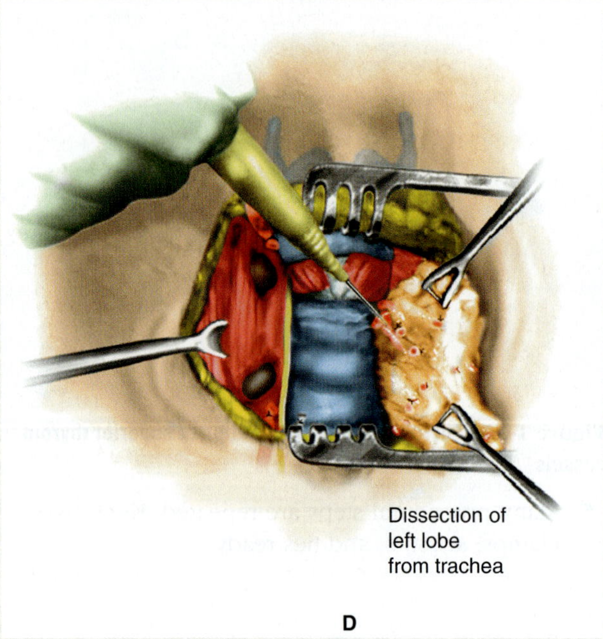

Figure 14-21 Thyroidectomy: (D) Dissection from trachea

8. Hemostasis is achieved after lobe or lobes removed. A drain may be placed. The wound is closed.

8. Sequence is irrigation, placement of wound drain, and closure. Initiate count.

Postoperative Considerations

Immediate Postoperative Care

- Check voice as soon as possible
- Transport to PACU
- Tracheotomy tray available

Complications

- Hemorrhage
- Wound infection
- Damage to nearby structures

Prognosis

- Return to normal activities
- Medications usually required for life

PEARL OF WISDOM

Maintain the integrity of the sterile field until the patient is extubated, breathing freely, and has been transported to the PACU. Emergency tracheotomy is a possibility.

ILLUSTRATIVE PROCEDURE: TRACHEOTOMY

Tracheotomy is performed to facilitate breathing and to protect damage to other structures (Procedure 14-14). The terms tracheostomy and tracheotomy are often used interchangeably. However, tracheostomy is the creation of a tracheal stoma, usually permanent. The mucus membrane of the trachea is sutured to the skin. Tracheotomy is the creation of an opening in the trachea, usually temporary, for placement of a tracheotomy tube.

Table 14-26 Indications for Tracheotomy

Indications for Tracheotomy
Upper airway obstruction with one or more of the following:
stridor, air hunger, chest retractions, obstructive sleep apnea, bilateral vocal cord paralysis, previous neck surgery, throat trauma, or previous irradiation to the neck
Other:
Prolonged intubation
Inability to manage secretions
Facilitation of ventilation
Inability to intubate
Adjunct to management of head and neck surgery or trauma

PEARL OF WISDOM

Check patency of the balloon on the tracheotomy tube prior to beginning the procedure.

PROCEDURE

14-14 Tracheotomy

Equipment

- Suction apparatus
- Electrosurgical unit with dispersive electrode
- Roll or thyroid rest to extend neck

Instruments

- Tracheotomy set

Supplies

- Prep set
- Basic pack
- Basin set
- Thyroid drapes
- Electrosurgical pencil
- Gloves
- Blades (#10, #15)
- Suture according to surgeon's preference
- Tracheotomy dressing
- Tracheotomy tubes
- Endotracheal suction catheters

(continues)

PROCEDURE 14-14 **Tracheotomy** *(continued)*

Operative Preparation

Anesthesia

- General (preferred)
- Local

Position

- Supine with neck extended

Prep

- Point of chin to mid-chest and laterally as far as possible

Draping

- Anticipated surgical area is outlined with towels secured with adhesive or towel clips
- Thyroid sheet

Practical Considerations

- Have tracheotomy tube on table before incision is made to ensure patency of the balloon
- Have a sterile plastic suction catheter opened
- Have respirator available
- Procedure may be performed in the ICU; all necessary equipment (e.g., electrosurgical unit) and supplies must be transported
- Entry into the respiratory tract and attachment of the ventilation device will cause contamination of the sterile field; maintain the best possible technique

Operative Procedure	Technical Considerations
1. A symmetrical, transverse incision following the Langer lines about two fingerbreadths above the clavicular head.	1. *Note:* Tracheotomies may be performed under emergency conditions. All critical instrumentation and the tracheotomy tube should be checked before the incision is made.
2. The incision is extended through the subcutaneous tissues and the platysma muscle is divided.	2. Hemostasis: • May or may not secure on the way in • Electrosurgical pencil or clamp and tie possible
3. The strap muscles are separated and the thyroid isthmus and trachea are exposed.	3. May use handheld or self-retaining retractor.
4. Thyroid isthmus is divided if necessary.	4. May use electrosurgical pencil.
5. Tracheal hook is placed on the tracheal ring and an incision is made into second tracheal ring. A spreader is placed in incision.	5. Sequence happens quickly: • Hand tracheal hook • Hand scalpel with #15 blade • Hand tracheal spreader • Hand trach tube with obturator in place
6. The tracheotomy tube is placed in the incision and the obturator is withdrawn. The inner cannula is placed and secretions are removed by suction.	6. Obturator is removed. Hand the inner cannula. Hand suction to clear the tube.
7. Endotracheal balloon is inflated. The tracheotomy tube is secured. The wound is closed.	7. May suture tracheotomy tube or use umbilical tape. Count.

PROCEDURE 14-14 **Tracheotomy** *(continued)*

Postoperative Considerations

Immediate Postoperative Care

- Transport to PACU

Prognosis

- Depends on response to primary condition

Complications

- Hemorrhage
- Wound infection
- Damage to nearby structures

CASE STUDY

Jesse is a student assigned to a Whipple procedure as the STSR with his preceptor. The preceptor told Jesse that he should be an expert at several procedures before the case was finished.

1. What did the preceptor mean?
2. What individual procedures comprise the Whipple procedure?
3. What instrument sets will be used?

QUESTIONS FOR FURTHER STUDY

1. Why is everyone concerned about a patient's voice following a thyroidectomy?
2. Name and describe all of the variations for small bowel anastomosis.
3. Imagine a gunshot wound that entered a patient's left chest and exited above the right iliac crest. How many structures can you name that the bullet could have passed through?
4. What is the meaning of the term *vascular steal?*
5. Describe the patient position that is necessary when a thoracoabdominal approach is planned.
6. Is the surgical technologist at risk for development of varicose veins? Why or why not? If so, what can be done to minimize the severity of the condition?

BIBLIOGRAPHY

Adams, R. D. (1997). Electrophysiologic testing and laboratory aids in the diagnosis of neuromuscular disease. In R. D. Adams et al. (Eds.), *Principles of neurology*. New York: McGraw-Hill.

Asensio, J. A., & Buckman, R. F., Jr. (1996). Duodenal injuries. In G. D. Zuidema (Ed.), *Shackelford's surgery of the alimentary tract* (4th ed.). Philadelphia: W. B. Saunders.

Ashley, S. W., & Reber, H. A. (1994). Cancer and other neoplastic disorders of the exocrine pancreas. In I. Gitnick et al. (Eds.), *Principles and practices of gastroenterology and hepatology*. Norwalk, CT: Appleton and Lange.

August, D. A., & Sondak, V. K. (1997). Breast. In L. J. Greenfield et al. (Eds.), *Surgery: Scientific principles and practice* (2nd ed.). Philadelphia: Lippincott-Raven.

Banks, P. A. (1998). Acute and chronic pancreatitis. In M. Feldman, M. H. Sleisenger, & B. F. Scharschmidt (Eds.), *Sleisenger and Fordtran's gastrointestinal and liver disease*. Philadelphia: W. B. Saunders.

Bannister, L. H. (1995). Alimentary tract. In P. L. Williams et al. (Eds.), *Gray's anatomy: The anatomical basis of medicine and surgery* (38th ed.). New York: Churchill Livingstone.

Bannister, L. H. (1995). Haemolymphoid system. In P. L. Williams et al. (Eds.), *Gray's anatomy: The anatomical basis of medicine and surgery* (38th ed.). New York: Churchill Livingstone.

Bannister, L. H. (1995). Integumental system. In P. L. Williams et al. (Eds.), *Gray's anatomy: The anatomical basis of medicine and surgery* (38th ed.). New York: Churchill Livingstone.

Barnett, J. L., & Raper, S. E. (1995). Anorectal disease. In T. Yamada et al. (Eds.), *Textbook of gastroenterology*. Philadelphia: J. B. Lippincott.

Beger, H. G., & Buchlet, M. W. (1995). Surgical management of chronic pancreatitis. In W. S. Haubrich, F. Schaffner, & J. E. Berk (Eds.), *Bockus' gastroenterology* (5th ed.). Philadelphia: W. B. Saunders.

Behar, J. (1995). Anatomy and anomalies of the biliary tract. In W. S. Haubrich, F. Schaffner, & J. E. Berk (Eds.), *Bockus' gastroenterology* (5th ed.). Philadelphia: W. B. Saunders.

Bell, R. H. (1997). Neoplasms of the exocrine pancreas. In L. J. Greenfield et al. (Eds.), *Surgery: Scientific principles and practice* (2nd ed.). Philadelphia: Lippincott-Raven.

Bennion, R. S., & Wilson, S. E. (1993). Hemodialysis and vascular access. In W. S. Moore (Ed.), *Vascular surgery: A comprehensive review*. Philadelphia: W. B. Saunders.

Bennion, R. S., Williams R. A., & Wilson, S. E. (1994). Principles of vascular access surgery. In F. J. Veith et al. (Eds.), *Vascular surgery* (2nd ed.). New York: McGraw-Hill.

Bergan, J. J. (1993). Varicose veins: Chronic venous insufficiency. In W. S. Moore (Ed.), *Vascular surgery: A comprehensive review*. Philadelphia: W. B. Saunders.

Berne, T. V., & Ortega, A. (1992). Appendicitis and appendiceal abscess. In L. M. Nyhus & R. J. Baker (Eds.), *Mastery of surgery* (2nd ed.). Boston: Little, Brown and Co.

Biancani, P., & Behar, J. (1995). Esophageal motor function. In T. Yamada et al. (Eds.), *Textbook of gastroenterology*. Philadelphia: J. B. Lippincott.

Bland, K. I., & Vezeridis, M. P. (1992). Anatomy of the breast. In L. M. Nyhus & R. J. Baker (Eds.), *Mastery of surgery* (2nd ed.). Boston: Little, Brown and Co.

Block, G. E., & Hurst, R. D. (1995). Complications of the surgical treatment of ulcerative colitis and Crohn's disease. In J. B. Kirsner & R. G. Shorter (Eds.), *Inflammatory bowel disease* (4th ed.). Baltimore: Williams and Wilkins.

Bockus, M. S. (1995). Anatomy of the small intestine. In W. S. Haubrich, F. Schaffner, & J. E. Berk (Eds.), *Bockus' gastroenterology* (5th ed.). Philadelphia: W. B. Saunders.

Britt, L. D., & Berger, J. (1992). Splenic repair and partial splenectomy. In L. M. Nyhus & R. J. Baker (Eds.), *Mastery of surgery* (2nd ed.). Boston: Little, Brown and Co.

Brophy, M. T., Fiore, L. D., & Deykin, D. (1996). Hemostasis. In D. Zakim & T. D. Boyer (Eds.), *Hepatology: A textbook of liver disease* (3rd ed.). Philadelphia: W. B. Saunders.

Brown, S. D., van Sonnenberg, E., & Mueller, P. R. (1999). Interventional radiology in the liver, biliary tract, and gallbladder. *Schiff's diseases of the liver*. New York: Lippincott-Raven.

Bubrick, M. P., & Rolstad, B. S. (1999). Intestinal stomas. In P. H. Gordon & S. Nivatvongs (Eds.), *Principles and practices of surgery for the colon, rectum, and anus*. St. Louis, MO: Quality Medical Publishing, Inc.

Camilleri, M., & Prather, C. M. (1998). Gastric motor physiology and motor disorders. In M. Feldman, M. H. Sleisenger, & B. F. Scharschmidt (Eds.), *Sleisenger and Fordtran's gastrointestinal and liver disease*. Phildelphia: W. B. Saunders.

Carey, L. C., & Ellison, E. S. (1992). Cholecystostomy, cholecystectomy, and intraoperative evaluation of the biliary tree. In L. M. Nyhus & R. J. Baker (Eds.),

Mastery of surgery (2nd ed.). Boston: Little, Brown and Co.

Carter, D. C. (1997). Pain-relieving procedures in chronic pancreatitis. In M. Trede, Sir D. C. Carter, & W. P. Longmire, Jr. (Eds.), *Surgery of the pancreas* (2nd ed.). New York: Churchill Livingstone.

Cello, J. P. (1998). Pancreatic cancer. In M. Feldman, M. H. Sleisenger, & B. F. Scharschmidt (Eds.), *Sleisenger and Fordtran's gastrointestinal and liver disease*. Philadelphia: W. B. Saunders.

Chang, A. E., & Sondak, V. K. (1999). Clinical evaluation and treatment of soft tissue tumors. In F. M. Enzinger & S. W. Weiss (Eds.), *Soft tissue tumors* (3rd ed.). St Louis: Mosby-Yearbook.

Chapman, W.C., & Newman, M. (1999). Disorders of the spleen. In G. R. Lee et al. (Eds.), *Wintrobe's clinical hematology* (10th ed.). Baltimore: Williams and Wilkins.

Condon, R. E. (1992). Iliopubic tract repair of inguinal hernia: The anterior inguinal canal approach. In L. M. Nyhus & R. J. Baker (Eds.), *Mastery of surgery* (2nd ed.). Boston: Little, Brown and Co.

Condon, R. E. (1995). The anatomy of the inguinal region and its relation to groin hernia. In L. M. Nyhus & R. E. Condon (Eds.), *Hernia* (4th ed.). Philadelphia: J. B. Lippincott.

Cotton, P. B., & Williams, C. B. (1996). *Practical gastrointestinal endoscopy* (4th ed.). New York: Blackwell Science.

Crist, D. W., & Gadacz, T. R. (1996). Anatomy, embryology, congenital anomalies, and physiology of the gallbladder and extrahepatic biliary ducts. In G. D. Zuidema (Ed.), *Shackelford's surgery of the alimentary tract* (4th ed.). Philadelphia: W. B. Saunders.

Daly, J. M. (1999). Abdominal wall, omentum, mesentery, and retroperitoneum. In S. I. Schwartz et al. (Eds.), *Principles of surgery*. New York: McGraw-Hill.

Dempsey, D. T., & Ritchie, W. P., Jr. (1996). Anatomy and physiology of the duodenum. In G. D. Zuidema (Ed.), *Shackelford's surgery of the alimentary tract* (4th ed.). Philadelphia: W. B. Saunders.

Dempsey, D. T., & Ritchie, W. P., Jr. (1996). Anatomy and physiology of the stomach. In G. D. Zuidema (Ed.), *Shackelford's surgery of the alimentary tract* (4th ed.). Philadelphia: W. B. Saunders.

Deveney, K. E. (1994). Hernias and other lesions of the abdominal wall. In L. W. Way (Ed.), *Current surgical diagnosis and treatment* (10th ed.). Norwalk, CT: Appleton and Lange.

Donegan, W. L. (1995). Staging and primary treatment. In W. L. Donegan & J. S. Spratt (Eds.), *Cancer of the breast*. Philadelphia: W. B. Saunders.

Dong-Weng Eu, & Oakley, F. R. (1997). Stoma construction. In R. N. Allan et al. (Eds.), *Inflammatory bowel diseases* (3rd ed.). New York: Churchill Livingstone.

Dozios, R. G., & Kelly, K. A. (1995). The surgical management of ulcerative colitis. In J. B. Kirsner & R. G. Shorter (Eds.), *Inflammatory bowel disease* (4th ed.). Baltimore: Williams and Wilkins.

Eastwood, G. L. (1995). Stomach: Anatomy and structural anomalies. In T. Yamada et al. (Eds.), *Textbook of gastroenterology*. Philadelphia: J. B. Lippincott.

Eisenbert, M. M., Fondacaro, P. F., & Dunn, D. H. (1995). Applied anatomy and anomalies of the stomach. In W. S. Haubrich, F. Schaffner, & J. E. Berk (Eds.), *Bockus' gastroenterology* (5th ed.). Philadelphia: W. B. Saunders.

Ellis, H. (1989). Cholecystostomy and cholecystectomy. In S. I. Schwartz & H. Ellis (Eds.), *Maingot's abdominal operations* (9th ed.). Norwalk, CT: Appleton and Lange.

Ellis, H. (1989). Incisions and closures. In S. I. Schwartz & H. Ellis (Eds.), *Maingot's abdominal operations* (9th ed.). Norwalk, CT: Appleton and Lange.

Ellis, H., & Nathanson, L. K. (1989). Appendix and appendectomy. In S. I. Schwartz & H. Ellis (Eds.), *Maingot's abdominal operations* (9th ed.). Norwalk, CT: Appleton and Lange.

Ellis, H. (1997). Incisions, closures, and wound management. In M. J. Zinner et al. (Eds.), *Maingot's abdominal operations* (10th ed.). Stamford, CT: Appleton and Lange.

Fazio, V. W., & Erwin Toth, P. (1995). Stomal and pouch function and care. In W. S. Haubrich, F. Schaffner, & J. E. Berk (Eds.), *Bockus' gastroenterology* (5th ed.). Philadelphia: W. B. Saunders.

Fazio, V. W., & Tjandra, J. J. (1996). The management of perianal disease. In J. L. Cameron et al. (Eds.), *Surgery*. St. Louis: Mosby Yearbook.

Feliciano, D. V. (1996). Trauma and the liver. In D. Zakim & T. D. Boyer (Eds.), *Hepatology: A textbook of liver disease* (3rd ed.). Philadelphia: W. B. Saunders.

Fernandez-del Castillo, C., Rivera, J. A., & Warshaw, A. L. (1997). Cystic tumors. In M. Trede, Sir D. C. Carter, & W. P. Longmire, Jr. (Eds.), *Surgery of the pancreas* (2nd ed.). New York: Churchill Livingstone.

Flesch, L. (1992). Care of stomas. In L. M. Nyhus & R. J. Baker (Eds.), *Mastery of surgery* (2nd ed.). Boston: Little, Brown and Co.

Fong, Y., & Blumgart, L. H. (1996). Surgical therapy of liver cancer. In D. Zakim & T. D. Boyer (Eds.), *Hepatology: A textbook of liver disease* (3rd ed.). Philadelphia: W. B. Saunders.

Frey, C. F., Wardell, J. W., & McMurtry, A. L. (1997). Injuries to the pancreas. In M. Trede, Sir D. C. Carter, & W. P. Longmire, Jr. (Eds.), *Surgery of the pancreas* (2nd ed.). New York: Churchill Livingstone.

Gabella, G. (1995). Cardiovascular system. In L. H. Bannister (Ed.), *Gray's anatomy: The anatomical basis of medicine and surgery* (38th ed.). New York: Churchill Livingstone.

George, J. N., & El-Harake, M. (1995). Thrombocytopenia due to enhanced platelet destruction by nonimmunologic mechanisms. In Beutler, E. Lichtman, B. S. Coller, & T. J. Kipps (Eds.), *Williams hematology* (5th ed.). New York: McGraw-Hill.

Goldstone, J. (1994). Veins and lymphatics. In L. W. Way (Ed.), *Current surgical diagnosis and treatment* (10th ed.). Norwalk, CT: Appleton and Lange.

Gordon, P. H. (1999). Anorectal abscesses and fistula-in-ano. In P. H. Gordon & S. Nivatvongs (Eds.), *Principles and practices of surgery for the colon, rectum, and anus.* St. Louis, MO: Quality Medical Publishing, Inc.

Gorelick, F. S. (1995). Acute pancreatitis. In T. Yamada et al. (Eds.), *Textbook of gastroenterology.* Philadelphia: J. B. Lippincott.

Green, R. M., & Ouriel, K. (1999). Venous and lymphatic disease. In S. I. Schwartz et al. (Eds.), *Principles of surgery.* New York: McGraw-Hill.

Grendell, J. H. (1995). Embryology, anatomy, and anomalies of the pancreas. In W. S. Haubrich, F. Schaffner, & J. E. Berk (Eds.), *Bockus' gastroenterology* (5th ed.). Philadelphia: W. B. Saunders.

Grendell, J. H., & Ermack, T. H. (1998). Anatomy, histology, embryology, and developmental anomalies of the pancreas. In M. Feldman, M. H. Sleisenger, & B. F. Scharschmidt (Eds.), *Sleisenger and Fordtran's gastrointestinal and liver disease.* Philadelphia: W. B. Saunders.

Guice, K. S. (1997). Acute pancreatitis. In L. J. Greenfield et al. (Eds.), *Surgery: Scientific principles and practice* (2nd ed.). Philadelphia: Lippincott-Raven.

Hacker, N. F. (1998). Breast disease: A gynecologic perspective. In N. F. Hacker & J. G. Moore (Eds.), *Essentials of obstetrics and gynecology* (3rd ed.). Philadelphia: W. B. Saunders.

Hays, A. P., & Younger, D. S. (1995). Muscle and nerve biopsy. In L. P. Rowland (Ed.), *Merritt's textbook of neurology* (9th ed.). Baltimore: Williams and Wilkins.

Hoover, H. C., Jr. (1996). Pancreatic and periampullary carcinoma nonendocrine. In G. D. Zuidema (Ed.), *Shackelford's surgery of the alimentary tract* (4th ed.). Philadelphia: W. B. Saunders.

Huibregtse, K., & Kimmey, M. B. (1995). Endoscopic retrograde cholangiopancreatography, endoscopic sphincterotomy and stone removal, and endoscopic biliary and pancreatic drainage. In T. Yamada et al. (Eds.), *Textbook of gastroenterology.* Philadelphia: J. B. Lippincott.

Jesseph, J. E., & Jesseph, J. M. (1986). Ancillary procedures and miscellaneous techniques for operations on the stomach and duodenum. In L. M. Nyhus & C. Wastell (Eds.), *Surgery of the stomach and duodenum.* Boston: Little, Brown and Co.

Jesseph, J. M. (1992). Open gastrostomy. In L. M. Nyhus & R. J. Baker (Eds.), *Mastery of surgery* (2nd ed.). Boston: Little, Brown and Co.

Joehl, R. J. (1996). Gastrostomy and gastroenterostomy. In G. D. Zuidema (Ed.), *Shackelford's surgery of the alimentary tract* (4th ed.). Philadelphia: W. B. Saunders.

Jones, A. L., & Aggeler, J. (1995). Structure of the liver. In W. S. Haubrich, F. Schaffner, & J. E. Berk (Eds.), *Bockus' gastroenterology* (5th ed.). Philadelphia: W. B. Saunders.

Kafie, F. E., & Wilson, S. E. (1998). Complications of vascular access surgery. In J. S. T. Yao & W. H. Pearce (Eds.), *Techniques in vascular and endovascular surgery.* Stamford, CT: Appleton and Lange.

Karan, J. A., & Roslym, J. J. (1989). Cholelithiasis and cholecystectomy. In S. I. Schwartz & H. Ellis (Eds.), *Maingot's abdominal operations* (9th ed.). Norwalk, CT: Appleton and Lange.

Kaunitz, J. D., Barrett, K. E., & McRoberts, J. A. (1995). Electrolyte secretion and absorption: Small intestine and colon. In T. Yamada et al. (Eds.), *Textbook of gastroenterology.* Philadelphia: J. B. Lippincott.

Keljio, D. J., & Squires, R. H., Jr. (1998). Anatomy and anomalies of the small and large intestines. In M. Feldman, M. H. Sleisenger, & B. F. Scharschmidt (Eds.), *Sleisenger and Fordtran's gastrointestinal and liver disease.* Philadelphia: W. B. Saunders.

Kirsner, J. B., & Shorter, R. G. (1995). *Inflammatory bowel disease* (4th ed.). Baltimore: Williams and Wilkins.

Kodner, I. J. (1999). Colon, rectum, and anus. In G. D. Zuidema (Ed.), *Principles of Shackelford's surgery of the alimentary tract* (4th ed.). Philadelphia: W. B. Saunders.

Kuster, G. G. R. (1995). The appendix. In W. S. Haubrich, F. Schaffner, & J. E. Berk (Eds.), *Bockus' gastroenterology* (5th ed.). Philadelphia: W. B. Saunders.

Lance, P. (1995). Tumors and other neoplastic disease of the small bowel. In T. Yamada et al. (Eds.),

Textbook of gastroenterology. Philadelphia: J. B. Lippincott.

Langnas, A. N., & Shaw, B. W., Jr. (1999). Surgical therapy for hepatocellular carcinoma. In E. R. Schiff, M. F. Sorrell, & W. C. Maddrey (Eds.), *Schiff's diseases of the liver.* New York: Lippincott-Raven.

Lavery, I. C. (1992). Technique of colostomy construction and closure. In L. M. Nyhus & R. J. Baker (Eds.), *Mastery of surgery* (2nd ed.). Boston: Little, Brown and Co.

Lefkowitch, J. H. (1996). Pathologic diagnosis of liver disease. In D. Zakim & T. D. Boyer (Eds.), *Hepatology: A textbook of liver disease* (3rd ed.). Philadelphia: W. B. Saunders.

Lin, E., Lowry, S. F., & Calvano, S. E. (1998). The systemic response to injury. In M. Feldman, M. H. Sleisenger, & B. F. Scharschmidt (Eds.), *Sleisenger and Fordtran's gastrointestinal and liver disease.* Phildelphia: W. B. Saunders.

Low, P. A. (1998). Diseases of the peripheral nerves. In R. J. Joynt & R. C. Griggs (Eds.), *Clinical neurology.* Philadelphia: Lippincott-Raven.

Lucas, C. E., & Ledgerwood, A. M. (1992). Treatment of the injured liver. In L. M. Nyhus & R. J. Baker (Eds.), *Mastery of surgery* (2nd ed.). Boston: Little, Brown and Co.

Martindale, R. G., & Gadacz, T. R. (1996). Open cholecystectomy and cholecystostomy. In G. D. Zuidema (Ed.), *Shackelford's surgery of the alimentary tract* (4th ed.). Philadelphia: W. B. Saunders.

Martindale, R. G., & Gadacz, T. R. (1996). Treatment of common duct stones. In G. D. Zuidema (Ed.), *Shackelford's surgery of the alimentary tract* (4th ed.). Philadelphia: W. B. Saunders.

McArthur, K. E. (1998). Hernias and volvulus of the gastrointestinal tract. In M. Feldman, M. H. Sleisenger, & B. F. Scharschmidt (Eds.), *Sleisenger and Fordtran's gastrointestinal and liver disease.* Philadelphia: W. B. Saunders.

McGuiness, A. M., et al. (2002). *Core curriculum for surgical technology* (5th ed.). Centennial, CO: Association of Surgical Technologists.

Minei, J. P., & Shires, G. T., III. (1999). Trauma of the liver. *Schiff's diseases of the liver.* New York: Lippincott-Raven.

Morrow, M. (1992). Segmental mastectomy and axillary dissection. In L. M. Nyhus & R. J. Baker (Eds.), *Mastery of surgery* (2nd ed.). Boston: Little, Brown and Co.

Mulholland, M. W. (1997). Chronic pancreatitis. In L. J. Greenfield et al. (Eds.), *Surgery: Scientific principles and practice* (2nd ed.). Philadelphia: Lippincott-Raven.

Mulholland, M. W., Moossa, A. R., & Liddle, R. A. (1995). Pancreas: Anatomy and structural anomalies. In T. Yamada et al. (Eds.), *Textbook of gastroenterology.* Philadelphia: J. B. Lippincott.

Nance, F. C. (1995). Diseases of the peritoneum, retroperitoneum, mesentery, and omentum. In W. S. Haubrich, F. Schaffner, & J. E. Berk (Eds.), *Bockus' gastroenterology* (5th ed.). Philadelphia: W. B. Saunders.

Neglen, P. (1997). Cosmetic excision and stripping of varices. In S. Raju & J. L. Villavicencio (Eds.), *Surgical management of venous disease.* Baltimore: Williams and Wilkins.

Nivatvongs, S. (1997). Anorectal disorders. In L. J. Greenfield et al. (Eds.), *Surgery: Scientific principles and practice* (2nd ed.). Philadelphia: Lippincott-Raven.

Nivatvongs, S. (1999). Hemorrhoids. In P. H. Gordon & S. Nivatvongs (Eds.), *Principles and practices of surgery for the colon, rectum, and anus.* St. Louis, MO: Quality Medical Publishing, Inc.

Nivatvongs, S. (1999). Pilonidal disease. In P. H. Gordon & S. Nivatvongs (Eds.), *Principles and practices of surgery for the colon, rectum, and anus.* St. Louis, MO: Quality Medical Publishing, Inc.

Nordestgaard, A. G., & Williams, R. A. (1994). Varicose veins. In F. J. Veith et al. (Eds.), *Vascular surgery* (2nd ed.). New York: McGraw-Hill.

Nyhus, L. M. (1992). Iliopubic tract repair of inguinal and femoral hernia: The posterior preperitoneal approach. In L. M. Nyhus & R. J. Baker (Eds.), *Mastery of surgery* (2nd ed.). Boston: Little, Brown and Co.

Osborne, M. P. (1998). Breast development and anatomy. In J. R. Harris et al. (Eds.), *Diseases of the breast.* New York: Lippincott-Raven.

Owhyang, C., & Levitt, M. D. (1995). Chronic pancreatitis. In T. Yamada et al. (Eds.), *Textbook of gastroenterology.* Philadelphia: J. B. Lippincott.

Pachter, H. M., & Hofstetter, S. (1998). The spleen: Splenic salvage procedures. In J. L. Cameron (Ed.), *Current surgical therapy.* St. Louis Mosby-Year Book.

Palovan, D. (1997). Intestinal problems in gynecologic surgery. In J. J. Sciarra (Ed.), *Gynecology and obstetrics.* New York: Lippincott-Raven.

Patino, J. E. (1995). A history of the treatment of hernia. In L. M. Nyhus & R. E. Condon (Eds.), *Hernia* (4th ed.). Philadelphia: J. B. Lippincott.

Patten, R. M., & Moss, A. A. (1995). Computed tomography. In W. S. Haubrich, F. Schaffner, & J. E. Berk (Eds.), *Bockus' gastroenterology* (5th ed.). Philadelphia: W. B. Saunders.

Pearl, R. K. (1995). Indications for and techniques of ileostomy. In C. Wastell, L. M. Nyhus, & P. E. Donahue (Eds.), *Surgery of the esophagus, stomach, and small intestine.* Boston: Little, Brown and Co.

Pellegrini, C. A., & Quan-Yang Duh (1995). Gallbladder and biliary tree: Anatomy and structural anomalies. In T. Yamada et al. (Eds.), *Textbook of gastroenterology*. Philadelphia: J. B. Lippincott.

Pollak, R. (1992). Miscellaneous surgical techniques for the small intestine. In L. M. Nyhus & R. J. Baker (Eds.), *Mastery of surgery* (2nd ed.). Boston: Little, Brown and Co.

Pratt, J. S., & Donegan, W. L. (1995). Surgical management. In W. L. Donegan & J. S. Spratt (Eds.), *Cancer of the breast*. Philadelphia: W. B. Saunders.

Ratych, R. E. (1995). Anorectal disease. In W. S. Haubrich, F. Schaffner, & J. E. Berk (Eds.), *Bockus' gastroenterology* (5th ed.). Philadelphia: W. B. Saunders.

Ratych, R. E., & Smith, G. W. (1996). Anatomy and physiology of the liver. In G. D. Zuidema (Ed.), *Shackelford's surgery of the alimentary tract* (4th ed.). Philadelphia: W. B. Saunders.

Read, R. C. (1992). Anatomy of abdominal herniation: The parietoperitoneal spaces. In L. M. Nyhus & R. J. Baker (Eds.), *Mastery of surgery* (2nd ed.). Boston: Little, Brown and Co.

Read, R. C. (1996). Basic features of abdominal wall herniation and its repair. In G. D. Zuidema (Ed.), *Shackelford's surgery of the alimentary tract* (4th ed.). Philadelphia: W. B. Saunders.

Read, R. C. (1996). Femoral hernia. In G. D. Zuidema (Ed.), *Shackelford's surgery of the alimentary tract* (4th ed.). Philadelphia: W. B. Saunders.

Read, R. C. (1996). Ventral herniation in the adult. In G. D. Zuidema (Ed.), *Shackelford's surgery of the alimentary tract* (4th ed.). Philadelphia: W. B. Saunders.

Redel, C. A., & Zwiener, R. J. (1998). Anatomy and anomalies of the stomach and duodenum. In M. Feldman, M. H. Sleisenger, & B. F. Scharschmidt (Eds.), *Sleisenger and Fordtran's gastrointestinal and liver disease*. Philadelphia: W. B. Saunders.

Rees, W. D. W., & Brown, C. M. (1995). Physiology of the stomach and duodenum. In W. S. Haubrich, F. Schaffner, & J. E. Berk (Eds.), *Bockus' gastroenterology* (5th ed.). Philadelphia: W. B. Saunders.

Romolo, J. L. (1996). Embryology and anatomy of the colon. In G. D. Zuidema (Ed.), *Shackelford's surgery of the alimentary tract* (4th ed.). Philadelphia: W. B. Saunders.

Rosch, T. (1997). Endoscopic ultrasonography. In M. Trede, Sir D. C. Carter, & W. P. Longmire, Jr. (Eds.), *Surgery of the pancreas* (2nd ed.). New York: Churchill Livingstone.

Roubenoff, R. (1995). The musculoskeletal system. In W. S. Haubrich, F. Schaffner, & J. E. Berk (Eds.), *Bockus' gastroenterology* (5th ed.). Philadelphia: W. B. Saunders.

Rout, W. R. (1996). Abdominal incisions. In G. D. Zuidema (Ed.), *Shackelford's surgery of the alimentary tract* (4th ed.). Philadelphia: W. B. Saunders.

Rout, W. R. (1996). Exposure of the thoracic alimentary tract. In G. D. Zuidema (Ed.), *Shackelford's surgery of the alimentary tract* (4th ed.). Philadelphia: W. B. Saunders.

Rubin, D. C. (1995). Small intestine: Anatomy and structural anomalies. In T. Yamada et al. (Eds.), *Textbook of gastroenterology*. Philadelphia: J. B. Lippincott.

Runyon, B. A., & Hillebrand, D. J. (1998). Surgical peritonitis and other diseases of the peritoneum, mesentery, omentum, and diaphragm. In M. Feldman, M. H. Sleisenger, & B. F. Scharschmidt (Eds.), *Sleisenger and Fordtran's gastrointestinal and liver disease*. Philadelphia: W. B. Saunders.

Sabiston, D. C., Jr. (1994). Hernias. In D. C. Sabiston, Jr. & H. K. Lyerly (Eds.), *Sabiston essentials of surgery* (2nd ed.). Philadelphia: W. B. Saunders.

Salmons, S. (1995). Muscles. In L. H. Bannister (Ed.), *Gray's anatomy: The anatomical basis of medicine and surgery* (38th ed.). New York: Churchill Livingstone.

Salvati, E. P., & Eisenstat, F. E. (1996). Hemorrhoidal disease. In G. D. Zuidema (Ed.), *Shackelford's surgery of the alimentary tract* (4th ed.). Philadelphia: W. B. Saunders.

Schaffner, F., & Thung, S. N. (1995). Liver biopsy. In W. S. Haubrich, F. Schaffner, & J. E. Berk (Eds.), *Bockus' gastroenterology* (5th ed.). Philadelphia: W. B. Saunders.

Schrock, T. R. (1994). Large intestine. In L. W. Way (Ed.), *Current surgical diagnosis and treatment* (10th ed.). Norwalk, CT: Appleton and Lange.

Schrock, T. R. (1996). Colon and rectum: Diagnostic techniques. In G. D. Zuidema (Ed.), *Shackelford's surgery of the alimentary tract* (4th ed.). Philadelphia: W. B. Saunders.

Schrock, T. R. (1998). Appendicitis. In M. Feldman, M. H. Sleisenger, & B. F. Scharschmidt (Eds.), *Sleisenger and Fordtran's gastrointestinal and liver disease*. Philadelphia: W. B. Saunders.

Schrock, T. R. (1998). Examination and diseases of the anorectum. In M. Feldman, M. H. Sleisenger, & B. F. Scharschmidt (Eds.), *Sleisenger and Fordtran's gastrointestinal and liver disease*. Philadelphia: W. B. Saunders.

Schwartz, S. I. (1998). The spleen: Anatomy and splenectomy. In L. M. Nyhus & R. J. Baker (Eds.), *Mastery of surgery* (2nd ed.). Boston: Little, Brown and Co.

Schwartz, S. I. (1998). The spleen: Splenectomy for hematologic disorders. In J. L. Cameron (Ed.), *Current surgical therapy*. St. Louis, MO: Mosby-Year Book.

Schwartz, S. I. (1999). Gallbladder and extrahepatic biliary system. In S. I. Schwartz et al. (Eds.), *Principles of surgery*. New York: McGraw-Hill.

Selub, S. E. (1995). Digestion and absorption: Water, electrolyte, and vitamin transport. In W. S. Haubrich, F. Schaffner, & J. E. Berk (Eds.), *Bockus' gastroenterology* (5th ed.). Philadelphia: W. B. Saunders

Sherlock, S., & Dooley, J. (Eds.). (1997). Anatomy and function. *Diseases of the liver and biliary system* (10th ed.). Oxford, England: Blackwell Science Ltd.

Sherlock, S., & Dooley, J. (Eds.). (1997). Gallstones and inflammatory disease. *Diseases of the liver and biliary system* (10th ed.). Oxford, England: Blackwell Science Ltd.

Sherry, R. M., & Gadacz, T. R. (1996). Cholelithiasis and cholecystitis. In G. D. Zuidema (Ed.), *Shackelford's surgery of the alimentary tract* (4th ed.). Philadelphia: W. B. Saunders.

Shires, G. T. (1999). Trauma. In G. D. Zuidema (Ed.), *Principles of Shackelford's surgery of the alimentary tract* (4th ed.). Philadelphia: W. B. Saunders.

Smith, D. L., & Meyer, A. A. (1996). Anatomy, immunology, and physiology of the spleen. In G. D. Zuidema (Ed.), *Shackelford's surgery of the alimentary tract* (4th ed.). Philadelphia: W. B. Saunders.

Solomon, T. E. (1995). Physiology of the exocrine pancreas. In W. S. Haubrich, F. Schaffner, & J. E. Berk (Eds.), *Bockus' gastroenterology* (5th ed.). Philadelphia: W. B. Saunders.

Stirling, M. C., & Orringer, M. B. (1996). Esophageal varices. In G. D. Zuidema (Ed.), *Shackelford's surgery of the alimentary tract* (4th ed.). Philadelphia: W. B. Saunders

Stolz, A. (1998). Liver physiology and metabolic function. In M. Feldman, M. H. Sleisenger, & B. F. Scharschmidt (Eds.), *Sleisenger and Fordtran's gastrointestinal and liver disease*. Phildelphia: W. B. Saunders.

Suchy, F. J. (1998). Anatomy, anomalies, and pediatric disorders of the biliary tract. In M. Feldman, M. H. Sleisenger, & B. F. Scharschmidt (Eds.), *Sleisenger and Fordtran's gastrointestinal and liver disease*. Phildelphia: W. B. Saunders.

Telford, G. L., & Condon, R. E. (1996). Appendix. In G. D. Zuidema (Ed.), *Shackelford's surgery of the alimentary tract* (4th ed.). Philadelphia: W. B. Saunders.

Tominaga, G. T., & Jakowatz, J. G. (1996). Placement of indwelling venous access systems. *Vascular access: Principles and practice* (3rd ed.). St. Louis, MO: Mosby-Year Book.

Trede, M. (1997). Approaches to the pancreas and abdominal exploration. In M. Trede, Sir D. C. Carter, & W. P. Longmire, Jr. (Eds.), *Surgery of the pancreas* (2nd ed.). New York: Churchill Livingstone.

Trede, M. (1997). Embryology and surgical anatomy of the pancreas. In M. Trede, Sir D. C. Carter, & W. P. Longmire, Jr. (Eds.), *Surgery of the pancreas* (2nd ed.). New York: Churchill Livingstone.

Trede, M. (1997). Technique of Whipple pancreatoduodenectomy. In M. Trede, Sir D. C. Carter, & W. P. Longmire, Jr. (Eds.), *Surgery of the pancreas* (2nd ed.). New York: Churchill Livingstone.

Trede, M. (1997). Approaches to the pancreas and abdominal exploration. In M. Trede, Sir D. C. Carter, & W. P. Longmire, Jr. (Eds.), *Surgery of the pancreas* (2nd ed.). New York: Churchill Livingstone.

Trede, M., & Carter, C. (1997). The complications of pancreatoduodenectomy and their management. In M. Trede, Sir D. C. Carter, & W. P. Longmire, Jr. (Eds.), *Surgery of the pancreas* (2nd ed.). New York: Churchill Livingstone.

Veith, F. J. (1994). Vascular surgical techniques. In F. J. Veith et al. (Eds.), *Vascular surgery* (2nd ed.). New York: McGraw-Hill.

Wanebo, H. J., & Koness, R. J. (1992). Pancreatic cancer. Surgical approach. In J. Ahlgren & J. MacDonald (Eds.), *Gastrointestinal oncology*. Philadelphia: J. B. Lippincott Co.

Wanless, I. R. (1998). Anatomy and developmental anomalies of the liver. In M. Feldman, M. H. Sleisenger, & B. F. Scharschmidt (Eds.), *Sleisenger and Fordtran's gastrointestinal and liver disease*. Phildelphia: W. B. Saunders.

Wantz, G. E. (1999). Abdominal wall hernias. In S. I. Schwartz et al. (Eds.), *Principles of surgery*. New York: McGraw-Hill.

Way, L. W. (1994). Biliary tract. In L. W. Way (Ed.), *Current surgical diagnosis and treatment* (10th ed.). Norwalk, CT: Appleton and Lange.

Weiss, L. (1995). The structure of the spleen. In Beutler, M. A. Lichtman, B. S. Coller, & T. J. Kipps (Eds.), *Williams hematology* (5th ed.). New York: McGraw-Hill.

Werner, J., & Warshaw, A. L. (1997). Pseudocysts, post-inflammatory cystic fluid collections, and other non-neoplastic cysts. In M. Trede, Sir D. C. Carter, & W. P. Longmire, Jr. (Eds.), *Surgery of the pancreas* (2nd ed.). New York: Churchill Livingstone.

White, R. A., & Fogarty, T. J. (1996). Devices and techniques for vascular access: Utility and limitations of current methods. In R. A. White & T. J. Fogarty (Eds.), *Peripheral endovascular interventions*. St. Louis, MO: Mosby-Year Book.

Wile, A. (1996). Indications and devices for chronic venous access. *Vascular access: Principles and practice* (3rd ed.). St. Louis, MO: Mosby-Year Book.

Wilson, S. E. (1996). Complications of vascular access procedures: Thrombosis, venous hypertension, arterial steal, and neuropathy. *Vascular access: Principles and practice* (3rd ed.). St. Louis, MO: Mosby-Year Book.

Wood, D. K. (1992). Liver biopsy techniques. In L. M. Nyhus & R. J. Baker (Eds.), *Mastery of surgery* (2nd ed.). Boston: Little, Brown and Co.

Wright, P. E., II. (1997). Hand infections. In S. T. Canale (Ed.), *Campbell's operative orthopaedics*. St Louis, MO: Mosby-Year Book.

Zucker, S. D., & Gollan, J. L. (1995). Physiology of the liver. In W. S. Haubrich, F. Schaffner, & J. E. Berk (Eds.), *Bockus' gastroenterology* (5th ed.). Philadelphia: W. B. Saunders.

CHAPTER 15

Obstetric and Gynecologic Surgery

Bob Caruthers
Gary Allen

CASE STUDY

Meredith is in labor for the first time. She had a normal pregnancy and good prenatal care. Labor proceeded normally until she was dilated to 4 centimeters. Since that point, no progress has taken place. It has been 12 hours; Meredith is tired and frustrated. The fetus demonstrates no stress as of yet. Meredith is scheduled for a cesarean section.

1. What is the term used to describe this condition?
2. Is the condition a common reason for cesarean section?
3. What are the procedural steps for a cesarean section?

OBJECTIVES

After studying this chapter, the reader should be able to:

A 1. Discuss the relevant anatomy and physiology of the female reproductive system.

P 2. Describe the pathology of the female reproductive system that prompts surgical intervention and the related terminology.

3. Discuss any special preoperative obstetric and gynecologic diagnostic procedures/tests.

O 4. Discuss any special preoperative preparation procedures related to obstetric/gynecologic procedures.

5. Identify the names and uses of obstetric and gynecologic instruments, supplies, and drugs.
6. Identify the names and uses of special equipment related to obstetric/gynecologic surgery.
7. Discuss the intraoperative preparation of the patient undergoing an obstetric or gynecologic procedure.

8. Define and give an overview of the obstetric/gynecologic procedure.
9. Discuss the purpose and expected outcomes of the obstetric/gynecologic procedure.
10. Discuss the immediate postoperative care and possible complications of the obstetric/gynecologic procedure.

S 11. Discuss any specific variations related to the preoperative, intraoperative, and postoperative care of the obstetric/gynecologic patient.

SELECT KEY TERMS

1. adnexa	7. curettage	13. fimbria	19. myoma
2. bony pelvis	8. delivery forceps	14. fistula	20. occiput anterior
3. breech	9. DUB	15. gravida	21. parity
4. cesarean section	10. dystocia	16. LEEP	22. perineum
5. corpus luteum	11. episiotomy	17. ligament	23. Pfannenstiel
6. CPD	12. exenteration	18. marsupialization	24. vestibule

INTRODUCTION TO OBSTETRIC AND GYNECOLOGIC SURGERY

Obstetric and gynecologic surgery is a specialty in the field of medicine. This specialty area focuses its attention on females after the beginning of menstruation. The obstetrician's attention is given to the pregnant patient and issues concerned with fertility. Gynecologists focus on the female reproductive system and related problems outside pregnancy. Traditionally and typically, a practicing physician in this specialty field sees patients for both obstetric and gynecologic reasons. However, physicians may narrow their focus to either an obstetric or gynecologic practice. Some subspecialties exist. For instance, some physicians may specialize in infertility and its related treatment modes. Some surgeons specialize in the treatment of gynecologic cancer. In some locales, nonreconstructive types of breast surgery are considered the domain of the gynecologist.

ANATOMY

An understanding of obstetric and gynecologic surgery requires a basic background in female reproductive anatomy, physiology, and endocrinology. Most of this section will focus on female reproductive anatomy. The anatomy applies equally to obstetric and gynecologic considerations.

PELVIS

The intestinal, urinary, and reproductive systems all exit through their own orifices in the pelvic floor and are intricately related in both function and support. The internal female organs (the vagina, uterus and cervix, fallopian tubes, and ovaries) are situated in the abdomen's "lesser pelvis." These organs are protected by the bones of the pelvic girdle (**bony pelvis**) and supported by the muscularity of the pelvic floor. The pelvic girdle consists of the ilia, ischia, and pubic bones and is attached to the vertebral column at the sacrum (Figure 15-1). The coccyx is fused below the sacrum.

The pelvic floor consists of the levator ani muscle and its three components: the iliococcygeal, pubococcygeal and puborectalis (Figure 15-2). The iliococcygeus is a thin sheet of muscle that arises from the pelvic sidewall along the ischial spine and inserts at the midline behind the rectum. The U-shaped puborectalis originates at the pubic bones and attaches to the lateral walls of the vagina and rectum, providing the latter with "sling-like" support. The pubococcygeus arises from the back of the

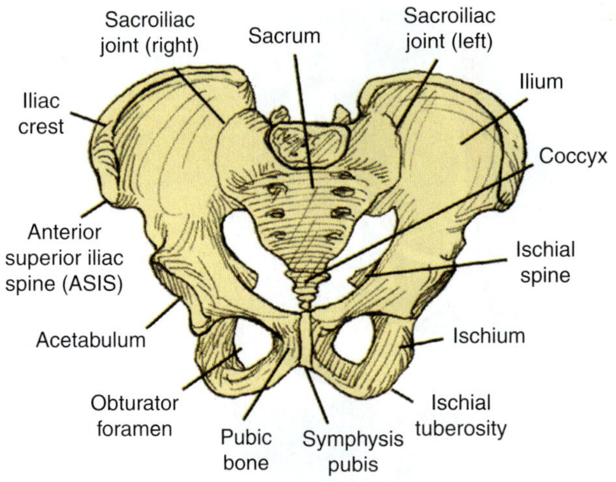

Figure 15-1 Bony pelvis

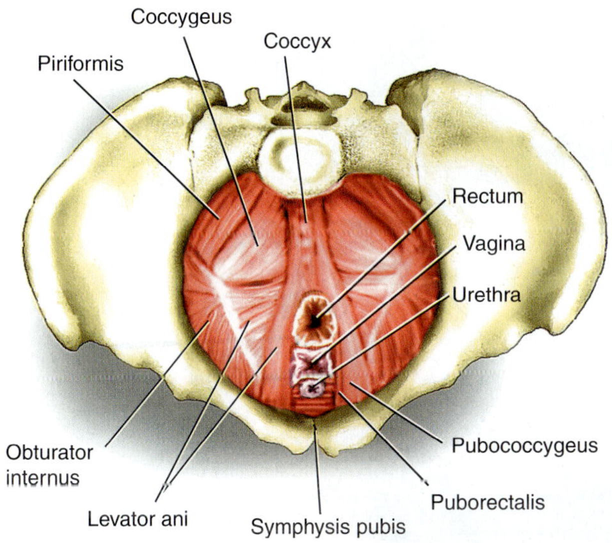

Figure 15-2 Muscles and bones of the pelvic floor

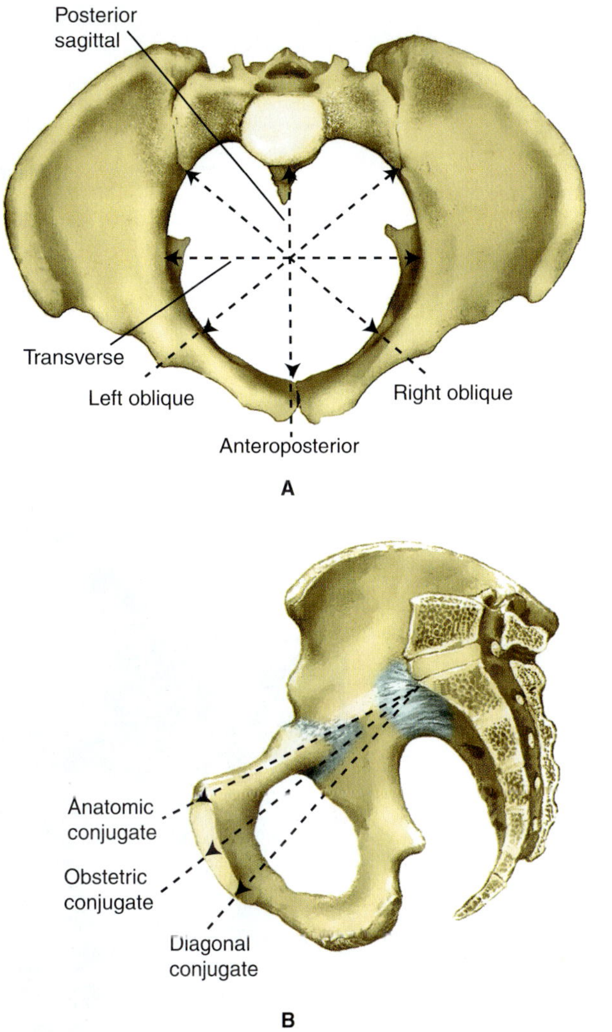

Figure 15-3 Pelvic girdle and diameters: (A) Inlet view, (B) lateral view

superior pubic ramus laterally as far as the obturator canal. The fibers pass posteriorly to converge behind the rectum and insert into the anococcygeal raphe and the coccyx. The iliococcygeus originates from the tendinous arch of the levator ani muscle and the ischial spine and inserts into the anococcygeal raphe and the coccyx.

The female pelvis varies from the male pelvis. The variations are related to the function of childbearing and are seen typically in the structures affecting the pelvic outlet. The pelvis is arranged in such a manner that two distinct cavities are created. The superior cavity is the "false pelvis," which bears little significance to gynecology and obstetrics other than its prominence as an attachment for pelvic musculature. The false pelvis can vary widely in size. The flared iliac bones (crests) are notable landmarks during surgery. The inferior cavity or "true pelvis" is bounded by the sacrum, ischia, pubis, and **ligaments**. The true pelvis has a pelvic "inlet" and pelvic "outlet" through which the fetus passes during childbirth. The pelvic inlet is rather round, while the outlet is more transversely oval. This shallower and wider outlet aids the process of fetal delivery (Figure 15-3).

The pelvic ligaments also lend support to the pelvic organs and help maintain the relative positions of the organs in the lesser pelvis. The pelvic ligaments, which include the cardinal, round, and infundibulopelvic ligaments, are loose configurations of areolar tissue, blood vessels, and muscle fibers that act as "moorings" for the uterus and vagina. Connective tissues, the "glue" of the human body, help to keep the structural integrity of the organs in stasis. Connective tissues are not static; they change with age, nutritional status, amount of exercise, and hormonal fluctuations (Figure 15-4).

Conditions arising from dysfunction of the pelvic musculature of concern in gynecologic surgery include prolapse of internal organs, such as the bladder or rectum, into the vaginal vault. Surgically, these organs are approached using various techniques by incision into the

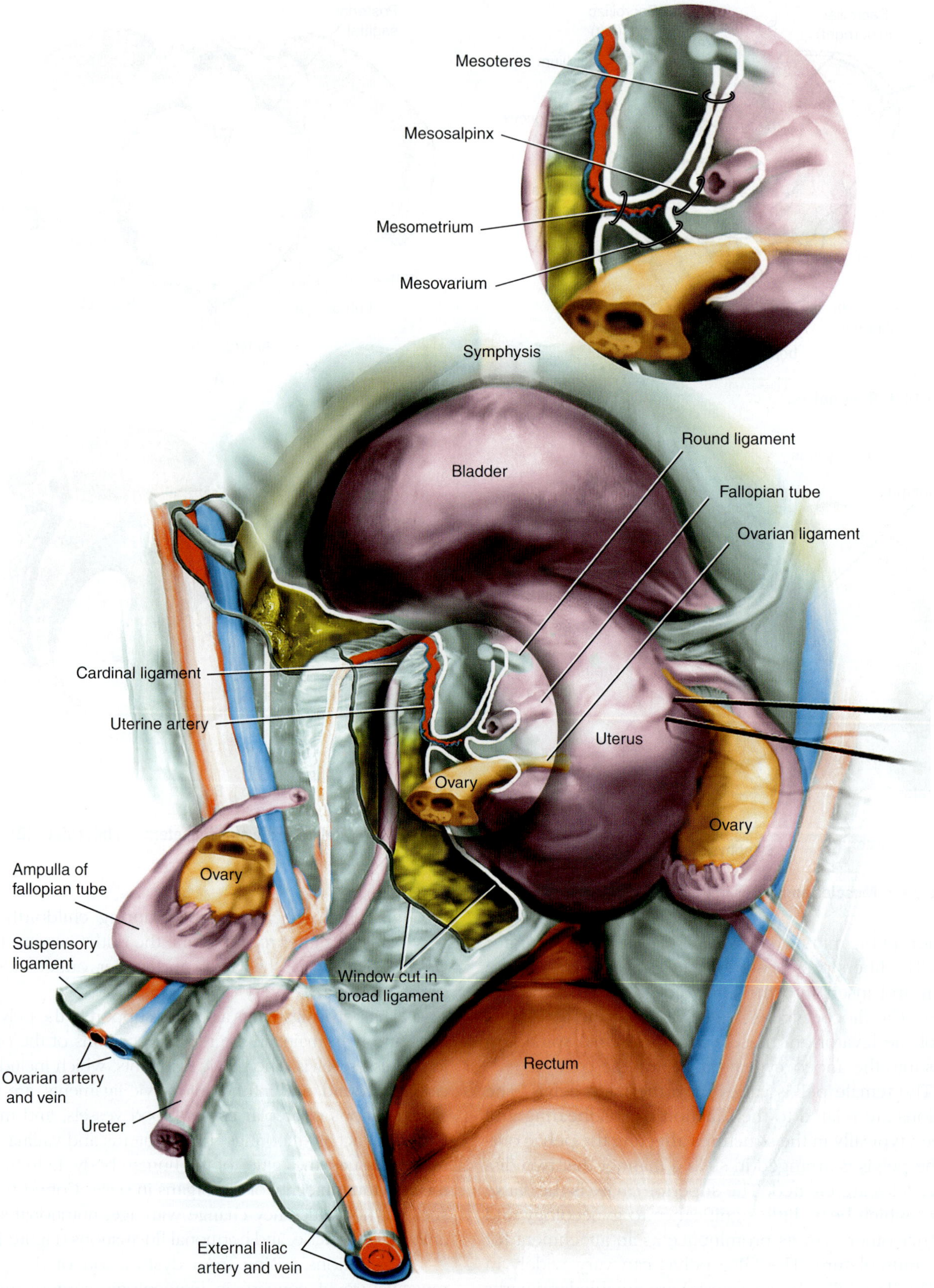

Figure 15-4 **Support structures of the female pelvis**

spaces that surround or divide them. These anatomical planes are termed the prevesical, vesicovaginal, vesicocervical, and rectovaginal spaces (Figure 15-5).

EXTERNAL GENITALIA

In addition to the internal organs, gynecology also addresses the external female genitalia, collectively known as the vulva. The vulva includes the mons pubis, the labia majora, labia minora, clitoris, Bartholin's glands, fourchette, and **perineum** (refer to Plate 2 in Appendix A). The external genitalia are vascularized and innervated by the clitoral, perineal, and inferior hemorrhoidal branches of the pudendal artery and nerve.

The mons pubis is a rounded eminence anterior to the symphysis pubis, the point at which the two pubic bones fuse. The mons pubis is formed by a mass of adipose tissue lying beneath the skin. The mons pubis is superior to the vaginal opening and is normally covered with coarse pubic hair following puberty.

The labia majora are two rounded, prominent, longitudinal flaps extending from the mons pubis to the perineum. The labia are thicker anteriorly and blend into the skin posteriorly. The labia minora are two flat, reddish cutaneous flaps lying between the labia majora. The labia minora bifurcate at the clitoris, passing below and above the clitoris. The labia minora contain sebaceous glands.

The clitoris is an erectile structure located directly above the urethral orifice and below the mons pubis. It is covered by a hood-shaped prepuce formed by the fused ends of the anterior labia minora.

The **vestibule** is the cavity between the labia minora, and it contains the urethral meatus, inferior to the clitoris, as well as the orifices of the vestibular glands (Bartholin's glands). The Bartholin's glands are paired structures about 0.5–1 cm in diameter that secrete a lubricating mucoid substance. The hymen, or hymenal ring, is a thin fold of mucous membrane located just inside the vaginal orifice, which, in virginal women, may appear completely closed.

The perineum in the female is the area between the inferior vaginal opening and anus. It is generally 2 to 3 cm in length and is supported by the pelvic and urogenital diaphragms, which consist of the levator ani, coccygeal, and deep transverse perineal muscles. The perineum is a sensitive area innervated by branches of the pudendal nerve originating at the second, third, and fourth sacral portions of the spinal cord. During delivery of the fetus, the perineum responds by stretching, but can be torn or otherwise damaged without sufficient care.

VAGINA

The vagina is a fibromuscular tube, continuous with the external genitalia, that increases in diameter in its internal

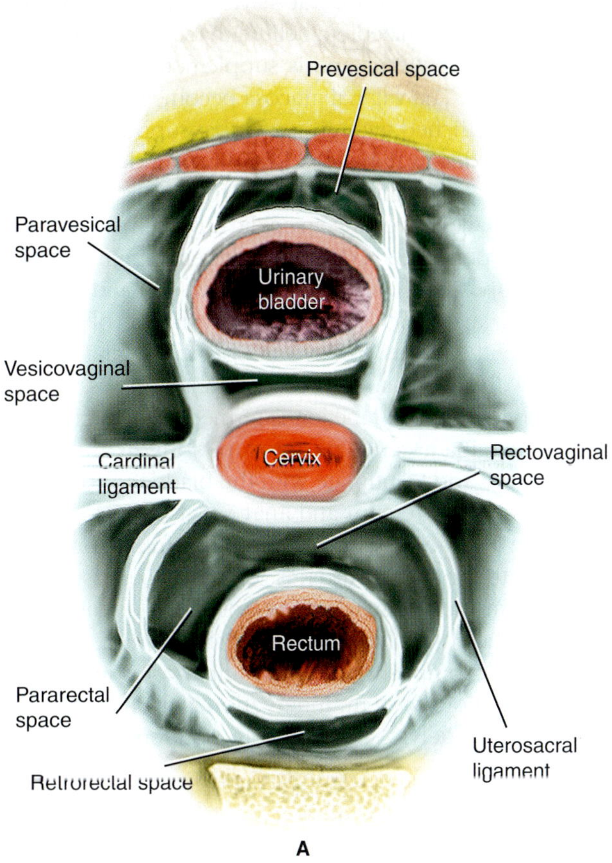

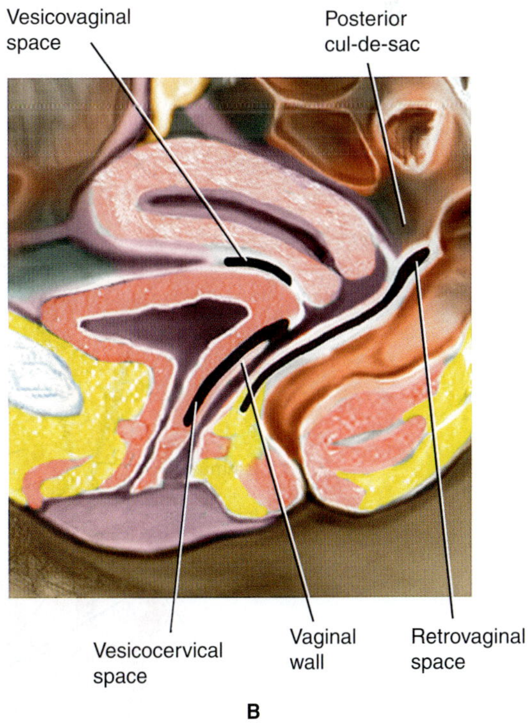

Figure 15-5 **Anatomical pelvic planes: (A) Cross section, (B) sagittal**

projection, becoming widest at its deepest region. Vaginal mucosa is nonkeratinized epithelium that changes little with adult menstrual patterns and is supplemented by mucous from the cervix. The vaginal mucosa becomes thicker at puberty and is enriched with glycogen that supports a normal flora that renders vaginal fluid acidic. Paradoxically, the vagina acts as a friendly receptacle for the male's semen during coitus while creating an acidic environment that kills most of the spermatozoa deposited therein. Vaginal muscularity is composed of an inner circular muscle and an outer longitudinal layer that is continuous with that of the myometrium of the uterus. In cross section, the vagina appears as a tube with an H-shaped cleft. The annular recess created by the cervical-vaginal junction is termed the fornix.

The vagina ascends posterosuperiorly in a gentle S-shaped curve and is intimate with the bladder and urethra anteriorly and the rectum and anal canal posteriorly. The ureters are also anterior to the vagina running somewhat laterally with the uterine arteries. A rich vascular supply is derived from the vaginal, uterine, internal pudendal, and middle rectal branches of the internal iliac arteries. Drainage is accomplished via the vaginal veins into the internal iliac venous system. Innervation is from the vaginal plexus and the pelvic splanchnic and pudendal nerves.

UTERUS

The uterus is a hollow, thick-walled and pear-shaped organ situated between the bladder and rectum (Figure 15-6). The uterine appendages (**adnexa**) are the fallopian tubes and ovaries. The normal uterus weighs 30–40 g, is approximately 7.5 cm long and 2.5 cm thick, and measures 5 cm at its widest point. The superior two-thirds of the organ is termed the corpus uteri, or body of the uterus, which narrows to a cylindrical lower section called the uterine cervix, or simply the cervix. The most superior portion of the uterus is termed the fundus. The uterine corpus lies entirely within the lesser pelvis while nearly all of the cervix extends into the vagina. At the junction between the corpus uteri and the cervix is an aperture termed the internal os; where the cervix ultimately opens into the vagina is the external os.

The uterus is lined with endometrium that varies in its consistency and sheds in accordance with phases of the menstrual cycle. At the internal os, the uterine lining becomes the mucous secreting tissue of the cervix. Several layers of muscle lie beneath the endometrium. The outermost layer is composed of longitudinal muscle; the innermost layer consists of fibers arranged both longitudinally and obliquely. Between these layers is a vascular layer of interlacing spiral configurations of smooth muscle and many blood vessels. This structure allows the uterus to secure hemostasis quickly by mechanical contraction of the muscle fibers encircling the blood vessels. Visceral peritoneum overlies the pelvic surface of the uterus.

Ligaments extending to the pelvic walls suspend the uterus. Laterally, these paired structures are the broad, the cardinal (anteriorly), the pubic (posteriorly), and the sacral (inferiorly) ligaments. The broad ligament, a result of peritoneal folds, contains the uterine (fallopian) tube, the round and ovarian ligaments, and various blood vessels, nerves,

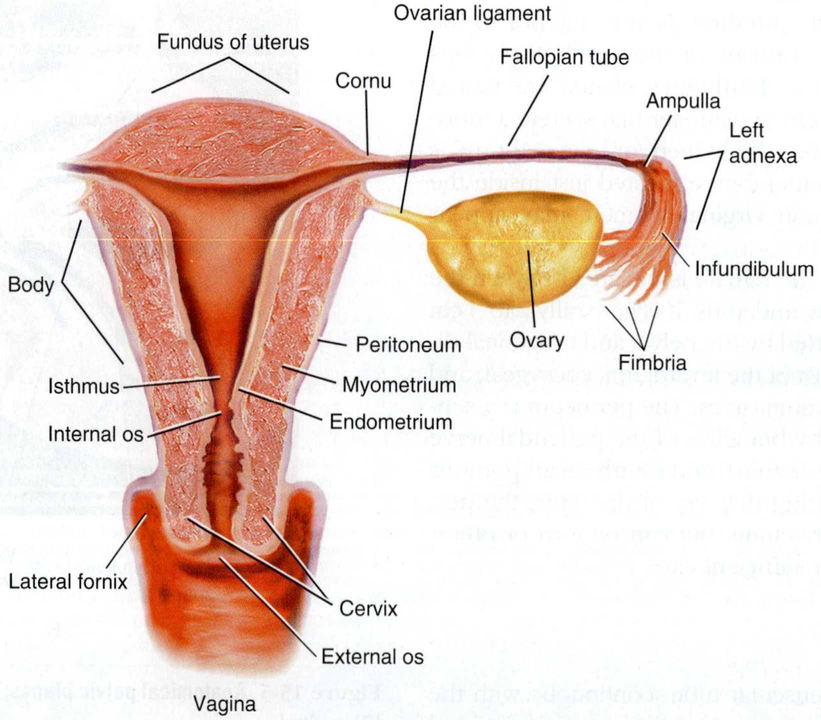

Figure 15-6 Uterus and adnexa

and lymphatics. The round ligament passes through the inguinal ring to the skin and connective tissue of the labia majora. The uterus is innervated by the ovarian and hypogastric plexuses, the twelfth thoracic and first lumbar spinal segments, and the second to fourth sacral spinal roots. Arterial supply is derived from the uterine branch of the paired internal iliac arteries. Venous drainage is accomplished by adjoining veins and the lymphatics course through the utero-ovarian pedicle to the external iliac area. Lymphatic drainage is arranged in four zones. The lymph nodes increase dramatically in size and number during pregnancy.

FALLOPIAN TUBES

The paired fallopian tubes, also called the uterine tubes or oviducts, are approximately 10 cm long and are divided into four portions: **fimbria** (infundibulum), ampulla, isthmus, and intramural region. Each fallopian tube is situated in the upper margin (the mesosalpinx) of the broad ligament. The fallopian tubes open into the uterus at the uterine os, in an area termed the cornu, where its lumen is narrowest at 1 mm. Likewise, the fallopian tube opens to the ovary at the abdominal os, which is about 3 mm wide and situated in the infundibulum.

The fimbria are finger-like projections at the terminal end of the fallopian tube that serve to "sweep" the pelvis in search of oocytes released by the ovaries and guide them into the tube's lumen. The ampulla is the largest and longest portion of the fallopian tube, measuring 5 or more cm in length and changing from a luminal diameter of over 1 cm at the fimbria to about 2 mm at the isthmus. The isthmus is nearly 2.5 mm in diameter, measures 2–3 cm in length, and is heavily muscled, acting as a "sphincter." This sphincter effect is important in the prevention of endometriosis. The isthmus opens to the intramural portion of the fallopian tube, which is that part within the wall of the uterus. The intramural portion communicates with the uterus at the cornu.

The fallopian tubes are lined with folded simple ciliated and secretory epithelium that changes in distribution with the portion of the tube. In fertility, the lining provides motility and lubrication for the captured oocytes on their journey to the uterus. The muscularis of the fallopian tubes is composed of both external longitudinal and internal circular layers of smooth muscle. The circular layer is at its thickest in the ampulla. The serosal, or outer, layer of the fallopian tube is continuous with the broad ligament.

Vascularity to the tubes is achieved by the ovarian and uterine arteries and their accompanying veins. Lymphatic drainage follows the upper edge of the broad ligament and joins the drainage from the uterus and ovary to the periaortic and lumbar nodes. Innervation of the fallopian tubes is via the sympathetic fibers from the tenth thoracic to second lumbar plexuses and the parasympathetic vagal fibers from the ovarian plexus, as well as the second to fourth sacral nerves.

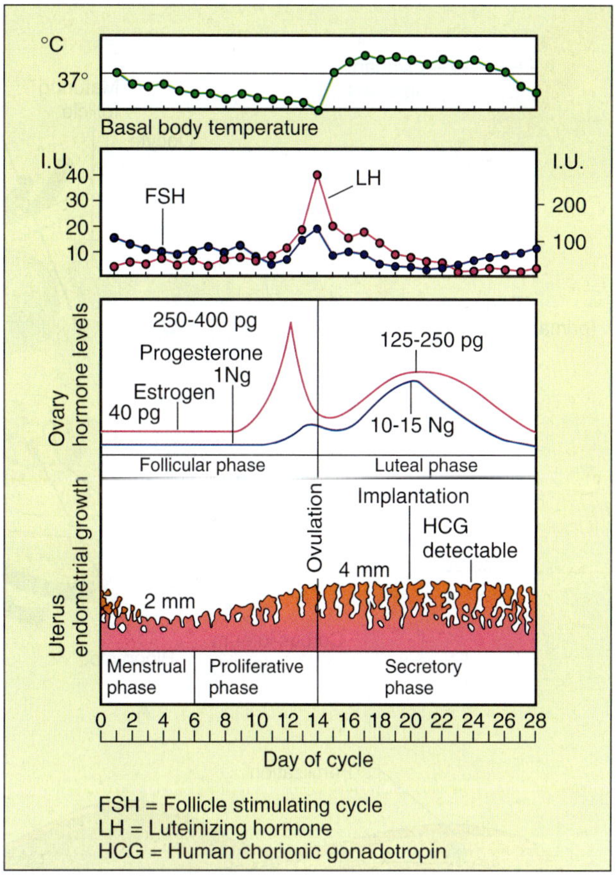

Figure 15-7 Menstrual cycle

OVARIES

The ovaries are paired, almond-shaped (amygdaloid) structures measuring approximately 3 cm × 1.5 cm × 1 cm with a volume of roughly 6 mL. They lie on either side of the uterus in the ovarian fossa of the lateral pelvic wall. Prior to puberty the ovaries exhibit a smooth surface, but thereafter demonstrate scarring from ovulatory activities. Mature ovaries are grayish pink but can appear bluish, yellow, or purple depending on the stage of ovulation. They may also exhibit cysts normally.

The function of the ovaries is the production and expulsion of oocytes (ova, or eggs) and the release of the hormones estrogen and progesterone. The ovarian cycle is stimulated by the release of luteinizing hormone (LH) and follicle stimulating hormone (FSH) from the pituitary gland (Figure 15-7). A "primary follicle" develops with influence from FSH and matures through several stages until it ripens under the influence of LH into a "Graafian follicle." The Graafian follicle then erupts, releasing the oocyte into the pelvis and the waiting fingers of the fimbria of the fallopian tube (Figure 15-8A and B). Within the ruptured ovarian follicle the anatomic structure known as the **corpus luteum** grows. It is a spheroid of yellowish tissue that reaches a maximum size of 2 to 3 cm in diameter. The corpus luteum

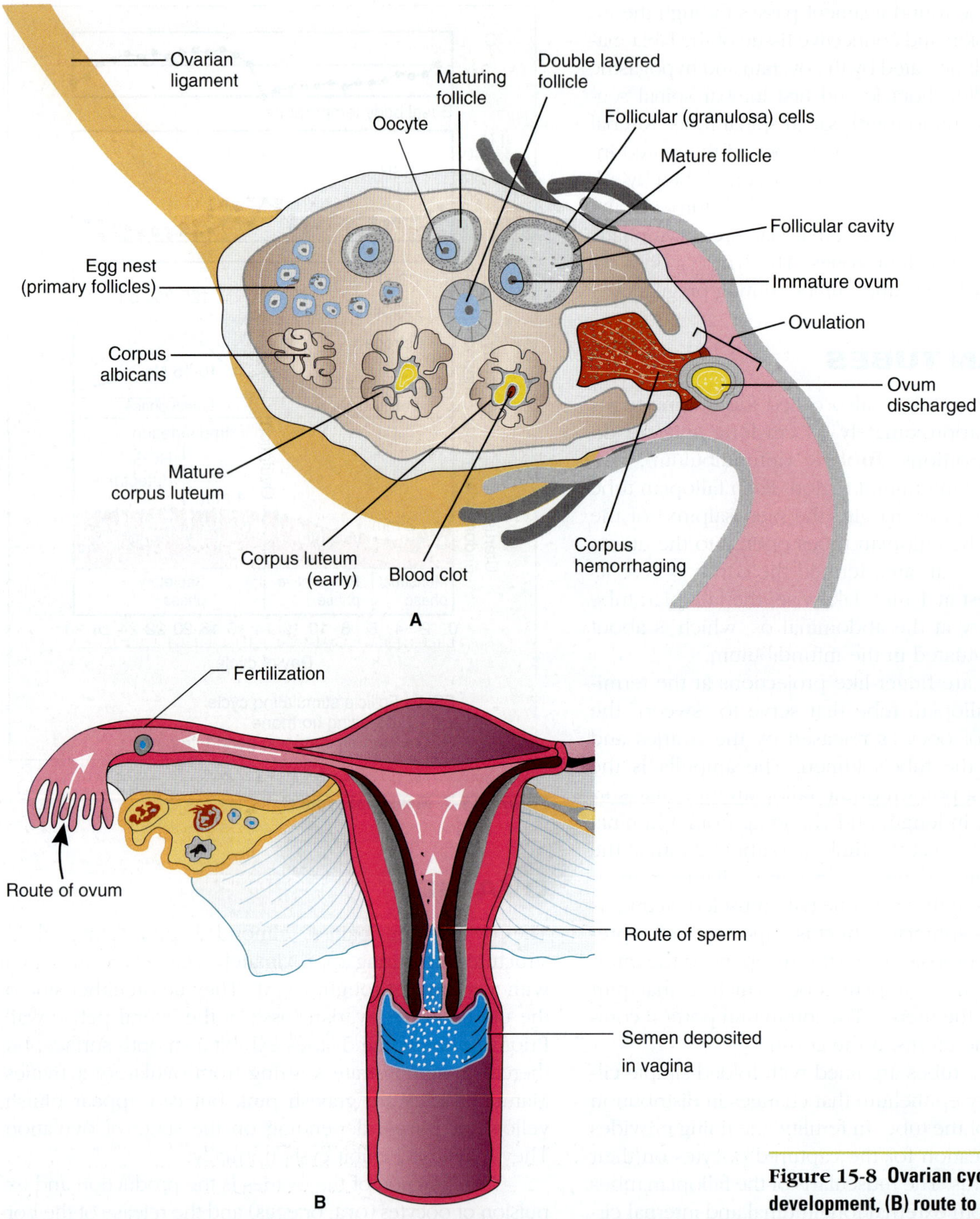

Figure 15-8 Ovarian cycle: (A) Ovum development, (B) route to fertilization

forms after every ovulation. It is actually a short-term endocrine gland that secretes the hormone progesterone that acts upon the endometrial layer of the uterine to maintain a vascular status in preparation of implantation of the oocyte. If conception takes place, it continues to grow and the secretion of progesterone increases. Maximum function occurs 10 to 12 weeks of gestation. After this period of time, the corpus luteum begins to shrink in size and function decreases until 6 months after gestation. If conception does not take place, approximately 2 weeks prior to menstruation the corpus luteum atrophies and degenerates until it is seen as a pale spot on the ovarian surface. The hormones estrogen and progesterone, produced by the ovary, influence this process.

The ovaries are supported at either end by ligaments. A fold of peritoneum arising near the overlying fimbria forms the suspensory ligament. The ovarian ligament, lying in the broad ligament, supports the bulk of the ovary. Blood arrives to the organs via the ovarian arteries branching from the aorta and follows ovarian veins back to the inferior vena cava. Lymph is drained to the lumboaortic and pelvic lymph nodes. Ovarian innervation is derived from postganglionic sympathetic, parasympathetic, and autonomic fibers of the ovarian plexus.

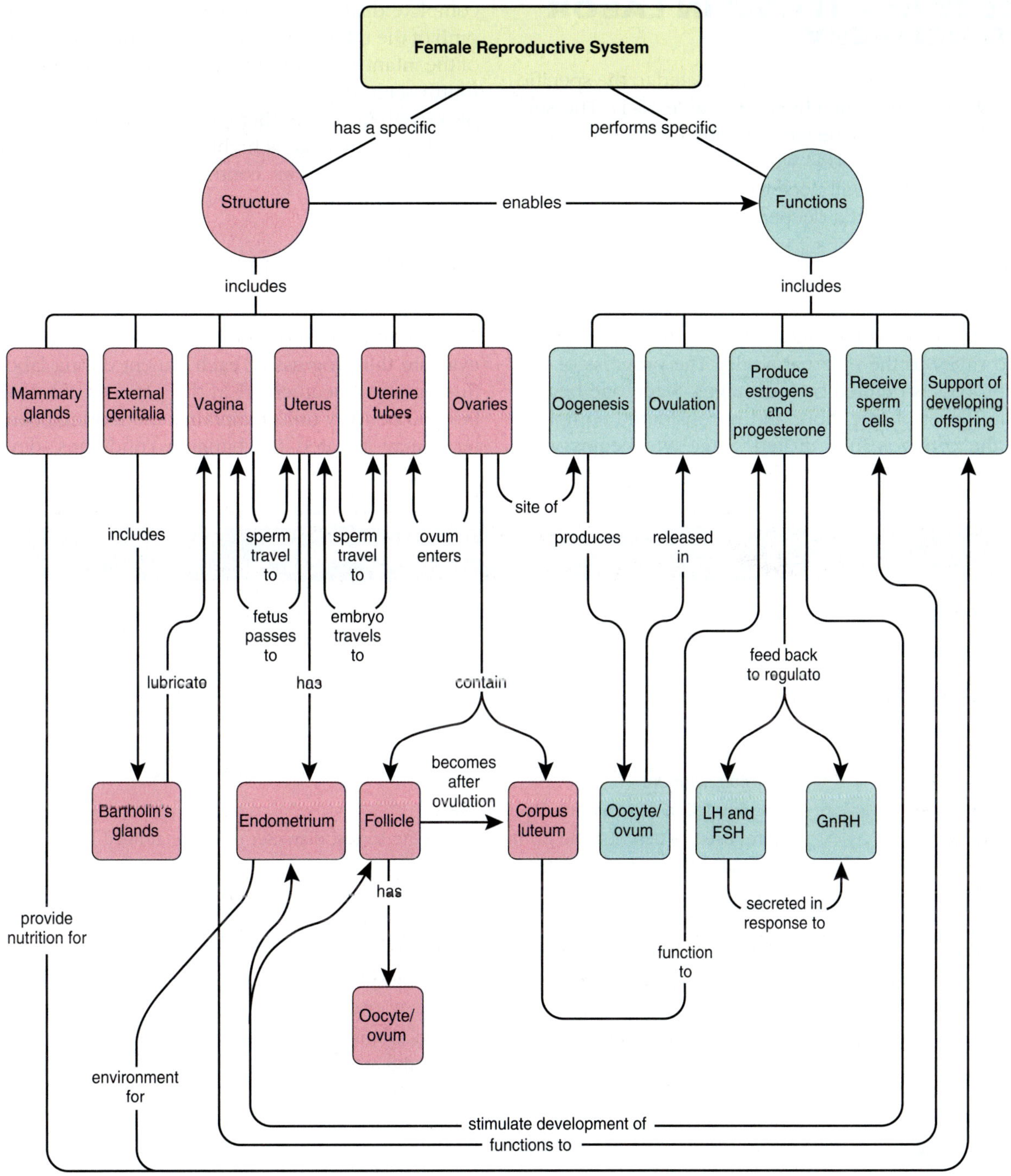

Figure 15-9 Female reproductive system concept map

A summary view of the female reproductive system provides a way for the student to conceptualize this complicated system (Figure 15-9).

PREGNANCY—A SPECIAL CONDITION

Surgery is an area of medicine that concerns itself mostly with gross structural pathology. The obstetrician performs surgery to facilitate or inhibit the natural state of pregnancy. Pregnancy brings changes to the female body and presents a condition that can lead directly to surgery or contribute to other conditions that lead to surgery. Obstetric surgery is significantly different from gynecologic surgery in its concerns. For that reason, the two areas will be separated in this chapter. The surgical technologist often assists with cesarean sections and, in larger facilities, may specialize in obstetrics, assisting with vaginal deliveries, cesarean sections, sterilization procedures, and other related procedures. This section will provide the student with a brief introduction to obstetric considerations.

SELECT KEY TERMS IN LABOR AND DELIVERY

Obstetrics has a language of its own related to the specific events of pregnancy and childbirth (Table 15-1). The surgical technologist must be familiar with the basic terms related to childbirth. Those who work in the labor and delivery department will need to understand the implications of these terms at a deeper clinical level.

LABOR

Labor is the process by which a fetus is moved from the uterine cavity to the external world. The progress of the labor process is defined by four stages. Stage one begins with the onset of true labor and is considered complete when the cervix is fully dilated. Stage two begins with complete dilatation of the cervix and terminates with the birth of the infant. The third stage is initiated with the birth of the infant and ends when the placenta is delivered. The fourth stage begins at that point and is considered completed when the mother's condition has stabilized. The length of each stage is highly variable under normal conditions. Many factors contribute to the length of labor (Table 15-2). Parity is one of these factors.

MONITORING THE PROGRESSION OF LABOR

The obstetrician and labor and delivery nurse routinely evaluate the progress of each patient during labor. Their findings are documented in the patient's chart. Many labor and delivery units maintain a monitoring board so the team may be alert to changing conditions, developing

Table 15-1 Key Terms in Labor and Delivery

Term	Definition
Braxton Hicks	"False" labor; normal contractions not associated with progressive cervical dilation
"Bloody show"	A term used to describe a small amount of blood-tinged mucus flowing from the vagina; may herald the onset of labor
Cervical dilation	A measurement of the opening available in the cervix for the passage of uterine contents (closed–8 cm in obstetric measurements)
Cervical effacement	A process in which the cervix softens and thins and is taken up into the lower uterine segment
Contractions	Muscular action of uterus to expel the fetus
Crowning	A term used to describe the event in which the largest diameter of the fetal head is encircled by the vulvar ring
Descent	Movement of the fetus through the pelvic canal caused by the force of uterine contractions
Expulsion	Delivery of the shoulders and body of the fetus
Extension rotation	Rotation of the fetal head back to its original position as the head passes over the perineum (after crowning)
Flexion	A change in the relative position of the cervical spine bringing the fetal head toward the chest; in the occipitoanterior position, the result is a smaller diameter of the presenting part; in the occipitoposterior, a larger diameter
Gravida	A term that indicates the number of times a woman has been pregnant
Internal rotation	Rotation of the fetal head as it meets the musculature of the pelvic floor; precise movements depend on initial position of the fetus relative to the pelvis
Lie	Relationship that exists between the long axis of the fetus and the long axis of the mother
Lightening	A term used to describe the settling of the fetal head into the brim of the pelvis
Parity	A term that indicates the number of times a woman has given birth; a multiple-birth experience is considered one birth
Position	Relationship between the presenting fetal part and the maternal body pelvis (most common is **occiput anterior** [OA])
Presentation	A term referring to the fetal part overlying the pelvic inlet (normally the fetal head but may be **breech** [buttocks] or compound [more than one part])
Station	A measurement of the descent of the presenting part of the fetus in relation to the ischial spines

Table 15-2 Normal Labor—Characteristics

EVENT OR CHARACTERISTIC	PRIMAPARA	MULTIPARA
Stage one—duration	6–18 hr	2–10 hr
Stage two—duration	0.5–3 hr	5–30 min
Stage three—duration	0–30 min	0–30 min
Stage four—duration	6 hr average	6 hr average
Cervical dilatation	1 cm/hr	1.2 cm/hr

Source: Adapted from *Essentials of Obstetrics and Gynecology,* 3rd ed., by N. F. Hacker and J. G. Moore, 1998, Philadelphia: W. B. Saunders.

problems, deliveries, or cesarean sections. The surgical technologist should be able to follow patients' progress and prepare delivery or operating rooms accordingly. A typical monitoring board contains the information illustrated in Table 15-3. Since the board may be open to public viewing, patients' names are often excluded.

NORMAL ROLE OF ST IN DELIVERY

Most deliveries occur in a natural and normative pattern. The surgical technologist is there as part of the team to assist the obstetrician, support the mother, and prepare for any developing problems. It is common to help with clamping and cutting the umbilical cord, collecting blood for cord gases, and assisting as needed. The surgical technologist working in the labor and delivery unit should be familiar with basic fetal monitoring equipment, infant resuscitation procedures, and signs of a developing crisis with either the mother or the fetus. An understanding of delivery techniques, including vacuum and forceps extraction, is mandatory. The most common surgical intervention in vaginal birth is the **episiotomy** and/or the repair of perineal lacerations, which are discussed later in this chapter.

SPECIAL INSTRUMENTATION, DRUGS, EQUIPMENT, AND SUPPLIES IN OBSTETRIC AND GYNECOLOGIC SURGERY

The basic instrumentation for obstetric surgery and cesarean section is the same as for general surgery (Chapter 14). Major abdominal sets are used for gynecologic laparotomy. Obstetrics requires unique instruments because of the purpose and the anatomical relationship between mother and fetus. Laparoscopic instrumentation is discussed in some detail in this chapter because of its historical roots in gynecologic surgery.

INSTRUMENTATION

Instrumentation varies. This is true with respect to geographic region, specific facility, and surgeon. Instrumentation may even vary from case to case. The instrumentation lists that follow are basic, relatively standard, and as generic as possible to give the student some insight into the equipment and instrumentation related to obstetric and gynecologic surgery. Some basic instrument sets are listed in Table 15-4 and illustrative examples are shown in the illustrations that follow (Figures 15-10, 15-11, 15-12, 15-13, and 15-14).

DRUGS

A number of drugs are used to treat infertility, prevent labor, induce labor, control uterine hemorrhage, and stimulate lactation (refer to Chapter 9). Three drugs that cause uterine contraction are discussed below.

Oxytocin (Pitocin, Syntocinon) is an oxytocic drug that may be used to induce or continue labor, contract the uterus following delivery thereby controlling hemorrhage, and stimulate lactation. It is also used to treat incomplete abortion, cause abortion, and control uterine bleeding following an abortion. Oxytocin is available in two forms: parenteral injection and nasal solution. The parenteral form may be given intravenously or injected directly into a muscle (including the myometrium). The nasal preparation is typically used to stimulate lactation.

Carboprost (Hemabate) is also an oxytocic drug available in parenteral form that is used to cause abortion by contracting the uterus and dilating the cervix. It is also used to control uterine hemorrhage following abortion and childbirth.

Side effects of oxytocic drugs include an increased risk of uterine rupture, irregular heartbeat (maternal), an increase in postpartum bleeding, and jaundice of the neonate and other effects that are more rare. The presence of certain medical conditions such as heart disease, hypertension, kidney disease, and jaundice may affect the use of oxytocics.

(Text continues on page 493)

Table 15-3 Sample Labor and Delivery Monitoring Board

ROOM	DOCTOR	GRAVIDA/PARITY	DILATION	EFFACEMENT	STATION	CARE NOTES
1	Johnson	3/2	8 cm	90%	0	Diabetes

Table 15-4 Examples of Basic Instrument Sets in Obstetric and Gynecologic Surgery

Set	Instruments
Vaginal Prep Set	(Commonly a disposable set)
	Graves vaginal speculum
	16 Fr urethral catheter
	Dressing forceps
	Sponge forceps
	Solution cups
Vaginal Delivery	Kelly hemostats
	Medium needle holder
	Tissue forceps with teeth
	Russian tissue forceps
	Straight Mayo scissors
	Curved Mayo scissors
	Placenta basin
	Cord clamps
	Cord blood tube
D&C	Knife handles, #3 and #4 long
	Dressing forceps, 8 in.
	Russian tissue forceps
	Towel clamp(s)
	Sponge forceps, 9.5 in.
	Bozeman dressing forceps, 10.5 in.
	Heaney needle holder
	Graves vaginal speculum
	Auvard weighted speculum
	Jackson vaginal retractor
	Hegar uterine dilator set
	Sims uterine sound
	Tenaculum forceps
	Sims uterine curette set
Basic Vaginal Set	Knife handles, #3 and #4
	Mayo scissors, several lengths
	Metzenbaum scissors, 7 in.
	Dressing forceps
	Tissue forceps, different lengths
	Kelly hemostats
	Rochester-Pean clamps
	Heaney clamps
	Kocher clamps
	Towel clamps
	Sponge forceps
	Vaginal retractors
	Deaver retractors
	Allis tissue forceps
	Auvard weighted speculum
	Tenaculum forceps
Gynecologic Abdominal	Basic laparotomy set plus:
	Mayo scissors, different lengths
	Jorgensen scissors
	Long and short tissue forceps with and without teeth
Gynecologic Abdominal *(continued)*	Long and short Russian tissue forceps
	Rochester-Ochsner clamps
	Heaney needle holders
	O'Sullivan-O'Connor retractor
	Tenaculum, triple toothed
	Heaney hysterectomy clamps
	Heaney-Ballantine hysterectomy clamps
Cesarean Section	Knife handles, #3
	Needle holders
	Tissue forceps, short and long Russian, with teeth, and Adson's
	Kelly hemostats, short and medium
	Rochester-Pean clamps
	Rochester-Ochsner clamps
	Mayo scissors
	Metzenbaum scissors
	Bandage scissors
	De Lee universal retractor or bladder blade from Balfour
	Richardson retractors
	Goelet retractors
	Cord clamps
	Cord blood tubes
	Bulb syringe
Laparoscopic	Basic laparotomy set (in room)
	"Minor" set open
	Graves vaginal speculum
	Auvard weighted speculum
	Sims uterine sound
	Cervical dilators
	Tenaculum forceps
	Camera and adapters
	Appropriate set of telescopes
	Trocar set or individual trocars
	Appropriate laparoscopic instruments
	Peritoneal scissors
	Hook scissors
	Grasping forceps
	Needle holder
	Atraumatic grasping forceps
	Knife electrode
	Veress needle
	Kleppinger
	Tubing for insufflator
	Cords and connectors for fiberoptics and ESU

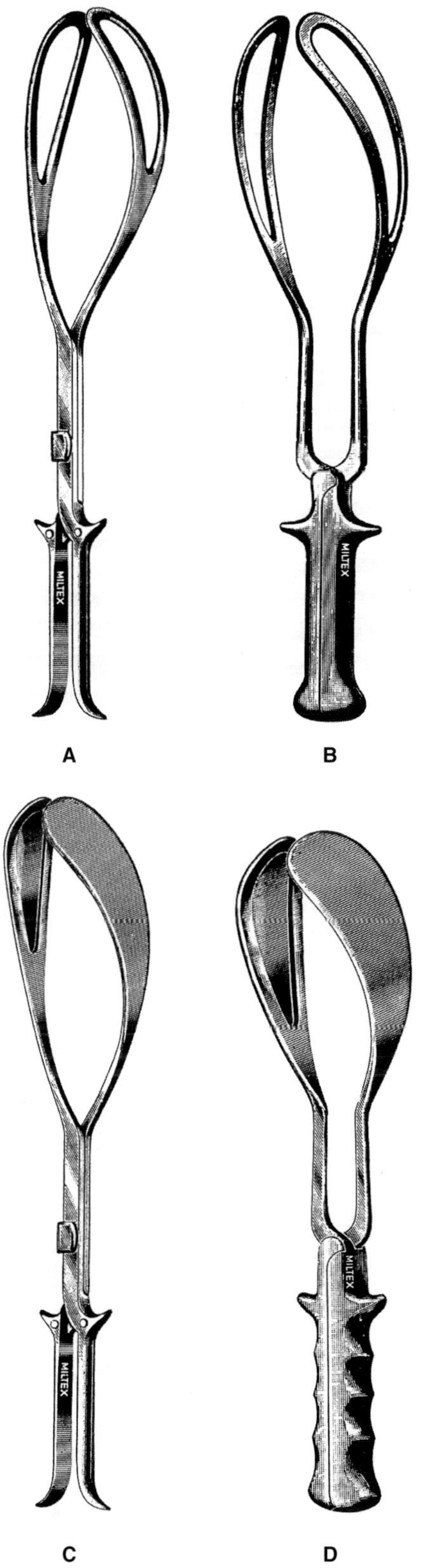

Figure 15-10 Delivery forceps: (A) Kielland, (B) De Lee, (C) Luikart, (D) Simpson-Luikart (Courtesy of Miltex Instrument Co., Inc.)

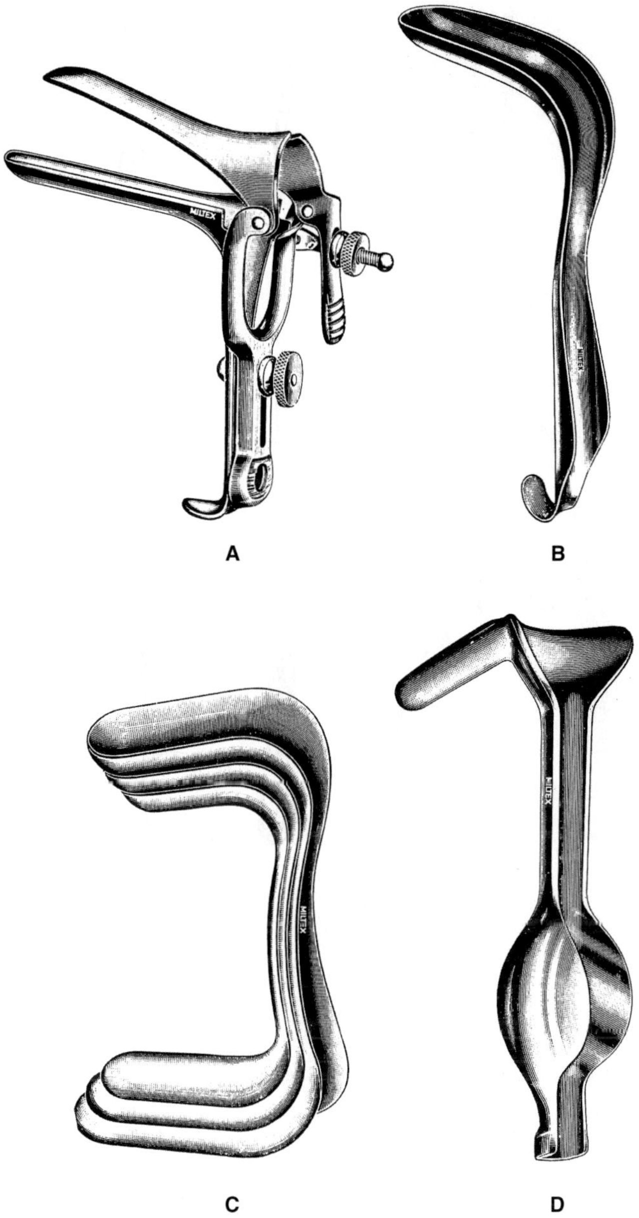

Figure 15-11 Vaginal retractors: (A) Graves vaginal speculum, (B) Sims vaginal speculum (single end), (C) Sims vaginal speculum (double end), (D) Auvard weighted vaginal speculum *(Courtesy of Miltex Instrument Co., Inc.)*

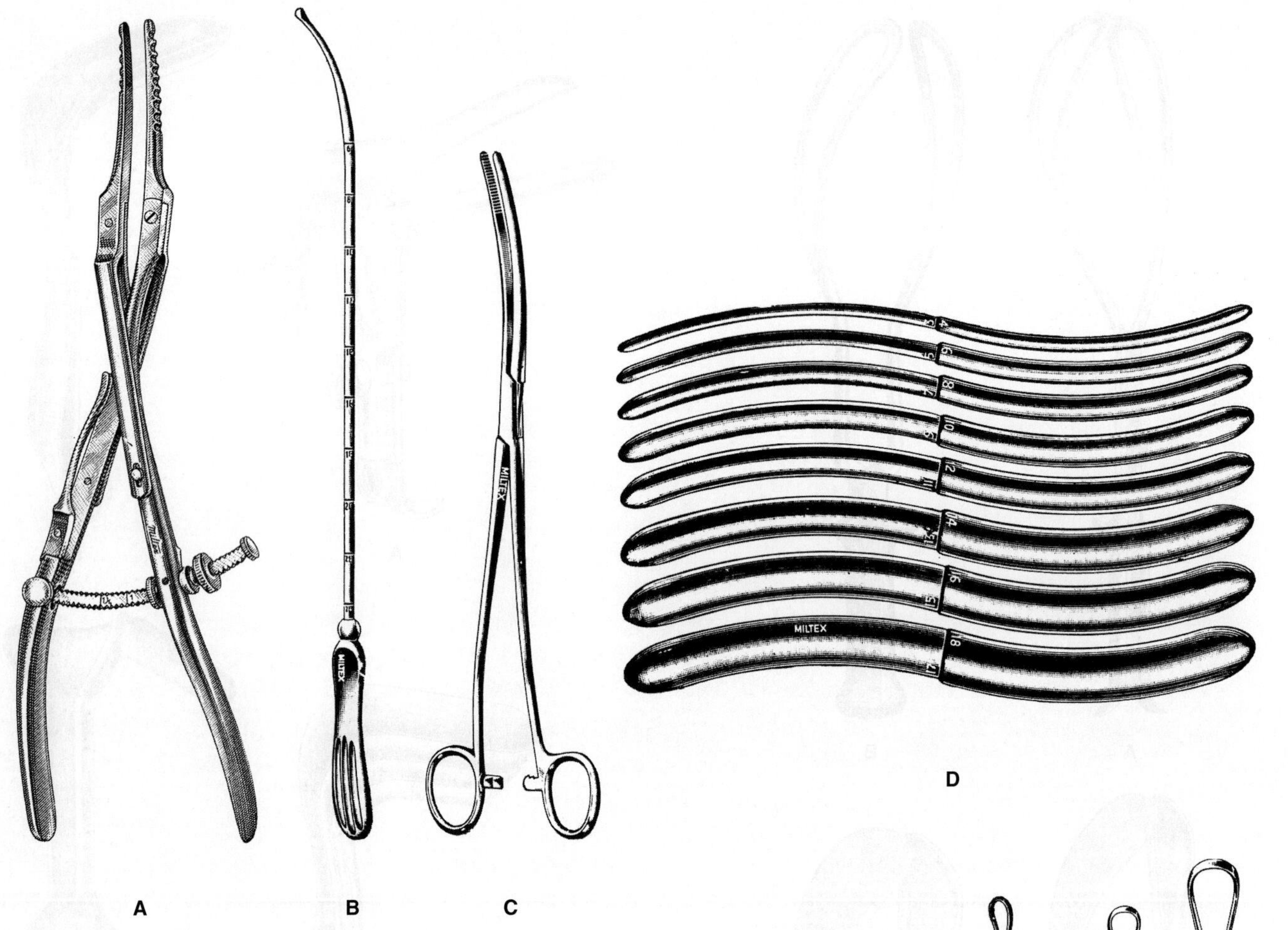

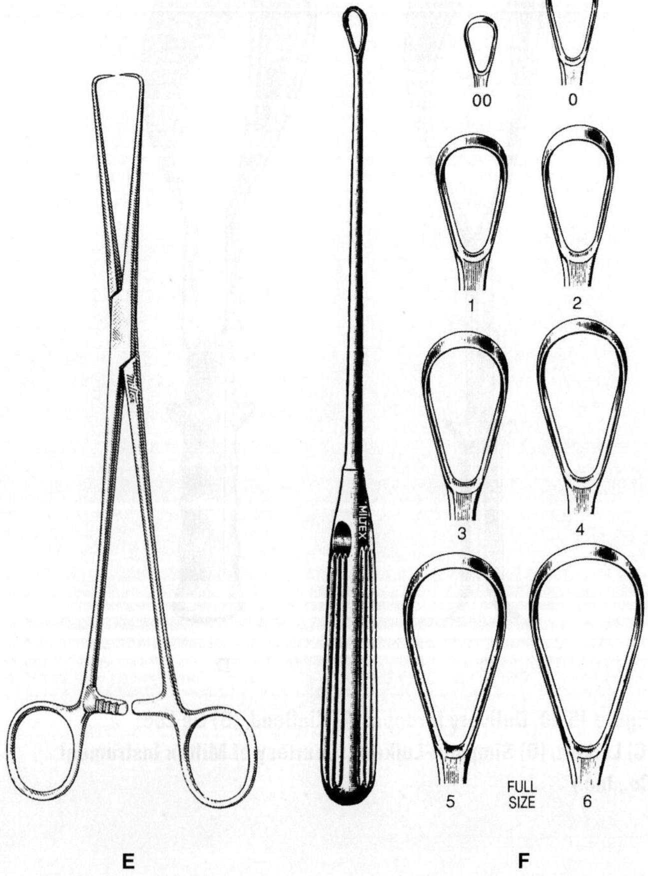

Figure 15-12 **Cervical and intrauterine instruments: (A) Goodell uterine dilator, (B) Sims uterine sound, (C) Bozeman uterine dressing forceps, (D) Hegar uterine dilators, (E) Schroeder-Braun uterine tenaculum, (F) Sims uterine curettes (sharp blades)** ***(Courtesy of Miltex Instrument Co., Inc.)***

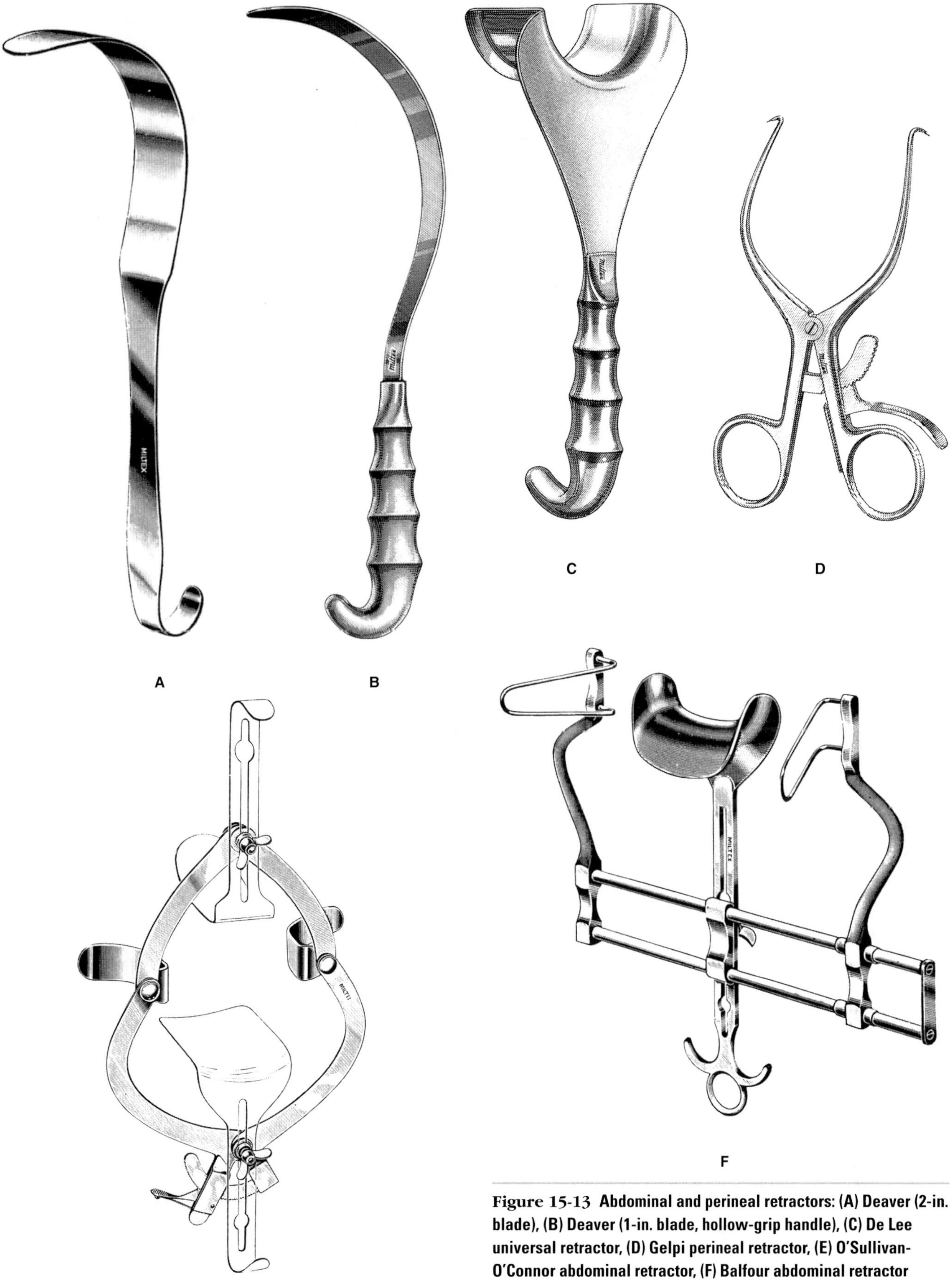

C D

A B

F

E

Figure 15-13 **Abdominal and perineal retractors: (A) Deaver (2-in. blade), (B) Deaver (1-in. blade, hollow-grip handle), (C) De Lee universal retractor, (D) Gelpi perineal retractor, (E) O'Sullivan-O'Connor abdominal retractor, (F) Balfour abdominal retractor (fenestrated blades)** ***(Courtesy of Miltex Instrument Co., Inc.)***

(continues)

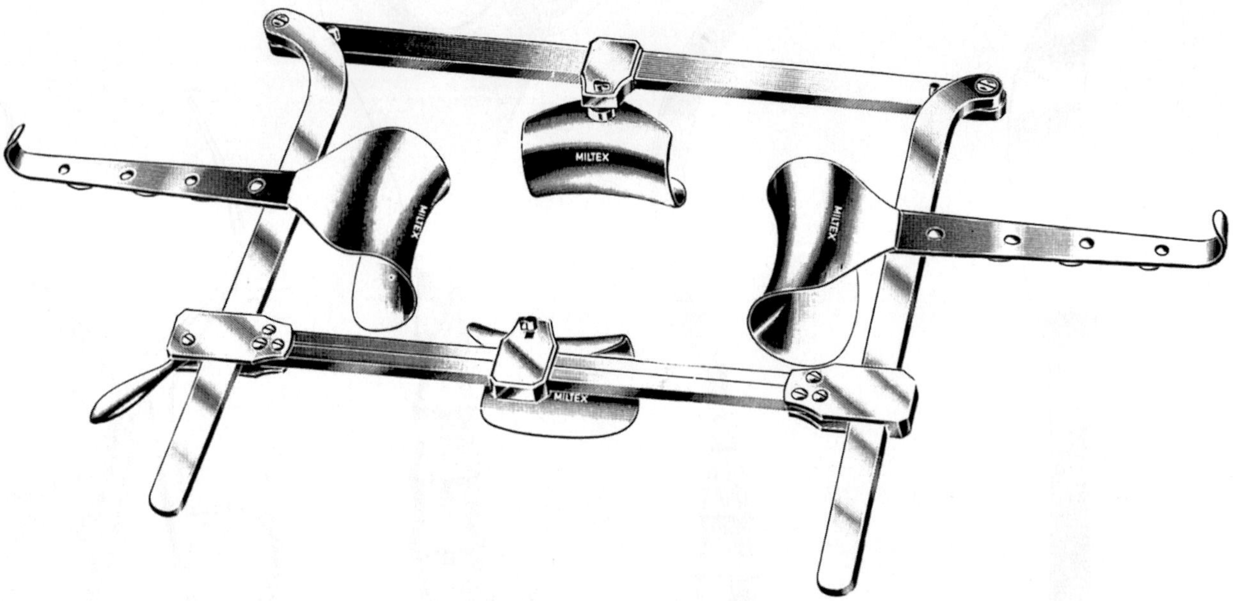

Figure 15-13 ***(continued)*** **(G) Franz abdominal retractor (interchangeable blades)** ***(Courtesy of Miltex Instrument Co., Inc.)***

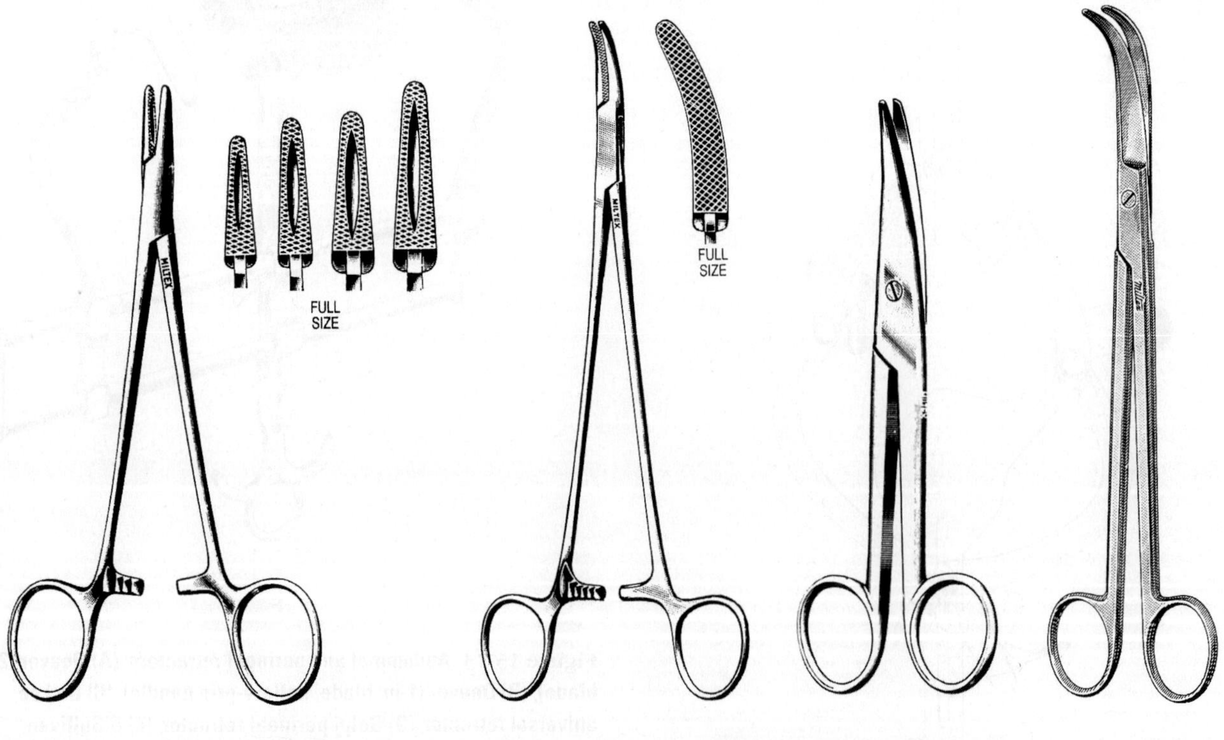

Figure 15-14 **General obstetric and gynecologic instruments: (A) Mayo-Hegar needle holder, (B) Heaney needle holder, (C) Mayo dissecting scissors (curved), (D) Jorgenson scissors** ***(Courtesy of Miltex Instrument Co., Inc.)***

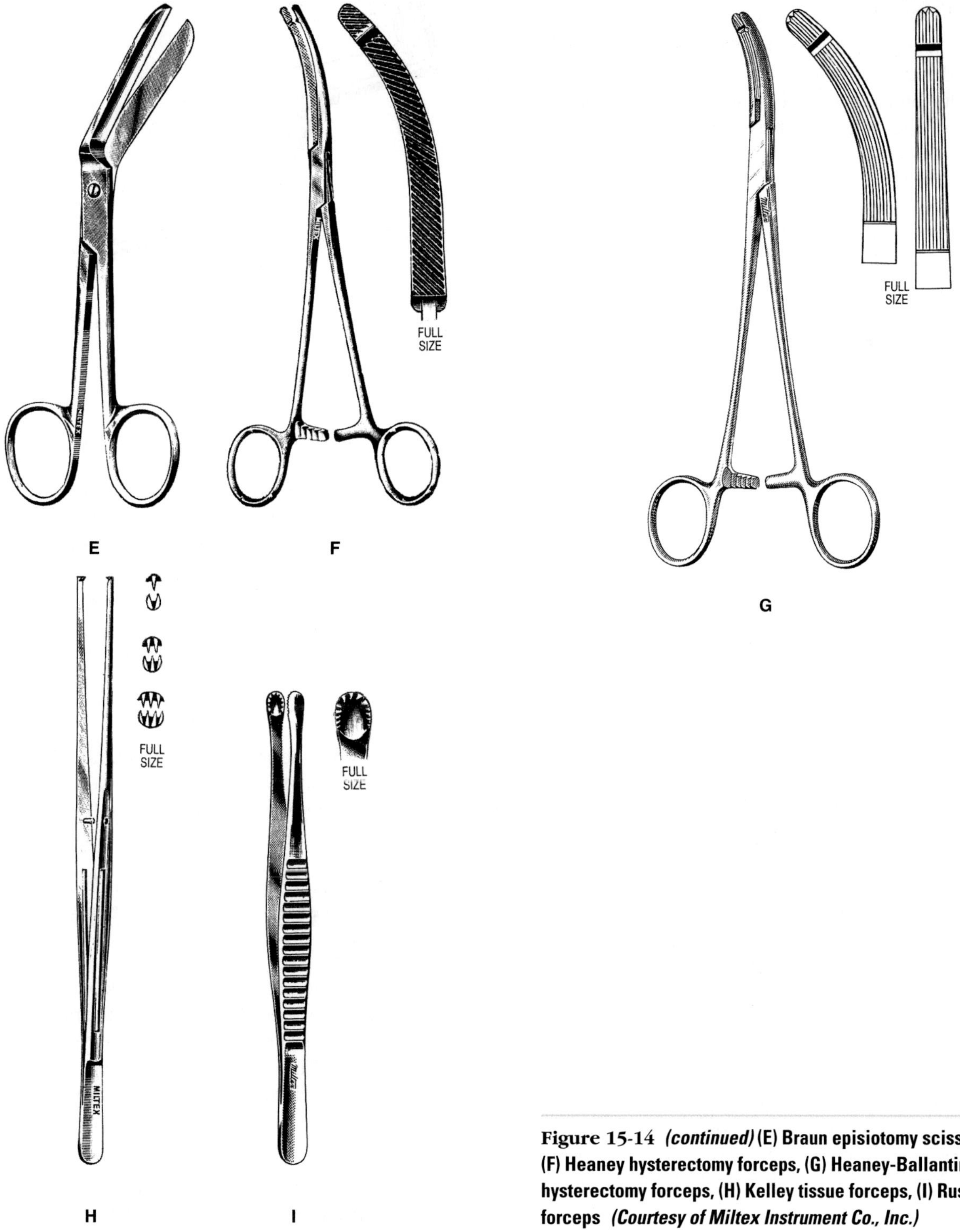

Figure 15-14 ***(continued)*** **(E) Braun episiotomy scissors, (F) Heaney hysterectomy forceps, (G) Heaney-Ballantine hysterectomy forceps, (H) Kelley tissue forceps, (I) Russian tissue forceps** ***(Courtesy of Miltex Instrument Co., Inc.)***

Ergonovine/methylergonovine (Ergotrate, Methergine) is an ergot alkaloid that is used following abortion or delivery to control hemorrhage by causing uterine muscle contraction. It is available in oral and parenteral preparations. Ergot alkaloids are known to pass into the breast milk and may cause serious neonatal effects such as vomiting, decreased circulation to the extremities, diarrhea, weak pulse, unstable blood pressure, and convulsions. Ergonovine/methylergonovine should not be used in conjunction with other drugs such as bromocriptine, other ergot alkaloids, nitrates, or any medication used to treat angina. Additionally, the presence of certain medical conditions such as heart disease (including angina), vascular disturbances, hypertension, history of stroke, infection, kidney disease, liver disease, or Raynaud's phenomenon may affect the use of this drug.

EQUIPMENT

In modern obstetric surgery, special beds are usually available in the delivery room. These beds function as a normal facility bed but have foot ends that separate or drop down for the delivery. These beds will accept one or more varieties of stirrups and other devices developed to accommodate the patient in various delivery positions. They may be electrically or manually operated.

The delivery room will also contain a fetal monitor and a warming bed for the fetus.

Gynecologic surgery requires the same equipment as the abdominal procedures of general surgery. Since many of the procedures are performed with the patient in the lithotomy position, various types of stirrups and leg holders will be used. Likewise, the high percentage of laparoscopic procedures will require the surgical technologist to be familiar with the video equipment and insufflators used in this type of surgery.

Lasers are used relatively frequently in obstetric and gynecologic surgery (Chapter 10). Use of a laser requires a corresponding smoke evacuator, goggles, and safety procedures.

SUPPLIES

Most of the supplies used in obstetric and gynecologic surgery are the same as those used in general surgery (refer to Chapter 14).

OR SETUP AND BASIC PATIENT POSITIONING AND DRAPING

For obstetric and gynecologic procedures, a standard operating table, with both Trendelenburg and foot-drop capability, is used. The table must accommodate sockets for leg holders such as "candy cane" or Allen stirrups. Because the patient's horizontal orientation may be changed frequently in some procedures, the surgical technologist must be intimately familiar with the operation of the operating table. Furthermore, the frequently used lithotomy position requires careful handling of both equipment and the patient's extremities. All equipment should be tested before the patient is placed on the operating table.

The anesthesia provider is invariably positioned at the head of the table. The OR should be arranged with this in mind. A Mayo stand is frequently used for abdominal approaches but may not be used for vaginal approaches. A back table of adequate size to accommodate the required instrumentation without clutter is necessary for all procedures and may be used alone for vaginal approaches. Suction devices (usually wall mounted), an electrosurgical unit (ESU) with the appropriate sterile hand piece(s), kick buckets, and sitting stools (if required) are basic components of any operation.

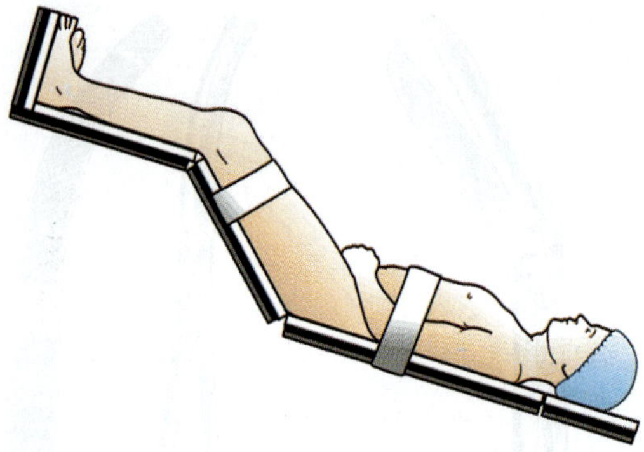

Figure 15-15 **Lithotomy position with Trendelenburg**

Draping for vaginal procedures includes an impervious drape to be placed under the buttocks. This drape may have a fluid catch bag with a suction port. Impervious leggings are used to cover the legs in the holders and a fenestrated perineal drape allows access to the vagina. A small impervious drape may be used to cover the lower abdominal area on vaginal procedures while a large, dual fenestrated drape may be used to cover the abdomen and chest on combination vaginal/abdominal procedures.

Positioning for abdominal cases is supine. Vaginal and combination procedures require the lithotomy position, usually with some degree of Trendelenburg (Figure 15-15).

SURGICAL PROCEDURES: OBSTETRICS AND FERTILITY RELATED

As mentioned above, obstetric and gynecologic surgery are part of the same specialty area of medicine, but they are significantly different enough to warrant special consideration for each. This chapter will present obstetric and fertility-related procedures and gynecologic procedures in separate sections.

PATHOLOGY AND SURGICAL CONDITIONS: OBSTETRICS AND FERTILITY RELATED

The obstetric patient presents an unusual situation in medicine. The "patient" exhibits a normal condition, pregnancy. The patient seeks medical support and help because the condition, while normal, may result in danger to the mother and/or fetus. Care, monitoring, and diagnosis of the pregnant patient begins at the physician's office. An outline of the routine obstetric visit is presented in Table 15-5. This model should help the student understand the broader picture of diagnosis. It begins with an overview of the patient's life and history.

VAGINAL DELIVERY

Pregnancy is as natural an event as it is possible to describe. Both personal joy and species survival are related to pregnancy. Pregnancy is also a physiologic condition that may place both mother and fetus in jeopardy. Many surgical technologists participate in cesarean sections even if they are not directly associated with a labor and delivery unit. Many others work full time in labor and delivery and assist with vaginal births (Procedure 15-1).

EPISIOTOMY AND PERINEAL LACERATIONS

Episiotomy is an intentional surgical incision (usually midline in the United States and mediolateral in Europe) in the vulva to ease the birth process or to protect the mother from uncontrolled perineal lacerations. Both surgical episiotomy and perineal laceration are classified according to the depth of the wound. The commonly used definitions are found in Table 15-6.

Episiotomy or perineal laceration is closed using absorbable suture (Figure 15-16). The patient is placed in the lithotomy or modified lithotomy position. Local anesthesia is used in the absence of general or regional anesthesia. The STSR should monitor the amount of local anesthetic used. It is common to use a handheld vaginal retractor for primary and secondary incisions or lacerations. Third- and fourth-degree episiotomies may

Table 15-5 Common Features of the Obstetric Examination

Obstetric history	
Previous pregnancies	
Time and place of delivery	
History of aborted pregnancies	
Duration of gestation	
Type of delivery	
Duration of labor	
Complications—maternal	
Weight—neonate	
Gender—neonate	
Complications—fetus or neonate	
Menstrual history	
Contraceptive history	
Medical history	
Surgical history	
Social history	
Physical examination	Speculum and bimanual examination
	External genitalia
	Vagina
	Cervix
	Pelvimetry
Cytologic specimens	Endocervix
	Ectocervix
Palpation	Cervix
	Uterus
	Adnexa
Vital signs	
Laboratory tests	Pregnancy test
	Routine labs

PROCEDURE

15-1 Vaginal Delivery

Equipment

- One neonatal bed per infant
- Fetal monitor
- Stirrups of choice
- Labor and delivery bed converted to delivery position

Instruments

- Vaginal delivery set
- **Delivery forceps** of choice

(continues)

PROCEDURE 15-1 Vaginal Delivery *(continued)*

Supplies

- Vaginal prep set
- Delivery pack
- Basin set
- Gloves
- Suture of choice (if necessary)
- Dressing: perineal pad
- Bulb syringe, one per infant
- Cord clamps, two per infant
- De Lee suction device available
- Amniotomy device
- Vacuum extractor device in room
- Cord blood tube, one per infant
- Cord blood gas set, one per infant

Operative Preparation

Anesthesia

- None
- Local
- Epidural
- Pudendal block

Position

- Variable
- Usually, low lithotomy with head raised slightly

Prep

- Vulva and inner thighs
- Predelivery one-time bladder catheterization usually performed

Draping

- Lithotomy most of the time
- Under-buttocks sheet or no drapes in some instances

Practical Considerations

- The room should be warm
- Check the neonatal bed for temperature and supplies
- Call neonatologist and related team members

Operative Procedure	Technical Considerations
1. (There may be no "surgical" action required.)	**1.** Everyone in the room should remain calm and relatively quiet. Support the mother with voice and action.
2. If required, episiotomy is performed during crowning.	**2.** Bandage scissors or straight Mayo scissors are used for this procedure.
3. Ritgen's maneuver is performed to keep the fetal head from ascending between contractions.	**3.** The obstetrician will need a folded towel for this maneuver.
4. Once the head is delivered, the oral cavity and nares are cleared of fluid.	**4.** A bulb syringe or De Lee suction is used to perform this action.
5. The obstetrician checks for a nuchal cord. If loose, the cord is slipped over the head. The head is maneuvered toward the floor delivering the upper shoulder.	**5.** If the cord is tight, the obstetrician may clamp and cut the cord immediately. Having done so, the fetus must be delivered quickly.
6. When the upper shoulder clears, the head is moved toward the ceiling, delivering the lower shoulder. The rest of the body follows quickly.	**6.** Pass the bulb syringe or De Lee suction catheter to the obstetrician to clear the mouth and nares a second time.
7. The cord is double clamped and cut. Cord blood is collected in a tube and the tube is sealed.	**7.** Cord clamp is placed on the fetal side and Kelly hemostat on the placental side. Blood will be collected in a test tube from the placental side. Blood for blood gas studies may be drawn from the artery within the umbilical cord.

PROCEDURE 15-1 Vaginal Delivery *(continued)*

8. The neonate is handed to the mother or to the pediatrician. The placenta is delivered and inspected. The cord is checked to verify the correct number of vessels.	**8.** Cord blood tubes always go to the laboratory. Placentas are usually sent to the laboratory.
9. If necessary, the episiotomy or vaginal tears are repaired.	**9.** Local anesthesia is typically used for episiotomy repair. Gelpi perineal retractors may be placed for third- and fourth-degree lacerations. The STSR will help with tissue retraction during most closures. Sponge count is required.

Postoperative Considerations

Immediate Postoperative Care

- Mother and infant bonding
- Monitor maternal blood pressure
- Transfer mother to postdelivery room if different from labor room
- Provide fluids and nourishment
- Neonate to nursery for examination

Prognosis

- Return to normal activities

Complications

- Hemorrhage
- Wound infection
- Retained placenta
- Rectal fistula
- Problems with neonate
- Coital pain

PEARL OF WISDOM

"Cord blood" is routinely collected and placed in a special tube. "Cord gases" are taken by physician's order. Blood is drawn from the cord artery in a prepared, heparinized syringe and sent immediately to the laboratory.

Table 15-6 Definitions: Perineal Lacerations and Incisions

First degree	Involves the vaginal mucosa or perineal skin
Second degree	Extends into the vaginal submucosa or perineum with or without the perineal body musculature being involved
Third degree	Involves the anal sphincter
Fourth degree	Involves the rectal mucosa

require the use of a Gelpi perineal retractor. Improperly closed wounds can lead to postpartum hemorrhage, sepsis, **fistulas**, and coital pain.

CESAREAN SECTION

Pregnancy is intended to terminate with a vaginal birth. The natural process can be interrupted or inhibited for structural and physiological reasons. **Cesarean section** is the surgical response to failure of the normal birthing process (Procedure 15-2). A common structural reason for cesarean section is cephalopelvic disproportion (**CPD**). The head of the fetus is too large to pass through the maternal birth canal. A physiologic reason for cesarean section might be severe eclampsia. Cesarean section may be performed due to problems with the fetus or with the mother. Cesarean section may to used to avoid potential complications, such as herpes, to the fetus arising from passing through the birth canal. There are many reasons (Table 15-7) for cesarean section; however, the most common remains "failure to progress," or prolonged labor.

(Text continues on page 503)

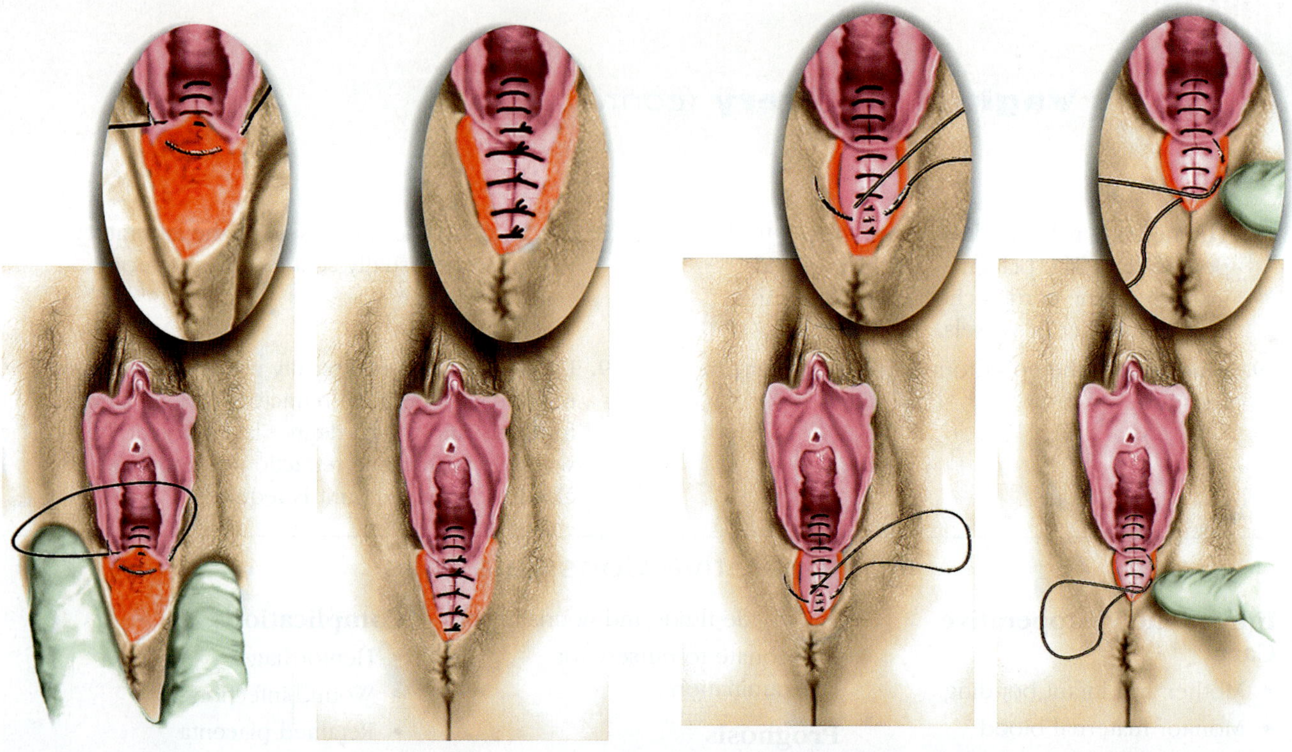

Figure 15-16 **Episiotomy repair: (A) Closure of vaginal epithelium from apex to hymenal ring, (B) interrupted sutures to close perineal fascia and levator ani muscles, (C) continuous closure of superficial fascia to the anal edge, (D) continuous closure of subcutaneous layer**

PROCEDURE

15-2 Cesarean Section

Equipment

- Fetal monitor
- Suction apparatus
- One neonatal bed per infant
- ESU

Instruments

- Cesarean section tray
- Surgeon's preference for bladder retractor
- Delivery forceps of choice (on back table or in room)

PROCEDURE

15-2 Cesarean Section *(continued)*

Supplies

- Prep set
- Cesarean section pack
- Basin set
- Gloves
- Bulb syringe, one per infant
- Cord clamps, two per infant
- De Lee suction device available
- Cord blood container
- Blood gas containers available
- Surgeon-specific sutures and dressings
- Suture of choice
- Dressings

Operative Preparation

Anesthesia

- Anesthesia of choice is an epidural anesthetic
- May be performed with general, spinal, or local anesthetic

Position

- Supine position with a roll placed under the right hip to keep uterine pressure off the vena cava

Prep

- Abdominal prep plus vagina and inner thighs
- Foley catheter inserted if not already in place

Draping

- Laparotomy (specialized C-section drape may be needed)

Operative Procedure	Technical Considerations
1. Skin incision may be midline or low transverse (Pfannenstiel). The most common incision is the low transverse. The incision is carried to the level of the fascia.	**1.** Initial steps vary with type of anesthesia. With an epidural or spinal anesthetic, the patient should be tested for sensitivity to skin pain prior to initiation of the incision. In the case of general anesthesia, all preoperative preparation should be completed prior to the induction. Once the patient is intubated, the procedure should progress rapidly.
2. The fascia is incised at the midline with a #10 blade and the incision is carried laterally using Mayo scissors. This is repeated on both sides.	**2.** Goulet or U.S. Army retractor is commonly used.
3. A longitudinal plane is developed in the midline by bluntly dissecting the posterior fascia from rectus abdominus muscle and cutting the aponeurosis superiorly to near the umbilicus and inferiorly to the symphysis pubis.	**3.** Two Kocher clamps are typically placed on the fascia near the midline during this phase. Mayo scissors are used in the horizontal plane for the sharp dissection.
4. A longitudinal peritoneal incision is made and extended the length of the facial opening.	**4.** Metzenbaum scissors are commonly used on the peritoneum.
5. The uterus is palpated to determine fetal placement and position.	**5.** Some fetal lies may require the use of delivery forceps.

(continues)

PROCEDURE 15-2 Cesarean Section *(continued)*

Operative Procedure

6. To perform the uterine incision, the line representing the bladder peritoneal reflection on the uterus is identified. The bladder is freed from the uterus and retracted inferiorly (Figure 15-17A).

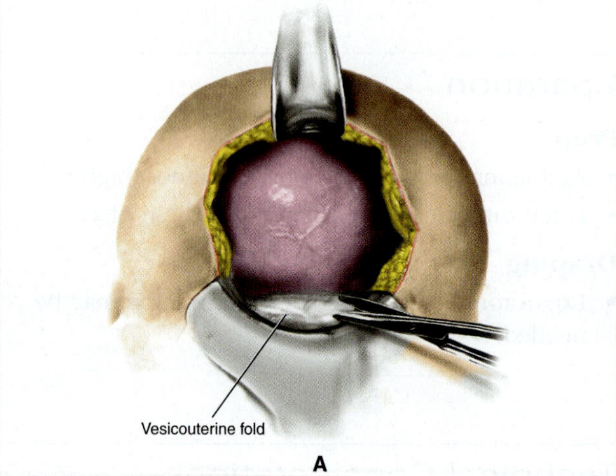

Figure 15-17 Cesarean section: (A) Creation of bladder flap at vesicouterine fold

7. A small transverse incision is made in the lower uterine segment and carried bilaterally with blunt or sharp dissection (Figure 15-17B).

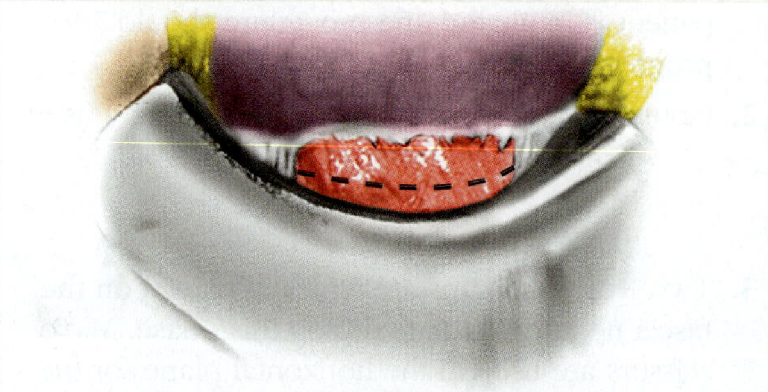

Figure 15-17 Cesarean section: (B) Bladder flap retracted and transverse incision made in lower uterine segment

8. The amniotic sac may or may not need incising.

Technical Considerations

6. The STSR should be prepared to assist with exposure using a bladder retractor of the surgeon's preference. (The bladder retractor is removed before the infant's head is elevated out of the uterus.)

7. The STSR should perform a visual double check at this time to be sure all supplies related to the infant are available and ready for use.

8. The STSR should note the nature of the amniotic fluid. Meconium-stained fluid may require suction with a De Lee suction catheter. The STSR should be prepared to keep the field clean of amniotic fluid if necessary.

PROCEDURE 15-2 Cesarean Section *(continued)*

9. The obstetrician places a hand inside the uterus and manipulates the fetus to draw it from the uterus. The nares and mouth of the fetus are suctioned immediately.

9. Once the head (typically) is controlled, all sharp and metal objects are removed from the field prior to elevating the infant's head.

10. The umbilical cord is clamped and cut. Cord blood sample is collected (Figure 15-17C).

10. Cord blood gases may or may not be drawn. In the case of multiple births, each cord is marked for individual identification. This can be accomplished by using a different type of clamp on each cord (e.g., straight clamp-neonate A).

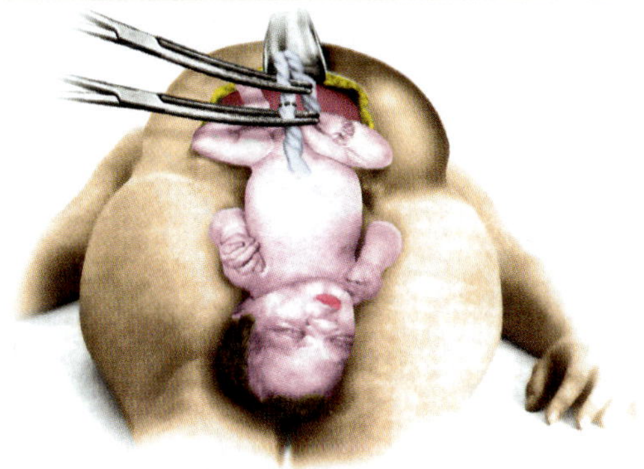

Figure 15-17 Cesarean section: (C) Delivery of infant with umbilical cord clamped

11. The neonate is passed to the pediatrician or neonatal nurse.

11. Be especially aware of the movements of the pediatrician and other nonsterile team members. Protect the sterile field and your Mayo stand.

12. The placenta is delivered, inspected, and removed to the back table (Figure 15-17D).

12. The placenta is placed in a designated basin. It may or may not routinely be sent to pathology.

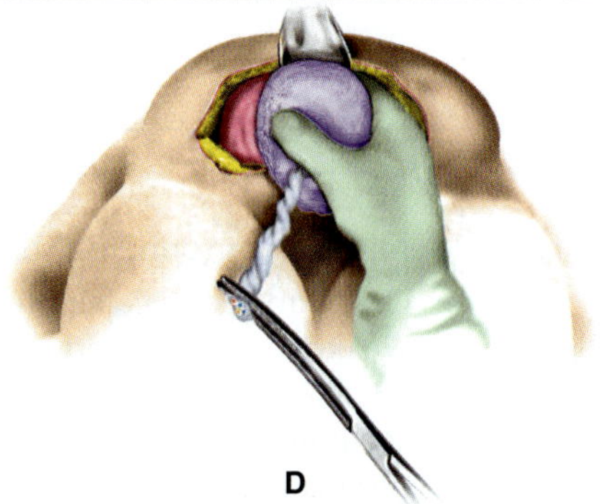

Figure 15-17 Cesarean section: (D) Dissection of the placenta from the uterine wall

13. The uterine interior may be cleaned with a laparotomy sponge, and oxytocin may be injected into the uterus to help with hemostasis secondary to contraction.

13. Sponge should be moist. Oxytocin is drawn up in advance.

(continues)

PROCEDURE 15-2 Cesarean Section *(continued)*

14. The uterus is usually closed in two layers using 2–0 or 0 absorbable suture (Figure 15-17E).

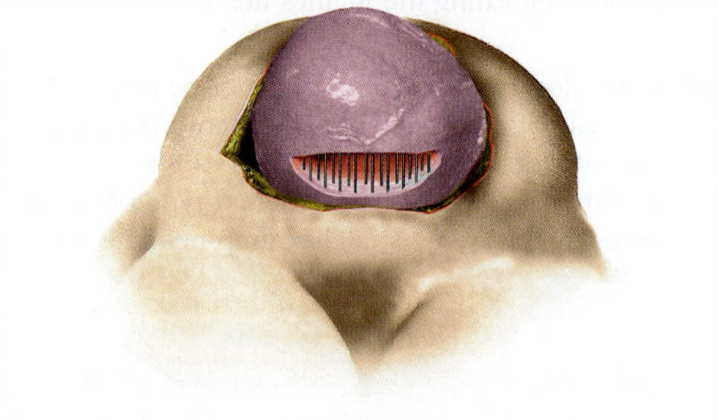

Figure 15-17 Cesarean section: (E) Uterine incision closed in two layers

14. The STSR may need to help with exposure during this phase. The STSR should request a "uterine count" as soon as the first suture is handed to the surgeon.

15. The bladder flap may be approximated or not. If approximated, a 3–0 nonabsorbable suture is commonly used.

15. There will be three counts on cesarean sections. A count is taken to cover the uterine cavity plus the normal abdominal closing counts.

16. The abdominal cavity should be examined for uncontrolled bleeding, sponges, and other potential problems. The abdominal cavity may be irrigated.

16. Prepare closing sutures during this time. Prepare for second count.

17. Closure of the abdominal wall and skin follow the usual procedure for low transverse incisions.

17. A subcuticular stitch or staples are commonly used for skin closure.

18. Blood clots are expressed from the uterus. The wound and vaginal area are cleaned and dressing and perineal pad applied.

Postoperative Considerations

Immediate Postoperative Care

- Routine laparotomy
- Bonding with infant if possible

Prognosis

- Maternal—return to normal activities
- Maternal—increased risk of future cesarean section
- Neonate—prognosis depends on nonsurgical factors

Complications

- Hemorrhage
- Sepsis
- Injury to surrounding structures
- Cesarean sections lead to a weakened uterus and may result in further cesarean sections associated with future pregnancies

PEARL OF WISDOM

Bulb syringes are normally used to suction the nares and mouth of neonates; however, a De Lee suction may be preferred in the presence of meconium. Be sure to know the surgeon's preference before the procedure begins.

Table 15-7 Cesarean Section—Indications

CATEGORY	INDICATION
Maternal	Diseases Eclampsia or severe preeclampsia Cardiac disease Diabetes mellitus Cervical cancer Herpes
	Prior surgery of the uterus Cesarean section (especially classical type) Previous rupture of the uterus Full-thickness myomectomy
	Obstruction to birth canal Fibroids Ovarian tumors
	Other Uterine rupture Failure to progress (etiology unknown) Maternal demise
Fetal	Fetal distress (sustained low heart rate)
	Prolapse of the umbilical cord
	Malpresentation Breech Transverse Brow
	Multiples (depends on number and presentation)
	Fetal demise
Maternal/Fetal	Dystocia Cephalopelvic disproportion Failed induction of labor Abnormal uterine action
Placental	Placenta previa
	Placental abruption

Cesarean section has significant risks. Maternal mortality is four to six times that associated with vaginal delivery. Anesthetic problems are the most significant cause of morbidity.

TUBAL OCCLUSION (STERILIZATION) PROCEDURES

Tubal occlusion (also referred to as ligation) is a relatively safe and simple procedure that has been used for more than a century and exhibits an extremely high rate of effectiveness in preventing pregnancy. The failure rate is below 1%. Because tubal occlusion is an entirely elective and often permanent procedure, careful patient counseling is necessary, and any contraindications, physical or psychosocial, should be ruled out. Tubal occlusion is done on an in-patient or out-patient basis, performed under general or local anesthesia, and may be achieved by vaginal colpotomy or abdominal minilaparotomy or laparoscopy (see descriptions below). Interruption of the fallopian tube's lumen may be accomplished by division, ligature, electrosurgery, or the application of silastic bands or clips.

The abdominal approach is via a minilaparotomy. This approach is common in the postpartum period. Once the abdomen is entered and the fallopian tubes are identified, several techniques are available to achieve sterilization, including the Irving, Pomeroy, Parkland, and Madlener techniques (Figure 15-18). In all cases, the fallopian tubes are grasped with a Babcock or similar instrument to gain control of them and to reveal the vascularity of the mesosalpinx. The tube is then divided or a portion of it is excised, and the free ends may be desiccated with electrosurgery per surgeon's preference. The Pomeroy technique is the most commonly utilized abdominal procedure. Although a portion of tube is excised, the potential for sterilization reversal, or tuboplasty, is excellent.

One procedure is directed at the fimbria: the Kroener fimbriectomy. In the Kroener approach, the tube is double ligated at the distal ampulla, the tube is divided at the ampulla, and the entire distal portion of the fallopian tube, with the fimbria, is removed.

Laparoscopy is commonly used when the procedure does not follow childbirth. The normal laparoscopic approach is followed by division, ligature, electrosurgical desiccation, or the application of silastic bands or clips.

Colpotomy is a considerably less common approach than minilaparotomy or laparoscopy but is nonetheless a good choice in select patients. This approach requires the patient to be placed in the lithotomy position. Proper exposure is attained by vaginal retractors. Instrumentation must be long in order to reach the required depth. With

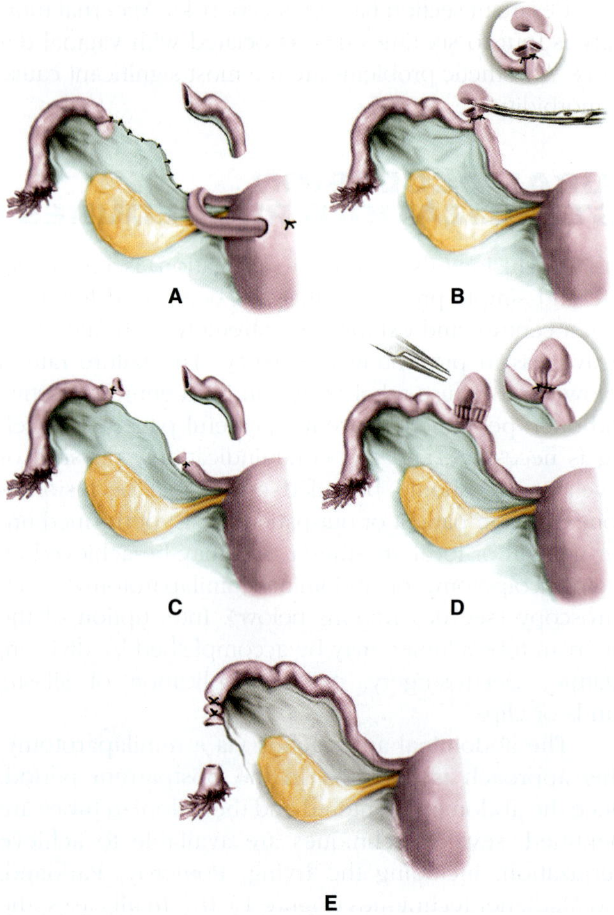

Figure 15-18 **Tubal occlusion techniques: (A) Irving, (B) Pomeroy, (C) Parkland, (D) Madlener, (E) Kroener fimbriectomy**

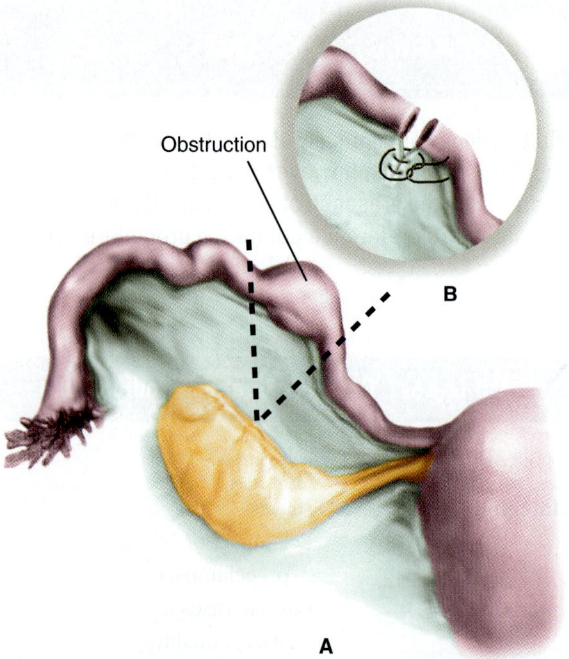

Figure 15-19 **Tuboplasty: (A) Obstruction must be removed. (B) Closure of mesosalpinx approximates the tubal segments; anastomosis is then accomplished with 7–0, 8–0, or 9–0 synthetic absorbable suture**

the colpotomy approach, the peritoneum is entered by either a transverse or vertical incision in the posterior vaginal fornix entering the cul-de-sac between the uterosacral ligaments. The fallopian tubes are then gently pulled into the surgical field with a Babcock or similar instrument. The appropriate technique is then utilized to occlude the tube and its vascularity. Since this approach increases the likelihood of infection, prophylactic antibiotics are routinely administered.

When segments of tubes are removed, they should be placed in separate containers, clearly labeled, and sent to the laboratory for identification.

Most complications of tubal sterilization occur secondary to the use of general anesthesia. Infection rates are very low due to the limited intervention and hemorrhage is usually easily controlled with additional sutures or direct pressure; however, the rare incidence of intra-abdominal bleeding may necessitate repeat laparotomy. The most persistent problem is pelvic pain following tubal ligation, which is usually resolved in a short period of time.

TUBOPLASTY

Tuboplasty is a term that refers to the microscopic resection and anastomosis of the fallopian tube (Procedure 15-3). It is the operative choice when infertility is secondary to tubal obstruction. Tuboplasty is a microsurgical procedure (Figures 15-19 and 15-20). Tubal anastomosis is primarily undertaken to reverse previous tubal ligation. Removal of silastic band and clip methods of sterilization have shown success rates of up to 87%, while those tubes sealed electrosurgically have revealed only 60% success rates. Resected and ligated fallopian tubes demonstrate variable success rates after tubal anastomosis depending on the segments involved in the repair. Tubal reanastomosis is classified according to anatomic location (e.g., isthmic-isthmic, or "midsegment," ampullary-ampullary, isthmic-ampullary, etc.). The highest rates of success have been realized with midsegment, or isthmic-isthmic reanastomosis, and this is likely due to the lack of luminal disparity found with other tuboplasties.

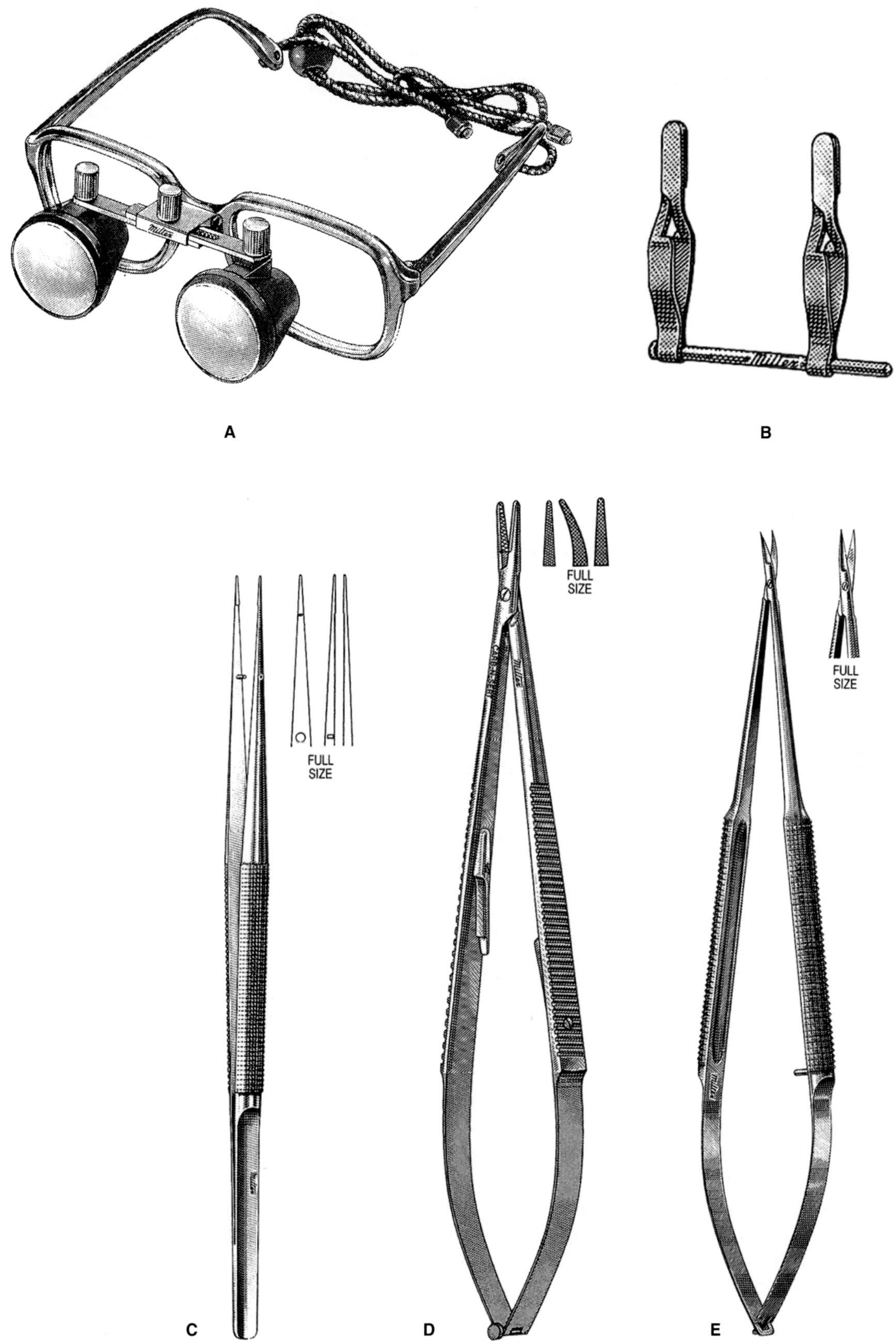

Figure 15-20 **Microsurgical instruments: (A) Binocular magnifying loupe, (B) micro approximation clips, (C) Rhoton micro forceps, (D) Jacobson microvascular needle holder, (E) micro surgery scissors** ***(Courtesy of Miltex Instrument Co., Inc.)***

PROCEDURE

15-3 Tuboplasty

Equipment

- Normal laparotomy equipment
- Operating microscope or operating loupes
- Electrosurgical unit with dispersive electrode
- Microscope drape
- Chairs for microscopic surgery

Instruments

- Laparotomy set
- Microsurgical instruments
- Bipolar coagulating forceps
- Lacrimal duct probes

Supplies

- Basic pack
- Basin set
- Gloves
- Blades, #10, #11
- Suture of choice
- Electrosurgical pencil
- Normal laparotomy supplies
- Microsurgical sutures
- 2–0 monofilament suture or stent to place in fallopian tube
- Tongue blade
- Variety of syringes, needles, and injection catheters
- Low molecular weight dextran
- Indigo carmine dye
- Dressings

Operative Preparation

Anesthesia
- General

Position
- Supine

Prep
- Normal laparotomy

Draping
- Laparotomy

Practical Considerations

- Secure diagnostic studies—hysterosalpingogram or tubal insufflation

Operative Procedure	Technical Considerations
1. Abdominal incision: Pfannenstiel or through a previous abdominal scar.	**1.** Be prepared for routine opening of the abdomen. Drape the microscope early.
2. The damaged portions of the fallopian tube are isolated. The tube is freed from its attachments to the mesosalpinx with careful dissection.	**2.** Dissection will require atraumatic tissue forceps and dissecting scissors.
3. Fallopian tube is transected with iris scissors or #11 blade against a tongue blade at a point that maintains as much length as possible while excising all damaged portions.	**3.** Be sure to identify the surgeon's preference prior to the procedure. If used, the tongue blade provides a cutting surface.
4. Proximal luminal patency is demonstrated by gentle probing with a lacrimal duct probe and injection of dye solution into the uterus.	**4.** Have indigo carmine dye ready in a syringe with the desired needle or catheter attached.

PROCEDURE 15-3 Tuboplasty *(continued)*

5. Distal tubal patency is also tested by probing, followed by cannulation with a pediatric catheter, or 18-gauge angiocatheter, and similar dye study that displays spillage through the fimbrial end.	**5.** Observe fimbria for evidence of dye.
6. The mesosalpinx is approximated to reduce tension on the tubal ends and an approximation clamp may be used to bring the tubal ends into close proximity.	**6.** Needle holders and needles will be very fine for the procedure. Handle them with extreme care. The surgeon may ask to have the needles loaded at a specific angle other than 90°.
7. A 2–0 monofilament suture (stent) may be threaded through the lumen to assist with approximation and protection of the lumen.	**7.** This suture is usually passed with a fine-eyed probe.
8. The sections of tube are sutured together at the 3-, 6-, and 9-o'clock positions with interrupted 8–0 synthetic absorbable suture. Sutures are placed in the muscularis only. No suture material should pass though the mucosa of the tube.	**8.** Remember that the surgeon and surgical assistant are looking through a microscope. Place instruments into their hands carefully and precisely. Do not pass instruments under the microscope lens.
9. The 2–0 monofilament stent is removed and a similar suture is passed at the 12-o'clock position.	**9.** *Note:* Hemostasis is critical in these procedures. Microscopic bipolar coagulation will usually be the method of choice.
10. A second layer of sutures is placed circumferentially in the serosa and outer muscle layer with 8–0 or 9–0 absorbable sutures.	**10.** Suture is loaded in advance if possible.
11. The area is then irrigated and the abdomen is closed.	**11.** Prepare for closure. Count is performed.

Postoperative Considerations

Immediate Postoperative Care

- Transport to PACU

Prognosis

- Return to normal activities
- Potential for fertility

Complications

- Hemorrhage
- Wound infection
- Ectopic pregnancy
- Continued infertility
- Adhesions

PEARL OF WISDOM

Low molecular weight dextran may be poured into the pelvic area like irrigation fluid but is left in place. The solution helps keep tissues separated for several days, thus reducing adhesions and scar tissue formation.

LAPAROSCOPIC RESECTION OF UNRUPTURED TUBAL PREGNANCY

Ectopic pregnancy refers to any pregnancy outside the uterine endometrial cavity. The vast majority of ectopic implantations, some 95%, are in the fallopian tube. Other sites include the peritoneal cavity, ovary, or uterine cervix. The most common causative mechanisms are alteration in the tubal transport mechanism prior to pregnancy and structural change to the fallopian tube. Factors that affect tubal structure or the alteration of the transport mechanism increase the likelihood of tubal pregnancy (Table 15-8).

Ruptured ectopic pregnancy is an emergency condition. Open abdominal surgical intervention is commonly used in this instance. Unruptured tubal pregnancy is amenable to treatment through laparoscopic means (Procedure 15-4).

Table 15-8 Risk Factors for Ectopic Pregnancy

- A history of pelvic inflammatory disease
- Previous ectopic pregnancy
- Pregnancy following sterilization procedure
- Prior tubal reconstructive surgery
- IUD usage
- Prolonged infertility
- Exposure to diethylstilbestrol

PROCEDURE 15-4 Laparoscopic Resection of Unruptured Tubal Pregnancy

Equipment

- Normal laparoscopic equipment
- Preferred stirrups

Instruments

- Laparotomy set in room
- Laparoscopic set
- Vaginal tray (may be combined with a D&C procedure)
- Specialty laparoscopic instruments as needed

Supplies

- Normal laparotomy supplies
- Defogging solution

Operative Preparation

Anesthesia

- Anesthesia of choice is a general anesthetic
- May be performed with local anesthetic

Position

- Modified lithotomy
- Hip flexion constrained to 45°
- Patient's buttocks must clear the operating table approximately 4 in.
- Grounding pad usually placed on thigh
- Trendelenburg position at about 15°

Prep

- Laparotomy plus vaginal prep

Draping

- Laparotomy plus lithotomy (combination drape may be used)
- One-time urethral catheterization performed prior to prep

Practical Considerations

- Check all equipment prior to the patient's arrival

Operative Procedure

1. Normal laparoscopic technique is employed.
2. The site of the tubal pregnancy is visually identified (Figure 15-21A).

Technical Considerations

1. Check all equipment in advance.
2. Visual confirmation is diagnostic. One critical goal is preservation of the tube.

PROCEDURE 15-4

Laparoscopic Resection of Unruptured Tubal Pregnancy *(continued)*

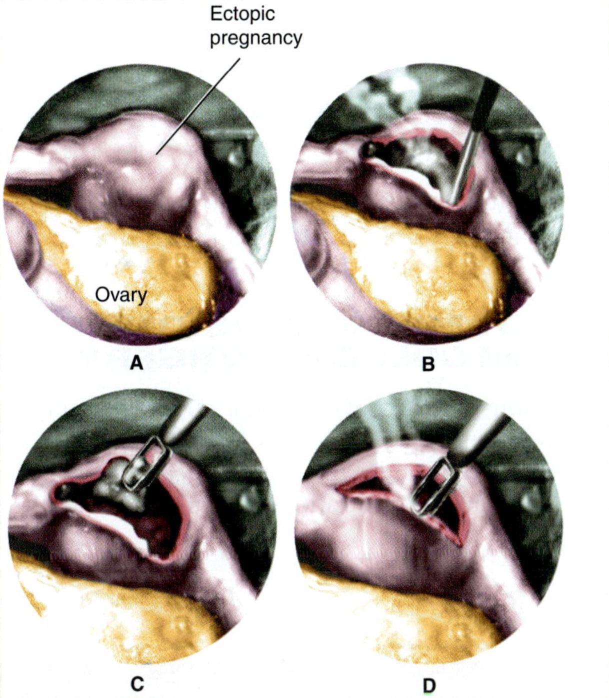

Figure 15-21 **Laparoscopic resection of unruptured tubal pregnancy: (A) Site of implantation identified, (B) longitudinal incision into fallopian tube, (C) removal of tissue, (D) hemostasis achieved**

3. A longitudinal incision is made in the tube electrosurgically (Figure 15-21B).
4. Grasping forceps are placed in the tube and the trophoblastic tissue is removed (Figure 15-21C).
5. Hemorrhage is controlled electrosurgically (Figure 15-21D).
6. The tubal incision is left open.
7. The laparoscopic procedure is terminated in the normal manner.

3. Pass the electrosurgical instrument through access port.
4. A laparoscopic Babcock is often used. Check patency of the tips before the procedure begins.
5. Smoke evacuator/suction may be needed.
6. Prepare for closure while hemostasis is being achieved.
7. Closure suture passed. Count is performed.

Postoperative Considerations

Immediate Postoperative Care

- Transport to PACU
- Psychological grief associated with lost fetus added to normal surgical reaction

Prognosis

- Return to normal activities

Complications

- Hemorrhage
- Wound infection
- Increased incidence of tubal pregnancy

PEARL OF WISDOM

Specific variations depend on the site of implantation. Pelviscopy with salpingostomy may be used if the ectopic pregnancy is unruptured and implantation is in the ampulla. Salpingotomy, resection of a tubal segment, expression of the fimbria, and salpingectomy are possible treatments.

SURGICAL PROCEDURES: GYNECOLOGIC PROCEDURES

Gynecology is the study of the female and particularly the female reproductive system. Gynecologic surgery is surgery on the female reproductive system. The distinction between gynecologic and obstetric surgery is that obstetric surgery is narrowly focused on childbirth. Gynecologic surgery refers to all other operative approaches to the female reproductive system.

GYNECOLOGIC PATHOLOGY

The gynecologic patient typically seeks medical help on the basis of a complaint. The patient has identified some symptom or set of symptoms that cause concern. The routine examination of the gynecologic patient is summarized in Table 15-9. The categories of conditions treated in gynecologic practice are found in Table 15-10 along with some diagnostic considerations.

SURGICAL INTERVENTION: OVERVIEW

Table 15-11 summarizes surgical interventions by anatomic area.

ABDOMINAL INCISIONS FOR GYNECOLOGIC SURGERY

Incisions used in gynecologic abdominal surgery fall into three basic categories: transverse, vertical, and oblique. Although transverse incisions provide the best cosmetic result and are nearly 30 times stronger

(Text continues on page 513)

Table 15-9 Common Features of the Gynecologic Examination

Gynecologic history	Present complaint	Abnormal vaginal bleeding
		Abdominal pain
		Amenorrhea
		Dysmenorrhea
		Other
Contraceptive history		
Obstetric history		
Marital history		
Medical history		
Review of systems	Head and neck	
	Breasts	
	Heart and lungs	
	Abdomen	
	Back	
	Extremities	
Physical examination	Vital signs	
	Pelvic examination	
	Rectal examination	
Laboratory test	Urinalysis	
	Complete blood count	
	Erythrocyte sedimentation rate	
	Blood chemistry	
	Other	

Table 15-10 Select Gynecologic Conditions, Symptoms, and Diagnostic Tests

CONDITION OR DISEASE	SYMPTOMS/SIGNS	TYPICAL DIAGNOSTIC TESTS
Genital anomalies	Symptoms Primary amenorrhea Dyspareunia Dysmenorrhea Cyclic pelvic pain Inability to achieve penile penetration Infertility Habitual abortion Spontaneous second trimester abortion Premature labor Postpartum hemorrhage Leakage with tampon in place Signs Vaginal mass Abdominal mass Absence of normal structures Ambiguous genitalia Fetal malpresentation Retained placenta	Physical examination, including pelvic examination Sonography Intravenous pyelogram Hysterosalpingogram Hysteroscopy Magnetic resonance imaging Examination under anesthesia Laparoscopic visualization
Benign lesions of the vagina		
Inclusion cysts	Usually asymptomatic	Visual examination
Endometriosis	Steel gray or black cysts that bleed at time of menses	Visual examination Biopsy
Gartner's duct cysts	Usually asymptomatic	Visual examination
Urethral diverticula	Recurrent urethral infection Dribbling of urine Dyspareunia (pain during intercourse) Dysuria	Visual examination Urethroscopy
Benign lesions of the cervix		
Chronic cervicitis	Persistent infections Leukorrhea Lower abdominal discomfort Dyspareunia	Visual examination Papanicolaou smear Colposcopy to rule out dysplasia or cancer
Cervical polyp	Pedunculated lesion	Removal and pathologic examination to rule out cancer
Benign lesions of the vulva	Five types Inflammatory vulvar dermatosis Vulvar dystrophies Benign cysts and tumors Dermatosis not unique to vulvar infections Infectious disease	Physical examination Biopsy of gross lesions

(continues)

Table 15-10 ***(continued)***

CONDITION OR DISEASE	SYMPTOMS/SIGNS	TYPICAL DIAGNOSTIC TESTS
Benign lesions of the uterus		
Leiomyomas	Majority are asymptomatic Symptoms Lower abdominal pain Pelvic pressure or congestion Menorrhagia Secondary dysmenorrhea Increased infertility Signs Abdominal mass	Bimanual examination Barium enema Intravenous pyelogram Computed tomographic scan Sonography X-ray Laparoscopic visualization
Endometrial hyperplasia	Postmenopausal bleeding Prolonged or irregular bleeding Anemia	Endometrial biopsy D&C to rule out carcinoma
Benign lesions of the ovaries and fallopian tubes		
Functional ovarian tumor	Usually asymptomatic Pelvic pain Peritoneal irritation Delayed menstrual period Rebound tenderness Acute abdominal pain Hemoperitoneum	Bimanual examination Regression of cyst after menstrual period Sonography Pregnancy test and erythrocyte sedimentation rate to rule out teratomas
Neoplastic ovarian tumor	Most are asymptomatic Symptoms Acute pain following torsion Increased abdominal girth Pelvic pressure/congestion Peritoneal irritation Signs Pelvic mass Dull percussion sound Abdominal rigidity Paralytic ileus	Sonography Serum CA 125 titer Laparoscopy
Endometriosis	Symptoms Dysmenorrhea Dyspareunia Dyschezia (difficult defecation) Signs Small, tender nodules Cystic abdominal mass Tender, fixed adnexal mass "Barb"-like uterosacral ligament pain	Symptom triad Bimanual examination Normal leukocyte count and erythrocyte sedimentation rate Slightly elevated CA 125 level Sonography Laparoscopy
Dysfunctional uterine bleeding (DUB)	During years around menarche and menopausal	Rule out other causes CBC Platelet count Coagulation studies Thyroid function studies Liver function studies Prolactin levels

Table 15-10 *(continued)*

CONDITION OR DISEASE	SYMPTOMS/SIGNS	TYPICAL DIAGNOSTIC TESTS
		Serum FSH levels Papanicolaou smear Endometrial biopsy Sonography Hysterosalpingography Hysteroscopy D&C
Genitourinary dysfunction Pelvic organ prolapse Urinary incontinence Infections	Symptoms and signs vary with condition. All are related to support structures in the pelvic area.	Bimanual examination Visual examination Urinary stress test Urethrocystoscopy Cystometrogram Sonography
Uterine cancer	Most common symptom—abnormal vaginal bleeding	Papanicolaou smear Endocervical curettage Endometrial biopsy
Cervical cancer	Usually asymptomatic Abnormal bleeding Vaginal discharge Abnormal Pap smear	Colposcopy Cervical conization Biopsy Endocervical curettage Schiller test
Ovarian cancer	Usually asymptomatic Symptoms Irregular menses Pelvic congestion Abdominal pain Signs Solid, irregular, fixed pelvic mass	Bimanual examination Papanicolaou smear Endometrial biopsy Endocervical curettage X-ray Sonography Barium enema CA 125
Vulvar cancer	Itching Visible abnormalities	Visual examination Collin's test
Vaginal cancer	Usually asymptomatic	Abnormal Papanicolaou smear in a woman post-hysterectomy Biopsy

after repair, they are relatively more time consuming and hemorrhagic than vertical incisions. Transverse incisions can compromise nerves, generally involve the division of muscles, and may limit access to the upper abdomen.

Vertical and oblique incisions are discussed in detail in Chapter 14. Transverse incisions are named for the surgeons who originally developed the technique. The three most commonly used are presented here: the **Pfannenstiel**, Maylard, and Cherney incisions (Table 15-12).

Closure of these incisions commonly begins with the fascia with a running #1 or #2 polyglycolic suture. In the Cherney technique, the peritoneum may be closed separately in similar fashion. Muscles are not usually sutured in the Maylard or Pfannenstiel approaches; however, they are reunited with the rectus tendon (the original point of division) in the Cherney technique using an adequate number of nonabsorbable sutures placed in an interrupted or horizontal mattress manner. The subcutaneous tissue is generally not closed and staples or subcuticular suture is used on the skin.

Table 15-11 Summary Information: Procedures in Gynecologic Surgery

STRUCTURE/ORGAN	PROCEDURE
Vulva and introitus	Biopsy of vulva
	Excision of vulvar skin—with STSG (split-thickness skin graft)
	Wide local vulvar excision—primary closure, secondary Z-plasty
	Vulvectomy
	Vulvar injection—alcohol
	Vulvar excision—LEEP (loop electrosurgical excision procedure)
	Vulvar injection—cortisone
	Excision of urethral caruncle
	Marsupialization—Bartholin's gland cyst
	Bartholin's gland biopsy
	Bartholin's gland excision
	Repair vaginal outlet stenosis
	Excision of vestibular adenitis
	Release of labial fusion
	Hymenectomy
Vagina and urethra	Anterior repair—cystocele
	Posterior repair—rectocele
	Vaginal repair—enterocele
	Vaginal suspension—sacrospinous ligament
	Vaginal evisceration
	Excision transverse vaginal septum
	Repair "double-barreled" vagina
	Sacral colpopexy
	Le Fort procedure
	Repair vesicovaginal fistula
	Repair rectovaginal fistula
	Repair urethrovaginal fistula
	Vaginoplasty for neovagina
	Urethral reconstruction
	Repair(s) of suburethral diverticulum
	Correction of urinary incontinence
	Sigmoid neovagina
Cervix	Biopsy
	Endocervical curettage
	Cervical cone—"cold"
	Cervical cone—LEEP
	Abdominal excision—cervical stump
	Correction—incompetent cervix
Uterus	Dilation and curettage
	Dilation and curettage—vacuum
	Dilatation and evacuation
	Cesarean section
	Myomectomy
	Correction—double uterus
	Hysteroscopy—diagnostic
	Hysteroscopy—intervention
	Vaginal hysterectomy
	Abdominal hysterectomy
	Laparoscopically assisted vaginal hysterectomy
Fallopian tubes and ovaries	Resection—unruptured tubal pregnancy
	Resection and hemorrhage control—ruptured tubal pregnancy (emergency)
	Ovarian biopsy
	Treatment—endometriosis
	Lysis of adhesions
	Sterilization procedures
	Salpingectomy
	Salpingo-oophorectomy
	Fimbrioplasty
	Tuboplasty
	Wedges resection—ovary
	Correction—torsion of ovary
	Ovarian cystectomy
Other	Bladder and ureter (see Chapter 20)
	Bowel, colon, abdominal wall (see Chapter 14)
	Malignant disease and special procedures

Table 15-12 Transverse Abdominal Incisions Used in Gynecologic Surgery

PFANNENSTIEL	MAYLARD	CHERNEY
Gently curved incision, 10–15 cm long at any level between the umbilicus and symphysis pubis.	Less curved incision between the crests of the anterior iliac spine.	Less curved incision between the crests of the anterior iliac spine.
Skin and subcutaneous fat are incised to the level of the anterior rectus sheath.	Skin and subcutaneous fat are incised to the level of the anterior rectus sheath.	Skin and subcutaneous fat are incised to the level of the anterior rectus sheath.
Fascia is incised transversely on either side of the linea alba.	Fascia is incised transversely.	Fascia is incised transversely.
Linea alba is then divided, joining the two incisions. Rectus sheath is separated from the underlying rectus muscle by blunt dissection.	Inferior epigastric vessels are located at the lateral edges of the incision and are ligated and cut.	Inferior epigastric vessels are located at the lateral edges of the incision and are ligated and cut.
Rectus muscles are separated in the midline.	Rectus muscle is divided, usually electrosurgically.	Rectus muscle is divided, usually electrosurgically at its insertion on the symphysis pubis.
Peritoneum is opened vertically.	Peritoneum is incised transversely.	Peritoneum is incised transversely.

SURGICAL INTERVENTION: LAPAROSCOPY

Certain steps in a laparoscopy are common to both diagnostic and interventional purposes. This section will review the basic steps of the laparoscopic approach in Procedure 15-5.

An operating laparoscope is shown in Figure 15-23.

PROCEDURE 15-5 Basic Laparoscopy

Equipment

- Camera
- Video monitor
- Insufflator
- Light source
- ESU
- Laser, if needed
- Preferred stirrups

Instruments

- Laparotomy set in room
- Laparoscopy set
- Vaginal tray (may be combined with a D&C procedure)
- Specialty laparoscopic instruments as needed

Supplies

- Normal laparotomy supplies
- Defogging solution

(continues)

PROCEDURE

15-5 Basic Laparoscopy *(continued)*

Operative Preparation

Anesthesia

- Anesthesia of choice is a general anesthetic
- May be performed with local anesthetic

Position

- Modified lithotomy
- Hip flexion constrained to 45°
- Patient's buttocks must clear the operating table by approximately 4 in.
- Grounding pad usually placed on thigh
- Trendelenburg position at about 15°

Prep

- Laparotomy plus vaginal prep

Draping

- Laparotomy plus lithotomy (combination drape may be used)
- One-time urethral catheterization performed prior to prep

Practical Considerations

- Check all equipment prior to the patient's arrival
- A separate field will be necessary if vaginal access is necessary

Operative Procedure	Technical Considerations
1. A handheld vaginal retractor is placed posteriorly in the vagina and the cervix is grasped with a tenaculum.	**1.** (*Note:* Vaginal steps do not apply to procedures in general surgery.)
2. A uterine manipulator of choice is placed on the cervix. The manipulator may be covered so it can be handled by the surgeon later.	**2.** The surgeon's top gloves should be removed and replaced using proper technique following the vaginal portion of the procedure. Instruments used vaginally must be isolated.
3. The anterior abdominal wall is elevated using two towel clips.	**3.** Techniques vary from surgeon to surgeon.
4. A Veress needle is placed into the midline at an angle 90° to the elevated body plane. The needle is stopped at the fascia and position verified. The abdominal cavity is then entered (Figure 15-22A).	**4.** Have a syringe ready to confirm entrance into the abdominal cavity. Check all cords and tubes for readiness.

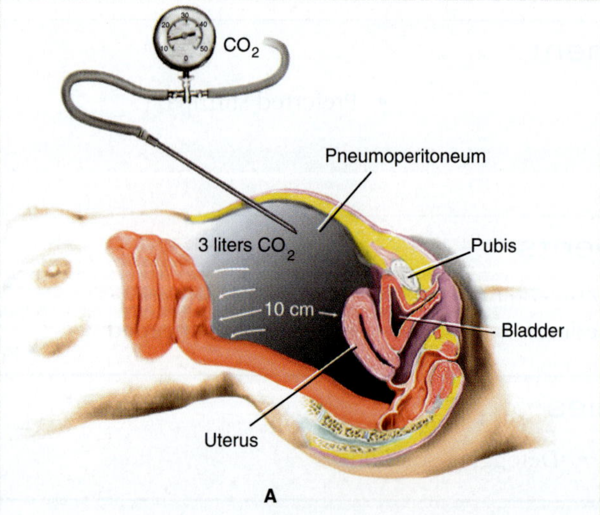

Figure 15-22 Basic laparoscopy: (A) Effects of CO_2 and proper position of Veress needle

15-5 Basic Laparoscopy *(continued)*

5. Sterile tubing is attached from the needle to a carbon dioxide insufflator and the carbon dioxide is allowed to enter to a pressure not exceeding 15 mm Hg.
6. The previous midline incision is extended from a small stab wound to approximately 1 cm length. A laparoscopic trocar and sleeve are placed into the abdominal cavity (Figure 15-22B).

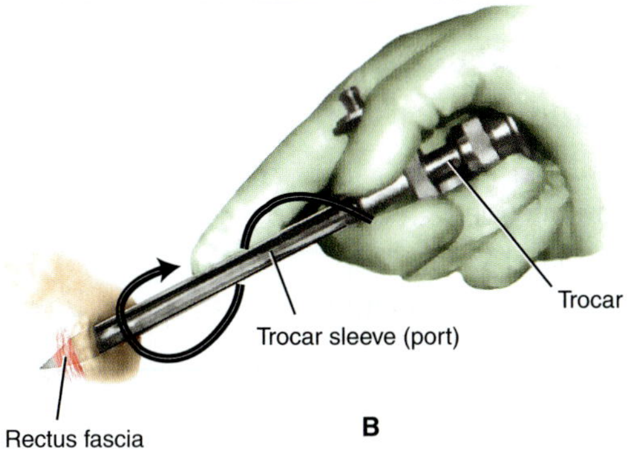

Figure 15-22 Basic laparoscopy: (B) Port with trocar entering the abdomen

5. If a clear flow is established, a pneumoperitoneum is produced. Pressure is monitored throughout the procedure by the circulator. Commonly 4–5 liters of carbon dioxide are used.
6. State the size of the sleeve as you hand it to the surgeon.

   Prepare telescope for passage to surgeon by applying defogging solution.

7. The trocar is removed from the sleeve and replaced with the telescope.
8. The carbon dioxide line is connected to a valve on the sleeve.
9. The telescope is connected to a camera and light source which, in turn, are connected to a monitor .
10. If the procedure is interventional in nature or requires internal manipulation of anatomical structures, other ports will be established for operating instrumentation (Figure 15-22C).

7. Assist with transfer of instruments.
8. Assist with transfer of CO_2 line if necessary.
9. The STSR should be familiar enough with all the equipment and connections to assist the team with troubleshooting if there are problems.
10. The precise placement of these ports depends on the surgical procedure to be performed. The size of the ports depends on their use.

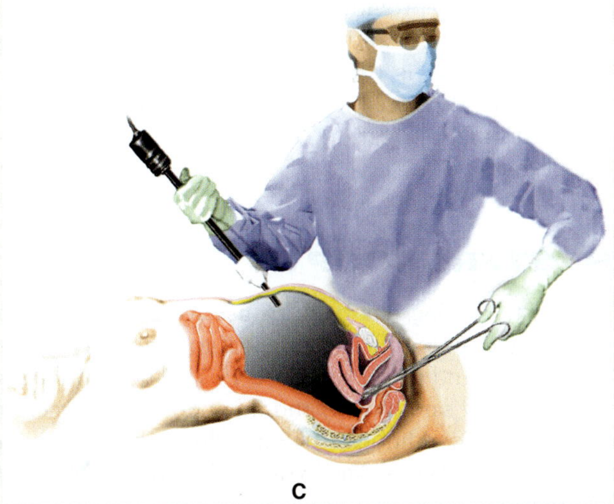

Figure 15-22 Basic laparoscopy: (C) Use of uterine manipulator and camera

(continues)

PROCEDURE

15-5 Basic Laparoscopy *(continued)*

11. Following the operative intervention, carbon dioxide is released from the abdomen and all ports removed. Some ports may require one or two sutures to close. Band-aids are usually applied.

11. Accept returned equipment and instrumentation. Pass prepared sutures. Prepare dressings.

Postoperative Considerations

Immediate Postoperative Care

- Transport to PACU

Prognosis

- Return to normal activities
- Prognosis according to diagnosis

Complications

- Hemorrhage
- Wound infection
- Perforation of viscus
- Damage to other structures

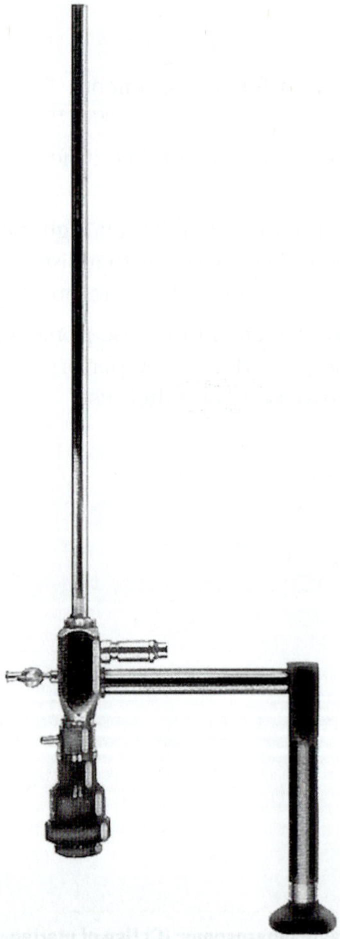

Figure 15-23 Operating laparoscope

PEARL OF WISDOM

The most common cause for failure of monitors or other equipment is the failure to plug the machine into the wall socket. Develop a system for checking all equipment before you scrub.

BASIC COLPOSCOPY

A colposcope is a binocular microscope that magnifies from 10–40X. It provides a stereoscopic view with centered illumination and a focal distance of 12–15 cm. The colposcope is used (colposcopy) to evaluate patients with abnormal Papanicolaou smear combined with a normal appearing cervix on visual examination (Procedure 15-6).

HYSTEROSCOPY

The hysteroscope has been in use for a long time, but modern technology has brought it to a new level of sophistication and use (Procedure 15-7). The approach offers relatively safe, quick, and inexpensive treatment for a number of conditions, such as adhesions, polyps, and submucous **myomas**. The hysteroscope may be of the rigid or fiberoptic type. Rigid telescopes vary from 2.9–4 mm

PROCEDURE 15-6 Basic Colposcopy

Equipment

- Colposcope
- Light source
- Camera

Instruments

- Vaginal tray

Supplies

- Normal vaginal procedure
- Slides or materials for collecting and preserving specimens

Operative Preparation

Anesthesia
- None for simple diagnostic view
- Biopsy or other action may require local or general anesthetic

Position
- Lithotomy

Prep
- Vaginal prep

Draping
- Lithotomy

Practical Considerations

- Check light source prior to the patient's arrival

Operative Procedure	STSR's Actions, Responses, Tips
1. A bivalve speculum is placed and opened to expose the cervix.	**1.** Unlike most surgical procedures, the basic colposcopy is not a sterile procedure. Back table is prepared for basic vaginal examination.
2. Cervical mucus and cellular debris are removed with a swab soaked in 3% acetic acid. This step may need repeating during the procedure.	**2.** Label all solutions.
3. The cervix is illuminated with white light. Illumination is centered and focal length is between 12 and 15 cm.	**3.** A green filter can be used to heighten the visibility of vascular changes associated with cervical pathology. Cameras can be attached to the colposcope for documentation purposes.
4. A biopsy may be required to rule out other conditions.	**4.** Specimen care according to physician orders and facility policy.

Postoperative Considerations

Immediate Postoperative Care
- Transport to room

Prognosis
- Return to normal activities dependent on findings

Complications
- Secondary to other procedures

PEARL OF WISDOM

Cervical intraepithelial neoplasia (CIN) is indicated by epithelium that appears white after the application of acetic acid. Patients with CIN may present with vascular "dots" referred to as punctuation or a mosaic of capillaries lying parallel to the surface of the cervix. Increased dilation and irregularity in punctuation and mosaicism indicate atypical tissue.

in diameter. Fiberoptic telescopes can be as small as 1.2 mm in diameter. Operating instruments are placed through operating channels. Hysteroscopy is used for both diagnostic and operative purposes. The most significant risks are perforation of the uterus, hemorrhage, and complications related to the use of the distension medium.

PROCEDURE 15-7 Hysteroscopy

Equipment

- Light source
- Camera
- Hysteroscopic pump or insufflator for distension media
- Laser, if required
- ESU, if required

Instruments

- Vaginal tray
- Hysteroscope

Supplies

- Normal vaginal procedure
- Slides or materials for collecting and preserving specimens

Operative Preparation

Anesthesia

- General anesthetic

Position

- Lithotomy

Prep

- Vaginal prep

Draping

- Lithotomy

Practical Considerations

- Check all equipment prior to the patient's arrival

Operative Procedure	STSR's Actions, Responses, Tips
1. A weighted speculum is placed in the vagina.	1. Hysteroscopy is not considered a sterile procedure. However, the best possible technique is used to prevent infection.
2. The cervix is grasped with a tenaculum and pulled toward the vaginal introitus.	2. Pass tenaculum with caution. The tip is pointed.

PROCEDURE

15-7 Hysteroscopy *(continued)*

3. A uterine sound is placed into the cervical canal to determine the direction and depth of the uterine cavity.
4. The cervix is dilated to the required diameter.
5. The hysteroscope is placed into the uterus via the cervix.
6. The uterus is distended with carbon dioxide, sorbitol or glycine, or dextran solution.
7. The uterus is explored visually. If biopsy or operative action is required, operative instruments will be used through the ports on the operative telescope.
8. At conclusion, all instruments are removed.

3. Instruments are arranged in order of use, typically from left to right. It may be necessary to lubricate the tips of the sound and dilators.
4. Hegar or Hank uterine dilators are commonly used.
5. Telescope is approximately 4 mm in diameter and may have a viewing angle of 0–30 degrees.
6. Complications are rare but cases involving distention medium are known. Rate of flow and total fluid volume should be monitored throughout the procedure.
7. Operative hysteroscopic sets include flexible instruments such as scissors and biopsy punches. These should be available on all procedures.
8. *Note:* If dextran solution was used for distention purposes, instruments will need to be cleaned immediately in warm water.

Postoperative Considerations

Immediate Postoperative Care

- Transport to PACU

Prognosis

- Return to normal activities
- Ultimate outcome dependent on findings

Complications

- Gas or air embolism
- Laceration of the cervix
- Specific complication secondary to intervention

PEARL OF WISDOM

All team members need to be aware of the type of distention medium used, the proper rate of flow, the maximum volume allowed, and the outflow rate.

MARSUPIALIZATION OF BARTHOLIN'S GLAND CYST

Obstruction of a Bartholin's gland duct commonly results from gonococcal infection, other various infections, or, most frequently, trauma, and can manifest as cyst formation. Cysts in this area usually display a mucoid and cloudy secretion. Most Bartholin's cysts are asymptomatic, although if the cyst becomes infected an abscess usually forms with symptomatic swelling, tenderness, and erythema. With larger cysts, the patient experiences pain during coitus and discomfort when walking or sitting. Incision and drainage bring almost immediate relief and can be performed under local anesthesia. **Marsupialization** (conversion of a closed cavity into an open pouch) may be required for permanent healing to occur (Procedure 15-8).

SIMPLE VULVECTOMY

Vulvectomy is performed for multifocal *in situ* neoplasia of the vulva. Conditions such as condylomata, Paget's disease, or those that involve areas that could be compromised through excision, such as the clitoris, are usually best treated with laser ablation. Wide local lesion excision, as well as medical therapy, is preferred prior to vulvectomy. Simple (conservative, or "skinning") vulvectomy

PROCEDURE

15-8 Marsupialization of Bartholin's Gland Cyst

Equipment

- Preferred stirrups
- ESU

Instruments

- Vaginal tray

Supplies

- Drains
- Culture tubes
- Surgeon-specific sutures and dressings

Operative Preparation

Anesthesia

- Local for incision and drainage
- General anesthetic for marsupialization

Position

- Lithotomy

Prep

- Vaginal prep

Draping

- Lithotomy

Practical Considerations

- The area may be very painful to touch prior to being anesthetized

Operative Procedure

1. Local excision of a Bartholin's gland cyst requires an elliptical incision created in the vaginal mucosa around the duct, as close to the gland as possible (Figure 15-24A).

Technical Considerations

1. The labia minor may be sutured to the skin to provide exposure. Have culture tube on field.

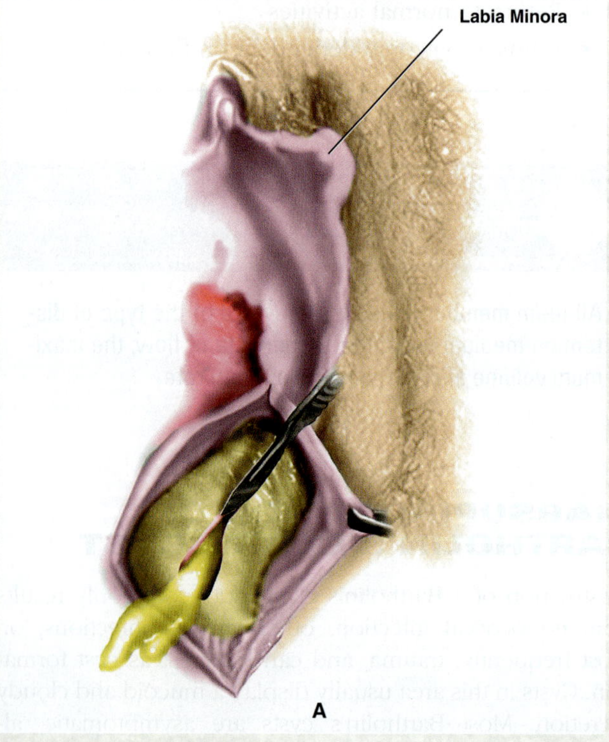

Figure 15-24 Marsupialization of Bartholin's gland cyst: (A) Retraction of labia minora and incision into infected cyst

PROCEDURE 15-8 Marsupialization of Bartholin's Gland Cyst *(continued)*

2. Dissection is begun bluntly but may require scissors to dissect the gland from its bed.
   - 2. Blunt dissection is often accomplished with a scalpel handle. Sharp dissection: Mayo scissors or knife blade.
3. If the cyst wall margins are unclear, it can be approached by incision into the cyst and dissection of it from the surrounding tissues.
   - 3. Complete removal of the gland tissue adherent to the cyst wall is essential.
4. After the cyst wall is opened, the cyst is drained.
   - 4. Fluid may be cultured. Have suction available.
5. The cavity created may be closed by approximating the vaginal wall tissues with fine, interrupted absorbable sutures.
   - 5. Pass sutures of choice. Have drain of choice available if needed.
6. The cyst wall lining is everted and sutured to the vaginal mucosa with interrupted 2–0 absorbable sutures (Figure 15-24B)
   - 6. Count. May need to remind surgeon to remove labial retraction sutures. Peri-pad dressing is applied.

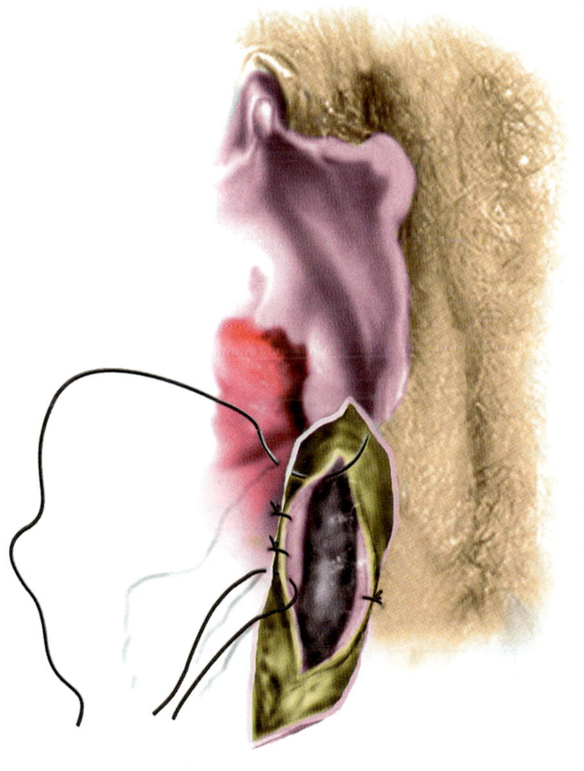

Figure 15-24 Marsupialization of Bartholin's gland cyst: (B) Marsupialization technique

Postoperative Considerations

Immediate Postoperative Care
- Transport to PACU
- Apply ice if indicated

Prognosis
- Return to normal activities

Complications
- Hemorrhage
- Wound infection

> **PEARL OF WISDOM**
>
> The vaginal mucosa may be closed in some cases using continuous or interrupted 3–0 absorbable stitches. When marsupialization is used, ice packs and drains are unnecessary because the created "pouch" is wide open.

is only used when these other treatments fail (Procedure 15-9). In any approach, the psychological needs of the patient following surgery must be addressed.

ANTERIOR AND POSTERIOR REPAIR (COLPORRHAPHY)

Cystoceles and rectoceles are prolapses of the bladder or rectum, respectively, into the vaginal vault. These may be caused by congenital defects but are most prevalent

PROCEDURE 15-9 Simple Vulvectomy

Equipment

- Preferred stirrups
- ESU

Instruments

- Vaginal tray

Supplies

- Drains
- Culture tubes
- Surgeon-specific sutures and dressings

Operative Preparation

Anesthesia
- General anesthetic

Position
- Lithotomy

Prep
- Vaginal and lower abdomen

Draping
- Lithotomy

Practical Considerations

- Patient usually has a Foley catheter

Operative Procedure	Technical Considerations
1. The area to be removed is usually outlined with a skin marker.	**1.** The area to be excised may encompass the entire vulvar area from the mons pubis to the perineum, extending laterally from the labia majora for several centimeters, or in a "butterfly" shape, sparing the clitoris and perineum.
2. Local injection of epinephrine may be used to reduce bleeding, but is sparingly used to avoid distorting anatomy.	**2.** Local is injected using a three-ring syringe. Report amount injected.
3. The incision with a #10 blade begins at the vaginal outlet so that the urethral borders can be identified (Figure 15-25A).	**3.** Be prepared to pass hemostatic instruments.

PROCEDURE

15-9 Simple Vulvectomy *(continued)*

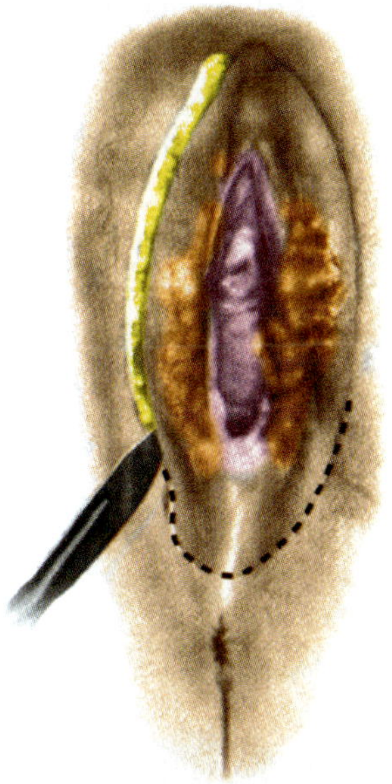

A

Figure 15-25 **Simple vulvectomy: (A) Skin incision**

4. The vaginal epithelium is undermined for a short distance.
5. The elliptical incision continues at the outer skin margins and minor bleeders are coagulated (Figure 15-25B).

4. Dissection may be sharp, blunt, or a combination of the two.
5. Considerable bleeding can occur in the area of the clitoris due to its high vascularity, and also at the lower one-third of the vulva where the Bartholin's ducts are located. These should be controlled with hemostatic sutures.

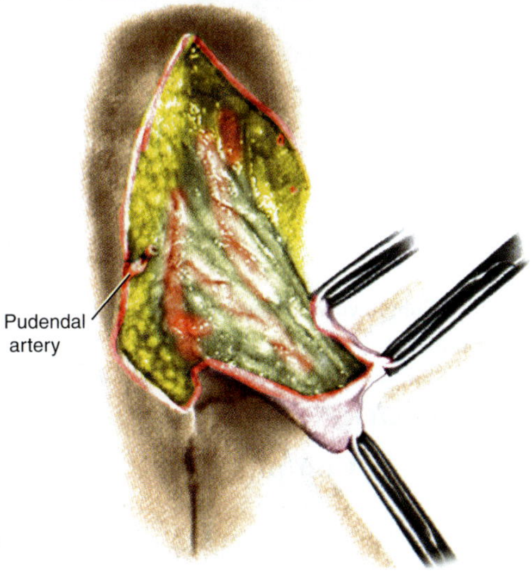

B

Figure 15-25 **Simple vulvectomy: (B) Pudendal artery ligated and cut**

(continues)

PROCEDURE 15-9 Simple Vulvectomy *(continued)*

6. The incision is carried almost to the anal orifice; care is taken in dissection to avoid the sphincters.

6. Knife will be used repeatedly.

7. Dissection continues into the adipose layer to facilitate closure but does not continue down to the deep fascia or muscles.

7. Various dissection techniques will be employed. Several hemostatic clamps will be used.

8. Hemostasis is achieved, tissues are approximated in layers with absorbable suture, and the skin edges are likewise approximated.

8. Specific variation: The area may also be left open to granulate, or, if considerable excision has occurred, it can require a split thickness or myocutaneous graft. Have skin graft set available in room.

9. A small drain is commonly placed in the lower end of the incision.

9. Drain and suture of choice are prepared in advance.

10. The vaginal epithelium is everted over the perineum to the level of the anal orifice to allow for satisfactory coitus (Figure 15-25C and D).

10. Count, if necessary. Prepare dressing.

11. Dressing is a firm pack applied over the entire area.

11. Held in place by panties.

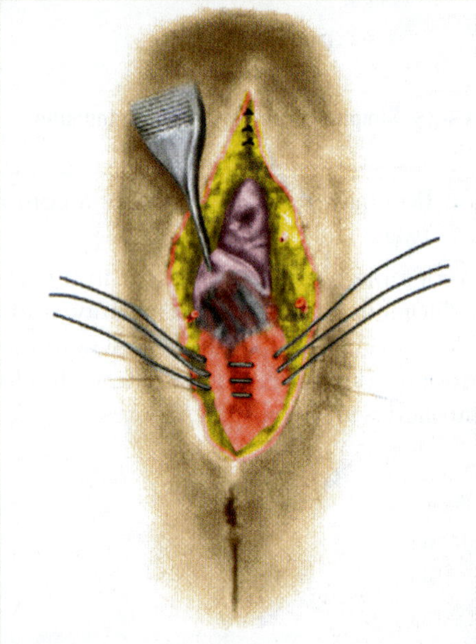

C

Figure 15-25 Simple vulvectomy: (C) Closure of levator ani muscles

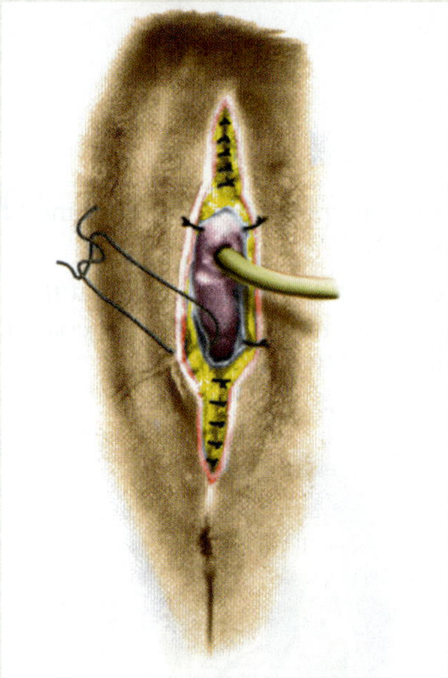

D

Figure 15-25 Simple vulvectomy: (D) Subcuticular closure (catheter in urethra)

Postoperative Considerations

Immediate Postoperative Care

- Transport to PACU
- Indwelling or suprapubic catheter is maintained for 4–6 days
- Ice packs applied to reduce swelling

Prognosis

- Return to normal activities

Complications

- Hemorrhage
- Wound infection

PEARL OF WISDOM

When using local anesthetics with epinephrine, be sure to state "with epinephrine" to the surgeon as you hand the medication. Be sure the anesthesia team knows that epinephrine is being given. Monitor the amount of local used.

in multipara women and result from stretching of the pelvic muscles or perineal tears during childbirth. Cystoceles are associated with urinary incontinence. Both cystoceles and rectoceles appear as bulges in the vaginal wall and in extreme cases present through the vaginal opening pushing the vaginal lining ahead of it. A cystocele will be evident in the anterior vaginal wall and a rectocele will be visible along the posterior vaginal wall (Procedure 15-10). Posterior presentation can also be due to enterocele and either condition can be due to previous hysterectomy. Repair of a rectocele incorporates perineorrhaphy to restore fecal continence and sexual competency of the vagina. Asymptomatic prolapses are not usually treated.

(Text continues on page 533)

PROCEDURE 15-10

Anterior (Cystocele) and Posterior (Rectocele) Colporrhaphy

Equipment

- Preferred stirrups
- ESU
- Headlamp

Instruments

- Vaginal hysterectomy set
- D&C set (if also performed)

Supplies

- Basic vaginal setup
- Surgeon-specific sutures and dressings

Operative Preparation

Anesthesia
- General anesthetic

Position
- Lithotomy

Prep
- Vaginal prep
- Indwelling catheter inserted

Draping
- Lithotomy

Practical Considerations

- Place catheter drainage bag where it can be monitored

Operative Procedure	Technical Considerations
1. **Anterior repair:** a transverse incision is made at the union of the vaginal mucosa and cervix and continued down to the pubovesical cervical fascia (Figure 15-26A).	1. The labia minora may be sutured to the skin to provide exposure. Cervical traction is maintained with a tenaculum.

(continues)

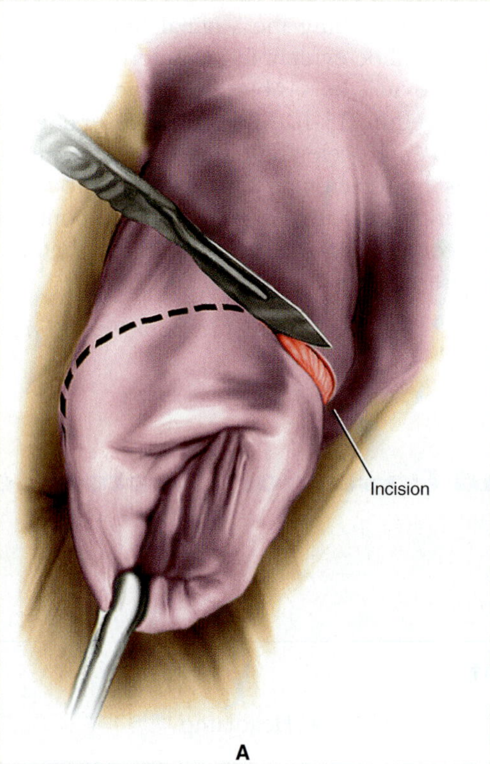

Figure 15-26 Anterior repair: (A) Transverse incision at the junction of the cervix and vaginal mucosa

2. The vaginal mucosa is dissected from the pubovesical and cervical fascia and opened in the midline (Figure 15-26B).

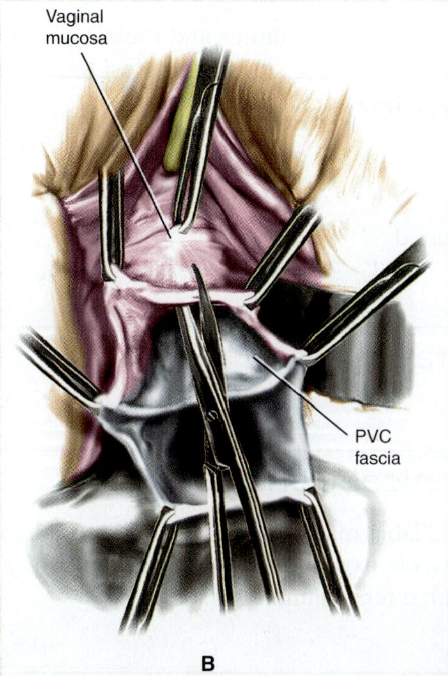

Figure 15-26 Anterior repair: (B) The vaginal mucosa is dissected from the pubovesical and cervical fascia. When dissection is complete, the vaginal mucosa is incised in the midline. *Note:* Hysterectomy has been completed in this case. This is not a necessary prerequisite for anterior repair

2. Careful positioning and manipulation of retractors are required for good visualization and tissue care.

Anterior (Cystocele) and Posterior (Rectocele) Colporrhaphy *(continued)*

3. Dissection continues with the vaginal mucosa being opened in the midline until a point is reached 1 cm from the urethral meatus. The pubovesical and cervical fascia is bluntly dissected from the vaginal mucosa (Figure 15-26C).

3. Allis clamps are applied as dissection progresses. The STSR should have an ample number on the field.

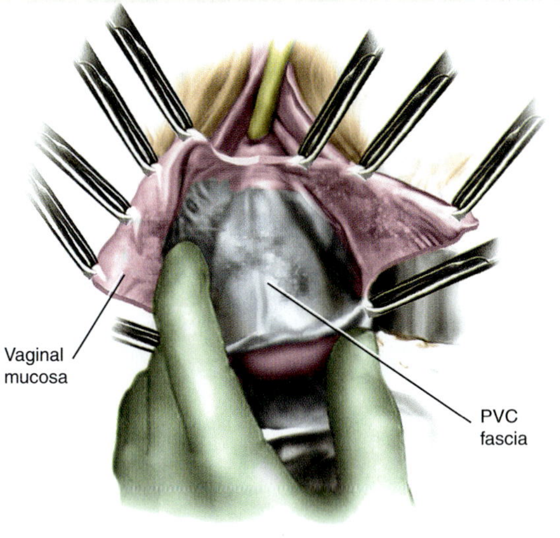

Figure 15-26 Anterior repair: (C) Blunt dissection of vaginal mucosa from pubovesical and cervical fascia

4. This dissection continues until the bladder and urethra are separated from the vaginal mucosa and the urethral vesical angle identified.
5. If a Kelly plication is performed to treat stress incontinence, a nonabsorbable suture is placed bilaterally to the urethra. A hemostat is placed so that the tissue is inverted as the suture is tied. Other sutures are placed as needed (Figure 15-26D).

4. Technique often used is blunt dissection with gauze wrapped around the index finger. *Note:* Use radiologically detectable sponge.
5. The presence of an excessive cystocele may warrant further bladder suspension techniques.

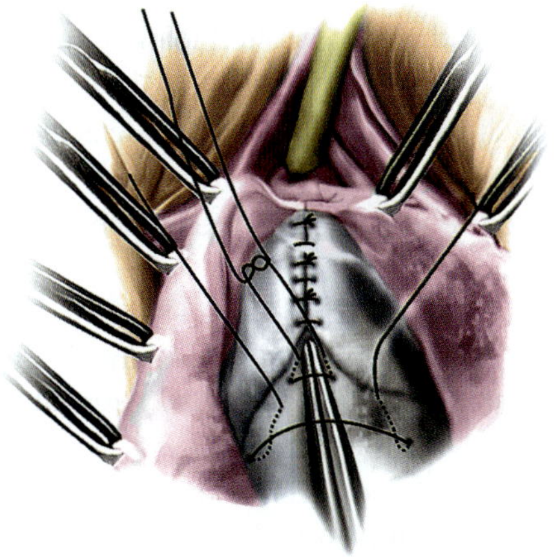

Figure 15-26 Anterior repair: (D) Completion of Kelly plication (not always required)

(continues)

PROCEDURE 15-10 Anterior (Cystocele) and Posterior (Rectocele) Colporrhaphy *(continued)*

6. The anterior repair begins as synthetic absorbable sutures are placed in the pubovesical and cervical fascia starting 1 cm below the urethral meatus.

6. The STSR should be prepared with enough sutures to complete multiple single mattress sutures.

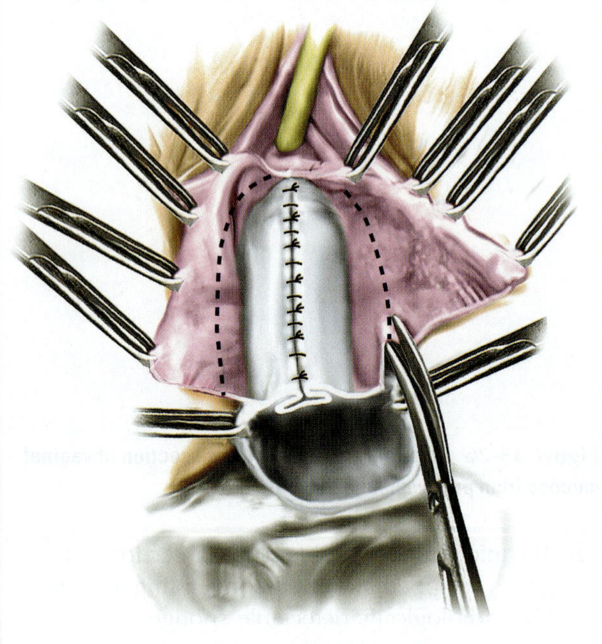

Figure 15-26 Anterior repair: (E) Excess vaginal mucosa is excised, lower portion shows vaginal cuff and plication technique used on pubovesical cervical fascia

7. The repair continues until the entire cystocele is reduced (Figure 15-26E).

7. Suture for this step is often loaded on control release needles. Keep close track of needles.

8. The excessive vaginal mucosa is removed.

8. This will usually be done with Metzenbaum scissors.

9. The vaginal mucosa is closed in the midline with interrupted 0 synthetic absorbable sutures to the level of the vaginal cuff.

9. Pass suture of surgeon's preference.

10. The edge of the vaginal cuff is sutured with a continuous 0 absorbable suture.

10. The STSR should quickly clean and reorganize instruments and be prepared to "repeat" the process posteriorly.

11. *Posterior repair:* Allis clamps are placed on the posterior vaginal mucosa and elevated to create a triangle (Figure 15-27A).

11. *Note:* Technical considerations are the same for the posterior repair.

PROCEDURE 15-10 Anterior (Cystocele) and Posterior (Rectocele) Colporrhaphy *(continued)*

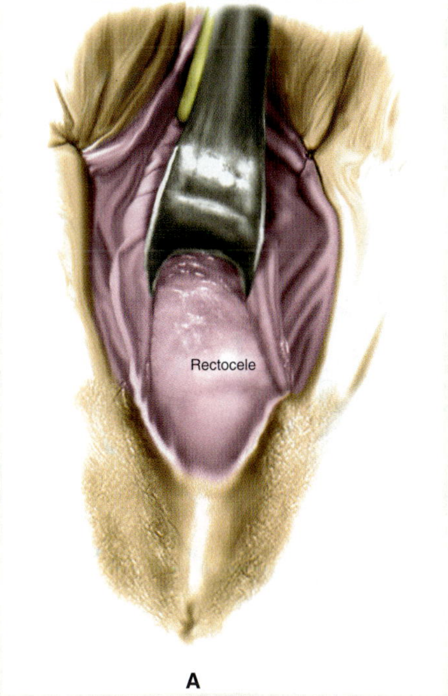

Figure 15-27 Posterior repair: (A) Elevation of posterior vaginal mucosa overlying rectocele

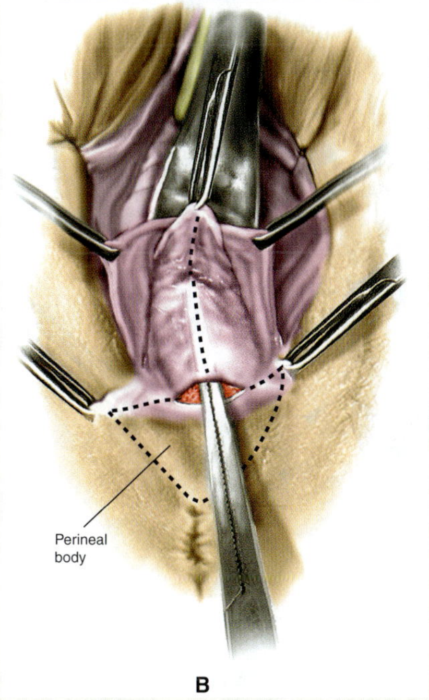

Figure 15-27 Posterior repair: (B) Blunt dissection of vaginal mucosa off perirectal fascia; intended incision lines noted

12. An Allis clamp is placed at the top of the rectocele in the midline. A transverse incision is made at the posterior fourchette. Blunt dissection is used to separate the posterior vaginal mucosa from the perirectal fascia.	**12.** Pass scalpel per facility policy. Have radiologically detectable sponge for blunt dissection prepared in advance of need.
13. A V-shaped portion of the mucosa is excised as determined by extent of repair required, and the levator ani muscles are observed below (Figure 15-27B).	**13.** Vaginal mucosa will be sent to pathology as specimen.
14. The bulbocavernosus muscle is exposed by an incision in the perineal body with removal of a triangular segment of perineal skin.	**14.** Sharp and blunt dissection is carried out.
15. A vertical incision is made in the posterior vaginal mucosa and the edges are retracted. The perirectal fascia is bluntly dissected from the posterior vaginal mucosa.	**15.** Several Allis clamps will be needed to retract the mucosal edges.
16. The rectocele is reduced with a finger, revealing the margins of the levator ani muscles. A 0 or 1 synthetic absorbable suture is placed at the margin of the levator ani to the posterior fourchette (Figure 15-27C).	**16.** Several of these sutures will be placed, progressively tied, and cut.

(continues)

PROCEDURE 15-10

Anterior (Cystocele) and Posterior (Rectocele) Colporrhaphy *(continued)*

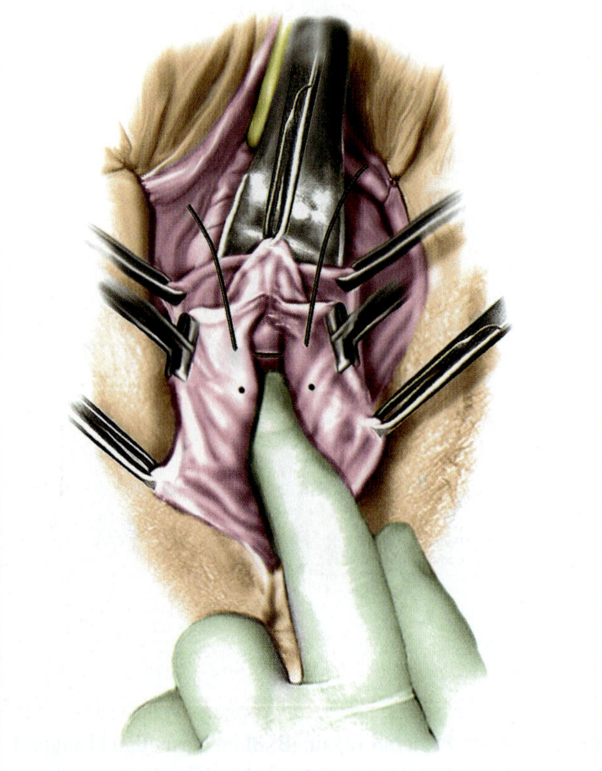

C

Figure 15-27 **Posterior repair: (C) Manual reduction of the rectocele allows margins of levator ani muscles and suture placement sites to be identified**

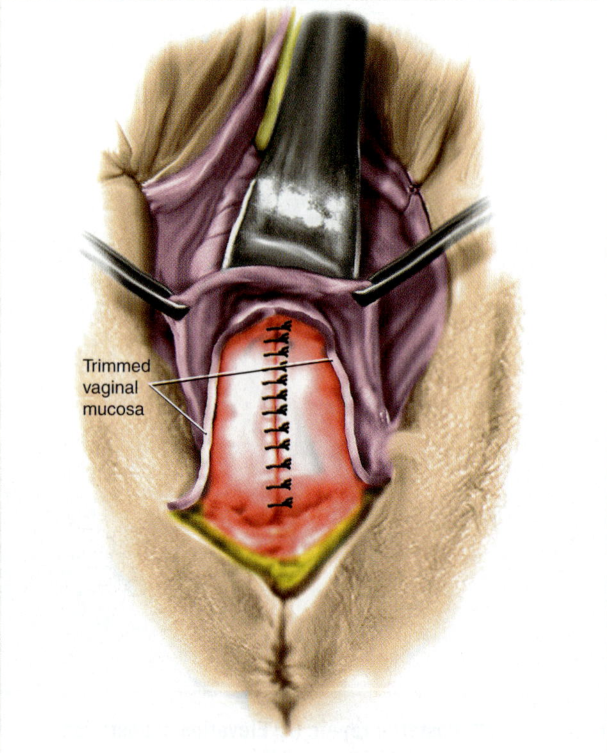

D

Figure 15-27 **Posterior repair: (D) Levator ani muscles sutured, excess posterior vaginal mucosa trimmed and prepared for closure**

17. The excessive posterior vaginal mucosa is excised and the perirectal fascia is closed with interrupted 0 synthetic absorbable suture.

17. The STSR should be prepared to supply suture for multiple stitches.

18. The posterior vaginal wall is closed to the posterior fourchette. The hymenal ring is reconstructed as is the perineal body (Figure 15-27D).

18. Additional sutures will be needed.

19. The subcutaneous layer and skin are closed with a subcuticular suture.

19. The STSR may be asked to "follow" the suture for subcuticular closure. Initiate count. Prepare dressings.

20. After closure, the repair is again assessed for integrity. The vaginal opening is reassessed to assure a two finger breadths space exists. Sutures are removed from the labia minora. The wound is then cleansed and a perineal pad dressing applied.

20. A vaginal pack may be used.

PROCEDURE 15-10 **Anterior (Cystocele) and Posterior (Rectocele) Colporrhaphy** *(continued)*

Postoperative Considerations

Immediate Postoperative Care

- Transport to PACU
- Observe color and amount of urine in urine drainage bag

Prognosis

- Return to normal activities

Complications

- Postoperative bleeding
- Hematoma
- Urinary tract infection
- Inability to urinate or stress incontinence
- Shortened or narrowed vagina
- Rectovaginal fistula
- Wound infection
- Recurrence of herniation

PEARL OF WISDOM

The posterior repair follows anterior because of potential contamination via the anus.

CERVICAL BIOPSY, CRYOTHERAPY, LASER TREATMENT, LEEP, AND CONIZATION

The Pap smear is a routine diagnostic modality used in most industrialized countries for the detection of cervical cancer. A swab specimen of the epithelial tissue of the cervix is taken, placed on a slide, and studied under the microscope for signs of unusual cellular growth. (A variation of this type of diagnostic study is the Pipelle.) An abnormal Pap smear can reveal several differing grades of cervical intraepithelial neoplasia (CIN) that are or may become cancerous. High-grade CIN is a precursor to invasive cancer if left untreated. Indications obtained from a Pap smear are followed by biopsy of suspected areas or obvious lesions, usually through colposcopy, which is also employed to evaluate the extent and nature of the disease.

Therapy is selected according to the lesion grade, its size and location, the size and contour of the cervix, and the patient's age and reproductive history. Therapy should aim to remove the disease safely and effectively and to prevent its recurrence without compromising cervical competency or producing other obstetrical or gynecological complications. Treatment modalities include punch biopsy, cryotherapy, and carbon dioxide (CO_2) laser treatment for smaller lesions, while loop electrosurgical excision (**LEEP**) and cervical conization are employed when the entire transitional zone (TZ) of the cervical mucosa cannot be observed.

Procedures can take place in the office or OR setting. Patient positioning is lithotomy and a standard D&C setup is usually used, although neither dilation nor **curettage** takes place. Acetic acid is applied to the operative area to "stain" the tissues white. This aids in determining the size and extent of the target lesion. A 3–5% acetic acid solution is applied to the target area with a cotton-tipped swab. It takes 30–60 seconds for whitening to occur, and the effect generally fades after 1–2 minutes. Therefore, repeat application of acetic acid may be necessary. Any mucous in the area should be swabbed to dry the tissue.

Punch biopsy is generally reserved for diagnostic confirmation, but can be used for the complete excision of small low-grade lesions via colposcopy (Figure 15-28). This procedure can be enhanced by curettage of the area biopsied. When punch biopsy is not permissible, these small lesions can be destroyed with cryotherapy or the CO_2 laser.

Cryotherapy utilizes either nitrous oxide or CO_2 as a refrigerant delivered by a flat silver cryoprobe that lowers tissue temperature to −22° centigrade, creating cell death by intracellular water crystallization. The refrigerant is applied to the cervical epithelium for a few minutes until the tissue is frozen 5 mm to 1 cm past the lesion. This may require one or two freeze-thaw cycles depending upon the size of the lesion. About 20% of patients experience a profuse watery discharge after

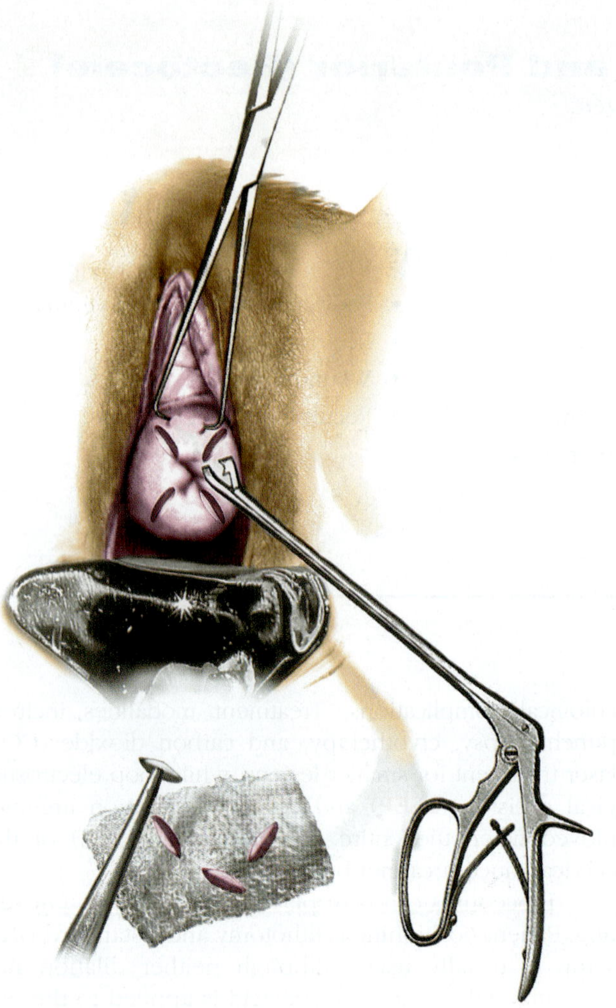

Figure 15-28 Cervical biopsy

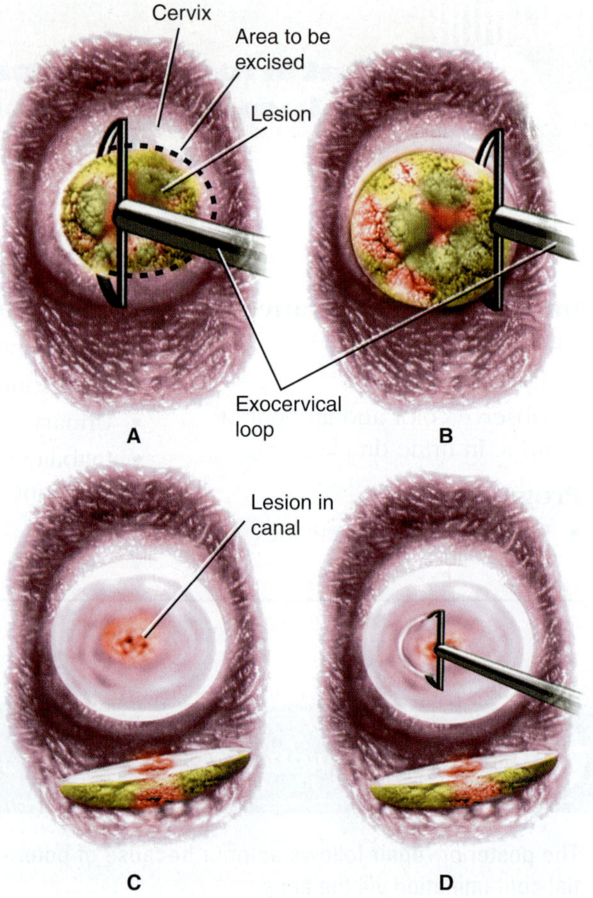

Figure 15-29 Cervical conization—LEEP technique: (A) Path of electrosurgical loop through distal cervix, (B) loop near completion of excision, (C) lesion identified in cervix, (D) loop excision of lesion

cryosurgery that can require use of a perineal pad; light bleeding can occur when the eschar begins to slough. Complications include cervical stenosis in 1–4% of patients and a recurrence rate of 10%. Fertility is not disturbed and healing is normally rapid.

CO_2 vaporization is accomplished by complete desiccation of the lesion by boiling the water within the cells until they explode. The laser can also be used as a knife to excise the lesion and a small area of tissue around it. With a laser the physician can either ablate or excise the tissue depending upon the laser's spot size and power density. Small lesions are ablated, while those extending into the cervical canal are usually excised using a conization technique. A CO_2 laser produces minimal side effects, and healing is rapid. There is also little vaginal discharge and no diminution of fertility.

Laser usage has declined steadily since the introduction of LEEP to North America in the early 1990s. LEEP requires an electrosurgical generator coupled to a loop electrode of tungsten or stainless steel measuring 2.5 mm wide and 7 mm deep to excise the lesion, or to a 5-mm ball-tipped electrode that is generally used for electrocoagulation of the defect (Figure 15-29). LEEP is performed in conjunction with colposcopy. "See and treat" is a modality that incorporates a colposcopic examination with LEEP as needed. This philosophy of treatment eliminates the patient's having to undergo punch biopsy and endocervical curettage.

LEEP begins with the patient placed in lithotomy position. A bivalve speculum is placed for proper exposure and the colposcope set for viewing. The cervix is stained with acetic acid and the whitened areas are observed. The lesion is then excised in a cuboid or bowl fashion or ablated using the properly sized electrode. LEEP is especially useful in ruling out early invasive carcinoma and in identifying unsuspected adenocarcinoma *in situ*. The area can be examined after excision to assure all margins of the lesion are removed. LEEP provides a specimen, unlike CO_2 or cryotherapy. Although LEEP provides limited morbidity, indiscriminate use of the electrode can cause irreversible cervical damage.

Cervical conization is performed for cervical neoplasms and for diagnosis in cases of suspected cervical cancer. Conization is performed on CIN lesions that extend into the endocervical canal or when the entire TZ cannot be observed. A suspected lesion is cut out in a cone fashion with a scalpel (or electrosurgically, not a true "cold knife"), leaving a conical crater extending into the cervical tissue; its apex is the center of the cervical os. Depth and wideness of excision is dependent upon the lesion size and location. Conization usually requires placement of sutures over an endocervical dilator to close the defect; hemostatic control can be significant.

Cryotherapy usually eliminates CIN. CO_2 laser provides less bleeding, less tissue damage and lower morbidity, and high effectiveness. Conization appears to be curative in most cases; however, complications such as uterine perforation, prolonged period of postoperative bleeding, and resultant incompetent cervix are a concern. A follow-up Pap smear is performed at 4 months.

DILATION AND CURETTAGE

Dilation and curettage (D&C) is utilized for both diagnostic and therapeutic purposes. Diagnostic indications for D&C include dysmenorrhea, collection of abnormal cytology to rule out endometrial disease, to rule out pregnancy prior to elective sterilization, and to determine a cause for infertility. Therapeutic usage includes removal of suspected pathology (such as polyps), treatment of postpartum bleeding or to evacuate retained secundines (placenta), retrieval of "lost" IUD, placement of radioactive carriers for the management of cervical or uterine malignancies, and treatment of polyps, incomplete abortion, or dysmenorrhea (Procedure 15-11). If the procedure is performed after the thirteenth week of pregnancy, it is termed dilation and evacuation (D&E).

PROCEDURE 15-11 Dilation and Curettage (D&C)

Equipment

- Stirrups of choice

Instruments

- Vaginal tray
- D&C set

Supplies

- Basic vaginal pack
- Telfa for specimen samples
- Perineal pad

Operative Preparation

Anesthesia

- General anesthetic preferred
- May be performed under regional block

Position

- Lithotomy

Prep

- Vaginal prep

Draping

- Lithotomy

Practical Considerations

- Preoperative sonography may be done

(continues)

PROCEDURE 15-11 Dilation and Curettage (D&C) *(continued)*

Operative Procedure

1. A pelvic exam is performed to determine the size, shape, and position of the uterus and to detect any masses.
2. An Auvard weighted speculum is placed in the posterior vagina and tucked under the external os of the cervix.
3. The cervix is grasped in the 12-o'clock position with a single-toothed tenaculum, and a uterine sound is placed into the external os (Figure 15-30A).

Technical Considerations

1. Set up vaginal exam tray as separate tray. Reglove surgeon after examination.
2. A sterile glove may be placed over the round weighted section of the speculum to catch any blood or tissue.
3. The STSR may hold the tenaculum. Care is taken not to tear the cervix.

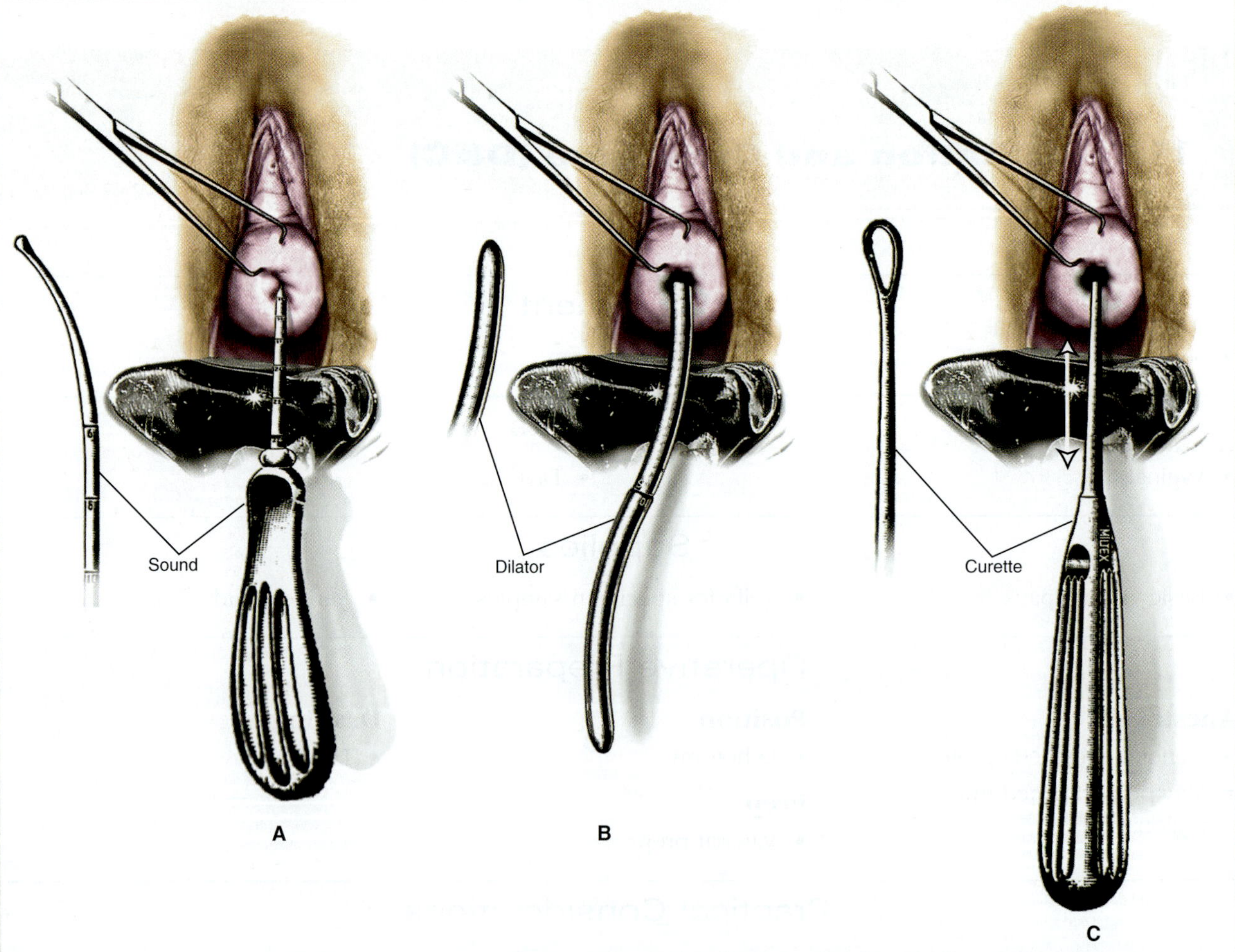

Figure 15-30 Dilation and curettage (D&C): (A) Tenaculum placement and sounding, (B) dilation of cervix, (C) curettage of uterus

PROCEDURE

15-11 Dilation and Curettage (D&C) *(continued)*

4. The sound is advanced through the internal os and to the fundus to determine the depth of the uterus, noted by the calibrations on the sound. After uterine depth is determined, the sound is withdrawn.

4. A piece of Telfa may be placed on the blade of the speculum to catch tissue specimens.

5. If an endocervical specimen is to be taken, a sharp narrow curette is placed into the external os and the cervical mucosa is scraped and extracted onto the Telfa.

5. Remove the Telfa and place the specimen in a predetermined container on the back table.

6. The cervix is dilated with a progressive series of dilators (Figure 15-30B).

6. Align dilators on the back table so sizes are sequential and progressive. A small amount of lubricant should be placed on each dilator before use. Provide a second Telfa for intrauterine (endometrial) specimen.

7. Randall forceps may be placed and the uterus explored for any polyps, fibroids, or remnants of pregnancy that may require removal.

7. STSR may be unable to pass instruments while providing exposure. Place instruments to allow surgeon to "help him- or herself."

8. Curette of choice is advanced into the uterus and the endometrium is scraped in the same manner as the cervix; the tissue extracted onto the Telfa is handed off as endometrial specimen (Figure 15-30C).

8. Examination with Randall forceps and curettage may be repeated several times.

9. The instruments are withdrawn, the weighted speculum removed.

9. The operative area is cleansed. A perineal pad dressing is applied.

Postoperative Considerations

Immediate Postoperative Care

- Transport to PACU

Prognosis

- Return to normal activities

Complications

- Perforation of uterus
- Laceration of the cervix
- Tear of the internal os
- Damage to other pelvic organs
- Excessive bleeding (monitored for 6 hours)
- Postoperative infection

PEARL OF WISDOM

Specimens may need special identification relative to location within the uterus. Have extra Telfa and specimen containers in the room. Keep a sterile marker on the back table to assist with identification. Multiple specimens require careful communication between STSR and the circulator.

SUCTION CURETTAGE

For this procedure, patient preparation, anesthesia, positioning, and instrumentation remains the same as for D&C. Although suction curettage is faster, safer, and does not require sharp curettage, sharp curettage may be necessary if sufficient tissue is not retrieved with the suction technique. Dilation of the cervix is required to accommodate the special cannula for the procedure. This may be achieved by using metal dilators, such as Pratt dilators, or accomplished by the use of a hygroscopic dilator, which causes less trauma to the tissues. Suction usually collects better quality tissue samples than sharp curettage, because extraneous tissue is not collected.

Various suction aspiration cannulas are available; all are plastic, single-use disposable, slightly curved to accommodate the shape of the uterus, and rounded at the tip with a portal along one aspect of the shaft. Variations include serrations at the tip to aid in gathering specimens, controllable suction rings, and several diameters (Figure 15-31). The smooth-tipped varieties are most commonly used. These cannulas are approximately 8 mm in diameter, with a sliding suction control ring at the operator's end. The cannula can be hooked up to a suction device with tubing going to a controlled suction unit or simply to a large syringe.

The cervix is dilated to a width to accommodate the cannula, which is then placed to the required depth. A 25 French dilator must place easily to accommodate an 8-mm curette. Controlled suction is applied and the cannula is rotated a full 360 degrees and moved in and out to loosen and collect the specimen. The suction apparatus may have a separate collection reservoir that traps and holds the specimen. The surgeon repeats the process until he or she is assured that the required sample is obtained. This is then examined to confirm presence of fetal tissue. The vagina is then cleansed and a perineal pad is applied as dressing. Postoperative care is similar to that for a D&C.

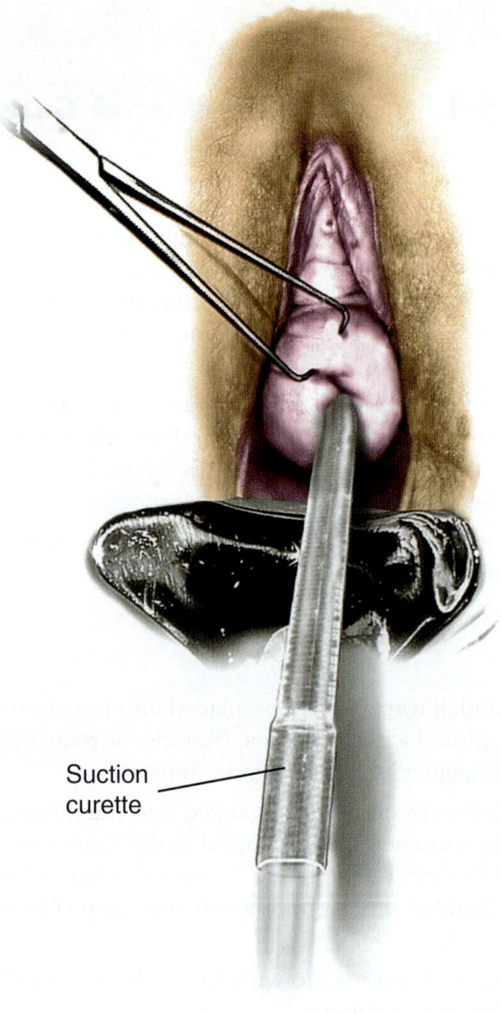

Figure 15-31 **Vacuum aspiration of the uterus, suction curette in place**

MYOMECTOMY

Myomectomy, the excision of uterine fibroids (leiomyomas or myomas) is a procedure with higher rates of morbidity and bleeding than hysterectomy. Indications for myomectomy include:

- Anemia secondary to uterine bleeding
- Chronic, severe pelvic pain
- Chronic secondary dysmenorrhea
- Fibroid preventing evaluation of adnexa
- Urinary tract symptoms secondary to fibroid
- Continued growth of fibroid postmenopause
- Infertility
- Rapid increase in size

The procedure is technically challenging, but it is one that is performed in select patients when preservation of the uterus is warranted. The size, number, and location of the myomas manifest as a variety of clinical signs and symptoms, although 50–80% may be asymptomatic. Myomectomy can be performed through pelviscopy or laparoscopy, and via abdominal and vaginal approaches. Fibroid resection is most often accomplished through abdominal procedures (Procedure 15-12).

PROCEDURE

15-12 Myomectomy (Abdominal Approach)

Equipment

- Normal laparotomy equipment
- ESU

Instruments

- Laparotomy set

Supplies

- Routine supplies for laparotomy

Operative Preparation

Anesthesia
- General anesthetic
- Spinal or epidural is possible

Position
- Supine

Prep
- Laparotomy

Draping
- Laparotomy

Practical Considerations

- Follow adhesion prevention procedures (see "Pearl of Wisdom," page 541)

Operative Procedure	Technical Considerations
1. Incision may be of the Pfannenstiel or vertical midline type.	**1.** Adapt initial routine to incision of choice.
2. The abdominal cavity is explored. A self-retaining retractor is placed. The bowel is packed cephalad with moist sponges.	**2.** Balfour and O'Sullivan-O'Connor retractors are commonly used. Warm, moist sponges to pack bowel. *Note:* STSR, the best practice is to count sponges as they are placed and have circulator record the number.
3. A vertical incision into the anterior surface of the uterus is made over the myoma.	**3.** There may be several incisions depending on the number of myomas.
4. The general strategy in myomectomy is to incise the pseudocapsule of the fibroid, expose the tissue planes (controlling the edges of the capsule with Allis clamps), and use blunt dissection, scissors, electrosurgical pencil, or laser, and peel the myoma from the capsule (Figure 15-32A).	**4.** Prepare for the specific approach to be used in advance. Use of the laser will require laser safety procedures to be in place.

(continues)

PROCEDURE 15-12 Myomectomy (Abdominal Approach) *(continued)*

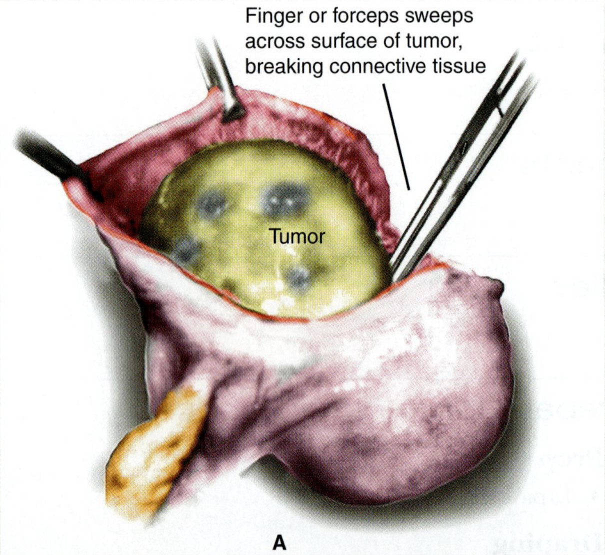

Figure 15-32 Myomectomy: (A) Longitudinal incision over myoma with blunt dissection

5. Once dissected free, the myoma is removed (Figure 15-32B).

5. Uterine bleeding is controlled with clamps and suture ligatures.

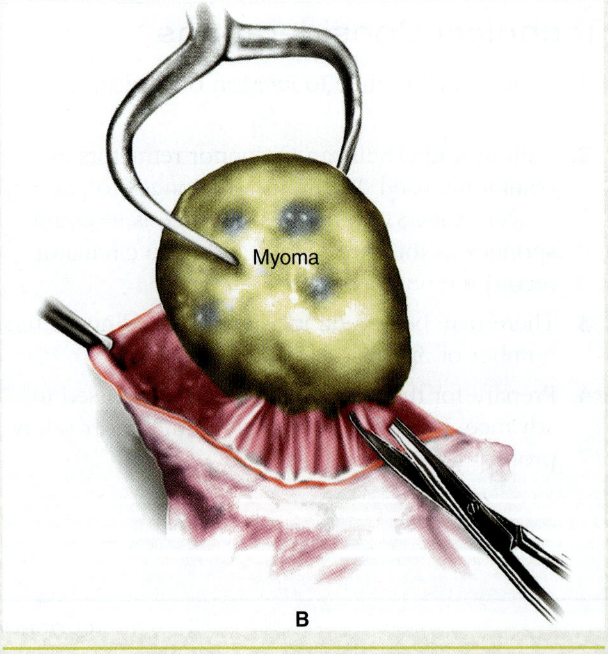

Figure 15-32 Myomectomy: (B) Excision of myoma

PROCEDURE 15-12 Myomectomy (Abdominal Approach) *(continued)*

6. The uterine incision is closed with 0 or 2–0 synthetic absorbable suture (Figure 15-32C).

6. Use of several sutures may be required.

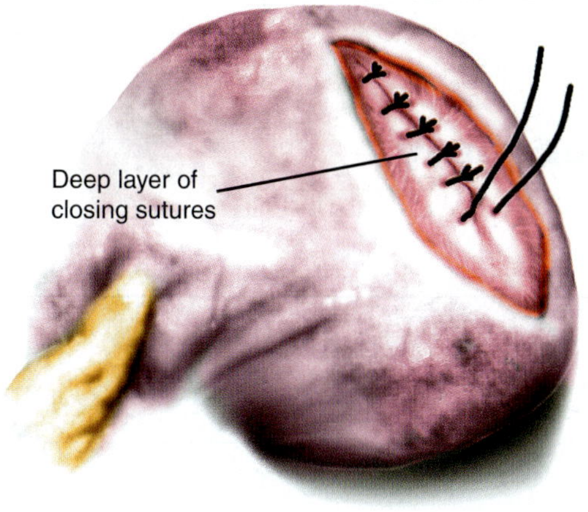

Figure 15-32 Myomectomy: (C) Uterine closure

7. The abdomen is closed in the usual manner.

7. Usual closure routine. Dextran may be instilled. Counts as needed.

Postoperative Considerations

Immediate Postoperative Care

- Transport to PACU

Prognosis

- Return to normal activities

Complications

- Bowel obstruction or damage
- Bladder injury
- Fallopian tube or ureter compromise
- Wound infection or dehiscence
- Approximately 20–25% of patients undergoing myomectomy will require additional pelvic surgery
- Infertility secondary to the procedure

PEARL OF WISDOM

The biggest problem following myectomy is adhesion formation. This can be reduced with gentle tissue handling, removal of talc from the operators' gloves, avoiding the posterior peritoneal surface of the uterus, incorporating various uterine suspension techniques, and using copious intraoperative irrigation of heparinized Ringer's lactate. Instillation of 100–200 mL of 10% dextran 70 can be used to provide a slippery surfactant between the organs, but is not common. Promethazine and corticosteroids, as well as intravenous Decadron (20 mg) and intramuscular Phenergan (25 mg) given every 4 hours for 48 hours, are also utilized to prevent adhesion formation postoperatively.

TOTAL ABDOMINAL HYSTERECTOMY WITH BILATERAL SALPINGO-OOPHORECTOMY (TAH-BSO)

Abdominal hysterectomy (Procedure 15-13) with bilateral salpingo-oophorectomy is a complex procedure, because it requires knowledge of the entire internal reproductive system. The procedure is also understandable as several independent, component procedures—hysterectomy, oophorectomy, and salpingectomy. The student should recognize that the steps of freeing the ovary or fallopian tube from the uterus are not required if the procedure is a TAH-BSO.

(Text continues on page 546)

PROCEDURE 15-13 Total Abdominal Hysterectomy

Equipment

- Normal laparotomy equipment
- ESU

Instruments

- Laparotomy set
- Self-retaining retractor of choice
- Gynecologic instruments such as Heaney and Heaney-Ballantine clamps

Supplies

- Routine supplies for laparotomy
- Passive and negative pressure drains

Operative Preparation

Anesthesia

- General anesthetic

Position

- Supine

Prep

- Abdominal and vaginal prep
- Probable placement of indwelling catheter

Draping

- Laparotomy

Operative Procedure	Technical Considerations
1. Following transverse or vertical entrance into the abdominal cavity, the abdomen is thoroughly explored for any unsuspected pathology, and the uterus and adnexa are assessed.	**1.** Adjust according to incision selected by the surgeon.
2. A self-retaining retractor is placed and the bowel is packed cephalad with moist lap sponges.	**2.** Balfour, O'Sullivan-O'Connor, Bookwalter are commonly used. Have full selection of blades available for Bookwalter. Warm, moist laps will be needed.
3. A tenaculum may be placed into the fundus of the uterus to facilitate control of the organ.	**3.** Most commonly, a multitoothed tenaculum is used to manipulate the uterus.
4. Ligament clamps are placed across each broad ligament at a position close to the cornu incorporating the round and ovarian ligaments.	**4.** Some of these clamps, after division of the ligament, will be left in place to aid with elevation and deviation of the uterus during its excision.

PROCEDURE

15-13 Total Abdominal Hysterectomy *(continued)*

5. The round ligaments are now divided electrosurgically or are suture ligated and cut developing anterior and posterior "leaves" of the broad ligament (Figure 15-33A).

5. Sutures are immediately placed on patient side of dissection. Dissection may be sharp, blunt, or combined.

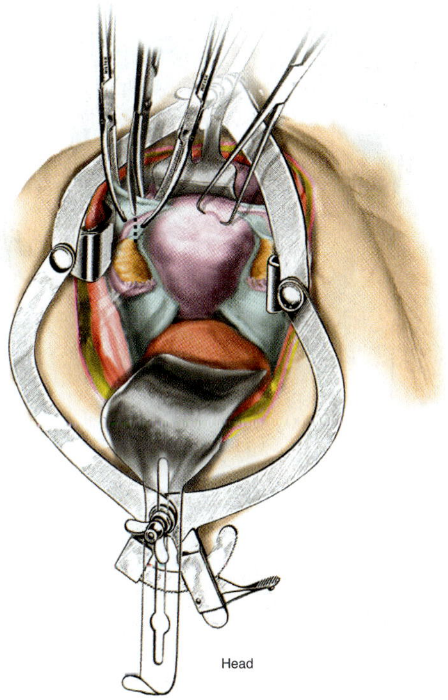

Figure 15-33 **Total abdominal hysterectomy (TAH): (A) Division of round ligament**

6. These are incised with Metzenbaum scissors, separating the peritoneum of the bladder from the lower uterus, and opening the retroperitoneum to expose the underlying iliac vessels and the ureters. These structures are properly identified and protected at all times for the remainder of the procedure.

6. Hysterectomies are methodical, and the same steps must be repeated bilaterally. The STSR should have an adequate supply of clamps and sutures throughout the procedure.

7. The peritoneal opening is enlarged to expose the infundibulopelvic ligament and uterine artery. A curved Ballantine or Heaney clamp is placed medial to the ovary and the infundibulopelvic ligament is double ligated and divided. (Figure 15-33B).

7. Classically, a hysterectomy procedure uses the "clamp, clamp, cut, tie" method. However, the tie is usually a "stick tie," a suture with a needle on a needle holder. Heaney needle holders are often used. The jaws are curved, and the needle is loaded with the point projecting behind the convex surface.

8. The bladder is bluntly dissected from the lower uterus and cervix along an avascular plane.

8. Usually blunt dissection requires "sponge on a stick."

(continues)

PROCEDURE 15-13 Total Abdominal Hysterectomy *(continued)*

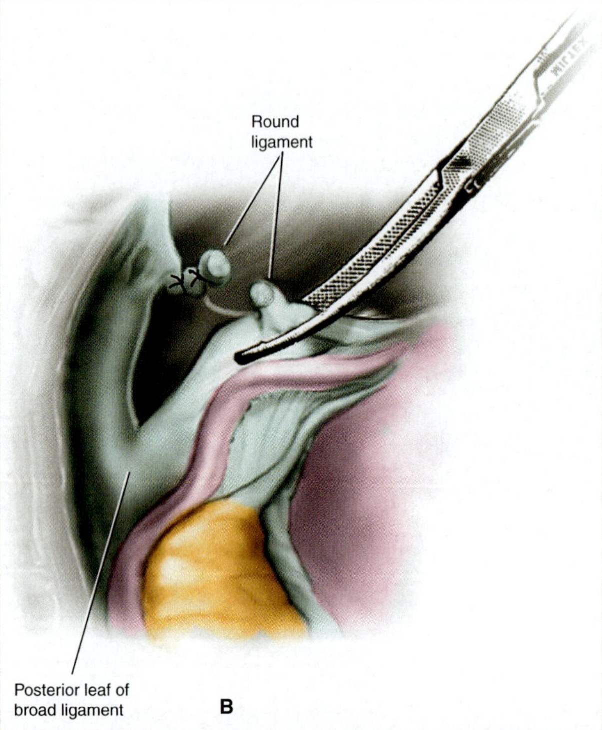

Figure 15-33 TAH: (B) Broad ligament—posterior and anterior leaves

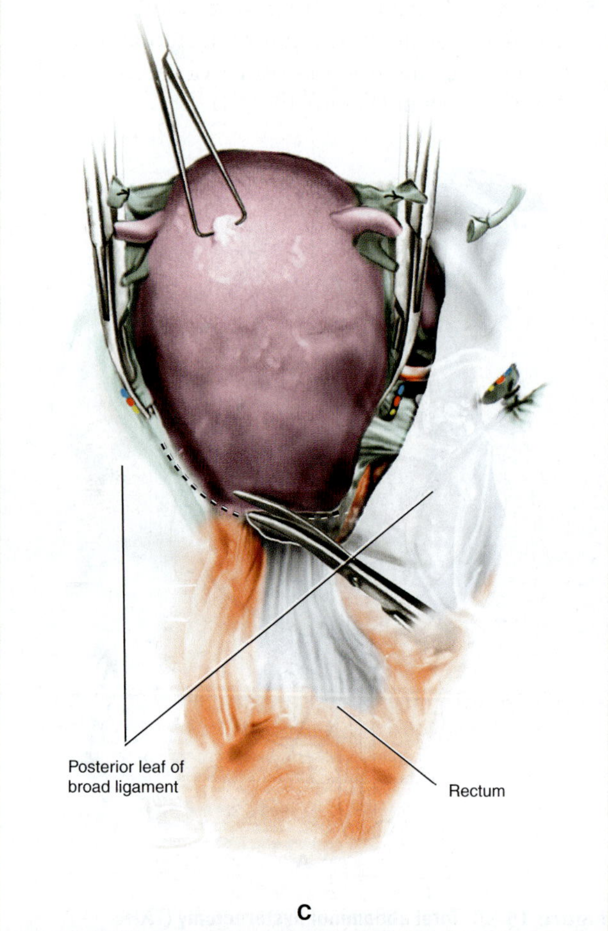

Figure 15-33 TAH: (C) Dissection line

9. The uterus in now retracted cephalad and deviated to one side, stretching the lower ligaments and facilitating exposure of the uterine vessels, which are then cross-clamped at the junction of the uterus and cervix, cut, and ligated.

9. Depending on the patient's pelvic anatomy, more caudal portions of the procedure may require extra-long instruments.

10. The rectum can now be mobilized from the posterior cervix and reflected inferiorly, out of the way (Figure 15-33C).

10. Long instruments are usually required.

11. The cardinal ligament is clamped, divided, and ligated on both sides.

11. Follow clamp, clamp, cut, tie routine.

PROCEDURE

15-13 Total Abdominal Hysterectomy *(continued)*

12. The uterus is again placed in cephalad traction and curved clamps are placed bilaterally, incorporating the uterosacral ligaments. The uterus is freed and removed.

12. Mayo or Jorgensen scissors are commonly used. Bring up a specimen container after passing the scissors.

13. The resulting vaginal "cuff" can now be closed with interrupted or running #1 or 0 absorbable suture or stapled. The peritoneum is closed over it in a similar manner (Figure 15-33D).

13. These instruments are considered contaminated since they may project into the vagina. They should be isolated or removed from the field following use.

14. The abdomen is thoroughly irrigated and drained and checked for hemostasis. The ureters are reassessed for position and integrity and to ensure they are not dilated. (If left behind, the ovaries may be sutured to the lateral pelvic walls.)

14. Various types of drains may be placed. Anticipate use of warm irrigation fluid. Prepare suture.

15. The abdomen is closed in the usual manner.

15. Usual closure routine. Counts as needed.

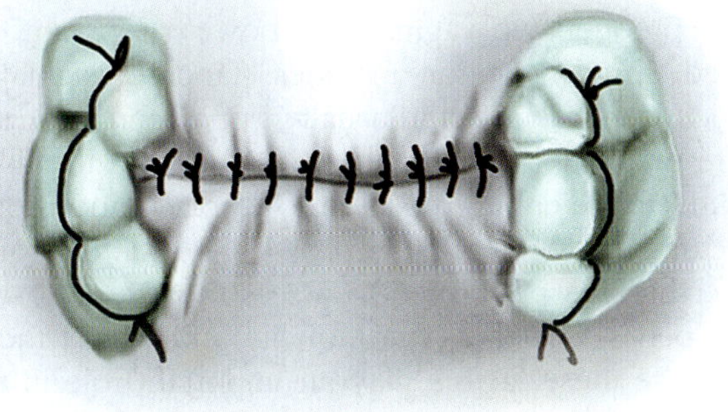
D

Figure 15-33 TAH: (D) Vaginal cuff closure

Postoperative Considerations

Immediate Postoperative Care

- Transport to PACU

Prognosis

- Return to normal activities

Complications

- Bowel obstruction or damage
- Bladder injury
- Wound infection or dehiscence
- Ureteral injuries
- Hemorrhage

PEARL OF WISDOM

Some surgeons complete actions on one side of the uterus then move to the other side; some alternate sides as they move caudally. The STSR must adjust to the pattern and be sure to have an adequate supply of hemostats.

SPECIFIC VARIATIONS WITH HYSTERECTOMY—TAH WITHOUT OOPHORECTOMY

Under certain conditions, the ovaries may be left behind for their hormonal value. To accomplish this, the uterus is retracted toward the symphysis pubis and to one side creating tension on the structures of the contralateral side. A window is created in the peritoneum of the posterior leaf of the broad ligament under the utero-ovarian ligament and fallopian tube. The fallopian tube and utero-ovarian ligament are then clamped with a curved Heaney or Ballantine clamp, cut, and ligated with both a free tie and a suture of #1 or 0 absorbable suture. This technique will separate the ovaries and tubes from the uterine specimen.

OOPHORECTOMY

The ovaries may be removed along with the uterus. Indications for oophorectomy are prophylaxis, ovarian malignancy, cystic ovaries, strangulated ovaries, infection and adhesions, and extensive endometriosis. The ovary is isolated, with moist lap sponges placed around the ovary to contain spillage of cystic ovaries. A window is created in the peritoneum of the suspensory ligament of the ovary, which is then double clamped, cut with Metzenbaum scissors, and ligated in a series until the specimen is free.

SALPINGECTOMY

Salpingectomy is removal of part or all of the fallopian tube. This can include tubal ligation procedures, but is usually indicated by other pathology, such as occlusive disease or ectopic (tubal) pregnancy. It is especially indicated when there is a desire to leave the associated ovary intact. Total salpingectomy requires an incision into the myometrium of the uterus to excise the cornu, and closure of the defect with a figure-of-eight, 0-sized suture. A window is created in the mesosalpinx of the leaf of the broad ligament between the fallopian tube and the round ligament. The fallopian tube is then separated along the entire length of its attachment by a succession of Kelly clamps applied on the mesosalpinx side and sharp division. Ties are then applied around the Kelly hemostats, attaining hemostasis along this line as they are tied. This division of the ligament proceeds toward the uterus and ovary until the fallopian tube is free. It is then excised from, or transected at an arbitrary point close to, the myometrium. The mesosalpinx is closed with interrupted 0 absorbable sutures. Complete hemostasis is achieved to avoid hematoma formation in the broad ligament.

VAGINAL AND LAPAROSCOPICALLY ASSISTED VAGINAL HYSTERECTOMY (LAVH)

A vaginal approach to hysterectomy under proper conditions has long been routine in gynecologic surgery. Modern advancements in technology allow other options. The laparoscopically assisted vaginal hysterectomy is a common procedure. In this approach, the hysterectomy is actually a vaginal hysterectomy but certain steps are performed through laparoscopic technique. This allows the surgeon to benefit from better visualization of the internal structures. The approach taken here is to describe the vaginal hysterectomy in its traditional form and then discuss the laparoscopic portion separately. The student should refer to the laparoscopy section in this chapter to review the initial steps in this technique.

The procedure requires general or spinal anesthesia and preoperative vaginal and bowel preps are encouraged. Instrumentation includes standard vaginal setup, electrosurgical unit, and usually 0 or #1 chromic catgut suture material. The patient is positioned in the lithotomy with Trendelenburg position to displace and protect the rectum and loops of pelvic bowel. An examination under anesthesia is performed to assess the size and shape of the pelvis as well as the mobility and size of the uterus because these factors play an important role in this approach. Retractors are positioned for optimal exposure and 1% lidocaine with 1:200,000 epinephrine may be injected in the vaginal mucosa to reduce bleeding.

VAGINAL HYSTERECTOMY

The procedure involves the same structures as the abdominal hysterectomy. The most significant difference is that the structures are encountered in the reverse order. The vaginal hysterectomy is outlined briefly below.

1. The cervix is grasped with a tenaculum and pulled downward.
2. A circumferential incision is made around the cervix.
3. The vaginal wall is dissected away from the cervix by sharp or blunt means until the peritoneal reflection in the posterior cul-de-sac and the vesicovaginal space are identified.
4. The bladder is advanced to prevent injury.

5. The peritoneum is now opened with curved Mayo scissors.
6. The ligament is clamped with a Heaney, incorporating the cardinal ligament in its tip.
7. The ligament is divided and the resultant pedicle is sutured.
8. The uterine vessels are now identifiable and are clamped and ligated.
9. The vesicovaginal space is entered and the bladder is advanced by retraction.
10. The uterus is delivered and the utero-ovarian and round ligaments identified.
11. These are then clamped, cut, and double sutured or ligated.
12. The uterus can now be removed.
13. Hemostasis is achieved on all pedicles and the vaginal "cuff" closed.
14. Upon completion of the procedure the bladder is drained, the operative field is cleansed, and a perineal pad is applied.

SPECIFIC VARIATION—LAVH

Use of the LAVH technique (Figure 15-34) has significant advantages: It allows potential abdominal hysterectomies to be converted to far less traumatic vaginal approaches, thereby shortening the patient's hospital stay considerably, while providing the visualization advantages of the abdominal procedure. The downsides to the LAVH may be greater cost and longer procedural time.

The LAVH may require as many as 4 portals, potentially one 12-mm, two 10-mm, and one 5-mm sites. The ovary and fallopian tube are grasped and moved medially exposing the infundibulopelvic ligament. The ureter is identified and an endosurgical linear cutting stapler is placed across the infundibulopelvic and round ligaments. The stapler is closed. Proper position is verified, and the stapler is activated, ligating and incising the enclosed structures. A similar procedure is followed on the broad ligament. This may take more than one step. Transection is stopped approximately 0.5 cm above the ureter and uterine artery. These steps must be repeated on the opposite side. The bladder peritoneum is elevated and endoscopic scissors are used to transect the peritoneum from the lower uterine segment. The surgeon then moves to the vaginal portion of the procedure. The surgeon may return to the laparoscope at the end of the procedure to verify hemostasis.

The immediate postoperative period requires fluid maintenance and pain relief. Nausea and a slowing of gastrointestinal activity is common; a liquid diet is suggested for the first 12–24 hours. The bladder should also be drained if spontaneous voiding does not occur. Complications of vaginal hysterectomy include hemorrhage, which can require an abdominal incision to resolve, injury to the bladder, bowel or rectum injury, wound infection, ureteral injuries, and the long-term complication of developing vesicovaginal or enterovaginal fistulas.

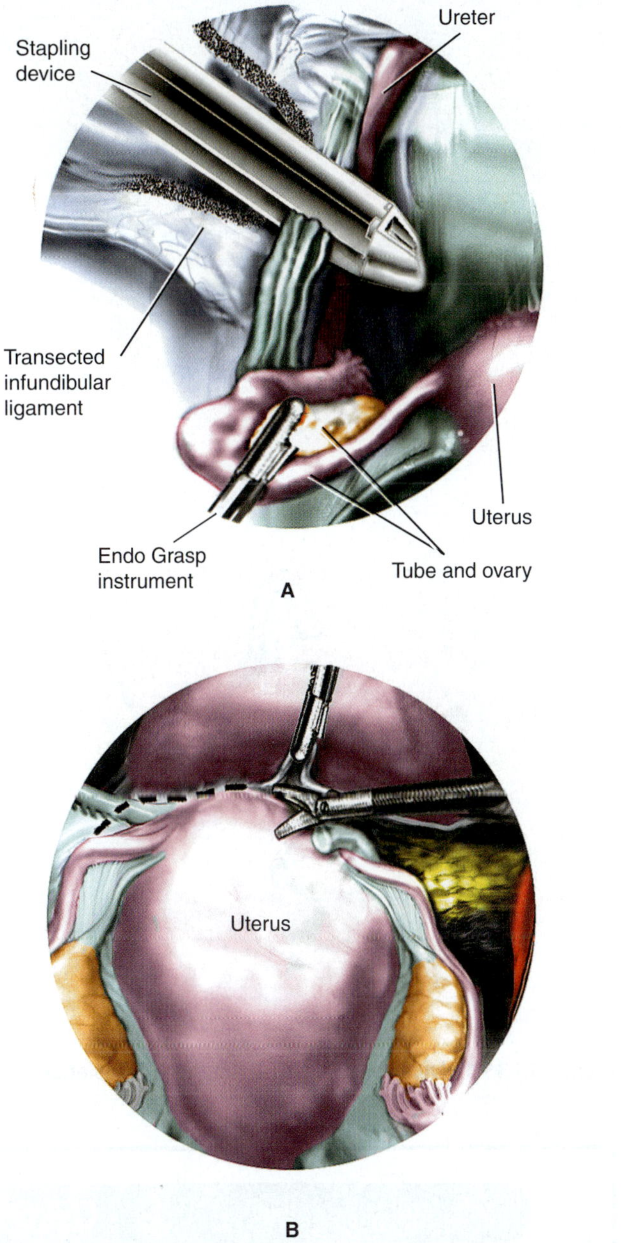

Figure 15-34 **Laparoscopically assisted vaginal hysterectomy (LAVH): (A) Use of stapling device on ligament, (B) uterovesical line of dissection with endoscopic scissors**

RADICAL CANCER SURGERY: TOTAL PELVIC EXENTERATION

Total pelvic **exenteration** is a radical procedure that involves the removal of the vagina, uterus and cervix, fallopian tubes, ovaries, bladder, and rectum (Figure 15-35).

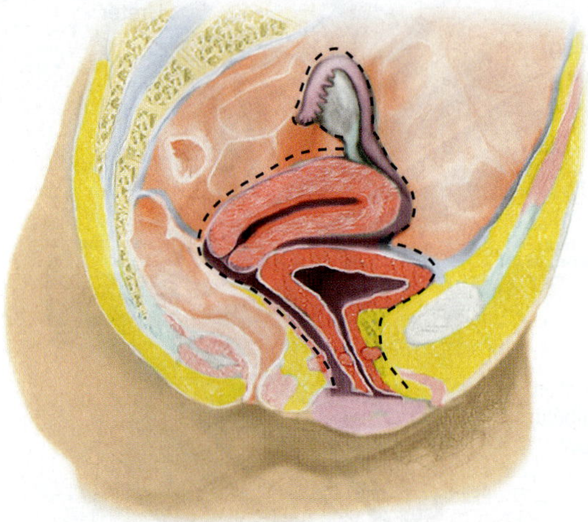

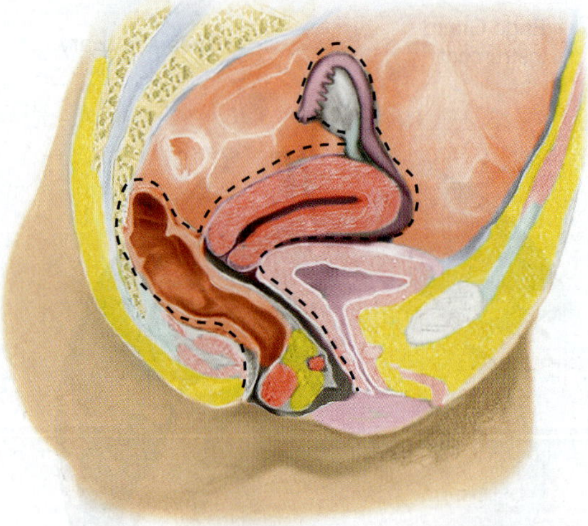

Figure 15-35 **Pelvic exenteration: (A) Anterior, (B) posterior**

Because of its complexity and overlap with procedures in general and genitourinary surgery, only a general description of the procedure will be presented here. The reader should refer to other illustrative procedures for technical details concerning the various components of the operation.

Total pelvic exenteration is the treatment of choice for recurrent squamous cell carcinoma of the cervix or vagina, recurrent adenocarcinoma of the cervix or endometrium, sarcoma in the pelvis, and in cases where carcinoma of the vulva has not responded to other therapies. The tissues adjacent to these structures, such as the bladder, urethra, and bowel, are commonly sites of metastasis and are therefore excised as well. Carcinoma of the ovary is an absolute contraindication to this route of treatment. Modifications of this procedure include either an anterior exenteration, involving the bladder and genitalia, or a posterior exenteration of the genitalia, and bowel. The former preserves the intestinal tract; the latter the urinary system.

Surgical risks must be weighed against the benefits of this procedure. Conditions such as patient age over 70, religious beliefs that do not allow the replacement of blood loss, gross obesity, and unrelated medical conditions that could pose intraoperative complications must all be considered and can be contraindications. The psychological ramifications of the procedure's drastic change to the patient's body must also be addressed by therapy preoperatively. The quality of life after pelvic exenteration is also important, as the patient will require either lifetime care or rehabilitation, depending upon the surgical outcome, including education and support for ostomy care.

CASE STUDY

Sandy, a 34-year-old female, went to see her gynecologist. She complained of a somewhat vague abdominal pain and said she "felt heavy down there." She was nulliparous and appeared to be in good health otherwise. The laboratory studies were normal. The bimanual pelvic examination revealed irregularly shaped nodules on the uterus. They felt rather firm and immobile. They moved when the uterus moved. Sonography confirmed the presence of tumors. After a period of conservative treatment, Sandy was admitted to the local facility for surgery.

1. Sandy's symptoms are consistent with what diagnosis?
2. This condition is treated with what surgical procedure when the patient hopes to bear children? What other procedure could be used for treatment?
3. What are the common complications of the procedure Sandy will undergo?

QUESTIONS FOR FURTHER STUDY

1. List five reasons for performing a cesarean section and state the most frequent reason for this procedure.
2. What steps performed in a traditional vaginal hysterectomy may be performed laparoscopically? What is the advantage of the laparoscopic approach?
3. Define and list the basic steps in a Pfannenstiel abdominal incision.
4. List the structures that will be removed during a total pelvic exenteration.
5. Name at least two medications that can be used to treat uterine hemorrhage following childbirth.
6. Briefly, describe how the sequence of events for an emergency cesarean section (e.g., prolapsed umbilical cord, placenta abruptio) may differ from a planned cesarean section.

BIBLIOGRAPHY

Allen, G. (1998). Infertility: Resolving the causal factors. *The surgical technologist 30*(8).

Anderson, J. R., & Genadry, R. (1996). Anatomy and embryology. In J. S. Berek, E. Y. Adashi, & P. A. Hillard (Eds.), *Novak's gynecology* (12th ed.). Philadelphia: Williams and Wilkins.

Baggish, M. S., & DeLeon, F. D. (1997). Lasers in gynecology. In J. J. Sciarra (Ed.), *Gynecology and obstetrics* (rev.). New York: Lippincott-Raven.

Bannister, L. H. (1996). *Gray's anatomy* (38th ed.). New York: Churchill Livingstone.

Brumsted, J. R., & Riddick, D. H. (1994). Menstruation and disorders of menstrual function. In J. R. Scott, F. H. Diasaia, C. Hammond, & W. Spellacy (Eds.), *Danforth's obstetrics and gynecology* (7th ed.). Phildelphia: J. B. Lippincott.

Butler, W. J. (1997). Normal and abnormal uterine bleeding. In J. A. Rock & J. D. Thompson (Eds.), *Te Linde's operative gynecology* (8th ed.). Philadelphia: Lippincott-Raven.

Caruthers, B. L. (1994). Pregnancy-induced hypertension as a precipitating factor for DIC, part 1. *The Surgical Technologist 26*(3).

Caruthers, B. L. (1994). Pregnancy-induced hypertension as a precipitating factor for DIC, part 2. *The Surgical Technologist 26*(4).

Caruthers, B. L. (1998). Ectopic pregnancy. *The Surgical Technologist 30*(12).

Caruthers, B. L. (1999). Fetal lung development. *The Surgical Technologist 33*(3).

Caruthers, B. L. (1999). Kidney development and function in the fetus. *The Surgical Technologist 31*(1).

Chez, R. A., & Mischell, D. R. (1994). Total control of human reproduction: Contraception, sterilization, and pregnancy termination. In J. R. Scott, F. H. Diasaia, C. Hammond, & W. Spellacy (Eds.), *Danforth's obstetrics and gynecology* (7th ed.). Phildelphia: J. B. Lippincott.

Clarke-Pearson, D. L., Olt, G. H., Rodriquez, G. C., & Boente, M. P. (1996). Preoperative evaluation and postoperative management. In J. S. Berek, E. Y. Adashi, & P. A. Hillard (Eds.), *Novak's gynecology* (12th ed.). Philadelphia: Williams and Wilkins.

Creasman, W. T. (1994). Disorders of the uterine corpus. In J. R. Scott, F. H. Diasaia, C. Hammond, & W. Spellacy (Eds.), *Danforth's obstetrics and gynecology* (7th ed.). Philadelphia: J. B. Lippincott.

Cromer, D. W. (1997). Postpartum sterilization procedures. In J. J. Sciarra (Ed.), *Gynecology and obstetrics* (rev.). New York: Lippincott-Raven.

Cruikshank, S. H. (1997). Vaginal hysterectomy. In J. J. Sciarra (Ed.), *Gynecology and obstetrics* (rev.). New York: Lippincott-Raven

Cunningham, F. G. (1997). *Williams obstetrics* (20th ed.). Stamford, CT: Appleton and Lange.

Daniels, R. K., & Terzis, J. K. (1997). *Reconstructive microsurgery*. Boston: Little, Brown.

De Cherney, A. H. (1990). Infertility: General principles of evaluation. In N. G. Kase, A. B. Weingold, & D. M. Gershenson (Eds.), *Principles and practices of clinical gynecology* (2nd ed.). New York: Churchill Livingstone.

DeLancey, J. O. L. (1994). Pelvic organ prolapse. In J. R. Scott, F. H. Diasaia, C. Hammond, & W. Spellacy (Eds.), *Danforth's obstetrics and gynecology* (7th ed.). Phildelphia: J. B. Lippincott.

DeLancey, J. O. L. (1997). Surgical anatomy of the female pelvis. In J. A. Rock & J. D. Thompson (Eds.), *Te Linde's operative gynecology* (8th ed.). Philadelphia: Lippincott-Raven.

DeLeon, F. D., & Peters, A. J. (1997). Reversal of female sterilization. In J. J. Sciarra (Ed.), *Gynecology and obstetrics* (rev.). New York: Lippincott-Raven.

Del Priore, G. (1997). Vulvar intraepithelial neoplasms. In J. J. Sciarra (Ed.), *Gynecology and obstetrics* (rev.). New York: Lippincott-Raven.

DiSaia, P. J. (1994). Disorders of the uterine cervix. In J. R. Scott, F. H. Diasaia, C. Hammond, & W. Spellacy (Eds.), *Danforth's obstetrics and gynecology* (7th ed.). Phildelphia: J. B. Lippincott.

DiSaia, P. J. (1994). Radiation therapy in gynecology. In J. R. Scott, F. H. Diasaia, C. Hammond, & W. Spellacy (Eds.), *Danforth's obstetrics and gynecology* (7th ed.). Phildelphia: J. B. Lippincott.

DiSaia, P. J. (1994). Vulvar and vaginal disease. In J. R. Scott, F. H. Diasaia, C. Hammond, & W. Spellacy (Eds.), *Danforth's obstetrics and gynecology* (7th ed.). Phildelphia: J. B. Lippincott.

DiSaia, P. J., & Creasman, W. T. (1997). *Clinical gynecology oncology*. New York: Mosby-Year Book.

DiSaia, P. J., & Walker, J. L. (1994). Perioperative care. In J. R. Scott, F. H. Diasaia, C. Hammond, & W. Spellacy (Eds.), *Danforth's obstetrics and gynecology* (7th ed.). Phildelphia: J. B. Lippincott.

Dorsey, J. H. (1997). Application of laser in gynecology. In J. A. Rock & J. D. Thompson (Eds.), *Te Linde's operative gynecology* (8th ed.). Philadelphia: Lippincott-Raven.

Dorsey, J. H. (1997). Application of laser in surgery. In J. A. Rock & J. D. Thompson (Eds.), *Te Linde's operative gynecology* (8th ed.). Philadelphia: Lippincott-Raven.

Droegmueller, W. (1996). Benign gynecological lesions. In D. R. Mishell, M. A. Stenchever, W. Droegemueller, & A. L. Herbst (Eds.), *Comprehensive gynecology* (3rd ed.). St. Louis, MO: Mosby-Year Book.

Eifel, P. J., Morris, M., Delclos, L., & Wharton, J. T. (1997). Radiation therapy for cervical carcinoma. In J. J. Sciarra (Ed.), *Gynecology and obstetrics* (rev.). New York: Lippincott-Raven.

Elkins, T. E., & Arrowsmith, S. (1997). Repair of urogenital and rectovaginal fistulas. In J. J. Sciarra (Ed.), *Gynecology and obstetrics* (rev.). New York: Lippincott-Raven.

Estes, M. E. Z. (1998). *Health assessment and physical examination*. Clifton Park, NY: Delmar Learning.

Gallup, D. G. (1997). Incisions for gynecologic surgery. In J. A. Rock & J. D. Thompson (Eds.), *Te Linde's operative gynecology* (8th ed.). Philadelphia: Lippincott-Raven.

Gallup, D. G., & Hoskins, W. J. (1997). Surgical principles in gynecologic oncology. In W. J. Hoskins, C. A. Perez, & R. C. Young (Eds.), *Principles and practices of gynecologic oncology* (2nd ed.). Philadelphia: Lippincott-Raven.

Gomel, V. (1997). Reconstructive tubal surgery. In J. A. Rock & J. D. Thompson (Eds.), *Te Linde's operative gynecology* (8th ed.). Philadelphia: Lippincott-Raven.

Gomel, V., & Wang, I. (1994). Laparoscopic surgery for infertility therapy. In *Current opinions in obstetrics and gynecology*. Vancouver: University of British Columbia.

Grifio, J. A., & DeCherney, A. H. (1997). Myomectomy. In J. J. Sciarra (Ed.), *Gynecology and obstetrics* (rev.). New York: Lippincott-Raven.

Grimes, D. A. (1997). Management of abortion. In J. A. Rock & J. D. Thompson (Eds.), *Te Linde's operative gynecology* (8th ed.). Philadelphia: Lippincott-Raven.

Grody, M. H. T. (1997). Posterior compartment defects. In J. A. Rock & J. D. Thompson (Eds.), *Te Linde's operative gynecology* (8th ed.). Philadelphia: Lippincott-Raven.

Guyton, A. C. (1998). *Textbook of medical physiology* (9th ed.). Philadelphia: W. B. Saunders.

Hacker, N. F. (1996). Vulvar cancer. In J. S. Berek, E. Y. Adashi, & P. A. Hillard (Eds.), *Novak's gynecology* (12th ed.). Philadelphia: Williams and Wilkins.

Hacker, N. F., & Moore, J. G. (1998). *Essentials of obstetrics and gynecology* (3rd ed.). Philadelphia: W. B. Saunders.

Hammond, C. B. (1994). Infertility. In J. R. Scott, F. H. Diasaia, C. Hammond, & W. Spellacy (Eds.), *Danforth's obstetrics and gynecology* (7th ed.). Phildelphia: J. B. Lippincott.

Hatch, K. D., & Hacker, N. F. (1996). Intraepithelial disease of the cervix, vagina, and vulva. In J. S. Berek, E. Y. Adashi, & P. A. Hillard (Eds.), *Novak's gynecology* (12th ed.). Philadelphia: Williams and Wilkins.

Herbst, A. L. (1992). Principles of radiation therapy and chemotherapy in gynecologic cancer. In A. L. Herbst & D. R. Mischell (Eds.), *Comprehensive gynecology*. St. Louis, MO: Mosby-Year Book.

Horbelt, D. V., & Delmore, J. E. (1997). Benign neoplasms of the vulva. In J. J. Sciarra (Ed.), *Gynecology and obstetrics* (rev.). Philadelphia: Lippincott-Raven.

Horowitz, I. R., Buscema, J., & Woodruff, J. D. (1997). Surgical conditions of the vulva. In J. A. Rock & J. D. Thompson (Eds.), *Te Linde's operative gynecology* (8th ed.). Philadelphia: Lippincott-Raven.

Hulka, J. F. (1997). Dilatation and curettage. In J. J. Sciarra (Ed.), *Gynecology and obstetrics* (rev.). New York: Lippincott-Raven.

Isaacs, J. H. (1997). Posterior colpoperineorrahpy. In J. J. Sciarra (Ed.), *Gynecology and obstetrics* (rev.). New York: Lippincott-Raven.

Isaacson, K. B., & Schiff, I. (1994). Surgery for infertility. In P. J. Morris & R. A. Malt (Eds.), *Oxford textbook of surgery*. New York: Oxford.

Kase, N. (1997). Infertility: General principles of evaluation. In J. A. Rock & J. D. Thompson (Eds.), *Te Linde's operative gynecology* (8th ed.). Philadelphia: Lippincott-Raven.

Lee, R. A. (1997). Combined compartment defects. In J. A. Rock & J. D. Thompson (Eds.), *Te Linde's operative gynecology* (8th ed.). Philadelphia: Lippincott-Raven.

Martin, D. C. (1990). Laser safety. In W. R. Keye, Jr. (Ed.), *Laser surgery in gynecology and obstetrics*. Littleton, MA: Year Book Medical Publishers.

Martin, D. G. (1996). Ovarian cystectomy. In *Endoscopic management of gynecologic disease*. Philadelphia: Lippencott-Raven.

McGuiness, A. M., et al. (2002). *Core curriculum for surgical technology* (5th ed.). Centennial, CO: Association of Surgical Technologists.

Miltex Instrument Co., Inc. (1996). *Miltex surgical instruments*. Lake Success, NY: Author.

Mischell, D. R., Jr. (1997). Family planning. In D. R. Mischell, Jr., W. Droegemueller, M. A. Stenchever, & A. L. Herbst (Eds.), *Comprehensive gynecology*. St. Louis, MO: Mosby-Year Book.

Morley, G. W., Hopkins, M. P., & Johnston, C. M. (1997). Pelvic exenteration. In J. A. Rock & J. D. Thompson (Eds.), *Te Linde's operative gynecology* (8th ed.). Philadelphia: Lippincott-Raven.

Muckle, C. W. (1997). Clinical anatomy of the uterus, fallopian tubes, and ovaries. In J. J. Sciarra (Ed.), *Gynecology and obstetrics* (rev.). Philadelphia: Lippincott-Raven.

Nichols, D. H., & Milley, P. S. (1997). Clinical anatomy of the vulva, vagina, lower pelvis, and perineum. In J. J. Sciarra (Ed.), *Gynecology and obstetrics* (rev.). Philadelphia: Lippincott-Raven.

Nichols, D. H., & Ponchak, S. F. (1997). Anterior and posterior colporrhaphy. In L. M. Nyhus, R. J. Baker, & J. E. Fischer (Eds.), *Mastery of surgery*. New York: Little, Brown.

Noller, K. L., & Wagner, A. L., Jr. (1997). Colposcopy. In J. J. Sciarra (Ed.), *Gynecology and obstetrics* (rev.). Philadelphia: Lippincott-Raven.

Partridge, E. E. (1997). Pelvic exenteration. In J. J. Sciarra (Ed.), *Gynecology and obstetrics* (rev.). Philadelphia: Lippincott-Raven.

Peterson, H. B., Pollack, A. E., & Warshaw, J. S. (1997). Tubal sterilization. In J. A. Rock & J. D. Thompson (Eds.), *Te Linde's operative gynecology* (8th ed.). Philadelphia: Lippincott-Raven.

Porges, R. F. (1997). Anterior colporraphy. In J. J. Sciarra (Ed.), *Gynecology and obstetrics* (rev.). Philadelphia: Lippincott-Raven.

Richart, R. M. (1997). Cervical cancer precursors and their management. In J. A. Rock & J. D. Thompson (Eds.), *Te Linde's operative gynecology* (8th ed.). Philadelphia: Lippincott-Raven.

Rock, J. A., & Damario, M. A. (1997). Ectopic pregnancy. In J. A. Rock & J. D. Thompson (Eds.), *Te Linde's operative gynecology* (8th ed.). Philadelphia: Lippincott-Raven.

Rock, J. A., & Keenan, D. L. (1997). Surgical corrections of uterovaginal anomalies. In J. J. Sciarra (Ed.), *Gynecology and obstetrics* (rev.). Philadelphia: Lippincott-Raven.

Sakala, E. P. (1997). *Obstetrics and gynecology, board review series*. Baltimore: Williams and Wilkins.

Schoeppel, S. L., & Lichter, A. S. (1997). The role of radiation therapy in the treatment of malignant uterine tumors. In J. J. Sciarra (Ed.), *Gynecology and obstetrics* (rev.). Philadelphia: Lippincott-Raven.

Sciarra, J. J. (1997). Surgical procedures for tubal sterilization. In J. J. Sciarra (Ed.), *Gynecology and obstetrics* (rev.). Philadelphia: Lippincott-Raven.

Scott, J. R. (1994). Early pregnancy loss. In J. R. Scott, F. H. Diasaia, C. Hammond, & W. Spellacy (Eds.), *Danforth's obstetrics and gynecology* (7th ed.). Phildelphia: J. B. Lippincott.

Siegler, A. M. (1997). Salpingotomy and salpingectomy: Indications and techniques for tubal pregnancy. In J. J. Sciarra (Ed.), *Gynecology and obstetrics* (rev.). Philadelphia: Lippincott-Raven.

Stovall, T. G. (1996). Hysterectomy. In J. S. Berek, E. Y. Adashi, & P. A. Hillard (Eds.), *Novak's gynecology* (12th ed.). Philadelphia: Williams and Wilkins.

Stubblefield, P. G. (1996). Family planning. In J. S. Berek, E. Y. Adashi, & P. A. Hillard (Eds.), *Novak's gynecology* (12th ed.). Philadelphia: Williams and Wilkins.

Thompson, J. D. (1997). Pelvic organ prolapse. In J. A. Rock & J. D. Thompson (Eds.), *Te Linde's operative gynecology* (8th ed.) Philadelphia: Lippincott-Raven.

Thompson, J. D. (1997). Vesicovaginal and urethrovaginal fistulas. In J. A. Rock & J. D. Thompson (Eds.), *Te Linde's operative gynecology* (8th ed.). Philadelphia: Lippincott-Raven.

Thompson, J. D., & Shull, B. L. (1997). Anterior compartment defects. In J. A. Rock & J. D. Thompson (Eds.), *Te Linde's operative gynecology* (8th ed.). Philadelphia: Lippincott-Raven.

Thompson, J. D., & Warshaw, J. S. (1997). Hysterectomy. In J. A. Rock & J. D. Thompson (Eds.), *Te Linde's operative gynecology* (8th ed.). Philadelphia: Lippincott-Raven.

Wall, L. L. (1996). Incontinence, prolapse, and disorders of the pelvic floor. In J. S. Berek, E. Y. Adashi, & P. A. Hillard (Eds.), *Novak's gynecology* (12th ed.). Philadelphia: Williams and Wilkins.

Wallach, E. E. (1997). The mechanism of ovulation. In J. J. Sciarra (Ed.), *Gynecology and obstetrics* (rev.). Philadelphia: Lippincott-Raven.

Walton, L. A., & Van Le, L. (1997). Reconstructive surgery following treatment of female genital tract malignancies. In J. J. Sciarra (Ed.), *Gynecology and obstetrics* (rev.). Philadelphia: Lippincott-Raven.

Wells, E. C. (1997). Abdominal hysterectomy and bilateral salpingo-oophorectomy. In J. J. Sciarra (Ed.), *Gynecology and obstetrics* (rev.). Philadelphia: Lippincott-Raven.

Wright, T. C., & Ferenczy, A. (1994). Precancerous lesions of the cervix. In R. J. Kurman (Ed.), *Blaustein's pathology of the female genital tract*. New York: Springer-Verlag.

Zaino, R. J., Robboy, S. J., Bentley, R., & Kurman, R. J. (1994). Diseases of the vagina. In R. J. Kurman (Ed.), *Blaustein's pathology of the female genital tract*. New York: Springer-Verlag.

CHAPTER 16

Ophthalmic Surgery

Jim Swalley
Ben D. Price
Paul Price

CASE STUDY

Heather has been referred to the ophthalmic surgeon because her symptoms have not improved after several weeks of more conservative treatment. She has been suffering pain in her left eye, and the area beneath her eye and next to her nose is red, painful, and inflamed. The area is sensitive to touch, and for several days a discharge has been present on the nasal side of the eye.

1. What must have been the diagnosis that caused the patient's doctor to refer her to a surgeon?
2. What will be the most probable surgical intervention?
3. What special anesthesia needs directly related to the particular surgical procedure will need to be met?

OBJECTIVES

After studying this chapter, the reader should be able to:

A 1. Discuss the anatomy of the eye.

P 2. Describe the pathology that prompts surgical intervention of the eye and related terminology.

3. Discuss any special preoperative ophthalmic diagnostic procedures/tests.

O 4. Discuss any special preoperative preparation procedures.

5. Identify the names and uses of ophthalmic instruments, supplies, and drugs.
6. Identify the names and uses of special equipment.
7. Discuss the intraoperative preparation of the patient undergoing an ophthalmic procedure.
8. Define and give an overview of the ophthalmic procedure.

9. Discuss the purpose and expected outcomes of the ophthalmic procedure.
10. Discuss the immediate postoperative care and possible complications of the ophthalmic procedure.
11. **S** Discuss any specific variations related to the preoperative, intraoperative, and postoperative care of the ophthalmic patient.

SELECT KEY TERMS

1. anterior chamber	7. enucleation	11. intracapsular cataract extraction	16. posterior chamber
2. BSS	8. extracapsular cataract extraction	12. iridotomy	17. retrobulbar
3. cataract	9. extrinsic muscles	13. kerato-	18. strabismus
4. chalazion	10. globe	14. lacrimal	19. trephine
5. dacryo-		15. ocutome	20. tunic
6. diathermy			

ANATOMY OF THE EYE

The eye is the sensory organ of sight (refer to Plate 3 in Appendix A). The main function of the eye is to convert environmental light energy into bioelectrical energy and to relay the information to the brain for processing. Much like the brain, the eye itself is substantially protected by surrounding bony structures.

ORBIT

Seven bones—the frontal, sphenoid, ethmoid, superior maxillary, malar (zygomatic), **lacrimal**, and palate—form the orbit of the eye (Figure 16-1). Three of these bones, the frontal, ethmoid and sphenoid, combine to form both orbits. Consequently, only 11 bones form the two cavities. Each orbital cavity presents a roof, floor, inner and outer wall, four angles, a circumference or base, and an apex. The roof is concave, is directed downward and slightly forward, and is formed in front by the orbital plate of the frontal bone. The lesser wing of the sphenoid forms posteriorly. This surface provides the depression for the cartilaginous pulley of the superior oblique muscle. The depression for the lacrimal gland is situated externally. The suture connecting the frontal and lesser wing of the sphenoid is positioned posteriorly.

The floor is directed upward and outward and is of less extent than the roof. It is formed chiefly by the orbital process of the superior maxilla, in front, to a small extent, by the orbital process of the malar bone, and behind, by the superior surface of the orbital process of the palate.

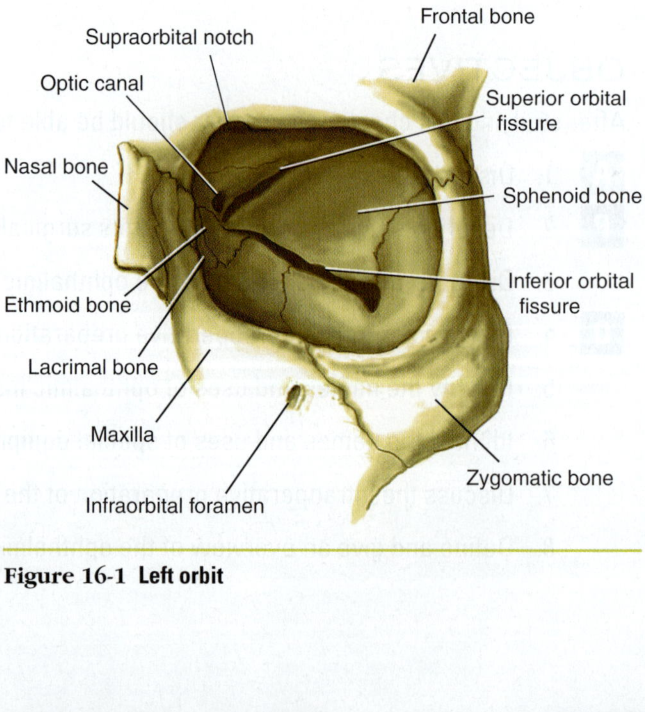

Figure 16-1 Left orbit

The orbital floor presents at its anterior and internal portion (just external to the lacrimal groove), a depression for the attachment of the inferior oblique muscle; externally, the suture between the malar and superior maxillary bones; near its middle, the infraorbital groove; and posteriorly, the suture between the maxilla and the palatine bones.

EXTRINSIC MUSCLES

The **extrinsic muscles** of the eye come from the bones of the orbit and are movable. Broad tendons attach to the eye's outer surface (Figure 16-2). Six muscles function to move the eye in various directions and, although any eye movement may involve more than one muscle, each muscle is associated with one primary movement.

The six extrinsic muscles of the eye and the primary function of each are:

- *Superior rectus:* rotates the eye upward and toward the midline
- *Inferior rectus:* rotates the eye downward and toward the midline
- *Medial rectus:* rotates the eye toward the midline
- *Lateral rectus:* rotates the eye away from the midline
- *Superior oblique:* rotates the eye downward and away from the midline
- *Inferior oblique:* rotates the eye upward and away from the midline

Two check ligaments (the lateral and medial check ligaments) limit the movement of the lateral and medial rectus. The motor units of these eye muscles contain the smallest number of muscle fibers (5 to 10) of any muscle in the body. Because of this, the eyes move together so that they are aligned when looking at something.

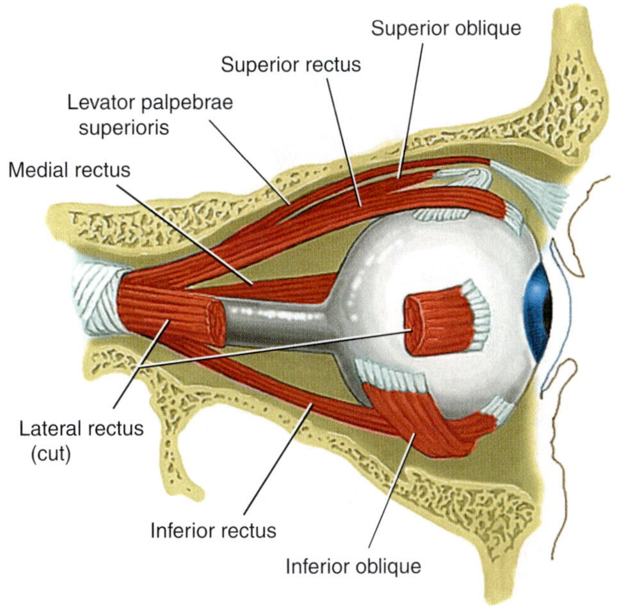

Figure 16-2 Extrinsic muscles of the eye

Both eyes "target" the desired scene so that the focused image falls onto the retina at the back of the eye at corresponding locations. Each retinal-receiving unit, called *rods* and *cones,* has a matching unit in the other eye. If the focused image falls on "corresponding" areas of each retina, the brain can use this information to perceive a stereoscopic image resulting in depth perception.

LACRIMAL SYSTEM

The lacrimal system consists of the lacrimal gland, which secretes the tears that keep the conjunctiva moist, and its excretory ducts, which convey the fluid to the surface of the eye (Figure 16-3). This fluid is carried away by the lacrimal canals into the lacrimal sac, and along the nasolacrimal duct into the cavity of the nose.

The lacrimal gland is located within the upper eyelid near the outer angle of the orbit, on the inner side of the external angular process of the frontal bone. It is oval in shape, about the size of an almond, and is connected by a few fibrous bands to the periosteum of the orbit. The surface rests upon the convexity of the eyeball and upon the superior and external recti muscles. Vessels and nerves enter at the posterior border, while the anterior margin is closely approximated to the back part of the upper eyelid where it is covered by a slight reflection of the conjunctiva. Six to 12 ducts exit the lacrimal gland and run obliquely beneath the mucous membrane. After a short distance, the ducts separate from one another and open through a series of minute orifices on the upper, outer portion of the conjunctiva near the reflection onto the globe. These orifices are arranged in a row, dispersing the secretion over the surface of the conjunctiva.

LACRIMAL CANALS

The lacrimal canals are located at the minute orifices called *punctum lacrimale* on the summit of a small conical

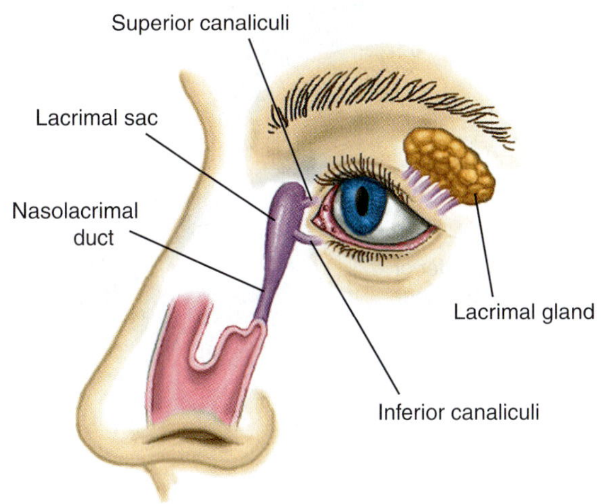

Figure 16-3 Lacrimal system

elevation called the *lacrimal papilla* on the margin of the lids at the outer extremity of the lacus lacrimalis. The superior canal is the smaller and shorter of the two; it ascends then bends at an angle then passes downward to the lacrimal sac. The inferior canal descends, then passes horizontally inward to the lacrimal sac.

LACRIMAL SAC

The lacrimal sac is a dilated segment of the nasal duct. It is positioned in a deep grove formed by the lacrimal bone and nasal process of the superior maxillary bone. Its shape is oval; the upper area is closed in and rounded then narrows into the nasolacrimal duct.

GLOBE

The **globe** is the eyeball in its entirety. The human eye is the organ of sight (Figure 16-4). It is often compared to a camera. Like a sophisticated camera, the eye has multiple parts which must function together properly to produce clear vision.

CONJUNCTIVA

The conjunctiva is the mucous membrane covering the eye. The conjunctiva lines the inner surface of the eyelid and reflects over the forepart of the sclera and the cornea. It is opaque and highly vascular. At the outer margin of the upper lid, the lacrimal ducts open onto the conjuncti-

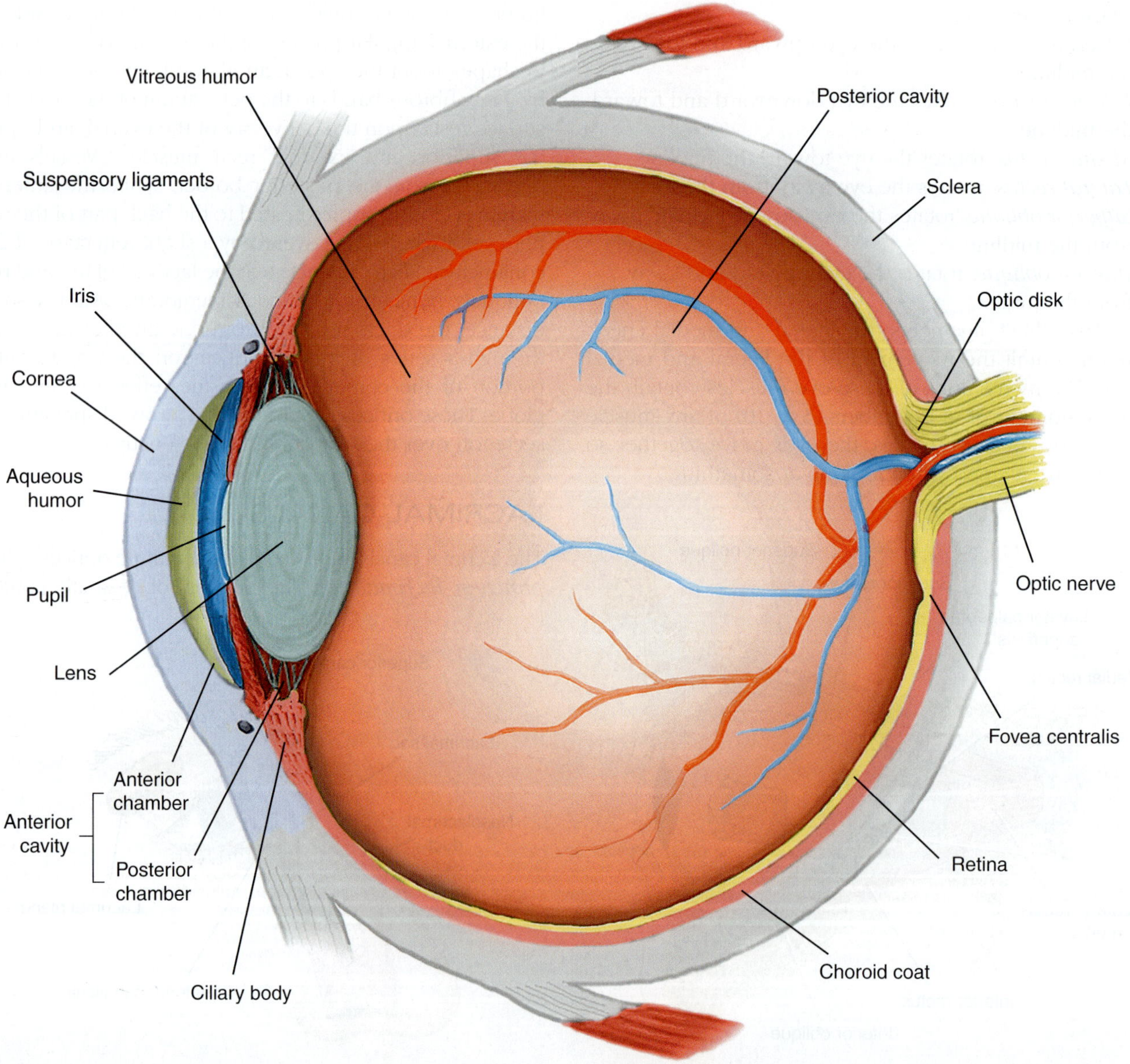

Figure 16-4 Sagittal section of the eye

val surface. On the sclera, the conjunctiva is loosely connected to the globe becoming thinner and transparent. The corneal surface consists only of epithelium.

SCLERA AND CORNEA

The sclera and cornea form the external **tunic** of the eye. Both are essentially fibrous in structure. The sclera is opaque, forming the posterior five-sixths of the globe. The cornea forms the remaining transparent sixth.

The sclera is a firm fibrous membrane that serves to maintain the form of the globe. The posterior portion is the thickest; it thins anteriorly. The external surface is white and smooth except at the points where the rectus and oblique muscles are attached. The conjunctiva covers the anterior portion.

The inner surface of the sclera is brown and marked by grooves, which contain the ciliary nerves and vessels. The sclera is loosely connected by a fine cellular tissue to the outer surface of the choroid.

The cornea is the transparent part of the external tunic of the eye and forms the anterior sixth of the globe. It is almost circular in shape. The degree of curvature of the cornea varies in individuals, and will vary at different periods of life. The cornea tends to be more prominent in youth and flattens with age. It is dense and of a uniform thickness throughout.

The cornea consists of four layers:

- Epithelial cells
- Substantia propria
- Elastic lamina
- Endothelial cells

CHOROID

The choroid is a thin, dark-brown, highly vascular membrane that makes up the posterior five-sixths of the eye. The choroid is pierced from behind by the optic nerve and is firmly adhered to the sclera. It is thicker behind than in front. The inner surface of the choroid attaches to the retina and consists mainly of a dense capillary plexus. The choroid, along with the ciliary body and the iris, makes up the middle tunic of the globe.

CILIARY BODY

The ciliary body is similar in structure to the choroid, but contains larger vessels. The ciliary processes are covered on the inner surface by two layers of black pigment cells, which are anterior continuations of the retina called the *pars ciliaris retinae.*

The ciliary (intrinsic) muscle consists of unstriped fibers that form a grayish, semitransparent, circular band approximately ⅛ in. wide on the outer surface of the forward part of the choroid. The ciliary body is thick anteriorly, gradually thinning posteriorly. It consists of two sets of fibers, one radiating and one circular. The radiating fibers are more numerous and arise from the junction of the cornea and sclera. The muscle fibers are attached to the choroid, opposite the ciliary processes, and follow a circular course around the attachment of the iris. They are sometimes called the *ring muscle.*

IRIS

The iris (meaning "rainbow") is named for its various colors. It is a thin, circular-shaped, contractile curtain suspended in the aqueous humor posterior to the cornea and anterior to the crystalline lens. It is perforated at the center by a circular aperture called the *pupil.* The pupil allows for the transmission of light. The iris is continuous with the ciliary body and connects to the posterior elastic lamina of the cornea by means of the pectinate ligament. The inner edge of the iris forms the margin of the pupil. The anterior surface of the iris is colored and marked by lines that converge toward the pupil. The posterior surface is a deep purple.

RETINA

The retina makes up the inner tunic and is the delicate nervous membrane on which images are received. When examined microscopically the retina is found to consist of 10 layers. The outer surface is in contact with the choroid and its inner surface with the vitreous body. Posteriorly, the retina is continuous with the optic nerve. The anterior portion extends nearly as far as the ciliary body, terminating at a margin called the *ora serrata.* Exactly in the center of the posterior part of the retina, corresponding to the axis of the eye and at a point where the sense of vision is the most accurate, is an oval yellowish spot called the *macula.* The macula has a central depression called the *fovea centralis,* an exceedingly thin area through which can be seen the dark color of the choroid. About one-eighth of an inch to the inner side of the macula and slightly raised is the optic nerve. The arteria centralis retina pierces its center. This is the only part of the retina from which vision is absent, and is called the *blind spot.*

CRYSTALLINE LENS

The crystalline lens is situated behind the pupil, in the *fossa patellaris,* in front of the vitreous body. It is encircled by the ciliary processes, which slightly overlap its margin. It is encapsulated in a transparent, highly elastic, and brittle membrane. Anteriorly, the lens contacts with the border of the iris, which recedes from it at the circumference, forming the **posterior chamber** of the eye. It is held in its position by the suspensory ligament. The lens is a transparent, biconvex body. The central points of its anterior and posterior surfaces are known as its anterior and posterior poles.

CAVITIES AND CHAMBERS OF THE EYE

The anterior cavity of the eye lies in front of the lens and contains two chambers: the **anterior chamber** is the space anterior to the iris, but posterior to the cornea; the posterior chamber consists of a small space directly posterior to the iris, but anterior to the lens. Both chambers of the anterior cavity are filled with a clear, watery fluid called *aqueous humor*. Aqueous humor helps to give the cornea its curved shape and is small in quantity (about four or five grains in weight). The fluid is alkaline and mostly composed of water. Less than 1⁄60th of its weight is solid matter (mainly chloride of sodium).

The posterior cavity of the eye is larger than the anterior cavity, since it occupies all of the space posterior to the lens, suspensory ligaments, and ciliary body. The posterior cavity contains a substance, with a consistency similar to soft gelatin, called *vitreous humor*. Vitreous humor helps maintain sufficient pressure inside the eye to prevent the eyeball from collapsing. The hyaloid membrane encloses the whole of the vitreous humor. In front of the *ora serrata* it is thickened by radial fibers and is termed the *zonule of Zinn* or *zonula ciliaris*.

OPHTHALMIC SURGICAL PATHOLOGY

Numerous conditions affect the ophthalmic system. Some of these may be systemic, as in diabetes mellitis. Some conditions are primarily neurological in nature, such as stroke and neoplasm. Trauma results in pathological conditions affecting the visual system. The most common conditions related to ophthalmic surgery are discussed below.

GLAUCOMA

As a review, the optic nerve is a bundle of thousands of nerve fibers that connects the retina with the brain. In the front of the eye is the space called the anterior chamber located between the cornea and iris. Aqueous fluid flows through the space to provide nourishment to the tissues of the eye and maintain the shape of the eye. The fluid exits the anterior chamber at the angle where the cornea and iris meet. At the angle is the trabecular meshwork through which the fluid travels to drain from the eye through small blood vessels. Hence the name *angle closure glaucoma,* which refers to the inability of the aqueous fluid to exit the eye at the correct angle due to blockage by the iris. This places extreme pressure on the optic nerve, creating a condition called *glaucoma*.

Glaucoma is a leading cause of blindness in the United States. It is an insidious disease that rarely causes any symptoms until it has reached advanced stages. Angle closure glaucoma is an emergency situation that presents with the following symptoms: sudden decrease in vision; eye pain, often severe; headache; sensitivity to light; nausea and vomiting; and a rapid increase in intraocular pressure.

CATARACT

The word **cataract** is used to describe a crystalline lens that has become opaque due to age or trauma. Cataracts are a condition affecting the eye, not a disease. As the lens gradually clouds, light is unable to pass through as well as it did when the lens was transparent. A cataract begins with a slight cloudiness and progressively grows more opaque. Cataracts are usually white, but may take on a yellow or brown color. As the cataract matures, less light is able to pass, blurring and distorting images received by the retina. Vision is gradually impaired; if untreated, a cataract can cause needless blindness.

The development of cataracts is a normal part of the aging process, but they can also result from a number of other reasons. Cataracts due to aging are a result of natural changes in the lens that coincide with other changes in the body, but traumatic cataracts may result from an injury or blow to the eye. Other causes of cataracts include the use of certain drugs or medications, exposure to harmful chemicals or excessive sunlight, and some diseases. Some infants are born with congenital cataracts.

SMALL RETINAL DETACHMENT

When a person develops a retinal detachment, flashes of light or large spots in the vision may occur. The flashes of light are caused by the tugging of the vitreous where it is attached to the retina. The brain interprets this pulling as flashing of light. As the vitreous pulls away from the retina, the fluid becomes somewhat condensed and stringy, forming strands, seen as spots.

Sometimes a small retinal detachment develops around a retinal tear. Frequently this can be repaired by either laser or cryotherapy alone. It may break through the scar, however, and develop a retinal detachment. This would be experienced as a loss of peripheral vision.

LARGE RETINAL DETACHMENT

When a tear occurs, the liquid in the vitreous cavity may pass through the tear and get under the retina, separating it from the back wall (choroid) of the eye. This separation is called a retinal detachment. Vision is lost wherever the retina becomes detached. A patient may notice a dark shadow, or a veil, coming from one side, above, or below. Eventually the entire retina will detach and all useful vision in the eye will be lost.

VITREOUS HEMORRHAGE

When a retinal tear occurs, blood vessels may also be torn and a vitreous hemorrhage may occur. Because of the tear, a detachment may also occur. A vitrectomy must be performed to remove the blood so the surgeon can see if there is a detachment.

PROLIFERATIVE VITREORETINOPATHY (PVR)

Excessive scar tissue causes scleral buckles to fail approximately 5–10% of the time. The scar tissue pulls on the retina, causing it to re-detach. The scar tissue also puckers the retina into stiff folds. The vitreous pulls on the retina, detaching it from the back wall of the eye. This condition is called proliferative vitreoretinopathy, or PVR.

TRACTION RETINAL DETACHMENT

When vitreous pulls on scar tissue, the retina may detach. This is called traction retinal detachment. When the detachment involves the macula, central vision is lost. Scar tissue may wrinkle the retina and cause visual loss. The vitreous and scar tissue are surgically removed from the surface of the retina, releasing the traction.

EPIRETINAL MEMBRANE

Scar tissue, which forms over the macula, is termed epiretinal membrane. This membrane may be removed surgically.

CORNEAL PATHOLOGY

To perform properly, the cornea must be clear and be of a proper curvature. If the cornea is not perfectly clear or if it is irregular or damaged, vision can be dramatically decreased. Replacing the cloudy or damaged cornea with healthy donor tissue via corneal transplant can make a dramatic improvement in vision. There are many causes of clouding of the cornea. They include:

- Eye injuries that leave a dense white scar on the cornea
- Severe corneal infection that leads to corneal scarring (various herpes viruses are known to cause such scarring)
- Corneal dystrophies
- Inherited diseases of the cornea
- Cataract or other eye surgery can prompt corneal clouding

CHALAZION

A **chalazion** is a small lump on the inner or outer surface of the eyelid. It is caused by an inflammatory reaction to material trapped inside an oil-secreting gland in the eyelid. A chalazion can develop when an eyelid gland becomes blocked. A red, swollen area of the eyelid often characterizes chalazion.

PTERYGIUM

A pterygium is a wedge-shaped fibrovascular growth of conjunctiva that extends onto the cornea. Pterygia are benign lesions that can be found on either side of the cornea. Prolonged exposure to ultraviolet light may contribute to the formation of pterygia, and they are often seen in people from tropical climates.

Most pterygia are asymptomatic and may not require treatment. However, some pterygia may become inflamed, and thick pterygia may feel like a foreign body in the eye. For inflammation, an ophthalmologist may recommend a mild steroid eye drop during acute flares. In some cases, surgical removal of the tissue is required if the pterygium is growing far enough onto the cornea to threaten vision or if inflammation is persistent. Some pterygia grow onto the cornea in such a way that they can pull on the surface of the cornea and change the refractive properties of the eye, causing astigmatism that requires surgical removal for correction.

For repair, the pterygium is carefully dissected away. To prevent regrowth of the pterygium, the surgeon may remove some of the conjunctiva and suture it into the bed of the excised pterygium.

DACRYOCYSTITIS

Dacryocystitis, an inflammation of the lacrimal sac, is often caused by an obstruction of the nasolacrimal duct. Typically, the area beneath the eye and adjacent to the nose becomes red and inflamed. The area is sensitive to touch and swollen. Occasionally, a mucous discharge may be seen from the opening at the nasal corner of the eye. Conservative treatment to treat infection may be recommended, but severe cases may require surgical intervention to clear the infection, open the blocked duct, and prevent recurrence.

STRABISMUS

Strabismus is a misalignment or deviation of the eyes that normally work simultaneously to track visual objects. Various forms of strabismus include "crossed eyes" (esotropia) and "wall eyes" (exotropia). For both eyes to be synchronized in their movements and positions, they require about the same vision and accommodative (focusing) ability. The six muscles that move each eye must work together in a coordinated fashion for stereoscopic vision and depth perception. The brain combines, into a single three-dimensional image, the images from each separate eye. If the eyes are not aimed in exactly the same direction, binocular vision is impossible. In a child, an eye that is turned may develop permanent loss of vision; the eye may become amblyopic, that is, a "lazy eye." The strabismus is called *comitant* when the amount of misalignment stays the same no matter which direction the eyes are pointed. Strabismus is called *incomitant* when the amount of misalignment changes as the eyes move to view objects in different directions. There are two basic types of incomitant strabismus: restrictive and paralytic. Variable misalignment is the defining symptom of incomitant strabismus. The eyes may work together normally or be only a little misaligned when looking in one direction, but be very deviated from one another when looking in another direction. *Diplopia* (double vision) may result.

OPHTHALMIC MEDICATIONS

Various drugs are used in preoperative, intraoperative, and postoperative phases of ophthalmic surgery to facilitate diagnosis and treatment of pathological conditions of the eye. The STSR is primarily concerned with the drugs used during the procedure, and must be aware of the various classifications of ophthalmic drugs and their actions.

Mydriatics and cycloplegic drugs cause mydriasis (pupil dilation) by paralyzing the iris of the eye. Mydriatics are used to dilate the pupil for examination of the retina, to prepare the eye for ophthalmoscopy, and to optimize removal of a diseased lens. Cycloplegic drugs paralyze the ciliary muscle. The difference between the two is that mydriatics allow the patient to focus after dilation, whereas cycloplegic drugs inhibit focusing. After these drugs are applied topically, the lacrimal gland must be compressed to prevent rapid absorption. Common mydriatic drugs include atropine sulfate (Atropisol) and phenylephrine (Neo-Synephrine). Common cycloplegic drugs include tropicamide (Mydriacyl) and cyclopentolate (Cyclogyl).

Viscoelastic agents are used to expand the anterior chamber and prevent injury to nearby tissues during cataract extraction, and they are also employed as a vitreous substitute. Chondroitin sulfate-sodium hyaluronate (Viscoat) is a commonly used viscoelastic agent.

Miotics are pupil-constricting agents that act on the sphincter of the iris, and include pilocarpine hydrochloride (Isopto Carpine) and carbachol (Carbacel). They may be administered by injection or topical application. These drugs also facilitate the drainage of aqueous humor through the canal of Schlemm, thus decreasing intraocular pressure. This is especially useful for the treatment of increased intraocular pressure due to glaucoma.

Miotics may be used intraoperatively when pupil constriction is necessary, as in laser iridectomy. Pilocarpine hydrochloride may be used following cataract extraction to maintain the position of the implanted lens.

Hyperosmotic drugs are diuretics that are used preoperatively to shrink the vitreous body, thus reducing intraocular pressure. They are also used intraoperatively to aid scleral closure during retinal detachment repair.

Anti-inflammatory agents include steroids and nonsteroidal anti-inflammatory agents (NSAIDs). Steroids are used in traumatic eye injuries to suppress the inflammatory response, while NSAIDs are used to control postoperative inflammation. Common steroids include prednisolone (PreMild), dexamethasone (Decadron), and betamethasone (Celestone suspension).

Ointment medications are an important part of ophthalmic treatment, especially for external ocular infections. Ophthalmic antibiotic ointments include the aminoglycosides gentamycin, neomycin, and tobramycin.

Lubricants are used to protect the cornea when the eye is unable to close or when natural lubrication of the eye is impaired. Lubricants such as Lacri-lube or Duratears are always used when general anesthesia is administered to prevent corneal drying.

Many ophthalmic procedures are done under local anesthesia. Tetracaine (Pontocaine) and proparacaine (Ophthaine) are the most commonly used local anesthetics. **Retrobulbar** anesthesia may be necessary for some procedures to block both sensory and motor sensations, and this type of anesthesia is accomplished by injecting the area around the optic nerve with lidocaine or bupivacaine. Hyaluronidase (Wydase) or epinephrine may be added to the solution to prolong the duration of the block.

Irrigating solutions are necessary during ophthalmic surgery to keep the cornea from drying out. Balanced salt solution (**BSS**), a sterile, physiologically balanced irrigating fluid, is the irrigant most frequently employed. The STSR will have bottles of 15 or 30 mL available on the sterile field for irrigating the exposed cornea during the procedure.

SPECIAL CONSIDERATIONS IN OPHTHALMIC SURGERY

The ability of the surgical technologist in the scrub role or the surgical technologist in the surgical assistant role—often one in the same in ophthalmic surgery—is very important. Although there may be little for the STSR or surgical assistant to actually do in these procedures, the manner in which things are done is very important, because of the delicate nature of the procedure. Many patients are under local anesthesia, and therefore the ability of the STSR to anticipate the needs of the surgeon will provide a quiet and more secure atmosphere for the patient. The STSR must be familiar with specialized equipment, such as the **diathermy** probe, and specialized microscopic instrumentation required for ophthalmic surgery.

SPECIAL EQUIPMENT

Eye surgeons typically develop a small set of favored instruments for their own personal use, and these may be modified to suit personal tastes. Every instrument should be examined by the STSR before the procedure to ensure that it is in perfect operating condition. Disposable instruments should be examined as they are opened.

Blades that are spotted or stained should be discarded. Scissors should be tested for proper alignment and ease of movement.

SUTURE NEEDLES

Standard needles used in ophthalmic surgery are listed in Table 16-1.

SUTURE MATERIALS

The standard suture materials used in ophthalmic surgery are listed in Table 16-2.

INSTRUMENTS

Instruments for eye surgery include various microsurgical instruments, and, as stated above, surgeons usually develop their own small sets to suit their own particular tastes. Commonly used instruments include:

Forceps

- Colibri forceps: for holding the edges of corneal and scleral incisions
- Nontoothed forceps: for holding skin edges in eyelid procedures and for holding the conjunctiva for suturing

Table 16-1 Suture Needles for Ophthalmic Surgery

TYPE	DESCRIPTION	USE
Round bodied	Available with plain collagen and polyglactin	Conjunctival closure
Round bodied with cutting tip (tapercut)	Initially cuts like cutting needle, minimal trauma	Lacrimal sac and nasal mucosa
Reverse cutting (micropoint)	Triangular needle with third cutting edge on the outside of curvature	Eliminates possibility of outward tearing while suturing
Spatula micropoint	Fine needles with thin flat profile	Corneal and corneoscleral suturing
Spatulated	Similar to spatula	Scleral passage in strabismus correction, retinal detachment repair

Table 16-2 Suture Materials for Ophthalmic Surgery

TYPE	DESCRIPTION	USE
Nonabsorbable		
Monofilament nylon	Strong monofilament; does not support bacterial growth	Corneal incision closure
Monofilament polypropylene	Supple nonabsorbable; ties well	Intraocular lens fixation
Polybutilate-coated braided polyester	Multifilament braided coated with polybutilate for lubrication and smooth passage	Scleral tissue, retinal surgery
Braided silk	Silk	Various
Absorbable		
Plain and chromic gut	Plain loses half strength in 5–7 days and all strength in 15 days; chromic loses half strength in 17–21 days and all strength in 30 days	Various
Extruded collagen	Bovine tendon; consistent in strength; absorbs at about the same rate as catgut	Various
Polyglactin (Vicryl)	Braided synthetic suture, less irritating than gut, absorbable coating; absorbs in 60–90 days, but retains strength for 30 days	Various

Needle Holders

- Castroviejo: locking needle holder
- Microsurgical needle holder: available with various shaped tips, locking needle holder

Scalpels

- Graefe cataract knife
- Keratomes (disposable): available in various angles
- Razor fragments: broken from razor blades and placed in holders
- Diamond knife
- Oscillating knife

Hooks and Retractors

- Scleral hooks: scleral retraction
- Kilner hook: reconstructive surgery
- Lid retractors
- Iris retractor

Scissors

- Westcott scissors, spring action microscissors: useful in strabismus and conjunctiva operations
- Small spring scissors: intraocular use

Diathermy Apparatus

- Used in surgical treatment of retinal detachment (although not as frequently as cryotherapy)
- Used to destroy extraocular neoplasms
- Bipolar diathermy (wet-field coagulator): miniaturized version of the bipolar electrocautery unit, used to achieve hemostasis

Cryotherapy Unit

- Used in treatment of retinal detachment
- Uses localized cold temperature to seal tears and holes much as a diathermy unit; CO_2 gas passed is under pressure through flexible tubes to the tip of a probe
- Controlled by foot switch

SURGICAL INTERVENTION

A variety of surgical procedures and approaches are available to the ophthalmic surgeon and patient.

SURGICAL REPAIR OF PTOSIS

Ptosis is a drooping of the upper eyelid and may be congenital or acquired. Congential ptosis is marked by a dystrophy of the levator muscle. The majority of cases are unilateral, but it can be bilateral with associated weakness of the superior rectus muscle. In terms of clinical characteristics, the eye may look smaller than normal due to the drooping eyelid. The lid crease is decreased or absent where the levator muscle would normally insert just below the skin surface. The levator muscle is replaced by fibrous tissue that does not allow the lid to move when gazing downward. This is referred to as *lid lag*. The child may attempt to compensate for lid lag by lifting the eyebrow or tilting the head upward. Acquired ptosis is due to either third cranial nerve palsy or a gradual weakness of the levator aponeurosis.

Surgery is performed to restore the function of the eyelid by creating an upper lid fold combined with elevation of the lid. Surgical procedures have been developed to correct muscles that are responsible for the elevating actions of the lid—levator aponeurosis, frontalis muscles, or combined levator and Muller's muscles.

Two popular procedures are the levator aponeurosis repair and frontalis suspension. Frontalis suspension requires the use of suspension material that is placed between the frontalis muscle and the tarsus of the eyelid. Suspension materials include suture, silicone rods, or fascia lata, either cadaver or autologous. The procedures are performed under local anesthesia unless autologous fascia lata is used. General anesthesia is necessary for the incision in the leg. The following is a description of a levator aponeurosis repair:

1. The eyelid region to be resected is identified by the surgeon with a sterile marking pen.
2. Local anesthesia is obtained by injecting lidocaine with epinephrine. (Some surgeons may combine this with Marcaine.)
3. A #15 knife blade is used to make the incision down to the preaponeurotic fat, and the levator aponeurosis is identified.
4. The tarsus is identified.
5. A plane is dissected through the orbicularis at the superior aspect of the tarsus and advanced to the inferior margin of the tarsus. This plane is also widened laterally, temporally, and nasally.
6. The surgeon will use a double-armed 6–0 nonabsorbable suture, usually silk, that is passed through the superior aspect of the levator aponeurosis and then passed through the tarsus.
7. The sutures are tightened to reattach the aponeurosis to the tarsus to achieve the desired level of lid elevation and contour.
8. The sutures are tied and cut.
9. To create the lid crease, 6–0 nonabsorbable suture (frequently Prolene) is used, incorporating the skin, orbicularis, and levator aponeurosis.
10. The skin incision is closed with simple running 6–0 nonabsorbable suture (again, frequently Prolene).

IRIDECTOMY

Iridectomy is the removal of a section of the iris (either surgically or by laser) to relieve the pressure buildup that occurs in individuals with glaucoma. Three types of iridectomy procedures are performed: peripheral, radial, and sector. The procedure is often performed at the same time as a trabeculectomy. As mentioned, a laser iridectomy can be performed for treating angle closure glaucoma. The laser beam creates a small hole in the peripheral portion of the iris to connect the posterior and anterior chambers of the eye. This permits the iris to fall back away from the trabecular meshwork, opening the angle of the anterior chamber to allow the outflow of the aqueous fluid through Schlemm's canal.

Common side effects of laser iridectomy are increased intraocular pressure and anterior uveitis. Occasionally, laser iridectomy cannot be performed due to a clouded cornea or uveitis, requiring a surgical peripheral iridectomy, described below:

1. The eyelid speculum is placed and the globe held in place with a 4–0 or 5–0 traction suture placed under the superior rectus and fastened to the drape with a mosquito hemostat.
2. One of two incisions will be employed: A slightly curved incision is made at the superior limbus, *or* a perpendicular incision is made in the cornea.
3. Small smooth forceps are used to grasp the peripheral edge of the iris, and it is drawn through the incision and excised using scissors or a small Beaver blade.
4. The iris is repositioned by gently rubbing the surface of the cornea with a small von Graefe hook.
5. The corneal incision is closed with a 10–0 or 11–0 nonabsorbable suture.
6. Antibiotic drops are placed and an eye pad is placed for dressing.

TRABECULOPLASTY

Open angle glaucoma (OAG) treatment is centered on lowering the pressure inside the eye to prevent damage to the optic nerve. Most treatment involves specific medications (eye drops or pills) or laser treatments. Laser and conventional surgical treatments create passages for quicker drainage of aqueous humor, while medications reduce its production.

Argon laser trabeculoplasty (ALT) uses evenly spaced burns in the trabecular meshwork with an argon laser to stimulate the drainage of aqueous humor. However, argon laser burns scar the trabecular meshwork, making any necessary retreatments difficult.

Selective laser trabeculoplasty (SLT) selectively targets pigmented cells in the trabecular meshwork instead of generally burning tissue as in ALT, reducing the amount of scarring. Therefore, SLT may potentially be repeated many times. SLT has also been found to be effective when ALT and other forms of treatment have failed.

STRABISMUS CORRECTION: RECESSION/RESECTION

Recession or resection of the muscles of the eye may be used to correct strabismus (Procedure 16-1). Recession is generally more effective when performed on the vertically acting muscles, and resection has a greater effect on the lateral rectus.

PROCEDURE 16-1 Strabismus Correction—Recession

Equipment

- Headrest
- Loupes
- Sitting stools

Instruments

- Basic eye muscle instrumentation set

(continues)

PROCEDURE 16-1 Strabismus Correction—Recession *(continued)*

Supplies

- Eye pack
- Basin set
- Gloves
- Disposable eye knife
- Adhesive-backed disposable aperture drape
- Adhesive backed sheet
- Suture:
  - 4–0 silk
  - 6–0 polyglactin
- Dressing
- Eye pad
- Antibiotic ophthalmic ointment
- Lidocaine with epinephrine
- BSS
- Cotton-tipped applicators
- Cautery, disposable
- Marking pen

Operative Preparation

Anesthesia

- General; sometimes local in adults

Position

- Supine
- Arm on affected side may be tucked and the other arm extended on an armboard

Prep

- Unilateral: Prep from hairline to inferior mandibular border, and from the anterior auricular border to beyond the midline. Cleanse the eyelid first, then the eyelashes, brow, and skin. Avoid pooling prep solution in the eye. Irrigate the eye using a bulb syringe filled with normal saline.
- Bilateral: Prep from the hairline to the inferior border of the mandible and laterally to the anterior auricular borders. Prep both eyes as above.

Draping

- Unilateral: Use disposable drapes. Adhesive-backed sheet placed across forehead. Split sheet placed with operative eye in the V of the drape, with adhesive-backed split sheet tails secured to the top of the head, and remainder of sheet over patient's body. Place adhesive-backed aperture drape over the affected eye.
- Bilateral: Adhesive-backed sheet placed across forehead. Split sheet placed so that the V of the drape fits over the bridge of the nose to expose both eyes. Adhesive-backed tails of split sheet secured to the top of the head; remainder of split sheet draped over patient's body. Place sterile adhesive-backed aperture drapes over each eye.

Practical Considerations

- Talking and movement in the room should be kept to a minimum, as the patient is often awake
- Retrobulbar block may be administered
- Eyes should be periodically irrigated using BSS; this task often falls to the STSR
- Powder is meticulously removed from gloves to prevent corneal irritation
- Extra care should be taken to keep lint off the instruments and the sterile field

PROCEDURE

16-1 Strabismus Correction—Recession *(continued)*

Operative Procedure

1. A speculum is inserted and 4–0 silk traction suture one placed at the 12- and 6-o'clock positions. Intermittently throughout the surgery, the cornea is moistened with drops of BSS.
2. A radial incision is made from the limbus level with the upper border of the affected muscle.
3. Westcott scissors are inserted through this incision to dissect free the conjunctiva from the limbus.
4. A second radial incision is made toward the lower border of the muscle (Figure 16-5).

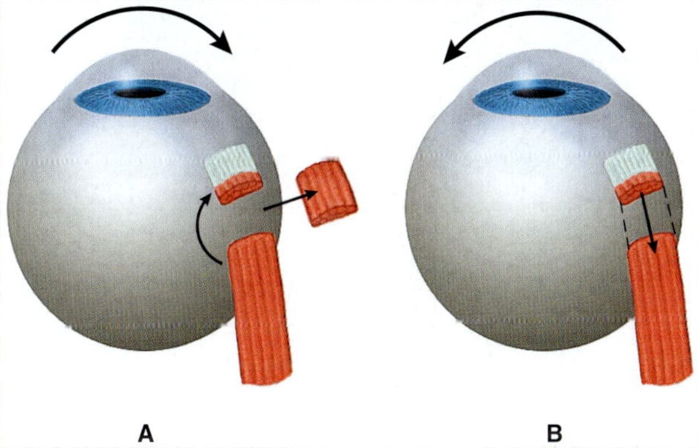

Figure 16-5 Strabismus correction: (A) Resection, (B) recession

5. A strabismus hook is introduced beneath the muscle insertion, and is swept backward, freeing the muscle from the sclera, and then forward.
6. Sutures are passed through the muscle for traction.
7. After this "flap" of muscle is further developed, the muscle is measured and marked at the points of recession.
8. The tendinous insertion is divided by scissors. Two absorbable sutures (6–0 polyglactin) may be placed at this point in the end of the muscles. These should be left untied with the needles attached.
9. The muscle is reattached at the new recession point.
10. The conjunctiva is closed using 6–0 absorbable or 8–0 silk sutures. Antibiotic drops are instilled into the eye, and usually no dressing is required.

Technical Considerations

1. Traction sutures are used to position and stabilize the eye, and the free ends of the suture may be clamped to the drape with a mosquito. Provide irrigation as needed.
2. Incision is made using a disposable eye knife of the surgeon's choice.
3. Care should be taken to keep the scissors lint free.
4. This second radial incision forms a flap of conjunctiva and Tenon's capsule that will be dissected further to expose the upper and lower borders of the muscle.
5. Provide muscle hook of surgeon's preference or according to the size of the muscle.
6. 4–0 silk sutures. Disposable cautery will be needed to control bleeding at this point.
7. A caliper may be used to measure the distance from the original point of insertion to the new one. The sterile marking pen may be used to mark the points of recession.
8. Westcott scissors are used to divide tendinous insertion. A straight mosquito hemostat may be used to compress small blood vessels in the muscle between the suture and the insertion.
9. 6–0 polyglactin suture with needle of surgeon's choice is used for reattachment.
10. Conjunctiva closed using 6–0 absorbable or 8–0 silk sutures with needle of surgeon's choice. Antibiotic drops may be instilled into the eye at this point.

(continues)

PROCEDURE

16-1 Strabismus Correction—Recession *(continued)*

Postoperative Considerations

Immediate Postoperative Care
- Eye patch dressing placed, if surgeon requires

Prognosis
- Stereoscopic vision restored

Complications
- Hemorrhage
- Infection

PEARL OF WISDOM

Limit the use of towels on the field to reduce the amount of lint present, and be sure all sterile team members remove the lubricant from their gloves.

ADJUSTABLE SUTURE SURGERY

An alternative addition to the method previously described is adjustable suture surgery. In adult strabismus, especially with diplopia, the adjustable suture technique allows more accurate alignment and placement of the field of vision is more exact.

When the muscle to be recessed has been isolated, the tendon is secured with a double-armed 6–0 polyglactin suture. This suture is attached to the free end of the muscle and to the sclera, the two ends are held vertical to the eye and tied together with a knot that slides up and down the muscle sutures. The desired recession is measured and marked and the muscle is allowed to fall back into position. The knot is slipped down to the sclera. The conjunctival incision is closed using 8–0 silk, leaving the slipknot exposed for later adjustment, and the two free ends of the muscle suture are tucked into the conjunctival fornix (Figure 16-6).

After the effects of anesthesia have completely worn off and the patient is completely awake, but not more than 24 hours after surgery, the adjustment is performed. Drops of 1% amethocaine are instilled into the conjunctival sac and a cotton applicator soaked in amethocaine is applied to the adjustment site. The sutures may now be adjusted to the proper recession while the patient reports vision status. When the proper visual alignment and depth of vision are achieved, the muscle sutures are tied and the ends cut. This technique gives the added benefit

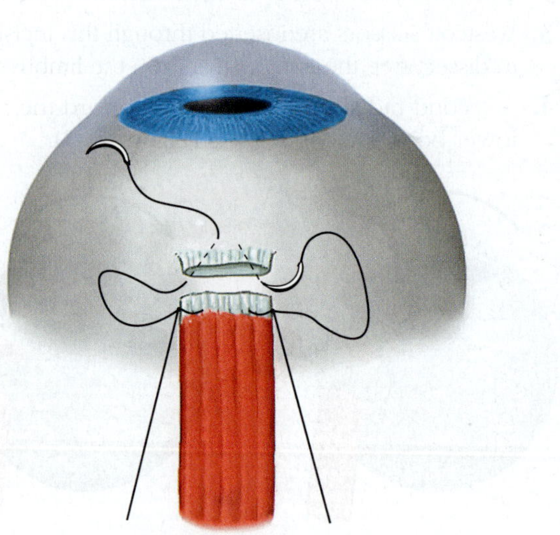
A

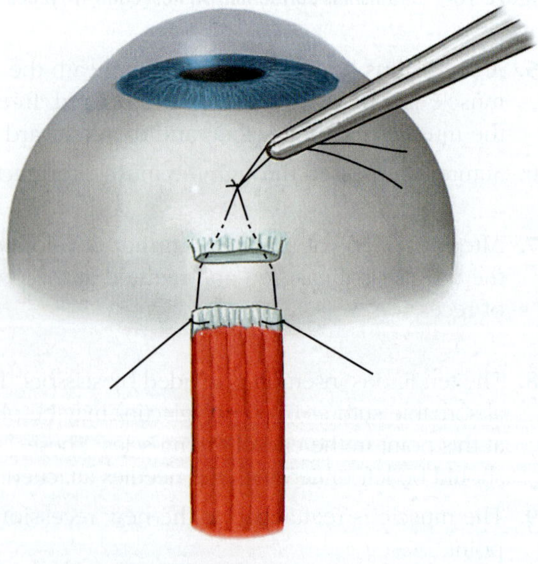
B

Figure 16-6 Recession by adjustable suture: (A) Suture placement, (B) adjustment

of precision, with the patient reporting proper or improper visual alignment as the sutures are adjusted.

The bulky knot may cause discomfort for several days, but the patient is usually discharged following surgery.

SCLERAL BUCKLE

Scleral buckle procedures have been in use for more than 30 years, and are still commonly used for retinal detachments, especially when there are no complicating factors (Figure 16-7). The procedure involves localizing the position of all retinal breaks, treating them with a cryoprobe, and supporting all retinal breaks with a scleral buckle. The buckle or "tire" is usually a piece of silicone sponge or solid silicone. The type and shape of the buckle varies depending on the location and number of retinal breaks. The buckle is sutured onto the sclera to create an indentation or buckle effect inside the eye. The buckle is positioned so that it pushes in on the retinal break and effectively closes the break. Postoperatively the patient can resume most activities within several days.

Several important terms related to this procedure include:

Buckle or tire: Silicone bolster that encircles the eye

Band: Silicone strip used to keep the buckle in place

Sleeve: Silicone band used to keep the two ends of the band in place

Cryo: Instrument used to freeze the sclera over the area of detachment

Diathermy: High-frequency electrosurgery used to mark the sclera over the area of detachment; edges of any sclerotomy made for drainage of subretinal fluid may also be coagulated

Indirect ophthalmoscope: Headlight used to view the retina with 20D and 28D handheld lenses

For the scleral buckle procedure, the patient is placed in the supine position, the skin is cleaned using an antiseptic solution and a sterile adhesive drape is applied. A speculum is inserted and the conjunctiva is opened using a limbal incision, which opens the conjunctiva. Blunt-ended scissors are used to separate the conjunctiva from the sclera, and a swab is used to clear any adherent tissue. The rectus muscles are tagged using 4–0 silk sutures, secured by mosquito forceps. All four recti are tagged so that the globe can be rotated in any direction during the procedure.

Using the tag sutures, the globe is steadied in the required position and OR lights are dimmed. The cryoprobe is used to seal to any tears. Diathermy may also be used for this same purpose, but cryotherapy has become the preferred method (Figure 16-8).

When cryotherapy or diathermy has been applied to all holes, an appropriate sized explant (silicone sponge or band) is chosen. This explant is sutured in place using double-armed 5–0 nonabsorbable polyester sutures on spatulated needles. After the local explant is attached, a "tire" or encircling band may be placed to support the buckle and to reduce the volume of the globe and thus to reduce vitreoretinal traction.

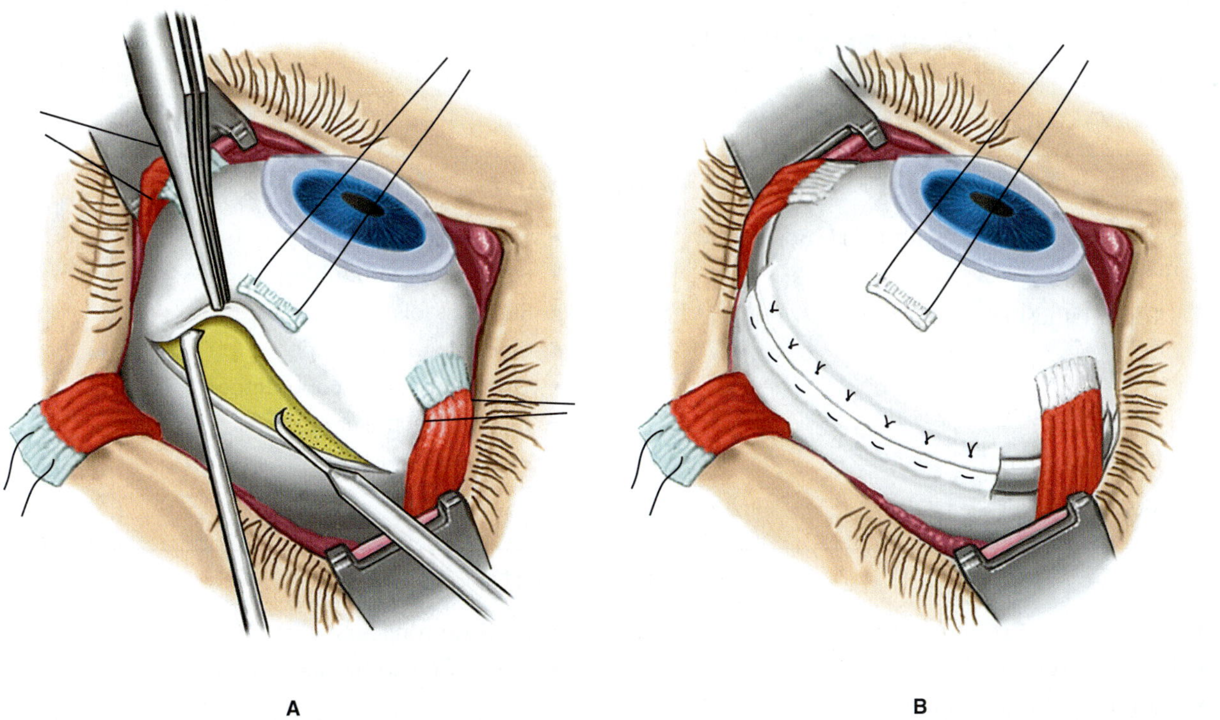

Figure 16-7 Scleral buckling for treatment of retinal detachment: (A) Preparation of sclera for buckle, (B) scleral buckle sutured in place

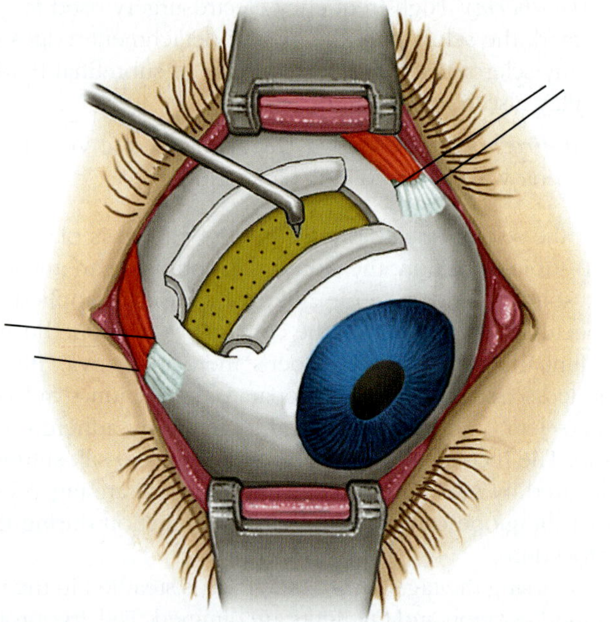

Figure 16-8 Diathermy electrode used to dot areas of retinal detachment

The strap is pulled under each rectus muscle in turn, and the free ends of the strap are positioned away from the other buckle elements. A mattress suture is placed in each quadrant to hold the band in place. At the end of the procedure, an antibiotic injection of 20 mg of gentamicin may be administered subconjunctivally, and a dressing is applied.

COMPLICATIONS

Complications that may arise after scleral buckling/encircling procedures include:

- Extraocular infection
- Anterior segment ischemia
- Uveitis: inflammation of the uveal tract, choroid
- Choroidal detachment leading to glaucoma

DACRYOCYSTORHINOSTOMY

Dacryocystorhinostomy is performed to assist in the drainage of tears and secretions from the lacrimal sac into the middle meatus of the nose by forming a short circuit through the lacrimal bone and the nasal mucosa. This procedure is performed when the nasolacrimal duct is obstructed by fibrous tissue or bone and has become impermeable, in order to establish a new communication pathway between the lacrimal sac and the nose (Procedure 16-2).

PROCEDURE 16-2 Dacryocystorhinostomy

Equipment

- Separate Mayo stand with nasal preparation materials
  - Topical anesthetic: 4% cocaine
  - Bayonet forceps
  - Nasal speculum
  - Packing material
  - Medicine cup
- Footboard, padded
- Suction set with tubing
- Sitting stools
- Operating microscope
- Operating microscope drape
- Bipolar electrosurgical unit

Instruments

- Minor set
- Basic eye set
- Dacryocystorhinostomy set
- Kerrison rongeurs
- Power drill with burs and cord

PROCEDURE

16-2 Dacryocystorhinostomy *(continued)*

Supplies

- Eye pack or basic pack
- Basin set
- Gloves
- Blades: #15, #11
- Adhesive-backed disposable aperture drape
- Split sheet
- Adhesive backed sheet
- Suture: surgeon's choice, 7–0 braided silk usually used for final closure
- Drains: catheter—10 Fr Robinson or infant feeding tube
- Iodoform- or petrolatum-impregnated gauze packing
- Eye pad
- Antibiotic ophthalmic ointment
- Topical anesthetic: cocaine 4 or 5% or phenylephrine 0.25% or 0.5%
- Thrombin
- BSS
- Cotton-tipped applicators
- Cautery, disposable
- Marking pen
- Gelfoam cut into pledgets

Operative Preparation

Anesthesia

- Surgeon performs initial nasal preparation including the administration of local, then general anesthetic is induced.
- Dacryocystorhinostomy is usually performed under general anesthetic, because the procedure is often long and tedious due to considerable bleeding and the resultant time needed to achieve hemostasis.
- To minimize bleeding, hypotensive anesthesia is utilized, and the patient is placed in a supine position with a head-up tilt.

Position

- Supine.
- Arm on the affected side may be tucked and the other arm extended on an armboard.
- Table in reverse Trendelenburg position; padded footboard used.
- Head positioned with the face turned slightly away from the side of the operation; table is tilted 15–20° with the head up and the feet down.

Prep

- From hairline to inferior mandibular border, and from the anterior auricular border to beyond the midline. Cleanse the eyelid first, then the eyelashes, brow, and skin.
- Avoid pooling prep solution in the eye.
- Irrigate the eye using a bulb syringe filled with normal saline.

Draping

- Adhesive-backed sheet placed across forehead.
- Split sheet placed with operative eye in the V of the drape, with adhesive tails secured to the top of the head, and remainder of sheet over patient's body.
- Place adhesive-backed aperture drape over the affected eye.

(continues)

PROCEDURE 16-2 Dacryocystorhinostomy *(continued)*

Practical Considerations

- Eyes should be periodically irrigated using BSS; this task often falls to the STSR
- Powder is meticulously removed from gloves to prevent corneal irritation
- Extra care should be taken to keep lint off the instruments and the sterile field
- The procedure is performed under an operating microscope
- The eye is protected using a gelatin sponge

Operative Procedure	Technical Considerations
1. After general anesthesia is induced, local anesthetic (tetracaine 1% with adrenaline 1:5000 two drops) is instilled into the conjunctival sac. Lidocaine 2% with adrenaline is injected at the beginning of the lacrimal crest, and lidocaine is sprayed into the anterior third of the nasal meatus. Lidocaine is injected into the mucoperiosteum after the insertion of a nasal speculum.	**1.** The local anesthetics help control bleeding intraoperatively, and provide some pain relief in the immediate postoperative phase.
2. A curved incision is made conforming to the anterior lacrimal crest and is deepened through the orbicularis muscle to expose the entire lacrimal crest.	**2.** Bleeding is controlled with bipolar coagulation.
3. Retractors are inserted on each side of this incision.	**3.** Usually these are rake retractors.
4. Using blunt dissection, the lacrimal sac is separated from the lacrimal fossa and is retracted, and the periosteum is dissected from the lacrimal fossa.	**4.** A freer elevator may be used for the dissection.
5. The anterior lacrimal crest to the entrance of the nasolacrimal duct is removed.	**5.** This is achieved using a rongeur.
6. An ostium is made using either punches, a small oscillating saw, or a bur.	**6.** When a saw is used, the eyelids are protected with sterile gauze. Irrigation is used to keep the field clear of debris and provide cooling of the tissues.
7. A window of bone is cut and then removed using bone forceps; a mucoperiosteal elevator is used to strip the nasal mucosa within. A sphenoidal punch is used to trim the edges of this opening.	**7.** A sphenoidal punch will be needed to trim the edges of this opening. The STSR should periodically irrigate the area (at the surgeon's request) and suction debris. Be sure to clean the tips of the punch of specimen after each use.

PROCEDURE

16-2 Dacryocystorhinostomy *(continued)*

8. A vertical cut is made in the anterior wall of the lacrimal sac, and a probe is passed into the lumen to verify the patency of the sac.	**8.** Care should be taken that the probe is free of lint.
9. The wall of the sac is slit horizontally, and the nasal mucosa is incised horizontally.	**9.** Provide cutting instrument of surgeon's choice.
10. The flaps of the nasal mucosa and lacrimal sac are then joined.	**10.** Flaps are joined using 6–0 polyglactin or 9–0 monofilament nylon sutures. This is done under the microscope.
11. The incision is closed using 5–0 absorbable sutures. The skin is closed using 7–0 interrupted braided silk.	**11.** Bleeding is controlled using gelatin sponges. Some surgeons suture a silicone tube using absorbable sutures to the anterior wall of the sac above and a nylon suture to the nasal septum at the nares.

Postoperative Considerations

Immediate Postoperative Care

- The incision is sprayed with an antibiotic solution.
- Eye protection is removed and an antibiotic is instilled in the conjunctival sac.
- A pressure dressing is applied.
- If used, the silicone tube is removed in approximately 2 weeks.

Prognosis

- The lacrimal system remains functional.
- The patient will have a permanent facial scar.

Complications

- Hemorrhage
- Infection

PEARL OF WISDOM

Local anesthesia with epinephrine may be used during the procedure to provide additional hemostasis. The STSR is expected to keep the drill and tissues cool by irrigating the area being drilled with saline. Care should be taken that all saline and bone fragments from drilling are suctioned out of the sterile field by the STSR.

ENUCLEATION AND EVISCERATION OF THE EYE (TRADITIONAL APPROACH)

Enucleation is indicated for excision of an eye due to malignant neoplasm, penetrating wounds, or if the eye has been so extensively damaged that no vision can be regained (Figure 16-9). In some cases, evisceration rather than enucleation may be performed, allowing retention of the shrunken remnants of the eye. Evisceration eliminates corneal sensitivity and allows the patient to wear a prosthetic eye that will have mobility and a better cosmetic result.

For enucleation a peritomy is made at the limbus circumferentially separating the conjunctiva and Tenon's capsule from the globe. The superior oblique tendon is grasped with a muscle hook and divided. The inferior oblique muscle is double clamped with hemostats for hemostasis and the muscle is cut. Hemostats are released after several minutes. All attachments to the globe are separated, permitting the globe to move freely. The eye is held steady by the medial rectus insertion. The location of the optic nerve is identified. The optic nerve is transected, the globe delivered, and the remaining attachments are separated. Hemostasis is achieved and a prosthetic sphere implant is sutured into Tenon's capsule. The conjunctiva is approximated and a conformer is placed over the sphere in the cul-de-sac. An intermarginal suture is placed to produce a mild pressure effect.

For *evisceration,* the patient is positioned in a supine position and draped after the induction of anesthesia. A speculum is inserted and the eye is fixed with forceps. A cataract knife is used to excise the cornea. Forceps and scissors are used to cut through the lower half of the corneal circumference. The cornea is detached and removed.

Hooks are inserted into the sclera at the 12-, 5-, and 9-o'clock positions and are retracted to give exposure of the intraocular contents. A scoop is used to scoop out the contents inside the sclera and to tear through the intraocular portion of the optic nerve. A cellulose sponge is used to sweep out uveal remnants. After the cavity is cleared, the inside is swabbed with chlorhexidine solution.

If no active inflammation of the eye is present, a small plastic or silicone ball may be placed within this scleral cavity to provide a good cosmetic result. The ball is placed in the scleral cavity and the sclera is sutured using interrupted absorbable sutures. Tenon's capsule is sutured with 6–0 polyglactin sutures and the conjunctiva with 8–0 polyglactin continuous suture.

Antibiotic drops are instilled and a gauze bandage is applied. Postoperatively, the sclera will shrink and contract around the ball, providing a good base on which a prosthesis may be fitted.

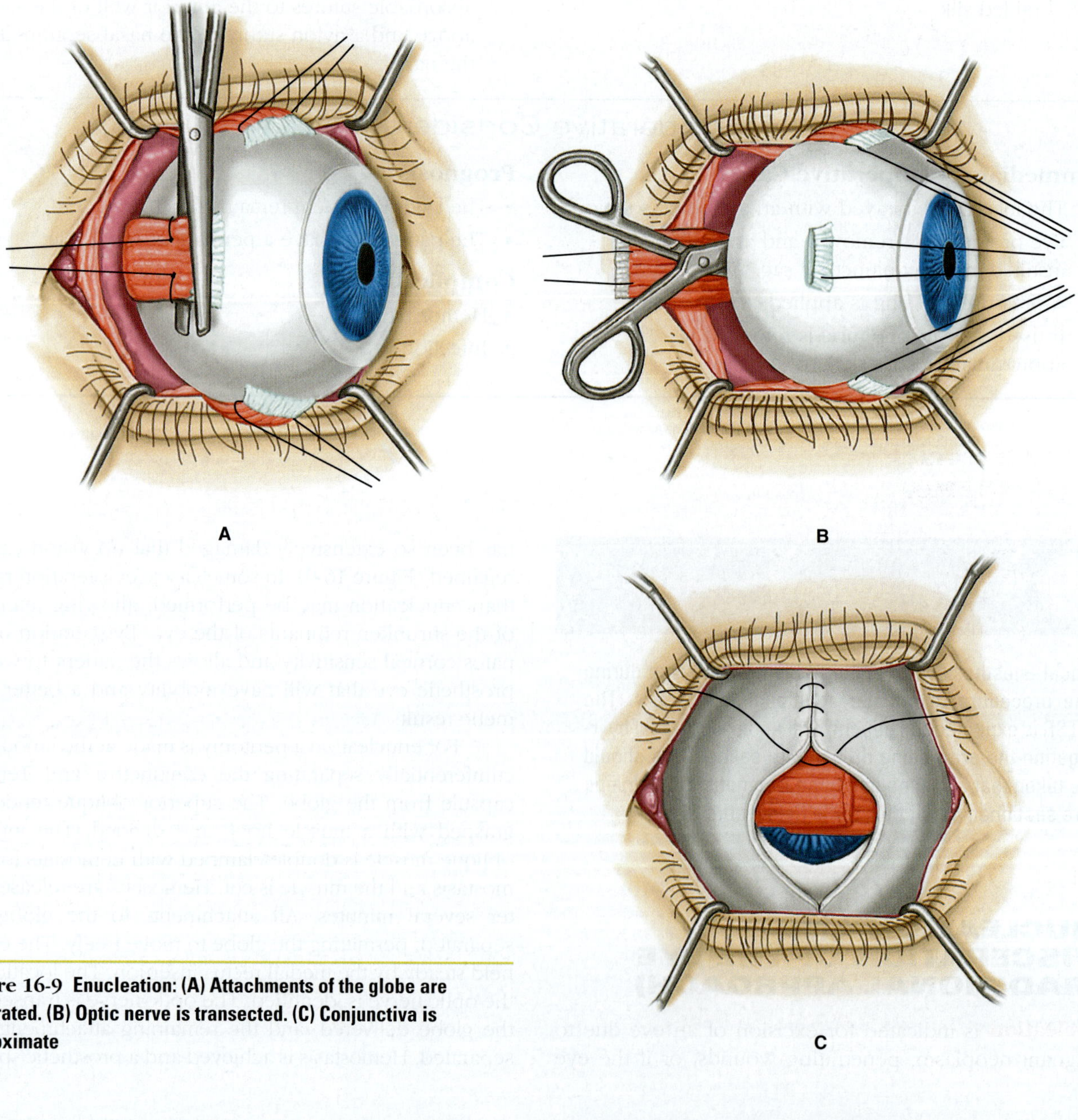

Figure 16-9 Enucleation: (A) Attachments of the globe are separated. (B) Optic nerve is transected. (C) Conjunctiva is approximate

ENUCLEATION OF THE EYE (HYDROXYAPATITE IMPLANT WITH PEGS)

Patient is positioned and anesthetized as above. Tenon's capsule is opened and all structures that pass through it are divided. The optic nerve is severed as far back as possible using scissors. The posterior layer of Tenon's capsule is preserved to prevent herniation of orbital fat and socket deformity. An implant may now be placed.

Ocular implants are used following enucleation to provide the patient with a base on which to place a prosthetic eye and to replace the volume lost by enucleation. Implants can be classified as integrated or nonintegrated. The integrated implants have the benefit of improving prosthetic motility, but in the past these became exposed through the conjunctiva. The resultant complications have forced physicians to rely on spherical implants, which are simple, nonintegrated, buried silicone or plastic spheres. The spherical implants reduce exposure complications but often become dislocated, resulting in limited motility of the implant. Spherical implants remain in use but in many instances they are being replaced by the hydroxyapatite implant. This type of implant has been used since 1985 and received FDA approval in September 1989.

Hydroxyapatite is a complex calcium phosphate (CA_{10} $[PO_4]_6$ $[OH]_2$) and a naturally occurring body substance. Porous hydroxyapatite is made from a genus reef-building coral, which is converted from calcium carbonate to calcium phosphate. This form of hydroxyapatite has a microstructure similar to cancellous bone with interconnecting channels. When implanted in soft tissue it becomes invaded by fibrovascular tissue.

The implant is coupled with the artificial eye by means of a peg that articulates with the posterior aspect of the artificial eye, fitting into a hole drilled through the conjunctiva and soft tissue directly into the buried implant. This hole fills in with fibrovascular tissue, which eliminates the problems associated with an exposed implant.

Two separate surgical procedures are involved. The initial implant insertion placement is done under local or general anesthesia. Approximately 6 months later (after formation of fibrovascular filling) a hole is drilled, under retrobulbar anesthesia, and a peg is fitted, on which the ocular prosthesis is placed. In 2–3 weeks, the patient is sent to the ocularist to have the peg fitted to the posterior surface of the artificial eye.

ENUCLEATION OF THE EYE (HYDROXYAPATITE IMPLANT WITH DONOR SCLERA)

This procedure utilizes the hydroxyapatite implant, but rather than using pegs, donor sclera is used. When the globe is removed, the lateral and medial rectus muscles are secured using silk sutures. The hydroxyapatite implant is then inserted and secured into donor sclera. The lateral and medial rectus muscles are then sewn to the surface of the donor sclera. The conjunctiva is closed and a conformer is placed.

KERATOPLASTY (CORNEAL TRANSPLANT)

The cornea is the anterior window to the eye. It allows light into the eye and bends (refracts) the light rays to help the lens focus them upon the retina. To perform properly, the cornea must be clear and of a proper curvature.

If the cornea is not perfectly clear, vision can be dramatically decreased. If the cornea is irregular or damaged, it will cause blurred vision. Replacing cloudy, damaged, or cone-shaped corneal tissue with healthy donor tissue through a corneal transplant can make a dramatic improvement in vision.

Many causes of clouding of the cornea exist, including:

- Eye injuries leave a dense white scar on the cornea. These injuries may include penetrating wounds from a sharp object, burns, or chemical contamination of the eye.
- Severe corneal infection may lead to corneal scarring. The infection may be bacterial, viral, or fungal in origin. Various herpes viruses are known to cause such scarring.
- Abnormal shapes of the cornea, such as occur with keratoconus, may scar the center of the cornea or distort vision so severely that glasses or contact lenses are of little help.
- Corneal dystrophies may cause clouding.
- Inherited diseases may damage the cornea.
- Cataract or other eye surgery may prompt corneal clouding.

During corneal transplant surgery, only the central part of the cornea is replaced. Corneal tissue used for transplant surgery comes from donors. An eye bank procures the tissue, examines it, and then stores and protects it until used. All tissue used for transplantation is extensively tested. It is screened for the presence of communicable diseases such as hepatitis and HIV.

In the following procedure, we will examine penetrating **kerato**plasty, in which a full thickness of the cornea is replaced. The donor material comes from the eye bank either as a whole eye from which the cornea may be taken, or as prepared and sized cornea buttons. These are stored for up to 30 days prior to use in a special refrigerated medium. The donor disk is punched 0.1 mm larger than the recipient opening to ensure proper fit. The procedure described will assume that the donor material is from an isolated cornea (Procedure 16-3).

PROCEDURE 16-3 Keratoplasty (Corneal Transplant)

Equipment

- Headrest
- Suction set with tubing
- Sitting stools
- Operating microscope
- Operating microscope drape

Instruments

- Basic eye set
- Corneal procedures set

Supplies

- Eye pack or basic pack
- Basin set
- Gloves
- Blades: #15, #64 disposable Beaver blade, #30 Superblade
- Adhesive-backed disposable aperture drape
- Split sheet
- Adhesive backed sheet
- Suture: surgeon's choice; 7–0 braided silk usually used for final closure
- Dressing
- Eye pad
- Antibiotic ophthalmic ointment
- Anesthetic for retrobulbar injection if necessary
- Antibiotic solution to wash donor corneal button
- Anti-inflammatory agent such as betamethasone
- BSS
- Cotton-tipped applicators
- Cautery, disposable or wet field
- Cellulose sponges
- Petri dish (for storage of donor corneal button)
- Fluorescein strip (to temporarily stain corneal epithelium)

Operative Preparation

Anesthesia

- General: tetracaine drops may be instilled after general anesthesia induced

Position

- Supine
- Arm on the affected side may be tucked and the other arm extended on an armboard

Prep

- Unilateral: Prep from hairline to inferior mandibular border, and from the anterior auricular border to beyond the midline at the sides. Cleanse the eyelid first, then the eyelashes, brow, and skin. Avoid pooling prep solution in the eye. Irrigate the eye using a bulb syringe filled with normal saline.

Draping

- Unilateral: Use disposable drapes. Adhesive-backed sheet placed across forehead. Split sheet placed with operative eye in the V of the drape, with adhesive-backed split sheet tails secured to the top of the head, and remainder of sheet over patient's body. Place adhesive-backed aperture drape over the affected eye.

PROCEDURE 16-3 Keratoplasty (Corneal Transplant) *(continued)*

Practical Considerations

- Powder is meticulously removed from gloves to prevent corneal irritation
- Extra care should be taken to keep lint off the instruments and the sterile field
- The procedure is performed under an operating microscope
- When a portable microscope is used, it should be brought over the patient from the side opposite the affected eye
- In some cases, the surgeon may request a separate sterile table for donor cornea preparation

Operative Procedure	Technical Considerations
1. The medium is poured into a sterile medicine glass and the donor tissue is placed on a punching block with a concavity that conforms to the anterior corneal curvature.	**1.** A portion of the medium is sent as a specimen for bacterial culture.
2. The endothelial surface is placed facing upward. The donor cornea is punched using a Cottingham punch to the correct size for placement. A punch of slightly greater diameter than the punch used for the patient's host eye is used for the donor cornea.	**2.** The donor cornea is stored in a safe place on the sterile field for later use.
3. The eyelids are retracted and 4–0 silk traction sutures are placed at the insertions of the superior and inferior rectus muscles and clamped to the surgical drape using a mosquito.	**3.** These sutures are used to fix and steady the eye while the graft bed is prepared. If a cataract is present, the surgeon can remove it in addition to the corneal transplant operation. If an artificial lens is already in place and it is believed to be responsible for the clouding of the cornea, the artificial lens can be replaced with a type of lens less likely to irritate the donor cornea tissue.
4. A **trephine** is placed on the cornea and is used to make the corneal cut around the cornea and into the anterior chamber (Figure 16-10).	**4.** If the trephine cut is complete, the cornea is removed; if incomplete, corneal scissors or a diamond knife is used to finish the cut.
5. The edge of the donor corneal disk is slid from its silicone base, laid in the trephine opening, and placed in position.	**5.** In some cases, temporary indirect sutures will have been placed prior to this step; they are now tensioned to hold the graft in place.
6. The transplant is gently held in place while 10–0 polyamide sutures are used to suture the graft in place.	**6.** The STSR may be asked to wet the suture with saline prior to passing it to the surgeon.
7. After the graft is sutured in place, BSS or acetylcholine solution is injected into the anterior chamber through a fine cannula at the graft margin.	**7.** This cannula is used to ensure that the wound is water-tight.
8. Antibiotic drops are instilled and the traction sutures removed. The eye is covered with antibiotic-impregnated gauze, an eye pad, and a shield.	**8.** Medication of choice and dressing are prepared in advance.

(continues)

PROCEDURE

16-3 Keratoplasty (Corneal Transplant) *(continued)*

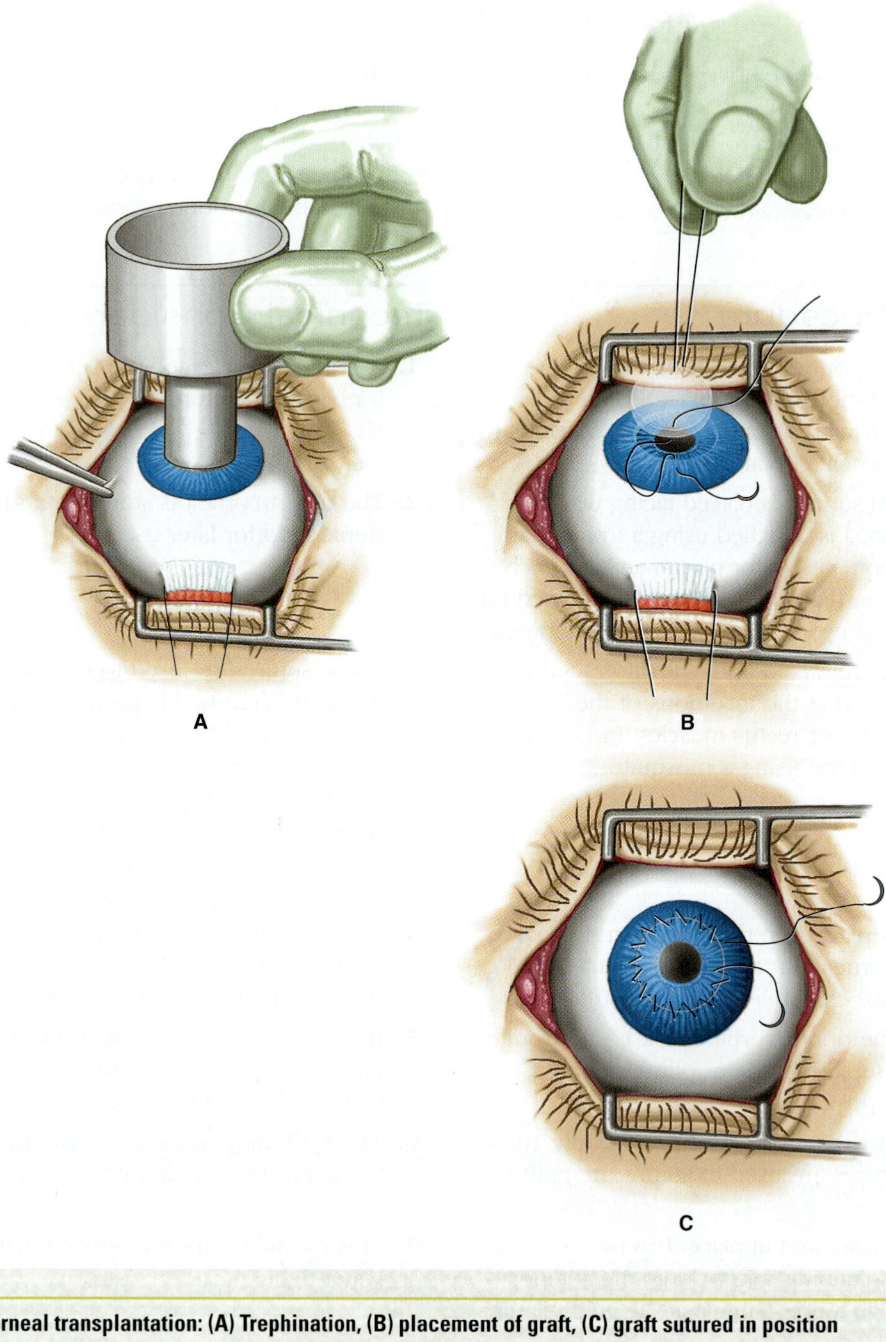

Figure 16-10 **Corneal transplantation: (A) Trephination, (B) placement of graft, (C) graft sutured in position**

PROCEDURE

16-3 Keratoplasty (Corneal Transplant) *(continued)*

Postoperative Considerations

Immediate Postoperative Care

- The eye is patched overnight and examined the next day.

Prognosis

- Usually there is little or no discomfort after surgery.
- Occasionally, further surgery may be required to minimize residual astigmatism.
- The success of transplantation surgery is often related to the original cause of the underlying corneal disease process. Transplant procedures resulting from abnormally shaped corneas due to keratoconus or for corneal clouding following cataract surgery typically have very high success rates. Conversely, transplants due to scarring of the cornea from infections, such as herpes, typically have a lower success rate.
- Although risks are present, the success rate of corneal transplantation is very high. It enjoys the highest success rate of any transplant procedures commonly performed.
- Corneal graft rejection rarely occurs within 2 weeks and may occur as late as 20 years following corneal transplant. Pain, light sensitivity, redness, and decreasing vision are warning signs of corneal tissue rejection and indicate the need for immediate medical attention. When started at the first signs of tissue rejection, steroids (drops, injections, and/or pills) may be effective in halting the rejection process. If the rejection process continues, the donor tissue becomes cloudy, resulting in blurry vision. Often, a repeat transplant may be performed.

Complications

- Hemorrhage
- Infection
- Rejection of the transplanted tissue can occur following corneal transplant surgery
- Permanent loss or impairment of vision
- Scarring
- Glaucoma
- Retinal swelling
- Retinal detachment
- Cataract formation
- Swelling of the donor graft

PEARL OF WISDOM

Prior to the induction of anesthesia, the STSR should always confirm that the donor cornea has arrived.

CATARACT EXTRACTION

Two methods of cataract extraction are commonly used. Extracapsular and intracapsular methods are available for removal of the opaque lens. With either method, an artificial lens may be inserted.

The **intracapsular cataract extraction** involves a large incision. The lens is picked up for extraction with forceps, suction, or a cryoprobe. The entire capsule is removed.

Extracapsular cataract extraction is performed through a small incision and the lens is expressed or removed manually or by phacoemulsification (Procedure 16-4). The phacoemulsification method uses ultrasonic energy to break up the lens; the lens material is irrigated and aspirated simultaneously. The posterior capsule remains.

INTRAOCULAR LENSES

Intraocular lenses (IOLs) are small prescription lenses placed inside the eye during cataract or clear lens replacement surgery. The lenses are designed to replace the eye's natural lens after a cataract has developed. Prior to the development of IOLs, cataract patients were forced to wear thick glasses or contact lenses after surgery, and they were unable to see without them.

Because of sophisticated formulas used to calculate the corrective prescription power of the lens, the IOL corrects the eye's existing refractive error, and the patient does not require glasses or contacts postoperatively.

Intraocular lenses may be foldable or hard. Foldable lenses are made of silicone or acrylic and can be rolled up and placed inside a tiny tube that is inserted through a very small incision (less than 2.5 mm in length). Once inside the eye, the IOL gently unfolds. Hard plastic lenses are used less often and, since they cannot be folded, must be inserted through a slightly larger incision.

Phakic lenses are a type of intraocular lens that are implanted without removing the eye's natural lens. These lenses are an option that will soon become available to young patients who may not be candidates for other refractive surgery options. Clear lens replacement surgery gives patients older than 40 years of age the option to improve their vision without glasses and to avoid cataract surgery later in life.

PROCEDURE 16-4 Cataract Extraction: Extracapsular Method

Equipment

- Intraocular pressure reducer cuff
- Lift sheet
- Headrest
- Sitting stools
- Microscope
- Microscope drape

Instruments

- Basic eye set
- Cataract extraction tray
- Intraocular lens implant (IOL)

Supplies

- Eye pack or basic pack
- Basin set
- Gloves
- Blades: #15, #64 disposable Beaver blade, #30 Superblade
- Adhesive-backed disposable eye drape
- Split sheet
- Sterile plastic adhesive drape
- Suture: surgeon's choice
- Dressing
- Eye pad dressing
- Antibiotic ophthalmic ointment
- Anesthetic for retrobulbar block: lidocaine 2% with epinephrine
- Anti-inflammatory agent: betamethasone drops
- Viscoelastic agent: Healon
- BSS
- Sterile medication labels
- Cautery: wet field or disposable
- Cellulose sponges

Operative Preparation

Anesthesia

- General (typically)
- Local may be used; should include a retrobulbar block

Position

- Supine
- Arm on the affected side may be tucked and the other arm extended on an armboard
- Head may be supported on a headrest

PROCEDURE 16-4

Cataract Extraction: Extracapsular Method *(continued)*

Prep

- Unilateral: Prep from hairline to inferior mandibular border, and from the anterior auricular border to beyond the midline. Cleanse the eyelid first, then the eyelashes, brow, and skin. Avoid pooling prep solution in the eye. Irrigate the eye using a bulb syringe filled with normal saline.

Draping

- Unilateral: Use disposable drapes. Adhesive-backed sheet placed across forehead. Split sheet placed with operative eye in the V of the drape, with adhesive-backed split sheet tails secured to the top of the head, and remainder of sheet over patient's body. Place sterile adhesive-backed aperture drape over the affected eye.

Practical Considerations

- Powder is meticulously removed from gloves to prevent corneal irritation
- The procedure is performed under an operating microscope
- When a portable microscope is used, it should be brought over the patient from the side opposite the affected eye

Operative Procedure	Technical Considerations
1. The lid is retracted.	**1.** Provide retractor of choice. Prepare bridle suture.
2. A superior rectus bridle suture, as in the previous procedures, is placed for manipulation of the globe.	**2.** Suture is clamped and attached to the surgical drape with a mosquito.
3. An incision is made, either corneoscleral or corneal.	**3.** A corneal incision is self-sealing.
4. The anterior chamber is entered with the knife.	**4.** Beaver blade preferred by surgeon will be needed.
5. The corneal incision is followed with **iridotomy** or iridectomy if the posterior capsule is not intact.	**5.** Iridotomy is preferred.
6. The anterior capsule is incised and the lens is expressed using method of surgeon preference.	**6.** Pass sharps carefully. The surgeon may not be willing to look away from the microscope. This is one situation in which the STSR may be required to accept sharps from the surgeon. The specimen may not be required to be sent to pathology according to facility policy.
7. An intraocular implant may be inserted below the iris.	**7.** The surgeon will select a lens prosthesis prior to surgery; the preselected lens is opened and prepared when requested.
8. Acetylcholine solution is injected into the anterior chamber to constrict the pupil, pulling the iris back into position.	**8.** Syringes are preloaded and labeled according to facility policy. Do not cover increment markings on the syringe with the label.
9. Sterile air is injected into the anterior chamber.	**9.** Be certain that correct syringe is passed. The room may be darkened to enhance the microscopic view.

(continues)

PROCEDURE 16-4 Cataract Extraction: Extracapsular Method *(continued)*

10. A previously placed 12-o'clock suture is tied, and two interrupted sutures are placed in the cornea.	**10.** If possible, prepare suture in advance. This may not be possible if the surgeon prefers a nonlocking needle holder.
11. The remainder of the incision is closed with continuous or interrupted 10–0 sutures.	**11.** Prepare Miochol according to manufacturer's instruction.
12. Air in the chamber is replaced with Miochol, and the wound is checked for leaks.	**12.** Air extraction syringe will be used first, followed immediately by the Miochol.
13. Antibiotic drops are instilled, and the superior rectus retention suture is removed.	**13.** Pass medication preferred by surgeon.
14. The speculum is removed and the eye dressed with antibiotic-impregnated gauze, an eye pad, and a shield.	**14.** Retrieve speculum and assist with dressing application as needed.

Postoperative Considerations

Immediate Postoperative Care

- Patient is transported to PACU for immediate postoperative period.
- Patient is discharged from facility the same day.

Prognosis

- The patient is expected to return to normal activities in 1–3 days.
- Vision is expected to be markedly improved. Corrective glasses should not be needed for normal activities, but may be required for reading.

Complications

- Hemorrhage
- Infection

> **PEARL OF WISDOM**
>
> For this procedure, positive pressure ventilation is very important, and dust-free adhesive drapes should be used. Miochol must be mixed on the field by the STSR immediately prior to use.

PHACOEMULSIFICATION

The phacoemulsification method is a variation of the irrigation/aspiration technique. A smaller incision is made (often requiring no stitches for closure), just large enough for the tip of the "phaco" handpiece to be inserted. Phacoemulsification uses ultrasonic energy to fragment the lens while simultaneously irrigating and aspirating the fragments. After the nucleus of the lens is removed, an irrigating/aspiration device is used to remove any remaining pieces of cortex. With newer "foldable" intraocular lens implants, a smaller self-sealing incision requires no stitches.

VITRECTOMY

Vitrectomy is a microsurgical procedure in which specialized microinstruments and techniques are used to repair retinal disorders, many of which were previously considered inoperable. The initial step in this procedure is usually the removal of the vitreous gel through small (1.4-mm) incisions in the eye wall. The vitreous is removed with a miniature handheld cutting device and replaced with a special saline solution similar to the liquid being removed from the eye. A high intensity fiberoptic light source is used to illuminate the inside of the eye.

Most vitreoretinal surgeons enter the globe through a part of the eye known as the pars plana, with the approach and procedure being referred to as trans pars plana vitrectomy. This approach avoids damage to the retina and the crystalline lens. This procedure may also be used when local buckling and cryosurgical repair of retinal holes has failed.

During vitrectomy surgery (Procedure 16-5), the retinal surgeon may use a variety of special techniques to achieve the desired results. They include:

- *Intraocular gases:* Usually either perfluoropropane (C_3F_8) or sulfur hexafluoride (SF_6); when mixed with sterile air, these gases have the property of remaining in the eye for extended periods of time (up to two months). The eye's own natural fluid eventually replaces them. Gas is useful for flattening a detached retina and keeping it attached while healing occurs. Gas injection is also used to close macular holes. It is frequently necessary for the patient to maintain a certain head position following surgery when gas is used. Possible complications of intraocular gas include progression of cataracts and elevated intraocular pressure.
- *Silicone oil:* This is sometimes used instead of gas to keep the retina attached postoperatively. Silicone remains in the eye until it is removed (often necessitating a second surgery). The technique is advantageous when long-term support of the retina is required. Unlike what they experience with gas, patients are still able to see through clear silicone oil. Positioning is less critical with silicone oil; therefore, it may be used with patients who are unable to position themselves appropriately postoperatively. Like gas, silicone oil may promote cataracts, cause glaucoma, and damage the cornea.
- *Endophotocoagulation:* This technique uses a laser to treat intraocular structures. This modality is often used to treat retina tears in the setting of retinal detachment and is frequently used to treat proliferative diabetic retinopathy as well.
- *Microsurgical instruments:* Forceps, scissors, and picks may be used to manipulate intraocular structures, such as in the removal of scar tissue and foreign bodies. Literally hundreds of vitrectomy instruments are available to assist in different surgical maneuvers. Most of these vitreoretinal tools have a diameter of less than 1 mm.
- *Lensectomy:* Lensectomy is the removal of the eye's crystalline lens during a vitrectomy procedure. This is sometimes performed when there is a cataract, which prevents the surgeon from adequately visualizing the internal structures. A lensectomy may also be necessary to gain access to and remove scar tissue during complicated retinal detachment or diabetic retinopathy procedures. The natural lens can be replaced with a clear lens implant at a later date or during the same surgical procedure. Lensectomy is usually performed using high-frequency ultrasound.

Some special terms used for vitrectomy procedures include:

Gas forced infusion: Method by which intraocular pressure is maintained.

Ocutome: Instrument with which vitreous is cut and aspirated. Variable cut and aspiration rates are controlled from the main panel.

Fragmatome: Ultrasonic instrument with aspiration used to remove a cloudy lens, which obstructs the view of the retina.

Membrane peeler/cutter (MPC): Microscissors used to cut and peel membranes from the retina. It has aspiration capability.

Endoilluminator: Fiberoptic microillumination for intraocular use.

Endo/exo cautery: Low current cautery for use inside or outside the eye. Different tips used for each.

Argon laser: Laser with either endo or indirect capability.

PROCEDURE 16-5 Vitrectomy

Equipment

- Headrest
- Sitting stools
- Microscope
- Microscope drape
- Endoilluminator light source
- Endocoagulator (bipolar or Wetfield)
- Ocutome

(continues)

PROCEDURE 16-5 Vitrectomy *(continued)*

Instruments

- Basic eye set
- Retinal procedures tray
- Forceps
  Curved and straight McPherson
  Lister
  Curved and straight Pierse-Hoskins Cryoprobe and cable
- Endocoagulator handpiece and cable
- Endoilluminator handpiece and cable
- Vitrectomy instruments
- Vitrectomy handpiece and tubing
- Caliper
- Infusion cannula
- Vitreous scissors
- Membrane pick
- Foreign body forceps

Supplies

- Eye pack or basic pack
- Basin set
- Gloves
- Blades: special vitrectomy blade and knife (disposable)
- Adhesive-backed disposable aperture drape
- Split sheet
- Adhesive backed sheet
- Suture: surgeon's choice
- Dressing
- Eye pad
- Antibiotic ophthalmic ointment
- Anti-inflammatory agent: betamethasone drops
- Sodium hyaluronate: Healon (vitreous replacement)
- Acetylcholine (with filter) for pupil constriction
- Amydricaine No. 2
- BSS
- Cotton-tipped applicators
- Cellulose sponges
- Sclerotomy plugs

Operative Preparation

Anesthesia

- General

Position

- Supine.
- Arm on the affected side may be tucked and the other arm extended on an armboard. The head may be supported on a headrest.
- The table is placed in slight reverse Trendelenburg position with the neck extended and supported on a rolled sheet.
- The head is stabilized using a headrest.
- Since reverse Trendelenburg is used, antiembolic hose should be applied. Pressure points should be padded.

Prep

- Unilateral: Prep from hairline to inferior mandibular border, and from the anterior auricular border to beyond the midline at the sides. Cleanse the eyelid first, then the eyelashes, brow, and skin. Avoid pooling prep solution in the eye. Irrigate the eye using a bulb syringe filled with normal saline.

Draping

- Unilateral: Use disposable drapes. Adhesive-backed sheet placed across forehead. Split sheet placed with operative eye in the V of the drape, with adhesive tails secured to the top of the head, and remainder of sheet over patient's body. Place adhesive-backed aperture drape over the affected eye.

PROCEDURE

16-5 Vitrectomy *(continued)*

Practical Considerations

- The procedure is performed under an operating microscope
- When a portable microscope is used, it should be brought over the patient from the side opposite the affected eye
- Vitrectomy handpiece will be attached to sterile tubing, which, in turn, is attached to the ocutome unit

Operative Procedure

1. The eyelids are retracted with a speculum and amydricaine No. 2 is injected subconjunctivally to dilate the pupil.
2. A small incision is made in the conjunctiva to expose the sclera.
3. A sclerotomy is made under the microscope.
4. This sclerotomy is placed 3–4 mm from the limbus. The blade is inserted until it is seen through the pupil; it is withdrawn and the infusion cannula is inserted through this sclerotomy (Figure 16-11).

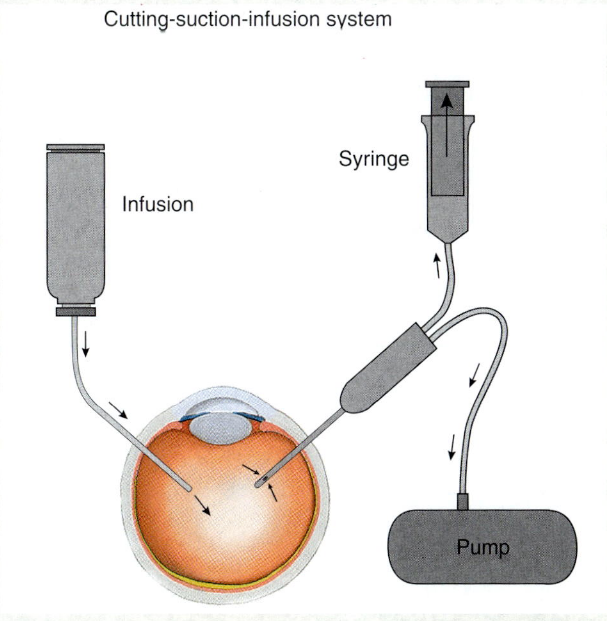

Figure 16-11 Vitrectomy

Technical Considerations

1. Provide lid retractor of surgeon's choice. Medication should be prepared and labeled in anticipation of need.
2. Provide Beaver blade of surgeon's choice. A 5–0 polyester suture is typically placed in advance to eventually support the infusion cannula.
3. A 20-gauge microvitreoretinal blade may be used for the sclerotomy.
4. The infusion cannula must be primed with solution of the surgeon's choice and air bubbles must be removed. The previously inserted suture is tightened to hold this cannula in place.

(continues)

PROCEDURE 16-5 Vitrectomy *(continued)*

5. Two more sclerotomies are made, one at the upper border of the lateral rectus muscle and one at the medial sides of the lateral rectus muscle. The endoilluminator is inserted through one of these sclerotomies and the Ocutome probe or other instruments are inserted through the final sclerotomy.

5. An irrigating contact lens may be placed on the eye. The surgical assistant moves this lens with the globe as the surgeon moves the globe. At this point, the STSR will have tested the suction vacuum and assessed the cutting function of the vitrector, and also ensuring that the unit rates have been set for proper infusion, cutting, and aspiration according to the surgeon's preference.

6. The vitrectomy is performed using the maximum cutting speed on the instrument.

6. The surgeon controls the vitrector via a foot switch. Be sure it is in a comfortable, easy-to-access location. Other instruments, such as intraocular scissors or foreign body forceps, may be introduced through the same sclerotomy to accomplish the surgical objective. Prior to removal of instruments from the eye, infusion should be stopped.

7. When the procedure is complete, the instruments are withdrawn and sclerotomy plugs are inserted if necessary.

7. The surgeon may request that cultures of the vitreous washings be sent to pathology.

8. The sclerotomies are closed using 9–0 nylon sutures, infusion site last. The conjunctiva is closed with 6–0 polyglactin suture.

8. Suture should be prepared in advance of need. A count may not be necessary according to facility policy.

9. A subconjunctival injection of betamethasone 4 mg and gentamicin 40 mg may be given.

9. Medication and dressing material are ready for use. Assist with dressing application as needed.

Postoperative Considerations

Immediate Postoperative Care

- An eye patch may be placed at the surgeon's request.
- Patient should not strain or cough, as this may increase intraocular pressure.

Prognosis

- Vision is expected to be improved.

Complications

- Hemorrhage
- Infection

PEARL OF WISDOM

Many pieces of complex equipment are required. Always check equipment function before the procedure begins.

CASE STUDY

John is a 73-year-old male. His vision has become progressively darker and more cloudy in his left eye. He has suffered no pain during this slow loss of vision, and states that the loss of vision has occurred equally across his entire left field of vision. John is diagnosed with a cataract in his left eye.

1. What surgical intervention will be performed?
2. What special large piece of equipment will be required in order to perform this procedure?
3. Why must powder be meticulously removed from the gloves for this procedure?

QUESTIONS FOR FURTHER STUDY

1. What type of energy is used during phacoemulsification?
2. List two possible complications of intraocular gas injection.
3. What is meant by the term *retrobulbar block*?

BIBLIOGRAPHY

Albert, D. M., & Brightbill, F. S. (Eds.). (1999). *Ophthalmic surgery: Principles and techniques*. Malden, MA: Blackwell Science Inc.

Azar, D. T. (1997). *Refractive surgery*. New York: McGraw-Hill.

Chignell, A. H., & Wong, D. (1998). *Management of vitreo-retinal disease: A surgical approach*. New York: Springer-Verlag.

Del Monte, M. A., et al. (1993). *Atlas of pediatric ophthalmology and strabismus surgery*. Woburn, MA: Butterworth-Heinemann.

Folk, J. C., & Pulido, J. S. (1997). Laser photocoagulation of the retina and choroid. *Ophthalmology Monographs*, 11.

Goldman, M. A. (1988). *Pocket guide to the operating room*. Philadelphia: F. A. Davis.

McGuiness, A. M., et al. (2002). *Core curriculum for surgical technology* (5th ed.). Centennial, CO: Association of Surgical Technologists.

Stallard, H. B. (1989). *Stallard's eye surgery*. London; Boston: Wright.

CHAPTER 17

Otorhinolaryngologic Surgery

Teri Junge

CASE STUDY

Theodore, a 16-month-old male, has been brought by his father to the otorhinolaryngologist's office. The parent states that Theo has a cold and is suffering from a runny nose. The discharge is yellow and has a foul odor. Theo was uncooperative during the exam, but the physician was able to visualize a foreign object lodged between the middle and superior turbinates in his left nostril. Surgical removal of the object is scheduled for the next morning at the local surgery center.

1. Theo's surgery is considered urgent rather than emergent. Why?
2. Why is surgical removal of the object necessary?
3. What special equipment and supplies will be required for the procedure?
4. Will the STSR be required to employ sterile technique for the procedure?

OBJECTIVES

After studying this chapter, the reader should be able to:

A 1. Discuss the relevant anatomy of the ear, nose, and upper aerodigestive tract.

P 2. Describe the pathology that prompts otorhinolaryngologic surgical intervention and the related terminology.

3. Discuss any preoperative otorhinolaryngologic diagnostic procedures/tests.

O 4. Discuss any otorhinolaryngologic preoperative and intraoperative preparation procedures.

5. Identify the names and uses of otorhinolaryngologic instruments, supplies, and drugs.
6. Identify the names and uses of special otorhinolaryngologic equipment.
7. Define and give an overview of the otorhinolaryngologic procedure.
8. Discuss the purpose and expected outcomes of the otorhinolaryngologic procedure.
9. Discuss the immediate postoperative care and possible complications of the otorhinolaryngologic procedure.
10. **S** Discuss any specific variations related to the preoperative, intraoperative, and postoperative care of the otorhinolaryngologic patient.

SELECT KEY TERMS

1. aerodigestive tract
2. apnea
3. carina
4. cholesteatoma
5. congenital
6. dynamic equilibrium
7. epiglottis
8. epistaxis
9. Gelfoam
10. glottis
11. hydrops
12. hypertrophy
13. laryngo-
14. myringo-
15. olfaction
16. oropharynx
17. oto-
18. pharyngotympanic tube
19. polyp
20. polysomnography
21. rhino-
22. -sclerosis
23. SMR
24. T&A
25. UPPP

ANATOMY OF THE EAR

There are three main regions of the ear: the outer, middle, and inner ear. (Refer to Plate 4B in Appendix A.)

OUTER EAR

The external ear is comprised of the pinna (auricle) and the external auditory canal (meatus). The auricle is the portion of the ear that is visible on each side of the head; it encircles the opening into the external auditory meatus. Muscles and ligaments attach it to the head. The pinna consists of flexible cartilage that is covered with thick skin. The superior rim is referred to as the helix. The lobule (earlobe) is located inferiorly and lacks cartilage. The cartilaginous projection located anterior to the opening of the canal is called the tragus.

The external auditory canal extends from the pinna to the tympanic membrane. It has an S-shape and is approximately 2.5 cm in length. It passes through the auditory meatus of the temporal bone. The canal is covered with epithelium, lined with fine hairs, and houses the ceruminous glands, which secrete a substance called cerumen (earwax).

TYMPANIC MEMBRANE

The tympanic membrane, or eardrum, is the separation between the outer and middle ear. It is comprised of three layers. The outer surface is covered with epithelium, the central layer is fibrous connective tissue, and the inner lining is mucous membrane. It is disk shaped, normally concave, and has a diameter of about 1 cm. The eardrum is normally pearly gray in color, translucent, and has a shiny appearance. It assumes an oblique position. Incidentally, a branch of the facial nerve that carries taste impulses from the tongue passes along the inner surface of the tympanic membrane.

There are several landmarks on the tympanic membrane. The fibrous ring surrounding the tympanic membrane is referred to as the annulus. The major portion of the membrane is taut fibrous tissue called the pars tensa. A small superior portion is less tense and is called the pars flaccida because it lacks the central fibrous connective tissue. The umbo is the point of maximum concavity. The handle and the short process of the malleus can often be visualized behind the membrane. The cone of light is a triangular reflection of light that can be seen on the inferior anterior portion of the tympanic membrane.

MIDDLE EAR

The middle ear (tympanic cavity) is an air-filled chamber located within the temporal bone. The tympanic cavity is lined with a mucous membrane, which is a continuation of the inner layer of the tympanic membrane. The lateral border of the tympanic cavity is the tympanic membrane; the cavity ends medially with the superior oval window and the inferior round window. There are two openings into the wall of the middle ear. The tympanic antrum opens posteriorly into the mastoid sinus and the eustachian (auditory or **pharyngotympanic**) **tube** connects the middle ear to the nasopharynx.

The tympanic cavity houses a series of three small bones called the auditory ossicles. They have been named according to their shape and are, from lateral to medial, the malleus (hammer), the incus (anvil), and the stapes (stirrup). The ossicles have movable (synovial) joints between them. Ligaments connect the ossicles to the wall of the middle ear and two tiny skeletal muscles control their movement. The handle and short process of the malleus are embedded in the tympanic membrane; the head and neck extend upward into the epitympanic space, or attic. The head of the malleus articulates with the body of the incus. The ossicular chain is completed with the connection of the incus to the head of the stapes. The footplate of the stapes rests upon the oval window.

MASTOID SINUS (AIR CELLS)

The air cells of the mastoid sinus are located behind the auricle within the mastoid process of the temporal bone. The mastoid sinus is contiguous with the middle ear through an opening called the tympanic antrum (aditus ad antrum) (Figure 17-1).

INNER EAR

The inner ear, or labyrinth, consists of two main sections: the bony (osseous or perilymphatic) labyrinth and the membranous labyrinth. Labyrinths are complex series of

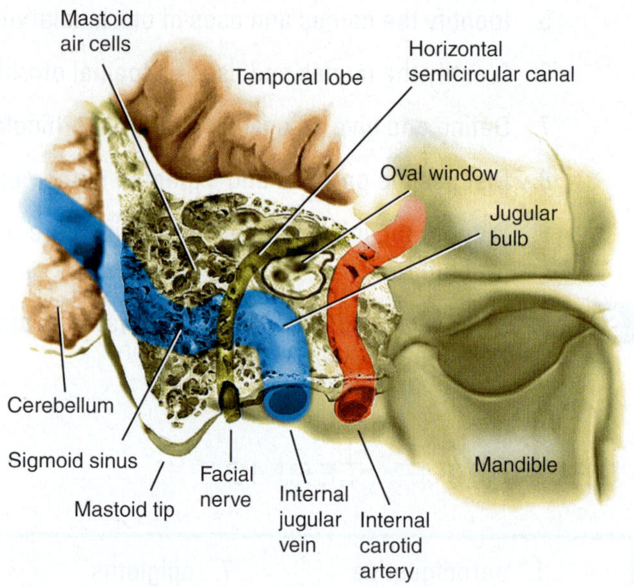

Figure 17-1 Mastoid sinus and related structures

canals and chambers located within the petrous portion of the temporal bone. A fluid called perilymph fills the spaces of the bony labyrinth, which is then lined by a thin membrane that houses another fluid called endolymph. The three compartments of the osseous labyrinth are the vestibule, the semicircular canals, and the cochlea, which are named according to their shapes.

The vestibule separates the cochlea from the semicircular canals and is centrally located. The vestibule contains two sacs called the utricle and the saccule, which are connected by the endolymphatic duct. The maculae possess sensitive hair cells, are contained within the sacs, and function in static equilibrium (stationary).

Three semicircular canals make up the lateral portion of the bony labyrinth. They are at approximate right angles to each other and are referred to by their positions: anterior, lateral, and posterior. The membranous labyrinth extends inside each of the semicircular canals; these extensions are referred to as semicircular ducts. The base of each canal has a small swelling called the ampulla. The ampullae come together to form the utricle. Each ampulla contains ridges called ampullary crests that possess cristae, which are clusters of sensitive hair cells embedded in a gelatin-like substance called cupula. **Dynamic equilibrium** (during movement) is controlled by the cristae.

The principal organ of equilibrium, the vestibular apparatus, is made up of the semicircular ducts including their ampullae, and the utricle and saccule of the vestibule. The vestibular branch of the eighth cranial (vestibulocochlear) nerve carries the information related to equilibrium to the cerebral cortex.

The organs of hearing (spiral organs or organs of Corti) are contained within the cochlea, a coiled portion of the bony labyrinth extending from the vestibule. Two membranes pass through the cochlea, dividing it into three chambers. The chamber between the membranes (vestibular and basilar membranes) is called the scala media, or cochlear duct. The cochlear duct is filled with endolymph and is considered the membranous labyrinth of the cochlea. It is believed that the endolymph is secreted from the wall of the cochlear duct. The chamber above the vestibular membrane is the scala vestibule, communicating laterally with the oval window, and continuing with the scala tympani, which is the chamber formed below the basilar membrane, at the cochlear apex called the helicotrema. The scala tympani terminate laterally at the round window. Both are filled with endolymph.

The organs of Corti are located along the length of the basilar membrane. They consist of a series of hair cells and supporting cells, which extend into the endolymph and touch a flexible gelatinous flap called the tectorial membrane that covers the organs of Corti. These hair cells within the basilar membrane directly contact the fibers of the cochlear nerve. The cochlear nerve is the branch of the eighth cranial nerve (vestibulocochlear nerve) that conducts the sound impulses to the auditory cortex of the temporal lobe of the brain.

PATHOLOGY OF THE EAR

Deafness is defined as any reduction of hearing, no matter how slight. Types of hearing loss are separated into the following seven categories: conduction-type deafness, sensorineural deafness, central deafness, mixed-type deafness, functional deafness, **congenital** deafness, and neonatal deafness. Types of hearing loss are outlined below.

- *Conduction-type deafness:* Occurs when there is an interference with the transmission of sounds from the external or middle ear, preventing sound waves from entering the inner ear. The causes are many. Some of these conditions will be described briefly in the following paragraphs. Many of the causes of conduction-type deafness are treatable with medication, surgery, or sound amplification.
- *Sensorineural deafness:* Also referred to as "nerve deafness." This condition involves the cochlear portion of the inner ear and/or the cochlear division of the acoustic (vestibulocochlear—eighth cranial) nerve. Little can be done to assist these patients, although some of the newer models of cochlear implants show great promise.
- *Central deafness:* Involves the acoustic center of the cerebral cortex.
- *Mixed-type deafness:* Involves both the conduction system and the nervous system. Generally, only the conduction portion of this condition is treatable.
- *Functional deafness:* Said to be of psychogenic nature. No conduction or nerve problem can be identified. Sometimes this condition is referred to as "selective" deafness.
- *Congenital deafness:* Present at the time of birth. This can be hereditary or due to the mother's exposure to disease (such as rubella) or toxic drugs during the pregnancy.
- *Neonatal deafness:* Occurs at the time of birth or shortly afterward. Prematurity, trauma, or Rh incompatibility can cause it.

PATHOLOGY AFFECTING THE OUTER EAR

The external auditory canal can easily become obstructed, especially in young children. Two common causes of obstruction are excess earwax (cerumen) and the presence of a foreign body. The patient may complain of loss of hearing, a feeling of fullness, dizziness, and tinnitus (ringing in the ear). Bony growths, called exostoses, and soft tissue growths, such as polyps, may also occur in the canal causing hearing impairment.

Infections and abscesses may affect the pinna and the canal. The patient may also suffer from otitis externa. This term applies to any general inflammation of the external auditory canal. One example of otitis externa is the common swimmer's ear. Swimmer's ear can be caused by stagnant water and wax in the ear or may be acquired from swimming in contaminated water. The inflammations can be either bacterial or fungal and cause the patient a great deal of pain. The condition is easily treated by keeping the ear canal dry and with antibiotics if necessary. Conditions of the external auditory canal are usually diagnosed using direct vision, possibly with the assistance of an **oto**scope.

PATHOLOGY AFFECTING THE TYMPANIC MEMBRANE

The tympanic membrane is easily ruptured. The perforation can be caused by either external trauma or excess pressure from within the middle ear. The patient's complaints may include pain, hearing loss, drainage, and dizziness. The presence of a tympanic defect will be confirmed with the use of an otoscope. The damage may be permanent or surgically repairable with a procedure called a **myringo**plasty (tympanoplasty). Occasionally, a small opening resolves spontaneously.

PATHOLOGY AFFECTING THE MIDDLE EAR

Damage to the ossicles of the middle ear can be a continuation of the previously mentioned trauma and perforation of the tympanic membrane. Fluid and microorganisms entering the middle ear cavity cause the damage. The patient's complaints will include pain, hearing loss, drainage, and dizziness. The extent of the damage can often be determined with the use of an otoscope. The type of myringoplasty to be performed will be determined by the extent of damage to the ossicular chain.

Otitis media is a very common acute inflammation of the middle ear, usually initiated by blockage of the eustachian tube causing an accumulation of fluid, which would normally be drained into the nasopharynx. The cardinal symptom of otitis media would be the patient's complaint of severe ear pain. The main sign of otitis media, observed by the clinician using the otoscope, is an inflamed, tense tympanic membrane. Generally, there is no permanent loss of hearing if the condition is treated immediately with systemic antibiotics. Decongestants may also assist in opening the eustachian tube, thereby facilitating drainage of the middle ear cavity. The tympanic membrane may rupture spontaneously or may require surgical incision. This procedure is called myringotomy.

Oto**sclerosis** occurs when there is a bony overgrowth of the stapes. Eventually the footplate of the stapes becomes fixed to the oval window, preventing the normal sound vibrations from entering the inner ear. This progressive disease is hereditary, affecting women more commonly than men and is diagnosed with the assistance of a tuning fork and audiometric exams. Surgical treatment to consider for this disorder would be stapedotomy or stapedectomy.

PATHOLOGY AFFECTING THE MASTOID

Mastoiditis is considered a complication of acute otitis media. The symptoms, which include pain and purulent discharge from the external auditory canal, generally develop 10–14 days following acute otitis media. Infection that has not been cleared from the middle ear may be forced into the mastoid air cells (sinus) through the antrum, causing destruction of the mastoid bone. The patient's complaints include earache, fever, purulent discharge from the ear, and inflammation of the mastoid process. Destruction of the mastoid bone is diagnosed with the use of computed tomographic scanning (CT scan) or magnetic resonance imaging (MRI). Mastoidectomy is the surgical intervention for mastoiditis, but only after extensive antibiotic therapy has failed. Mastoiditis that extends beyond the mastoid sinus can lead to meningitis or encephalitis and can be catastrophic.

Cholesteatoma is a benign cyst or tumor that fills the mastoid cavity and erodes the mastoid air cells. This process can also damage the ossicles. Cholesteatoma is formed when epithelial cells that would normally be shed through the eustachian tube are unable to migrate out of the middle ear cavity due to a blockage of the auditory tube. Earache, headache, purulent discharge from the ear, hearing loss, dizziness, and weakness of the facial muscles due to damage to the seventh cranial nerve are evidence of cholesteatoma (Figure 17-2). Surgical intervention is the only option to correct this condition; the procedure is called mastoidectomy. If the disease has damaged the ossicles, ossicular reconstruction may be useful in restoration of auditory function.

PATHOLOGY AFFECTING THE INNER EAR

Menière's syndrome patients suffer from fluctuating hearing loss, vertigo, tinnitus, and a feeling of fullness in the ear. It is caused by a dilatation (**hydrops**) of the endolymphatic spaces and is thought to be a failure of the membrane to reabsorb the endolymphatic fluid. The syndrome can affect the cochlea, vestibule, or both. Menière's syndrome is usually treated conservatively with lifestyle changes and medication. Surgical treatment, if necessary, is an endolymphatic shunt procedure to relieve the pressure and possibly severing of the auditory nerve.

DIAGNOSTIC PROCEDURES/TESTS FOR THE EAR

The tuning fork is a small two-pronged metal device that emits clear tone of a fixed pitch when tapped. The tuning fork is used as a diagnostic tool to perform an initial assessment of a patient's level of hearing, and may be used

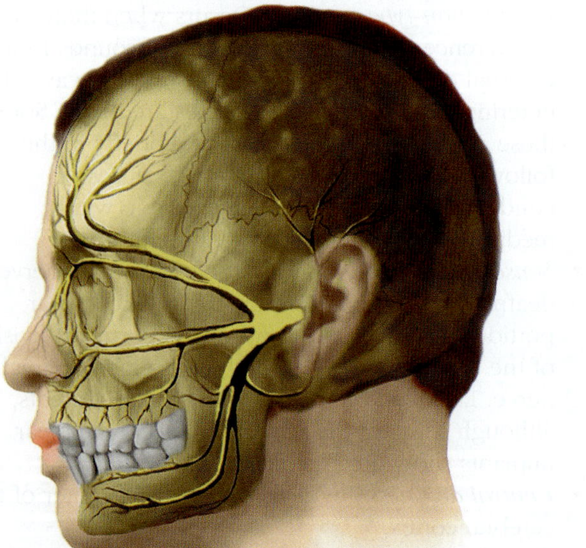

Figure 17-2 **Seventh cranial nerve**

intraoperatively on a patient under local anesthesia to determine improvement in his or her condition.

Audiometry is a more sophisticated method of testing a patient's hearing. The audiometer is a machine capable of emitting a tone at several different pitches and volumes. The patient indicates to the examiner which sounds are heard. The patient must be of an age and mental capacity to cooperate with the examiner. The patient may wear headphones for this examination or be placed in a sound-proof room to eliminate distractions. The audiogram can be helpful in determining the amount of damage to the sound conduction system, and very valuable in determining the type of hearing aid that will be most helpful to the patient. The results are generally reported in graph form.

The otoscope is a handheld, lighted instrument for viewing the external auditory canal (Figure 17-3). A speculum is inserted in the patient's ear by placing gentle traction on the pinna to straighten the canal. Many conditions of the middle ear may also be visualized with the use of the otoscope. The translucent tympanic membrane is regarded as a window to the middle ear. With very few exceptions, diseases of the middle ear manifest themselves with alterations in the color, position, and integrity of the tympanic membrane.

Computed tomography (CT scan), also known as computed axial tomography (CAT scan), and magnetic resonance imaging (MRI) are two specialized noninvasive methods of viewing the inside of the body. CT scans are very accurate in defining bony structures; MRI more accurately defines the soft tissues.

Tympanogram measures the vibrations of the eardrum by placing a probe against the tympanic membrane.

Electronystagmogram (ENG) is an exam that tests the balance mechanism in the inner ear. Cool, then warm liquid is introduced into the ear canal. The sudden temperature changes stimulate rapid eye movements which, when recorded, indicate the functioning of the balance mechanism.

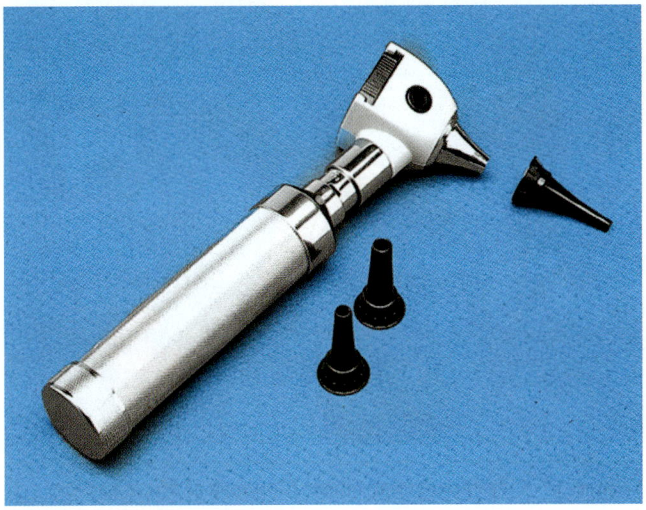

Figure 17-3 Otoscope

PREOPERATIVE CONSIDERATIONS

The operating room and equipment are prepared prior to the arrival of the patient. For procedures on pediatric patients, the temperature of the operating room may be raised and specialized anesthesia equipment employed.

If the use of a microscope is planned, the following preparatory steps should be taken:

- Clean according to facility standards
- Transport to OR from storage area
- Arrange eyepiece configuration according to the surgeon's preference
- Apply the proper magnification lens
- Position in advance

Generally, when a microscope is in use, the sterile team members are seated. Team members will need to gather and position the necessary number of adjustable stools.

Often for ear surgery, the operating table is reversed. The patient's head is placed at the foot of the table, allowing space under the foot portion of the table to accommodate the seated team member's legs and to allow for equipment placement (Figure 17-4).

Nitrous oxide causes expansion of the middle ear and can cause dislocation of a tympanic membrane graft. Nitrous oxide use is therefore restricted during reconstructive ear surgery.

For most ear procedures, the patient will be placed in the supine position and given a general endotracheal

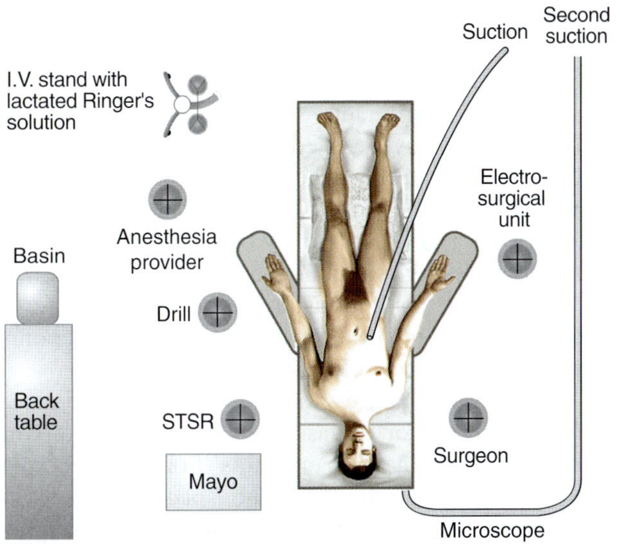

Figure 17-4 Sample operating room setup for head and neck procedures

anesthetic. A headrest is often used and the operative ear is turned upward. Steps should be taken to protect the unaffected ear from pressure. The arms are tucked at the patient's side after special consideration is given to pad and protect the ulnar nerve. A pillow under the knees will ease stress on the lower back.

A turban style head drape is commonly used to restrain the hair. A small area is shaved according to the surgeon's preference. The skin prep extends from the hairline to the shoulders and from the midline of the face to well behind the operative ear. Prep solution should not be allowed to contact the patient's eyes or pool in or near the eyes and ears (a cotton ball may be useful).

Draping of the patient may be extensive (according to the type of procedure to be performed) and include a head wrap and body drape. The final adjustments to the microscope should be made and the sterile microscope drape applied at the time of draping.

A solution containing epinephrine may be injected for its vasoconstrictive properties.

SPECIAL INSTRUMENTS, SUPPLIES, AND DRUGS

Delicate microscopic instrumentation should be handled carefully. When expecting a microscope to be used, the oculars and controls should be adjusted in advance according to the surgeon's preference. The use of specially designed sterile drapes or sterile handles may be employed. It may be helpful for the STSR to guide the instrumentation into the surgeon's field of vision under the microscope.

The argon laser is especially useful in the middle ear for stapedectomy and stapedotomy procedures.

A speculum holder may be used to free the surgeon's hands. The speculum holder attaches to the rail at the side of the operating table for stability.

A nerve stimulator should be available for identification of the facial and vestibulocochlear nerves.

Powered instruments, such as a rotating drill (osteon, ototome), may be used. It may be powered electrically or pneumatically. These complex instruments involve several components. All parts should be inspected and tested prior to use. A variety of burrs (cutting and diamond or polishing) should be available for selection by the surgeon. A continuous irrigation system may be needed in addition to the power equipment for cooling the tissue and removal of debris.

Several options are available for repair or replacement of damaged or diseased ossicles or the tympanic membrane. These may be autografts (from the same person), homografts (from the same species), xenografts (from animals), or allografts (synthetic). A variety of prosthetic graft materials is available. The surgical technologist must be certain that graft material from a source other than the patient has been secured in advance. The most commonly used autograft for tympanoplasty is the temporalis fascia because it is easily accessible and provides a thick, well-vascularized graft that easily epithelializes.

A variety of pharmaceutical agents may be used during ear surgery, including local anesthetics (with or without epinephrine according to the surgeon's preference), epinephrine, **Gelfoam**, bone wax, antibiotics (systemic and topical—wound irrigation, ointment, drops, or suspension), and anti-inflammatory agents.

The ear dressing may be a very simple dressing, such as cotton ball inserted in the external ear canal; or quite complex, such as a mastoid (Shea or a modification thereof) dressing. A mastoid dressing consists of antibiotic ointment, a nonadherent pad, fluffed gauze, and gauze that is wrapped around the patient's entire head.

EAR PROCEDURES

Many surgical options are available to correct deformities of the ear and restore function.

MYRINGOTOMY

Myringotomy or tympanotomy is an incision into the tympanic membrane for removing accumulated fluid, as is often seen with otitis media (Procedure 17-1). Myringotomy is often accompanied by the insertion of polyethylene ventilation tubes, or pressure equalizing (PE) tubes, to maintain the pressure equalization (Figure 17-5). The procedure is performed under general inhalation anesthesia for pediatric patients. A sample myringotomy instrument set is shown in Figure 17-6.

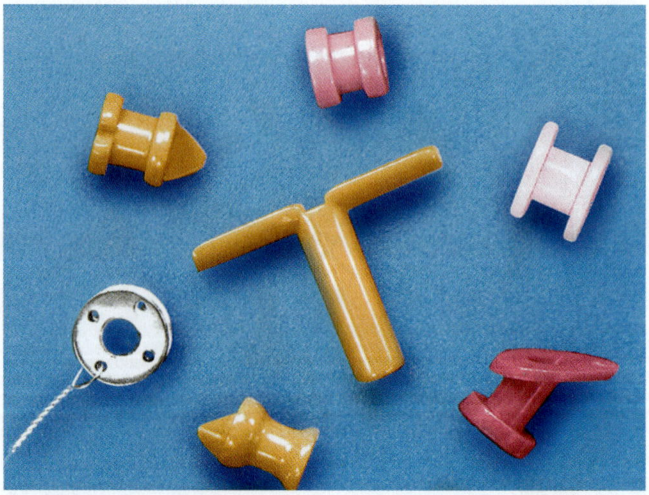

Figure 17-5 **Tympanostomy tubes** ***(Courtesy of Micromedics, Inc.)***

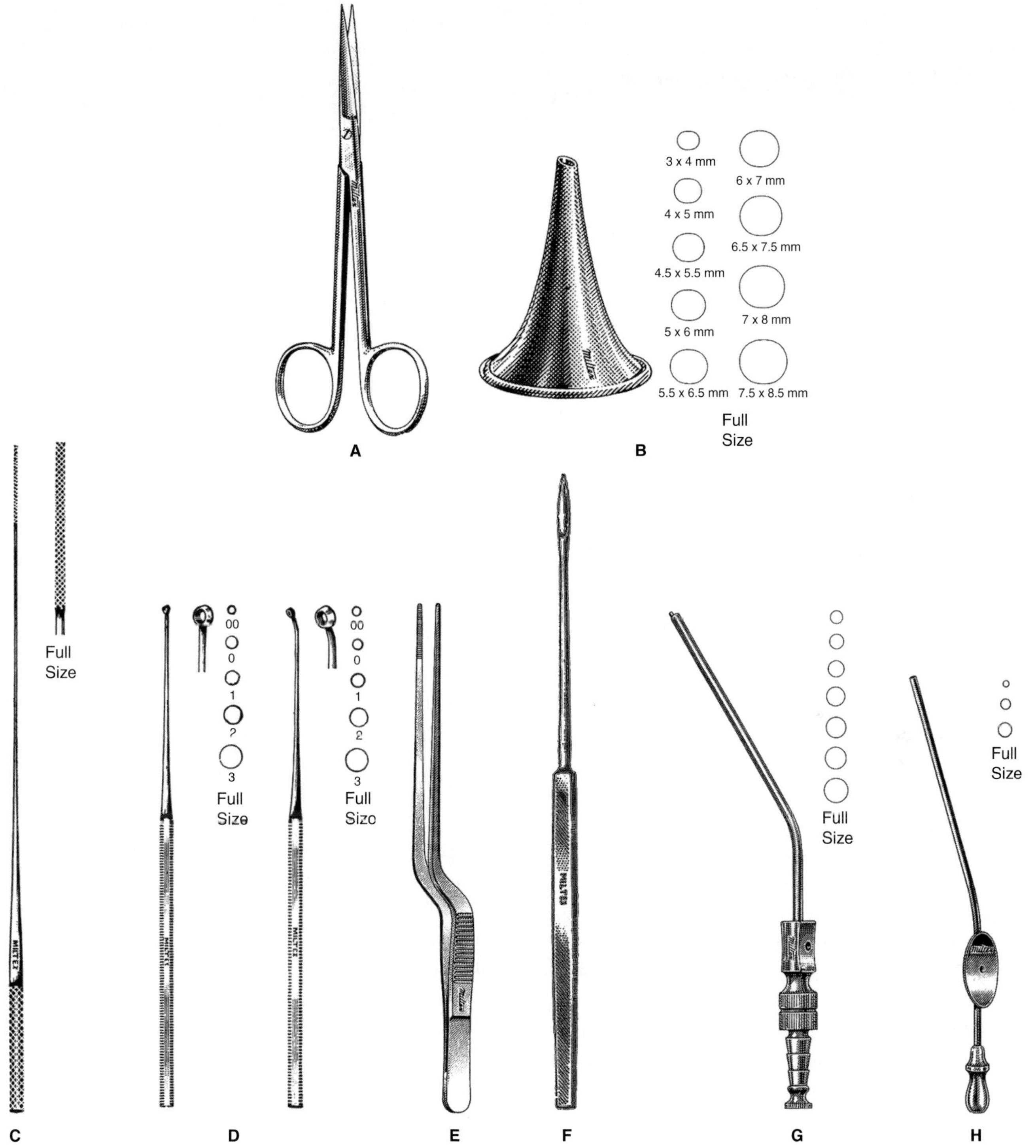

Figure 17-6 Myringotomy instrumentation: (A) Iris scissors (straight), (B) Farrior ear specula, (C) Brown applicator, (D) Buck ear curettes (straight and angled), (E) Adson bayonet dressing forceps, (F) Sexton ear knife, (G) Frazier Ferguson suction tip, (H) Baron suction tip *(Courtesy of Miltex Instrument Co., Inc.)*

PROCEDURE 17-1 Myringotomy

Equipment

- Operating microscope
- Suction apparatus
- Sterile microscope hand grips (available)
- Sitting stool for the surgeon

Instruments

- Myringotomy tray

Supplies

- Mayo stand cover
- Suction tubing
- Gloves
- PE tubes: size and style according to surgeon's preference
- Fenestrated drape sheet
- 4 × 4 gauze
- Disposable myringotomy knife
- Small basin with water
- Pharmaceuticals according to surgeon's preference

Operative Preparation

Anesthesia

- General
- Special equipment may be necessary for the pediatric patient

Position

- Reverse the operating table to accommodate seated surgeon and equipment
- Supine, with head turned to expose operative side
- Arms tucked at patient's side; protect ulnar nerves

Prep

- The hair may be restrained. Usually the cap is sufficient; occasionally an elastic band may be used
- The surgeon may not require that the skin be prepped

Draping

- Drapes may not be required
- Small fenestrated sheet may be used

Practical Considerations

- The PE tubes are considered implants and must be documented as such according to facility policy
- Sterile gloves are used, but a gown usually is not
- A Mayo stand is used for the procedure; a back table may not be necessary
- The surgeon is seated for the procedure
- Special accommodations may be needed for the pediatric patient
- Myringotomy is not a sterile procedure; use the best technique possible

Operative Procedure

1. Following placement of a fenestrated drape, a speculum is placed in the external auditory canal. Any visible wax accumulation will be removed with a curette.

Technical Considerations

1. Assess the diameter of the patient's ear canal and present the surgeon with the appropriate size speculum. The STSR should be prepared to clean the wax curette with gauze between uses.

PROCEDURE 17-1 Myringotomy *(continued)*

2. An incision is made in the inferior posterior portion of the tympanic membrane with a disposable myringotomy knife.

2. Prepare to pass myringotomy knife. The surgeon may not be willing to look away from the operative site, so it may be helpful for the STSR to guide the surgeon's hand into the field of vision. Fluid may be collected for culture and sensitivity. Suction will be used to remove excess fluid. Keep the suction apparatus patent by suctioning water through it or using the stylet. The fluid from the middle ear is thick.

3. A PE tube is placed into the tympanic incision.

3. The STSR will grasp the PE tube in the jaws of an alligator forceps or appropriate applicator (without touching it to prevent powder contamination) and carefully pass it to the surgeon.

4. Final positioning of the tube is achieved (Figure 17-7).

4. An instrument, such as a pick, may be used to aid in the final positioning of the tube.

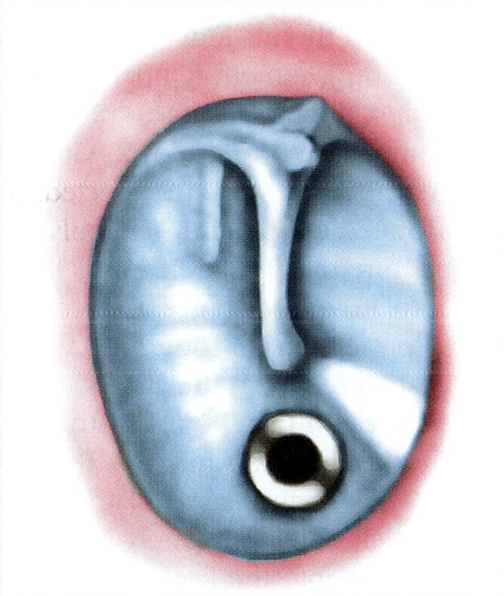

Figure 17-7 Myringotomy incision with PE tube in place

5. The speculum is removed. If desired, antibiotic/anti-inflammatory solution or suspension, such as Cortisporin, may be placed in the canal and the canal may then be packed with cotton.

5. Have antibiotic solution and/or cotton ready for use. Count may not be necessary, according to facility policy.

6. If the procedure is planned to be bilateral, the patient's head will be repositioned, the surgical team members will switch sides, and the sequence repeated.

6. Prepare to switch sides of the table with the surgeon if bilateral myringotomy is planned.

(continues)

PROCEDURE 17-1 **Myringotomy** *(continued)*

Postoperative Considerations

Immediate Postoperative Care

- Patient is expected to be released from the health care facility within an hour after the procedure is completed.
- Ear canal must be kept dry until PE tubes fall out or are removed and the tympanic membrane is healed.

Prognosis

- Patient is expected to return to normal activities within a few hours.
- Hearing is expected to return to normal.

Complications

- Recurrent infection
- Occasionally, patient may require a second procedure to remove a retained tube

PEARL OF WISDOM

Be sure that the microscope has been set up in advance of the procedure to the surgeon's specifications. The STSR may have to change the lens and/or the eyepieces. In addition, the oculars may need to be adjusted specifically for the surgeon's eyes.

MYRINGOPLASTY/ TYMPANOPLASTY

Myringoplasty is a type of tympanoplasty. Tympanoplasty is employed as a solution to a variety of conditions affecting the tympanic membrane and the ossicular chain. There are five classifications for tympanoplasty, which are determined by the extent of the damage to the eardrum and the middle ear:

- *Type I:* The damage is limited to the tympanic membrane. All contents of the middle ear are intact. A soft tissue graft is used to replace or repair the damaged eardrum.
- *Type II:* The destructive process extends beyond the damaged tympanic membrane to include the malleus. The entire malleus or the diseased portion is removed. The tympanic membrane graft is placed directly against the remaining portion of the malleus or the incus.
- *Type III:* In addition to the damaged tympanic membrane, both the malleus and incus have been affected. The replacement tympanum is placed directly against the intact stapes, permitting the transmission of sound to the oval window.
- *Type IV:* All of the ossicles are affected, in addition to the perforated tympanum. The only remaining natural structure of the middle ear is the intact and mobile footplate of the stapes. Only an air pocket remains as protection for the round window, as the graft rests directly on the stapes footplate. The ossicular chain may be reconstructed.
- *Type V:* This situation is similar to Type IV with one exception. The remaining footplate of the stapes is fixed. All ossicles are completely removed. A window is made into the horizontal semicircular canal and the tympanic graft seals off the middle ear and provides protection for the oval window.

Often the disease affecting the middle ear has extended into the mastoid sinus. This will require a combination procedure consisting of a tympanoplasty and a mastoidectomy. Tympanoplasty will be used as an illustrative procedure for the student (Procedure 17-2). Any major ear case will follow this basic sequence, with minor adjustments for the specific procedure. Many of the technical considerations are the same, although the procedures are designed to provide the patient with completely different results. Mastoidectomy will be described separately later in this chapter.

PROCEDURE 17-2 Myringoplasty/Tympanoplasty

Equipment

- Operating microscope
- Sitting stools for sterile team members
- Suction apparatus
- Ear drill if mastoidectomy is also planned
- Electrosurgical unit with dispersive electrode

Instruments

- Ear instrumentation set
- Sterile components of ear drill

Supplies

- Prep set
- Basic pack
- Basin set
- Gloves
- Head and neck drapes
- Fenestrated adhesive plastic drape
- Microscope drape
- Ossicular implants if requested
- Gelfoam
- Micro wipe
- Specialized knife blades per surgeon's preference
- Pharmaceuticals according to surgeon's preference
- Bone wax
- Suture according to surgeon's preference
- Dressing materials according to surgeon's preference

Operative Preparation

Anesthesia

- General (preferred)
- Lubricate and protect patient's eyes
- Local anesthetic with epinephrine may be used in addition to the general anesthetic to reduce intraoperative bleeding and to promote postoperative comfort

Position

- Reverse operating table to accommodate seated team members and equipment
- Supine, with head turned to expose operative side; donut, foam head rest, or head holder may be used
- Arms tucked at patient's sides; protect ulnar nerves

Prep

- A small area behind the ear may need to be shaved
- The hair is restrained with an elastic band or tape
- The entire side of the head is prepped. Prevent prep solution from pooling near the eye. Dry

Draping

- A turban-style head wrap or three towels arranged triangularly may be used
- Remove protective paper from disposable drapes with adhesive edges
- The adherent plastic fenestrated drape, if used, is applied first
- Place the bar drape across the patient's forehead and allow the remainder of the drape to fall toward the floor covering the head of the operating table
- Situate the U-drape on the patient's cheek. Bring the edges of the U up along both sides of the patient's ear. Extend the remainder of the drape to cover the patient's body

(continues)

PROCEDURE

17-2 Myringoplasty/Tympanoplasty *(continued)*

Practical Considerations

- Tympanoplasty is considered a sterile procedure
- The patient, under local anesthesia, should be advised that any movement could cause permanent disability and that any noise (especially use of a drill) in the operating room will seem amplified

Operative Procedure

1. The surgeon may choose either a transaural or a retroauricular (postauricular) approach. If a mastoidectomy is also planned, or the possibility of a temporalis fascia graft exists, the retroauricular approach is preferred.
2. If the surgeon is planning to use an autograft, the specimen is taken at the beginning of the procedure, so that the sometimes-lengthy graft preparation process can begin.
3. The tympanic membrane and the ossicular chain are assessed. A variety of microinstruments may be necessary for the exploration and dissection.
4. Diseased tissues and damaged ossicles are removed.

Technical Considerations

1. Communicate with the surgeon about the specific variances for this particular patient. Assist with draping the patient and equipment. Assist with placement of sterile equipment. Be sure that powder is removed from the gloves of all team members. Once seated, remain seated.
2. Pass #15 blade for postauricular incision. Electrosurgery and Senn retractors will be utilized next. The STSR will likely be expected to hold the retractors. Have the scissors and tissue forceps in a position such that the surgeon can "help him- or herself" to facilitate the dissection. Once secured, the graft will need special attention according to surgeon's preference. Graft tissue, when allowed to air dry, becomes thin and light (like tissue paper). Be sure that it is in a secure location so that an air current doesn't carry it to the *floor!*
3. Provide the appropriate size ear speculum. Install the speculum holder if its use is intended. Instrumentation for the middle ear is often stored in a rack. The rack is also designed for intraoperative use. This is an advantage for the STSR, in that it keeps the Mayo stand organized, but it also presents a hazard, as the tips of the instruments are pointed upward. Use extreme caution. Take great care when handling the delicate microinstrumentation. Use a micro wipe to clean the instruments rather than gauze to keep the items free of lint.
4. The room is often darkened to enhance the surgeon's view of the operative site—keep safety measures in mind. Keep the most used microinstruments on the Mayo stand in the rack and *always* return them to their original location for organizational purposes. Suggestion: Use

PROCEDURE

17-2 Myringoplasty/Tympanoplasty *(continued)*

alphabetical order to organize the "ringed" instruments (e.g., "a" alligator, "b" Bellucci scissors, "c" cupped forceps). To save time, use one hand to take the used instrument from the surgeon and the other to pass the requested instrument. It may be helpful for the STSR to guide the instrumentation into the surgeon's field of vision. Removed ossicles may be repositioned. *Do not* pass off the field until the end of the case.

5. If necessary, the mastoidectomy would be performed at this point.	**5.** The ear drill and suction/irrigation system should be connected, turned on, and tested. Be sure that an adequate amount of irrigation fluid is constantly available during drilling to prevent bone necrosis. Bone wax may be requested. A variety of cutting burs for the drill will be necessary. Typically, the surgeon starts with a large bur and progressively changes to smaller sizes as the nerve is approached. Diamond burs are used for smoothing and reducing bleeding. The STSR should be able to change the bur quickly and efficiently. Use the safety mechanism on the drill to prevent injury. Epinephrine may be instilled to reduce bleeding.
6. Ossicular reconstruction using materials of the surgeon's choice is performed, if possible.	**6.** A previously removed ossicle may be reinserted (it may be necessary to refashion it with the drill). An ossicle holder will be necessary. Other types of reconstruction materials may be implanted.
7. Small Gelfoam pledgets may be packed into the tympanic cavity to temporarily stabilize the contents of the middle ear and to make a bed on which the new tympanic membrane may rest.	**7.** Gelfoam is packaged in a large sheet; pledgets will need to be cut and possibly compressed. It may be used dry or moistened with saline or antibiotic solution.
8. The graft is placed under the remnant of the existing eardrum. Additional packing of Gelfoam or Vaseline gauze may be placed in the external auditory canal. The retroauricular wound, if used, is sutured.	**8.** The graft is fragile. Handle with caution. Small scissors may be needed to tailor the graft to fit the ear canal. More packing will be needed. Suture should be ready—pass with an Adson tissue forceps. Suture scissors next. Count.
9. A protective dressing is applied.	**9.** Application of the dressing can be a complex process. The STSR will likely be asked to hold the patient's head while the surgeon applies the dressing. Have all supplies laid out in the anticipated order of use. Be certain that the patient's airway is not disturbed when manipulating the head.

(continues)

PROCEDURE

17-2 Myringoplasty/Tympanoplasty *(continued)*

Postoperative Considerations

Immediate Postoperative Care

- Patient is instructed not to blow his or her nose forcefully until healing has occurred.
- Patient is instructed to keep ear dry.

Prognosis

- Patient may resume normal activity in about two weeks.
- In most cases full hearing is restored.

Complications

- Hemorrhage
- Infection
- Failure to restore full hearing

PEARL OF WISDOM

DO NOT disturb the microscope or operating table once the procedure has begun. Do not use it as a foot or armrest.

MASTOIDECTOMY

Mastoidectomy is the removal of the bony partitions that form the mastoid air cells. Mastoidectomy would be indicated for cholesteatoma or mastoiditis. Mastoidectomy may be performed in conjunction with other procedures for hearing restoration, such as tympanoplasty. Great care is taken to preserve the facial nerve, which passes through the temporal bone near the mastoid sinus. There are three types of mastoidectomy.

Simple mastoidectomy is the removal of the mastoid air cells only. This is accomplished through a postauricular incision. The mastoid sinus is eradicated with a bur. Prior to wound closure, a drain may be placed.

Modified radical mastoidectomy is the removal of the posterior and superior walls of the external auditory canal, as well as the eradication of the mastoid air cells. The middle ear remains intact.

Radical mastoidectomy involves the removal of the mastoid air cells, as well as the tympanic membrane and the malleus and incus. The middle ear and mastoid cavity are combined. The stapes remains in place; it is usually covered by a temporalis fascia graft. The tensor tympani muscle is used to occlude the eustachian tube. Occasionally, the cavity is left to heal by second intention.

Complications of mastoidectomy may include damage to the facial nerve, hearing loss, vertigo, and meningitis.

STAPEDECTOMY

Stapedectomy is the surgical intervention of choice for patients with otosclerosis. This procedure is often performed under local anesthetic with a compliant patient so that the surgeon using either voice commands or a tuning fork may immediately assess hearing restoration. Stapedectomy involves the removal of the fixed stapes through a transaural or retroauricular incision. Stapedectomy may be either total or partial. Several types of prostheses are available for reconstruction of the ossicular chain (Figure 17-8). The final determination of the type and size of prosthesis necessary will be made after the surgeon has assessed the damage under direct visualization with the microscope. If necessary, prior to insertion of the prosthesis, a soft tissue graft is positioned over the oval window. The wound is closed and the canal may be packed with Gelfoam. Stapedectomy is usually an out-patient procedure. The patient may be kept overnight if nausea or dizziness is a problem. The patient is advised not to make any sudden movements to avoid these symptoms. The patient is expected to return to normal activities, including work, in approximately 2 weeks. The success rate with stapedectomy is greater than 80%. Stapedectomy patients may also benefit from hearing aids. Complications may include dizziness, taste disturbances, loss of hearing, eardrum perforation, and temporary weakness of the facial muscles.

STAPEDOTOMY

Stapedotomy is an alternate procedure to stapedectomy. A small opening is created in the fixed stapes footplate with a small drill or a laser. This allows for transmission of sound waves or placement of the prosthesis.

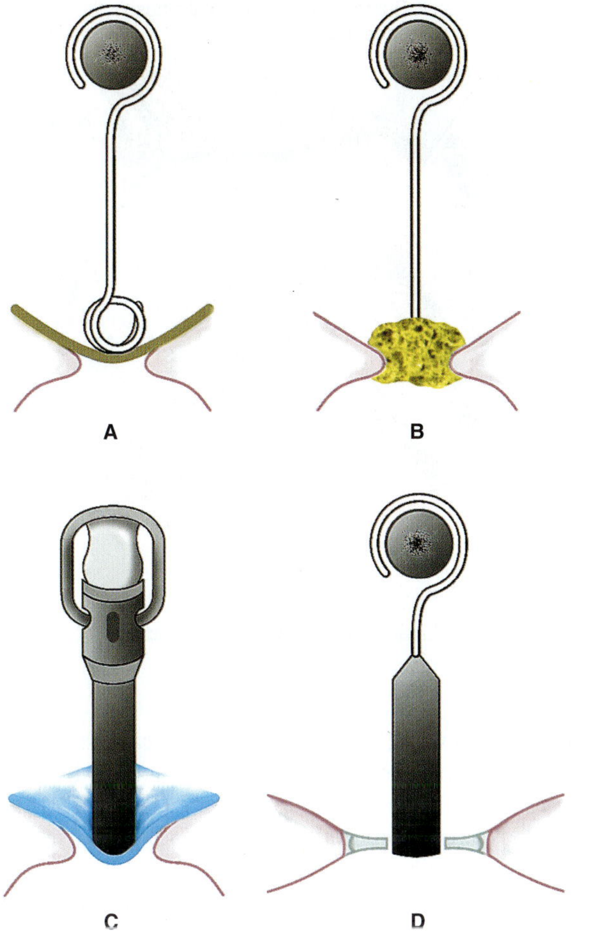

Figure 17-8 **Stapes prosthesis in place: (A) Wire and absorbable sponge, (B) wire and fat graft, (C) piston-type and vein or fascia graft, (D) piston-type without graft**

COCHLEAR IMPLANTS

A cochlear implant is a prosthetic replacement for the cochlear portion of the inner ear (Figure 17-9). This type of prosthesis is beneficial for individuals with sensorineural deafness. The device has two components. The first is an internal component that possesses several electrodes which enter and circle around inside the cochlea. This is implanted under the patient's skin behind the ear. The electrodes receive signals transmitted from the external portion of the device to the cochlea activating the fibers of the eighth cranial nerve to transmit the signal to the brain for interpretation. The second part of the device is external and consists of a microphone, a speech processor that converts sound into electrical impulses, and connecting cables.

ANATOMY OF THE NOSE AND SINUSES

The nose is a facial feature that serves as the organ for the sense of smell and as the upper portion of the respiratory

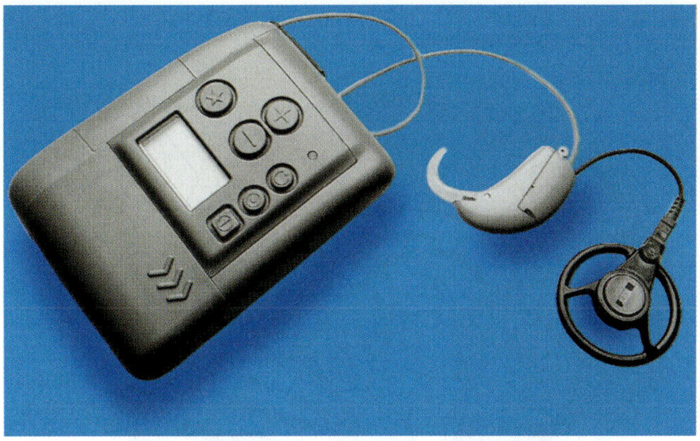

Figure 17-9 **Cochlear prosthesis** ***(Courtesy of Cochlear Corporation)***

system (Figure 17-10). A pair of nasolacrimal ducts enters the nasal cavity near the inferior meatus and is part of the tear drainage system.

EXTERNAL NOSE

Several terms are used to describe the outer, skin covered, aspects of the nose (Figure 17-11). The tip is referred to as the apex. The base includes the openings or nares and the root joins the nasal bones to the skull superiorly. The flared lateral wings of the external nose are referred to as ala. The dorsum is between the root and the tip, with the bridge being the upper portion of the dorsum.

Two nasal bones are located just inferior to the frontal bone and provide support to the dorsum. Only the upper third of the nasal projection is bony, the lower two thirds is cartilaginous. Upper lateral (lateral nasal) cartilages provide support for the middle third of the nose. Lower lateral (major alar) cartilages flare from the septum to form the tip of the nose. A series of minor alar cartilages give the shape to the lateral edges of the ala.

INTERNAL NOSE

The nasal cavity is the interior chamber of the nose and is lined with mucous membrane. Its two outside openings or nostrils are referred to as the external nares. The internal nares are the openings from the nasal cavity into the pharynx. The hard and soft palate, respectively, form the anterior and posterior floor of the nasal cavity. The ending of the soft palate is the uvula.

The nasal cavity is divided into two chambers by the nasal septum (Figure 17-12). Anteriorly, the septum is cartilaginous; posteriorly, the septum has bony attachments to the ethmoid and vomer bones. The septal cartilage is also known as the quadrilateral cartilage.

Each nasal cavity, or fossa, has a series of four bony projections called conchae or turbinates. The conchae are osseus ridges on the lateral walls of the cavity. Their names are indicative of their location—supreme, superior,

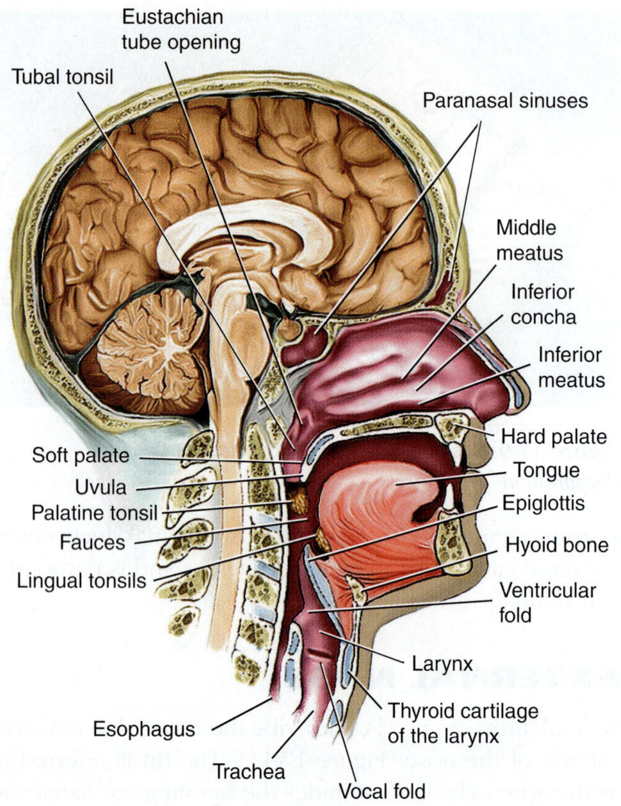

Figure 17-10 Paranasal sinuses and related structures

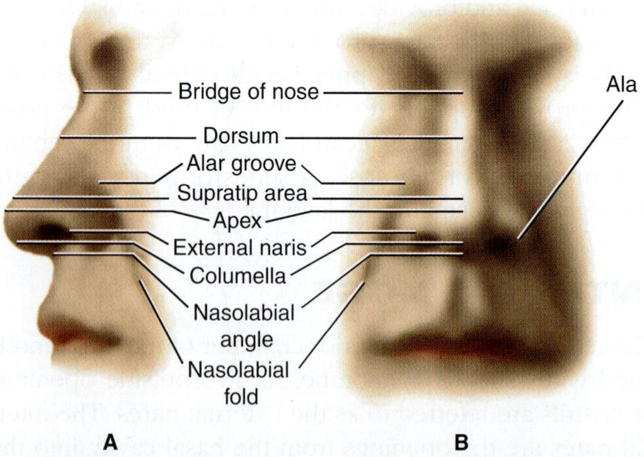

Figure 17-11 External nose: (A) Lateral view, (B) anterior view

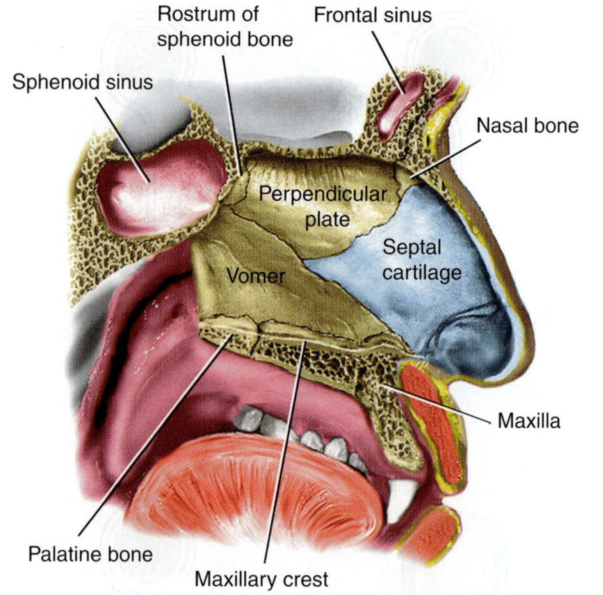

Figure 17-12 Nasal septum and related structures

middle, and inferior. The orifice of each eustachian tube enters the nasal cavity posterior to the turbinates.

PARANASAL SINUSES

A series of ducts called ostia lead to the paranasal sinuses, which are air cavities in the bone surrounding the nasal cavity. The sinuses are lined with mucous membrane that is contiguous with the lining of the nasal cavities. There are four pairs of paranasal sinuses. Each is named by location according to the bone that encloses it (Figure 17-13). The four pairs are frontal, ethmoid, sphenoid, and maxillary. They are located as follows:

- Frontal sinuses are located within the frontal bone behind the eyebrows, and may be one cavity or divided.
- Ethmoid sinuses, numbering 10–15, are located between the eyes and have a honeycomb appearance.
- Sphenoid sinuses are located directly behind the nose at the center of the skull and may be one cavity or divided.
- Maxillary sinuses are located below the eyes and lateral to the nasal cavity.

BLOOD SUPPLY TO THE NOSE

Branches of both the internal and external carotid arteries provide the blood supply to the nose (Figure 17-14). The main source is the internal maxillary artery, which is one of the terminal divisions of the external carotid. The internal maxillary artery, specifically the sphenopalatine branch, serves most of the posterior nasal septum and the posterior lateral walls of each nasal cavity. The ethmoidal arteries are branches of the ophthalmic artery, which is an extension of the internal carotid artery. The ethmoidal arteries mainly supply the anterior septum and anterior lateral walls of the cavity. Kiesselbach's plexus is the terminal end of the anterior ethmoid artery and the corresponding veins in the anterior septum and is a common site for **epistaxis** (nosebleed).

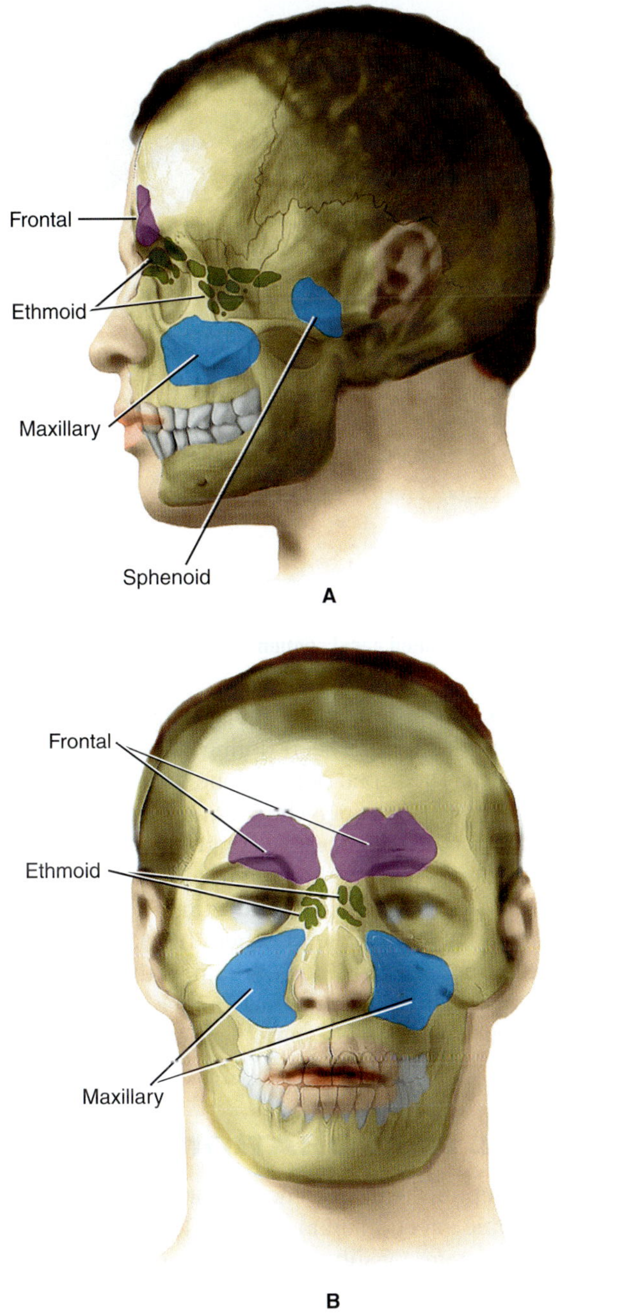

Figure 17-13 Paranasal sinuses: (A) Lateral view, (B) anterior view

OLFACTION

The sense of smell is called the olfactory sense. The chemoreceptors for **olfaction** are located in the olfactory epithelium in the most superior region of each nasal cavity just above the superior turbinate near the cribriform plate of the ethmoid bone. The olfactory nerve fibers pass through the cribriform plate in the roof of the nose, where they integrate with the olfactory bulb. The olfactory bulb is the tip of the first cranial nerve. The sense of smell is processed in the olfactory cortex of the temporal lobe.

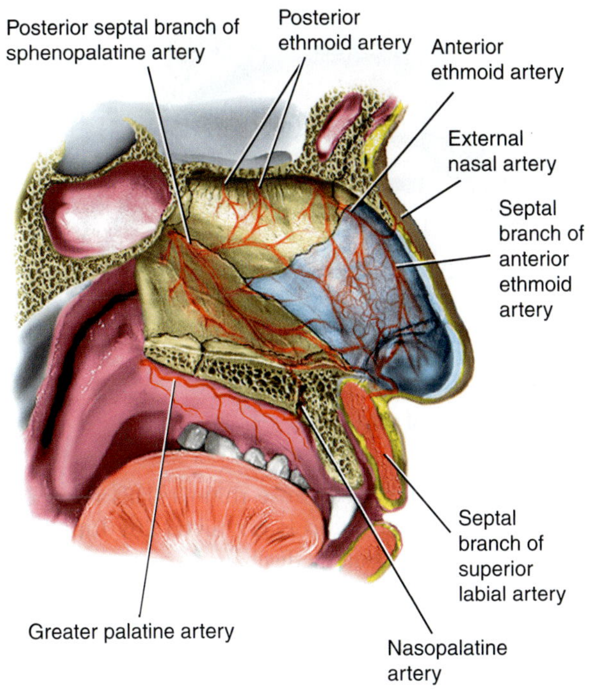

Figure 17-14 Blood supply of the nose

PATHOLOGY OF THE NOSE AND PARANASAL SINUSES

The nose and paranasal sinuses are prone to suffer several types of pathological conditions. These are reviewed below.

RHINITIS/SINUSITIS

Rhinitis is inflammation of the nasal mucosa, usually evidenced by excessive mucous production or **rhino**rrhea. Sinusitis is inflammation of the mucosal lining of the paranasal sinuses. Sinusitis is considered serious when it becomes chronic and suppurative causing permanent changes in the tissues of the sinus. Rhinitis and sinusitis are closely linked. If the cause of rhinitis is not solved, the inflammation can easily extend to the nasal mucosa and to the paranasal sinuses. Rhinitis and subsequent sinusitis can be attributed to several causes.

The most common cause of rhinitis is the virus that causes the common cold. Treatment for the cold is symptomatic; antibiotic or surgical intervention is not recommended.

Allergic rhinitis, or hay fever, may be acute or chronic. The usual symptoms are itchy eyes and nose, tearing, nasal discharge, and headache caused by nasal obstruction. Allergic rhinitis can be seasonal due to pollens, or it can be perennial, caused by sensitivity to dust or other substances constantly present in the environment. Treatment may include antihistamines for mild cases and can include steroids for the more severe. In all cases, the substance causing the allergy should be identified; the patient may possibly need immunotherapy for desensitization.

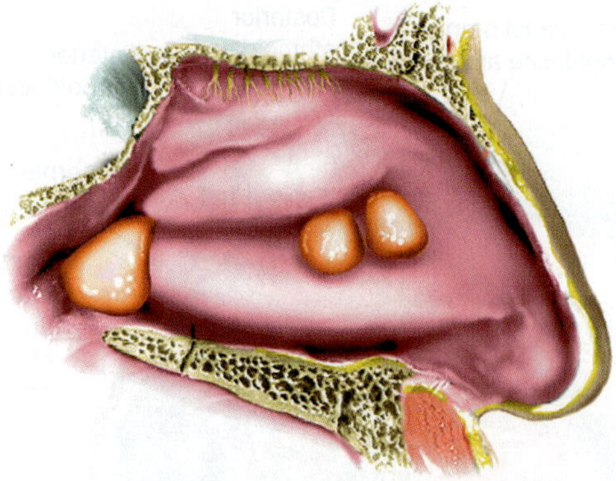

Figure 17-15 Nasal polyps

Foreign bodies also cause rhinitis. This is generally unilateral rhinitis and often is not given any further consideration until a purulent discharge appears. The clinician is usually able to diagnose the presence of a foreign body with direct vision. Removal is necessary, and in a small child, the use of an anesthetic may be necessary.

NASAL POLYPS

Polyps are growths that originate from mucous membrane (Figure 17-15). Often the polyps arise from the walls of the sinuses or the ostia and protrude into the nasal passageway. Most often nasal polyps develop in patients suffering from allergic rhinitis. The recurrent inflammatory process eventually causes a small swelling that enlarges with each subsequent episode. The polyp is connected to the mucous membrane by a pedicle. Polyps can be multiple and in some cases, the size and number may cause complete obstruction of the nose. The sense of olfaction is often impaired. In many cases, polyps reoccur following treatment. Nasal polyps are usually diagnosed by direct vision. Conservative treatment with steroids can cause temporary shrinkage of the polyps, but surgical removal usually becomes necessary.

HYPERTROPHIED TURBINATES

Permanent enlargement of the turbinates or nasal conchae may occur as a result of chronic rhinitis. Because of recurring inflammations, the turbinate loses its normal elastic ability. This can be severe enough to cause nasal obstruction. The hypertrophic turbinate can be seen during a visual examination of the nasal cavity. Occasionally the size of the turbinate can be reduced electrosurgically or with the use of a sclerosing agent. Often the affected turbinate must be excised.

DEVIATED NASAL SEPTUM

The nasal septum is typically straight at birth. During aging, the septum tends to deviate to one side or the other.

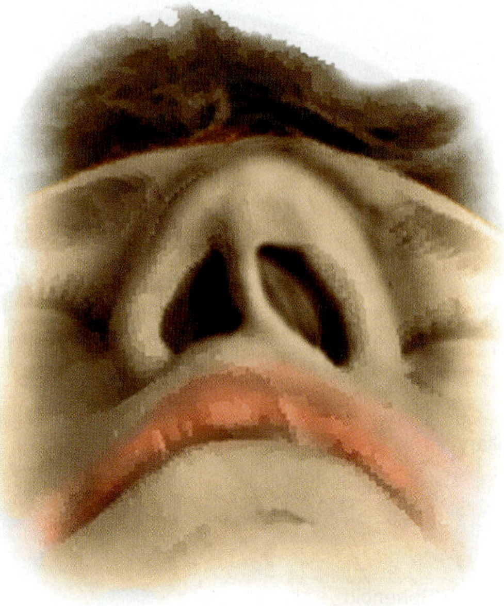

Figure 17-16 Deviated nasal septum

The septum may also become deviated due to trauma. A deviated nasal septum is seen during visual examination (Figure 17-16). The septal defect alone does not cause the patient to be symptomatic. There is no related pain, unless soft tissue damage occurs in conjunction with trauma. If the deviation is severe, the patient may experience difficulty breathing due to the obstruction. The patient may also suffer sinusitis because of ostium blockage, resulting in failure of the affected sinus to drain. If the septum has been traumatically displaced, it may be manually reduced. An anesthetic may be necessary. Surgical repair of a deviated nasal septum is common.

SEPTAL PERFORATION

The nasal septum may become perforated due to carcinoma, chronic infection, intractable picking, occupational chemical exposure, or substance (cocaine) abuse. The patient with septal perforation may complain of a whistling noise during respiration and the defect is obvious on visual examination. The perforation rarely occurs in the bony septum. The defect may be allowed to close by second intention, or may require surgical intervention.

EPISTAXIS

Trauma is the main cause of nosebleed. Excess drying of the nasal mucosa, over-blowing, picking, hypertension, and chronic inflammation can also be contributing factors to epistaxis. Most nosebleeds originate at the Kiesselbach's plexus located in the anterior portion of the nasal septum. Anterior nosebleeds are easily controlled by direct pressure. Posterior bleeding is more profuse and more difficult to control. Packing and electrosurgery may be initial treatments, with internal maxillary artery ligation becoming necessary in only the most severe cases.

DIAGNOSTIC PROCEDURES/TESTS

Diagnostic approaches to nasal and paranasal sinus pathology include direct vision, mirror examination, and radiography.

DIRECT VISION

The most common and highly effective method of examining the interior of the nose is direct vision. Excellent illumination is imperative. This is often accomplished with the use of a lamp affixed to the examiner's head. The direction and the intensity of the light beam is adjustable on most of these devices. A nasal speculum may be used to spread the nares.

MIRROR EXAMINATION

Another approach is mirror examination of the nasopharynx and posterior nasal cavity. The patient is instructed to open the mouth and the tongue is gently retracted. A small mirror is warmed to prevent fogging, inserted into the **oropharynx**, and directed upward. With good illumination, the examiner is able to view the posterior nares, the turbinates, the posterior end of the vomer bone, and the outlet of the maxillary sinus.

RADIOGRAPHY

Standard radiography is still a very valuable tool in diagnosing nasal and sinus disorders (Figure 17-17). Simple X-ray can easily show fractures and occluded sinuses. Four basic views make up a "sinus series": the Waters view, Caldwell view, lateral view, and submental view. Each is specifically valuable in viewing the four main sinuses.

Computed tomography is rapidly replacing the use of standard radiography. CT scanning makes a very clear delineation between bony and soft tissue structures. The computer-generated views are able to produce projections of otherwise inaccessible anatomical structures. Magnetic resonance imaging does not clearly define the bony structures; for this reason, it is of little value in diagnosing sinus disorders.

Angiography is used to demonstrate blood flow. This can be useful in determining the exact location of hemorrhage in case of traumatic injuries or epistaxis.

PREOPERATIVE CONSIDERATIONS

If a local anesthetic is planned, and an anesthesia provider will not be in attendance, the presence of a second circulator may be requested for patient monitoring. The patient may be given a local anesthetic in addition to a general anesthetic to help provide hemostasis, shrink the nasal mucosa, and minimize postoperative pain.

Preoperative patient teaching is very important with all nasal procedures. In this instance, patients should be forewarned that nasal packing will be inserted as part of the procedure. The packing may be uncomfortable and will require breathing through the mouth. Nose and sinus surgery is generally done on an out-patient basis. Patients should be instructed to have a responsible person available to drive them home and to stay with them for the next 24 hours. A visit to the doctor's office the first or second postoperative day is usually necessary for removal of the packing.

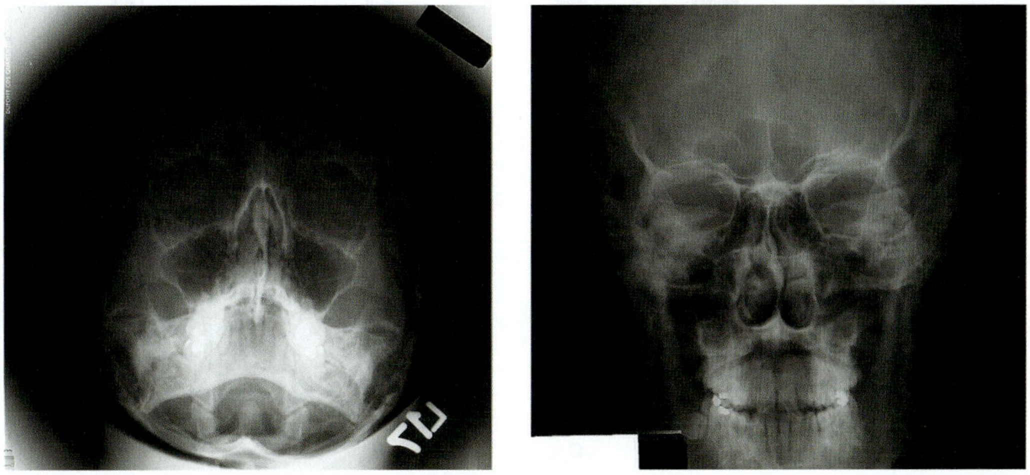

A B

Figure 17-17 Radiographic views of sinuses: (A) Waters, (B) Caldwell

Procedures performed through the nose are not considered sterile procedures. However, great care should be taken to use the best possible technique to prevent introducing an infectious agent to the area.

The patient is placed on the operating table in the supine position. The table may be flexed for patient comfort. The head is placed on a headrest and may be raised to reduce bleeding and prevent edema. The arms should be restrained at the patient's sides, with the ulnar nerve well padded and the fingers protected. A pillow under the knees will reduce lumbar strain.

Removal of facial hair is usually not necessary. The prep, if requested, should begin at the upper lip and extend to the hairlines and beyond the chin. Caution must be used not to allow prep solution to enter the patient's eyes or ears.

Draping may include a turban-style wrap to restrain the hair. Three wound towels may be placed in a triangular arrangement, then a bar sheet placed across the forehead, with a split sheet encircling the face and covering the body.

SPECIAL INSTRUMENTS, SUPPLIES, AND DRUGS

Instrumentation for rhinoplasty (often considered "plastic surgery") differs from the instrumentation for internal nasal and sinus surgery. Endoscopic sinus surgery requires specialized instrumentation and auxiliary equipment, for which special care and handling will be necessary. A sample nasal instrument set is shown in Figure 17-18.

In addition to standard operating lamps, the surgeon may use an additional illumination device. The use of a headlight should be planned. This may be a direct light beam or it may be reflected.

The use of a small table (prep stand) or second Mayo stand may be requested to hold the supplies necessary for administering the local anesthetic. Suggested supplies for this "clean" setup include:

- Two medicine cups
- Two local (Luer-lock, control) syringes
- Two 25- or 27-gauge × 2-in. needles
- Long cotton-tip applicators

(Text continues on page 609)

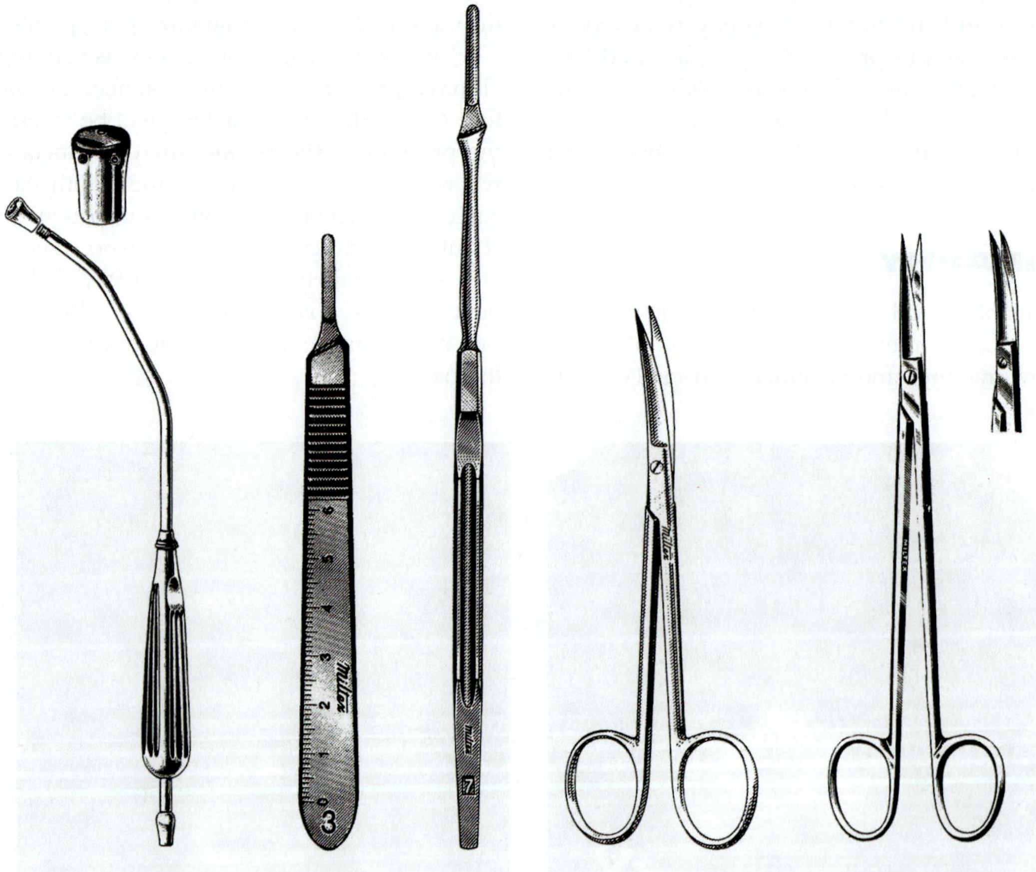

Figure 17-18 **Nasal instrumentation: (A) Yankauer suction tip, (B) #3 scalpel handle, (C) #7 scalpel handle, (D) plastic surgery scissors (curved—sharp point), (E) Joseph nasal scissors (straight and curved—sharp point)** ***(Courtesy of Miltex Instrument Co., Inc.)***

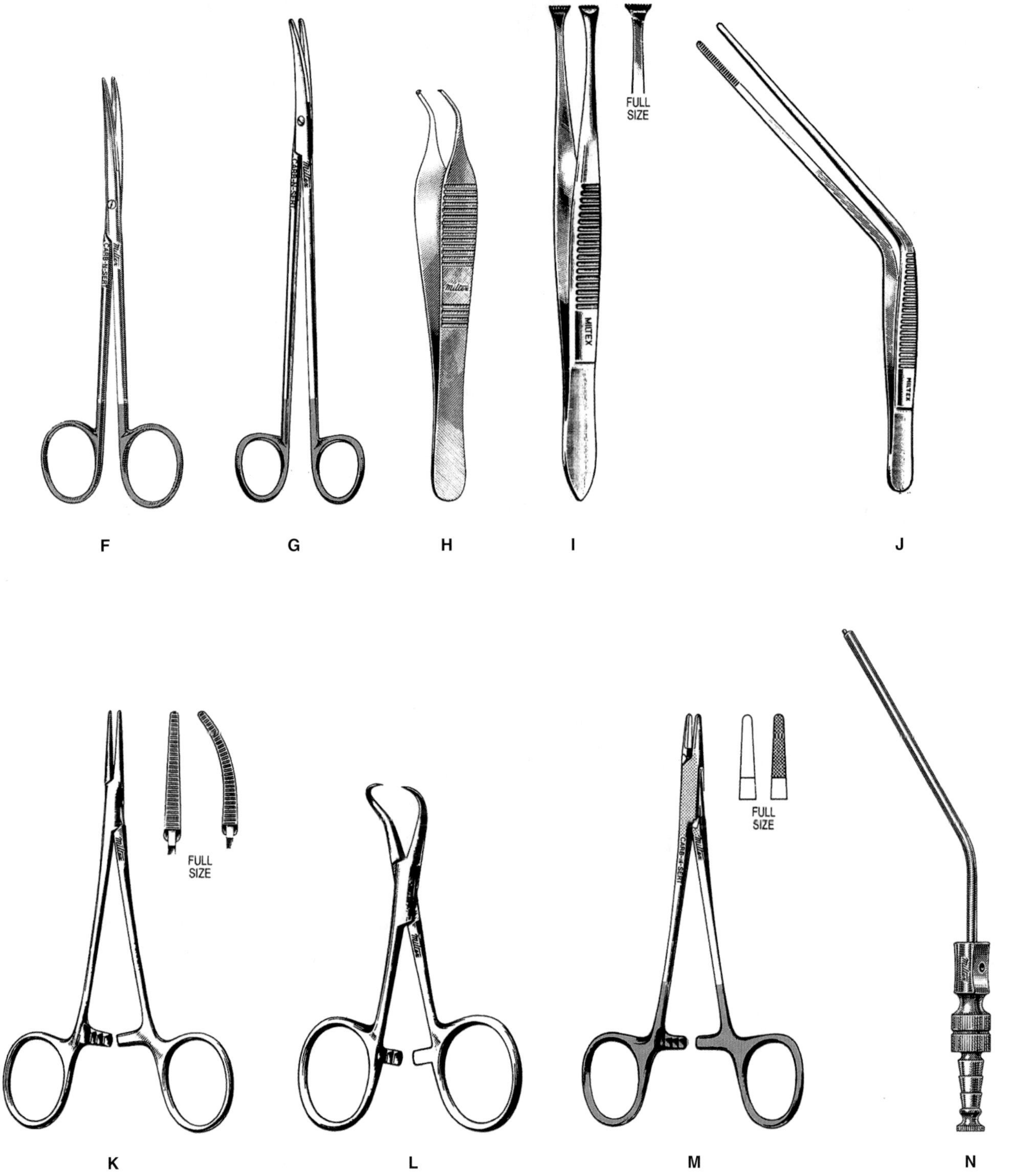

Figure 17-18 *(continued)* **(F) Metzenbaum scissors (delicate pattern 5½ in.), (G) Metzenbaum scissors (delicate pattern 7 in.), (H) Adson tissue forceps (with teeth—angled), (I) Graefe tissue forceps, (J) Wilde dressing forceps, (K) Halsted mosquito forceps (straight and curved), (L) Backhaus towel clamp (3½ in.), (M) Halsey needle holder, (N) Frazier Ferguson suction tip** ***(Courtesy of Miltex Instrument Co., Inc.)***

(continues)

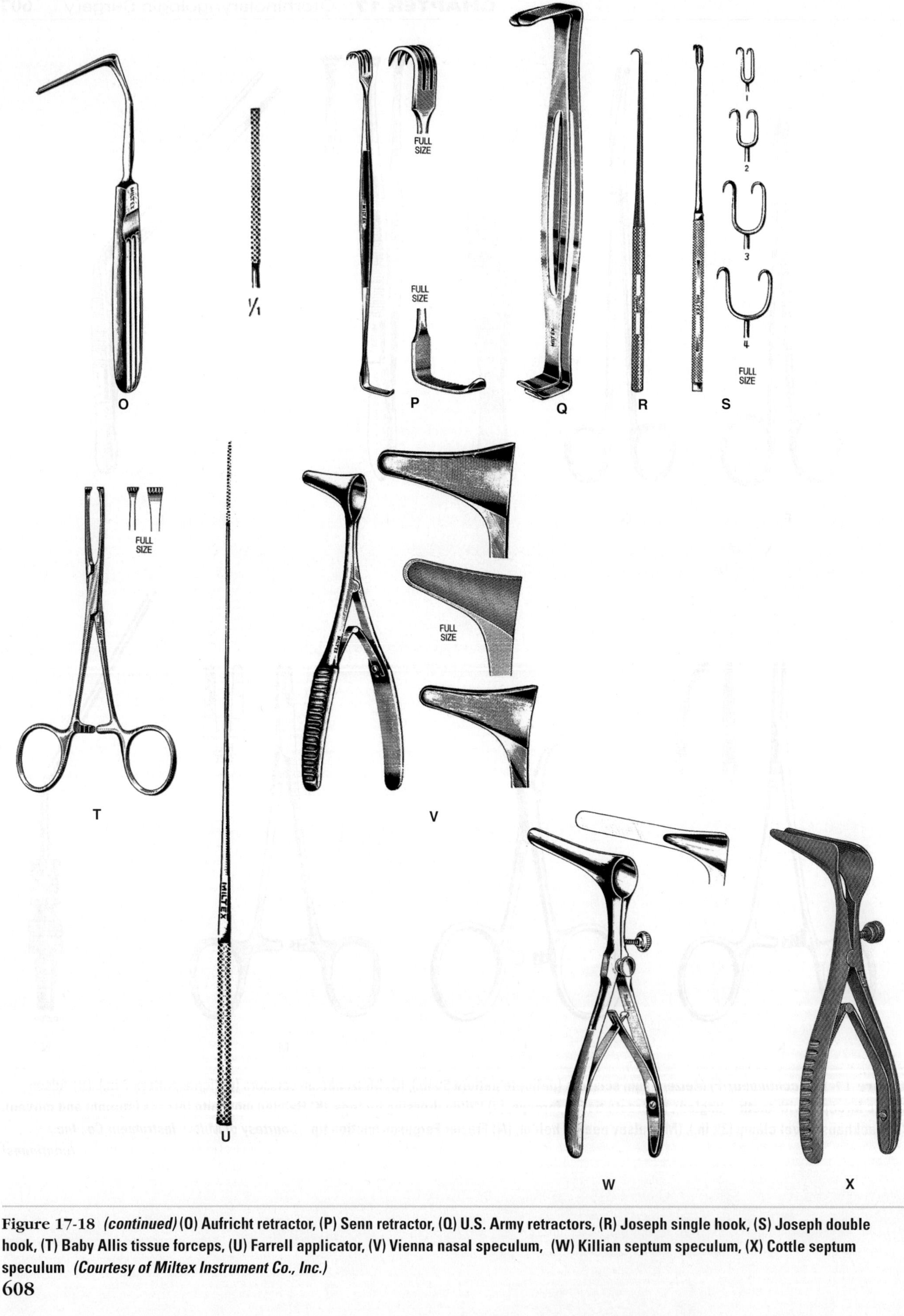

Figure 17-18 *(continued)* (O) Aufricht retractor, (P) Senn retractor, (Q) U.S. Army retractors, (R) Joseph single hook, (S) Joseph double hook, (T) Baby Allis tissue forceps, (U) Farrell applicator, (V) Vienna nasal speculum, (W) Killian septum speculum, (X) Cottle septum speculum *(Courtesy of Miltex Instrument Co., Inc.)*

- Packing material (½-in. gauze strips, cotton, or ½-in. × 3-in. cottonoids)
- Local anesthetic, with or without epinephrine
- Topical anesthetic (cocaine 4%)
- Nasal speculum
- Bayonet forceps
- Small scissors for trimming nasal hair, if necessary

Provisions to protect and prevent drying of the patient's eyes should be made. Protective eyewear should be available for the patient. The eyewear may be sterile, allowing an awake patient to open his or her eyes during the procedure without danger of injury. It should also adhere and conform to the patient's face so that fluids are restricted from entering and damaging the eye. A cooperative patient may have ointment instilled into the eyes to provide moisture, then be asked to keep the eyes closed during the procedure.

Following nasal procedures, the nose may be packed with gauze. This packing may be dry or impregnated with ointment, such as antibiotic or Vaseline, to prevent crusting and infection, and to aid in removal. Internal and external splint materials may be used as well. The patient is usually provided with a mustache-style dressing that may be secured with tape or tied behind the patient's head.

Hemostasis may be achieved in several ways. The common methods include the conventional unipolar electrosurgical pencil, an insulated electrosurgical device with a suction attachment, or a bipolar unit.

NASAL PROCEDURES

Procedures of the nose performed by the otorhino**laryngo**logist are most often done to restore function.

Rhinoplasty is considered cosmetic and is performed by the plastic/reconstructive surgeon to change the external appearance of the nose. One or a combination of remodeling steps may be taken. The tip of the nose may be remodeled, a hump may be removed, the nose may be narrowed, or a septoplasty may be performed. This surgery is tailored to the individual patient's need or desire. If the patient desires to change other features, or if multiple trauma is a factor, additional plastic and reconstructive procedures may be performed at the same time.

SUBMUCOUS RESECTION (SMR)

As the name implies, submucous resection (**SMR**) indicates that the mucous membrane lining the nasal cavity will be incised, and the underlying perichondrium or periosteum lifted. The structures underlying the mucous membrane will be removed to help restore normal breathing. The mucous membrane is then laid back into position and held there with nasal packing material. An absorbable suture may be placed at the incision site.

SMR/SEPTOPLASTY

Septoplasty is most often done to straighten a deviated nasal septum, although it is also used to repair a perforated septum or one damaged by trauma (Procedure 17-3). A submucosal approach is used. The cartilaginous or osseous portion of the septum causing nasal obstruction is removed, readjusted, or reinserted. Care must be taken not to perforate the septum or cause a weakness of the septum that could lead to a future deformity. Internal nasal splints may be inserted and sutured in place. Septoplasty is often done in conjunction with rhinoplasty.

PROCEDURE 17-3 SMR/Septoplasty

Equipment

- Headlamp
- Suction apparatus
- Electrosurgical unit with dispersive electrode

Instruments

- Nasal/sinus instrumentation set

(continues)

PROCEDURE 17-3 **SMR/Septoplasty** *(continued)*

Supplies

- Prep set
- Basic pack
- Basin set
- Gloves
- Head and neck drapes
- #15 knife blade
- Insulated electrosurgical device with suction attachment
- Pharmaceuticals according to surgeon's preference
- Suture according to surgeon's preference
- Packing and dressing material according to surgeon's preference

Operative Preparation

Anesthesia

- Local or general (preferred)
- Lubricate and protect patient's eyes
- Topical/local anesthetic will be used alone or in conjunction with general anesthesia to reduce bleeding, shrink mucous membranes, and minimize postoperative pain

Position

- Supine, with head tilted back; a donut or foam headrest may be used to stabilize
- Head of operating table may be slightly elevated
- Flex hips and knees
- Arms tucked at patient's sides; protect ulnar nerves

Prep

- Shave usually not necessary even if the patient has a mustache
- Face may be prepped with a mild antiseptic. Prevent prep solution from pooling in or near the eyes and ears. The interior of the nose is usually not prepped

Draping

- A turban-style head wrap or three towels arranged triangularly may be used
- Remove protective paper from disposable drapes with adhesive edges
- Place the bar drape across the patient's forehead and allow the remainder of the drape to fall toward the floor covering the head of the operating table
- Situate the U-drape on the upper lip. Bring the edges of the U lateral to the nose and eyes. Extend remainder of the drape to cover the patient's body

Practical Considerations

- Patient may be awake—keep noise to a minimum
- Advise the awake patient to remain still and to anticipate vibrations caused by bone remodeling (e.g., mallet and osteotome)
- Keep drapes away from the face of an awake patient to minimize feeling of claustrophobia and facilitate respiration
- Nasal surgery is not considered sterile; use the best technique possible
- Set up topical/local anesthetic on a separate clean surface for preoperative use

Operative Procedure	Technical Considerations
1. Cocaine-soaked cottonoids placed preoperatively are removed.	1. Speculum and bayonet will be needed to remove preoperative packing. Count cottonoids to be sure all have been removed.

PROCEDURE

17-3 SMR/Septoplasty *(continued)*

2. Nostril on affected side is opened with a speculum and incision made in mucous membrane and perichondrium.	**2.** Provide surgeon with nasal speculum of appropriate size. Cottle clamp may be used to aid in incision process. Use #15 blade on #7 knife handle for incision.
3. Cartilage is incised and mucous membrane is elevated.	**3.** Provide suction as needed. Freer elevator has a sharp and blunt end—most likely the sharp end will be used.
4. Deviated structures or bone spurs of the septum, vomer, and/or ethmoid are reduced or removed.	**4.** Continue to provide suction as needed. A chisel and mallet may be used. The STSR may be asked to "tap" the chisel held by the surgeon with the mallet. *This can be an extremely dangerous maneuver and in some areas may be considered a task "outside the scope of practice" for the STSR. Check the regulations in your state and at your facility prior to performing this task.* Bayonet or Takahashi forceps will be needed to extract tissue remnants. Bone and cartilage may be refashioned and reinserted in the nasal cavity to provide strength to weakened areas.
5. Hemostasis is achieved.	**5.** Have suction, hemostatic agents, and/or electrosurgical pencil available.
6. The incision may be sutured or the tissue replaced and held in position with packing material.	**6.** Provide suture or packing according to surgeon's preference. Count.
7. Internal splints may be used.	**7.** Have splint material ready. Splint may need to be cut to fit the individual patient. Heavy scissors will be needed. The splint may be sutured into place.
8. Dressing that may include an external splint is applied.	**8.** Provide "mustache" dressing and external splint if requested.
9. Secretions are removed from the pharynx to reduce the risk of aspiration.	**9.** Provide Wieder retractor and Yankauer suction tip.

Postoperative Considerations

Immediate Postoperative Care

- The patient should be aware in advance that nasal packing will prevent breathing through the nose.
- Bruising and swelling around the nose and eyes is expected. Advise application of ice packs.
- Patient will have the packing removed in the physician's office 1–3 days postop.

Prognosis

- Patient is expected to return to normal activities in approximately 7 days.
- Full restoration of nasal function is expected.

Complications

- Hemorrhage
- Infection

> **PEARL OF WISDOM**
>
> If any cocaine is left at the end of the procedure, be sure that it is irretrievably discarded. For legal reasons and accountability, the STSR should ask the circulator to observe the discard process.

SMR/TURBINECTOMY

Turbinectomy is used to remove a hypertrophic turbinate, usually the inferior. Turbinectomy is also achieved with a submucosal approach. The nasal mucosa along the edge of the affected turbinate is incised. All or some of the bones of the turbinate are removed. The mucosa is repositioned and held in place with intranasal packing material. The patient should be observed carefully for postoperative hemorrhage.

POLYPECTOMY

Nasal polyps usually require surgical removal. During polypectomy, the polyp is grasped with a forceps, encircled by a snare wire, and amputated, or a polyp forceps may be used for removal (Figure 17-19). If necessary, the electrosurgical unit will be used to achieve hemostasis. Occasionally, a recurrent polyp attached within the sinus may require more extensive surgery (within the sinus) to prevent regrowth.

INTRANASAL ANTROSTOMY

Antrostomy is performed to treat sinusitis or remove recurrent polyps that originate from within the maxillary sinus. Intranasal antrostomy is an opening into the maxillary sinus through the nasoantral wall of the maxilla just below the inferior turbinate. The incision is made over the inferior turbinate. The mucosa is elevated and the wall of the nasal cavity is punctured with an antrum trocar or an antrum rasp that has a trocar tip (Figure 17-20). The opening into the sinus may be enlarged with the use of a small rongeur. The cavity is inspected under direct vision. Purulent material is aspirated and possibly cultured. Any polyps or diseased tissue is removed with antrum curettes that are specifically angled for exactly this purpose. It may be necessary to irrigate the sinus with saline or antibiotic solution. The small defect in the maxilla is not repaired. The mucosa is returned to the normal location and is held in place with packing material. If greater exposure is needed, a Caldwell-Luc procedure may be necessary.

REMOVAL OF FOREIGN BODY

Removal of a foreign body is usually done without anesthesia under direct vision in the doctor's office. This only becomes an OR procedure if the patient requires a general

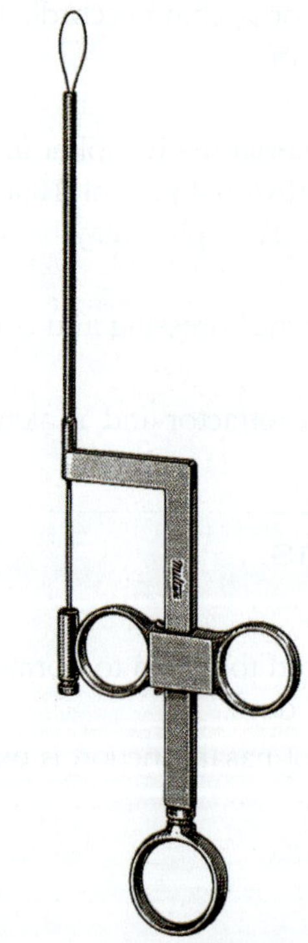

Figure 17-19 Polyp snare ***(Courtesy of Miltex Instrument Co., Inc.)***

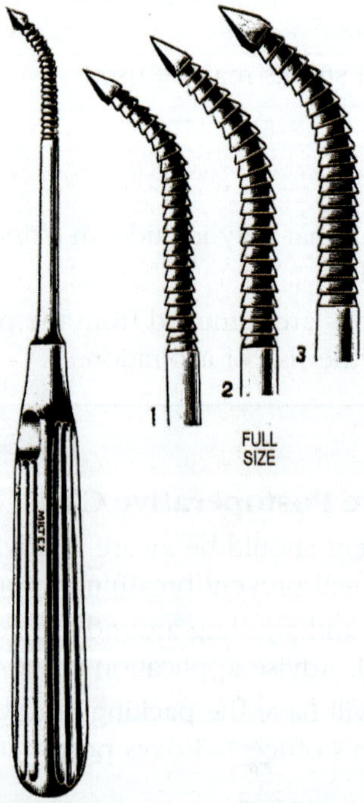

Figure 17-20 Nasal antrostomy rasp ***(Courtesy of Miltex Instrument Co., Inc.)***

anesthetic because of an inability to cooperate due to age or disability, or if the object has penetrated the wall of the nasal cavity and the procedure must be more extensive.

INTERNAL MAXILLARY ARTERY LIGATION

Ligation of the internal maxillary artery is a "last resort" type of procedure, as most cases of severe epistaxis can be controlled with internal packing or electrosurgery. The maxillary sinus is exposed via an antrostomy, either intranasal or through the canine fossa (as in Caldwell-Luc; refer to Procedure 17–4). The artery is isolated, and a ligating clip is applied using an applicator designed specifically for this purpose (Figure 17-21). A microscope may be needed.

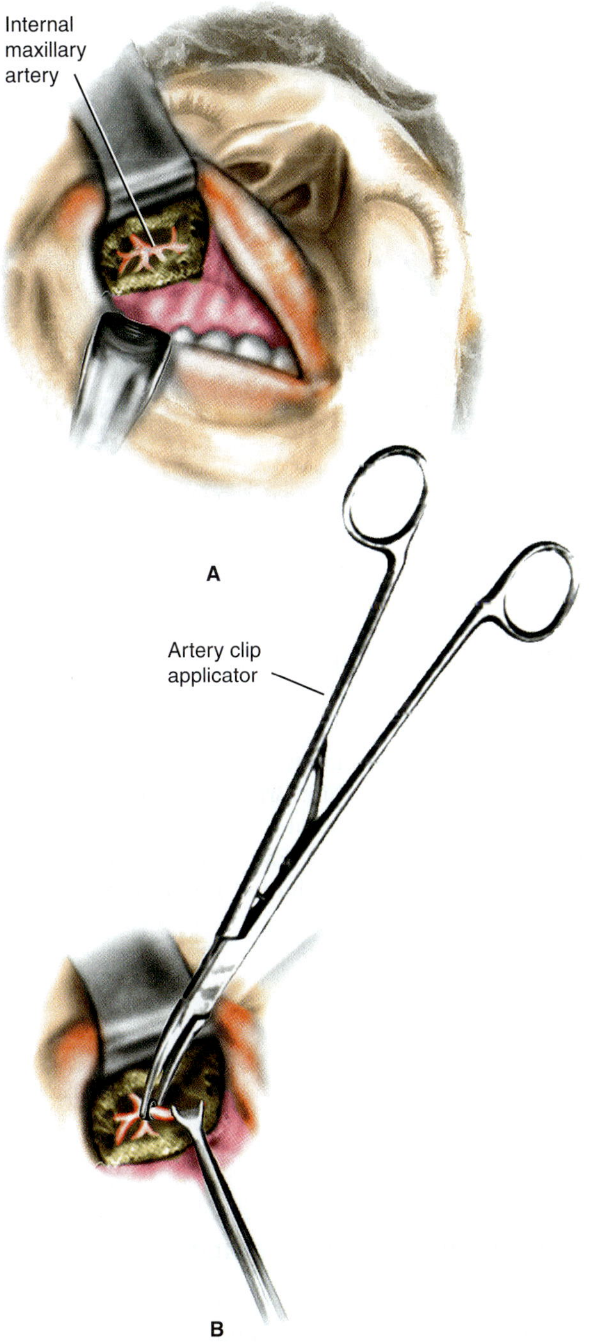

Figure 17-21 Internal maxillary artery clip application: (A) Artery exposed via transoral incision, (B) clip applied

SINUS PROCEDURES

Recurrent sinusitis that may require surgical attention can occur in any of the paranasal sinuses. Each sinus, because of its individual location, may have one or more surgical approaches. Complications are rare, but can be serious. Neurologic evaluation of the postoperative patient should be routine.

CALDWELL-LUC

The Caldwell-Luc procedure is a more radical type of antrostomy and is performed when intranasal antrostomy alone does not provide adequate visualization (Procedure 17-4). The approach into the maxillary sinus for this procedure is through the canine fossa (Figure 17-22). The purpose of Caldwell-Luc is to remove diseased portions of the antral wall, evacuate sinus contents, and establish drainage through the nose. Even if the patient is under general anesthesia, a local anesthetic containing a vasoconstrictor may be injected under the upper lip on the affected side.

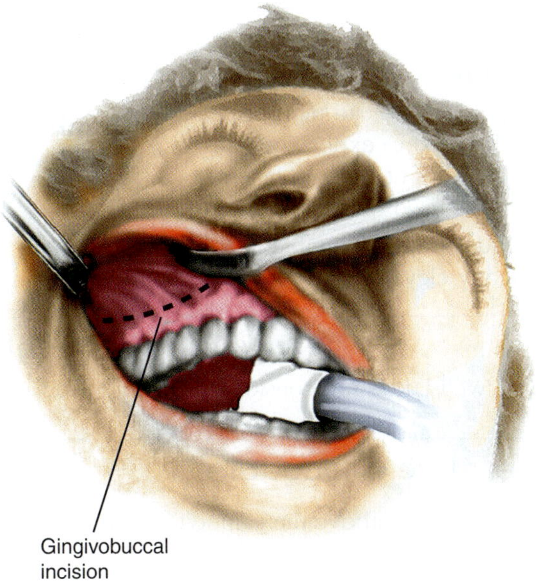

Figure 17-22 Caldwell-Luc

PROCEDURE 17-4 Caldwell-Luc

Equipment

- Electrosurgical unit with dispersive electrode
- Suction apparatus
- Drill if requested to puncture maxilla

Instruments

- Nasal/sinus instrumentation set
- Caldwell-Luc retractor

Supplies

- Prep set
- Basic pack
- Basin set
- Gloves
- Head and neck drapes
- Insulated electrosurgical device with suction attachment
- #15 knife blade
- Pharmaceuticals according to surgeon's preference
- Suture according to surgeon's preference

Operative Preparation

Anesthesia
- General anesthesia preferred
- Lubricate and protect patient's eyes
- Local anesthetic with epinephrine may be used alone or in conjunction with general anesthesia to reduce bleeding and minimize postoperative pain

Position
- Supine, with head tilted back and turned to expose operative side. A donut or foam headrest may be used to stabilize
- Head of operating table may be slightly elevated
- Flex hips and knees
- Arms tucked at patient's sides; protect ulnar nerves

Prep
- Shave usually not necessary even if the patient has a beard or mustache
- Face may be prepped with a mild antiseptic. Prevent prep solution from pooling in or near the eyes and ears

Draping
- A turban-style head wrap or three towels arranged triangularly may be used
- Remove protective paper from disposable drapes with adhesive edges
- Place the bar drape across the patient's forehead and allow the reminder of the drape to fall toward the floor covering the head of the operating table
- Situate the U-drape on the chin. Bring the edges of the U lateral to the mouth, nose, and eyes. Extend the remainder of the drape to cover the patient's body

Practical Considerations

- Caldwell-Luc is not considered a sterile procedure; use the best technique possible

Operative Procedure	Technical Considerations
1. The gingiva above the canine tooth and second molar is incised.	1. Provide the Caldwell-Luc retractor and the #15 blade. Provide suction as needed.

PROCEDURE

17-4 Caldwell-Luc *(continued)*

2. The periosteum of the inferior wall of the maxilla is elevated and the infraorbital nerve is identified and carefully retracted.	2. Have electrosurgical device available for hemostasis. Freer elevator will be needed for the periosteal dissection. Observe incisional site for nerve. Caldwell-Luc retractor will be repositioned.
3. The bone is perforated with an osteotome or a small drill bit.	3. Present drill or osteotome and mallet.
4. The opening into the maxillary sinus is enlarged with a small rongeur.	4. Have Kerrison rongeur ready. Continue to provide suction. Suction apparatus is easily clogged by purulent diseased material; prepare to change suction tips frequently and clean with water or stylet as needed.
5. The sinus is evacuated of any purulent matter and polyps or diseased tissue is removed.	5. Coakley curettes or Takahashi will be needed to remove tissue. All tissue removed is saved as specimen.
6. If necessary, an opening is made into the nasoantral wall below the inferior turbinate.	6. Antrum trocar/rasp will be needed to create nasoantral window. Anticipate the use of the antral suction tip and place on tubing.
7. Hemostasis is achieved and the nose and sinus may be packed.	7. Have hemostatic agents or insulated electrosurgical suction apparatus ready. Prepare packing material according to surgeon's preference.
8. The gingiva is sutured with absorbable suture material.	8. Pass suture loaded on needle holder and tissue forceps followed by suture scissors. Count.

Postoperative Considerations

Immediate Postoperative Care

- Bruising and swelling inside the mouth, on the upper lip, and around the nose and eyes are expected. Advise application of ice packs and soft diet.

Prognosis

- Patient is expected to return to normal activities within 7 days.
- Normal respiratory function is expected, but may take several weeks.

Complications

- Hemorrhage
- Infection

PEARL OF WISDOM

The Caldwell-Luc retractor is a specialty retractor that may need to be sterilized prior to the case. Be sure this and all other necessary instruments are available.

Caldwell-Luc is contraindicated in children prior to the descent of the permanent teeth.

ETHMOIDECTOMY

Either one of two approaches can be used to perform ethmoidectomy. The ethmoid sinus may be entered through the nose, or an incision can be made near the inner canthus of the eye on the affected side.

If the intranasal approach is used, the mucosal incision is made at the level of the middle turbinate. The turbinate may be partially removed. Once the sinus is entered, the ethmoid air cells are destroyed and all affected tissue is removed. The frontal and sphenoid sinuses may be additionally accessed as a continuation of this approach.

The external approach is the preferred method because the increased exposure allows for more complete exenteration. The incision is carefully placed in the existing folds of the facial skin, leaving very little visible scar. The orbital contents may be gently retracted, the wall of the sinus punctured, and the cavity visualized. Any necessary surgery can be performed through this incision.

SPHENOIDECTOMY

The sphenoid sinus may be approached externally or intranasally. Either approach involves passing through the ethmoid sinus, then entering the sphenoid sinus to allow for drainage. Incidentally, a transphenoidal approach may be used for hypophysectomy. A rhinologist will work in conjunction with the neurosurgeon to provide access for removal of the pituitary using this approach.

DRAINAGE OF THE FRONTAL SINUS

The frontal sinus is drained through an external incision. The incision follows the inferior edge of the eyebrow along the anterior and lateral aspects of the nasal bone. The periosteum is elevated and the lacrimal apparatus identified and protected. First, the ethmoid sinus is entered, and then the window is extended to expose the frontal sinus. All diseased membrane is obliterated. A fistula for drainage is created at the level of the middle turbinate to facilitate drainage. A drain may be placed to maintain the nasofrontal passage. The external wound is closed cosmetically.

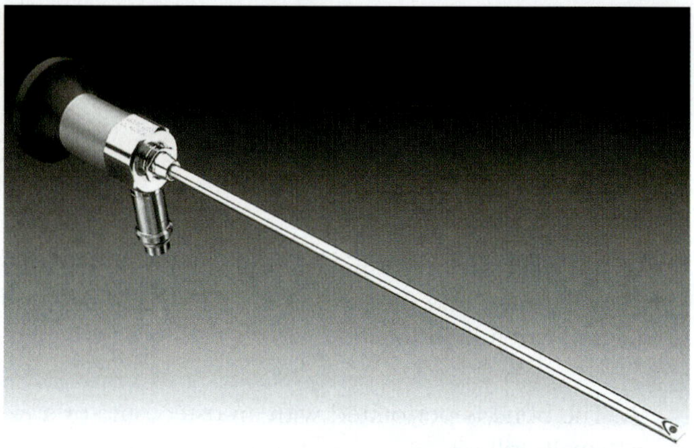

Figure 17-23 SharpSite™ Ac autoclavable endoscope for sinus endoscopy from Xomed Surgical Products, Inc.

SINUS ENDOSCOPY

Sinoscopy can be used as a diagnostic procedure, or can be considered functional (Procedure 17-5). The paranasal sinuses can be accessed with the endoscope using an intranasal approach or the external incisions previously described for each of the sinuses (Figure 17-23). The main advantage to sinus endoscopy is that the surgery can be focused on the area of concern without damaging the surrounding tissue. The individual ostia of each sinus can be clearly visualized with the specialized equipment. The image may be magnified and displayed on a monitor for all team members to view. In addition to advanced optics, many accessories are available to enhance the use of the endoscope.

PROCEDURE 17-5 Rigid Sinus Endoscopy

Equipment

- Headlamp
- Suction apparatus
- Video equipment
- Fiberoptic light source

Instruments

- Nasal/sinus instrument tray
- Sinoscopy instrumentation

PROCEDURE

17-5 Rigid Sinus Endoscopy *(continued)*

Supplies

- Prep set
- Basic pack
- Basin set
- Gloves
- Head and neck drapes
- Antifog solution
- Pharmaceuticals according to surgeon's preference
- Mustache dressing

Operative Preparation

Anesthesia

- Local or general (preferred)
- Lubricate and protect patient's eyes
- Topical/local anesthetic will be used alone or in conjunction with general anesthesia to reduce bleeding, shrink mucous membranes, and minimize postoperative pain

Position

- Supine, with head tilted back. A donut or foam headrest may be used to stabilize
- Arms tucked at patient's side; protect ulnar nerves

Prep

- Shave usually not necessary even if the patient has a mustache
- Face may be prepped with a mild antiseptic. Prevent prep solution from pooling in or near the eyes and ears. The interior of the nose is usually not prepped

Draping

- A turban-style head wrap or three towels arranged triangularly may be used
- Remove protective paper from disposable drapes with adhesive edges
- Place the bar drape across the patient's forehead and allow the remainder of the drape to fall toward the floor covering the head of the operating table
- Situate the U-drape on the upper lip. Bring the edges of the U lateral to the nose and eyes. Extend the remainder of the drape to cover the patient's body

Practical Considerations

- Sinoscopy is not considered a sterile procedure; use the best technique possible
- Set up topical/local anesthetic on a separate clean surface for preoperative use

Operative Procedure	Technical Considerations
1. The endoscope is introduced into the nose.	**1.** Verify that all equipment is connected and in working order. Prior to insertion of the endoscope, the antifog solution is applied. The process is repeated every time the scope is extracted and reinserted.
2. The ostia to the individual sinus is visualized and enlarged to provide access to the sinus.	**2.** Provide suction as needed. The lens will be changed as needed to provide the necessary angle for viewing—be sure antifog solution has been applied. A spoon or antrum punch will be needed to enlarge the ostium.

(continues)

PROCEDURE 17-5 **Rigid Sinus Endoscopy** *(continued)*

3. Diseased tissue is visualized and removed.	**3.** Provide straight or angled Blakesley forceps for removal of tissue. Continue to provide suction as needed. Maintain patency of suction apparatus by irrigating suction tip or using stylet.
4. Biopsy may be performed and polyps are removed.	**4.** Provide biopsy forceps or polypectomy instruments. Several specimens may be obtained.
5. For ethmoidectomy, the frontal recess is entered and the diseased tissue removed.	**5.** Continue to alternate between Blakesley forceps and suction. This can be a long and tedious procedure especially in a darkened room—remain alert. Lens changes may be necessary for enhanced viewing. Instrumentation is very delicate. Use caution especially when changing lenses.
6. Scope is removed; antibiotic ointment may be applied.	**6.** Suturing and packing are not necessary. Have antibiotic ointment drawn up in a syringe for internal application. Count may not be necessary—according to facility policy.
7. Mustache dressing is applied.	**7.** Have dressing materials prepared.

Postoperative Considerations

Immediate Postoperative Care

- Some bruising and swelling around the nose and eyes is expected. Advise application of ice pack.

Prognosis

- Patient is expected to return to normal activities in approximately 5 days.
- Normal respiratory function is expected, but may take several weeks.

Complications

- Hemorrhage
- Infection

PEARL OF WISDOM

Once functional endoscopic sinus surgery (FESS) has been performed, a second FESS becomes more difficult because the anatomical landmarks may be destroyed.

ANATOMY OF THE UPPER AERODIGESTIVE TRACT

The upper **aerodigestive tract**, known to the general population as the throat, is, in actuality, several individual and specialized structures that work in harmony to facilitate respiration and ingestion of food. The pharynx, larynx, trachea, and esophagus all contribute to this complex anatomical region.

PHARYNX

The pharynx, commonly referred to as the throat, is a tubular structure approximately 13 cm (5 in.) in length (Figure 17-24). The pharynx serves the respiratory tract by receiving air from the nose and mouth, and the digestive system as a passageway for food and liquids. The pharynx is lined with mucous membrane and is contiguous with the nose superiorly and the larynx and esophagus inferiorly. The pharynx lies anterior to the vertebrae in the midline of the neck. The pharynx begins at the internal nares and terminates posterior to the larynx at the level of the esophagus. The pharynx is divided into three regions according to location: the nasopharynx, the oropharynx, and the laryngopharynx. The lymphoid elements (pharyngeal, palatine, and lingual tonsils, and the pharyngeal band) contained within the pharynx are collectively known as Waldeyer's ring.

NASOPHARYNX

The nasopharynx is the most superior portion of the pharynx, located posterior to the nasal cavity. Beginning at the posterior nares, the nasopharynx extends inferiorly to the uvula. The eustachian tubes enter the nasopharynx, and it houses the pharyngeal tonsils.

Eustachian Tubes

The eustachian (auditory or pharyngotympanic) tubes enter the nasopharynx from the middle ear. The function of the eustachian tube is to equalize the pressure on both sides of the tympanic membrane, preventing rupture of the tympanic membrane. The eustachian tube opens during yawning, chewing, swallowing, and blowing of the nose.

Pharyngeal Tonsils

The pharyngeal tonsils are located on the posterior wall of the nasopharynx. When the pharyngeal tonsils are enlarged, they are referred to as the adenoids. The pharyngeal tonsils are a single mass of lymphatic tissue embedded in the mucous membrane of the nasopharynx. These tonsils provide protection against pathogens entering the nose. The lymphatic tissue of the tonsils usually begins to shrink in size after about age 7.

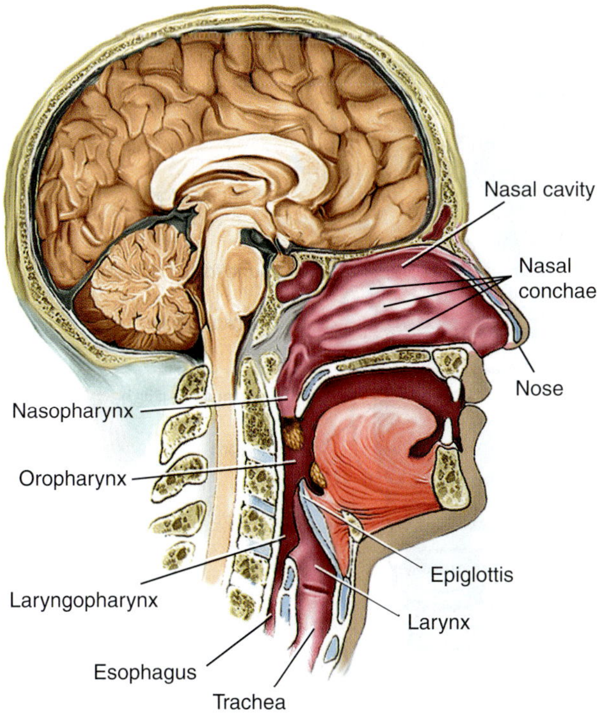

Figure 17-24 Three sections of the pharynx and related structures

OROPHARYNX

The oropharynx is the middle portion of the pharynx, located posterior to the oral cavity, and it houses the palatine and lingual tonsils. The oropharynx begins at the uvula, communicating superiorly with the nasopharynx and extends to the level of the hyoid bone. The anterior opening to the oropharynx is the mouth (refer to Plate 6).

The fauces is the opening between the mouth and the oropharynx. The mouth or buccal cavity opens anteriorly through the lips. The vestibule is the space between the lips (extending along the cheeks) and the teeth. The gums, teeth, tongue, and floor of the mouth are contained within the buccal cavity. Secretions from the salivary glands are received here as well. The roof of the mouth consists of two segments, which are collectively referred to as the palate. The anterior segment is referred to as the hard palate and is supported by extensions of the maxillary and palatine bones. The soft palate is posterior and consists of connective tissue and muscle. The soft palate terminates with a projection of lymphoid tissue called the uvula. During swallowing the nasopharynx is protected by the soft palate, which moves upward to seal off the nasopharynx, directing food and liquids downward.

Palatine Tonsils

The palatine, or faucial, tonsils are the two oval masses of lymphoid tissue commonly called "the tonsils." The palatine tonsils are located at each edge of the fauces within the folds of two bands of tissue that descend from the soft palate to the base of the tongue, called the tonsillar pillars. Each tonsil has an anterior and a posterior pillar. Behind each posterior tonsillar pillar is a pink band of lymphoid tissue called the lateral pharyngeal band. The tonsils produce lymphocytes. Each of the palatine tonsils contains 10–20 crypts or dips that help trap bacteria.

Lingual Tonsils

The lingual tonsils are a pair of lymphoid areas located on the posterior surface of the tongue near the base.

LARYNGOPHARYNX

The laryngopharynx, or hypopharynx, is the inferior portion of the pharynx. It begins at the level of the hyoid bone and extends to the lower margin of the larynx.

LARYNX

The larynx, commonly called the voice box, is located between the pharynx and the trachea (Figure 17-25). The larynx is approximately 5 cm long; nine laryngeal cartilages and the hyoid bone form its rigid framework. There are three pairs of cartilages: two arytenoid, two corniculate, and two cuneiform, and three individual cartilages: the thyroid cartilage, the cricoid, and the **epiglottis**. Muscles and ligaments connect the nine cartilages to one another. The larynx has ligamentous attachments to the hyoid bone.

The largest and most superior of the single cartilages is the thyroid cartilage. It consists of a pair of shield-like plates that are fused in the front, projecting forward to form what is commonly known as the "Adam's apple." The cricoid cartilage is the only cartilage in the upper aerodigestive tract to form a complete circle and is found at the base of the larynx. It is the most inferior of the laryngeal cartilages and attaches to the trachea. Unlike the other laryngeal cartilages, which are hyaline cartilage, the epiglottis is elastic cartilage. The epiglottis is an elongated leaf-like structure. The base of the epiglottis is attached inferiorly to the thyroid cartilage. The posterior aspect is located in the laryngopharynx. During swallowing, the superior movable portion of the epiglottis folds over the opening into the larynx, called the **glottis**, to prevent liquids and food from entering the larynx. The epiglottis then returns to its upright or erect position, allowing for the passage of air and sound.

The arytenoid cartilages are the largest of the paired laryngeal cartilages. They are pyramid shaped and attach to the superior posterior edges of the cricoid cartilage. The arytenoid cartilages also attach to the posterior ends of the vocal folds and move them during sound production. The smaller cuneiform and corniculate cartilages attach to the arytenoids. The cuneiform is the attachment of the arytenoid cartilages to the epiglottis.

The superior opening into the larynx is the glottis. Two pairs of ligaments extend to the posterior surface of the thyroid cartilage from the arytenoid cartilages. The uppermost are referred to as the false vocal cords or the ventricular folds. Along with the epiglottis, they help keep food and fluids out of the respiratory tract. The lower pair is the true vocal cords that are capable of vibration when air passes through them during exhalation to produce sound (Figure 17-26). The pitch of the sound is determined by the tension of the cords. More tension leads to a higher pitched sound. The force of the air

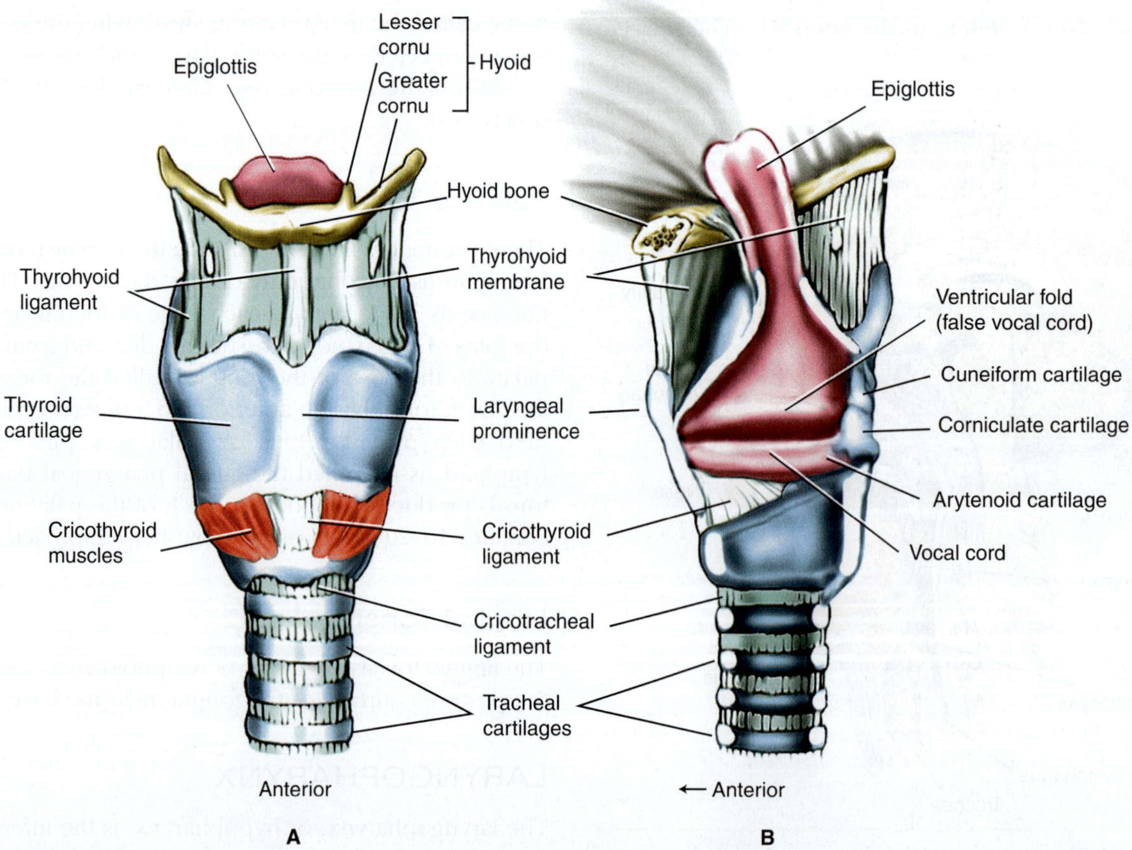

Figure 17-25 Larynx and related structures: (A) Anterior view, (B) lateral view

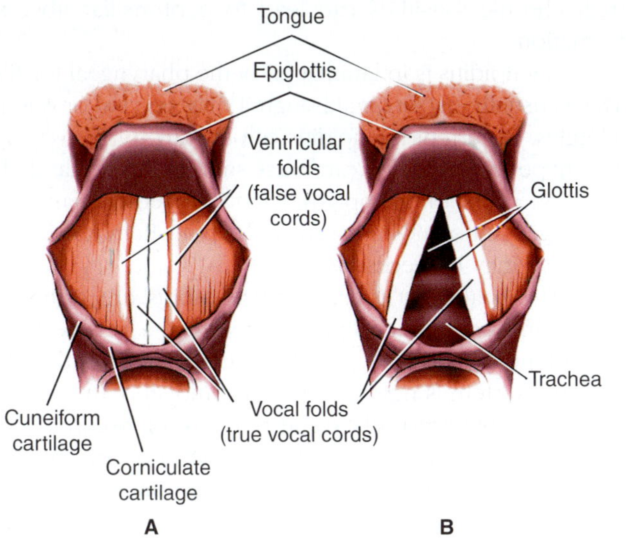

Figure 17-26 Vocal cords and related structures: (A) Closed, (B) open

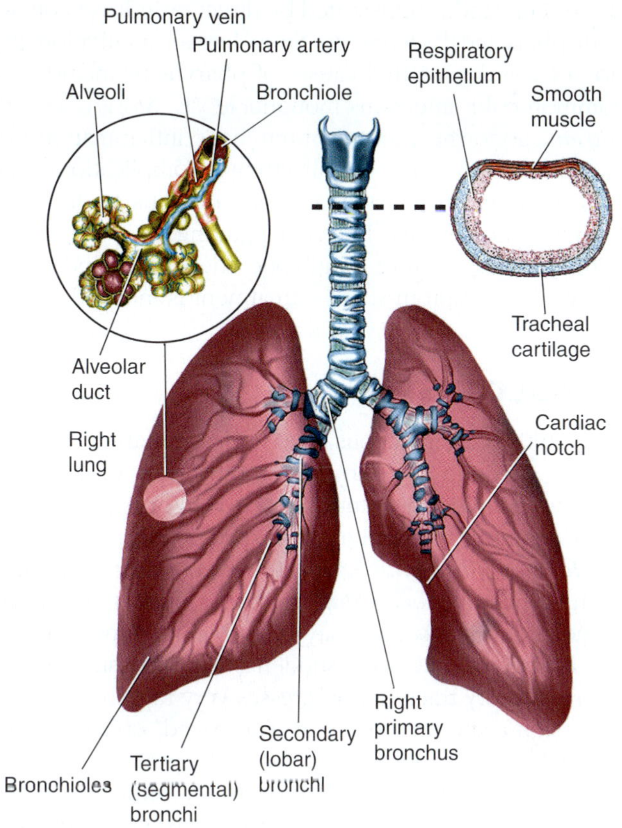

Figure 17-27 Trachea and lungs

moving through the larynx determines loudness of the sound.

TRACHEA

The trachea, or windpipe, is approximately 11 cm in length, 2.5 cm in diameter, and located anterior to the esophagus (Figure 17-27). The upper half of the trachea is located in the midline of the neck; as it descends, it enters the superior mediastinum. The trachea joins the cricoid cartilage of the larynx to the main stem or primary bronchi leading to each lung. There are 15–20 C-shaped pieces of hyaline cartilage supporting the anterior and lateral tracheal walls. These cartilages keep the trachea from collapsing due to any pressure changes. The posterior wall of the trachea is closed with smooth muscle and connective tissue. This allows for expansion of the esophagus during swallowing. The most inferior tracheal cartilage is called the **carina**, which bifurcates into the two primary bronchi.

BRONCHI AND LUNGS

Cartilaginous rings similar to those protecting the trachea also support the right and left main-stem bronchi. The right main-stem bronchus is larger in length and diameter than the left. There is also less of an angle of deviation from the trachea toward the right, making the right lung more inviting to foreign bodies. Each lung is divided into lobes. The right lung has three lobes (upper, middle, and lower); the left has only two (upper and lower). Each lobe is further divided into segments. At the distal end of the bronchial tree are the alveolar sacs, which contain the functional tissue of the lungs. This is where the exchange of gases occurs.

ESOPHAGUS

The esophagus is inferior to the laryngopharynx and posterior to the larynx in the mediastinum. It is approximately 25 cm in length. The esophagus passes through the diaphragm at the level of the hiatus and is joined to the stomach by the lower esophageal, or cardiac, sphincter. The esophagus is encircled with muscle tissue that produces peristaltic contractions to propel a bolus of food toward the stomach.

PATHOLOGY AFFECTING THE UPPER AERODIGESTIVE TRACT

The upper aerodigestive tract may be affected by several conditions ranging from minor inflammation to malignancy. Some of the more common disorders will be described.

PHARYNGITIS

A very common inflammation of the throat is acute pharyngitis, which may be either viral or bacterial in origin. Streptococcal pharyngitis ("strep throat") is the most common type. Strep is highly communicable during the acute stage and is transmitted by direct or indirect contact with pharyngeal secretions. Strep has an incubation period of 2–5 days. Other causes of pharyngitis include the common cold, infectious mononucleosis, *Staphylococcus aureus,* gonorrhea, and post-traumatic inflammation, for example following a tonsillectomy. Complications that may occur as a result of pharyngitis are otitis media, mastoiditis, and sinusitis. Bacterial pharyngitis is diagnosed with a throat culture. Antibiotic therapy, if indicated, along with symptom-specific treatment is initiated.

EPIGLOTTITIS

Epiglottitis is an infectious disease that can affect any age group, although it is most commonly seen in the 2- to 5-year-old child. Epiglottitis may be viral or bacterial. The most common bacterial agent responsible for epiglottitis is *Haemophilus influenzae.* However, other organisms such as pneumococci, *Staphylococcus aureus,* and beta-hemolytic *Streptococcus* may be to blame. Acute epiglottitis is characterized by a sudden onset of obstruction of the respiratory tract that progresses very rapidly. The cardinal sign is the presence of a "cherry-red" epiglottis. Additionally, the patient is often in respiratory distress, which is apparent by inspiratory stridor, retraction of the chest, and cyanosis. If epiglottitis is suspected and the epiglottis is not easily visible under direct visualization, it is recommended that the examiner *not* make any attempt at viewing the epiglottis with the use of any instrument including a tongue blade. Any manipulation of the area may increase the inflammation or induce a laryngospasm causing total airway occlusion. Immediate treatment will include inspiration of humidified air and antibiotic therapy. If the airway becomes obstructed, endotracheal intubation or tracheotomy may be indicated. Failure to diagnose and respond quickly to this condition results in a 20% death rate.

TONSILLITIS

Tonsillitis may affect the pharyngeal, palatine, or lingual tonsils. Tonsillitis usually refers to the palatine tonsils and it is the palatine tonsils that are removed during the procedure commonly called "tonsillectomy."

Tonsillitis of the palatine tonsils may be acute or chronic. Most often tonsillitis is caused by a streptococcal organism. Acute tonsillitis is an inflammation of the tonsils and their crypts. On visual examination, the tonsils appear enlarged and dusky in color. Purulent matter may be seen in the tonsillar crypts. The tonsils may enlarge to the point of being obstructive. Antibiotic therapy is initiated. Repeated attacks of acute tonsillitis may indicate that removal is necessary. Chronic tonsillitis is evidenced by a persistent sore throat, foul breath, and enlarged cervical lymph nodes. Removal may become necessary. Failure to treat chronic tonsillitis can lead to peritonsillar abscess formation.

Adenoiditis is inflammation of the pharyngeal tonsils. This is usually bacterial, although it may be viral or due to allergies. Recurrent adenoiditis can lead to **hypertrophy**. This hypertrophic tissue can cause snoring due to nasal obstruction or hearing impairment due to eustachian tube blockage. Antibiotics are usually helpful. Removal of the adenoids may be necessary.

The (palatine) tonsils and adenoids are often removed in a combination procedure called a tonsillectomy and adenoidectomy (**T&A**). Research has shown that the immune system is not impaired by removal of the tonsils.

The lingual tonsils are also at risk of becoming inflamed. Antibiotics and saline irrigations are recommended initial treatments. If the infection is recurrent, lingual tonsillectomy can be performed. This is often accomplished with the use of the carbon dioxide laser.

PERITONSILLAR ABSCESS

Peritonsillar abscess formation is a major complication of tonsillitis, resulting from a failed antibiotic therapy or chronic tonsillitis. Typically the abscess forms between the tonsil and the fascia covering the pharyngeal constrictor muscle and is quite visible when the mouth is opened (Figure 17-28). The patient is in extreme pain and may experience difficulty breathing and referred pain to the ear on the affected side. Antibiotics may be helpful, but surgical intervention may be necessary. An incision and drainage (I&D) is performed. The tonsils are usually

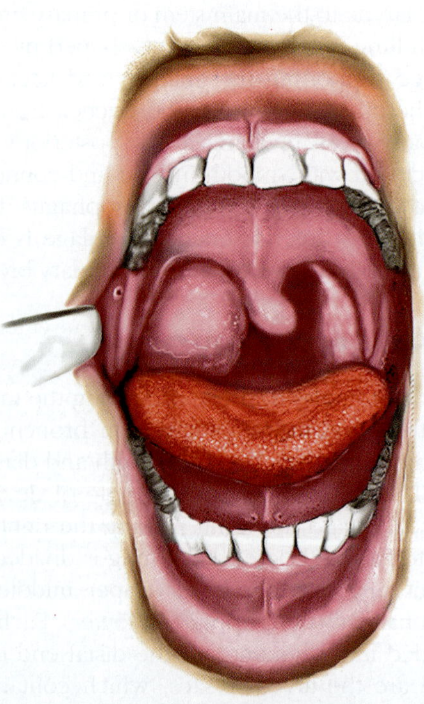

Figure 17-28 Right peritonsillar abscess

removed when all evidence of infection has subsided. The infection from a peritonsillar abscess may quickly spread throughout the neck and chest, causing complications such as pericarditis, which can be fatal.

SLEEP APNEA

Sleep **apnea** affects approximately 18 million Americans. The victim suffers numerous (as many as 20–30 per hour), brief interruptions in respiration during sleep, leaving the patient feeling sleepy during the day. All age groups and both genders may suffer from sleep apnea, although it is more common in men. Sleep apnea is a potentially life-threatening disorder that has been linked to serious complications including irregular heartbeat, high blood pressure, heart attack, and stroke. Two common tests for sleep disorders are **polysomnography** and the Multiple Sleep Latency Test, discussed later.

Sleep apnea has two known causes. Central sleep apnea is the less common type and occurs when the brain fails to signal the muscles controlling respiration. Obstructive sleep apnea occurs when a problem with the upper respiratory tract prevents movement of air through the nose or mouth even when respiratory effort is attempted. Victims of sleep apnea generally have a family history of the disorder, are overweight, snore, have high blood pressure, and may have a physical abnormality of the upper airway. Drug and alcohol use increase the frequency and duration of apneic episodes.

The structural problems causing the airway obstruction can be varied. A natural relaxation of the muscles of the throat and tongue can cause the tongue and soft palate to sag into the airway causing obstruction. The supine position assumed during rest periods can also be a contributing factor. In obese individuals, an excess amount of tissue in the upper airway can cause obstruction.

Treatment must be tailored to suit the individual. Pharmacologic treatment has been found ineffective. Oxygen administration under pressure may be tried, but this involves the use of appliances and mechanical equipment that may be cumbersome.

Behavioral therapy may be helpful. The patient may be advised to avoid the use of drugs, tobacco, and alcohol, lose weight if necessary, and to try sleeping in a semisitting or side-lying position. Surgical procedures to achieve weight loss (bariatrics), to correct a defect (septoplasty or polypectomy), or to enlarge the airway (adenoidectomy, tonsillectomy, or uvulopalatopharyngoplasty) may be recommended. In extreme life-threatening cases, the patient may require a tracheotomy.

LARYNGITIS

Laryngitis is an inflammation of the vocal cords usually caused by a virus and is rarely seen in children. The normal voice quality is usually altered due to localized erythema and edema, but the airway is not compromised. The larynx may be observed for inflammation by indirect laryngoscopy (mirror examination). The disease usually resolves spontaneously. The patient is advised to rest his or her voice, avoid respiratory irritants (such as tobacco smoke), and breathe humidified air. Laryngitis may become chronic but the treatment remains the same.

POLYPOID CORDITIS OR VOCAL CORD POLYPS

Polypoid corditis can result from chronic laryngitis (Figure 17-29). The patient complains of persistent hoarseness, but exhibits no other symptoms. Indirect laryngoscopy shows edema so extensive that the true vocal cords take on the appearance of having "water bags." Vocal cord polyps are an extension of polypoid corditis. Treatment is usually surgical removal of the polyps.

VOCAL CORD NODULES

Vocal cord nodules generally result from vocal abuse. They may be seen in a child or adult who does a considerable amount of screaming or in the adult singer. The only symptom is prolonged hoarseness. Nodules usually appear at the junction of the upper and middle third of the cord and on both true vocal cords simultaneously. The nodules do not increase in size, nor are they considered precancerous. There is no danger of airway obstruction. Behavior modification techniques and voice therapy may help to resolve the situation. Otherwise, surgical intervention is advisable.

VOCAL CORD GRANULOMAS

Vocal cord granulomas develop at the edge of the arytenoid cartilages and can become ulcerative, spreading to

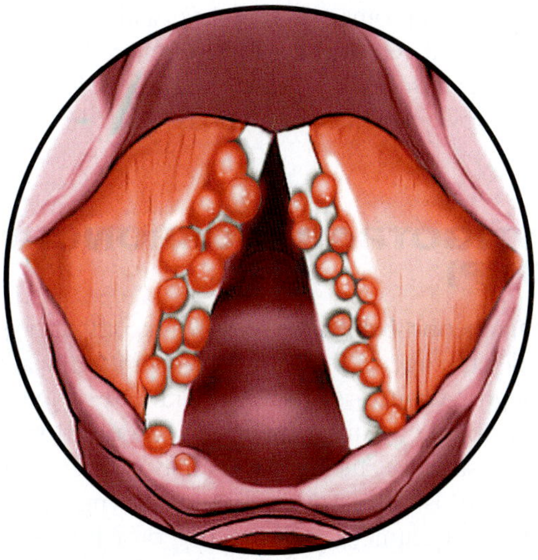

Figure 17-29 Vocal cord polyps

the free edge of each vocal cord. Secondary infection may result. The patient experiences hoarseness that may be accompanied by pain if infection is present. This disease may be from mechanical irritation (such as an endotracheal tube) and is often seen in singers and teachers. Many treatment options are available including steroid injections and surgery. There is a strong possibility of recurrence.

LARYNGEAL NEOPLASMS

Laryngeal neoplasms may be benign or malignant. Evidence of neoplasms may include changes in voice quality and pain. The neoplasm may arise from any structure within the larynx and is not limited to the vocal cords. Persons who smoke are at greater risk for developing laryngeal neoplasms. The larynx is examined indirectly by mirror or directly by rigid or fiberoptic laryngoscopy. The size and location of the neoplasm are noted and a biopsy may be taken to determine the etiology of the neoplasm. Several varieties of benign neoplasms have been identified. Most of these can be treated laryngoscopically and the use of the carbon dioxide laser may be employed. Malignant lesions are classified according to their location: supraglottic, glottic, and subglottic. Generally, malignant tumors require a more extensive procedure, such as laryngectomy. Additionally, if the lymph system in the neck is involved, it may be recommended that the patient undergo a radical neck dissection. Radiation therapy may also be used.

TRACHEITIS AND BRONCHITIS

Tracheitis and bronchitis are similar in the fact that either may be acute (usually caused by a virus) or chronic (caused by an irritant, such as air pollutants, including tobacco smoke). Both disorders can affect all age groups. The patient will notice an increase in clear secretions due to the inflammation of the airway. The secretions will become yellow or green if a secondary bacterial infection is present. The symptoms may improve with increased humidification and removal of any irritants. The airway is rarely compromised. Occasionally it may become necessary to remove aspirated secretions with the use of a bronchoscope.

LARYNGOTRACHEOBRONCHITIS (CROUP)

Laryngotracheobronchitis, or "croup," mostly affects children under the age of 3. The major symptom is a "barking" cough. Croup is usually viral in origin with adenovirus being the most common. Examination is usually not possible because a small child is often noncompliant. There is also some fear of laryngospasm on examination. Treatment includes use of a humidifier. In severe cases, one or more treatments with aerosolized epinephrine may be administered.

FOREIGN BODIES

A person of any age can be the victim of a foreign body in the upper respiratory tract. In adults, the situation is generally associated with talking and laughing while eating. Alcohol ingestion can also be a factor. Children under the age of 2 are most commonly found to have airway obstruction due to the presence of foreign bodies, with nuts being the most common, although any small object can pose a potential hazard. If the obstruction is complete, the patient will be unable to make any sound; he or she will become cyanotic and eventually unconscious. Emergency maneuvers to clear the airway should be carried out at once. If the obstruction is partial, the patient will have a persistent nonproductive cough; there may be inspiratory and expiratory stridor. The mucosa surrounding the foreign object may become inflamed and edematous, which may further impair the airway. Immediate surgical removal is necessary. Rigid bronchoscopy is considered the safest method.

PATHOLOGY AFFECTING THE ESOPHAGUS

The esophagus may be affected by several inflammatory and mechanical disorders.

ESOPHAGITIS

Inflammation of the esophagus can have many causes. Among adults, the most common cause is reflux of stomach acid into the esophagus, leading to what is commonly called "heartburn." Esophagitis is usually treated with diet modification, stress reduction, and antacid therapy. Presence of a hiatal hernia should be ruled out. Repeated episodes of esophageal inflammation or an injury such as ingestion of a caustic agent may cause scar tissue formation in the esophagus. This can ultimately lead to the formation of a stricture, which may require surgical intervention.

ULCERATION OF THE ESOPHAGUS

Ulceration of the esophagus is typically seen in longtime alcohol abusers. This behavior may also cause varices in the esophagus, which may become hemorrhagic. Often, these problems are handled endoscopically with the use of sclerosing agents.

NEOPLASMS AFFECTING THE ESOPHAGUS

The esophagus can be the site of neoplasms. Benign tumors are rare, but lipomas or fibromas may be found. These are usually asymptomatic unless they become obstructive. Malignancies are more common and can occur in any segment of the esophagus. Most are squamous cell carcinomas. The patient may complain of difficulty swallowing (dysphagia), hoarseness, and pain. Tumors may be diagnosed endoscopically; treatment options include surgery, radiation, and chemotherapy.

FOREIGN BODIES

Children are often the victims of foreign bodies in the esophagus, with coins being the most common. Foreign bodies in the esophagus do not present as serious a danger as foreign bodies in the respiratory tract, unless the object is lodged near the laryngopharynx, which presents the possibility of aspiration into the larynx or trachea. An esophagoscopy is performed to remove the object. The rigid technique is preferred.

ZENKER'S DIVERTICULUM

A diverticulum is an out-pouching of the wall of the intestinal tract. Occasionally, a diverticulum can occur in the esophagus. An esophageal diverticulum is referred to as Zenker's diverticulum. The diverticulum often occurs just above a stricture. The patient usually complains of dysphagia, or difficulty swallowing. The diverticulum can be seen on X-ray (with contrast) or endoscopically.

DIAGNOSTIC PROCEDURES/TESTS

Any patient assessment should include a full history given by the patient, if possible. Any medication allergies should be noted. This should include any symptoms that the patient is experiencing and any exposure to disease that the patient may have recently had. The examiner should take the patient's temperature, as this can be a reliable indicator of an inflammatory process under way. The physical exam should include special attention to the suspected target of the disorder, but should not be limited. Nearby lymph nodes should be palpated for any abnormalities.

DIRECT VISUALIZATION

Direct visualization is the most efficient method of examining the pharynx. The examiner uses direct lighting, which may be in the form of a flashlight, headlamp, or gooseneck lamp. The patient is asked to open his or her mouth for the examination. A tongue blade maybe used for soft tissue manipulation.

INDIRECT VISUALIZATION

In addition to direct visualization, the use of a mirror can be employed to view the nasopharynx and laryngopharynx. The mirror should be treated with a commercial antifog preparation or warmed to prevent fogging. A light is directed toward the mirror and refracted into the area to be viewed. The image of the structures is revealed in the mirror. If the vocal cords are visible, the patient may be asked to imitate certain sounds so that the examiner can better view the vocal cords and assess the quality of the sound produced.

LABORATORY TESTS

The following laboratory examinations are useful in the diagnosis of disorders of the throat:

- *Culture and sensitivity:* If the presence of a microorganism is suspected, any tissue or body fluid can be cultured. The area of the body that is suspected of hosting a microorganism is rubbed with a sterile swab. The collected fluid is placed in a culture medium and incubated. Growth of the invading organism is encouraged under these circumstances. When sufficient growth has occurred, the organism can be identified. Cultures are usually obtained to determine the presence of bacteria, although tuberculosis, fungi, and some viruses can also be identified this way. Once the infective agent has been identified, the susceptibility (sensitivity) to various antibiotics can be evaluated so that eradication of the causative organism will be achieved. A throat culture is very common and takes only a few seconds to obtain. It is relatively painless. If *Streptococcus* is suspected, a rapid strep test may be performed.
- *Blood count:* A complete blood count may be ordered. This is useful in determining anemia, a tendency to bleed, and the presence of infection. The white blood cells (WBCs) are the cells that usually fight infection. The normal range for WBCs is from 4,000 to 10,000. A WBC count over 10,000 may indicate the presence of an infection.

RADIOLOGIC EXAMINATIONS

The following radiographic examinations are useful in the diagnosis of disorders of the throat:

- *X-rays:* Routine radiographic examinations are very useful in determining pathology of the larynx and trachea. The only bony structure in the larynx is the hyoid, but the cartilaginous structures of the upper respiratory tract are clearly visible on X-ray, as are some of the more dense soft tissue structures, such as the epiglottis. Contrast media, such as barium, may be introduced into the area to enhance visualization. The use of barium is especially helpful in determining pathology of the esophagus. Great care must be taken to prevent aspiration of the liquid. Fluoroscopy may be helpful in tracking the flow of the barium.

- *CT scans:* Computed tomography allows comparison of the soft tissue structures of the neck to the other structures. Gross changes in the structure can be detected with CT.
- *MRI:* Magnetic resonance imaging provides superb viewing of the soft tissue structures of the neck.

VIDEOSTROBOSCOPY

Videostroboscopy is used for precise analysis of endolaryngeal tissue during speech. The strobe equipment is introduced into the larynx via a flexible laryngoscope. The exact movement of the vocal mucosa can be studied and pathological changes easily noted.

POLYSOMNOGRAPHY

Polysomnography is an examination used to diagnose sleep apnea and determine its severity. The test is used to record vital body functions such as heart rate, respiration, air flow, and blood oxygen levels during sleep, as well as brain activity, eye movement, and muscle activity.

MULTIPLE SLEEP LATENCY TEST (MSLT)

The Multiple Sleep Latency Test measures the amount of time that it takes an individual to fall asleep. The average time is 10–20 minutes. Those who fall asleep in less than 5 minutes are considered to have some type of sleep disorder.

PREOPERATIVE CONSIDERATIONS

The operating room and equipment are prepared prior to the arrival of the patient. Special considerations for pediatric patients may need to be made in advance. If a local anesthetic is planned, and an anesthesia provider will not be in attendance, the presence of a second circulator may be requested for patient monitoring.

If the use of a local or topical anesthetic is planned, a small table or second Mayo stand may be requested specifically for the administration of the anesthetic. This should be prepared in advance of the patient entering the operating room. Suggested supplies for this "clean" setup are:

- Medicine cups
- Syringes and needles
- Cotton tip applicators
- Anesthetic of choice
- Atomizer
- Tongue blades
- Laryngeal mirror
- Small basin of warm water for defogging the mirror
- Gauze sponges

Preoperative patient teaching should be carried out. The patient should be aware of what to expect before, during, and after the procedure. Most likely the patient will be on a restricted diet of liquid or soft foods for several postoperative days. Cold foods may help with pain control and minimize swelling. An external ice collar may also be recommended. If the patient is expected to rest the voice following the procedure, he or she should be made aware in advance what type of communication will be used postoperatively. Many procedures of the upper aerodigestive tract are performed on an out-patient basis. The patient should make arrangements in advance for transportation and assistance for at least the first 24 hours.

The STSR may work directly from the back table instead of using a Mayo stand if this arrangement is more convenient for the procedure. It may be helpful for the STSR to guide the instrumentation into the endoscope when assisting with endoscopic procedures. Although procedures performed through a normal body opening are not considered sterile, great care should be taken to use the best possible technique to prevent infection. Procedures done through the nose or mouth usually do not require a prep to be performed and sterile drapes are not used. A clean sheet may be spread over the patient for prevention of cross-contamination.

The position of the patient will depend on age, the type of surgery, and the type of anesthetic that is planned for the procedure. Often, the local anesthetic will be applied while the patient is in the sitting position and the procedure will be performed while the patient is supine. If the patient is in the supine position, the arms are usually tucked at the patient's side with the ulnar nerve carefully padded. A rolled towel may be placed under the patient's shoulders to extend the neck to provide better exposure. Adult tonsillectomies are often done with the use of a local anesthetic and while the patient is sitting up. Endoscopies with flexible endoscopes may also be accomplished with the patient in the sitting position.

SPECIAL INSTRUMENTS, SUPPLIES, AND DRUGS

Tonsillectomy and adenoidectomy (T&A) instrumentation sets are very site specific. Historically, little has changed with the T&A instrument set, although there are several techniques for removal of the tonsils and adenoids.

The operating microscope is a critical part of laryngeal surgery (Figure 17-30). Great care should be used when relocating the microscope. The microscope should be brought into the operating room and set up in advance of the surgery. An $f = 400$ lens is commonly used. For laryngeal procedures, a sterile microscope cover is not usually used. A laser may be attached to the microscope to enhance microlaryngeal surgery.

Laser surgery is becoming very common in procedures involving the larynx and oropharynx. The most

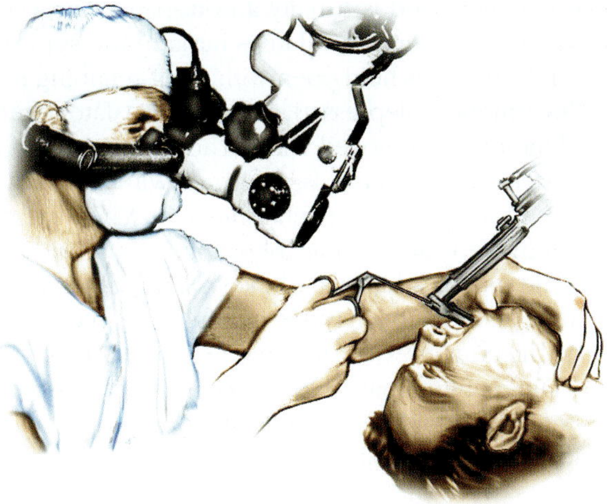

Figure 17-30 **Operating microscope set up for microlaryngoscopy**

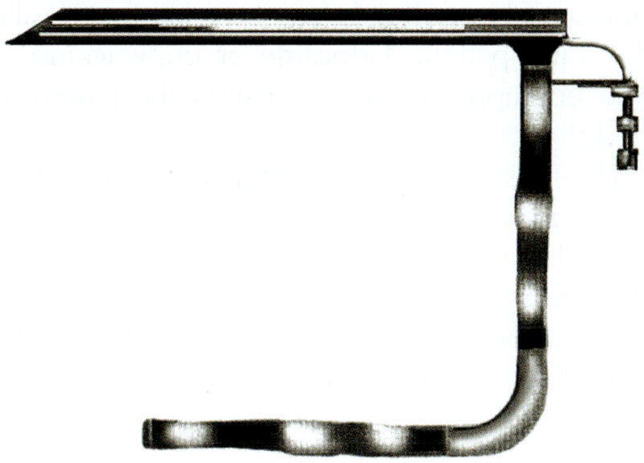

Figure 17-31 **U-shaped laryngoscope**

Figure 17-32 **Rigid esophagoscope**

popular laser for this application is the carbon dioxide laser. The carbon dioxide laser can be used in conjunction with the operating microscope to focus the beam.

As with any surgical procedure, proper illumination is essential. A variety of illumination devices are available. Each surgeon will have a preference for the type of device that he or she finds most effective.

Sitting stools should be available, especially when the use of a microscope is anticipated.

A #12 knife blade is often used in oropharyngeal surgery. The special feature of the #12 knife blade is that it is curved with the cutting surface on the inner aspect of the curve. Because of its extended length and slim handle, the #7 knife handle is often used as well.

A variety of endoscopes are used for oral (or transnasal) endoscopy. These instruments may be flexible or rigid. Each structure to be viewed has its own set of specialized scopes and correlating instrumentation.

There are three common varieties of laryngoscopes:

- An L-shaped, battery-operated laryngoscope is the instrument of choice for endotracheal intubation. The battery is located in the handle of the instrument. A variety of interchangeable oral blades are available to assist with intubation of patients of all sizes and shapes.
- Flexible laryngoscopes are available for assisting with a difficult intubation, diagnosis, or may be used for obtaining a biopsy.
- Rigid U-shaped laryngoscopes are used for biopsy, removal of a foreign body, or vocal cord procedures (Figure 17-31). The rigid laryngoscope is often suspended on a holding apparatus to maintain its position and to free the surgeon's hands. Microscopic and laser procedures are performed using the rigid laryngoscope.

Bronchoscopes are also available in flexible and rigid styles and come in a variety of sizes for use in infant, pediatric, and adult patients. A rigid bronchoscope can be differentiated from the rigid esophagoscope because the distal portion is relatively straight and it houses the ventilation holes. Flexible bronchoscopes are small in diameter and are longer than laryngoscopes. If the patient will require oxygen therapy, a special adapter must be used to make the connection with the oxygen source.

The esophagoscope, as with the other styles of endoscopes, may be either flexible or rigid. Because the esophagus is a collapsible structure, the rigid esophagoscope is flared at the distal end for better visibility (Figure 17-32). Often the flexible gastroscope is used when the esophagoscopy is performed as part of a more comprehensive procedure called esophagogastroduodenoscopy or EGD, where the gastroenterologist inspects not only the esophagus, but the stomach and duodenum as well. There is a flexible esophagoscope available but it is not often used alone.

Video equipment may be used in conjunction with the microscope and a variety of endoscopes. This is useful in enhancing the view for the surgeon and allows team members to anticipate the progress of the case.

An insulated electrosurgical device with a suction attachment may be used. The suction device is a flexible modification of a neuro suction tip. It is insulated and may have a thumb control for the suction. The active electrode is at the very tip of the instrument and is usually controlled with a foot pedal. It is capable of suction and coagulation at the same time. The length of the instrument makes it very useful in the pharynx.

A histological stain may be used to differentiate abnormal cells. This is especially useful in the esophagus and larynx. An example of one of these stains is toluidine blue.

Topical anesthetics may be used for oral endoscopy. The anesthetic agents may include Cetacaine spray or cocaine. Local anesthetics may be used for tonsillectomy on the adult patient. Lidocaine or bupivacaine, with or without epinephrine, may be used. The patient may be sedated.

The Lukens tube, sometimes referred to as the Lukens trap, is incorporated into the suction apparatus by attaching it between the suction tip and the suction tubing. It uses gravity to capture fluid (secretions or fluid instilled to obtain cell washings) to be sent for laboratory analysis. The tube must be maintained in the upright position during specimen collection to prevent the fluid from entering the suction tubing.

AERODIGESTIVE TRACT PROCEDURES

Some of the basic aerodigestive tract procedures will be described in the following section.

ADENOIDECTOMY

Adenoidectomy is the removal of the pharyngeal tonsils, which have become enlarged. This is typically done on a pediatric patient and is usually an out-patient procedure. The patient is under general anesthesia in the supine position. The mouth is held open with a self-retaining mouth gag. The tongue is depressed and the soft palate retracted. The adenoids are removed with an adenotome or an adenoid curette. Hemostasis is achieved with packing that may be left in place for several minutes. When the packing is removed, any visible bleeding points are coagulated. The use of an insulated electrosurgical device with a suction attachment may be helpful. The nasopharynx may be rinsed with water to remove loose tissue or blood clots. The patient may experience some postoperative bleeding. The adenoidectomy is often performed in combination with the tonsillectomy.

TONSILLECTOMY

Tonsillectomy is the removal of the palatine or faucial tonsils. Tonsillectomy is usually done on an out-patient basis. The palatine tonsils and the pharyngeal tonsils are often removed simultaneously in a combination procedure called tonsillectomy and adenoidectomy, or T&A (Procedure 17-6).

PROCEDURE 17-6 Tonsillectomy and Adenoidectomy

Equipment

- Headlamp
- Suction apparatus
- Electrosurgical unit with dispersive electrode

Instruments

- T&A instrumentation set

Supplies

- ½ sheet × 2
- 4 × 4 X-ray detectable sponges
- Tonsil sponges
- Towels
- Gowns
- Gloves
- Small basin
- Suction tubing
- #12 knife blade
- Electrosurgical pencil with extension
- Insulated electrosurgical device with suction attachment
- 2–0 plain tonsil needle
- Syringe for irrigation of nasopharynx (available)
- Additional supplies will be necessary if local anesthesia is planned (anesthetic, syringe, tonsil needle)

PROCEDURE 17-6 Tonsillectomy and Adenoidectomy *(continued)*

Operative Preparation

Anesthesia
- General
- Oral endotracheal tube used
- Lubricate and protect eyes

Position
- Supine, with neck hyperextended by a roll placed under the shoulders
- A donut or foam headrest may be used for stabilization
- Arms tucked at patient's sides; protect ulnar nerves
- For the comfort of the surgeon, a small patient may be placed closer to the side of the operating table at which the surgeon will be standing

Prep
- None needed

Draping
- Not required; a head wrap and/or cover sheet may be used

Practical Considerations

- An adult patient may receive a local anesthetic and will be placed in the sitting position
- Surgeon preference will dictate the order of the procedure. In a combination procedure, some surgeons prefer to perform the tonsillectomy first while others will remove the adenoids first
- The surgeon may stand at the patient's side or sit at the head of the table. Make the necessary equipment adjustments and arrange the OR accordingly
- T&A is not a sterile procedure; use the best technique possible

Operative Procedure	Technical Considerations
1. The mouth is held open with a self-retaining mouth gag. The tongue is retracted with a Wieder tongue depressor.	**1.** If using a Jennings mouth gag, it will be necessary for the anesthesia provider to disconnect the ET tube from the anesthesia circuit for insertion of the retractor and then reconnect it. The anesthesia provider will position the oral ET tube on the nonoperative side. Be sure ET tube is not dislocated or occluded with the retractor. The STSR will likely hold the tongue depressor after placement by the surgeon and provide suction. Have all other supplies within reach of the surgeon.
2. The tonsil is grasped and the mucosa of the anterior pillar incised.	**2.** Tonsil tenaculum or long Allis will be needed to put tension on the tonsil. Pass scalpel and follow with electrosurgical pencil or scissors.
3. The tonsil is dissected free of its mucosa.	**3.** Pass pillar dissector and continue to provide suction.
4. The tonsil may be amputated with a snare, a guillotine, or electrosurgically removed from its fossa.	**4.** If the use of a snare is planned, it should be loaded in advance.
5. Once the tonsil is amputated, pressure may be applied to the fossa with a tonsil sponge for a few minutes.	**5.** Tonsil sponge is loaded on a long instrument for temporary placement in the tonsil fossa.

(continues)

PROCEDURE 17-6 Tonsillectomy and Adenoidectomy *(continued)*

6. Hemostasis is achieved.	**6.** Hemostasis is usually achieved electrosurgically. Have tonsil hemostats and suture available if hemostasis is not achieved electrosurgically.
7. The procedure is repeated contralaterally.	**7.** The anesthesia provider will move the ET tube to the contralateral side of the mouth. Quickly reorganize the supplies to facilitate removal of the second tonsil. The surgeon generally does not switch sides.
8. The uvula is retracted to expose the nasopharynx.	**8.** The soft palate retractor is positioned by the surgeon and held in position by the STSR. Provide suction as needed.
9. Adenoids are removed with an adenotome or curette.	**9.** Provide instrument of choice.
10. Pressure is applied to control bleeding.	**10.** Provide tonsil sponge loaded on a long instrument.
11. Hemostasis is achieved electrosurgically.	**11.** Provide pillar retractor and electrosurgical pencil to surgeon. Suction as needed. It may be necessary to change from electrosurgical pencil to the electrosurgical device with the suction attachment.
12. The nasopharynx may be irrigated to be sure all clots and tissue have been removed.	**12.** Have irrigation supplies ready according to surgeon's preference. STSR may be asked to instill irrigation fluid through the nose.
13. A final inspection of all sites is performed and hemostasis verified.	**13.** Continue to provide retraction and suction as needed. Count.
14. Retractors are removed.	**14.** Anesthesia provider will disconnect ET tube if necessary for retractor removal. Do not dislocate ET tube. Clean patient's face if needed.

Postoperative Considerations

Immediate Postoperative Care

- Once extubated, the patient should be placed on his or her side to prevent aspiration.
- Elevate the head of the bed slightly to reduce postoperative swelling.
- Provide cold fluids to aid in comfort and prevent swelling.

Prognosis

- Patient is expected to return to normal activities in 2 weeks.
- Incidence of "sore throats" should be greatly reduced.

Complications

- Bleeding is the most common postoperative complication and can occur up to 10 days after surgery.
- Infection.

PEARL OF WISDOM

The tonsils and adenoids may be sent to pathology in the same container per facility policy. If it is necessary to distinguish the right from the left, the STSR should make the necessary adjustments.

INCISION AND DRAINAGE OF A PERITONSILLAR ABSCESS

A peritonsillar abscess may be surgically drained. An incision is made into the abscess and the pocket of pus is removed with suction. The patient usually undergoes tonsillectomy after the infection has been resolved with antibiotics, although recent studies show that it may be safe to remove the tonsils at the time of the acute infection.

UVULOPALATOPHARYNGO-PLASTY

Uvulopalatopharyngoplasty, or **UPPP** (also known as UP3), is the definitive treatment for intractable snoring and obstructive sleep apnea (Procedure 17-7). UPPP is performed on adults and is done under general anesthesia. Redundant tissue of the fauces, the tonsils (if present), and a portion of the soft palate including the uvula are removed (Figure 17-33). If necessary, an adenoidectomy may be included with this procedure. The tissue is usually removed en bloc. The procedure can be accomplished with standard surgical techniques or with a carbon dioxide laser. The success rate is roughly 50%. Postoperative complications include apnea and bleeding.

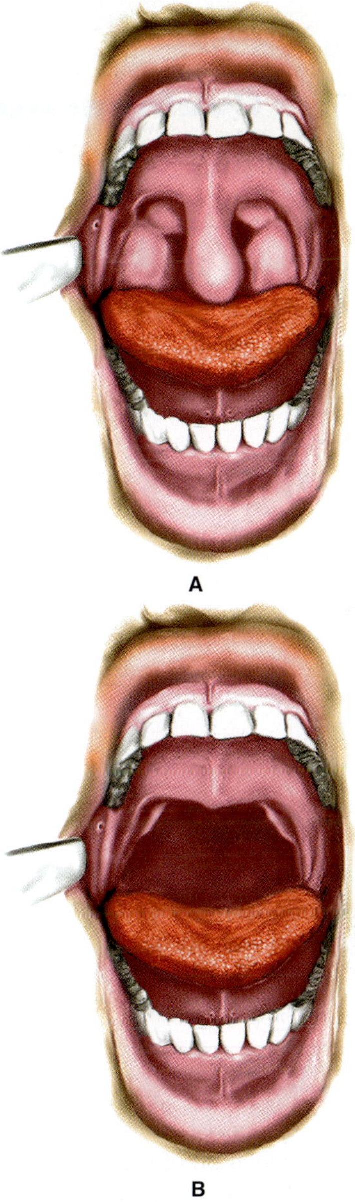

Figure 17-33 **UP3: (A) Preoperative view—redundant tissue (fauces, tonsils, and soft palate), (B) postoperative view**

PROCEDURE 17-7 Uvulopalatopharyngoplasty

Equipment

- Headlamp
- Suction apparatus
- Electrosurgical unit with dispersive electrode
- Carbon dioxide laser and protective attire

(continues)

PROCEDURE 17-7 Uvulopalatopharyngoplasty *(continued)*

Instruments

- T&A instrumentation set

Supplies

- ½ sheet × 2
- 4 × 4 X-ray detectable sponges
- Tonsil sponges
- Towels
- Gowns
- Gloves
- Small basin
- Suction tubing
- #12 knife blade
- Electrosurgical pencil with extension
- Insulated electrosurgical device with suction attachment
- Suture according to surgeon's preference
- Bulb syringe
- Sterile components for laser
- Tracheotomy supplies

Operative Preparation

Anesthesia

- General
- An oral or nasal endotracheal tube may used
- Systemic steroids may be initiated to prevent edema

Position

- Supine, with neck hyperextended by a roll placed under shoulders
- A donut or foam headrest may be used for stabilization
- Arms tucked at patient's sides; protect ulnar nerves

Prep

- None needed

Draping

- Not required; a head wrap and/or cover sheet may be used

Practical Considerations

- Obesity is often a contributing factor in sleep apnea. Consideration of the patient's size may be necessary when planning and positioning equipment and supplies
- A tracheotomy may be performed in advance of the UPPP to ensure patent airway (an extra long trach tube may be necessary)
- If a tracheotomy is not planned in advance, the possibility of an emergency tracheotomy exists. All equipment and supplies should be readily available
- The patient may be difficult to intubate; additional supplies and personnel may be needed
- UPPP is not a sterile procedure; use the best technique possible
- Tonsillectomy will be performed in conjunction with UPPP if tonsils are present
- Adenoids may also be removed
- If use of a laser is anticipated, all safety measures must be followed

Operative Procedure	Technical Considerations
1. Self-retaining mouth gag is inserted.	1. ET tube should not be dislocated or occluded with the retractor. Provide suction as needed.
2. An outline of the tissue to be resected may be made with a scalpel or the electrosurgical pencil.	2. Provide #12 blade on a #7 knife handle or electrosurgical pencil.

PROCEDURE 17-7 Uvulopalatopharyngoplasty *(continued)*

3. Tonsils, if present, will be included in en bloc dissection.	**3.** Provide tonsil tenaculum or Allis clamp. Metzenbaum scissors, electrosurgical pencil, or laser and tissue forceps will be used for dissection.
4. Dissection progresses to include the soft palate on the operative side, uvula, and continues with the soft palate on the contralateral side. It is completed with the second tonsil, if present.	**4.** Dissection will continue with instrument of surgeon's choice. Continue to provide suction as necessary.
5. The specimen will be extracted and hemostasis achieved.	**5.** Prepare to accept the tissue specimen. Tonsil clamps and suture may be needed for hemostasis. Prepare to switch back and forth between the electrosurgical pencil and the electrosurgical device with the suction attachment or the laser.
6. Oral cavity and pharynx are irrigated to remove blood clots or tissue remnants.	**6.** Bulb syringe should be prefilled with irrigation solution. Suction is necessary.
7. The mucosal edges are sutured with a running stitch.	**7.** Provide absorbable suture according to surgeon's preference and long tissue forceps. Suture scissors as needed.
8. Adenoidectomy is performed if necessary.	**8.** Refer to Procedure 17-6 for technical considerations.
9. Mouth gag is removed.	**9.** Count. Do not dislocate ET tube.

Postoperative Considerations

Immediate Postoperative Care

- When fully awake, the patient may be provided with cold liquids for comfort and prevention of swelling.
- The patient should be instructed not to use a straw for fluid intake.
- Tracheotomy may become necessary, if not already implemented.

Prognosis

- Patient may remain hospitalized for several days and is expected to return to normal activities in 2 weeks.
- Sleep disorders and episodes of hypoxia should be reduced or eliminated.

Complications

- Hemorrhage
- Infection
- Airway obstruction due to swelling

PEARL OF WISDOM

A tongue blade should not be used for postoperative inspection of the surgical site to prevent disruption of the suture line.

LARYNGOSCOPY

Laryngoscopy may be performed to remove a foreign body, obtain a diagnosis, or treat a condition of the vocal cords, such as removal of a nodule (Procedure 17-8).

PROCEDURE 17-8 Rigid Laryngoscopy

Equipment

- Microscope, if planned
- Laryngoscopy holder, if suspension laryngoscopy
- Fiberoptic light source
- Sitting stool for surgeon
- Suction apparatus
- Laser and protective devices, if requested

Instruments

- Laryngoscopes: size according to patient; style according to surgeon's preference
- Laryngeal suction tips
- Fiberoptic light cord
- Tooth protector
- Laryngeal mirror
- Laryngeal knives (variety)
- Laryngeal biopsy forceps (variety)
- Foreign body forceps
- Nonpiercing towel clamp

Supplies

- ½ sheet × 2
- Towels
- Gloves
- Suction tubing
- 4 × 4 gauze sponges
- Small basin
- Lukens trap
- Lubricant
- Specimen container(s)
- Additional supplies will be needed if local anesthesia is planned

Operative Preparation

Anesthesia
- General preferred
- Lubricate and protect eyes

Position
- Supine, with neck hyperextended by a roll placed under the shoulders
- Patient is situated on operating table with his or her head as far as possible toward the head of the table
- Operating table will be turned 90° to allow surgeon to be positioned directly above patient's head
- A donut or foam headrest may be used for stabilization
- Arms tucked at patient's sides; protect ulnar nerves

Prep
- None needed

Draping
- Not required; a head wrap and/or cover sheet may be used

Practical Considerations

- Oral assessment is necessary. Removal of dentures is required. Teeth can be damaged
- Laryngoscopy is not a sterile procedure; use the best possible technique
- Safety measures must be employed if laser use is intended

Operative Procedure	Technical Considerations
1. Surgeon is seated.	**1.** Table is turned and equipment positioned once surgeon is seated.

PROCEDURE

17-8 Rigid Laryngoscopy *(continued)*

2. The rigid scope of choice is inserted.	**2.** Light cord and suction are passed off the field and connected to the corresponding equipment. The tooth protector is inserted into the patient's mouth to protect the upper front teeth. Provide laryngoscope of choice. Lubricate if requested to do so.
3. The scope may be suspended for better visualization.	**3.** Assist in suspending the laryngoscope.
4. A microscope may be used to enhance visualization.	**4.** The microscope is prepared in advance with the magnification lens and eyepiece configuration of surgeon's preference.
5. Tissues are inspected.	**5.** Provide suction as needed.
6. Fluid may be aspirated for pathological examination.	**6.** Connect Lukens trap to suction apparatus if necessary. Prepare to accept fluid aspiration specimen. During aspiration Lukens trap must remain in an upright position.
7. Biopsy may be taken.	**7.** Continue to provide suction as needed. Pass biopsy forceps of choice. Prepare to accept tissue samples. A hypodermic needle may be useful to gently remove tissue specimens from delicate biopsy forceps. Multiple specimens may be obtained—it is essential that no error in specimen handling is made.
8. Benign lesions may be removed with the use of a laser.	**8.** Have laser components ready and employ all safety measures.
9. Lesions may be removed with traditional surgical techniques.	**9.** Pass instrumentation of preference. Prepare to accept specimen. Anticipate the repeated use of suction.
10. Hemostasis is verified and the scope extracted.	**10.** Count may not be necessary—according to facility policy. Cleanse face if necessary.

Postoperative Considerations

Immediate Postoperative Care

- This is normally an out-patient procedure.
- Patient is not discharged until he or she is able to demonstrate control of the gag reflex and retain fluids taken orally.

Prognosis

- Patient is expected to experience a sore throat and a raspy quality to the voice that should resolve in a few days.
- According to diagnosis, may need more extensive treatment.

Complications

- Hemorrhage
- Infection
- Raspy voice quality that does not resolve

PEARL OF WISDOM

It is helpful to direct the suction tip into the opening of the laryngoscope so that the surgeon does not have to look away from the operative site.

BRONCHOSCOPY

Bronchoscopy is accomplished in much the same way as laryngoscopy and is performed for the same reasons. If the flexible bronchoscope is to be used, the patient is often given a topical anesthetic and remains in the sitting position for the procedure. For rigid bronchoscopy, general anesthesia is the treatment of choice. The oxygen connector should be checked to ensure that it corresponds with the type of bronchoscope being used. Maintenance of the patient's airway is of utmost importance.

ESOPHAGOSCOPY

Esophagoscopy may be either diagnostic or for removal of a foreign body. Foreign bodies are most often removed with the use of a rigid esophagoscope with the patient supine and under general anesthesia. Most diagnostic procedures are done with sedation in the endoscopy laboratory with a gastroscope as part of a more extensive procedure.

PANENDOSCOPY

The term *panendoscopy* refers to a procedure that may involve inspection of several portions of the upper aerodigestive tract. This may be done with the use of a flexible scope, several specific rigid instruments, or an endoscope with a wide-angle lens.

RADICAL NECK DISSECTION WITH MANDIBULECTOMY

A radical neck dissection is generally performed unilaterally (Procedure 17-9). The following structures of the lateral neck are removed: cervical lymph nodes, jugular vein, and sternocleidomastoid muscle (SCM). While performed alone to treat metastatic squamous cell carcinoma, this type of neck dissection is also done in conjunction with mandibulectomy for metastatic lesions of the mouth and jaw. For both psychological and physiological reasons, the ensuing defect caused by such extensive resection necessitates immediate reconstruction, involving (in part) the use of a composite graft. Several body structures would make viable composite grafts for mandibular reconstruction; the fibula, and its adjoining vessels, is commonly used. An approach employing two surgical teams working concurrently is recommended.

PROCEDURE 17-9 Radical Neck Dissection with Mandibulectomy

Team A: Neck Dissection and Mandibulectomy

Equipment

- Headlamp
- Electrosurgical unit with dispersive electrode
- Power source and accessories for drill(s)
- Suction apparatus

Instruments

- Standard neck instrument set
- Tracheotomy set
- Standard dental instrument set
- Microdrill, with assortment of burs
- Mini-driver and Synthes facial fracture set

PROCEDURE 17-9 Radical Neck Dissection with Mandibulectomy *(continued)*

Supplies

- Prep set
- Basic pack
- Basin set
- Gloves
- Head and neck drapes
- Anode endotracheal tube
- Tracheotomy tube (size and style may vary)
- Several #15 scalpel blades
- Electrosurgical pencil, with both blade and needle electrodes
- Facial nerve stimulator
- Suture according to surgeon's preference
- Assortment of free ties: 2–0, 3–0, and 4–0 silk; 2–0, 3–0, and 4–0 Vicryl (or chromic gut)
- Assortment of stick ties: 2–0 and 3–0 silk on both cutting and tapered needles; 2–0, 3–0, and 4–0 Vicryl on both cutting and tapered needles; 3–0 and 4–0 nylon on cutting needles (for skin closure)
- Several 10-cc syringes, with 25-gauge 1-in. and ½-in. hypodermic needles
- Pharmaceuticals according to surgeon's preference (e.g., bupivacaine with epinephrine)
- Skin staples

Team B: Composite Graft Procurement

Equipment

- Headlamp
- Electrosurgical unit with dispersive electrode
- Power source and accessories for drill
- Microscope
- Suction apparatus

Instruments

- Minor instrument set
- Minor orthopedic instrument set
- Standard microinstrument set
- Small vascular instrument set
- Variety of bone-holding clamps
- Microdrill/sagittal saw
- Mini-driver

Supplies

- Prep set
- Basic pack
- Basin set
- Gloves
- Medium-large stockinette
- Impervious U-drape
- Extremity drape sheet
- Several #10 scalpel blades
- Electrosurgical pencil
- Vessel loops
- Suture according to surgeon's preference
- 2–0, 3–0, and 4–0 silk ties; 2–0, 3–0, and 4–0 Vicryl ties; 2–0 and 3–0 Vicryl on tapered needles (for closure)
- 7–0 and 8–0 Prolene or nylon for vascular anastomosis
- Assortment of 3-cc, 5-cc and 10-cc syringes, with heparin (olive-tipped) needles
- Pharmaceuticals according to surgeon's preference (e.g., Heparin-saline solution)
- Microscope drape

(continues)

PROCEDURE

17-9 Radical Neck Dissection with Mandibulectomy *(continued)*

Operative Preparation

Anesthesia

- General
- Lubricate and protect eyes

Position

- Supine, with neck hyperextended by a roll placed under the shoulders
- Head is turned to expose operative side and may be secured on a donut or foam headrest
- Arms tucked at patient's sides; protect ulnar nerves

Prep

- Both sites may need to be shaved
- Both sites will require skin preps; it is helpful to have two circulators to facilitate the dual procedure

Draping

- Towels and the respective specialty sheets are placed

Practical Considerations

- Because this is a multiple-part procedure, it is necessary to have two STSRs, with each assisting one team and responsible for one surgical site. It should be noted that the team working in the mouth is not considered sterile. Therefore, everyone should be diligent in preventing contamination of the sterile areas of the operative field (e.g., no passing instruments or supplies between the two areas, etc.).
- For our purposes, "Team A" will be considered the nonsterile team handling the upper body procedures and "Team B" will be considered the sterile team responsible for graft procurement.
- Ordinarily, once the graft is harvested and the donor site sutured and dressed, there is no need for the second team.

Operative Procedure	Technical Considerations
1. Team A will start by creating a tracheotomy. Once the opening is made into the trachea, the anesthesia provider will slowly remove the endotracheal tube.	**1.** Follow procedural guide for tracheotomy in Chapter 14.
2. As the ET tube is withdrawn, the surgeon will begin inserting the anode tube into the trachea. On satisfactory placement, the proximal end is connected to the anesthesia circuit (and is thus considered contaminated). The tube is then stabilized by inflating the balloon cuff at its distal end (within the trachea) with a 10-cc syringe, and held in place by suturing the external segment to the chest with a 2–0 silk.	**2.** Prepare anode tube in advance—be certain that balloon is patent. Provide anode tube and syringe for balloon inflation at appropriate time. Pass 2–0 silk on needle driver and tissue forceps followed by suture scissors.
3. To aid in hemostasis, the surgeon may start by injecting the operative site with a local anesthetic (e.g., bupivacaine) containing epinephrine.	**3.** Solution for injection should be drawn up in advance. Notify anesthesia provider of epinephrine injection.

PROCEDURE

17-9 Radical Neck Dissection with Mandibulectomy *(continued)*

4. The neck dissection is initiated. The incision begins at the mastoid tip (below the ear), and continues distally to approximately 2 cm inferior to the mandible, and around to the area immediately below and lateral to the chin.	**4.** Intended incision line may be outlined with a sterile marking pen. Pass #15 scalpel blade on #7 knife handle. Anticipate the use of the electrosurgical pencil. Provide instruments for retraction; a green retractor is commonly used.
5. The subcutaneous tissues are separated from the underlying structures, creating a flap, which can be anchored out of the way by folding it over and tacking it with a 2–0 silk suture.	**5.** Metzenbaum scissors and tissue forceps will be used for the dissection. Have peanut sponges loaded on clamps for blunt dissection. Provide suction as needed. Be sure fresh 4 × 4s are available throughout—expect the use of several packages. Blood vessels will be coagulated or double clamped, cut, and ligated. Prepare retraction suture in advance. Pass suture and tissue forceps when needed; follow with suture scissors.
6. Through careful and tedious dissection, the internal neck structures are identified. The nerve stimulator is used frequently in an effort to identify—and preserve—vital nerves, such as the lingual and hypoglossal.	**6.** Nerve stimulator should be ready for intermittent use; sharp component requires caution. Dissection will continue with Metz and tissue forceps or electrosurgical pencil. Hemostasis will be achieved as vessels are encountered.
7. Continuing the dissection, the sternocleidomastoid (SCM) muscle is divided at the point of its inferior insertion.	**7.** The electrosurgical pencil will likely be used to divide the SCM.
8. The internal jugular vein is located and subsequently ligated with a 0 silk stick tie. Smaller vessels are ligated with either a 2–0 or 3–0 silk or a 2–0 or 3–0 Vicryl free tie.	**8.** Provide two clamps for the jugular vein. Prepare 0 silk in advance—vessel may be ligated prior to separation. Vessel will be cut. Any peripheral vessels will be clamped, cut, and ligated, or hemoclips may be applied and then the vessel cut.
9. The nodes along the cervical lymph tree are then freed from the surrounding tissues, and the entire contents of the neck dissection is removed en bloc.	**9.** Prepare to accept and process the first specimen. The surgeon may request that the pathologist verify that the margins are cancer free, possibly requiring a frozen section.
10. The mandibulectomy is initiated. The original incision, which terminated at the contralateral submental area, is extended superiorly over the chin, through the midline of the bottom lip, bisecting it.	**10.** Skin knife will be needed again. Anticipate use of the electrosurgical pencil.
11. The soft tissues are retracted with double-prong skin hooks as the surgeon continues his incision through the oral mucosa and gingiva, along the superior aspect of the affected portion of mandible. If there are any teeth remaining in this section of the mandible, they are extracted at this time.	**11.** Provide skin hook retractors; use caution—tips are pointed. Scissors and tissue forceps or the electrosurgical pencil will be needed to continue the dissection. Have tooth extraction tools available.

(continues)

PROCEDURE 17-9 Radical Neck Dissection with Mandibulectomy *(continued)*

12. Finally, once the mandible is exposed, the bone is cleaned of soft tissue with a periosteal elevator, and the involved section is excised, using a sagittal saw. *Note:* To maintain function of the jaw following reconstruction, excision of the mandible will ordinarily stop short of the temporomandibular joint.	**12.** Provide periosteal elevator. Anticipate the use of the sagittal saw and prepare in advance. Provide irrigation fluid to cool bone. Prepare to accept final specimen. Follow physician's orders concerning specimen care; it may be needed as a template to tailor the graft.
13. While Team A is completing the neck dissection and mandibulectomy, Team B will begin work on harvesting the fibular composite graft. First, a linear incision is made on the lateral aspect of the leg, beginning approximately 5 cm distal to the knee, and continuing to approximately 5–10 cm proximal to the ankle. (The exact length of the incision will be determined by the length of fibula needed for reconstruction.)	**13.** Pass skin knife. Anticipate the use of the electrosurgical pencil. Provide retractors as needed.
14. The dissection continues through the subcutaneous tissues, fascia, and muscle layers, until the fibula is exposed.	**14.** Scissors and tissue forceps or the electrosurgical pencil may be used for dissection.
15. At this point, the dissection becomes slow and deliberate, in order to identify and preserve the blood vessels supplying the fibula. Some of these vessels are quite small, necessitating the use of a microscope.	**15.** If use of microscope is anticipated, drape and position in advance of need. Switch to more delicate instrumentation if necessary.
16. Once adequate venous and arterial conduits are located, the vessels are cannulated with a small-gauged angiocatheter and heparinized to prevent thrombus formation. (Sometimes papaverine is also used, to prevent vasospasm.)	**16.** Provide heparinized saline in syringes with angiocatheter attached. Have other pharmaceuticals on the field, labeled, and prepared for use.
17. A small vascular clamp, such as a bulldog, is applied proximal to the cannulation point, and the vessel is then ligated with an appropriate-sized free tie. This process is repeated for each vessel.	**17.** Pass vascular clamp and appropriate suture or clips for ligation. Prepare to repeat this process as many times as necessary.
18. Once the integrity of the fibular blood supply is preserved, the section of fibula is removed by using the sagittal saw. The proximal and distal stumps of the remaining fibula may need to be filed, in order to prevent any rough edges from damaging the surrounding tissues.	**18.** Prepare sagittal saw in advance. Rasp may be needed.
19. The donor site is then closed using 2–0 Vicryl for the deep layers; 3–0 Vicryl for the subcutaneous layers, and staples for the skin.	**19.** Have wound irrigation ready if requested. Follow closure routine including count. Be sure wound is dressed prior to introduction of mandibular template onto field.

PROCEDURE

17-9 Radical Neck Dissection with Mandibulectomy *(continued)*

20. The composite graft will be prepped for transplant. Using the excised section of mandible as a template, the bony portion of the graft is contoured with a micro bur to approximate size and shape.

20. A work space should be set aside for preparation of the graft. Anticipate the necessary instrumentation and have it available at the work space.

21. Under the microscope, the venous and arterial vessels of the fibula are anastomosed to their counterparts in the graft site, with the 7–0 and 8–0 Prolene or nylon.

21. The graft is transferred to Team A for insertion in the jaw. The microscope and microinstrumentation may be transferred to Team A to facilitate the implant of the composite graft. This completes Team B's participation in the procedure.

22. The bony portion of the graft is anchored to the remaining (unaffected) portion of the mandible, as well as the temporomandibular joint on the affected side, using plates and screws from the Synthes facial fracture set.

22. Have a variety of plates and screws available for fixation of the fibula to the mandible. Drill with appropriate size drill bits should be ready, along with any necessary guides, taps, etc.

23. The gingiva and oral mucosa are then closed with a running 3–0 chromic (or Vicryl) suture.

23. Anticipate the use of irrigation fluid. Provide the total amount of all irrigation fluid used during the procedure to the anesthesia provider. Prepare for closure by loading suture and obtaining appropriate size drain(s). Pass suture and tissue forceps when requested; follow with suture scissors when needed. Count.

24. A Jackson-Pratt drain is placed in the inferior portion of the neck dissection and covered by the skin flap.

24. Pass drain. When appropriate, connect drain to suction device/reservoir.

25. The wound edges are then approximated and stabilized with 3–0 Vicryl sutures, placed subcutaneously. For skin closure, a staple gun can be used from the portion of the incision beginning at the mastoid tip, and extending to the submental area. However, for the area between the chin and the external portion of the bottom lip, a soft, nonabsorbable suture (such as 3–0 silk) is preferable.

25. Continue to provide closing materials and support as needed. Prepare dressing materials.

26. Following skin closure, the anode tube is removed by the surgeon, and replaced with an appropriate-sized tracheotomy tube. (*Note:* the STSR should verify patency of the balloon cuff prior to giving the tracheotomy tube to the surgeon.) The anesthesia circuit is then attached to the tracheotomy tube, and ventilation is resumed.

26. Communicate with surgeon in advance concerning preference for tracheotomy tube style and size. Obtain tube of choice. Assemble tube and ensure patency of balloon, if there is one. Assist with airway as needed—suction will be necessary.

(continues)

PROCEDURE 17-9 Radical Neck Dissection with Mandibulectomy *(continued)*

Postoperative Considerations

Immediate Postoperative Care

- Patient may require intensive care and remain hospitalized for several days.
- Patient will need wound care instruction.
- Patient may have a tracheotomy.

Prognosis

- According to diagnosis, may need more extensive treatment.
- Tracheotomy (if present) may be permanent.

Complications

- Hemorrhage
- Infection
- Recurrence of cancer
- Failure of graft to *take* (rejection)

PEARL OF WISDOM

Naturally, it is necessary to have at least two separate setups, as well as separate "counts," for each portion of this procedure. Both STSRs will need to be extremely vigilant with the countable items. Extreme care must also be taken to keep the two fields separate.

CASE STUDY

Beth, a 26-year-old female, was involved in an automobile accident in which the air bag of her vehicle deployed. She states that she feels very fortunate that a nasal septum fracture was her only injury. Beth is scheduled for a septoplasty under local anesthesia and is fearful that she may feel pain during the procedure.

1. What is septoplasty?
2. What steps will be taken to ensure that Beth's surgical site is adequately anesthetized?
3. What medications and supplies should the STSR expect the surgeon to use to provide Beth's anesthesia?
4. What reassurances, if any, can the surgical team members offer Beth to alleviate her fears?

QUESTIONS FOR FURTHER STUDY

1. What special preparations should be made in advance of the pediatric patient's arrival into the OR?
2. What type of anesthesia will the pediatric patient undergoing foreign body removal from the nose most likely receive? Will an IV be necessary?
3. Outline the draping sequence for exposure of the face.
4. What position will the patient be placed in for an adenoidectomy?
5. What bone houses the tympanic cavity?
6. What is the function of the turbinates?

BIBLIOGRAPHY

Applegate, E. (1995). *The anatomy and physiology learning system*. Philadelphia: W. B. Saunders.

Atkinson, L. J., & Fortunato, N. (1996). *Berry and Kohn's operating room technique* (8th ed.). St. Louis, MO: Mosby.

Beckett, B. J. (1997). *Identifying surgical instruments* (2nd ed.). Thousand Oaks, CA.

Bess, F. H., & Humes, L. E. (1990). *Audiology: The fundamentals*. Baltimore: Williams & Wilkins.

Gaudin, A. J. (1989). *Human anatomy & physiology* (2nd ed.). Ft. Worth, TX: Saunders College Publishing.

Georgiade, G. S., et al. (1992). *Textbook of plastic, maxillofacial and reconstructive surgery* (2nd ed.). Baltimore: Williams & Wilkins.

Goldman, M. A. (1996). *Pocket guide to the operating room* (2nd ed.). Philadelphia: F. A. Davis.

Intermountain Laser Institute. (1998). [Online]. Available from *http://cfwurstermd.com/laser_surgery_for_sleep_apnea.htm*

Jackson Gastroenterology. (1998). [Online]. Available from *http://www.gicare.com/pated/eiegmced.htm*

Lehigh Valley Hospital And Health Network. (1998). [Online]. Available from *http://www.lvhhn.org/healthy_you/body/respiratory/apnea*

Lowe, J. (1997). *Histotechnology technical methods*. University of Nottingham Medical School [Online]. Available from *http://www.ccc.nottingham.ac.uk/~mpzjlowe/protocols/tolbluehelm.html*

Mayo clinic family health 3.0 [CD-ROM]. (1996). Minneapolis: IVI Publishing.

Mayo clinic family pharmacist 2.0 [CD-ROM]. (1996). Minneapolis: IVI Publishing.

McGuiness, A. M., et al. (2002). *Core curriculum for surgical technology* (5th ed.). Centennial, CO: Association of Surgical Technologists.

Raney, R. W., (1995). *Myringoplasty and tympanoplasty*. Grand Rounds Archive at Baylor. [Online]. Available from *http://www.bcm.tmc.edu*

Riley, M. K. (1987). *Nursing care of the client with ear, nose, and throat disorders*. New York: Springer.

Schuller, D. E., & Schleuning A. J., II, (1994). *DeWeese and Saunders' otolaryngology head and neck surgery* (8th ed.). St. Louis, MO: Mosby-Year Book.

Sleep Apnea Society of Alberta. (1996). [Online]. Available from *http://www.sleep-apnea.ab.ca/treat.html*

Taylor, E. J. (Ed.). (1995). *Dorland's pocket medical dictionary* (25th ed.). Philadelphia: W. B. Saunders.

CHAPTER 18

Oral and Maxillofacial Surgery

Amy Croft

CASE STUDY

Alan is a 23-year-old male who has been admitted to the emergency department following his involvement in a motorcycle accident. Alan was not wearing a helmet at the time of his injury.

Alan is awake and alert, but is having difficulty breathing. He states that he is experiencing double vision.

1. Why may Alan be experiencing respiratory distress and what steps, if any, should be taken to protect his airway?
2. Which diagnostic examinations may be ordered by the team of emergency specialists treating Alan?
3. Is surgery a possibility in Alan's case and, if so, is it an emergency?

OBJECTIVES

After studying this chapter, the reader should be able to:

A 1. Discuss the anatomy relevant to oral and maxillofacial surgery.

P 2. Describe the pathology that prompts oral and maxillofacial surgery and the related terminology.

3. Discuss special preoperative diagnostic procedures/tests pertaining to oral and maxillofacial surgery.

O 4. Discuss special preoperative preparation procedures related to oral and maxillofacial surgery.

5. Identify the names and uses of oral and maxillofacial instruments, supplies, and drugs.

6. Identify the names and uses of special equipment used for oral and maxillofacial surgery.

7. Discuss the intraoperative preparation of the patient undergoing an oral or maxillofacial procedure.
8. Define and give an overview of oral or maxillofacial procedures.
9. Discuss the purpose and expected outcomes of oral and maxillofacial procedures.
10. Discuss the immediate postoperative care and possible complications of oral and maxillofacial procedures.
11. **S** Discuss any specific variations related to the preoperative, intraoperative, and postoperative care of the oral and maxillofacial surgical patient.

SELECT KEY TERMS

1. alveolar process	7. dentition	13. maxillofacial	19. ramus
2. arthroscopy	8. glenoid fossa	14. meniscus	20. reduction
3. calvarial	9. gnath-	15. mouth prop	21. sagittal
4. condyle	10. labia	16. orbicular	22. symphysis
5. coronal flap	11. malar bone	17. osteotomy	23. TMJ
6. craniosynostosis	12. malocclusion	18. pan-	

ANATOMY OF THE ORAL CAVITY

The oral, or buccal, cavity consists of the lips, teeth, palate, cheeks, and tongue (refer to Plate 6 in Appendix A). It also receives the ducts from the salivary glands. The lips surround the mouth. The teeth are rooted in the alveolar processes of the maxilla and mandible. The hard and soft palates comprise the roof of the mouth. The cheeks form the lateral walls of the oral cavity. The tongue is the muscular organ that forms a portion of the floor of the mouth and lies along the bottom of the oral cavity.

LIPS

The lips, or **labia**, are the anterior entry to the oral cavity. Thermal receptors in the lips protect the mouth from burns from hot food or liquids. The lips also contain muscles that aid in facial expression, food retention, and mastication. The space between the lips (extending to include the cheeks) and the teeth is referred to as the vestibule.

TEETH

Humans have two **dentitions**, deciduous and permanent, classifying them as diphyodonts. The primary, or deciduous, teeth begin to appear around 6 months of age and the process continues until 2 to 4 years of age. The primary teeth for each jaw are as follows: two central incisors, two lateral incisors, two cuspids or canines, and four molars. The loss of primary teeth usually follows the order of initial eruption. The secondary, or permanent, set of teeth push the primary teeth out beginning at about the age of 6. The third molars, or wisdom teeth, can appear between the ages of 17 and 25. The permanent teeth for each jaw are as follows: two central incisors, two lateral incisors, two cuspids, four bicuspids, and six molars.

The teeth lie in each jaw in a semicircular fashion. The side of the tooth that lies closest to the lips is referred to the labial; the tongue side is lingual, and the cheek side is buccal. Each individual tooth is imbedded in a socket of the **alveolar process** of each jaw. The alveolar maxillary process contains the upper teeth while the mandibular process contains the lower teeth.

The teeth aid in speech and the breakdown of food. There are four different types of teeth. The four front teeth of each jaw are the *incisors*. Incisors have sharp cutting edges that tear food. The *cuspids* are located lateral to the incisors and are stronger; their purpose is to grasp and shred food. The *bicuspid* teeth are distal to the cuspid teeth. They, along with the flat topped *molar* teeth, grind the food into smaller portions.

The tooth can be divided into three main regions. The portion of the tooth above the gumline is the crown, the portion below the gum is considered the root, and the junction of the two is referred to as the neck.

The crown of the tooth contains several areas. Enamel covers the outer portion of the crown. Made of calcium salts, it is the hardest part of the tooth. The enamel wears with age and injury and is not replaced. The dentin forms the majority of the tooth. Dentin is harder than bone and encases the pulp. Within the pulp cavity lie the blood vessels, nerves, and connective tissue.

The root of a tooth projects below the gumline and is held in place by the periodontal ligament. The periodontal ligament, made of thick bundles of collagenous fibers, connects the bony alveolar process and cementum of each tooth. The cementum is a bone-like substance that covers the tooth from the termination of the enamel at the neck to the thickest region at the apex of the root.

PALATE

The roof of the mouth is called the palate. The anterior portion is called the hard palate and is formed by the maxillary and palatine bones. The posterior portion is referred to as the soft palate; it consists of muscle and fat that has a mucous membrane lining. The uvula is the posterior portion of the soft palate and is considered to be lymphoid tissue. The soft palate separates the mouth from the nasopharynx; it rises during swallowing to prevent food from entering the nasal cavity.

CHEEKS

The cheeks form the lateral walls of the oral cavity. They consist of skin, fat, the major muscles of mastication, and an inner lining of mucous membrane.

TONGUE

The tongue is a thick muscular organ covered with a mucous membrane that contains the chemoreceptors for taste. It is attached to the floor of the buccal cavity by a structure called the lingual frenulum. The muscles of the tongue are both intrinsic and extrinsic. The intrinsic muscles are contained within the tongue and give the tongue its ability to change shape. The extrinsic muscles originate from the temporal bone, the mandible, and the hyoid bone and provide the mobility of the tongue. Together these two sets of lingual muscles function in speech and in propelling food through the oral cavity and swallowing.

ANATOMY OF THE FACE AND CRANIUM

The skull is comprised of 22 bones that are divided into two categories: facial and cranial (refer to Plate 7).

The 14 facial bones, most of which occur in pairs, include:

- 2 nasal
- 2 maxillary
- 2 lacrimal
- 2 zygomatic
- 2 palatine
- 2 inferior nasal turbinate
- 1 mandible
- 1 vomer

The arrangement of the facial bones forms the cheeks, nose, mouth, and the lower rim of the orbit.

The bones of the cranium enclose and protect the brain. There are eight of them:

- 1 frontal
- 1 occipital
- 1 sphenoid
- 1 ethmoid
- 2 parietal
- 2 temporal

The pair of nasal bones come together to form what is commonly known as the "bridge" of the nose. They are located in the middle, superior portion of the face. Each nasal bone articulates with the frontal, ethmoid, maxillary, and the opposite nasal bone. In the anterior view, the nasal bones are bordered laterally by the maxilla and superiorly by the frontal bone. Cartilage attaches to the anterior portion of the small nasal bones to form the tip of the nose.

The maxillary bones meet inferior to the nasal septum to form the upper jaw. The joining is referred to as the intermaxillary suture. The maxillary bones articulate with the following facial bones: inferior turbinate, lacrimal, nasal, palatine, vomer, and zygomatic. The frontal and ethmoid bones articulate with the maxillary bones. Each of the maxillary bones contains a sinus, referred to as a maxillary sinus. The sinuses are cavities within the bone that are lined with mucous membrane and open into the nasal cavity. The upper teeth are also located in the maxillae. Each tooth is individually housed in its own alveolus, or bony socket. The alveoli, in turn, are located in the alveolar process, part of the maxilla. The hard palate, or roof of the mouth, is the palatine process of the maxilla. The infraorbital foramen, found below the eye, contains the infraorbital nerve and artery. It is important to note that the maxilla articulates with all of the facial bones, excluding the mandible.

The smallest of the facial bones, the lacrimal bones, articulate with the frontal, ethmoid, maxillary, and inferior turbinate. Their name derives from the Latin word for tear, *lacrima*. These bones form the "corner of the eye." More specifically, they are located lateral and posterior to the nasal bones within the orbital wall.

The zygomatic (also called **malar**) **bones** form the prominences of the cheeks and a portion of the inferior and lateral wall of the orbit. These bones do not articulate with one another, but they do join with the frontal, sphenoid, temporal, and maxillary bones. Each zygomatic bone has a temporal process that proceeds posteriorly to meet the zygomatic process of the temporal bone. This articulation is referred to as the zygomatic arch.

The L-shaped palatine bones help to form several portions of the face. They articulate, not only with each other, but also with the sphenoid, ethmoid, maxillary, inferior turbinate, and the vomer. The horizontal plates of the palatine bones form the anterior (hard) portion of the palate. The palate separates the nasal and oral cavities. Consequently, they form the floor and lateral wall of the nasal cavity. They contribute somewhat to the orbital floor.

The inferior nasal turbinates are also referred to as the inferior nasal conchae. They articulate with the ethmoid, maxillary, lacrimal, and palatine bones. They partly create the lateral wall of the nasal cavity. They enter the cavity below the superior and middle nasal conchae of the ethmoid. Although the whole of the conchae work in conjunction to filter and circulate air before it proceeds to the lungs, the inferior nasal conchae are considered separate bones.

The vomer contributes to the posterior and inferior portion of the nasal septum. It is surrounded by the sphenoid, the ethmoid, both maxillary, and both palatine bones. It is singular and triangular, lending to its name: *vomer* means "plowshare" in Latin.

The largest and strongest facial bone is the mandible, or lower jaw. The mandible articulates with the **glenoid fossa** of each temporal bone to form a synovial joint. The joint is referred to as the temporomandibular joint, or **TMJ**. The mandible consists of several portions. The first portion, the body of the mandible, lies horizontally and contains the alveolar process for the lower teeth. The mental foramen is located on the body and below the first molar tooth. The mental protuberance is commonly known as the chin. The second portion of the mandible is the **ramus**. The rami each project upward at an angle from the posterior part of each mandibular body. The condylar process is the posterior projection of the ramus. The temporomandibular joint contains the condylar process of the mandible and two parts of the temporal bone, the mandibular fossa, and the articular tubercle. The coronoid process is the anterior projection of the ramus. The temporalis muscle attaches here. The depression between these two processes is the mandibular notch. Located on the medial surface of the rami, the mandibular foramen contains the inferior alveolar nerve along with its vessels. The mental foramen, like the mandibular foramen, is used by dentists for the injection of anesthetics. The last area of the mandible that will be mentioned is the angle. The angle connects each ramus to the body.

ORBIT

The bones of the orbit support and protect the eyes. Each orbit comprises the following seven craniofacial bones:

- Frontal
- Lacrimal
- Ethmoid
- Maxilla
- Zygomatic
- Sphenoid
- Palatine

The orbit also contains fat to protect the eye from shock, connective structures to retain the eyeball and allow for its motion, blood vessels, and nerves, the most important being the optic, or second cranial, nerve.

FACIAL MUSCLES AND INNERVATION

The principal facial muscles will be discussed here (Figure 18-1). These muscles lead to such various facial movements as smiling, frowning, chewing, and speaking. The innervation of these muscles is by two of the cranial nerves. The seventh cranial nerve is the facial nerve. The facial nerve innervates all of the facial muscles that will be discussed except for the muscles of the lower jaw. Different branches of the trigeminal, or fifth cranial nerve, innervate these four muscles.

The epicranius is a large muscle that is divided into two parts. The occipitalis muscle covers the occipital bone and connects to the frontalis portion of the epicranius through the galea aponeurotica. The occipitalis draws the scalp backward, while the frontalis draws the scalp forward, wrinkles the brow, and raises the eyebrows.

The **orbicular**is oculi covers a circular path around the eye. The root *ocul* is derived from the Latin word for eye. The action of this muscle closes the eye.

Two muscles work in conjunction to produce smiling or raising of the upper lip. The levator labii superioris runs along the zygomatic arch just above the zygomaticus major muscle. Specifically the levator labii superioris elevates the upper lip while the zygomaticus major pulls the corner of the mouth up and out. Both insert at the orbicularis oris, allowing for smiling and laughing. The orbicularis oris surrounds the mouth, compressing, closing, and protruding the lips. These actions aid in speech.

The primary muscles of the cheek and chin that aid in facial expressions are the buccinator, mentalis, depressor labii inferioris, and platysma. The buccinator extends horizontally across the cheek and is responsible for cheek

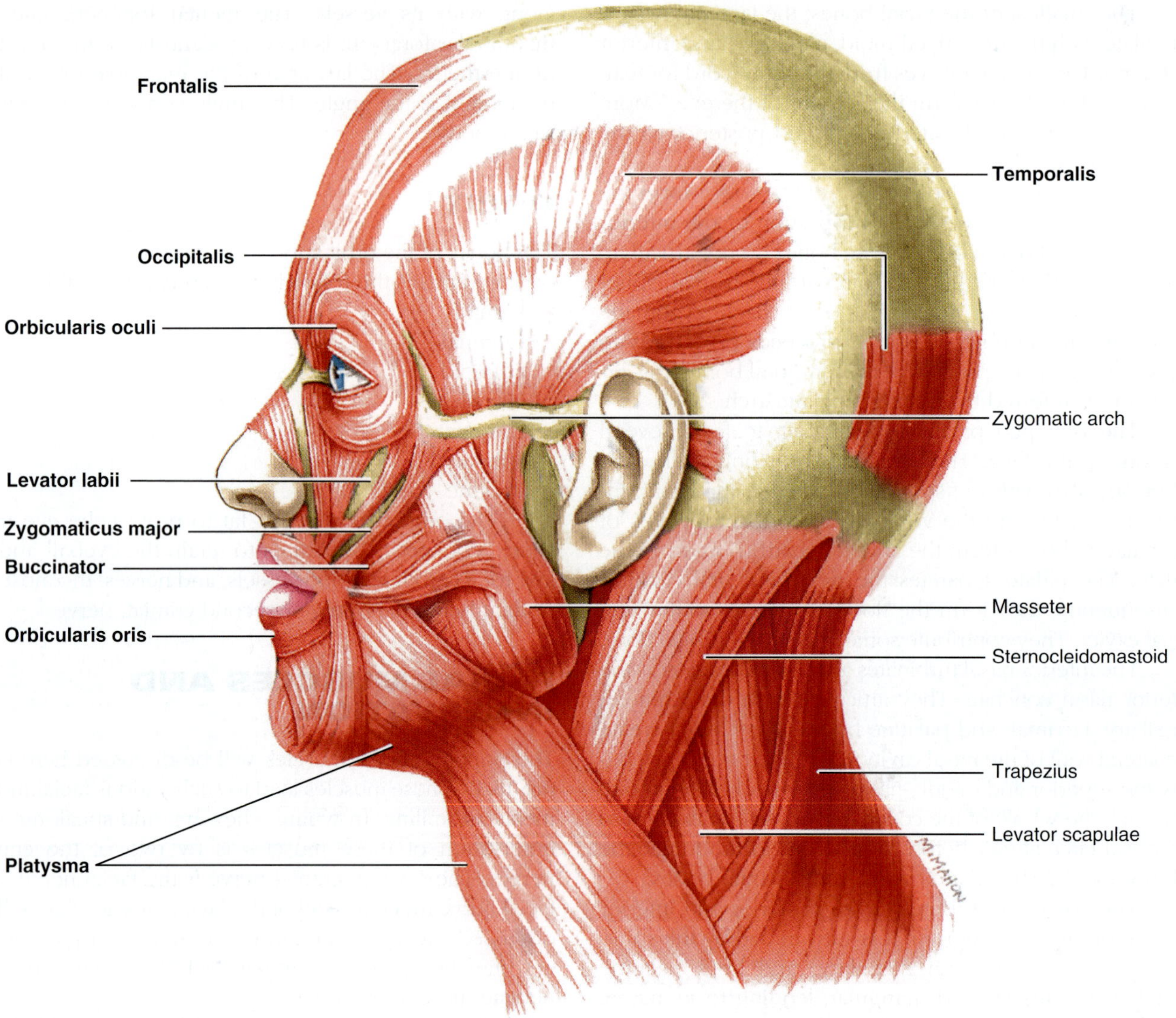

Figure 18-1 Facial muscles

compression and sucking. The mentalis resides on the chin below the bottom lip. It raises and protrudes the lower lip. The depressor labii inferioris also aids in lowering the bottom lip. Although the platysma lies over the neck and reaches up to the chin and edge of the mouth, it still helps the other muscles to lower the mandible and turn the outer corners of the mouth out and down.

Movement of the lower jaw is achieved by the following four muscles: masseter, temporalis, medial pterygoid, and lateral pterygoid. The masseter in action closes the mouth and protrudes the chin. The temporalis muscle elevates and retracts the mandible. The medial and lateral pterygoid muscles work together to elevate, protrude, and move the mandible side to side.

The temporalis muscle is innervated by the temporal nerve, which derives from the mandibular branch of the trigeminal (fifth cranial) nerve. The remaining muscles are innervated by the mandibular branch of the trigeminal nerve.

EMBRYOLOGIC DEVELOPMENT OF THE FACE

Anatomical development of the face occurs along with the development of the cranium around the sixth week of embryologic life. At this point, the primitive cranium forms a cartilaginous shell around the already-developing brain.

The facial bones arise from the five pairs of branchial arches. One of the arches is known as the mandibular arch. The mandibular arch is considered to have two parts, the mandibular and maxillary processes. These two processes grow and ossify to form the mandible and maxillary process. During their growth, the oral sinus, later known as the mouth, is formed.

The primary teeth develop between 14 and 19 weeks *in utero* and continue to develop after birth. Permanent tooth development begins after birth. The root is the last portion to develop in both sets of teeth.

PATHOLOGY OF THE ORAL CAVITY

The teeth are subject to much use and abuse throughout their existence. They can be fractured through such actions as chewing on hard objects or trauma to the mouth. Lack of proper oral hygiene can lead to dental caries and gingivitis. In addition, teeth can develop improperly in the jaw, leading to many other problems.

Fractures of the teeth are classified into four categories. Class I consists of fractures to the enamel cap of the crown. Class II fractures are those that extend into the dentin of the tooth, but do not expose any pulp. Class III fractures cause extensive damage to the coronal portion of the tooth and expose the pulp. Class IV fractures occur at or below the cementoenamel junction of the tooth. Diagnosis and classification of fractured teeth can be accomplished through dental X-rays and visual examination.

Treatment of the fractured tooth depends on the type of fracture and condition of the root, tooth, and surrounding alveolus. If the root, tooth, and alveolus are healthy, then the tooth can be repaired using restoration techniques. If restoration cannot be done, then dentures or implantation can be considered following extraction.

Dental caries is the decay of tooth enamel. The metabolic activity of bacteria in the mouth, such as *Streptococcus mutans,* creates an acidic environment, lowering the pH. Once oral pH has fallen below the normal range of 6.5–7.5, the enamel begins to demineralize, or dissolve, and decay begins. When the pH rises, remineralization can occur. Remineralization depends on the remaining crystalline structure of the enamel and the presence of fluoride, calcium, and phosphate ions. The ions remineralize using the existing enamel as a framework. The newly formed area is more resistant to acidic conditions, however, the cyclic rise and fall of pH wears down the enamel, allowing for the formation of caries (cavities).

Cavities can be diagnosed with the use of X-rays and oral examinations. The examination should consist of both a visual and manual inspection with a gingival probe. Signs of periodontal disease are inflamed bleeding gums, receding gum line, pus pockets, and discolored teeth. Treatment of the diseased tooth depends on the condition of the tooth, root, and alveolar process. Restoration can be performed on teeth that have not reached the advanced stages of periodontal disease. Those teeth that cannot be restored are extracted.

MOUTH

The mouth is subject to conditions such as cysts and cancer. Biopsies of suspicious sites can be done to determine pathology. Extensive resection of the mouth, which can involve removal of all or portions of the tongue, palate, and mandible, may be required for treatment. A radical neck dissection may also be needed (refer to Procedure 17-9).

JAW BONES

The bones of the jaw can be congenitally deformed or traumatically injured. In either case, **malocclusion** can occur. Malocclusion refers to a misalignment of the alveolar process of the jawbones resulting in overbite or underbite. Orthodontics and osteotomies of the jaw are used to correct malocclusion. Acquired deformities can develop from ear infections, disease processes, or trauma. Congenital deformities due to Paget's disease or acromegaly can cause developmental disturbances in the jaw. Paget's disease causes an overgrowth of bone in the cranium, maxilla, and mandible.

Several types of jaw deformities exist. Micro**gnath**ia, meaning small jaw, can affect either the upper or the lower jaw. This arises in Pierre Robin syndrome and in conjunction with other congenital defects. The affected jaw appears to be thrust inward. The appearance of micrognathia can be due to several things. The jawbones can be in abnormal relation to one another, with one of the bones smaller, or the mandibular angle can be steep.

Macrognathia, or large jaw, usually involves both jaws. The enlargement can be due to acromegaly or Paget's disease. Prognathism is also referred to as mandibular protrusion. Both angles of the mandible are of a wider degree leading to an outwardly thrust lower jaw.

Retrognathism is the underdevelopment of the mandible. Congenital hypoplasia and childhood rheumatoid arthritis can cause retrognathism. Laterognathism is asymmetry with respect to each side of the jaw. This can be due to unilateral ankylosis or acromegaly, among other conditions.

MANDIBULAR FRACTURES

Mandibular fractures can occur anywhere along the mandible (Figure 18-2). The techniques involved to fixate mandibular fractures are the primary use of mandibulomaxillary fixation and subsequent **reduction** and fixation of the fracture site with rigid fixation. The four categories of mandibular fractures will be described here, along with appropriate incision sites.

Symphysis and parasymphyseal fractures occur along the mandible between the bicuspid teeth (Figure 18-3). Most of these fractures do not dislocate. Hematomas can form sublingually due to damage along the floor of the mouth. These fractures can be fixated intraorally. An incision into the anterior gingivobuccal area provides adequate exposure for reduction and placement of rigid fixation devices.

Horizontal ramus fractures occur along the lateral portion of the mandible between the bicuspid teeth and the molars. The mental foramen lies underneath the bicuspid

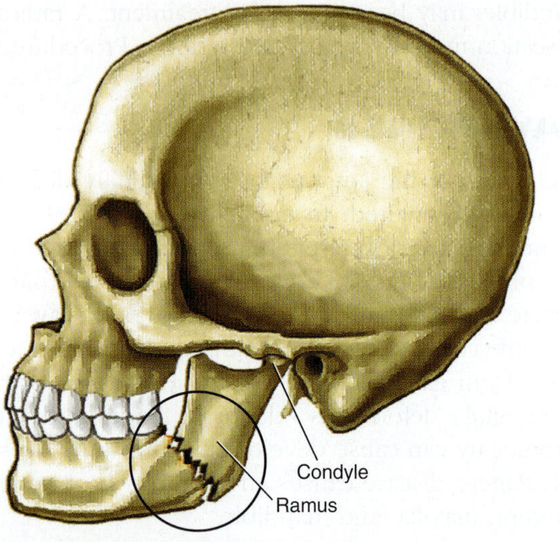

Figure 18-2 Mandibular fracture

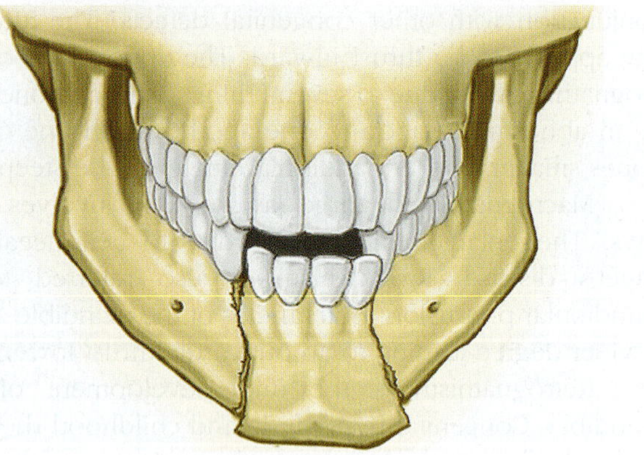

Figure 18-3 Symphysis fracture

teeth. The mental nerve and vessels exit through the foramen, so care should be taken to avoid damage to them. The degree of fracture dictates the type of incision. Most fractures can be approached through an intraoral incision. Heavily comminuted fractures may require a transbuccal approach.

Mandibular angle fractures occur from the second molar to the ascending ramus. Few fractures of this nature can be fixated intraorally. The awkward location of the fracture, along with mandibulomaxillary fixation, makes an extraoral incision a better option. The site can be reached with submandibular or preauricular incisions. The mandibular branch of the facial nerve should be preserved when submandibular approaches are used. Preauricular incisions require the preservation of the frontal branch of the facial nerve.

The **condyle** and subcondylar area of the mandible can also be fractured. Condylar fractures occur within the capsular head of the mandible. Subcondylar fractures are below the capsule. Condylar and subcondylar fractures can be approached through submandibular and preauricular incisions, or a combination of the two. The treatment of these fractures can involve mandibulomaxillary fixation alone if the fracture is not dislocated. Otherwise, the standard rigid fixation is used.

FRONTAL FRACTURES

The frontal bone contains a sinus cavity that is irregular in shape. A median view of the frontal bone will show the anterior and posterior walls of the frontal sinus. Frontal fractures are detected with plain X-rays, specifically the Waters view. CT (computed tomography) scans also show abnormalities of the frontal bone. Physical signs such as cerebrospinal rhinorrhea may indicate a posterior table fracture that has torn the dura. Denting of the forehead could indicate a displaced frontal fracture, but as with most facial fractures, swelling can obscure this characteristic.

The anterior wall of the frontal sinus lies closest to the muscles and skin of the face, while the posterior wall is near the brain. The categories of frontal sinus fractures are based on the involvement of the sinus walls. If the walls of the frontal sinus are referred to as tables, a fracture on the anterior wall is referred to as an anterior table fracture. Fractures occurring on the posterior wall, are posterior table fractures. Nasofrontal duct fractures occur along the duct that communicates the frontal sinus with the nose. Each of these fractures can be displaced or nondisplaced.

ORBITAL FRACTURES

Orbital fractures are usually classified in two ways: floor fractures or orbital blowouts involving one or more of the numerous bones of the orbit (Figure 18-4). Trauma caused by auto accidents, fights, and falls commonly results in these fractures. The orbital floor separates the eye from the maxillary sinus. The floor is a thin extension of the maxillary and zygomatic bones. Orbital fractures may appear unilaterally, bilaterally, alone, or in conjunction with other facial fractures.

Orbital fractures have several characteristics. Diplopia (double vision) and enophthalmos (sagging of the eye) are the most common. The periorbital fat and muscles may be pinched in the fracture line or they may actually herniate into the maxillary antrum. Swelling and bruising will occur. Preoperative CT scans and X-rays help in the diagnosis of orbital floor fractures, and they should be available for reference during surgery.

ZYGOMATIC FRACTURES

Due to the dense nature of the zygomatic (malar) bone, true fractures are rarely seen (Figure 18-5). More commonly, fractures are seen in the arch of the zygoma, or at one or more of the three suture lines. Fractures of the arch are usually depressed. Separation of the bones can occur at the zygomaticofrontal, zygomaticotemporal, or zygo-

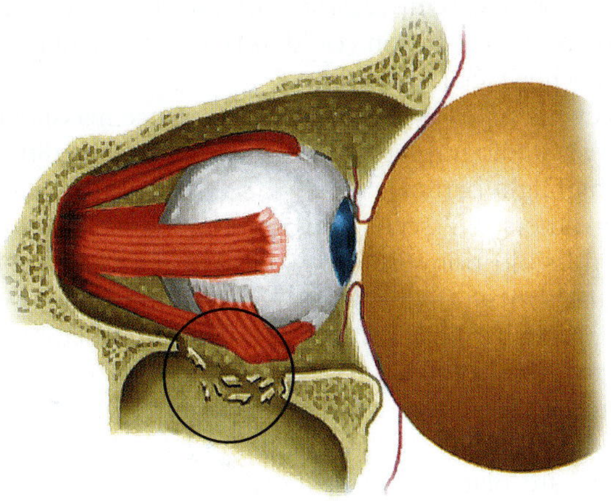

Figure 18-4 Orbital floor fracture

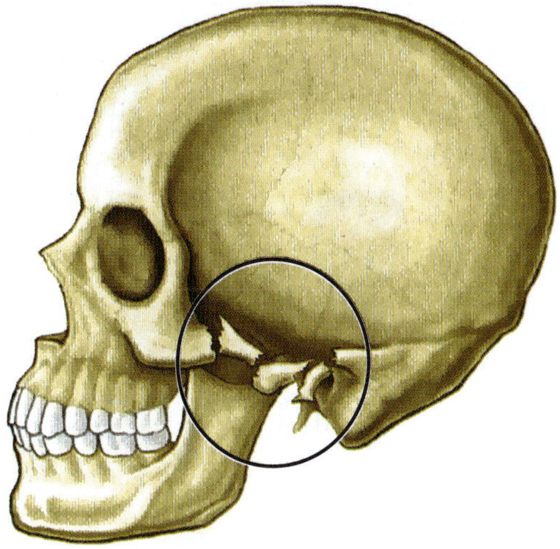

Figure 18-5 Zygomatic arch fracture

maticomaxillary suture lines. Combination of all three suture-line fractures is referred to as a tri-malar fracture.

Zygomatic fractures can be diagnosed visually, by palpation, and with the use of X-rays. Visual findings that indicate malar fractures include dimpling of the skin above the cheek, depressed level of the eyeball, and scleral or nasal hemorrhage. CT scans and plain films can show the actual fracture, and rule out other facial fractures.

MIDFACIAL FRACTURES

To understand midfacial fractures, extensive knowledge of the facial bones is a necessity. The midface includes the following bones: two maxilla, two palatine, and the medial and lateral pterygoid processes of the sphenoid bone. Fractures can involve several combinations of those bones. In the early 1900s, Rene Le Fort categorized midfacial fractures into three basic classifications (Figure 18-6). Although actual fractures may not exactly fit these classifications, they still provide a means of describing similar fractures. A Le Fort I fracture is the most common type of midfacial fractures. The alveolar process of the maxilla is horizontally separated from the base of the skull. The upper jaw can be floating free in the oral cavity. Le Fort II fractures may be triangular or pyramidal in shape. The vertical fracture line extends upward to the nasal and ethmoid bones. Le Fort II fractures can be unilateral or bilateral in nature. Le Fort III fractures are located high in the midface. The fracture line extends transversely from the zygomatic arches, through the orbits, and to the base of the nose. These fractures can exist unilaterally, bilaterally, alone, or in conjunction with other facial fractures.

A study was conducted on 64 patients with Le Fort fractures. The findings showed 53% of these fractures were received in automobile accidents, 39% were from blunt trauma, and 8% were the result of gunshot injuries. The occurrence of other facial fractures accompanying Le Fort fractures was 75%.

Diagnosis of midfacial fractures can be made through examination of X-rays and the physical examination of the patient. X-rays and CT scans can show the fracture lines, although nondisplaced fractures may not be visualized as well. Evidence of midfacial trauma can be seen, such as malocclusion, movable alveolar process, and flattened facial features. However, edema can hide the characteristics of midfacial fractures. X-rays provide evidence of a fracture and are a useful guide for reconstruction. Other items such as pretrauma photographs and dental records can aid the surgeon in determining the proper placement of fractured facial bones.

CRANIOFACIAL DEFORMITIES

Craniofacial problems can occur from several disorders, such as **craniosynostosis** or Crouzon's disease. Reconstruction procedures involve corrections of the cranial vault and maxilla. They can be accompanied by orthognathic procedures as well. These procedures also involve specialists other than **maxillofacial** surgeons. Plastic, ophthalmic, and neurosurgeons may work in conjunction with the maxillofacial surgeon.

DIAGNOSTIC TESTS

For the patient with possible maxillofacial defects, various diagnostic tests can be administered. To begin, a complete history should be gathered from the patient if possible. When the patient is unable to communicate, a relative, observer, or other professional (such as paramedics or emergency department personnel) should relay any vital information. This information will aid physicians and surgical team members to form an appropriate treatment plan. For example, in a trauma situation, the type of injury and direction of impact may help the physician to ascertain the extent of injuries the patient has suffered.

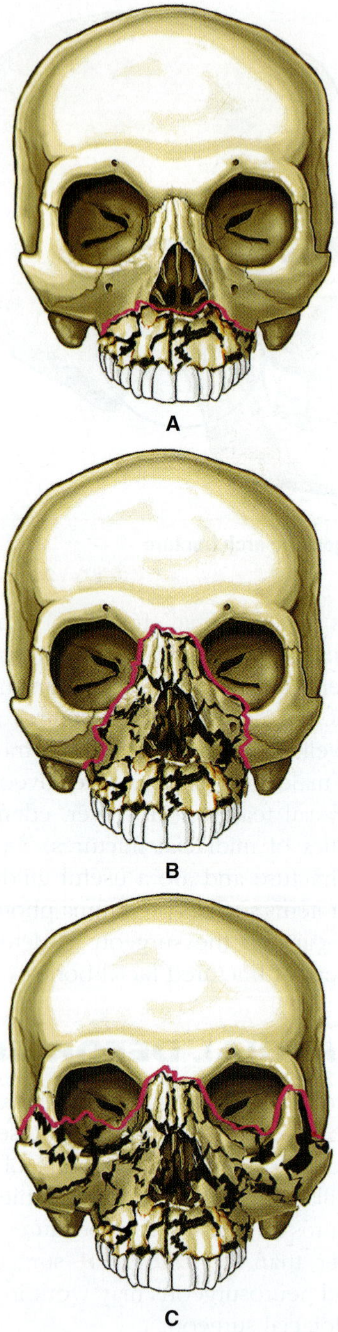

Figure 18-6 Le Fort fractures: (A) Le Fort I, (B) Le Fort II, (C) Le Fort III

A physical examination should be done for the facial trauma patient. This exam should be done carefully, especially in a suspected maxillary fracture. Movement of the fracture could cause any number of repercussions from dural tears and nerve injury to infection. Obvious signs like bleeding, bruising, lacerations, and swelling may indicate an underlying fracture. Other signs such as cerebrospinal fluid leaking from the ears (cerebrospinal otorrhea) or nose (cerebrospinal rhinorrhea) may indicate dural tears. Malocclusion could also indicate dental, alveolar, or other facial fractures.

Several types of imaging help diagnose maxillofacial fractures. Radiographic techniques involving different views highlight particular bony facial structures while obscuring others. CT scans provide important information about possible bony defects. MRI scans provide details about the surrounding soft tissues of the face.

For plain films, several options are available. The suspected type of fracture dictates the type of view or views to be taken. The Waters view requires the patient to sit or stand upright and hyperextend the neck. The nose and chin are placed against the X-ray cassette while the film is taken. The facial bones are shown in best detail in this position. Specifically, the infraorbital rims, frontal and maxillary sinuses, maxillary alveolar arch, and zygomas can be observed. The Caldwell view is similar to the Waters view. Both are anteroposterior projections, but in this case, the nose and forehead are placed against the cassette (Figure 18-7). This view shows the hard palate, nasal septum, orbital floor, and zygoma. The lateral facial view is mainly used for anatomical orientation of the face. The basal view shows zygomatic fractures. A **pan**oramic X-ray shows on one film the alveolar processes, mandible, posterior maxillary sinuses, and the zygomas.

CT scans of the head show the facial structures in different planes. Some of the important planes for maxillofacial abnormalities are the hard palate, mid-maxillary, and mid-orbital. The hard palate plane shows the entire palate and pterygoid plates. The zygomatic arch, temporal bone, nasal septum, and turbinates can be seen in the mid-maxillary plane. Finally, the mid-orbital plane displays the globe, lens, and optic nerve.

MRI scans best define soft tissue injuries or congenital defects. Since an MRI scan consumes a vast amount of time that a trauma victim may not have, its uses are limited to those patients who are deemed stable or receiving elective maxillofacial treatments.

Three-dimensional imaging can also be used for reconstructive procedures. The imaging involves the use of computers with three-dimensional programming and CT scans. The patient's CT scans can be projected onto the computer screen in a three-dimensional fashion. Any anatomy that interferes with viewing can be eliminated. Before and after models can be generated on the computer to aid the surgeon. This is an invaluable resource for reconstruction.

ORAL PROCEDURES: GENERAL CONSIDERATIONS

For the patient about to undergo oral surgery, several preoperative factors need to be considered. Fear of surgery

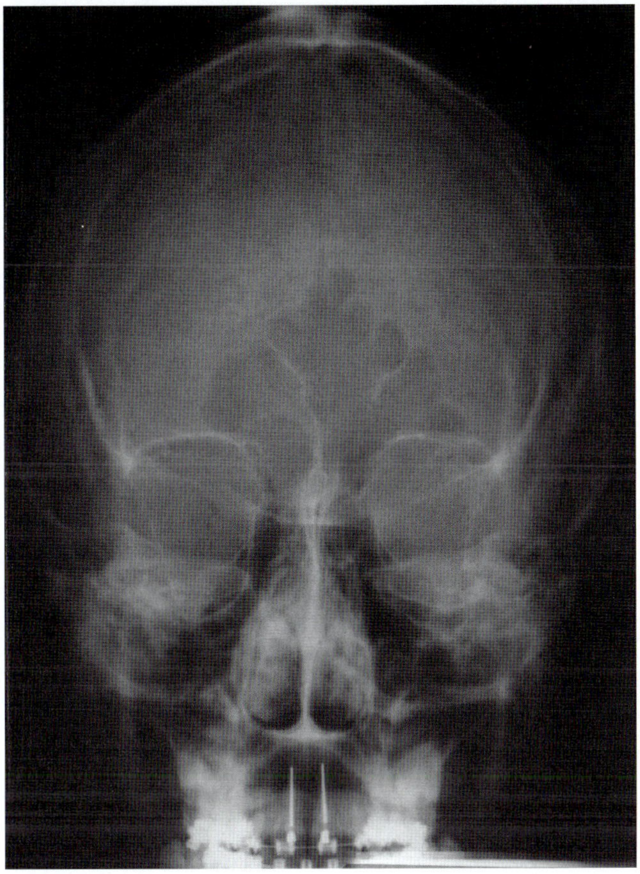

Figure 18-7 Caldwell view of the skull (anteroposterior nasal bones)

is a common patient concern. Many patients will be concerned about the aesthetic outcome of their surgery. Others will be worried about the amount of pain the procedure will produce. Each patient's concerns should be addressed properly. Patient education about the entire process from transportation to the OR to the recovery process will help to alleviate any fears.

Many patients who come to the OR for oral procedures will have special needs. Children requiring extensive dental work may be brought to the OR. Patients already in the hospital for other concerns, such as transplant recipients, may come to the OR for dental work. The surgical team should be prepared to deal with each situation.

Each patient should be interviewed and the chart examined with specific regard to the history, physical, NPO status, allergies, diagnostic, and laboratory results. This evaluation will help the surgical team provide accurate, efficient assistance for every case. X-rays are a vital part of oral surgery, and all relevant films should be readily available to the team. Consultation with the surgeon in advance of the procedure about the specific procedural details and possible variations will help the team prepare for the wide range of possibilities.

TOOTH EXTRACTION/ODONTECTOMY

Extraction of teeth involves the removal of a tooth or teeth that cannot be salvaged by restoration, or those that interfere with occlusion (Procedure 18-1). Simple extraction is removal of the tooth from the alveolar socket with an extraction forceps. Odontectomy involves resection of the soft tissue and excision of the bone surrounding the tooth prior to removal of the tooth. X-rays, along with a visual and digital inspection of the area, aid in the diagnosis of ectopic, diseased, or fractured teeth. For impacted teeth, the technique varies a little. Impacted teeth have not erupted through the gumline. Other erupted teeth or the impacted tooth's position in the jaw can prevent eruption. To remedy this painful situation, the tooth may need to be removed. The gum surrounding the affected area may have advanced stages of gingivitis, or swelling and lacerations due to the fractured tooth. Contents of a typical dental instrumentation set are listed in Table 18-1.

Table 18-1 Contents of a Typical Dental Instrumentation Set
Mouth prop—A rubber wedge available in a variety of sizes. A mouth prop (bite block) is placed between the upper and lower teeth of the unaffected side to maintain the patient's mouth in an open position during surgical intervention to facilitate visualization and prevent injury to the surgical staff (Figure 18-8).
Plastic cheek retractor—A plastic cheek retractor can be used to keep the cheeks and lips from falling into the operative field (Figure 18-9).
Assorted periosteal elevators
Assorted extraction forceps—Several styles of extraction forceps are available. The styles range in varying degrees of curvature and different jaw styles to enhance visualization and ease removal. The jaw, or grasping end of the instrument, is individually shaped for each type of tooth. Therefore, the tooth to be extracted dictates the type of forceps to be used.
Mirror
Gingival probe
Minnesota retractor (Figure 18-10)
Wieder tongue depressor
McGill
Probe
Frazier suction tip with stylet
Yankauer suction tip
#7 knife handle
Needle holders
Tissue forceps with and without teeth
Scissors (assortment—straight and curved)
Towel clips
Straight and curved hemostats

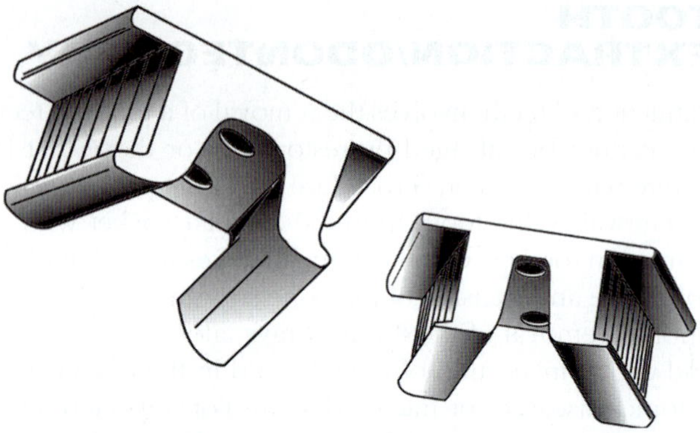

Figure 18-8 Mouth props

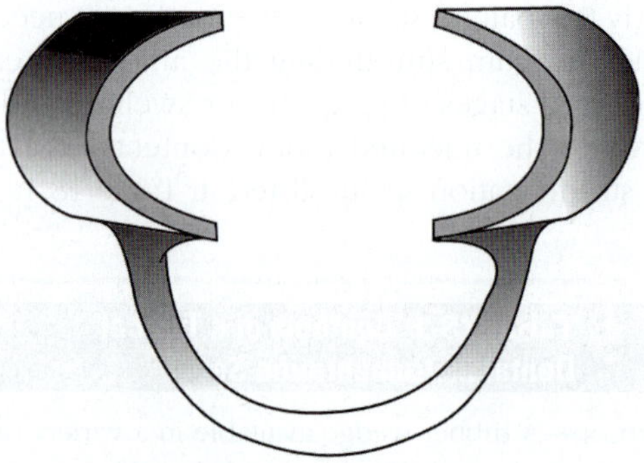

Figure 18-9 Plastic cheek retractor

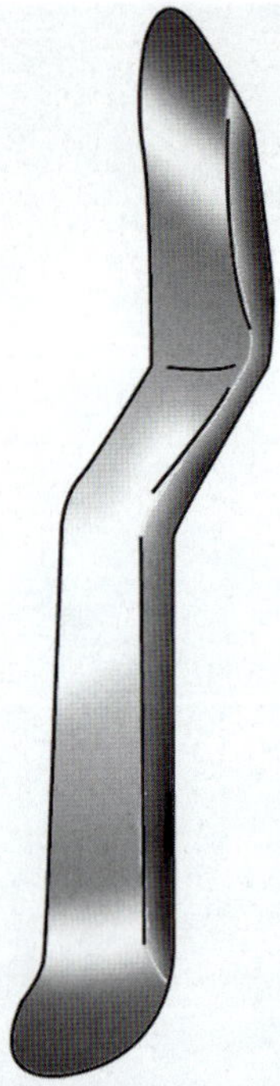

Figure 18-10 Minnesota retractor

PROCEDURE

18-1 Tooth Extraction/Odontectomy

Equipment

- Dental drill with energy source
- Suction system
- Irrigation system

  Note: Often the drill, suction, and irrigation systems are combined into one piece of specialized equipment
- Headlamp

Instruments

- Dental instrumentation set

Supplies

- Pack: basic
- Basin: small
- Gloves
- Blades: #15
- Drapes: ½ sheet × 2
- Suture: according to surgeon's preference
- Drains: none
- Dressings: none
- Drugs: according to surgeon's preference

PROCEDURE

18-1 Tooth Extraction/Odontectomy *(continued)*

- Miscellaneous:
  - Sterile components of drill system including an assortment of bits
  - Suction tubing
  - Irrigation fluid
  - Throat pack
  - Gauze sponges
  - Dental rolls
  - Antifog solution for mirrors
  - Two 10-cc syringes with 25-gauge 1½-in. needles for local injection
  - Two 20-cc syringes with 19-gauge 1½-in. blunt needles for irrigation

Operative Preparation

Anesthesia

- General preferred
- Lubricate and protect patient's eyes
- Local anesthetic with epinephrine may be used alone or in conjunction with general anesthesia to reduce bleeding and minimize postoperative pain
- Anesthesia circuits should be long enough to accommodate the position of the OR table

Position

- Supine, with head tilted back to provide exposure
- A donut or foam headrest may be used for stabilization
- Arms tucked at patient's sides; protect ulnar nerves

Prep

- May not be required
- Brush teeth or swab inside of mouth with an oral antiseptic
- Face may be prepped with a mild antiseptic. Protect eyes and ears from contact with prep solution

Draping

- May not be necessary
- A ½ sheet may be placed across the patient's body to provide a clean surface on which to rest equipment and supplies
- A turban style head wrap may be used to restrain the hair

Practical Considerations

- Oral procedures are not considered sterile; use the best technique possible
- If the surgeon plans to be seated during the procedure, the table should be assembled in a fashion that allows chair access under the head of the table. The table should be placed where operating room lights illuminate the field properly. Fluoroscopy and X-ray machines should be able to enter the area without disturbing the field. The table may be angled to allow access
- During lengthy oral procedures, the patient's lips may dry and crack. To alleviate this problem a cream or ointment may be applied to the lips

Operative Procedure	Technical Considerations
1. Insert mouth prop.	**1.** Have appropriate size mouth prop ready. Provide suction with Yankauer tip as needed.
2. A throat pack may be placed.	**2.** Prepare throat pack for use. A dressing forceps or McGill may be used to aid in the insertion of the throat pack.

(continues)

PROCEDURE 18-1 Tooth Extraction/Odontectomy *(continued)*

3. Additional exposure is achieved.	**3.** Anticipate the use of the Minnesota retractor or mirror for cheek/tongue retraction. Precoat mirror with antifog solution.
4. The site may be injected with a local anesthetic using a control syringe.	**4.** Local anesthetic should be prepared in advance according to surgeon's preference. Inform anesthesia provider of epinephrine use.
5. To determine the amount of damage to the surrounding gingiva, a probe with graduated marks is inserted into the gumline.	**5.** Switch suction tip to Frazier.
6. The gingiva is removed from the surface of the tooth with an elevator.	**6.** Periosteal elevator of surgeon's preference will be needed for gingival dissection.
7. The tooth is removed from the alveolar socket; the socket may be packed with gauze.	**7.** Choose extraction forceps according to the type of tooth to be removed and surgeon's preference. 2×2 gauze may be used to temporarily pack the socket.
8. The alveolar socket is inspected and irrigated to ensure that no debris remains. Direct pressure may be applied to the site for a short time and chromic or gut sutures may be placed as needed.	**8.** Irrigation fluid should be preloaded in the syringe with the blunt needle attached. (Provide two irrigation systems so that one can be refilled while the other is in use.) Provide suction as needed. Suture of choice is loaded on needle holder in anticipation of use. Count.
9. If the tooth scheduled for extraction is impacted, odontectomy is performed. The gumline is incised with a #15 blade.	**9.** A #15 blade is loaded on the #7 knife handle.
10. The soft tissue is dissected to expose the impacted tooth.	**10.** Provide periosteal elevator of choice.
11. A dental drill may be required to remove any bone preventing exposure of the tooth.	**11.** Dental drill is assembled in advance and the bit of surgeon's preference inserted and locked into position. Be sure to pass power tools with the safety mechanism in use. Suction and irrigation will be needed every time the drill is used.
12. The tooth may be removed as a whole or require splitting with the drill or an osteotome so that it can be removed in sections.	**12.** Provide extraction forceps of choice. Change drill bit if necessary and provide suction and irrigation. An osteotome must be accompanied by a mallet for use.
13. The area is inspected for debris, rinsed, and closed with a 4–0 chromic or silk on a cutting needle.	**13.** Provide suction and irrigation if needed. Suture of choice is loaded and passed. Count.
14. Pharynx is suctioned and throat pack removed.	**14.** Switch suction tip to Yankauer. Provide Wieder retractor. The instrument that was used to insert the throat pack will be needed again for extraction.

PROCEDURE 18-1 Tooth Extraction/Odontectomy (continued)

Postoperative Considerations

Immediate Postoperative Care

- Following any oral procedure, the surgical team should be prepared to assist with extubation. A suction setup is necessary. Occasionally, reintubation is necessary and a laryngoscope and ET tube should be readily available.
- Bruising and swelling of the lips and cheeks may occur. The patient should be advised to apply ice.
- Out-patients must be able to tolerate a liquid diet prior to discharge.

Prognosis

- Patient is expected to return to normal activities in 3–5 days.
- No visible scarring is expected.

Complications

- Hemorrhage
- Infection
- Malocclusion

PEARL OF WISDOM

The throat pack consists of rolled gauze that contains a radiopaque marker. It is moistened and any excess fluid is squeezed out prior to insertion. The throat pack should be included in the formal count. To reduce the risk of aspiration, a throat pack is used to prevent oral secretions, irrigation fluid, blood, and bone or tooth fragments from becoming lodged in the pharynx. It is imperative to provide suction to the pharynx and remove the throat pack prior to extubation.

TOOTH RESTORATION

Restoration of teeth involves the removal of diseased or broken portions of a tooth and refurbishing the tooth into a working element. X-rays and an oral examination are needed to determine extent of the damage and the possibility of restoration.

A **mouth prop** is placed and the cavity is removed using the dental drill. Once the majority of the diseased area is removed, a small dental curette can be used to remove the remaining cavity. If the nerve to the tooth is exposed, a liner may be inserted to protect the nerve from the filling. The filling can be either amalgam (an alloy of two or more metals, one of which is mercury) or a composite of resin. The filling material is prepared as needed and placed into the space created by the drill. Composite resin fillings require light to harden. Once hardened, either type of filling may be contoured with the drill. If no cavity is present, the cap or crown is fabricated and fixed in position. Proper occlusion of the teeth will be verified and adjustments made if necessary.

IMPLANTATION

Implantation is a series of treatments that results in permanent placement of a prosthetic tooth or teeth. The process involves placing a fixture, or titanium root, into the alveolar process. The bone surrounding the fixture forms a strong bond to it through a process known as osseointegration. An abutment, or connecting piece, attaches the prosthetic tooth to its fixture. Several phases are required to achieve a final working prosthetic implant. These phases can take anywhere from 3 to 6 months to complete.

First, an in-depth visual oral examination is performed and the type of implant is determined. Following the visual examination, photographs, a series of full mouth/panoramic X-rays, and dental impressions are obtained. From the dental impression, temporary dentures and a metal framework are made in the dental laboratory. The dentures are used until osseointegration of the fixture takes place. The metal framework allows for a trial run of the planned prosthesis prior to its actual fabrication. Also, any nonviable teeth should be removed and allowed to heal before the next phase.

Next, the implants are placed into the jaw. This step may be performed in an out-patient setting. The process can take from one to several hours, depending on the number of implants. Even if the patient is under general anesthesia, the intended incision site is injected with local anesthetic containing epinephrine and the mucosa is incised with a #15 blade to form a mucoperiosteal flap. A periosteal elevator is used to further expose the bone. The implant site is prepared using a series of drill bits with increasing diameters. Once the implant is positioned, a cover screw is placed to keep scar tissue from forming in the hollow of the fixture. The site is closed using a 3 or 4–0 chromic suture. The patient uses the temporary removable dentures during the healing phase.

Three to 6 months later, once the osseointegration process is complete, the fixture is uncovered by making a small incision injected with local anesthetic in an office setting. The correct abutment is selected and connected to the fixture and sutures are placed. The metal framework is seated to ensure proper fit and a new series of X-rays and impressions are made. The metal framework is removed and sent to the laboratory along with the new impressions for fabrication. The temporary dentures are converted to attach to the abutments; this device is now referred to as a conversion prosthesis.

When the permanent prosthesis is completed, the patient returns for placement. This final phase can also be accomplished in the office setting. The permanent prosthetic teeth are placed onto the abutments and any final adjustments are made. Proper occlusion is verified and X-rays are taken.

MAXILLOFACIAL PROCEDURES: GENERAL CONSIDERATIONS

As with all cases, the chart should be reviewed for pertinent information. Many times a maxillofacial injury can prohibit speech. If the patient is unable to communicate verbally, relevant information is obtained through the history and physical report, emergency personnel, observers, relatives, or with the use of a pencil and paper.

Any facial imaging studies, dental impressions, or preoperative photographs should accompany the patient to the operating room.

Maxillofacial procedures can be lengthy. Adequate precautions should be taken to ensure the patient's comfort and safety. These precautions may include the use of warming devices and insertion of a Foley catheter. Any bony areas, such as heels, elbows, sacrum, and shoulders, should be padded.

Blood loss should be measured closely, especially in children. Scales and volumetric suction devices can be employed to estimate blood loss. Blood and blood products should be ordered in advance and made available as needed.

Maxillofacial surgery involves manipulation of the bones near the patient's airway. Both elective and traumatic procedures can endanger the airway status. Determination of the patient's NPO status is vital. Vomiting can lead to aspiration, but in the maxillofacial trauma patient, it can also lead to infection that may interfere with fracture/wound healing.

Surgical personnel should be prepared to handle a variety of situations concerning airway management. The trauma patient may arrive with a tracheotomy, nasal endotracheal, or oral endotracheal tube already in place. Intubation (oral or nasal) may prove to be difficult due to a distortion of the bony anatomy or soft tissues due to congenital abnormalities, disease, or trauma. The patient may require implementation of a rapid induction technique, an awake intubation, or a tracheotomy. Several types of intubation aids are available and may be stored in a central location or on a portable cart for emergency use. In addition to the rigid laryngoscope, McGill forceps, and stylets, the difficult airway supplies should include a variety of shapes and sizes of blades for the rigid laryngoscope and a flexible fiberoptic laryngoscope. The flexible fiberoptic laryngoscope will allow the anesthesia provider to advance an oral or nasal endotracheal tube under indirect visualization.

Because maxillofacial procedures are done in the region of the endotracheal tube delivering the oxygen to the patient, care should be taken to avoid an intraoperative fire. Sparks from the electrosurgical unit can cause ignition of oxygen from the ventilation system. A closed ventilation system, use of a fire retardant ET tube, and careful use of the electrosurgical unit can reduce the potential for fire.

The surgical site is prepared by carefully removing any gross debris such as glass or dirt. Facial hair is removed if necessary; however, eyebrows and lashes should never be shaved or removed. The lashes may be trimmed if the surgeon deems necessary. The area is washed with the prep solution preferred by the surgeon. If trauma is present, care must be taken to avoid further soft tissue damage or dislocation of fractured bone during the skin prep.

Maxillofacial reconstructions usually involve several procedures. The surgical technologist should be prepared to deal with a number of possibilities. Communication between the surgeon(s), anesthesia provider, and surgical team is vital. Trauma reconstruction patients have possibly received other injuries in addition to facial fractures. These can include brain injury and dural tears. A dural tear may be repaired by the maxillofacial surgeon by placing a suture or sealing off the CSF leak with a fat, fascia, or muscle graft. Maxillofacial fractures can be treated at the same time other injuries are repaired if the patient's condition allows. Open reduction techniques often require the use of internal fixation devices and can involve a variety of graft materials. All implanted metals must be of the same type to prevent electrolytic reactions. Grafts may be obtained from the patient or secured from another source.

GRAFT MATERIALS

Graft material can be used in several situations. It can fill defects from bone loss, fill cavities to promote osteogenesis, or support a weak reduction. Graft material can be autogenous (from one part of the patient's body to another), homogenous (also referred to as allograft—from the same species), heterologous (also referred to as xenograft—from a dissimilar species), or synthetic.

Autogenous bone grafts are harvested from the patient. Iliac crest, ribs, and **calvarial** bone are often harvested for use in maxillofacial surgery.

Calvarial bone is an excellent choice because of its density, and the fact that it can often be harvested from the same operative field. Calvarial bone graft harvesting requires the chosen area of the skull to be shaved and prepped. A craniotomy set is necessary. A small skin incision is made or a coronal flap that has already been implemented is extended. A drill with a perforator attachment is used to create a bur hole (refer to Chapter 24). Then, a footed attachment with a cutting blade is inserted into the bur hole. This attachment creates the bone flap by cutting out a segment of the skull. A right-angle dural dissector placed in the bur hole elevates the bone flap. A Penfield #1 is used to dissect the dura off the bone, and a heavier elevator, for example, a Langenbeck, is used to remove the bone flap from the skull. The bone flap is split transversely into anterior and posterior tables. The posterior table is placed back into the site and affixed with plates and screws. The anterior table, containing the cortical bone, is shaped into the needed form. The bone flap may be temporarily stored on the back table in a sterile container. It may be kept dry, moistened with saline, or treated with antibiotic solution.

Rib grafts are harvested from a small incision over the chosen rib. A chest set should be used to obtain the graft. The area over the rib is prepped and draped separately from the face. The incision is made with a #10 blade and the chosen rib is exposed. The periosteum is removed with a periosteal elevator. The rib is then cut with rib cutters and preserved on the back table. Hemostasis is achieved and the wound closed. If the pleura is inadvertently entered, it will be necessary to insert a chest tube.

Homogenous bone, such as a fibular strut, usually from a cadaver, is procured from a bone bank. Xenograft material, such as coral, is gaining popularity. Synthetic material, Silastic for example, may be used, and a variety of implantable rigid fixation devices are available as well.

REPAIR OF MANDIBULAR/ MAXILLARY FRACTURES

To properly repair many of the following fractures, several basic techniques will be used repeatedly: placement of arch bars, wires, and plates and screws, and/or the use of graft material. Several techniques may be used in the correction of one problem.

Rigid fixation by plates and screws, or screws alone, is the most common repair technique for mandibular fractures. Many plating systems have specially designed plates for mandibular fixation. These plates range in thickness from 1.0 to 3.0 mm. The design of the plates may vary; plates can be straight, angled, or contoured. Most fractures require a combination of plates and screws for proper fixation. For example, a 4-hole 2.0 miniplate and 4-hole 2.4 direct compression plates can be used together to fixate a symphyseal fracture. Two 2.4-mm lag screws, without a plate, can also be employed to fixate the same fracture. The fracture and surgeon's discretion dictate how each one should be fixated.

APPLICATION OF ARCH BARS

Arch bar fixation is used to immobilize the jaw following mandibular and/or maxillary fracture (Procedure 18-2).

PROCEDURE 18-2 Application of Arch Bars

Equipment

- Headlamp
- Suction system

Instruments

- Stainless steel arch bars (appropriate size—pediatric or adult)
- Stainless steel wire (24 and 26 gauge)

(continues)

PROCEDURE 18-2 Application of Arch Bars *(continued)*

- Wire cutters
- 6-in. wire twister × 2
- Bayonet tissue forceps without teeth
- Mouth prop
- Freer elevator
- V-shaped probe
- Yankauer suction tip
- Frazier suction tip
- Wieder retractor
- Minnesota retractor
- Plastic cheek retractor
- Tonsil hemostat × 2

Supplies

- Pack: basic
- Basin: small
- Gloves
- Blades: #15
- Drapes: ½ sheet × 2
- Suture: none
- Drains: none
- Dressings: none
- Drugs: according to surgeon's preference
- Miscellaneous:
  - Suction tubing
  - Irrigation fluid
  - Throat pack
  - Gauze sponges
  - Two 10-cc syringes with 25-gauge 1½-in. needles for local injection
  - Two 20-cc syringes with 19-gauge 1½-in. blunt needles for irrigation

Operative Preparation

Anesthesia

- General preferred
- Nasal intubation if possible
- Lubricate and protect patient's eyes
- Local anesthetic with epinephrine may be used alone or in conjunction with general anesthesia to reduce bleeding and minimize postoperative pain

Position

- Supine, with head tilted back to provide exposure
- A donut or foam headrest may be used for stabilization
- Arms tucked at patient's sides; protect ulnar nerves

Prep

- May not be required
- Brush teeth or swab inside of mouth with an oral antiseptic
- Face may be prepped with a mild antiseptic. Protect eyes and ears from contact with prep solution

Draping

- May not be necessary
- A ½ sheet may be placed across the patient's body to provide a clean surface on which to rest equipment and supplies
- A turban-style head wrap may be used to restrain the hair

Practical Considerations

- Oral procedures are not considered sterile; use the best technique possible
- Wire used to attach arch bars to the teeth must be precut and prestretched to prevent stretching of the wire intraoperatively and postoperatively, ensuring the security of the arch bars. To prepare the wire, cut segments slightly longer than needed—approximately 10 cm. Place cut ends of wire in jaws of two wire twisters and secure. Twist each instrument half a turn and pull to stretch.

PROCEDURE

18-2 Application of Arch Bars *(continued)*

Remove the instruments and trim the crimped ends. Time permitting, several wires are prepared in advance. Plan to use at least one wire for each viable tooth. Allow extra in the event that some wires fall to the floor or break

- Wire is tightened in a clockwise manner during application and removed by twisting in the opposite direction. Adherence to this method facilitates both the application and removal of wires
- During oral procedures, the patient's lips may dry and crack. To alleviate this problem a cream or ointment may be applied to the lips

Operative Procedure	Technical Considerations
1. Insert mouth prop and plastic cheek retractor.	**1.** Have appropriate-size mouth prop and retractor ready for insertion.
2. Insert throat pack.	**2.** Prepare throat pack for insertion and present instrument for insertion.
3. The arch bars are measured, shaped, and cut to size.	**3.** Have two (one for the mandible and one for the maxilla) appropriate-size arch bars ready along with the wire cutter
4. The arch bar is attached to the maxilla with prestretched wires to the individual viable teeth.	**4.** Prepare wire as previously instructed. Place one end of wire in jaws of wire twister and secure. Pass wire with caution—the exposed ends can easily puncture.
5. Ten-centimeter segments of wire are placed around the neck of each tooth securing the bar to the tooth.	**5.** As soon as wire is passed, hand the wire twister and the V-shaped probe to position the wire during tightening.
6. A probe facilitates placement of the wires. The wire twisters are used to tighten the wires using a clockwise motion.	**6.** Wire cutter will be needed next. Provide suction and retraction as needed.
7. Another arch bar is secured to the mandible with wire.	**7.** The wire, probe, cutter sequence will be repeated until the arch bars are secured to each tooth in both mandible and maxilla.
8. If a throat pack was used, it must be removed prior to fixation of the mandible and maxilla to one another.	**8.** Provide bayonet to remove throat pack. Count. Anticipate use of irrigation and suction.
9. The upper and lower jaws are then stabilized to each other.	**9.** Additional wire or elastic bands may be used. Loops of precut, prestretched, preshaped wire may be fashioned beforehand to facilitate the procedure.
10. Wire or elastic loops can now be placed over the hooks of the arch bars and tightened to immobilize the jaw (Figure 18-11).	**10.** Variations of mandibulomaxillary fixation are used according to surgeon's preference and patient's needs.

(continues)

PROCEDURE

18-2 Application of Arch Bars *(continued)*

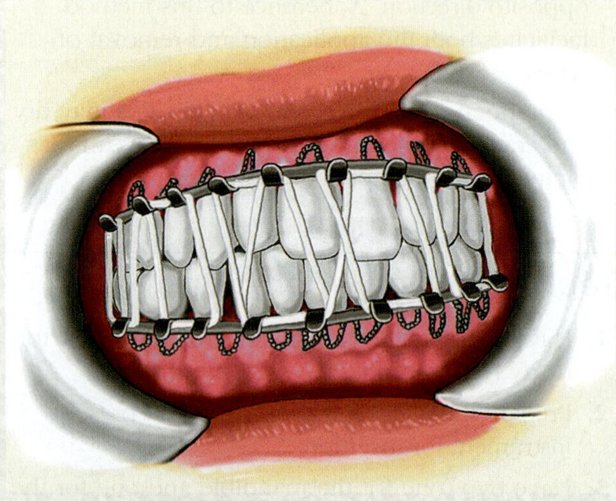

Figure 18-11 Maxillomandibular fixation

11. A final rinse of the oral cavity is performed and all fluid and debris removed.	**11.** Provide irrigation fluid and Yankauer suction tip.
12. Retractors are removed.	**12.** Be sure all loose wire is retrieved and disposed of properly.

Postoperative Considerations

Immediate Postoperative Care

- Scissors or wire cutter should accompany the patient to the postanesthesia care unit. It may be necessary to open the mouth in case vomiting or respiratory distress occurs.
- Tracheotomy may become necessary secondary to airway obstruction due to swelling.
- Bruising and swelling of the lips and cheeks may occur. The patient should be advised to apply ice.

Prognosis

- Bone healing is expected in 4–6 weeks. The jaw will remain immobilized for the entire time.
- Removal of the arch bars is usually an office procedure.
- Special consideration is given to the patient's nutritional needs. Patient will only be allowed liquids until fixation device is removed.

Complications

- Hemorrhage
- Infection
- Misalignment/malocclusion

PEARL OF WISDOM

Arch bars are thin strips of metal that have small intermittently placed hooks. The strips are malleable and the hooks should be placed pointing downward on the lower jaw and upward on the upper jaw. This placement allows for mandibulomaxillary elastic band or wire fixation.

WIRE FIXATION

Wires can be used to approximate bone fragments or for suspension. For example, a fracture along the mandibular body can be reduced using wire fixation. This technique involves drilling a pilot hole slightly larger than the wire gauge. Instruments for incision and exposure will be needed according to the incision type that is planned. The incision may be intraoral or on the exterior of the face or chin. For placement of wires into bone, a microdrill and power source, appropriately sized drill bit, 24- or 26-gauge prestretched wire, wire cutters, and 6-in. Berry wire twisters are required.

Exposure is achieved and the periosteum is stripped from the bone. Pilot holes, slightly larger than the wire gauge, are placed on either side of the fracture. The wire is passed through one hole, behind the fracture line, and back through the other hole forming a loop. The ends of the wire are pulled taught, reducing the fracture, and twisted. The wire is trimmed, and the sharp cut ends are turned in or placed into the existing drill hole, reducing the amount of irritation the sharp edges cause on surrounding soft tissue.

PLATE AND SCREW FIXATION OF MANDIBULAR FRACTURE

Plates and screws may be the method of choice in the fixation of craniofacial fractures (Procedure 18-3). Advanced plate design, screw type, and new implant material make this a versatile system. Bone plates are available in L, Y, H, and T shapes, among others, and range in thickness from 0.5 to 0.9 mm. Wire screens and specially designed orbital plates are available. The screws come in diameters of 1.0 to 4.0 mm. The smaller screws are designed for the delicate facial bones; the larger diameter screws are for placement in the mandible. Implant materials can be absorbable or nonabsorbable. Research perfecting the use of absorbable implants is on the rise. Absorbable implants are of great value in pediatric cases, but other applications are limited. Nonabsorbable implants are most commonly used for facial fractures in adults. Titanium is a strong, lightweight, noncorrosive metal that is used almost exclusively in craniofacial implants. Advances in rigid fixation instrumentation have decreased the necessity for and/or amount of time arch bars are required.

PROCEDURE 18-3 Plate and Screw Fixation of Mandibular Fracture

Equipment

- Power equipment with energy source
- Electrosurgical unit with dispersive electrode
- Suction system
- Headlamp
- Lead shields if use of X-ray is anticipated

Instruments

- Internal fixation system of surgeon's preference
- Maxillofacial instrumentation set

Supplies

- Pack: basic
- Basin: double
- Gloves
- Blades: #15
- Drapes: head and neck
- Suture: according to surgeon's preference
- Drains: none
- Dressings: none if intraoral incision used, or according to surgeon's preference
- Drugs: according to surgeon's preference
- Miscellaneous:
  - Sterile components of power system including bits
  - Suction tubing with Yankauer tip
  - Irrigation fluid
  - Electrosurgical pencil
  - Throat pack (if intraoral procedure)
  - Gauze sponges
  - Two 10-cc syringes with 25-gauge 1½-in. needles for local injection
  - Two 20-cc syringes with 19-gauge 1½-in. blunt needles for irrigation
  - Sterile X-ray cassette cover available

(continues)

PROCEDURE 18-3 Plate and Screw Fixation of Mandibular Fracture *(continued)*

Operative Preparation

Anesthesia
- General preferred
- Lubricate and protect patient's eyes
- Local anesthetic with epinephrine may be used alone or in conjunction with general anesthesia to reduce bleeding and minimize postoperative pain

Position
- Supine, with head positioned to provide maximum exposure
- A donut or foam headrest may be used for stabilization
- Arms tucked at patient's sides; protect ulnar nerves

Prep
- Shave if necessary
- May not be required if intraoral procedure
- Brush teeth or swab inside of mouth with an oral antiseptic
- Face, chin, and neck may be prepped with a mild antiseptic. Protect eyes and ears from contact with prep solution. Do not dislocate breathing tube

Draping
- The operative area may be outlined with towels, the towels may be secured with towel clips, skin staples, or suture
- A turban-style head wrap may be used
- Remove protective paper from disposable drapes with adhesive edges
- Place bar drape across patient's forehead, allowing remainder to cover head of operating table
- Situate the U-drape under patient's chin. Bring the edges of the U lateral to the head. Extend the remainder of the drape to cover the patient's body

Practical Considerations

- Oral procedures are not considered sterile; use the best technique possible
- The procedure will be performed using sterile technique if an external incision is planned
- Arch bars may be placed
- Notify scheduling clerk in radiology department of possible need for intraoperative X-rays

Operative Procedure	Technical Considerations
1. Local anesthetic with epinephrine is injected.	1. Local anesthetic of choice is preloaded in syringe with needle attached. Follow facility policy for passing sharps. Refill the syringe in anticipation of use on contralateral side. Notify anesthesia provider of epinephrine use.
2. An incision is made anterior to the angle of the mandible and any bleeding controlled.	2. A #15 blade will be needed. Anticipate use of electrosurgical pencil.
3. Wound edges are retracted.	3. Retractor(s) of choice will be needed. Provide suction as needed.

PROCEDURE 18-3 Plate and Screw Fixation of Mandibular Fracture *(continued)*

4. Periosteum is stripped from the bone.	**4.** Periosteal elevator such as a freer will be used.
5. Bone edges are manipulated into position and steadied by the surgical assistant or with a bone-holding clamp.	**5.** Stabilize patient's head during manipulation. Be sure breathing tube does not become crimped or dislocated. Bone clamp may be needed.
6. A plate of appropriate thickness, length, and design is chosen and customized for the patient.	**6.** Provide a variety of plates for selection. Plates can be customized to the area by curving the plate using bending irons.
7. The plate is placed against the bone bridging the fracture site and secured in position.	**7.** Provide plate-holding clamp to secure plate to bone. Load drill with correct size bit.
8. A hole is drilled with the correct diameter drill bit.	**8.** A drill guide may be used. Have depth gauge ready.
9. The depth of the hole is measured and tapped if necessary.	**9.** Present correct size tap. Retrieve requested size screw and load onto insertion device.
10. The proper screw is placed into the predrilled hole.	**10.** Reset the drill and organize insertion tools for reuse.
11. The sequence is repeated until the plate is firmly affixed to the bone.	**11.** Record the pertinent information about the implants for the patient's permanent operative record.
12. The procedure is repeated on the contralateral side, if necessary.	**12.** Reorganize tools for reuse.
13. Proper reduction/fixation is ensured by visual inspection of the area. Intraoperative X-rays may be useful.	**13.** Prepare to accept X-ray cassette into sterile field if requested. Prepare irrigation fluid and suture for closing.
14. The wound is irrigated and closed.	**14.** Count.
15. Dressings are applied.	**15.** Prepare dressing material for use.

Postoperative Considerations

Immediate Postoperative Care

- If arch bar fixation was also performed, scissors or wire cutter should accompany the patient to the postanesthesia care unit.
- Bruising and swelling of the lips and cheeks may occur. The patient should be advised to apply ice.
- Patient should be observed for airway difficulties secondary to swelling.

Prognosis

- Complete recovery is expected in 4–6 weeks.

Complications

- Hemorrhage
- Infection
- Misalignment/malocclusion

PEARL OF WISDOM

The same sequence of events is employed for attachment of the plate to the bone with most fixation systems (Figure 18-12).

1. A plate of appropriate thickness, length, and design is chosen.
2. Plates can be customized to the specific anatomy by contouring the plate using bending irons provided with the fixation set for that purpose.
3. Correct diameter drill bit is chosen and applied to the drill.
4. A drill guide may be used.
5. The depth of the hole is then measured.
6. The drill hole may be tapped. Tap use reduces the amount of torque applied during screw placement. Self-tapping screws are available.
7. The correct screw is selected and measured by the STSR and loaded onto the insertion device.
8. The screw is placed through the plate and into the predrilled hole in the bone.
9. The sequence is repeated until the plate is firmly affixed to the bone.
10. The implants are permanently recorded in the operative record.
11. Verification of fracture reduction and prosthesis placement is verified visually or with the use of X-ray.

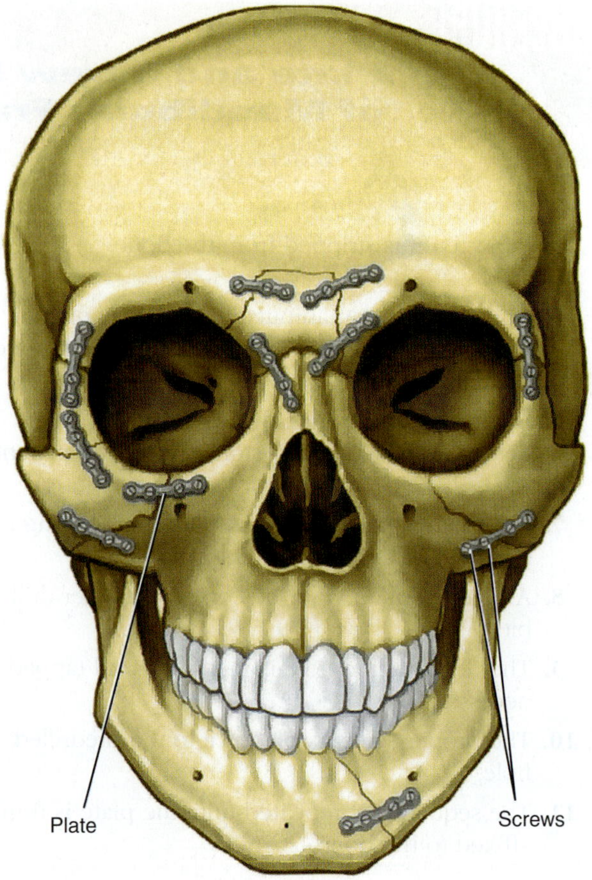

Figure 18-12 Miniplates and screws

FRONTAL FRACTURE REPAIR

Repair of a frontal sinus fracture depends on its type. Nondisplaced anterior table fractures showing no evidence of nasofrontal duct fractures usually do not require surgery. Displaced table fractures, occurring together or separately, do require an invasive procedure. If the nasofrontal duct is injured, the duct is checked for patency using dye. A nonfunctional duct indicates the necessity for frontal sinus obliteration to prohibit later infection due to blockage. The extent of the fracture will dictate the invasiveness of the procedure. For small fractures, exploration can be done through an existing laceration or small incision. Larger fractures and those involving the nasofrontal duct are best approached through a coronal incision.

Frontal sinus repair is often approached as a craniotomy, requiring a craniotomy setup. (Refer to Chapter 24.) The patient will be anesthetized and intubated and the eyes lubricated and taped shut or shielded. The operating table may be positioned at an angle for better access. The patient's hairline will be shaved if necessary, and the remaining hair should be swept out of the field and restrained. The forehead should be prepped to these margins: laterally behind the ears, inferiorly to the mouth, superiorly to the coronal suture. Care must be taken to avoid displacing the breathing tube or placing too much pressure on the fracture site.

A coronal incision is made following the patient's natural hairline; it can be extended anterior to the tragus, if needed (Figure 18-13). The coronal incision can be positioned further back into the hairline if desired. The intended incision line may be outlined with a marking pen and injected with local anesthetic. As the incision is made, pressure is applied to the skin edges to reduce the amount of blood loss. Raney scalp clips will be placed on both edges of the incision to achieve hemostasis. A Langenbeck periosteal elevator is used to free the soft tissue flap subgaleally and subperiosteally. The supraorbital nerve should be identified and protected as the dissection continues. The dissection will end about 2 cm above the orbital rim. Laterally, the dissection continues, taking care to avoid damaging the frontal branch of the facial nerve. The zygomatic arch is exposed if needed.

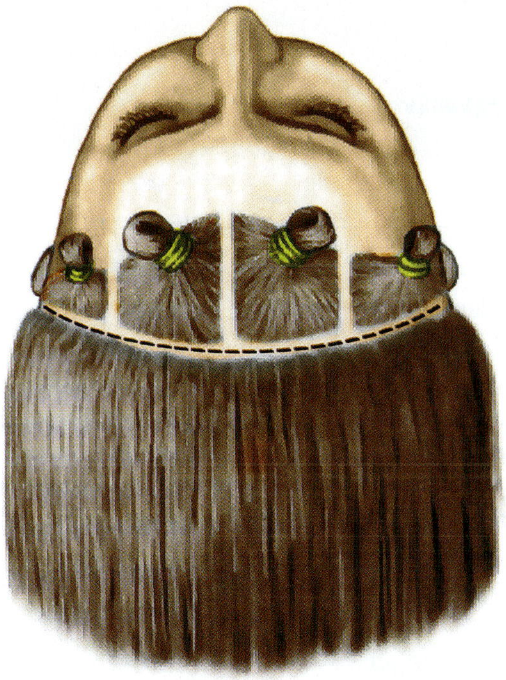

A

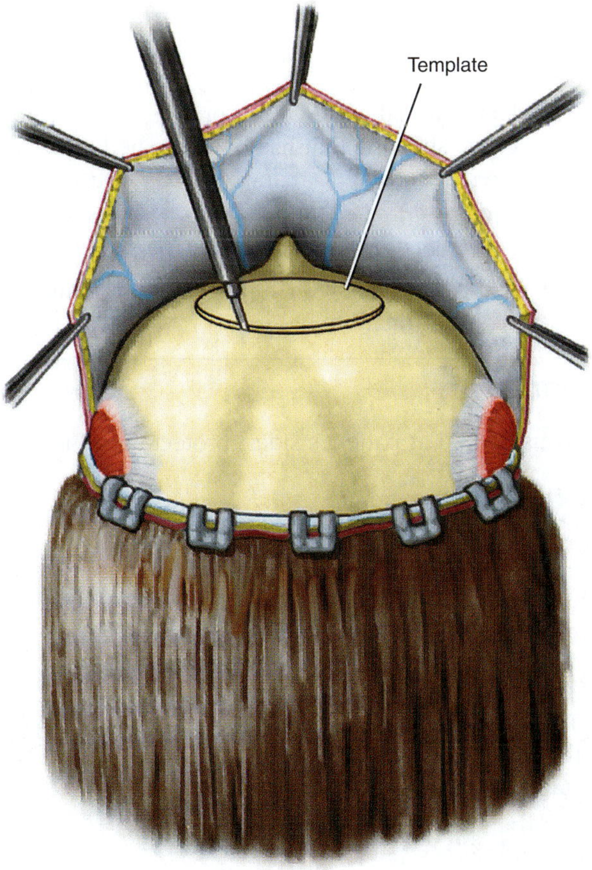

B

Figure 18-13 Coronal flap: (A) Intended incision site is exposed, (B) flap dissected

The **coronal flap** is retracted, using the surgeon's preferred method, and kept moist. The anterior table of the frontal bone is explored and any bone fragments removed and preserved for possible reimplantation. To visualize the posterior table and sinus cavity, it may be necessary to temporarily remove a segment of bone, which will be set aside and later reimplanted. The frontal sinus is entered, the mucosa removed using a curette, and the intrasinus bone cortex is drilled away. The posterior table can now be inspected for damage. Any dural leaks should be repaired at this time. A dural tear may be repaired by the maxillofacial surgeon by placing a suture or sealing off the CSF leak with a fat, fascia, or muscle graft. If the posterior table is fractured, it can be repaired with rigid fixation or supported with the bone graft packing. After irrigating the sinus cavity, the calvarial bone graft, if needed, can be shaped and placed over the nasofrontal duct or other areas requiring bone grafts. The sinus cavity can now be filled with the remaining particulate bone matter.

After the posterior table has been repaired and the sinus cavity filled, any anterior table fractures can be fixed. Previously removed bone fragments or calvarial bone graft can be incorporated into the repair. If the anterior table is unsuitable for use, then a piece of calvarial bone graft can be shaped to take the place of the fractured wall. Rigid fixation, if necessary, is achieved with a plate and screw system. Plates can be customized for placement along the forehead. Screws can be placed intermittently as needed.

Sometimes the posterior table fracture is too comminuted to repair. In those cases, cranialization is an option. Cranialization involves the removal of the posterior table of the frontal sinus. Obliteration of the remaining mucosa and placement of a galeal-frontalis muscle flap is performed prior to replacement of the anterior table. The frontal lobes will eventually expand to fill the vacant space.

On satisfactory reduction and fixation of the frontal fractures, the coronal flap is closed. Use of a closed drainage system may be indicated. The galea is approximated using interrupted absorbable suture and the skin closed with nylon. Each wound is dressed according to the surgeon's preference. A typical example of the wound dressing includes antibiotic ointment, Telfa, and 4 × 4s, placed over the incision, which are secured by wrapping the head with two 4-in. Kerlix rolls. When wrapping the head, caution is necessary to ensure patency of the airway and that the dressing is neither too tight nor too loose.

ORBITAL FLOOR FRACTURE REPAIR

The floor of the orbit consists of thin bones. It is susceptible to fractures from many forms of facial trauma. Fracture of the orbital floor allows the contents of the eye to herniate. These fractures are repaired surgically (Procedure 18-4).

PROCEDURE 18-4 Orbital Floor Fracture Repair

Equipment

- Power equipment with energy source
- Suction system
- Electrosurgical unit with dispersive electrode
- Headlamp
- Lead shields if use of X-ray is anticipated

Instruments

- Maxillofacial instrumentation set
- Orbital retractors
- Internal fixation system of surgeon's preference

Supplies

- Pack: ophthalmic
- Basin: double
- Gloves
- Blades: #15
- Drapes: head and neck
- Suture: according to surgeon's preference
- Drains: none
- Dressings: eye pad
- Drugs: according to surgeon's preference
- Miscellaneous:
  - Sterile components of power system, including bits
  - Suction tubing with Frazier tip
  - Irrigation fluid
  - Electrosurgical pencil
  - Sterile marking pen
  - Cotton swabs or Weck cell sponges
  - Gauze sponges
  - Corneal shield
  - Implant material of surgeon's preference (Teflon or Silastic sheeting that has been washed and sterilized according to manufacturer's instruction)
  - Two 10-cc syringes with 25-gauge 1½-in. needles for local injection
  - Two 20-cc syringes with 19-gauge 1½-in. blunt needles for irrigation

Operative Preparation

Anesthesia

- General preferred
- Lubricate and protect patient's eyes; corneal shield may be used
- Local anesthetic with epinephrine may be used alone or in conjunction with general anesthesia to reduce bleeding and minimize postoperative pain

Position

- Supine, with head positioned to provide maximum exposure
- A donut or foam headrest may be used for stabilization
- Arms tucked at patient's sides; protect ulnar nerves

Prep

- Shave if necessary
- Entire face is prepped with mild antiseptic. Protect eyes and ears from contact with prep solution. Do not dislocate breathing tube

Draping

- The operative area may be outlined with towels; the towels may be secured with towel clips, skin staples, or suture
- A turban-style head wrap may be used

PROCEDURE

18-4 Orbital Floor Fracture Repair *(continued)*

- Remove protective paper from disposable drapes with adhesive edges
- Place bar drape across patient's forehead, allowing remainder of drape to cover head of operating table
- Situate the U-drape on patient's nose. Bring the edges of the U lateral to the head. Extend the remainder of the drape to cover the patient's body

Practical Considerations

- Preoperative X-rays will be displayed in the operating room for referral during the procedure
- Notify scheduling clerk in radiology department of possible need for intraoperative X-rays
- Do not rest hands, instruments, or supplies on patient's face
- All implanted items must be recorded

Operative Procedure	Technical Considerations
1. The planned incision is marked and injected with a local anesthetic containing epinephrine.	**1.** Provide sterile marking pen. Medication is obtained and drawn into the syringe in advance. Notify anesthesia provider of epinephrine use.
2. Incision is made with a #15 blade underneath the lower eyelid on the affected side and hemostasis is achieved.	**2.** Cotton swabs or Weck cell sponges are used to blot away blood and irrigation solution around the incision. Keep an ample supply readily available. Present electrosurgical pencil, if needed. Provide suction as needed.
3. A traction stitch may be placed between the lower eyelashes and incision site to aid in exposure.	**3.** Traction stitch is preloaded on needle holder. It may either be tied and cut or secured with a hemostat. Dull Senn or vein retractors may be needed to provide additional exposure.
4. Curved tenotomy scissors and Adson tissue forceps are used for dissection through the infraorbital fat to expose the infraorbital rim.	**4.** Pass scissors to surgeon's dominant hand and tissue forceps to the opposite. Electrosurgical pencil may be used intermittently.
5. The periosteum is incised with a #15 blade and elevated with the use of a freer.	**5.** New #15 blade will be needed. Pass freer elevator. Be sure to present sharp or dull end as specified by surgeon.
6. A moistened orbital retractor or Teflon-coated malleable brain spatula may be placed to gently retract the eye, superiorly exposing the orbital floor.	**6.** Have premoistened retractor of choice available.
7. The periorbital fat and any other entrapped tissues are released and retracted.	**7.** Freer elevator or scissors and tissue forceps may be needed repeatedly.
8. The fracture site is exposed and bone fragments are manipulated into position.	**8.** Be sure eye is protected during reduction of bone fragments.

(continues)

PROCEDURE 18-4 Orbital Floor Fracture Repair *(continued)*

9. Any loose bone fragments are repositioned and the wound irrigated.

9. Irrigation fluid of surgeon's choice is preloaded in syringe with blunt needle. Pass irrigation fluid along with Frazier tip suction. A kidney basin placed at the side of the face may be useful in containing excess irrigation fluid.

10. If the reduction is stable, Silastic sheeting may be inserted over the fracture site to prevent entrapment of the orbital contents in the fracture and support the globe.

10. Sheeting must be prepared and sterilized according to manufacturer's instructions. Sheeting will be customized—have straight scissors ready.

11. If the reduction is not stable, a rigid fixation device may be implanted, followed by the insertion of Silastic sheeting.

11. Communicate additional needs with other team members. Secure any necessary additional supplies.

12. Reduction may be verified radiographically.

12. Provide necessary supplies to facilitate X-ray.

13. Once adequate stable reduction is achieved, the traction suture is removed and the wound closed.

13. Provide closing suture of surgeon's choice. Count.

14. If used, the corneal protector is removed and the dressing applied.

14. Provide dressing materials. Ice may be needed.

Postoperative Considerations

Immediate Postoperative Care

- Bruising and swelling may occur around the eyes and nose. Advise patient to apply ice.
- Patient may experience temporary vision disturbances due to swelling.

Prognosis

- A small visible scar will remain.
- Complete recovery is expected.

Complications

- Hemorrhage
- Infection
- Vision disturbance due to trauma to the eye

PEARL OF WISDOM

The STSR may also be expected to fill the role of the surgical assistant. Be sure that the instruments and supplies are organized so that the surgeon may obtain instruments independently if the STSR is using both hands to provide retraction.

REDUCTION OF ZYGOMATIC FRACTURES

Reduction of zygomatic fractures can be accomplished in one of two ways. First, a closed reduction may be attempted. This type of reduction elevates the depressed bone, placing it into the proper anatomical position. No fixation is required. Second, an open reduction with internal fixation can be done for severe fractures. This reduction will require direct fixation through wires, pins, or a screw and plate system.

Both types of reduction require the patient to be in a supine position. Adequate access to the head is a necessity. The patient's head may be placed on a donut-shaped pillow and turned so the affected side is up. The OR table may be rotated, depending on room design and the surgeon's preference.

For closed reduction procedures, few instruments and supplies are needed. A mini-plastic set, along with the surgeon's choice of reduction instruments, will be necessary. A zygoma hook, Kelly hemostat, or Van Buren sound can all be used to reduce the fracture. The necessary supplies include gown, gloves, head and neck drape pack, suction, electrosurgical pencil, #15 blade, gauze sponges, and 4–0 suture or skin closure tapes.

After prepping and draping the appropriate area, a small incision is made superior to the fracture. The reduction instrument is slid through the incision and placed under the depressed bone. Reduction of the fracture is achieved by elevating the zygoma to its proper position. The incision site may be closed with suture or Steri-Strips. The reduction can be maintained as long as no direct pressure is placed on it. The patient should avoid lying on the affected side.

For open reduction internal fixations, the above instruments and supplies are needed in addition to the chosen fixation system. There are several ways a zygoma fracture can be fixated after reduction. If the surgeon has decided to wire the fracture, a set containing 26-, 28-, and 30-gauge wires, wire cutters, and wire twisters will be needed. Kirschner wires can be used to stabilize the fracture as well. Wire cutters, benders, and driver such as a microdrill will be used for placement. More commonly, a miniplate and screw system can be used for fixation. The appropriate system and power drill with power source are required for this type of fixation.

The procedure begins with placement of a corneal shield to protect the patient's eye from injury. Local anesthetic can be injected at this time. For zygomaticomaxillary and zygomaticofrontal suture fractures, an incision is marked and placed below the lower eyelid. Zygomaticotemporal suture line fractures require an incision along the lateral portion of the eyebrow. The fracture site or sites are exposed. Vein or Senn retractors can be used to hold skin and subcutaneous fat away from the fracture site. The fractured zygoma is elevated using the surgeon's choice of tools. The zygoma may then be fixated in one or a combination of the following ways. Wiring of the broken portions involves drilling holes to either side of the fracture. The wire is passed through the holes and twisted together tightly. The excess is trimmed off, and the remaining wire is placed where the surrounding tissues will not be irritated. Kirschner wires may be used for additional stabilization. Using miniplates and screws is yet another form of fixation. First, a plate of appropriate thickness, length, and design is chosen. The plate is bent to follow the contour of the bone, and fixated to the site after the periosteum has been removed. Proper fixation is ensured by direct inspection of the area along with intraoperative X-rays.

Drugs used for zygomatic fractures are local anesthetic, antibiotics, and ointment. Local anesthetics containing epinephrine will aid in hemostasis. Antibiotics for irrigation or in the form of ointment help reduce the chance of infection.

LE FORT I FRACTURE REPAIR

Fractures to the maxilla are relatively common (Figure 18-14). Le Fort fractures are bilateral horizontal fractures of the maxilla. These fractures are repaired surgically (Procedure 18-5).

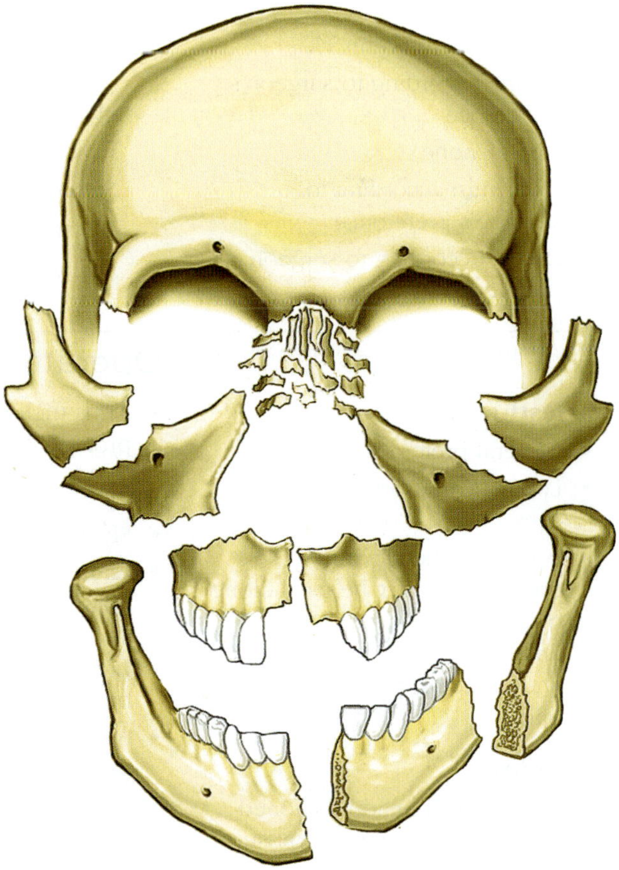

Figure 18-14 Maxillofacial injury

PROCEDURE

18-5 Le Fort I Fracture Repair

Equipment

- Power equipment with energy source
- Suction system
- Electrosurgical unit with dispersive electrode
- Headlamp
- Lead shields if use of X-ray is anticipated

Instruments

- Maxillofacial instrumentation set
- Internal fixation system of surgeon's preference

Supplies

- Pack: basic
- Basin: double
- Gloves
- Blades: #15
- Drapes: head and neck
- Suture: according to surgeon's preference
- Drains: none
- Dressings: according to surgeon's preference
- Drugs: according to surgeon's preference
- Miscellaneous:
  - Sterile components of power system including bits
  - Internal fixation device of choice
  - Suction tubing with Frazier and Yankauer tips
  - Irrigation fluid
  - Sterile marking pen
  - Electrosurgical pencil
  - Gauze sponges
  - Two 10-cc syringes with 25-gauge 1½-in. needles for local injection
  - Two 20-cc syringes with 19-gauge 1½-in. blunt needles for irrigation

Operative Preparation

Anesthesia

- General preferred
- Lubricate and protect patient's eyes
- Local anesthetic with epinephrine may be used alone or in conjunction with general anesthesia to reduce bleeding and minimize postoperative pain

Position

- Supine, with head positioned to provide maximum exposure
- A donut or foam headrest may be used for stabilization
- Arms tucked at patient's sides; protect ulnar nerves

Prep

- Shave if necessary
- Entire face is prepped with mild antiseptic. Protect eyes and ears from contact with prep solution. Do not dislocate breathing tube
- Avoid excessive pressure during prep to minimize movement of fractured segments of bone

Draping

- The operative area may be outlined with towels; the towels may be secured with towel clips, skin staples, or suture
- A turban-style head wrap may be used
- Remove protective paper from disposable drapes with adhesive edges
- Place bar drape across patient's forehead, allowing remainder of drape to cover head of operating table
- Situate the U-drape on patient's nose. Bring the edges of the U lateral to the head. Extend the remainder of the drape to cover the patient's body

PROCEDURE 18-5

Le Fort I Fracture Repair *(continued)*

Practical Considerations

- Several procedures may need to be accomplished prior to fracture reduction and stabilization. Tracheotomy may be performed. Arch bars may be applied. Dental impressions may be made. Debridement of the area may be necessary
- Preoperative photographs, dental records, and X-rays should be available for the surgeon's reference during the procedure
- Notify scheduling clerk in radiology department of possible need for intraoperative X-rays
- Do not rest hands, instruments, or supplies on patient's face
- All implanted items must be recorded

Operative Procedure

1. A gingivobuccal sulcus incision provides adequate exposure of the maxilla; actual prosthesis placement will depend on the fracture site. The gingiva may be injected with local anesthetic with epinephrine prior to incising with a #15 blade. Hemostasis is achieved.
2. Exposure of the operative site is attained.
3. The fracture line is exposed by dissecting the gingiva from the alveolar process with a small periosteal elevator.
4. The fracture is reduced using caution not to disrupt the breathing tube.
5. If wire fixation is anticipated, sites for the drill holes are identified.
6. A drill hole is made on each side of the fracture line.
7. A single wire is passed through each hole and pulled taut, reducing the fracture.
8. The wire is twisted clockwise, cut, and the ends of the wire imbedded in the drill hole. The wire technique can also be used to apply traction by simply placing the wires through the holes and pulling the impacted maxilla up and forward.
9. Plate and screws can also be employed to fixate the maxilla. The plate is placed over the fracture line and secured to the bone by the compressive force of the screw. Both the wiring and plating techniques can be utilized several times throughout the procedure, often in conjunction with one another.

Technical Considerations

1. Anticipate retractor use for exposure of incision site. Medications are obtained in advance and prepared for use. Notify anesthesia provider of epinephrine use. Pass #15 blade on #7 knife handle. Anticipate the use of the electrosurgical pencil and suction with appropriate tip.
2. Retractors may be replaced or repositioned.
3. A Freer or slightly larger elevator will be used to expose the fracture site.
4. Reduction of the fracture may be achieved with the use of an elevator or manually.
5. Drill with appropriate-size bit is preassembled and connected to the power source.
6. Suction and irrigation fluid will be necessary to cool the drill site.
7. Precut, prestretched lengths of wire of appropriate size are loaded onto the wire twister and passed to the surgeon.
8. Anticipate the use of the wire cutter. The fracture may require placement of more than one wire for stabilization.
9. Be prepared for a combination procedure that employs wire, screw, or plate and screw fixation. Refer to Procedure 18-3 for related technical considerations.

(continues)

PROCEDURE 18-5 Le Fort I Fracture Repair *(continued)*

10. Fracture reduction and stabilization may be verified with the use of intraoperative X-rays (Figure 18-15).

10. Prepare to accept X-ray cassette into sterile field if requested. Anticipate closure as next step. Prepare irrigation fluid and suture.

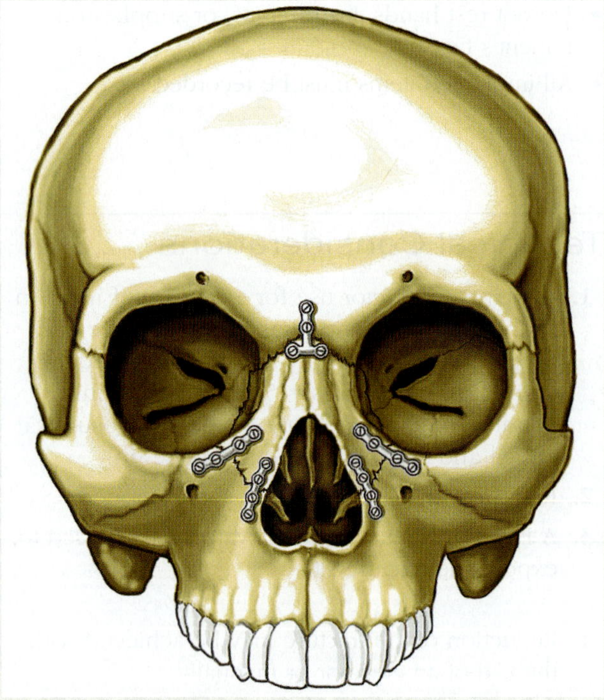

Figure 18-15 Repaired Le Fort I fracture

11. The wound is irrigated and closed.

12. Retractor is removed.

11. Count.

12. Dressing is not needed with intraoral approach.

Postoperative Considerations

Immediate Postoperative Care

- Patency of the airway may be compromised due to postoperative hemorrhage and swelling.

Prognosis

- Exact visual identity may not be restored. Further reconstructive surgery may be necessary.
- Scars will be visible.

Complications

- Hemorrhage
- Infection
- Malocclusion

PEARL OF WISDOM

The controls on the power equipment must be in the "safe" position when preparing the tool for use or when it is not in operation.

LE FORT II AND III FRACTURE REPAIR

Le Fort II and III fractures can be referred to as panfacial fractures, due to the extensive nature of the injuries. Injuries to the eyes, nose, and skull base can involve a specialist in each area. Still, the management of the fractures remains the same; the occlusion should be corrected first.

These fractures are typically approached using a coronal incision. This incision gives great exposure to the fracture sites and allows access to calvarial bone for grafting. Other incision options are the infraorbital and upper blepharoplasty incisions.

Once a decision is reached about the best incision, the exposure of the fractures is carried out as detailed earlier. After the occlusion is corrected, the remaining fractures can be reduced and fixated in the usual manner.

CRANIOFACIAL RECONSTRUCTION

Craniofacial reconstruction is an intricate solution to craniofacial deformities. Reconstruction of craniofacial deformities can be divided into three groups: anterior cranial expansion, posterior cranial expansion, and total cranial expansion. Anterior cranial expansion can be done to correct unilateral or bilateral coronal synostosis and metopic synostosis. Posterior cranial expansions correct unilateral or bilateral lambdoidal synostosis. Total cranial expansions correct **sagittal** synostosis.

Patient positioning will vary according to the exact type of reconstruction that is planned. The patient may be placed in a semisitting position with the head in a Mayfield head holder. Alternate positions depend on the patient's pathology and the surgeon's preference. In the semisitting position, special attention should be paid to the patient's comfort. The patient's head and chest will be raised and the knees flexed. Adequate padding should be placed around the scapula, olecranon, popliteal, and calcaneal areas to prevent injury. The arms may be placed and secured across the abdomen. The safety strap should be in place 2 inches proximate to the knees. The head will be placed in a three-point fixation system like the Mayfield head holder. A craniotomy setup should be used for these procedures.

For most craniofacial reconstructions, the best approach is the coronal flap. The patient's hair is removed from the surgical site. The remaining hair should be kept out of the surgical field. The area is prepped from the posterior portion of the head, laterally behind the ears, forehead, and face. Care should be taken around the ears and eyes.

ANTERIOR CRANIAL EXPANSION

Anterior cranial expansion begins with the development of a flap that extends from one temporal region to another, and horizontally across the frontal bone (Procedure 18-6). Osteotomies are done along each orbital roof, lateral zygoma, and the nasofrontal suture. Additional osteotomies may be performed depending on the patient's age and deformity.

(Text continues on page 678)

PROCEDURE 18-6 Anterior Cranial Expansion

Equipment

- Power equipment with energy source
- Craniotome with energy source
- Headlamp
- Electrosurgical unit with dispersive electrode
- Bipolar electrosurgical unit
- Headlamp
- Suction system
- Protective attire if the use of intraoperative X-ray is anticipated

(continues)

PROCEDURE 18-6 **Anterior Cranial Expansion** *(continued)*

Instruments

- Craniotomy instrumentation set

Supplies

- Pack: craniotomy
- Basin: double and single
- Gloves
- Blades: #10, 15, and 11
- Drapes: craniotomy
- Suture: according to surgeon's preference
- Drains: Jackson-Pratt × 2
- Dressings: adaptic, 4 × 4s, fluffs, rolled gauze × 2, paper tape
- Drugs: according to surgeon's preference
- Miscellaneous:
  - Sterile components of craniotome, including bits
  - Sterile components of power system, including bits
  - Internal fixation device of choice
  - Suction tubing × 2
  - Irrigation fluid
  - Sterile marking pen
  - Electrosurgical pencil
  - Bipolar cord and tips
  - Gauze sponges
  - Lap sponges
  - Cottonoid sponges
  - Peanut sponges
  - Raney clips
  - Two 10-cc syringes with 25-gauge 1½-in. needles for local injection
  - Two 20-cc syringes with 19-gauge 1½-in. needles for irrigation

Operative Preparation

Anesthesia

- General
- Lubricate and protect patient's eyes
- Anesthesia circuits must be long enough to accommodate table position
- Additional monitoring and vascular access devices may be used

Position

- Semi-Fowler's
- Be sure all bony prominences are well padded
- A donut, foam headrest, or the Mayfield headrest may be used for stabilization

Prep

- Hair will be removed first with clippers and then the head shaved
- Entire head, face, and neck are prepped with antiseptic. Protect eyes and ears from contact with prep solution. Do not dislocate breathing tube, vascular access devices, or monitors

Draping

- The operative area may be outlined with towels; the towels may be secured with adhesive, towel clips, skin staples, or suture
- Craniotomy incise drape is applied to expose the anterior portion of the skull
- The patient's body is covered with a ¾ sheet
- It may be necessary to create a barrier between the anesthesia provider and the sterile field with additional sheets

PROCEDURE 18-6 Anterior Cranial Expansion *(continued)*

Practical Considerations

- Notify scheduling clerk in radiology department of possible need for intraoperative radiography
- Foley catheter insertion may be necessary due to the length of the procedure or the need to monitor fluid balance
- Special considerations for pediatric patients will be necessary
- Preoperative radiographic studies should be displayed in the operating room
- A second setup may be needed to obtain an autologous bone graft
- If commercial implant materials have been requested, be sure they are available prior to the patient's arrival in the OR

Operative Procedure	Technical Considerations
1. A coronal incision is made.	**1.** A #10 blade on a #3 knife handle will be used.
2. Hemostasis is achieved with the use of the electrosurgical unit and Raney clips.	**2.** Electrosurgical pencil will be used. Raney clips should be preloaded on applier. 4 × 4 gauze may be used to line the incision prior to Raney clip placement.
3. The soft tissue flap is developed with the use of a periosteal elevator.	**3.** A key or similar elevator will be used.
4. The soft tissue flap is wrapped in a moist lap sponge and folded back and secured in position.	**4.** Moist sponge is prepared in advance. Provide retention device for soft tissue flap according to surgeon's preference.
5. The wound edges are lined with cottonoid sponges.	**5.** Provide premoistened cottonoids in a variety of sizes for the surgeon to select from.
6. The predetermined number of bur holes are created.	**6.** Craniotome with perforator attachment is prepared and tested in advance. Irrigation fluid and suction will be needed when power equipment is in use.
7. Hemostasis is achieved.	**7.** Small portions of bone wax may be placed on the raw bone edges. Present the bone wax on a Penfield or freer and follow with a peanut sponge secured on a heavy clamp.
8. Dural adhesions are separated from the cranium.	**8.** Dural separator will be needed.
9. The bone flap is developed using a drill with a footed attachment.	**9.** Power equipment must be changed to drill with footed attachment. The surgeon may wish to save bone chips for grafting later in the procedure—provide a container for collection.
10. Osteotomies are performed along the suture lines according to the patient's age and deformity.	**10.** Power equipment will be used repeatedly. Continue to provide irrigation fluid and suction.
11. Osteotomies may be incomplete, allowing for flexibility of the bone.	**11.** Osteotomes of various sizes/configurations and a mallet may be needed in addition to the power equipment.
12. The bone flap(s) is elevated with a periosteal elevator or right-angle dural elevator.	**12.** Provide elevator of surgeon's choice.

(continues)

PROCEDURE 18-6 Anterior Cranial Expansion *(continued)*

13. The bone flap may be completely removed, contoured, and repositioned. (Contouring the bone flap may involve placement of several small osteotomies, allowing "green-sticking" of the bone.)	**13.** Provide a work surface for bone contouring.
14. The flap is fixed into its new position with miniplates and screws.	**14.** Provide fixation system of choice. Provide power equipment and correct size drill bits. (Refer to Procedure 18-3 for technical considerations.)
15. If necessary, graft material is inserted.	**15.** A separate procedure may be necessary to obtain bone for grafting. Other commercially available graft material may be inserted.
16. Prosthesis placement may be radiographically verified.	**16.** Prepare to receive X-ray cassette into sterile field.
17. Drains are inserted if necessary.	**17.** Present drains for use—expect exit through bur holes and skin incision. Additional suture may be necessary to secure drains.
18. The flap is closed in the usual manner.	**18.** Prepare suture in advance. Count.
19. Dressing is applied.	**19.** Organize dressing material in advance. Assist with dressing placement. Protect and maintain the sterile field until the patient has been transported to the postanesthesia care unit.

Postoperative Considerations

Immediate Postoperative Care

- Neurologic status of the patient is assessed.

Prognosis

- Further surgery may be necessary to accommodate growth.
- Scar will be camouflaged by hair.

Complications

- Hemorrhage
- Infection

PEARL OF WISDOM

There are several methods for securing the soft tissue flap in position:

- Suture may be used.
- The flap may be weighted with instruments such as Dandy clamps.
- Towel clips may be used.
- Towel clips may be used in combination with elastic bands and Allis clamps to secure the flap to the drape while exerting only mild tension on the tissue.

POSTERIOR CRANIAL EXPANSION

Posterior cranial expansions expand the cranium through parietal and occipital bone flaps. The posterior skull is shaved and prepped, and a biparietal incision is made. The flap is developed using a periosteal elevator. The area is retracted in the same fashion as frontal flaps. Osteotomies are made in two portions using the bur hole and bone flap extension method. The first **osteotomy** starts several centimeters above the left lambdoidal suture and curves to the right lambdoidal suture. Another osteotomy is made inferior to the transverse sinus. An additional osteotomy can be made splitting the two bone flaps in half. A periosteal elevator can be used to ease the bone flap from the cranium. The flaps are contoured as needed and fixated with the 1.3 miniplating system.

COMPLETE CRANIAL EXPANSION

Complete cranial expansions are done for those patients over 2 years of age who cannot be reconstructed using other methods. Each flap is dissected in the previously discussed manner. The scalp may even be dissected further to allow for skin closure over the expanded region. Posterior and anterior osteotomies can be performed in varying combinations to correct the deformity. The same technique of contouring the bone flap and then fixating the flap is performed. Once the bone flap is fixated, the scalp is closed in proper fashion. The usual head dressing is applied.

CORRECTION OF RETROGNATHISM OR PROGNATHISM

Orthognathic (gnath = jaw) surgery involves correction of jaw deformities. The correction of jaw deformities involves direct manipulation. The mandible can be split and projected anteriorly, or it can be reduced in length and brought inward. At times, the maxilla can be manipulated through osteotomies and fixated with miniplates. Additionally, chin or cheek implants may be used to enhance the patient's facial features.

The method of reconstruction is determined by several factors, such as the type of deformity and the patient's status. A treatment plan for each patient is developed according to physical evaluation, dental casts, X-rays, photographs, and facial measurements. Several surgeries may be required before the desired outcome is achieved.

A sagittal split osteotomy may be performed to correct retrognathism or prognathism. An intraoral, gingival incision is made using a #15 blade on each mandibular ramus. Throughout the procedure, the mental nerve should be protected from possible injury. The horizontal ramus is exposed and the periosteum removed with a small periosteal elevator. A horizontal cut with a sagittal saw is made along the ascending ramus. The vertical cut is placed between the first and second molars. The split can be completed using a small osteotome. The jaw is moved into the new forward or backward position. The new position is held through rigid fixation. A variety of plates and screws can be used. The incision is closed with absorbable suture.

Genioplasties are performed to shorten the anterior portion of the mandible. An intraoral approach can be managed for this procedure. The vestibule is incised using a #15 blade and the mucosa is removed from the chin. The anterior mandible is cut horizontally with a sagittal saw. The bone is shortened and replaced onto the mandible. Rigid fixation is achieved. The mucosa is closed with absorbable suture.

PROCEDURE 18-7 Temporomandibular Joint Arthroscopy

Equipment

- Video tower, including monitor, VCR, color printer, camera, light source
- Bipolar electrosurgical unit
- Arthroscopic shaver control unit
- Fluid infusion system
- Electrosurgical unit with dispersive electrode
- Suction system

Instruments

- TMJ instrument set
- Small joint shaver
- Camera
- Light cord
- 0-, 30-, and 70-degree lenses

Supplies

- Pack: basic
- Basin: single
- Gloves
- Blades: #11 blade
- Drapes: head and neck
- Suture: according to surgeon's preference
- Drains: none

(continues)

PROCEDURE 18-7

Temporomandibular Joint Arthroscopy *(continued)*

- Dressings: adhesive bandage
- Drugs: according to surgeon's preference
- Miscellaneous:
  - Suction tubing
  - 30-in. extension tubing
  - Stopcock
  - Incise drape with fluid collection pouch
  - Gauze sponges
  - Assorted syringes
  - Lactated Ringer's solution (1000-cc bag)
  - 18-gauge 1½-in. needle

Operative Preparation

Anesthesia

- General
- Oral or nasal intubation may be performed
- Lubricate and protect the patient's eyes

Position

- Supine, with head turned to expose operative side
- Donut or foam headrest may be used for stabilization
- Arms tucked at patient's sides; protect ulnar nerves

Prep

- Hair is removed or restrained
- Face, chin, and neck are prepped with mild antiseptic. Protect eyes and ears from contact with prep solution. Do not dislocate breathing tube

Draping

- The operative area may be outlined with towels; the towels may be secured with adhesive, towel clips, skin staples, or suture
- A turban-style head wrap may be used
- Remove protective paper from disposable drapes with adhesive edges
- Place bar drape across patient's forehead, allowing remainder of drape to cover head of operating table
- Situate the U-drape under patient's chin. Bring the edges of the U lateral to the incision site. Extend the remainder of the drape to cover the patient's body
- Remove protective paper from incise drape. The mouth and nose will be covered and the area over the TMJ will be exposed. The fluid collection pouch will be in a dependant position

Practical Considerations

- TMJ arthroscopy may be performed bilaterally. Both sides of the face may be prepped and draped simultaneously according to the patient's size and surgeon's preference
- Preoperative X-rays will be displayed in the operating room

Operative Procedure	Technical Considerations
1. Irrigation solution is injected into the joint space to distend the capsule.	1. Lactated Ringer's solution is preloaded in syringe with needle attached.
2. A small stab incision is made (Figure 18-16).	2. A #11 blade on the #7 handle will be used.
3. The trocar/cannula assembly is inserted, the trocar removed, and the lens inserted.	3. Trocar/cannula is preassembled. Expect return of trocar. Be prepared to assist with the connections of video equipment.

PROCEDURE

18-7 Temporomandibular Joint Arthroscopy *(continued)*

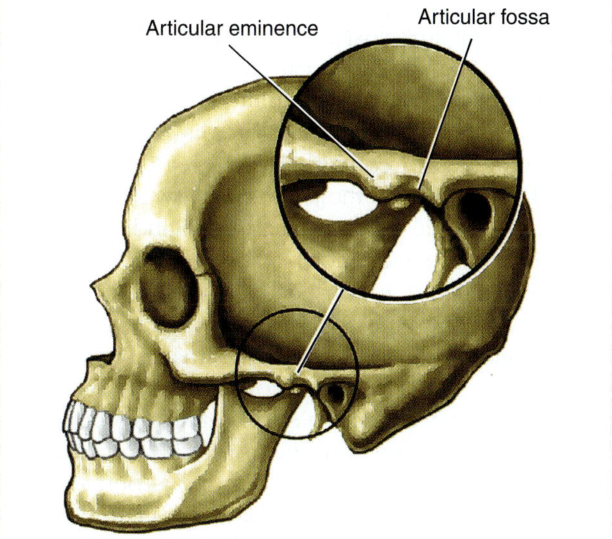

Figure 18-16 Temporomandibular joint

4. Irrigation solution is infused into the joint.	**4.** Lactated Ringer's solution is connected to the cannula via extension tubing.
5. The joint is examined.	**5.** Prepare to operate remote control for still photographs.
6. If functional surgery is required, a second stab wound is made.	**6.** Pass skin knife. Prepare additional equipment (probe, shaver, or grasper may be used).
7. Final visual inspection is performed.	**7.** Additional photos may be taken.
8. Cannulae are removed and excess fluid removed.	**8.** Prepare for closure. Count.
9. Wound is closed and dressing placed.	**9.** Pass suture of preference. Prepare dressings. Reorganize equipment and supplies if procedure is bilateral.
10. Procedure may be repeated on contralateral side.	**10.** Repeat previously described steps.

Postoperative Considerations

Immediate Postoperative Care

- Range of motion of the jaw may be limited. Extubation may be difficult. Suction and emergency airway supplies should be readily available.
- Application of ice may help reduce postoperative pain and swelling.
- Patient may be placed on a liquid or soft diet for several days postoperatively.

Prognosis

- Expected outcome is good.
- Recurrence is possible if contributing behavior is not resolved (e.g., grinding or clenching of teeth).

Complications

- Hemorrhage
- Infection
- Recurrence

PEARL OF WISDOM

This is one of those procedures where the STSR may be involved in numerous activities not commonly involved with the scrub role. The activities are technology driven. The STSR must understand the principles, procedures, and troubleshooting steps for all equipment involved in this procedure.

TEMPOROMANDIBULAR JOINT PROCEDURES

The temporomandibular joint can undergo several procedures. **Arthroscopy**, meniscal repairs, and joint replacements are the most common (Procedure 18-7).

MENISCUS REPAIR

The **meniscus** lies over the mandibular condyle. The meniscus is attached to the condyle by the external pterygoid muscle and the capsule. Due to stress on the joint, the meniscus can fray and tear. The meniscus can be reattached surgically and the frayed edges trimmed.

The patient is placed with the affected side up, the hair restrained, prepped, and draped. A preauricular incision is made with a #15 blade. The joint is exposed with Metzenbaum scissors and Adson-Brown pickups. Hemostasis is achieved. A Freer elevator can be used to gain additional exposure. Senn or Weitlaner retractors may be employed. The meniscus is examined and any perforations are closed with a 4–0 or 5–0 chromic or silk suture on a small cutting needle. The incision is closed and the wound dressed.

JOINT REPLACEMENT

The temporomandibular joint can be replaced with an artificial joint. These procedures are usually limited to severe cases of ankylosis. The replacement can involve bone graft. The bone graft can be an autogenous rib graft or homogenous fibular strut graft.

The affected side of the face is exposed and any hair is removed or contained. The area is prepped from behind the ear, down the jaw, and outward to the cheek. Inside, the auricle is gently cleansed. Mandibulomaxillary fixation (arch bar fixation) is used intraoperatively. A preauricular incision is used for joint replacement. This incision is made with a #15 blade and can be extended submandibularly if necessary. The area is dissected and retracted in the usual fashion. The condyle of the mandible is excised with a small sagittal saw. According to the patient's condition, the coronoid process may be resected as well. Once the ostectomy is performed, the prosthesis can be placed. The prosthesis can be of varying length, depending on the pathology of the patient. If the mandible is fractured or is diseased, a prosthesis with a longer body may be required. If a bone graft is utilized, the graft will be contoured to fit the patient's existing anatomy with a burr. The graft and/or prosthesis are positioned in the glenoid fossa, and the plate portion of the prosthesis is fixated to the mandible. The wound is closed and dressed; the mandibulomaxillary fixation is removed.

CASE STUDY

Gina is a young child. During her development her mother became concerned that "her head didn't look exactly right." She took Gina to her pediatrician. Gina was found to have bilateral coronal synostosis. Surgery has been scheduled to correct the condition.

1. What type incision will be used for this procedure?
2. What instrument sets will be required?
3. What is a craniotome and why is it on the instrument list?

QUESTIONS FOR FURTHER STUDY

1. Does the surgeon always stand while performing oral and maxillofacial procedures? If not, how does the choice to sit or stand affect patient positioning?
2. What is the particular danger created by operating in the area of the endotracheal tube? How is it minimized?
3. What graft materials can be used in maxillofacial surgery?
4. Describe the condition known as Pierre Robin syndrome.
5. What intraoperative measure may be taken to prevent drying and cracking of the patient's lips?
6. Why are rubber bands applied to arch bars?

BIBLIOGRAPHY

Alling, C. C., & Osborn, D. B. (1988). *Maxillofacial trauma*. Philadelphia: Lea & Febiger.

American Association of Oral and Maxillofacial Surgeons. (1998). *AAOMS news* [Online]. Available from *http://www.aaoms.org*

Blaustein, D. I., & Heffez, L. B. (1990). *Arthroscopic atlas of the temporomandibular joint*. Philadelphia: Lea & Febiger.

Borror, D. J. (1960). *Dictionary of word root and combining forms*. Mountain View, CA: Mayfield Publishing Co.

Boyne, P. (1997). *Osseous reconstruction of the maxilla and the mandible: Surgical techniques using titanium mesh and bone material*. Carol Stream, IL: Quintessence Books.

Gray, H. (1977). *Gray's anatomy* (16th ed.). New York: Bounty Books.

Kruger, G. O. (1984). *Oral and maxillofacial surgery* (6th ed.). St. Louis, MO: Mosby.

McGuiness, A. M., et al. (2002). *Core curriculum for surgical technology* (5th ed.). Centennial, CO: Association of Surgical Technologists.

Meeker, M. H., & Rothrock, J. C. (1991). *Alexander's care of the patient in surgery* (10th ed.). St. Louis, MO: Mosby.

Prein, J. (1998). *Manual of internal fixation in the cranio-facial skeleton*. New York: Springer.

Prosthodontics Intermedica. (1998). [Online]. Available from *http://www.members.aol.com/PITEAM/implants/index.html*

Riden, K. (1998). *Key topics in oral and maxillofacial surgery*. Oxford, UK: Bios Scientific.

Shier, D., Butler, J., & Lewis, R. (1996). *Hole's human anatomy and physiology* (7th ed.). Dubuque, IA: Wm. C. Brown.

Tortora, G. J., & Anagnostakos, N. P. (1987). *Principles of anatomy and physiology* (5th ed.). New York: Harper and Row.

Will, L. A. (1995). *Transverse maxillofacial deformities: Diagnosis and treatment*. Dallas, TX: University of Texas Southwestern Medical School.

CHAPTER 19

Plastic and Reconstructive Surgery

Teri Junge

CASE STUDY

Adriana was born just a few minutes ago. She has been diagnosed with cheiloschisis.

1. How was the diagnosis made?
2. Her mother views her as a "monster." What help can be provided for the family?
3. How will Adriana be nourished?
4. Is immediate surgery necessary?

OBJECTIVES

After studying this chapter, the reader should be able to:

A 1. Discuss the relevant anatomy and physiology of the skin and its underlying tissues.

P 2. Describe the pathology that prompts plastic/reconstructive surgical intervention and the related terminology.

3. Discuss any special preoperative plastic/reconstructive diagnostic procedures/tests.

O 4. Discuss any special preoperative preparation procedures related to plastic/reconstructive surgical procedures.

5. Identify the names and uses of plastic/reconstructive instruments, supplies, and drugs.
6. Identify the names and uses of special equipment related to plastic/reconstructive surgery.
7. Discuss the intraoperative preparation of the patient undergoing a plastic/reconstructive procedure.

8. Define and give an overview of the plastic/reconstructive procedure.
9. Discuss the purpose and expected outcomes of the plastic/reconstructive procedure.
10. Discuss the immediate postoperative care and possible complications of the plastic/reconstructive procedure.

S 11. Discuss any specific variations related to the preoperative, intraoperative, and postoperative care of the plastic/reconstructive patient.

SELECT KEY TERMS

1. aesthetic	7. dermatome	13. poly-	19. STSG
2. arthrodesis	8. elliptical	14. radial hypoplasia	20. syndactyly
3. augmentation	9. ganglion cyst	15. replantation	21. synthesis
4. carpal tunnel	10. gynecomastia	16. rhinoplasty	22. xenograft
5. cheilo-	11. integumentary	17. -schisis	
6. cleft	12. MPJ	18. sebum	

ANATOMY

The word *plastic* has its origins in the Greek *plastikos,* meaning to "mold or shape with one's hands." Plastic, or cosmetic, and reconstructive surgery refers to those procedures that have as a primary goal the restoration of appearance or function to a particular body structure. Unlike other surgical specialties that are restricted to specific anatomical systems (e.g., cardiovascular), plastic surgery encompasses a wide spectrum of many systems and structures, and often includes elements of other surgical specialties, such as vascular and orthopedics. Therefore, the surgical technologist participating in plastic/reconstructive surgery must have a strong foundation in human anatomy, as well as a working knowledge of the specialized instruments and supplies needed for the specific procedure.

SKIN AND UNDERLYING STRUCTURES

As the outer covering of the body, the skin, or cutaneous membrane, has several major responsibilities. These include:

- Protection from extrinsic forces, such as ultraviolet rays
- Defense against disease
- Preservation of fluid balance
- Body temperature maintenance
- Excretion of waste via sweat
- Sensory input through receptors for temperature, pain, touch, and pressure
- **Synthesis** of vitamin D

The **integumentary** system consists of two main layers. The outer layer is called the epidermis and the inner is the dermis (Figure 19-1).

EPIDERMIS

Depending on the location on the body, the epidermis consists of four to five layers called strata. The epidermis consists entirely of epithelial cells and contains no blood vessels or nerves. From innermost to outermost the layers are:

1. *Stratum basale:* This is the reproductive layer that derives its nourishment by diffusion from the capillaries of the dermis. Melanin, the pigment responsible for skin and hair color, is produced in this layer.
2. *Stratum spinosum:* This layer receives the daughter cells produced by mitosis in the stratum basale. These cells have a spiny or prickly appearance.

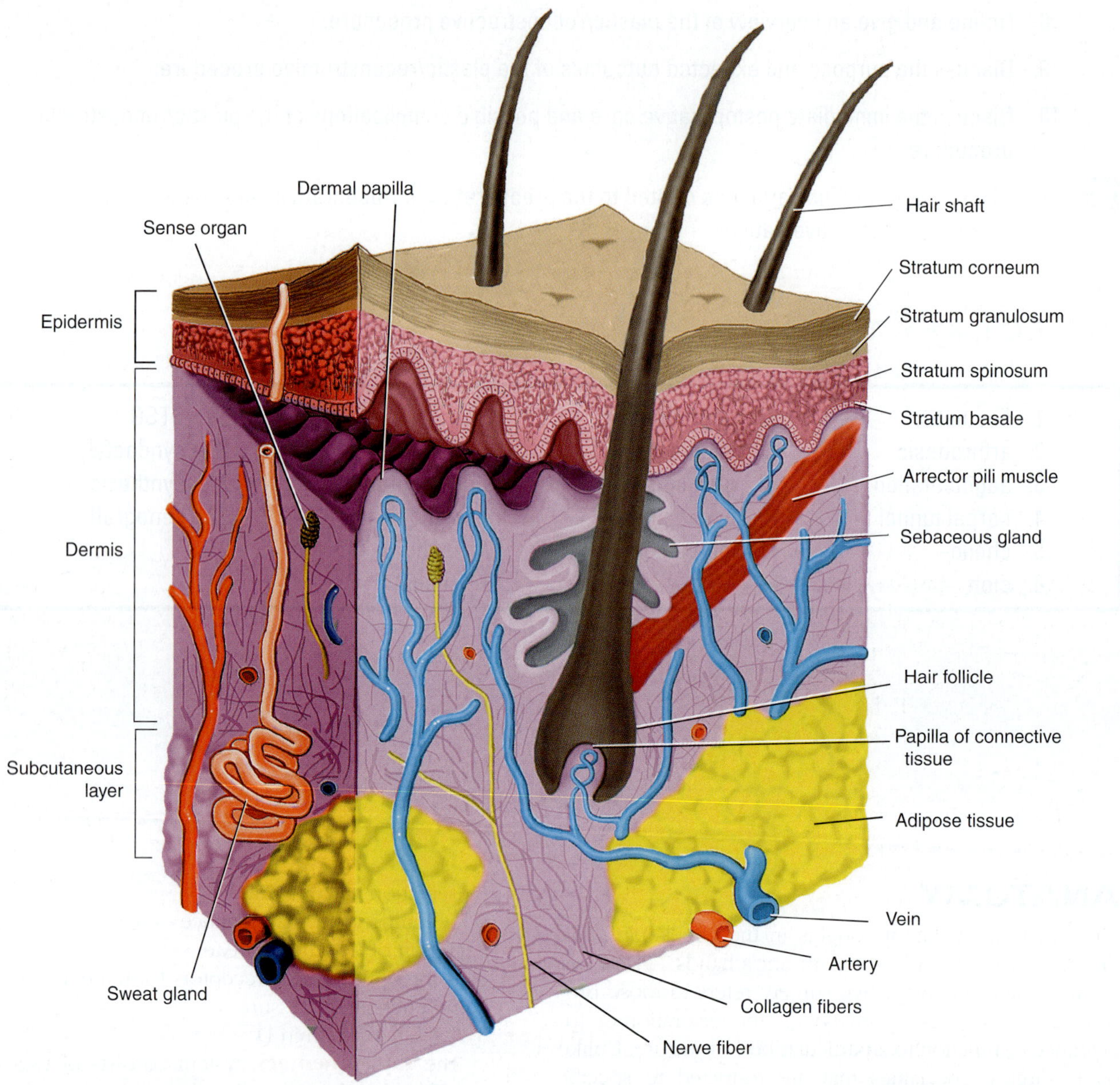

Figure 19-1 Structure of the skin

3. *Stratum granulosum:* As the spiny cells move toward the outer surface of the body, they begin to flatten and take on a granular shape. The process of keratinization begins in this layer. Keratin is a hard, fibrous, waterproof protein that is found in the hair, nails, and epidermis.
4. *Stratum lucidum:* This layer is present only in thick skin areas such as the palms of the hands and soles of the feet.
5. *Stratum corneum:* This layer consists of approximately twenty layers of cells in various stages of disintegration. As the cell dries and becomes scaly, the keratin remains. The cells of the stratum corneum are pressed tightly together; as they reach the body surface they are shed or sloughed.

The epidermis is constantly proliferating and shedding. The newly formed epithelial cells are pushed to the body surface and shed by the thousands each day. The entire process takes approximately 5 weeks.

DERMIS

The dermis, or stratum corium, is connective tissue that is located under the epidermis. The nerves and blood vessels that supply the skin, along with hair follicles, nails, and certain glands, are embedded in the dermal layer. The dermis has two distinct divisions.

1. *Reticular layer:* This is the thick, deep layer that provides collagen for strength and elastin for pliability of the skin.
2. *Papillary layer:* This layer is named for its papilla, or projections, which are the groundwork for fingerprints.

SUBCUTANEOUS LAYER

The subcutaneous layer is not actually considered part of the skin, but serves to anchor the skin to the underlying structures. The subcutaneous layer, or hypodermis, consists of adipose (fat) and loose connective tissue providing insulation and protection to the internal organs.

ACCESSORY STRUCTURES TO THE INTEGUMENTARY SYSTEM

The hair, nails, and certain glands are referred to as accessory structures to the integumentary system. They all are derived from the stratum basale of the epidermis and are found embedded in the reticular layer of the dermis.

Hair is found on most body surfaces. The exceptions are the palms of the hands, soles of the feet, distal portions of the fingers and toes, parts of the external genitalia, nipples, and lips. The hair itself is made up of dead keratinized epithelial cells. The hair extends from a shaft that is embedded in the dermis and extends through the epidermis.

The nails are composed of an extremely hard type of keratin that is a thin plate of dead stratum corneum. The nails cover the dorsal surfaces of the distal ends of the toes and fingers. Stratum basale in the nail bed is responsible for its production.

Sebaceous glands are the oil-producing glands. The oil that is produced is called **sebum** and reaches the skin surface through ducts that enter the hair follicle. Sebum helps with fluid regulation and also acts to keep the skin and hair soft and pliable. Sebaceous gland activity is stimulated by sex hormones, which explains the lack of sebum in children, the dramatic increase in production at puberty, and the gradual decrease that occurs during the aging process.

The sudoriferous glands are the sweat glands. There are two main types of sudoriferous glands. Merocrine sweat glands are distributed over most of the body and open directly to the skin surface through small openings called pores. This type of sweat gland secretes primarily water with some salts. The merocrine glands are stimulated to produce sweat or perspiration by heat or emotional stress.

Apocrine sweat glands are larger than the merocrine glands; their location is limited to the external genitalia and the axillae. The ducts of the apocrine glands open through the hair follicles into these regions. The secretion from this type of sweat gland consists of water and some salts, but also includes some organic compounds (proteins and fatty acids). Apocrine glands become active at puberty and are stimulated by pain, emotional stress, and sexual arousal.

The third type of sweat gland, the ceruminous gland, is a specialized version found only in the external auditory canal. The secretion, called cerumen, is commonly known as earwax.

The few locations that have no sweat glands are portions of the external genitalia, nipples, and lips.

PALATE

The palate is the roof of the mouth. The anterior portion, which is referred to as the hard palate, consists of the palatine processes of each maxilla and the palatine bones. The hard palate is covered with mucous membrane. The posterior portion is referred to as the soft palate, and is composed of muscle, fat, and mucous membrane. The soft palate terminates with the uvula at the fauces, or opening into the oropharynx. The function of the palate is to separate the nose from the mouth. This is important in swallowing and speech.

DEVELOPMENT OF THE LIP AND PALATE

Fetal development of the nose and mouth occurs during the first trimester of intrauterine life. The lips and palate develop from three prominences of the baby's developing face. The forehead, nose, palatine processes of the maxillary bone, and middle portion of the upper lip develop from the central or frontal nasal prominence. The left and right maxillary prominences form the lower face, upper lip, and the remainder of the upper jaw (Figure 19-2). During normal development, these three prominences move toward the center of the face to form the nose, upper lip, maxillary ridges (including the palatine processes), and the palate.

NOSE

For a comprehensive review of nasal anatomy, refer to Chapter 17.

HAND

The hand is made up of three regions: the wrist, the palm, and the fingers. Specific directional terms are also used in reference to the hand. Using the anatomical position, palms forward, the terms are as follows:

- *Volar surface:* palm of the hand
- *Dorsal surface or dorsum:* back of the hand

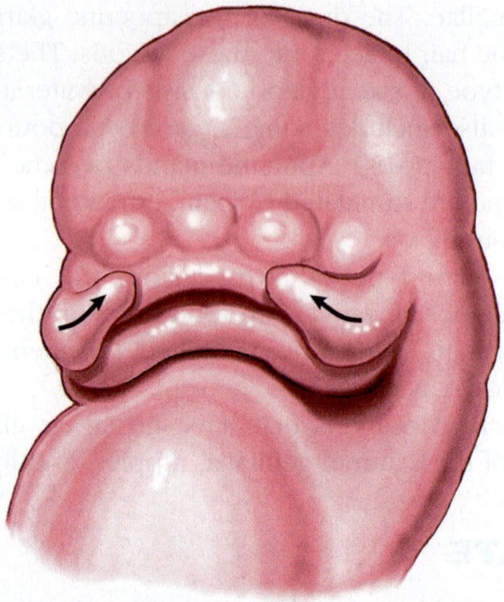

Figure 19-2 Development of the face

- *Radial:* refers to thumb side of the hand
- *Ulnar:* refers to the medial side of the hand

BONES OF THE HAND

Eight carpal bones compose each wrist, or carpus. They are arranged in two rows (proximal and distal) consisting of four bones each. From lateral to medial, the scaphoid, lunate, triquetral, and pisiform bones compose the proximal row. Listed from lateral to medial, the bones in the distal row are the trapezium, trapezoid, capitate, and the hamate. Proximally, the carpal bones articulate with the distal radius and the distal radioulnar joint, commonly known as the wrist (Figure 19-3).

The metacarpals are the bones of the palm, or metacarpus. There are five metacarpal bones in each hand. They are numbered I through V, the first correlating with the thumb. The metacarpals are long, cylinder-

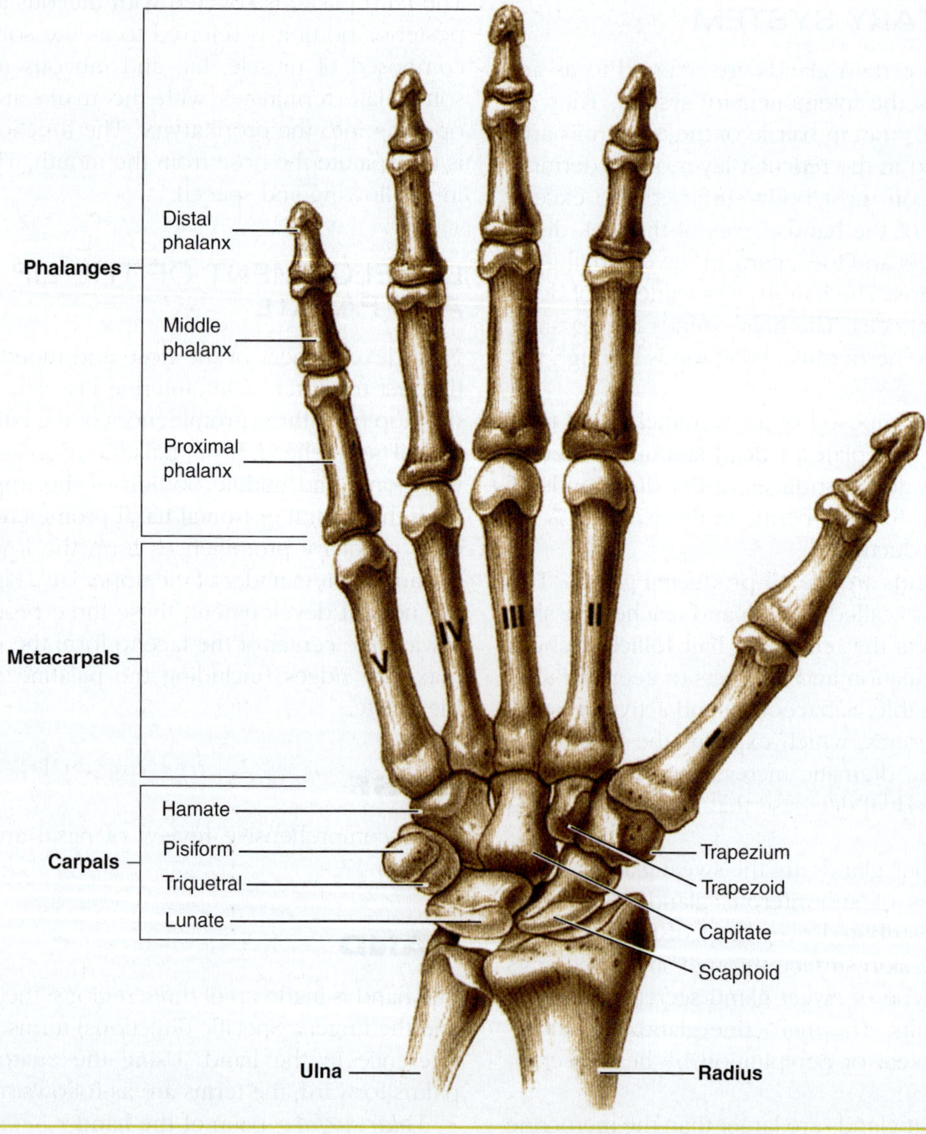

Figure 19-3 Bones of the hand

shaped shafts. The proximal end is referred to as the base and the distal portion forms the head.

Each digit, or finger, is made up of a series of phalanges. There are 14 phalanges in each hand. Each digit has 3 phalanges, with the exception of the thumb, which only has 2. The phalanges are named according to the order of their placement. The phalanx closest to the metacarpal is called the proximal, next is the medial, and the farthest is referred to as distal. As with the metacarpals, the digits are numbered, the thumb being called the first digit.

The head of each metacarpal articulates with one of the phalanges. These joints are considered *diarthroses,* or freely movable joints, and are synovial hinge-type joints called metacarpophalangeal joints (**MPJ**), which are commonly referred to as the knuckles. The same type of joint is formed between the phalanges and is called an interphalangeal joint (IPJ). Refer to Chapter 21 for a complete description of the types of joints.

INNERVATION OF THE HAND

The nerves that serve the forearm and the hand are all branches of nerves from the brachial plexus. The three nerves that we will be concerned with are the radial, median, and ulnar (Figure 19-4).

The radial nerve travels along the radius and provides feeling to the skin of the forearm and hand and also innervates the extensor muscles of the forearm.

The median nerve branches into two main sections that innervate the skin of the lateral two-thirds of the hand, flexor muscles of the forearm, and several intrinsic muscles of the hand.

The ulnar nerve provides feeling to the skin of the medial third of the hand and some of the flexor muscles of the hand and wrist.

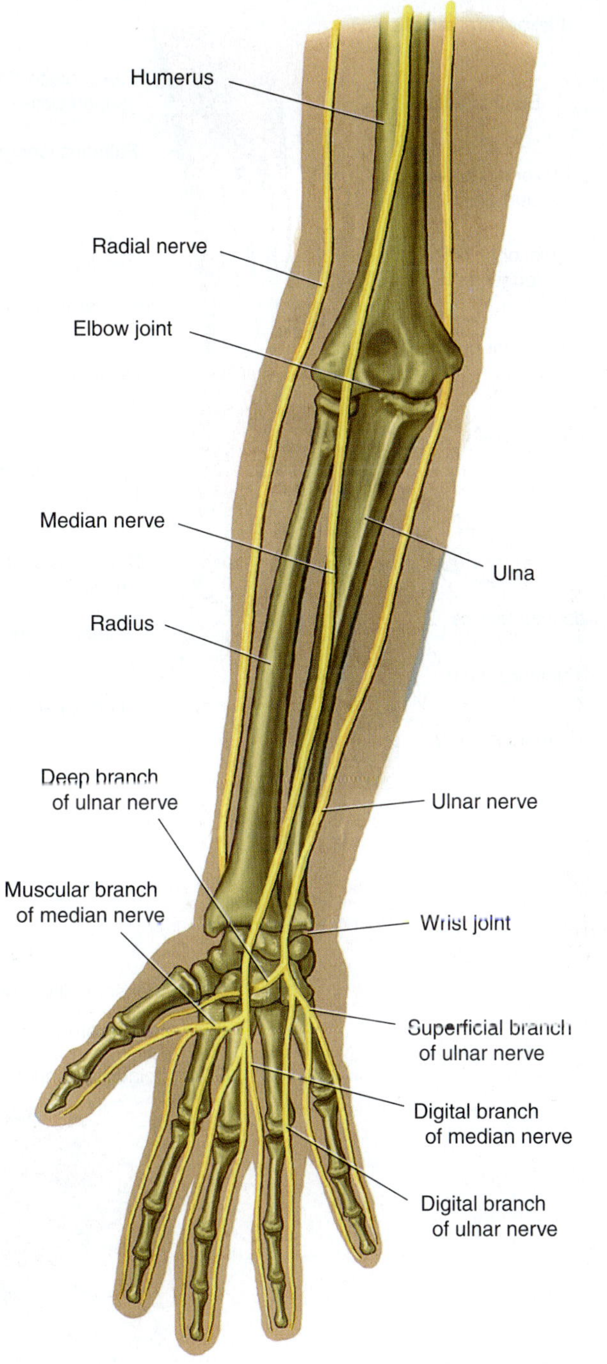

Figure 19-4 Innervation of the hand

MUSCLES AND TENDONS OF THE HAND

Almost 40 muscles and their coordinating tendons are responsible for movement of the wrist, hand, and fingers (Table 19-1). Most of the muscles on the anterior aspect of the hand are responsible for flexion; those located posteriorly control extension (Figure 19-5).

COMPARTMENTS/TUNNELS

On the anterior, or palm, side of the hand there is one main compartment or tunnel. This is the passageway in the wrist that is surrounded on three sides by the carpal bones and covered anteriorly by the transverse carpal ligament. Nine flexor tendons and the median nerve pass through this tunnel (Figure 19-6).

Dorsally, there are six compartments. The tendons for the muscles that extend the fingers and thumb and dorsiflex the hand separate and pass through these tunnels. The compartments are lined with synovial membrane. The synovium secretes a fluid that lubricates the compartment to reduce friction. The *dorsal carpal ligament* collectively covers the compartments.

TENDON SHEATHS/PULLEYS

The tendons of the fingers and thumbs are contained in a protective covering called a tendon sheath. The tendon

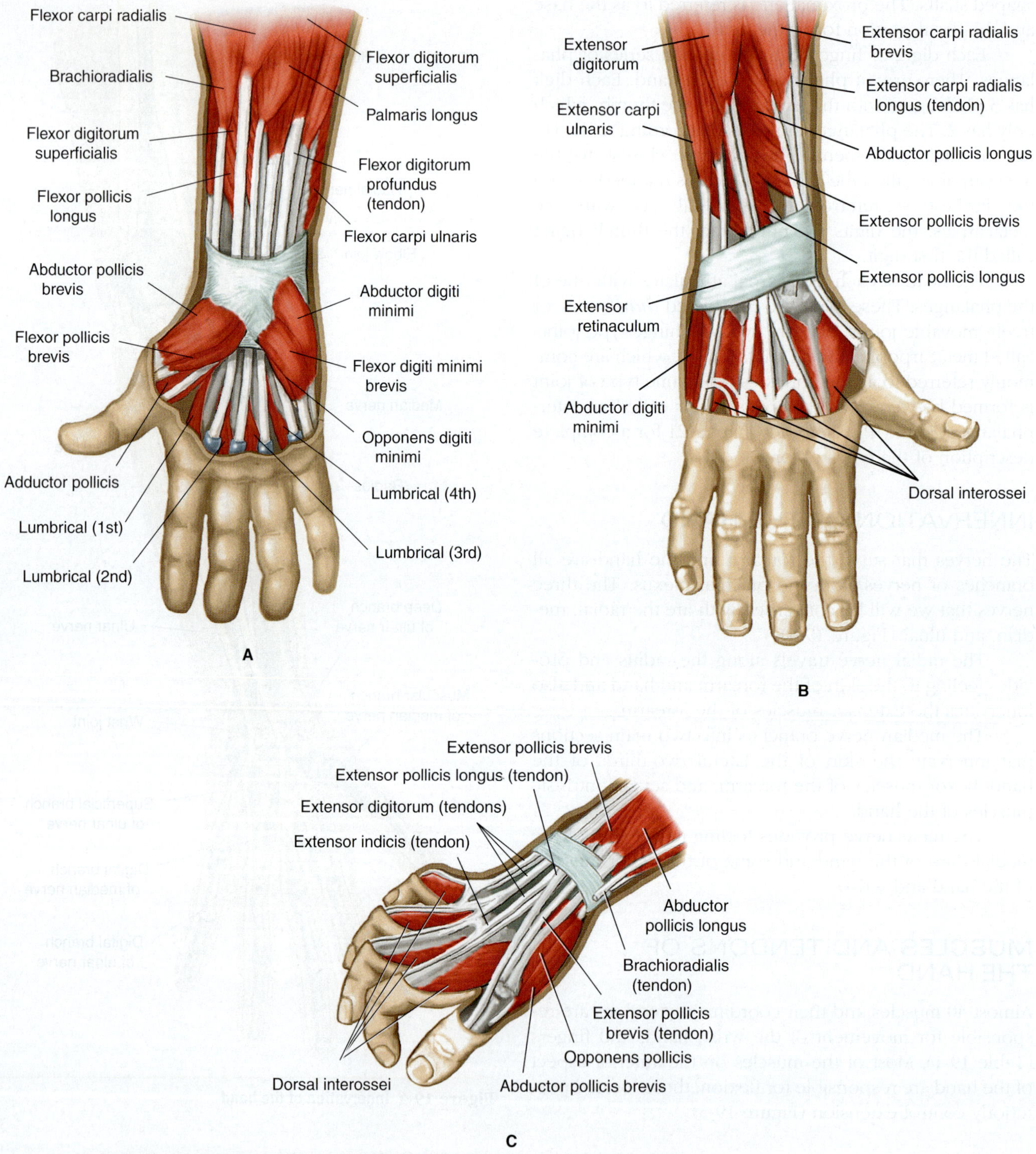

Figure 19-5 Muscles of the forearm and hand: (A) Anterior view, (B) dorsal view, (C) posteromedial view

Table 19-1 Muscles and Tendons of the Hand

NAME	ACTION	INNERVATION
DEEP AND SUPERFICIAL FLEXOR MUSCLES LOCATED IN THE FOREARM		
Flexor carpi radialis	Abducts and flexes hand at wrist	Median nerve
Palmaris longus	Flexes hand at wrist	Median nerve
Flexor carpi ulnaris	Adducts and flexes hand at wrist	Ulnar nerve
Flexor digitorum superficialis	Flexes IPJs and MPJs of medial four digits Flexes hand at wrist	Median nerve
Flexor digitorum profundus	Flexes distal IPJs of medial four digits Assists in flexion of proximal IPJs of medial four digits Flexes hand at wrist	Ulnar and median nerves
Flexor pollicis longus	Flexes IPJ and MPJ of thumb Assists in flexion of hand at wrist	Median nerve
DEEP AND SUPERFICIAL EXTENSOR MUSCLES LOCATED IN THE FOREARM		
Extensor carpi radialis longus	Extends and abducts hand at wrist	Radial nerve
Extensor carpi radialis brevis	Extends and abducts hand at wrist	Radial nerve
Extensor digitorum	Extends digits at IPJs and MPJs Extends hand at wrist	Radial nerve
Extensor digiti minimi	Extends MPJ and IPJs of fifth digit	Radial nerve
Extensor carpi ulnaris	Assists in extension and adduction of hand at wrist	Radial nerve
Abductor pollicis longus	Abducts and extends thumb at carpometacarpal joint	Radial nerve
Extensor pollicis brevis	Extends thumb at carpometacarpal and metacarpophalangeal joints	Radial nerve
Extensor pollicis longus	Extends metacarpophalangeal and IPJ of thumb Assists in abduction and lateral rotation of extended thumb	Radial nerve
Extensor indicis	Extends second digit at MPJ Assists in extension of hand at wrist	Radial nerve
MUSCLES OF ROTATION		
Pronator teres	Pronates forearm; assisted by pronator quadratus	Median nerve
Pronator quadratus	Pronates forearm; assisted by pronator teres	Median nerve
Supinator	Supinates forearm	Radial nerve
INTRINSIC MUSCLES OF THE HAND (20)		
Adductor pollicis	Adducts thumb	Ulnar nerve
Muscles of the Thenar Eminence (prominence on lateral, or thumb, side of palm)		
Abductor pollicis brevis	Abducts thumb	Median nerve
Opponens pollicis	Opposes thumb	Median nerve
Flexor pollicis brevis	Flexes thumb at carpometacarpal and metacarpophalangeal joints	Median nerve
Muscles of the Hypothenar Eminence (prominence on medial, or little finger, side of palm)		
Abductor digiti minimi	Abducts fifth digit	Ulnar nerve
Flexor digiti minimi brevis	Flexes fifth digit at metacarpophalangeal joint	Ulnar nerve
Opponens digiti minimi	Brings fifth digit into opposition with thumb	Ulnar nerve
Palmaris brevis	Deepens hollow (cup) of palm	Ulnar nerve
Lumbrical Muscles (4)		
Lumbricals	Flexes medial four digits at MPJs	Median and ulnar nerves
Interossei Muscles		
Dorsal interossei (4)	Abducts medial four digits	Ulnar nerve
Palmar interossei (4)	Adducts medial four digits	Ulnar nerve

Source: From *Human Anatomy and Physiology,* 2nd ed., by E. Solomon, R. Schmidt, and P. Adragna, Eds., 1990, Ft. Worth: Saunders College Publishing.

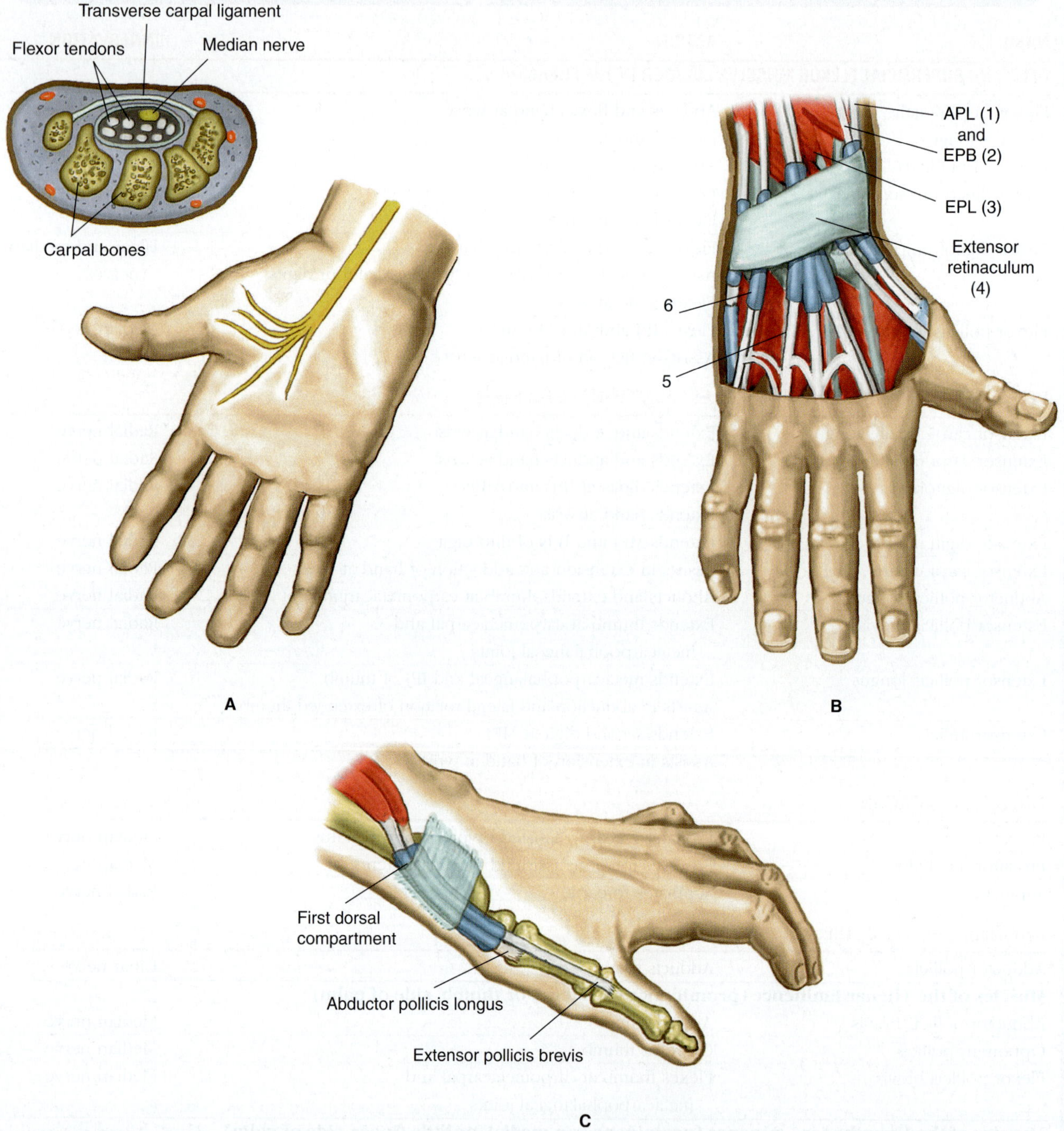

Figure 19-6 Compartments of the hand: (A) Anterior compartment with transverse section, (B) dorsal compartments (six), (C) first dorsal compartment

sheaths are lined with synovium. Pulleys or annular bands are attached to the bones at intervals along the tendon sheath. Their purpose is to hold the tendons in approximation to the bones they pass over (Figure 19-7).

CIRCULATION OF THE HAND

Two main arteries serve the distal portion of the upper extremities. The brachial artery divides to form the radial and ulnar arteries just distal to the elbow joint. The radial artery travels along the radius and serves the lateral aspect of the forearm. The ulnar artery provides arterial blood to the medial side of the forearm and descends along the ulna. Branches of these two arteries anastomose at two levels forming the deep palmar and superficial palmar arches. The individual arteries that serve each of the digits arise from these arches. The blood then travels through the capillary network and returns via the venous network.

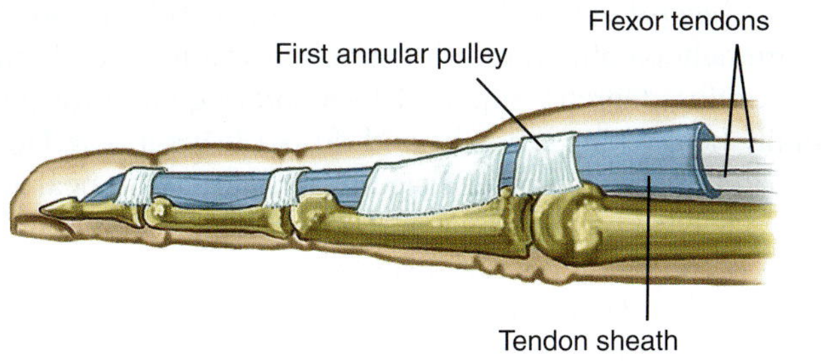

Figure 19-7 Tendon sheath and pulleys

The venous network is slightly more complex than the arterial delivery system. The names of the major veins in the hand and forearm directly correlate with the arteries (Figure 19-8).

DEVELOPMENT OF THE HAND

Embryological development of the human hand begins on the 26th day after conception with the formation of a small arm bud that protrudes from the upper torso. This

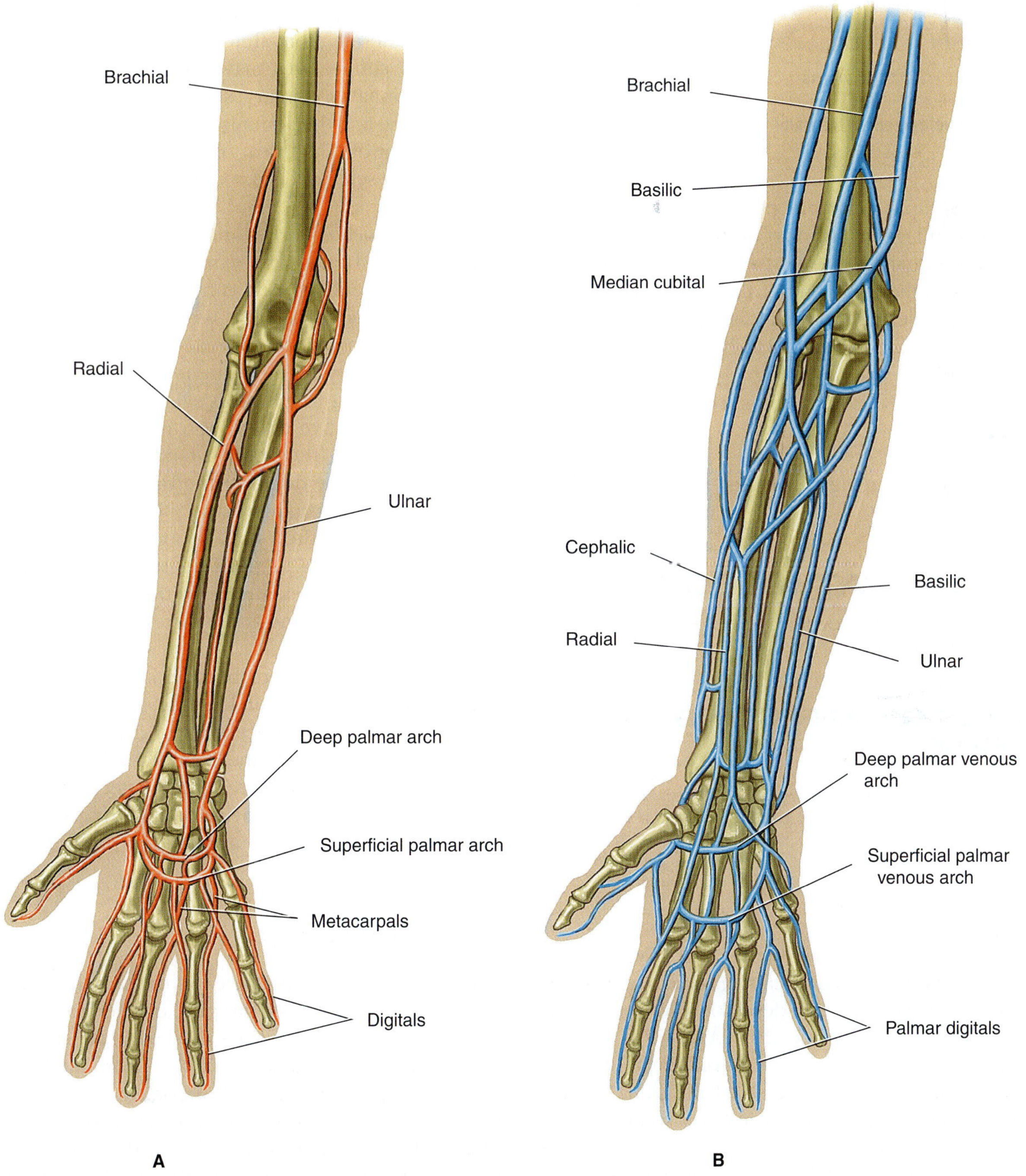

Figure 19-8 Blood vessels of the forearm and hand: (A) Arteries, (B) veins

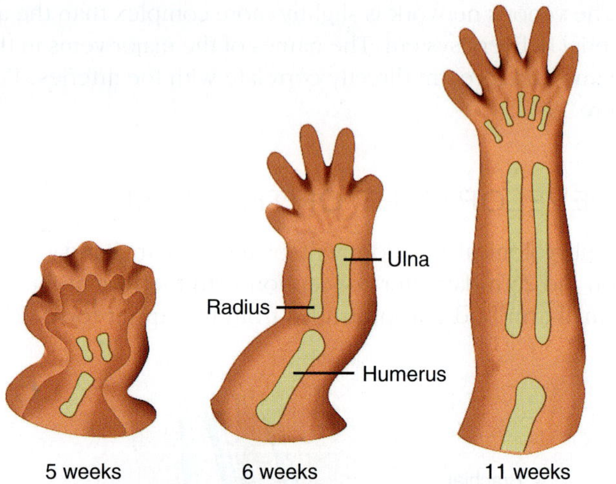

Figure 19-9 Development of the hand

bud undergoes rapid enlargement, neurovascular development, and cartilage formation. On the 33rd day, a paddle that will eventually represent the palm and individual digits appears on the distal end of the emerging arm. By the 54th day of development the individual digits are separated. The upper limb is complete by the 8th week *in utero* (Figure 19-9).

BREAST

For a comprehensive review of breast anatomy, refer to Chapter 14.

SURGICAL PATHOLOGY

Here we will examine specific pathologies leading to plastic surgical intervention.

PATHOLOGY AFFECTING THE SKIN

Several normal and pathological conditions of the skin may cause the patient to seek plastic and/or reconstructive surgery.

BURNS

A burn is an injury that can be derived from several sources. Heat, radiation, chemicals, gases, or electricity may cause tissue damage. The depth of a burn is classified according to degree (Figure 19-10A).

First-degree burns affect just the epidermis. They are characterized by erythema (redness of the skin) but do not blister. Healing takes place in about a week and no scar tissue formation is expected. The patient may desire to treat the affected area with a topical ointment to help control the mild pain and keep the area from drying.

Second-degree burns are those that blister and are extremely painful. Second-degree burns affect the dermis to varying degrees. Superficial second-degree burns generally heal within 2 weeks and do not leave a scar. Deep second-degree burns take significantly longer to heal and often leave a hypertrophic scar. Debridement and grafting may be recommended if healing is delayed.

Third-degree burns completely penetrate the full thickness of the skin and often affect the underlying structures. Permanent tissue damage occurs. Third-degree burns may be very painful or may be considered painless if the nerves are destroyed. Third-degree burns appear charred or pearly white; they are referred to as *eschars*. Patients suffering from third-degree burns that cover a large body surface area may need respiratory support if there is an inhalation injury, shock management with fluid replacement, and the administration of narcotic analgesics for pain control. The threat of infection is great. Debridement of the eschar and subsequent skin grafting is usually necessary.

Fourth-degree burns are referred to as char burns. Fourth-degree burns often damage blood vessels, nerves, muscles, and tendons, and can even affect bone density. Surgery to remove necrotic tissue is almost always required and reconstruction is extensive.

The severity of the patient's condition is also assessed according to the Abbreviated Burn Severity Index (ABSI). The five criteria for this assessment are the age of the patient, the sex of the patient, presence of inhalation injury, the depth of the burn (according to degree), and the percentage of total body surface burned. There are two ways to estimate body surface area (BSA) affected by second- or third-degree burns. The Lund-Browder method uses a chart with variables according to age. The rule of nines uses increments of 9% BSA, as shown in Table 19-2.

Patients with severe burns will require immediate intensive therapy to sustain life. They will also most likely need several surgical procedures to debride the wounds and provide coverage to the denuded areas by means of skin grafting, and even more surgery later to restore function and appearance. Individuals suffering from severe burns may also benefit from long-term physical and psychological therapy.

ACNE VULGARIS

Acne is an inflammatory disease of the skin that causes the formation of pustules, or pimples, on the face, neck, and upper body. The adolescent is most often affected; the disease progression is associated with hormonal changes, diet, and stress. Increased hormone activity causes an increase in the secretion from the sebaceous glands. Sebum and dead skin cells may block the exit to the skin from the gland. Bacteria infect the blocked passageway and cause the pustule formation. *Corynebacterium acnes,*

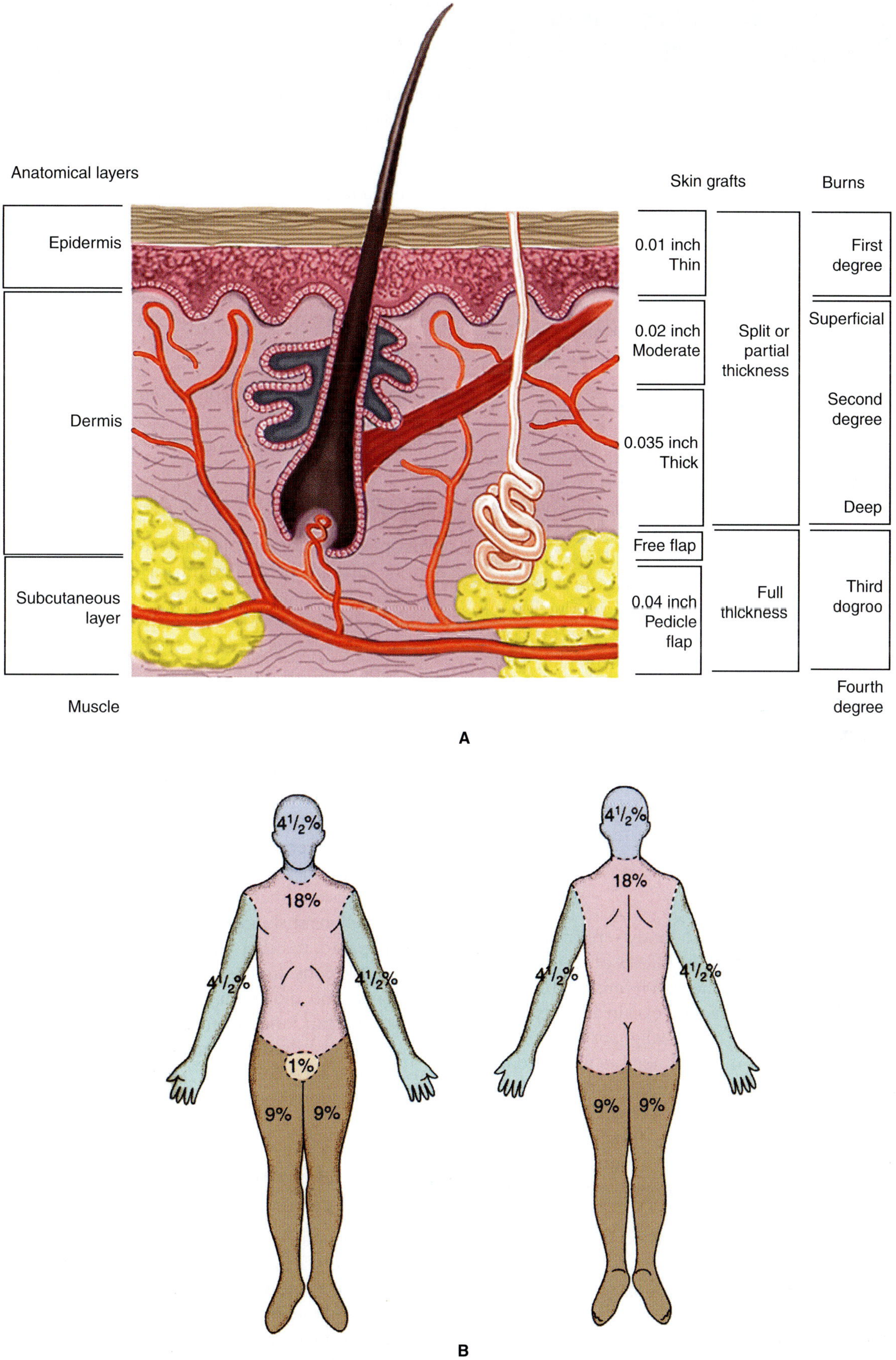

Figure 19-10 (A) Burn depth, (B) rule of nines

Table 19-2 Rule of Nines
Head and neck—9%
Anterior and posterior trunk—18% each
Upper extremity—9%
Lower extremity—18%
Perineum—1%

Staphylococcus albus, and *Pityrosporon ovale* are the three main causative agents. Unfortunately, the pustules leave deep pits and scars on the skin. Acne can be controlled with lifestyle adjustments as well as medication. Surgical intervention may be desired to remove pits and scars.

AGING

Signs of aging are seen throughout all body systems, but are externally noticeable primarily on the skin and especially on the face. As the patient ages, elastic fibers decrease in number and adipose tissue is lost, causing wrinkling and sagging; collagen fibers are lost, slowing healing; the mitotic activity of the stratum basale slows and the skin becomes thinner; and glandular production of sweat and sebum decreases causing drying. Patients complain of several problems. The four main complaints seem to be loose skin, fine lines, exaggeration of normal features, and bagginess around the eyes. These conditions may cause severe impairment for the patient. For example, dermachalasis may restrict vision. Or, the patient may desire to change his or her appearance. A wide range of options, from conservative (nonsurgical) to radical (highly invasive), are available to solve some of these problems.

Sun Exposure

Exposure to sunlight speeds the body's normal aging process and also has some serious effects of its own. Exposure to sunlight thickens the epidermis and causes damage to the elastin. The damaged elastin allows for the formation of premalignant and malignant cells. Fair-skinned individuals are far more vulnerable to skin damage from the sun than those with darker complexions.

The damaging component of sunlight is ultraviolet (UV) radiation. There are three types or bands of ultraviolet radiation, which are measured in nanometers (nm):

- *Type A (UVA 320–400 nm):* potentially as harmful as type B
- *Type B (UVB 290–320 nm):* associated with sunburn and skin cancer
- *Type C (UVC 200–290 nm):* danger increases as ozone layer diminishes

Prevention with sunscreen is the best form of treatment, although sun-damaged skin can be resurfaced pharmaceutically or surgically.

Eyelids

Several conditions affecting the eyelids may require surgical intervention for functional or cosmetic reasons. A limited list of examples follows.

Blepharochalasis is a lack of tone or relaxation of the skin of the eyelid causing the lid to appear thin and wrinkled. This often occurs in young people; the result of surgical intervention is usually poor.

Dermachalasis is relaxation and hypertrophy of the eyelid skin. Often in association with dermachalasis is the relaxation of the fascial bands that connect the skin to the orbicularis muscle causing a "bag." This disorder has been linked to sun exposure and age. The condition is easily corrected with surgery.

Ptosis is a drooping of the lid due to weakness or paralysis of the levator oculi. A muscle-shortening procedure is done to repair the ptosis. A blepharoplasty may be performed at the same time.

NEOPLASMS

A neoplasm is any type of new or abnormal growth; it may be benign, premalignant, or malignant. Neoplasms can be congenital or acquired; acquisition may be through direct contact or indirectly from exposure to certain chemicals or to the sun. Several types of neoplasms may appear on the skin.

Examples of benign skin lesions are warts, cysts, moles, granulomas, and hypertrophic scars. The incidence of noncancerous lesions is common and removal simple. The methods used for removal may include chemicals, lasers, and minor surgery.

Premalignant lesions may become malignant over time. Surgical removal is necessary for diagnostic purposes. Dysplastic nevi and actinic keratosis are two examples of lesions that fall into this category.

A malignant skin lesion has the potential to metastasize, or spread, to other parts of the body. Some common malignant lesions are basal cell carcinoma, squamous cell carcinoma, and melanoma. The treatment for cancerous skin lesions can range from simple excision with no further treatment to radical removal (which may lead to reconstructive surgery) along with supportive treatments such as radiation therapy and/or chemotherapy.

CLEFT LIP AND PALATE

A **cleft** is a split or a gap between two structures that are normally joined. **Cheilo**schisis (cleft or hare lip) and palato**schisis** (cleft palate) are two congenital deformities that can occur individually and are often seen in conjunction with one another (Figure 19-11). The cleft can be unilateral or bilateral. When a disruption in normal fetal development causes the three prominences that should fuse to form the midface to remain separated, a "cleft" oc-

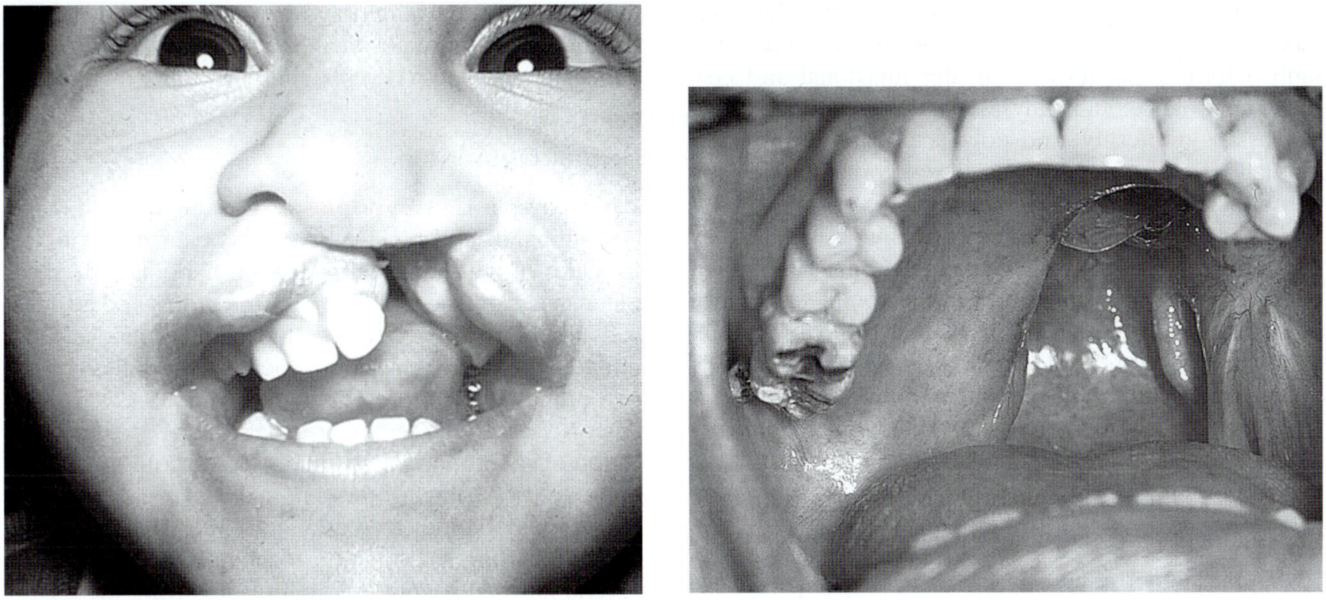

A B

Figure 19-11 Cleft lip and palate: (A) Unilateral cleft lip, (B) unilateral cleft palate ***(Courtesy of Dr. Joseph L. Konzelman, School of Dentistry, Medical College of Georgia)***

curs. The cleft may affect just the upper lip, just the palate, or a combination of both structures, depending on which stage of fetal development was affected. Cleft lip and palate occur as often as 1 in every 500 live births. It has been determined that only 20% of cleft deformities are genetic. The remaining 80% are attributed to maternal age and certain environmental factors that may include cigarette smoking, drug and alcohol abuse, infection, and vitamin deficiencies. Often palliative treatment, such as the use of special nipples for feeding, is implemented. This allows the definitive surgery to be delayed until the infant is older and stronger. This condition may be accompanied by other more severe congenital problems that may require immediate intervention. Cheiloplasty and palatoplasty can be performed in combination to correct the deformities. The surgical repairs are often planned when the child is between 7 and 18 months of age, depending on the individual situation. The infant with this type of deformity may suffer from difficulty sucking, swallowing, and eventually forming proper sounds. A variety of appliances is available to seal the defect, allowing the patient to suck prior to repair. Following corrective surgery, the child will most likely need speech therapy and orthodontia. Nasal deformities are often a result of this condition, and rhinoplasty may be considered when the nose has matured.

PATHOLOGY AFFECTING THE HAND

Congenital deformities, disease, or trauma may cause changes to the appearance and/or impairment of the function of the hand. Some of the more common problems will be discussed in this chapter. You will find information on **carpal tunnel** syndrome in Chapter 24.

CONGENITAL ANOMALIES OF THE HAND

Congenital limb deformities are often seen in association with a number of other nonrelated abnormalities. Two acronyms are used to describe this "family" of birth defects (Table 19-3).

Patients who fall into these categories generally have seven to eight abnormalities each. Fortunately, central nervous system disorders and mental retardation seldom accompany these syndromes. Often the limb deformity is considered a minor problem in the whole

Table 19-3 Birth Defects

VACTERL	VATER
V—vertebral	V—vertebral, vascular
A—anal atresia	A—anal atresia
C—cardiac	T—tracheoesophageal fistula
T—tracheoesophageal fistula	E—esophageal atresia (± tracheoesophageal fistula)
E—esophageal atresia	R—renal anomalies, radial dysplasia
R—renal anomalies	
L—limb anomalies	

scope of things at the time of birth, but as the child gets older and other more severe problems are solved, the limb deformity becomes of greater functional and cosmetic importance. Radial dysplasia, thumb and radial hypoplasia, **syndactyly**, and polydactyly are all disorders that fall into this category. For more information, see the website at www.vaterconnection.org.

Congenital hand deformities fall into a wide variety of categories. The spectrum may range from a simple partial duplication of a single digit to the complete absence of an entire structure. The anomaly may be an isolated incident or may be related to a larger systemic problem or generalized syndrome. The International Federation of Hand Societies has classified congenital upper limb deformities in the following manner:

1. Failure of formation of parts (arrested development)
2. Failure of differentiation (separation) of parts
3. Duplication of parts
4. Overgrowth (giantism or hyperplasia)
5. Undergrowth (hypoplasia)
6. Congenital constriction band syndrome
7. Generalized skeletal abnormalities

The incidence of hand deformities has shown little change in number over the past few decades. Depending on the type of deformity, the frequency of congenital hand anomalies varies greatly. Duplication of digits has been recorded in as many as 1 in 300 births, while major skeletal absences appear in as few as 1 out of 100,000.

The cause of some deformities remains unknown, while others represent well-documented environmental or genetic problems. Some environmental factors include maternal exposure to an infection (such as rubella) during the pregnancy and ingestion of certain medications (such as thalidomide that was prescribed in the 1950s for nausea associated with the first trimester of pregnancy) or chemical substances (such as alcohol). Chromosomal defects causing certain syndromes, such as Down syndrome, often have related anomalies of the upper extremity.

Surgical intervention may be required to correct congenital defects of the hand. Often, more than one surgical procedure and long-term physical therapy may be necessary for the patient to achieve maximum function. Adaptive equipment, such as the use of prosthetic devices, will frequently be a necessary adjunct to surgical intervention. The extent of correction possible, as well as the timing of the surgery, is affected by several variables, including:

- Age of the patient
- Neurovascular involvement
- Involvement of adjoining structures
- Relationship of defect to epiphyseal (growth) plates
- Ability of the patient to perform specific gross and fine motor tasks

An individual suffering from a congenital defect determined to be chromosomal in nature may wish to seek genetic counseling when planning his or her own family.

Radial Dysplasia

Radial dysplasia or **hypoplasia** is commonly referred to as "clubhand" and is often seen in conjunction with deformities of the thumb ranging from hypoplasia to complete absence. Due to a failure of the radius and adjacent soft tissues to fully develop, the hand is medially deranged. The degree of derangement is determined by the size of the radius, if present at all (Figure 19-12).

Neonatal intervention is usually limited to the application of splints and passive range-of-motion exercises to improve or maintain the baseline level of function. Surgery may be indicated at a later time. This may be as simple as using a distraction technique, or may require several intricate surgical procedures involving the elbow, wrist, and hand.

Syndactyly

Syndactyly, or webbed digits, occurs when the digits of the hands or feet fail to separate. Any combination of two or more digits may be partially or completely connected and the condition may affect one or more extremities. This may be a simple connection of the skin or may be more complex involving conjoined bone and fingernails (Figure 19-13).

Web deformities are usually surgically separated creating individual digits. Skin grafting may be required.

Polydactyly

A duplication of the digits is referred to as **poly**dactyly. This can be a partial or complete additional digit or digits, it may affect the hands and/or feet, and it may be unilateral or bilateral. Involvement of the metacarpal or metatarsal bones is rare. The condition usually involves just the phalangeal bones. Or the duplication may consist

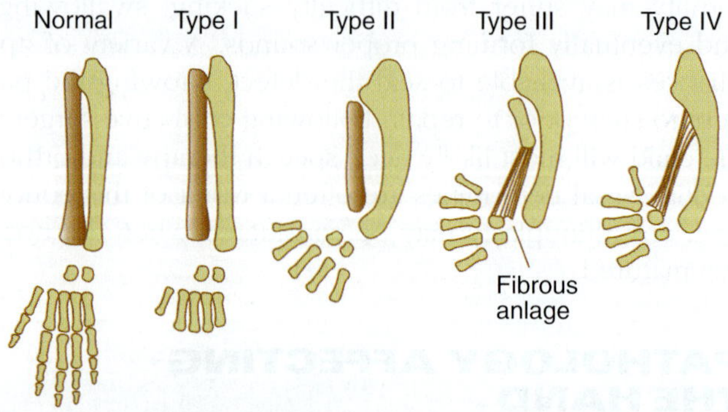

Figure 19-12 Radial dysplasia

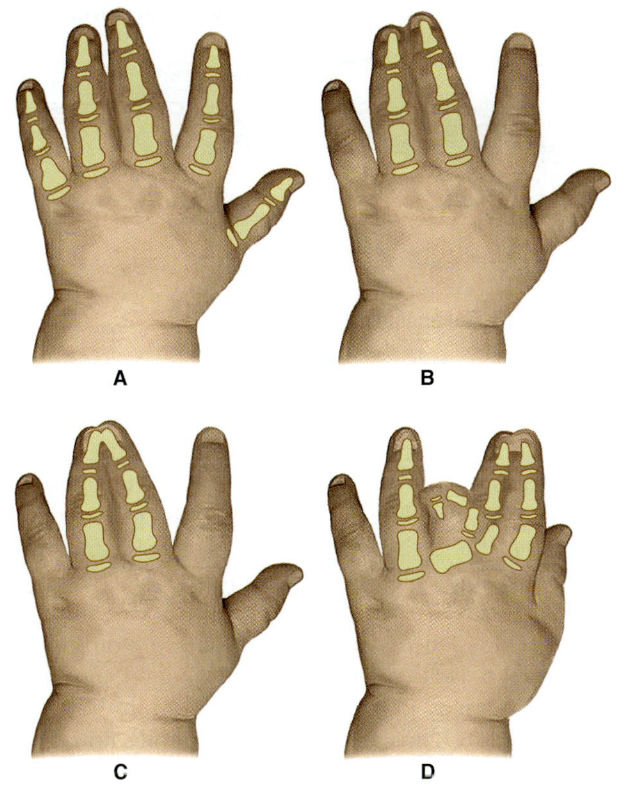

Figure 19-13 Syndactyly: (A) Simple, incomplete, (B) simple, complete, (C) complex, (D) complicated

simply of soft tissue. Fifth finger duplications are the most common type (Figure 19-14).

Surgical removal is usually indicated for cosmetic reasons. Reconstruction may involve the creation of a single digit from two that are underdeveloped.

DISEASES AFFECTING THE HAND

Certain diseases affect the hand such that surgical intervention becomes necessary.

De Quervain's Disease

De Quervain's stenosing tenosynovitis was once referred to as "washer woman's sprain." Fritz de Quervain of Switzerland first described the disease in 1895. It most often affects women between the age of 30 and 50. People who are involved in activities that require sideways motion of the wrist while gripping with the thumb (some examples of this type of motion include skiing and hammering) are prone to acquiring this disease.

De Quervain's stenosing tenosynovitis is a painful condition caused by inflammation of the tendons in the first dorsal compartment of the wrist. The first dorsal compartment is the housing at the lateral base of the thumb that allows passage of the tendons for the abductor pollicis longus and the extensor pollicis brevis muscles. Along with pain on the thumb side of the wrist, the patient will experience a weak grip.

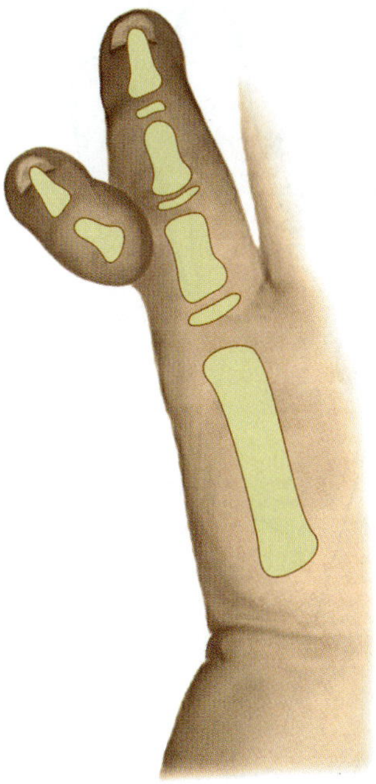

Figure 19-14 Polydactyly

Conservative treatments for De Quervain's disease may include the use of oral anti-inflammatory medications, local steroid injections, and the use of a splint. If conservative treatment is unsuccessful, surgery to release the tendons may be indicated. The condition seldom recurs following surgical intervention.

Trigger Finger

Trigger finger is another type of stenosing tenosynovitis that affects the digits. The patient experiences painful snapping or locking of the fingers or thumb. Trigger finger is caused by inflammation of the synovial sheath, enlargement of the tendon, or narrowing of the annular band or pulley.

Surgery is only recommended if the digit is in a locked position; otherwise, conservative treatments including local or systemic anti-inflammatory medications or the use of a restrictive device may be implemented.

Dupuytren's Disease

Baron Guillaume Dupuytren, a French surgeon, first described this type of contracture in 1831. The cause is unknown, but the disease seems to attack individuals of northern European descent and often is related to trauma of the hand.

Dupuytren's disease may present itself in one of three ways: a nonpainful nodule in the palm of the hand

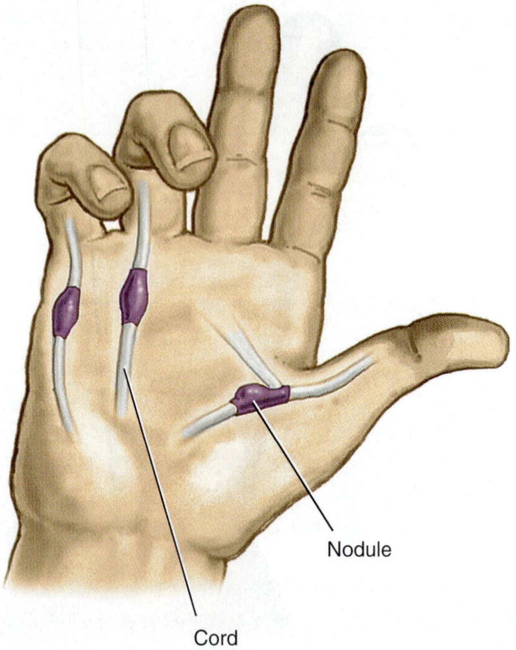

Figure 19-15 **Dupuytren's contracture**

near the fourth or fifth digit, a dimpling or pit in locations just described, or finally as a longitudinal fibrous band or cord extending from the palm toward the fingers (Figure 19-15). All of these primary signs are caused by contraction of the palmar fascia. Occasionally the patient may experience tenderness over an existing nodule. When the contracture causes restricted movement and impaired function, surgery is indicated. The surgery can be very complex and restoration of full function and normal appearance may not be possible.

Ganglion Cyst

A **ganglion cyst** is a benign lesion and is the most common mass developed in the hand. A ganglion is a cyst filled with synovial fluid that can arise from almost any tendon sheath or joint in the hand or wrist. Ganglion formation may be a result of trauma or tissue degeneration. The patient may feel slight discomfort or notice a reduced range of motion at the affected site, and the appearance of the cyst may be unsightly (Figure 19-16).

A variety of treatment options is available. Many of the cysts are spontaneously resolved. Aspiration of the fluid from the cyst is another option for positive diagnosis of the type of cyst and for treatment, although 50% of the time the cyst recurs. Surgical removal of a ganglion cyst is also an option.

Rheumatoid Arthritis

Rheumatoid arthritis (RA) is an autoimmune disease that affects approximately 3% of Americans. Three out of four persons suffering from RA are women and 90% of RA patients have upper limb involvement. It is the most common disorder of the connective tissues. The cause of RA remains unknown at this time, although a viral or bacterial protein is suspected. The disease attacks the synovial tissues causing the typical symptoms of inflammation: redness, pain, swelling, stiffness, and loss of function of the joint. As the disease progresses, damage can occur to the cartilage and bone within the affected joint, leading to severe deformity, pain, and loss of function. The patient may also experience some generalized symptoms that include fatigue, lack of appetite, and low-grade fever. The patient may enjoy periods of remission from the disease or suffer severe flare-ups. There is currently no cure for rheumatoid arthritis (Figure 19-17).

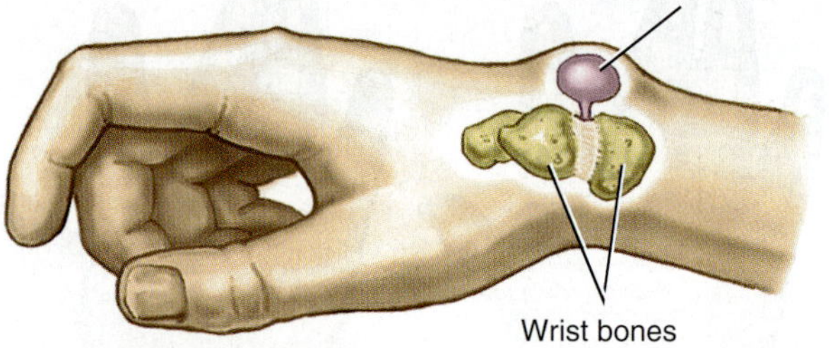

Figure 19-16 **Ganglionic cyst**

Initial standard treatment of RA is the administration of anti-inflammatory medications and lifestyle modifications. Surgery may become necessary to stabilize weakened joints or replace damaged structures.

HAND TRAUMA

Trauma to the hand can take many forms: cuts, sprains, fractures, burns, crush injuries, or amputation. No matter what the injury involves, there are two goals in surgical intervention: restoration of appearance and function of the hand to its preinjury state, with the emphasis on function.

Accidents resulting in the loss of any digit, and the thumb in particular, can have a profound impact on the ability of the hand to perform many functions. While most individuals will learn to compensate for the loss, the debility can be significant. **Replantation** of the severed digit carries the best chance for restoration of full function. Several factors will affect the viability of replantation, including:

- Type of injury (clean cut vs. crush or avulsion)
- Location of the amputation on the affected structure
- Extent of damage to underlying structures (blood vessels, nerves, tendons)
- Care of the severed part (immediate access to ice)
- Time elapsed between accident and initiation of replantation

Recent improvements in the area of microvascular techniques makes this a very hopeful time for those who have suffered severe injury to their hands. Such advancements have allowed for the replantation of severed digits, toe-to-hand transfers for lost digits, and even complete hand transplants. While revascularization is vital for the sur-

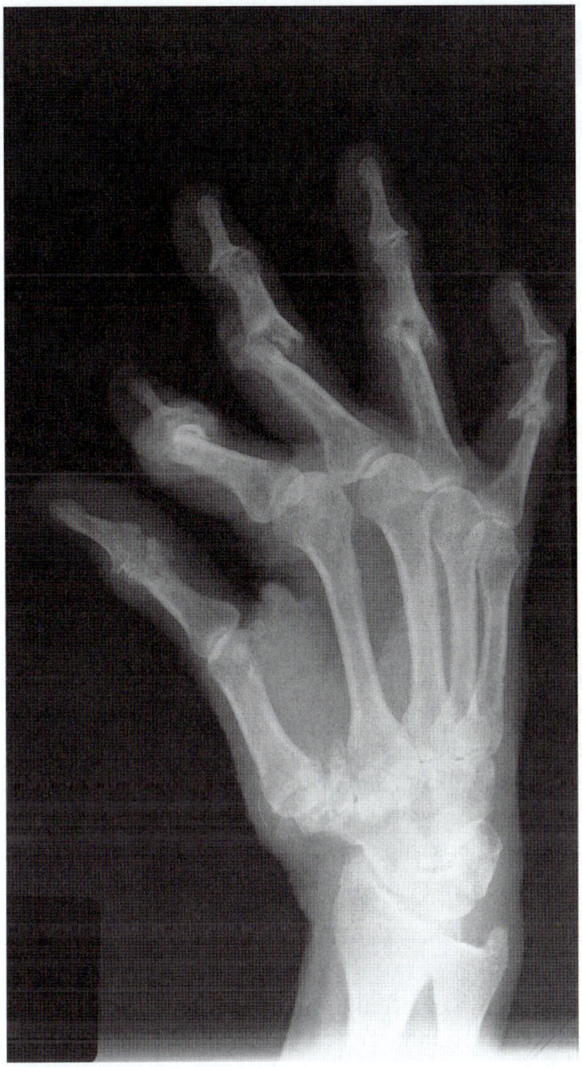

Figure 19-17 **X-ray of rheumatoid hand** ***(Courtesy of the Arthritis Foundation)***

vival of a severed digit, it has been the advancements in microneuroplastic techniques that have restored function.

PATHOLOGY AFFECTING THE BREAST

MALE BREAST

The term **gynecomastia** finds its roots in the Greek language and means "woman-like breasts." This is referring to excess development of the male breast, which can progress to the functional state. Breast enlargement in the male affects as much as 40% of the population. The cause may be physiological or pathological. Often, gynecomastia is seen at the time of puberty and usually regresses without treatment. Other causes include heredity, tumors, hormone imbalances, and the use of certain drugs.

Treatment for gynecomastia varies according to the extent of the disease and the desire of the patient. Medical treatment such as modification of the patient's medications may be indicated, or surgery may be recommended. Surgical interventions range from liposuction to mastectomy.

FEMALE BREAST

From a purely physiological standpoint, the primary function of the female breast is to produce milk, which provides nutrition and vital immunities to the newborn and infant. In most cultures throughout time, this ability to lactate has been intimately linked to a woman's femininity. Today, however, especially in Western society, this symbol of femininity has less to do with the functionality of the breast, than with its **aesthetic** qualities. For many women, the societal perception of what constitutes physical perfection—and how they measure up to that standard—has a profound impact on self-esteem. Thus surgery to improve the appearance of the breasts can have great psychological importance. The patient may desire to have the size of her breasts changed for medical or aesthetic reasons. Mammoplasty may be recommended following surgical removal of the breast (mastectomy) due to cancer or other disease, or to correct a congenital deformity.

DIAGNOSTIC PROCEDURES AND TESTS

Diagnosis of conditions that may require plastic/reconstructive surgery is often accomplished by visual examination. The patient may have a desire to change his or her appearance by altering physical features. A physician may recommend surgery due to a disease process or deformity that may be congenital or acquired.

Radiologic examination is often used to determine the type and severity of a condition of the bones, especially of the hand. CT scanning is useful in providing information regarding craniofacial problems.

SPECIAL INSTRUMENTATION, SUPPLIES, DRUGS, AND EQUIPMENT

Of course, instrument sets will vary from institution to institution. Additional instrumentation will have to be added to accommodate other body systems undergoing modification. A typical plastic set for use on the skin and immediate underlying tissues is shown in Table 19-4.

NASAL SET

A nasal instrumentation set for **rhinoplasty** is especially tailored to suit the plastic surgeon's needs. A rhinoplasty tray will contain just the instruments used in reshaping the nose. It may be used in addition to a plastic set or may contain a modification of the previously mentioned instruments. Please keep in mind that the following list is to be used as a general guideline and may not exactly match

Table 19-4 Typical Plastic Instrumentation Set

Qty	CLAMPS
4	Towel clips, 3½ in.
4	Micropoint mosquitos, curved
4	Halstead mosquitos, curved
2	Halstead mosquitos, straight
4	Crile hemostats
2	Allis clamps, 6 in.
	SCISSORS
1	Littler scissors
1	Iris scissors, curved
1	Stevens tenotomy scissors, curved
1	Suture scissors, small
1	Metzenbaum scissors, fine tip, 5½ in.
1	Metzenbaum scissors, blunt tip, 5½ in.
1	Metzenbaum scissors, 7 in.
1	Mayo scissors, straight
1	Mayo scissors, curved
1	Bandage scissors
	NEEDLE HOLDERS
1	Regular, 4¾ in.
1	Padgett, 4⅜ in.
2	Crile wood, 6 in.
1	Crile wood, 7 in.
	FORCEPS
2	Adson tissue forceps with teeth
2	Adson tissue forceps, smooth
1	Adson-Brown
1	Bishop-Harmon
2	DeBakey, 6 in.
	RETRACTORS
2	Skin hooks, double-prong, medium
2	Skin hooks, double-prong, large
2	Skin hooks, single-prong
2	Senn retractors
2	Spring retractors
2	Army-Navy retractors
	MISCELLANEOUS
2	Knife handles, #3
1	Knife handle, #7
2	Beaver knife handles
2	Medicine cups
2	Freer elevators
2	Key elevators, small
2	Frazier suction tips, 8 Fr, angled with finger cut-off

the tray at any specific facility. Suggested instrumentation for a rhinoplasty set is shown in Table 19-5.

DERMATOME

A **dermatome** is an instrument used to cut thin slices of skin for grafting. Several types and brands of dermatomes are available to the surgical team. These instruments vary from specialized handheld knives to powered machinery. The most common type of powered dermatome is the oscillating-blade-type dermatome (Figure 19-18).

OSCILLATING-BLADE-TYPE DERMATOME

Electricity or nitrogen may power the oscillating-blade-type dermatome. In either case, the STSR will have a cord that will need to be partially passed from the sterile field to the circulator for connection to the power source. It is important to locate and secure the cord on the sterile field so that its presence does not interfere with either of the operative sites (even though it will only be used at the donor site). For the safety of the STSR, it is recommended that the dermatome not be connected to the power cord until the blade has been loaded. Be sure that the safety switch is engaged.

A sterile disposable blade is used for each patient, or, if several grafts are to be procured, several blades may be used for one patient. Use extreme caution when removing the blade from the package and inserting it into the dermatome so that the blade is not damaged and injury is prevented. Once the blade is positioned within the dermatome, the surface of the blade, except for the cutting edge, is covered with one of four guard plates. This guard plate retains the blade and allows for the width of the skin graft to be procured. The width of the graft is determined by a "gap" in the edge of the plate. The gaps range in size from one to four inches. The blade and the retention plate are secured with screws. A screwdriver should be provided with the dermatome.

The thickness of the graft is determined by adjusting a small lever on the side of the dermatome, which has numbered markings (in tenths of a millimeter). This will be set according to the surgeon's preference and the patient's situation. Some surgeons prefer to insert the blade and select the settings themselves.

Prior to its use, the STSR should test the dermatome in a safe environment to ascertain that it is connected to the power source and functioning properly.

In addition to the dermatome, the surgeon may desire lubricant, such as sterile mineral oil, for the patient's skin. A device to stretch the skin while the dermatome is

Table 19-5 Typical Rhinoplasty Instrumentation Set

RETRACTORS	
1	Vienna nasal speculum, small
1	Vienna nasal speculum, medium
1	Vienna nasal speculum, large
2	Single-prong skin hooks
2	Cottle or Joseph double-prong skin hooks
1	Fomon retractor
1	Cottle retractor
1	Converse alar retractor
1	Cottle knife guide and retractor
1	Aufricht nasal septum retractor
BONE INSTRUMENTS	
1	Cottle osteotome, 4 mm
1	Cottle osteotome, 7 mm
1	Cottle osteotome, 9 mm
1	Cottle osteotome, 12 mm
1	Cinelli osteotome, double guards, 10 mm
1	Silver osteotome, single guard, right
1	Silver osteotome, single guard, left
1	Freer septum chisel, straight, 4 mm
1	Freer septum chisel, curved, 4 mm
1	Ballenger V-shaped chisel, 4 mm
1	Ballenger swivel knife, 4 mm
1	Mead mallet, 8 oz. head
1	Joseph nasal saw, straight
1	Joseph nasal saw, bayonet, right
1	Joseph nasal saw, bayonet, left
1	Joseph rasp, cross serrations
1	Maltz rasp, double-ended, forward & backward
MISCELLANEOUS	
1	Cushing tissue forceps with teeth, bayonet
1	Jansen bayonet dressing forceps
1	Takahashi forceps
1	Freer septum knife
1	Cottle septum elevator
1	Joseph periosteal elevator
1	Cottle cartilage crusher

being used may also be requested. A sterile tongue blade works well for this purpose.

OTHER TYPES OF DERMATOMES

Three types of handheld knife dermatomes are used: Ferris-Smith, Watson, and Weck. The Ferris-Smith dermatome is used to obtain free-hand skin grafts. The depth of the graft is controlled by the surgeon. A sterile straight razor blade is used. The Watson knife has an adjustable roller for the surgeon to control the desired thickness of graft. The Weck knife also uses a straight razor blade with

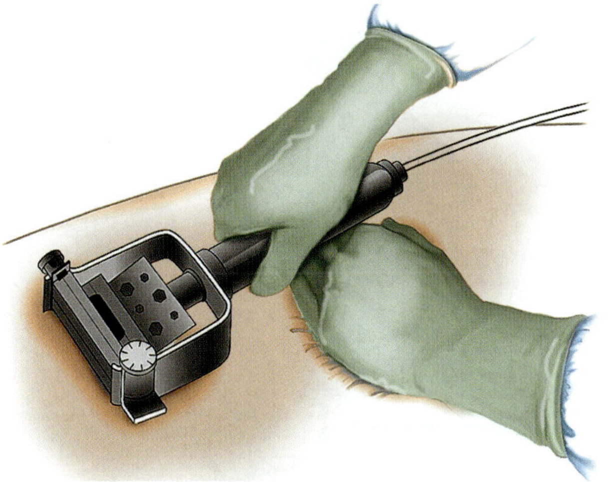

Figure 19-18 Oscillating-blade-type dermatome

various sizes of guards to control the depth of graft. The Weck is primarily used to obtain small skin grafts and for debridement of burns.

Padgett and Reese drum-type dermatomes are occasionally used to obtain skin grafts. They are hand operated, not power, and consist of one-half of a metal drum in which the skin surface is fixed. A metal handle goes through the center of the drum and has an arm on each end. The arms hold the bar that contains the skin graft blade. The bar swings around the drum to cut the skin graft. The size and width of the graft are determined by the size of the drum. The knife blade moves from side to side as the drum is rotated. Sterile dermatome tape must be used with the Reese dermatome. The tape has adhesive on each side and this must be exposed by the STSR by peeling the paper backing off. Remove the paper backing from one side and carefully apply the tape to the drum, making sure the edges of the tape line up with the edges of the drum. The second paper backing is removed from the other exposed side of the tape, and the drum is placed against the skin, which adheres to the adhesive. Due to the bulky size of drum-type dermatomes, their use is limited to large, flat areas of the body because they cannot follow contours of the body.

PEARL OF WISDOM

When placing the blade in an oscillating-blade-type dermatome, make sure the power, whether electrical, air, or nitrogen, is not connected to prevent inadvertent starting of the dermatome and severe injury. When handling a drum-type dermatome, always hold the blade carrier to prevent it from swinging around the drum and causing a severe injury.

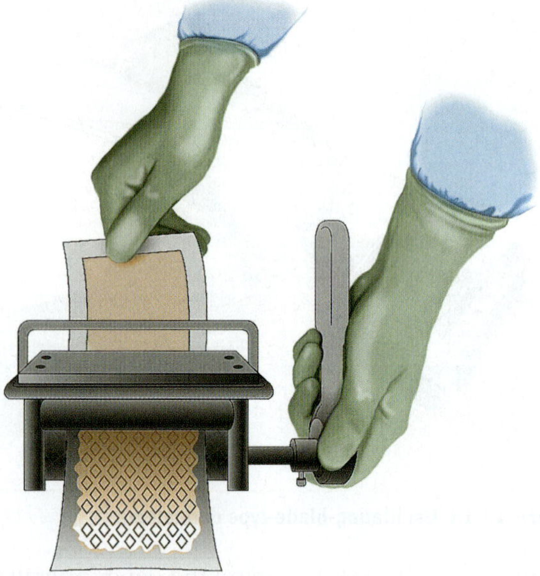

Figure 19-19 Mesh graft device

MESH GRAFT DEVICE

A mesh graft device is often used in conjunction with a split-thickness skin graft to expand the size of the skin that has been procured. The device is a manually operated "roller" with sharp raised surfaces that create evenly spaced slits in the graft. The harvested skin is placed on a plastic "carrier" prior to insertion in the mesh graft device. The purpose of the derma-carrier is to keep the graft flat and allow it to pass through the mesh graft device. The carrier has a smooth side and a ridged side. The ridges determine the size of the slits to be placed in the skin. Derma-carriers are available in a variety of sizes, which are expressed in ratios. For example, if the packaging of the derma-carrier states that the ratio is 3:1, the expanded graft will cover three times the area that it would have prior to being meshed. When stretched, the slits in the expanded graft will take on a diamond shape resembling a fishing net (Figure 19-19).

SURGICAL INTERVENTION

Here we examine several of the different types of plastic surgical intervention.

RHYTIDECTOMY

Rhytidectomy is commonly known as a face-lift and is often done in combination with other facial procedures, such as blepharoplasty and liposuction, to provide the patient with the optimal desired cosmetic effect (Procedure 19-1).

PROCEDURE 19-1 Rhytidectomy

Equipment

- Headrest
- Bipolar unit
- Electrosurgical unit
- Sitting stools

Instruments

- Basic plastic set
- Deaver retractors, 2 small

Supplies

- Pack: basic pack
- Basin: basin set
- Gloves
- Blades: several #15 scalpel blades
- Drapes: head drapes
- Suture: surgeon's preference
- Drains: Hemovac or Jackson-Pratt (optional)
- Dressings: surgeon's preference
- Drugs:
  - Local, according to surgeon's preference
  - Antibiotic ointment, surgeon's preference
- Miscellaneous:
  - Sterile skin marking pen with ruler
  - Electrosurgical pencil with needle electrode
  - Syringes: Luer-lock control with 25- or 27-gauge needles

PROCEDURE 19-1 Rhytidectomy *(continued)*

Operative Preparation

Anesthesia

- Local, sometimes supplemented with mild sedation, or
- General

Position

- Supine; arms may be tucked at the sides or on padded armboards

Prep

- Hair is secured away from the operative site. A shave is not usually done
- Skin is prepped according to surgeon's preference regarding solution to be used. The face, ears, and neck are cleansed from the hairline to the shoulders, and down to the table at the sides of the neck

Draping

- Head is wrapped turban-style with sterile towels, and head drape sheets are affixed

Practical Considerations

- Surgeon may outline the planned incision lines with a sterile marking pen
- Several vital structures, including the facial nerve, must be avoided during retraction. Retractors should not be placed if STSR is unsure of the location of these structures or cannot visualize the field

Operative Procedure

1. Incision is initiated within the hairline in the temporal region of the scalp, approximately 5 cm above the ear (Figure 19-20).

Technical Considerations: 1. The surgeon uses a #15 scalpel blade for the initial incision.

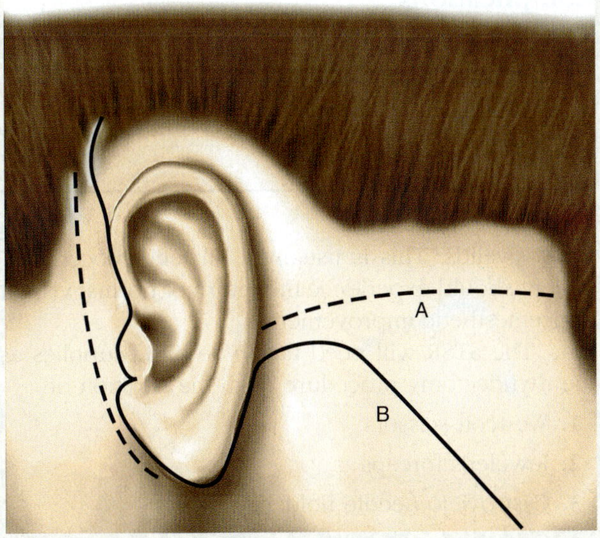

Figure 19-20 Rhytidectomy incision options: (A) Primary, (B) secondary

2. The incision is continued to just below the earlobe and then back up and around the ear.

Technical Considerations: 2. Incision follows natural creases in the skin to camouflage scarring.

(continues)

PROCEDURE 19-1 Rhytidectomy *(continued)*

3. The subcutaneous tissue in the preauricular area is undermined.

3. Tenotomy scissors are used for this step.

4. Moving inferiorly to the jaw line and superiorly to the lateral aspect of the nose, the subcutaneous tissue is separated (dissected) from the platysma below.

4. The STSR or STSFA uses double-prong skin hooks and progresses to larger retractors, as the situation allows, to hold tension along the wound edges and facilitate dissection.

5. Wound edges of the developed flap are pulled taut to determine the amount of redundant skin to be excised. The opposite side of the face will be referred to during this stage to maintain symmetry and create a natural appearance.

5. "Tacking" sutures may be placed temporarily to hold the skin in place until the desired level of tension is achieved.

6. Redundant tissue is excised and wound is closed using suture of surgeon's choice. A Jackson-Pratt drain may be placed to help eliminate dead space and reduce the risk of hematoma.

6. Excision is done with new #15 scalpel blade.

7. This process is duplicated contralaterally.

7. Reorganize and repeat steps.

Postoperative Considerations

Immediate Postoperative Care

- Incisions may be bathed in antibiotic ointment.
- A dressing is usually not applied.
- Patient should keep the head elevated and apply cold compresses to the area.
- Patient will return to the physician's office in 3–5 days for suture removal, and should avoid the use of makeup for 7–10 days postoperatively.

Prognosis

- Swelling and bruising are expected.
- Complications are rare, recovery is fast, and the patient is usually satisfied with the result.

Complications

- Hematoma
- Scarring
- Hemorrhage
- Infection

PEARL OF WISDOM

Even if the patient is under general anesthesia, the operative site will most likely be infiltrated with the local-epinephrine combination to cause vasoconstriction that will aid in hemostasis.

BLEPHAROPLASTY

The word *blepharoplasty* means surgical repair of the eyelid and can be used to describe just about any procedure involving the eyelid. The procedure is performed to remove excess skin or fat deposits of either the upper or lower eyelids. This is usually a bilateral procedure. The patient should experience the return of normal vision and notice aesthetic improvement.

The STSR will need the same basic supplies as for the rhytidectomy procedure, with the addition of:

1. Westcott scissors
2. Jeweler's forceps
3. Castroviejo needle holder
4. Caliper
5. Cotton tip applicators or spear sponges
6. Ophthalmic antibiotic ointment according to surgeon's preference

This procedure is usually done under local anesthesia. The patient is placed in a supine position on the operating table and may be sedated. The circulator preps the facial skin with a mild topical solution using great care to keep the solution from entering the patient's eyes to prevent the solution from burning the cornea. A turban-style head drape that exposes both sides of the face is applied along with a body drape. The sterile marking pen is used to mark the intended incision lines prior to the injection of the local anesthetic. If the anesthetic were injected first, the anatomy would become distorted. Ointment may be instilled into the eye to prevent corneal drying. Great care should be exercised to prevent accidental corneal abrasion.

Blepharoplasty of the upper lid begins with an **elliptical** incision along the ciliary margin following the natural curve of the eyelid possibly concealed within one of the normal folds. Using a jeweler's forceps and the Westcott scissors, a flap is developed and any redundant tissue, including the medial and central fat pads, may be removed. Great care is used to prevent damage to the levator muscle. If desired, a laser may be used for this purpose. The STSR is responsible for dabbing the incisional area as needed with the applicators, providing the surgeon with a dry visual field. Hemostasis is achieved by cauterization. If a wedge of skin is to be excised, the second incision is made at this time. It is arched above the primary incision and connected at the medial and lateral edges. A caliper may be used to ensure that the incisions on both eyelids are equal in size and to prevent the removal of too much tissue, which could cause a complication whereby the patient is permanently unable to close the eyelids (Figure 19-21).

The surgeon may desire to use the Castroviejo needle holder for closure. The underlying tissue will most likely be sutured with absorbable suture and the skin closed with monofilament nonabsorbable suture. Prolene is often used because its blue color differentiates it from the eyelashes at the time of removal. If bilateral blepharoplasty is to be performed, as is generally the case, the procedure is repeated on the opposite side. The same position, prep, drapes, and instruments are used.

The procedure for blepharoplasty of the lower lid is similar and is performed at this time if desired. There is no dressing, although an antibiotic ointment may be applied. The patient is expected to return home the same day. Bedrest with the head of the bed elevated is recommended. Cold compresses should be applied to the eyelids to reduce swelling and provide comfort. Oral analgesics should provide adequate pain control. Bruising is expected. The sutures are removed in 3–5 days. It is recommended that the patient refrain from wearing makeup for 7–10 days postoperatively. Most patients are satisfied with the result.

SUCTION LIPECTOMY

In its most literal sense, suction lipectomy, or liposuction, is the process by which unwanted and unsightly fat deposits are vacuumed from specific areas of the body (Figure 19-22). A variety of other plastic surgical procedures, such as abdominoplasty, may be performed along with liposuction to enhance the patient's body image. A commonly held misconception is that liposuction is an alternative to weight loss. It is not. For those who wish to lose weight, the normal treatment of diet modification and the implementation of an exercise program remain the only option. Liposuction provides a means of contouring those areas of the body that have not responded to changes in diet and exercise. Liposuction may be performed on virtually any problem area of the body. There are several variations to traditional liposuction.

Liposuction requires minimal preparation time for the surgical technologist and utilizes very few instruments. Certain specifics, such as drapes and positioning of the patient, will vary, depending on the operative site or sites and the amount of tissue to be removed. The following list of supplies, in addition to the supplies for the rhytidectomy procedure, should serve as a general guideline. A basic plastic set will not be necessary if the following instruments are gathered individually:

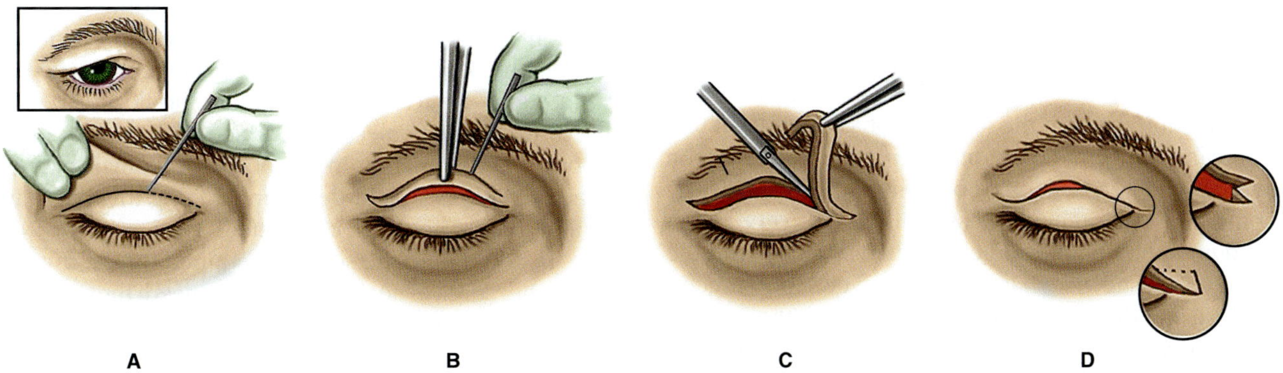

Figure 19-21 Blepharoplasty: (A) Inferior incision line is marked, (B) superior incision line is marked, (C) wedge of redundant removed, (D) closure

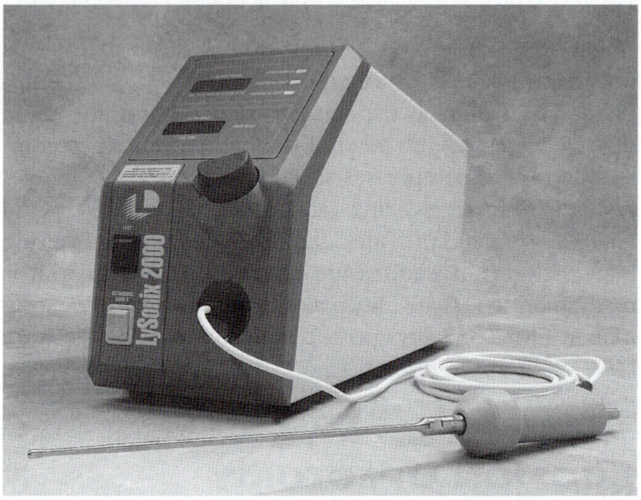

Figure 19-22 Liposuction equipment ***(Courtesy of Lysonix)***

1. #3 Knife handle
2. Several #15 scalpel blades
3. Needle holder
4. Adson tissue forceps with teeth
5. Suture scissors
6. Drapes appropriate for surgical site(s)
7. Large-bore suction tubing
8. Suction (Mercedes) cannulae, various sizes (3–10 mm)
9. Dressing material

Traditional liposuction usually is performed with the patient under general anesthesia. The area to be suctioned may be marked in advance with indelible marker. The patient will be positioned for maximum exposure of the operative site(s). Keep in mind that if the situation requires multiple incision sites, the patient may need to be repositioned during the procedure. Shaving is usually not necessary. The skin is prepped and the surgical site draped. A small incision is made in the most inconspicuous area possible. The smallest cannula that is practical is inserted into the established wound and strong vacuum is applied. The surgeon makes several jabbing passes parallel to the skin with the cannula through the surrounding adipose tissue. This blunt dissection technique loosens the fat globules, which are then removed by the suction through the fenestrations at the distal end of the cannula. Depending on the situation, the surgeon may graduate to a larger suction cannula, continuing the jabbing and suctioning process. This can be very physically demanding on the surgeon. When satisfied with the amount of tissue that has been removed, the surgeon will close and dress the wound. According to the amount of tissue that has been removed, the dressing may be as simple as a self-adherent bandage or a more complex pressure dressing may be applied to reduce dead space and decrease postoperative edema. This process is repeated in as many areas as necessary. The suctioned material is collected in a graduated cannister. Close monitoring of the volume of adipose extracted is of paramount importance, because excessive suctioning (greater than 1000 cc) can cause hypovolemia and other fluid/hemodynamic complications.

Tumescent liposuction involves injecting a mixture of local anesthetic, epinephrine, Wydase, and saline. The medications contained in this mixture serve many purposes. The presence of the local anesthetic may allow the patient to be awake with mild sedation rather than under general anesthesia and may provide some immediate postoperative pain control. The vasoconstrictive properties of the epinephrine provide intraoperative hemostasis. The mixture also helps to liquefy the fat, making suctioning easier.

Using traditional or tumescent liposuction techniques, laser or ultrasound may be added to enhance the procedure. Laser liposuction is accomplished by passing a laser probe through the cannula and vaporizing rather than extracting the fat. Ultrasonic liposuction uses ultrasound waves applied with a titanium probe to break down the walls of the fat cells, liquefying them for easier removal with the suction. Both of these methods may decrease the patient's risk for hemorrhage and reduce postoperative pain, swelling, and bruising.

With all types of liposuction, the patient is expected to be released from the health care facility the same day. Moderate pain (which should be controlled with oral analgesics), swelling, and bruising are expected. Mild edema may be persistent for several weeks, delaying the patient's appreciation for the new body contour. In cases where the skin does not conform to the new body shape, additional minor surgery to remove the excess may be desired.

ABDOMINOPLASTY

Abdominoplasty, or "tummy tuck," is often requested by the patient for the purposes of thinning the upper abdominal fat, tightening the abdominal muscles, and removing fat and excess skin from the mid to lower abdomen. Abdominoplasty may be performed in conjunction with other procedures, such as liposuction, to provide the patient with optimal results. This procedure is not a substitute for weight loss and should not be confused with panniculectomy, which is removal of the apron of abdominal fat in the obese. A woman planning to bear children should delay undergoing this procedure until all pregnancies are complete.

In addition to the supplies required for the rhytidectomy, the surgical technologist will need the following items to prepare for this type of surgery:

1. Fiberoptic retractor set
2. Laparotomy sponges
3. Umbilical template

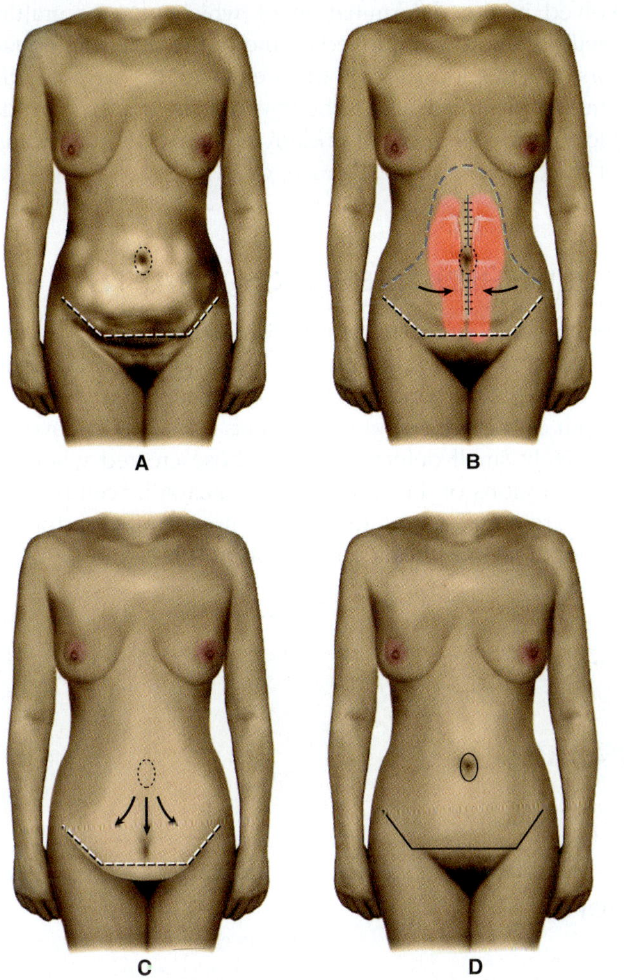

Figure 19-23 Abdominoplasty: (A) Primary incisions, (B) dissection and muscle tightening, (C) secondary incisions—panniculectomy, (D) closure, final effect

4. Abdominal drapes
5. Electrosurgical pencil with blade tip and extension blade tip

The extent of the surgery will dictate what type of facility the procedure will be performed in and the type of anesthetic used. A general anesthetic and an overnight hospital stay are required for a full abdominoplasty. Full abdominoplasty is considered major surgery and can take between 2 to 5 hours to complete. The patient is placed in the supine position on the operating table. The pubic hair should be removed and an extensive prep performed by the circulator. The skin prep should extend from mid-chest to mid-thighs and the entire width of the patient. The entire abdomen (not just the incision site) is then outlined with towels and a laparotomy sheet placed. The surgeon may mark the planned incision lines with the sterile marking pen (Figure 19-23).

A low transverse incision is made down to the level of the fascia (rectus sheath) and may extend the entire width of the patient. Bleeding is controlled, as it becomes evident, with cauterization. Much of the dissection may be accomplished with the use of the electrosurgery in either the cut or blend mode. A small inferior flap is created. Next, dissection begins on the superior flap that extends beyond the level of the umbilicus. The second incision is made around the umbilicus using the template, commonly called the "cookie cutter," to ensure that the incision is a perfect circle. The umbilicus is freed from the skin and subcutaneous tissue, allowing it to remain attached to its pedicle, or base. The flap dissection continues superiorly to the level of the outline of the ribs bilaterally. A variety of retractors is used as the dissection evolves. Some retractors may be enhanced with the use of fiberoptics.

The superior flap is retracted to reveal the rectus abdominis muscle. The vertical muscle, along with its fascia, or sheath, is pulled together and sutured to firm the abdominal wall and accentuate the waistline. The skin flap is then pulled down, the new location for the umbilicus is marked, and the excess tissue is removed. An opening is created for the umbilicus using the "cookie cutter" template and the structure is sutured into position. The operating table may be flexed at this point to facilitate closure. The wound is closed in layers. One or two closed wound drainage systems may be placed to evacuate any fluid and eliminate any dead space. The drains may be extruded through the lateral wound edges. Staples may be used on the skin. A light dressing is applied over the umbilicus, and a pressure dressing to the main wound. The surgeon may request the use of an abdominal binder or girdle.

The patient will most likely be hospitalized, at least overnight, and will probably receive hypodermic injections of narcotic pain medication for the first 24 hours. The patient's bed should be flexed to provide maximum comfort. Although it will be difficult for the patient to stand erect, ambulation is encouraged as soon as possible. The drain remains in place for 2–3 weeks after the patient is discharged from the hospital. Patient education regarding wound and drain care is necessary. The patient should have an appointment with the surgeon approximately 1 week postoperatively to have the external sutures or staples removed and another week or two later for extraction of the drains. It may take several weeks for the patient to return to normal activities. A lengthy horizontal scar will be quite evident, although regrowth of the pubic hair should provide some cover; the incision line should be low enough to be hidden in the patient's undergarment or bathing suit.

SKIN GRAFTS

You will recall that the body's first line of defense against infection is the skin. The skin is also vital in regulating body temperature and shielding the internal structures from damaging external forces, such as ultraviolet radiation.

Thus, whenever the integrity of the skin is compromised—whether through trauma or disease process—the homeostasis of the whole body is threatened. If a defect in the integrity of the skin is large and/or deep, replacement in the form of a skin graft to the affected area becomes necessary.

Skin grafts may be autologous (from one's self), or may come from another source. These options include homografts (obtained from the same species, such as from another person or a cadaver) and heterografts or **xenografts** (obtained from a dissimilar species, such as pig or calf skin). Skin grafts fall into two different categories: full-thickness skin grafts (commonly abbreviated as FTSG) and split-thickness skin grafts (**STSG**). Both types of grafts, if done autologously, involve the use of a "donor" site, the place where the tissue to be moved is taken from. The site of the defect that is to be covered is referred to as the "recipient" site. Several factors are involved in the determination of which type of grafting method is to be employed. Some of the determining factors are the location of the defect to be covered, the amount of surface area to be covered, the depth of the defect and involvement of underlying tissues, and the cause of the defect (trauma, disease, or heredity).

FULL-THICKNESS SKIN GRAFTS

As its name suggests, a full-thickness skin graft is composed of the epidermis and all of the dermis, and may include the underlying subcutaneous tissue. Because of the depth of this type of graft, its use is restricted to covering relatively small defects, such as those created when excising lesions of the skin, such as squamous cell or basal cell carcinoma. Often, this type of graft can be performed under local anesthesia with sedation (Procedure 19-2).

PROCEDURE 19-2 Full-Thickness Skin Graft

Equipment

- Electrosurgical unit

Instruments

- Basic plastic set

Supplies

- Pack: basic pack
- Basin: basin set
- Gloves
- Blades: several #15 scalpel blades
- Drapes: suitable for both operative sites
- Suture: surgeon's preference
- Drains: none
- Dressings: surgeon's preference
- Drugs:
  - Local anesthetic of surgeon's preference
  - Antibiotic ointment of surgeon's preference
- Miscellaneous:
  - Sterile skin marking pen with ruler
  - Electrosurgical pencil with needle-tip electrode
  - Extra prep tray
  - Syringes: Luer-lock control with 25- or 27-gauge needles

Operative Preparation

Anesthesia

- Local, sometimes supplemented with mild sedation, or
- General

Position

- Supine; arms may be tucked at the sides or on padded armboards

PROCEDURE 19-2 Full-Thickness Skin Graft *(continued)*

Prep

- Shave is carried out if necessary
- Both areas are prepped according to procedure for prepping that particular area of the body
- Normally the donor site is prepped first and is considered to be "clean"
- The recipient site, if it is an open wound or potentially contains cancer cells, is prepped last and is considered to be "dirty"

Draping

- Draping will vary according to the body parts affected

Practical Considerations

- Surgeon may outline the planned incision lines with a sterile marking pen
- If the recipient site is an open wound, two separate areas must be created on the sterile field, and the instrumentation and supplies for each part of the procedure must be segregated to prevent contamination of the donor site or "seeding" of cancer cells at the donor site
- It may also be necessary for the sterile team members to change their gloves during the procedure

Operative Procedure	Technical Considerations
1. The lesion is excised using a #15 scalpel blade and tenotomy or iris scissors.	**1.** Hemostasis is achieved by cauterization.
2. If the situation allows, the surgeon may use the excised lesion as a template for sizing the amount of tissue to be procured from the donor site by placing it on the skin and tracing around it with a sterile marking pen.	**2.** Surgeon will place the excised tissue on the skin and mark around it with the sterile marking pen.
3. Specimen is immediately sent to the pathology lab to be examined for margins (to ascertain that all of the malignant tissue has been excised, along with a "buffer" of normal tissue).	**3.** While waiting for the pathologist's report, it is advisable to place moistened gauze on the open wound to protect the tissues from drying out.
4. It may be necessary at this time for the sterile team members to change their gloves and for the surgical technologist to switch over to the "clean" instruments.	**4.** Have the second set of gloves in correct sizes for all team members readily available.
5. The next step is to excise the full-thickness skin graft from the donor site using technique similar to that used for preparing the recipient site.	**5.** Following removal, the graft is wrapped in moistened gauze and stored in a safe place on the back table.
6. If necessary to decrease tension on the wound edges, the subcutaneous tissue immediately surrounding the incision may be undermined using Metzenbaum or tenotomy scissors.	**6.** Again, these should be from the second setup.
7. The donor site is sutured closed and the sterile dressings applied.	**7.** Suture and dressings of surgeon's choice.
8. The graft and recipient site may each be modified in shape for proper "fit." The graft is positioned and secured with suture or stapled in place.	**8.** Any dressing used here must be dry.

(continues)

PROCEDURE 19-2 Full-Thickness Skin Graft *(continued)*

Postoperative Considerations

Immediate Postoperative Care

- A dry, sterile dressing with a nonadherent contact layer is applied.

Prognosis

- The patient is expected to have full function at both operative sites.
- Formation of scar tissue at both locations is expected.

Complications

- Scarring
- Hemorrhage
- Infection

PEARL OF WISDOM

When switching from the "dirty" setup to the "clean" setup, it is very important that the STSR change gloves first, or the gloves of all successive team members will be contaminated.

SPLIT-THICKNESS SKIN GRAFTS

Split-thickness skin grafts involve removing the epidermis and approximately half of the dermis for relocation to another part of the body. This type of graft is employed when a relatively large surface area needs to be covered, such as in the case of a burn. The surgeon's choice of the donor site is influenced by many factors, including:

- Age, sex, and general health of the patient
- Location of the wound to be grafted
- Body surface area to be covered
- Condition of potential donor sites

Ideal donor sites include:

- Lateral and ventral aspects of the thighs
- Back
- Abdomen
- Chest

Procurement of a STSG requires the use of a dermatome and often a mesh graft device. Because of the body surface area affected, the patient will most likely be under general anesthesia.

The surgical technologist will need the supplies used in a full-thickness skin graft and will also need the following:

1. Dermatome
2. Mineral oil
3. Sterile tongue blades
4. Mesh graft device
5. Derma-carrier (appropriate ratio)
6. Topical adrenalin or thrombin solution according to surgeon's preference

A debridement of the recipient site may be done prior to placement of the STSG. Debridement is the removal of foreign bodies or necrotic and infected tissue from the wound. This prepares the wound bed to accept the graft. Minimal capillary bleeding is desirable because it shows viability of the underlying tissue.

Prior to removing the tissue from the donor site, the area may be lubricated with sterile mineral oil. This serves to reduce friction and helps provide a smooth surface to allow for an even excision of skin. While the STSR provides traction on the skin to be harvested, the surgeon activates the dermatome, presses the blade against the skin surface, and guides the instrument along the surface area of skin to be removed. As the instrument is moved forward, the harvested skin comes through the top of the dermatome in a single strip. A #15 scalpel may be used to sever the remaining skin edge from the patient. This is done as many times as is necessary to acquire the amount of tissue needed. It may be necessary to change the dermatome blade if it becomes dull or damaged. The harvested skin should be placed in body temperature saline while awaiting meshing or application to the recipient site. Following removal of the graft, topical adrenalin or thrombin is often applied to the donor site to assist with hemostasis. Once hemostasis is achieved, the donor site may then be dressed with nonadherent gauze such as Adaptic or Xeroform and 4 × 4s, or may be covered with an occlusive material, such as Tegaderm or OpSite.

If meshing of the graft is desired, the harvested skin is placed on the derma-carrier and inserted into the mesh graft device. If more than one strip of skin is to be meshed, each should be placed on a new carrier. After the graft has been meshed, it is applied to the recipient site and sutured or stapled into position. A dry sterile dressing is applied and movement of the affected area may be restricted. The newly applied skin will derive its blood supply from capillary ingrowth from the recipient site; any disruption may cause the graft to be sloughed (shed). The patient may require physical therapy to help regain maximum function. Scarring is expected, especially if the graft was meshed (this leaves the skin with a "waffle-like" appearance).

A patient may have a congenital deformity in which the external ear abnormally protrudes from the side of the head due to the absence of the antihelical fold. The goal of the surgery is to create an antihelical fold that brings the external ear back against the side of the head in a normal anatomical position. In children the procedure is usually performed before they start school.

Besides a plastic instrument set, the STSR will also need calipers, a 22-gauge needle, methylene blue, cotton-tipped applicators, and mineral oil. The patient is placed in the supine position with the arms tucked at the sides and the head turned to expose the affected ear.

The surgeon will use a finger to bend the ear backward, and an antihelical fold is created. The antihelical fold position is marked by placing the 22-gauge needle through the ear, anterior to posterior, marking the tip of the needle with methylene blue and withdrawing the needle. This is usually done three to four times. Next the surgeon excises an elliptical-shaped portion of skin from the posterior of the ear. The cartilage is incised near what will be the antihelical fold and scored to allow the cartilage to bend backward. Several sutures are placed to hold the cartilage in the new anatomical position. The posterior skin incision is closed with suture and a bulky dressing usually consisting of a nonadherent dressing and fluffs is placed over the incision.

DERMABRASION

Dermabrasion is the planing of the skin, either mechanically or chemically, to smooth a skin surface that has been damaged by scars, most often those caused by acne vulgaris. Occasionally dermabrasion is used for the removal of body tattoos and to smooth facial skin wrinkles even though success is low for these circumstances. The goal of the surgery is to plane or sand down the irregular high points on the skin so that the low points appear even. The procedure removes the epidermal layer and part of the dermis. Healing occurs in the portion of the dermal layer that is spared from removal.

The STSR will need a plastic instrument set, dermabrader, and marking pen. The newer type of high-speed dermabrader is powered by compressed nitrogen. It has a rotating head in which different types of tips covered with diamond dust can be placed, such as burs or a tip that has flat sides. The speed of rotation is regulated by the pressure from the nitrogen gas tank. General or local anesthesia will be used. The patient position and draping depends on the area to be dermabraded. The surgeon will use the sterile marking pen to mark the areas to be dermabraded. On completion of the procedure, a single layer of dressing will be placed on the site of dermabrasion.

Some surgeons prefer to use chemicals, such as phenol, alpha-hydroxy acid, or trichloracetic acid to produce dermal peeling. After the chemical procedure, the patient should avoid direct sun exposure to the site for at least 6 months. The use of chemical dermabrasion is contraindicated in patients with dark, oily complexions because the chemicals decrease the melanin in the skin causing discoloration; patients with fair complexions have better results.

Dermabrasion can also be accomplished by laser resurfacing with the use of a CO_2 laser. Advantages include the fact that the depth of the beam can be precisely controlled by the beam's focus and skin color and texture can be uniformally maintained.

SCAR REVISION

Individuals with scars, acquired through a traumatic accident or surgically, can opt to have a plastic surgeon perform a scar revision procedure. The goal of the procedure is to remove the scar, realign the wound edges, and perform a closure in which, once healed, the cosmetic appearance will be improved.

Several techniques are used such as W-plasty, M-plasty, and Y-V-plasty; however, the Z-plasty is the most frequently used technique. The Z-plasty allows the surgeon to ensure that the primary portion of the Z-shaped incision is in the same direction of the natural skin line, thus making the scar less noticeable.

A plastic instrument set will be required with a marking pen for the surgeon to outline the Z-shaped incision. The procedure can be performed with the patient under general anesthesia or local anesthetic. As previously mentioned, the surgeon makes an incision in which the primary line is over the scar to be revised. The top and bottom portions of the Z incision are made equal in length and are at right angles to the primary line. The two skin flaps are then transposed; thus, the original Z incision is rotated and reversed. The surgeon may or may not apply a dressing depending on the extent of the procedure.

CHEILOPLASTY AND PALATOPLASTY

Cheiloplasty (lip repair) and palatoplasty (palate repair) can be performed as individual procedures or in combination with one another, if both types of correction are necessary. Often the lip and anterior palate defects are corrected at the same time, with the posterior palate repair done later. Because of the patient's age, the procedure is usually done under general anesthesia, although a local anesthetic may by injected to assist with hemostasis and postoperative pain control. This is considered a clean, rather than a sterile procedure because the aerodigestive tract is entered. None the less, scrupulous technique must be used to reduce the risk of infection. The circulator may perform an external skin prep, but an internal prep is seldom done.

The surgical technologist will need the basic supplies described for rhytidectomy as well as:

1. #15 scalpel blade
2. Oral instrumentation set
3. Dingman mouth gag with an assortment of retractor blades
4. 2-in. × 2-in. gauze for dressing

Two methods of cheiloplasty are commonly used. The first and more commonly used technique is called "rotation advancement." Incisions are made on both sides of the cleft and extend from the lip into the nostril. The edges are excised and the skin is dissected from the underlying tissues. Tissue from the cheek is rotated into position to eliminate the defect. The mucous membrane layer of the upper lip is closed first with absorbable sutures. The orbicularis oris muscle is then approximated and sutured together to restore its function. The skin is sutured last with every attempt made to create the "cupid's bow" formation of the upper lip (Figure 19-24).

The second and less commonly used repair is called the "triangular flap" method. It imitates the Z-plasty technique (zigzag incisions used to repair a skin defect or relax a contracture—two triangular-shaped flaps are transposed) used in other types of plastic surgery. This method provides for additional height and length of the lip if there is a minimum of tissue available. Again, incisions are made on either side of the defect and the medial tissue is removed. Following closure of the mucous membrane layer and the muscle tissue, the skin flaps are overlapped and interlocked to close the defect.

The wound may be dressed with a small bandage affixed to the outer upper lip that may be referred to as a "mustache" dressing. Both types of cheiloplasty will leave a permanent exterior scar that will partially fade over time. The shadow from the nose and lip is thought to help obscure it. Adult males may choose to grow a mustache to conceal the scar.

Palatoplasty is done to form the absent roof of the mouth. A triangular-shaped incision is made on both sides of the defect. A small amount of tissue is removed. The remaining tissue is undermined and brought toward the midline. The musculature of the palate is sutured together. The mucous membrane is closed over the top (Figure 19-25).

Postoperatively the patient should be observed for signs of bleeding and edema. Occasionally edema can become so severe that the airway is obstructed. If the patient is an infant, the use of restrictive devices on the arms may be employed to prevent accidental wound disruption.

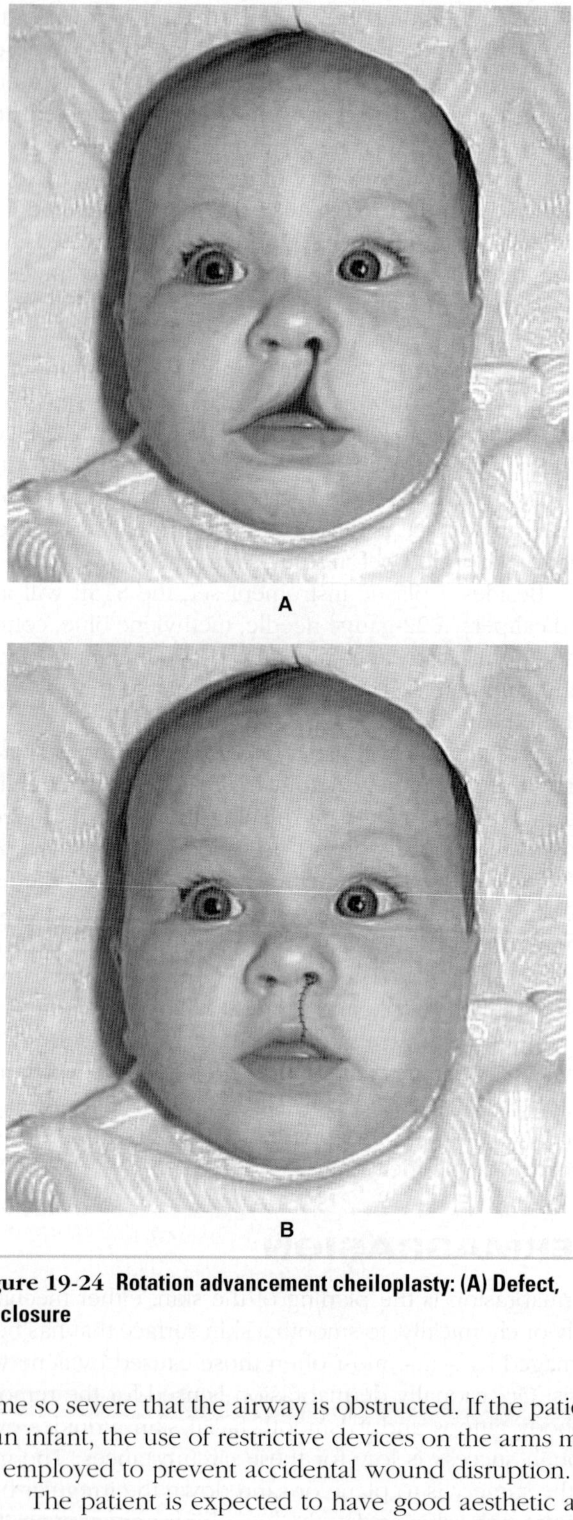

Figure 19-24 Rotation advancement cheiloplasty: (A) Defect, (B) closure

The patient is expected to have good aesthetic and functional results from both cheiloplasty and palatoplasty, but this is by no means the end of the treatment. Speech therapy, orthodontia, and nasal reconstruction are all options to be considered for the future.

RHINOPLASTY

Rhinoplasty is the reshaping of the nose. This is considered to be a plastic surgery procedure because no func-

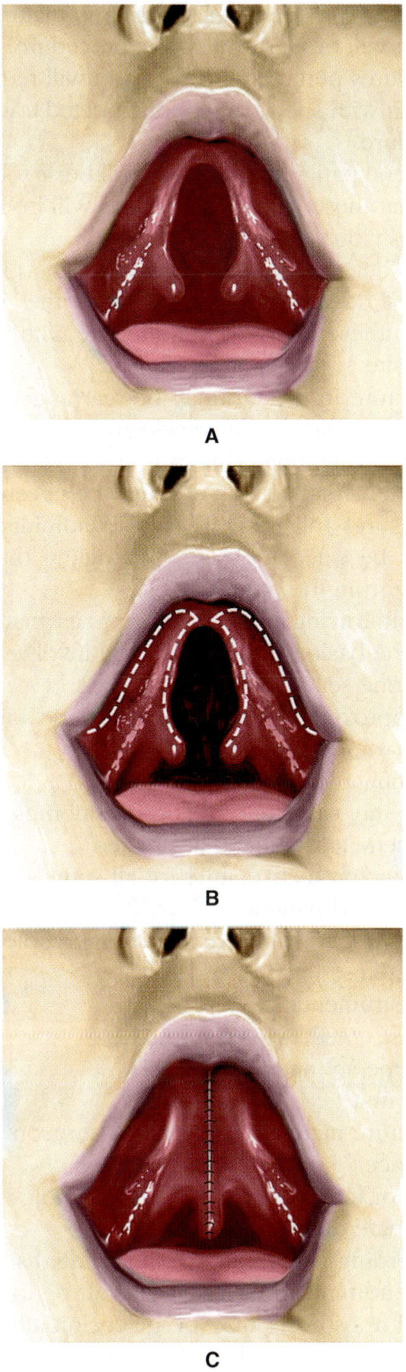

Figure 19-25 **Palatoplasty: (A) Bilateral defect, (B) dissection, (C) closure**

tional changes are made to the interior nasal passageways. Rhinoplasty may be done for reconstructive reasons or to meet a person's aesthetic goals. Rhinoplasty is often done in collaboration with other nasal procedures to restore function of the upper respiratory tract, especially in the post trauma patient. The patient may also desire to have some other facial features altered at the same time. Often mentoplasty (plastic surgery of the chin) and rhinoplasty are done together to improve the patient's overall appearance. The patient should be interviewed carefully to be certain that expectations of the surgery are realistic.

Several aspects of the nose may be altered or restored, including:

- Increase or reduce overall size
- Remodel shape of tip or bridge
- Change span between nostrils
- Change angle between nose and upper lip

Rhinoplasty may be performed in the hospital setting, ambulatory surgery center, or the physician's office. In any case, the patient is expected to go home the same day. The procedure is usually done under local anesthesia. Sedation may be provided. Even when a general anesthetic is planned, the local anesthetic may still be administered to aid in hemostasis, reduce the size of the nasal membranes, and reduce immediate postoperative pain.

The surgical technologist will need the supplies described for rhytidectomy (less the basic plastic set) as well as:

1. Nasal instrumentation set
2. Cocaine (% according to surgeon's preference)
3. ½-in. × 3-in. cottonoid sponges
4. Suction electrosurgery apparatus
5. Opti-Guard (available)
6. Headlamp
7. Packing material (available)
8. External nasal splint
9. 2-in. × 2-in. gauze for dressing

Often the surgeon will administer local anesthetic to the patient as a separate procedure prior to prepping and draping to allow the medication to take effect. This will require the use of a separate small table or Mayo stand. The surgical technologist should have the following items available for the surgeon:

- Nasal speculum
- Bayonet forceps
- Local anesthetic
- Syringe and needles for the local
- Cocaine
- ½-in. × 3-in. cottonoid sponges

Because rhinoplasty involves entry into the respiratory tract, it is considered to be a clean rather than a sterile procedure. If rhinoplasty is being performed in conjunction with another procedure, the sterile procedure should be done first. A male patient with a mustache generally is allowed to retain it. The surgeon may not require that a skin prep be performed. Minimal drapes are applied.

The incisions are usually created within the nose but may be made externally at the base of the nostrils or along the columella (Figure 19-26).

The rhinoplasty will be designed to meet the individual patient's needs. A hump may be removed with the use of a chisel or a rasp. The size and shape of the nose

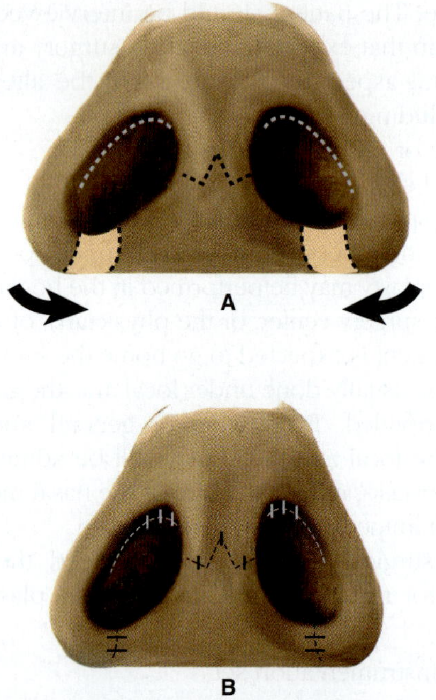

Figure 19-26 Rhinoplasty: (A) Preoperative, (B) postoperative

may be altered using a variety of techniques; tissue may be removed, relocated, or reshaped; or synthetic implants may be placed. Any minor bleeding is controlled with the use of cauterization. Internal nasal splints and packing usually are not necessary. Often an external splint is applied to help the nose maintain its new shape. Gauze may be taped over the nares to catch any drops of blood that may escape. A small amount of bleeding is expected. The patient should be on bedrest for the first day with the head of the bed elevated. The use of cold compresses will help reduce pain and edema. Oral analgesics should be adequate for pain control. The patient should avoid blowing his or her nose and vigorous face washing for approximately 1 week. Bruising and swelling for approximately 2 weeks postoperatively is normal. Some nasal stuffiness and minor swelling may persist for several weeks. The patient will not be able to recognize the final result immediately.

HAND SURGERY

Some health care professionals consider hand surgery part of many specialties. Median nerve surgery may be performed by the neurosurgeon, fractures may be cared for by the orthopedist, while a plastic/reconstructive surgeon may be called for certain conditions and injuries. Others consider surgery of the hand a specialty in its own right with practitioners who focus their expertise specifically on caring for the hands. Hand surgeons may further specialize by directing their practice toward those with congenital deformities or those with rheumatoid arthritis.

Surgery of the hand is performed for three main reasons: congenital deformities, disease, and trauma. From the perspective of the surgical team, no matter what type of surgeon will be performing the procedure, most surgical procedures pertaining to the hand will require similar preparation with special attention directed toward the exact procedure.

General patient preparation will be as follows. Keep in mind that these general guidelines will be modified to suit the individual patient's situation.

Consideration should be given to the placement of the patient identification band and the intravenous catheter so these items do not interfere with the planned operative site.

Furniture in the OR may be rearranged to provide more space on the operative side and to make better use of the existing lighting. This can be accomplished before the patient enters the room or it may be necessary to take these measures following anesthesia administration. Often this is best accomplished by angling the operating table away from the operative side.

The following is a list of supplies that should be added to the basic set if the case will involve the bones:

- Small bone set
- Bone approximation instrumentation including K-wires
- Small power equipment set
- Preoperative X-rays
- Sterile X-ray cassette covers or positioning aids for the cassette and patient, as needed
- Radiologic protective attire for all surgical team members and patient

If the case will involve microsurgery, please add the following items:

- Microinstrumentation set
- Microinstrument wipe
- Spear-type sponges (Weck cell)
- Bipolar unit
- Microsuture material according to surgeon's preference
- Loupes or microscope with sterile handles or appropriate drape

According to the patient's individual situation, the anesthetic administered may be local, regional, or general. Local anesthesia may be given initially, or the injections may be delayed until after the prep is complete and drapes are in place. Regional and general anesthetics are normally administered prior to prepping and draping.

SURGICAL CORRECTION OF DISEASES OF THE HAND

Here we examine the excision of a ganglionic cyst as an illustrative case. Setups and supplies for other hand cases are similar.

Excision of a ganglionic cyst is the removal of a dilation of the capsule of a joint or tendon sheath (Procedure 19-3). This dilation contains synovial fluid.

PROCEDURE

19-3 Excision of Ganglionic Cyst

Equipment

- Tourniquet and insufflator
- Suction
- Sitting stools
- Electrosurgical unit
- Hand table attachment for operating table

Instruments

- Minor orthopedic tray
- Minor plastic set
- Hayes metacarpal retractors
- Pediatric Deaver retractor

Supplies

- Pack: basic pack
- Basin: basin set
- Gloves
- Blades: several #15 scalpel blades
- Drapes: Hand/arm drapes consisting of:
  - Half sheet
  - Appropriate size stockinette
  - Impervious split sheet
  - Three-quarter sheet
  - Extremity sheet
- Suture: surgeon's preference
- Drains: none
- Dressings: surgeon's preference
- Drugs: local anesthetic of surgeon's choice if used
- Miscellaneous:
  - Sterile skin marking pen with ruler
  - Syringes: Luer lock control with 25- or 27-gauge needles
  - Bulb syringe
  - Esmarch bandage
  - Webril for tourniquet (non-sterile)
  - Suction tubing
  - Elastic bandage

Operative Preparation

Anesthesia

- Local, sometimes supplemented with mild sedation or
- General

Position

- The patient is placed in the supine position. The arm table attachment may already be in place or may need to be positioned after the patient is on the table. Initially, the affected hand should be supinated on the hand table to prevent injury to the ulnar nerve; it may be repositioned later to facilitate the surgery, taking care to protect the ulnar nerve

Prep

- If requested by the surgeon, the correct size tourniquet with appropriate padding should be positioned, but not inflated. It is permissible to ask the patient to lift the arm, if possible, to facilitate placement of the tourniquet by the circulator. A plastic adherent drape may be placed around the tourniquet to keep the padding underneath dry and to protect the tourniquet from the prep solution
- If the patient's arm is extremely large, the circulator may request assistance with holding it
- The arm is raised and prepped circumferentially to the level of the tourniquet
- The subungual spaces are cleaned first and the prep proceeds proximally along the surface of the arm toward the tourniquet
- Special attention is given to any existing wounds of the hand
- Once the prep is complete, the circulator is committed to holding the arm until a sterile team member can accept it into the sterile field that is being created

(continues)

PROCEDURE

19-3 Excision of Ganglionic Cyst *(continued)*

Draping

- The surgeon will accept the hand into the rolled stockinette (the circulator must not release the extremity until told to do so), keeping the arm elevated and away from the hand table attachment
- The STSR will place the half sheet over the hand table attachment, keeping the sterile gloved hands within the cuffed edge of the drape
- Place the impervious split sheet on top of the sterile field just created with the half sheet
- Unfold the split sheet and remove the paper covering the adherent edges of the drape
- Assist the surgeon to unroll the stockinette
- Place the covered arm on the prepared split sheet and wrap the adherent edges around the upper arm
- Place the three-quarter sheet over the patient's lower body and feet
- Pull the hand and arm through the fenestration in the extremity sheet and unfold the sheet. The distal edge of the extremity sheet should be unfolded first, the sterile hands protected, and edges transferred to the non-sterile team members to create a barrier between the anesthesiologist and the sterile field
- If the use of a tourniquet is planned, the arm will be elevated and wrapped with the Esmarch. Padding may be placed in the palm of the hand while the Esmarch is applied. The circulator will inflate the tourniquet to a predetermined pressure setting when requested to do so by the surgeon. The hand and arm will remain elevated with the Esmarch in place during the inflation process. When the surgeon is satisfied that the tourniquet is properly inflated, the Esmarch will be removed and the arm returned to the sterile hand table, the stockinette is cut to expose the operative area, and the hand positioned for the procedure

Practical Considerations

- Draping the hand table attachment and accepting the extremity into the sterile field *can* be accomplished by the STSR alone, but it is considered better technique for two sterile team members (usually the STSR and the surgeon) to work together to accomplish this task
- Some surgeons prefer that the arm remain elevated to facilitate exsanguination prior to tourniquet inflation
- All furniture and equipment should be positioned prior to the STSR sitting down. Keep safety in mind when attempting to sit on a wheeled stool. The circulator may steady the stool while the sterile team member sits down. Once seated, all sterile team members should remain seated until the end of the procedure to prevent contamination of the sterile field
- The surgeon may outline the necessary landmarks and the anticipated incision lines with the sterile marking pen
- The location of the ganglion will determine the type of anesthesia to be administered and the style incision to be made

Operative Procedure	Technical Considerations
1. An incision is made directly over the cyst.	**1.** Remove skin blade (#15) from field after use. Do not reuse.
2. Soft tissues are retracted to the side.	**2.** STSR may be called on to provide retraction using small rakes at this point. Often, only the surgeon and STSR are scrubbed for these cases.
3. An attempt is made to excise the cyst intact, taking care not to damage nerve branches.	**3.** The cyst may be sent to pathology as a specimen.

PROCEDURE

19-3 Excision of Ganglionic Cyst *(continued)*

4. Care is taken to identify the site of origin and destroy any causative agent, such as an osteophyte.	**4.** The wound may be irrigated.
5. The tendon sheath is repaired if necessary.	**5.** Suture should be on hand. Check the surgeon's preference card.
6. The wound is closed.	**6.** Many surgeons irrigate with antibiotic irrigation at this point.

Postoperative Considerations

Immediate Postoperative Care

- An elastic bandage is applied.
- Patient's activities are restricted only until suture removal.
- Movement of the affected area is encouraged immediately.

Prognosis

- The patient is expected to have full recovery with restoration of normal function.

Complications

- Hemorrhage
- Infection
- Scar tissue
- Recurrence of ganglion

PEARL OF WISDOM

The STSR must often function in the role of the surgical first assistant during a hand case. This requires an extra measure of concentration and skill. The STSR must not only anticipate the instrument needs of the surgeon, but the need to provide retraction, follow suture, and so on.

De Quervain's Disease

Surgical treatment for De Quervain's disease involves a longitudinal incision over the first dorsal compartment. The dorsal carpal ligament is cut to expose the tendons. Each tendon is identified and the passive motion of each is verified. The wound is closed and a bulky restrictive dressing is applied. This is an out-patient procedure. Pain is expected to be minimal and controlled with an oral analgesic. The bulky dressing is removed in 2–3 days and an exercise program implemented. Complications and recurrence are rare.

Trigger Finger Release

Local anesthetic is often chosen for the release of a trigger finger so that the patient will be able to actively demonstrate motion intraoperatively. A zigzag or transverse incision is made at the base of the affected digit. Most often the first annular band or pulley is cut, relieving the constriction of the tendon as it passes through the sheath at this level. The patient should be able to demon strate motion at this time. If the synovium surrounding the tendon appears thickened, a tenosynovectomy may be performed. The small wound is closed and a light dressing applied. The dressing should allow for passive and active range-of-motion activities. The patient is expected to return to normal activities in approximately 7–10 days, following removal of the sutures.

Release of Dupuytren's Contracture

A variety of procedures exists for the treatment of Dupuytren's disease. Subtotal palmar fasciectomy will be described here.

One or more incisions are made on the volar or palmar surface of the hand according to the extent of the disease (Figure 19-27). A zigzag-style incision is often used so that the existing tissue can be manipulated to cover the flattened palm. In extreme cases a skin graft may be necessary. The palmar incisions should extend toward the fingers that may be affected. The contracted fascia is carefully dissected away from the underlying nerves, blood vessels, and tendons. This dissection can be very tedious and time consuming if the disease is advanced. Drains

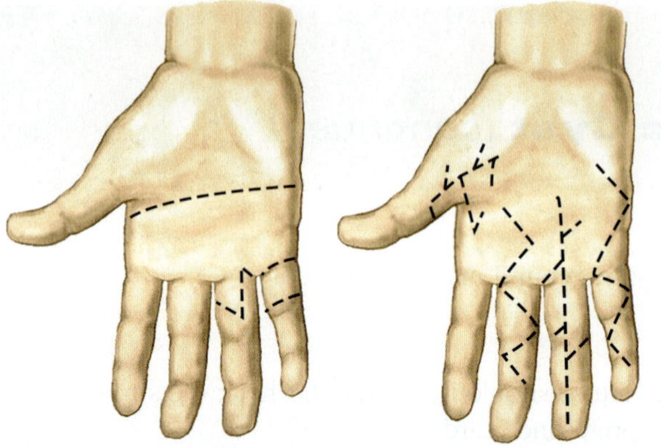

Figure 19-27 Possible incisions for treatment of Dupuytren's disease

may be placed prior to closure. Numerous stitches may be required to successfully stretch the existing skin to add the length necessary for closure. If skin is not available to cover a small surface of the palm, the wound may be left open to heal by second intention. A bulky dressing is applied, which will be left in place for several days. Pain and swelling are expected. Oral analgesics should be adequate for pain control. Physical therapy is introduced in about a week and is quite painful at first. Minor wound disruptions are not uncommon, forcing the patient to wear a dressing for an extended period of time. Therapy may last several months and full range of motion may never be achieved. This is especially true if the disease had progressed to the level of the second finger (PIP) joint. Following subtotal palmar fasciectomy the disease is likely to recur.

Joint Replacement

Joint replacement in the hand is usually done to correct the deformities and reduce the pain caused by rheumatoid arthritis. It may be performed on any one or all fourteen finger joints on each hand. Surgery on both hands is usually not accomplished on the same day, allowing the patient some autonomy in taking care of his or her own basic needs. The more severely affected hand is generally operated on first and, if necessary, the second about 3 months later.

With the patient under general anesthetic, the affected joint is opened and the diseased tissue is removed. The bone on either side of the area is hollowed to accept the silicone implant. Additionally, the bones may be realigned and the hand strengthened by tendon transfer. The wound is irrigated and closed. Drains may be placed. A local anesthetic may be injected to help with postoperative pain control. A bulky dressing is applied and the patient is expected to be hospitalized for 2–3 days. It is important to keep the hand elevated. Prior to discharge from the hospital, the drains are extracted and the bulky dressing removed and replaced with one that will need to allow for minimal movement. Permanent scars will remain on the hand. The patient will need to undergo intense physical therapy and is expected to return to normal activities in approximately 8 weeks. An improvement should be noted in the quality of life.

REPAIR OF TRAUMATIC INJURIES TO THE HAND

Traumatic amputation is the most severe type of injury that can be incurred by the hand. Replantation of a digit involves the implementation of every type of procedure that would be used to correct any traumatic injury to the hand. Therefore it will be used here to illustrate:

- Closure of a simple laceration
- Tenorrhaphy
- Neurorrhaphy
- Restoration of vasculature
- Bone approximation

The surgical technologist will be required to draw upon his or her general knowledge to suit the specific situation.

Replantation of a Digit

Due to the detail of the structures involved, the process of replantation is tedious and can take upwards of 12 hours to complete. This procedure is usually performed under general anesthesia because of the length of time required.

Digital replantation involves soft tissue repair, bone approximation, tendon repair, as well as micronerve and blood vessel repairs. The surgical technologist will need all of the supplies listed for Procedure 19-3 to prepare for this type of surgery.

The affected limb is positioned, prepped, and draped in the routine fashion described for Procedure 19-3.

If the availability of personnel allows, two workstations are set up simultaneously within the sterile field. While one surgeon is debriding the proximal stump and identifying the structures to be anastomosed, another is doing the same on the severed part. This is frequently done with the use of loupes or under the operating microscope. The structures to be anastomosed are often "tagged," meaning marked with suture or other materials. "Tagging" serves two main purposes; it eases future identification of the tendons, blood vessels, and nerves planned for reconnection and it prevents retraction of the structures into the deeper tissues. If two surgeons are not available, the severed part is kept cold and the surgeon first deals with the stump (Figure 19-28). In some unfortunate situations, a determination will be made that the stump will not be able to receive the severed part and the wound is closed at this point. Once the stump

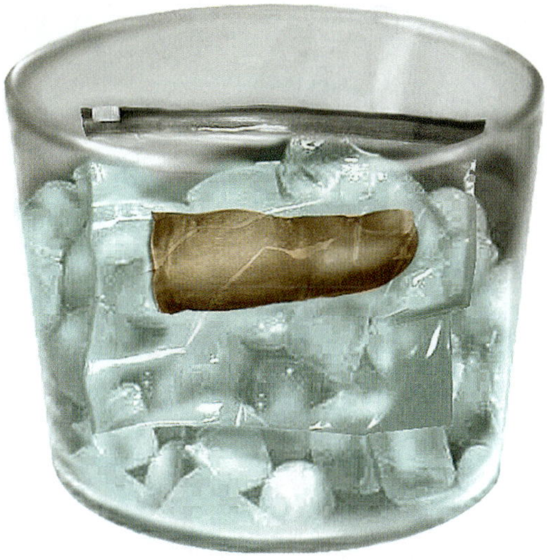

Figure 19-28 Preservation of a digit for replantation

has been prepared, the severed digit is removed from the ice and the processes of debridement and identification are repeated. Often, it is necessary to trim the ends of the structures to facilitate anastomosis.

Replantation begins with bone-to-bone attachment. This is accomplished with either intraosseous placement of K-wires or the use of plates and screws. The tendons are reconnected next by simply suturing the proximal and distal ends together. Following stabilization of the supportive structures, reanastomosis of the blood vessels is performed. Heparin may be used to irrigate the vessels prior to anastomosis to ensure patency. Because of the size of the vasculature, it is often necessary to perform this step under a microscope; it involves the use of very small suture material. The repair of at least one artery and vein will be necessary for viability. Papaverine may be used to prevent or relax vasospasm. The final structures to be repaired are the nerves. In some situations nerve grafting may be necessary.

Prior to final closure, the wound may be irrigated with antibiotic solution. To allow for expected edema and to prevent ischemia of the underlying structures, the soft tissues and skin are closed with a loose nonabsorbable suture. Drains may be placed if necessary. The dressing will most likely begin with a nonadherent gauze and progress to a bulky restrictive bandage. The use of a splint may be employed. If possible, the fingertips should remain exposed so that they may be checked for circulation and feeling. The arm should be kept elevated postoperatively to minimize edema. Frequent inspections should be made to ensure that proper circulation is maintained. The first few postoperative hours are critical to the success of the replantation. It is possible that the attempt at reattachment may fail and that the digit will eventually have to be removed. This is very disheartening, especially for the patient and family, but for the entire patient care team as well.

Toe-to-Hand Transfer

The loss of a thumb can create a significant disability, especially if the trauma has occurred to the dominant hand. Without an opposable thumb, the patient will be unable to perform such tasks as pinching and grasping. In cases of an avulsion, or crush-type injury, successful replantation may not be possible. In such situations, a toe-to-hand transfer may be a viable option. The great toe is selected because of its proximity in size and shape to the thumb.

In addition to the supplies needed for general hand surgery, the surgical technologist will need to gather draping materials for the leg and a second prep tray.

If possible, two surgical teams work together to accomplish this procedure. One team is responsible for the procurement of the great toe and the other for preparation of the stump on the hand to accept the graft.

The "harvest" of the toe requires careful dissection of the soft tissues to preserve the integrity of the blood vessels, tendons, and nerves. The structures are carefully tagged. Following soft tissue dissection, the toe is disarticulated at the metatarsophalangeal joint. Once hemostasis is achieved, the wound is closed and dressed.

Following acquisition of the toe, the procedure for toe-to-hand transfer becomes much like that for replantation of a digit. Some adjustments to the toe may be necessary prior to fixation to accommodate the minor structural differences.

An alternative to the toe-to-thumb transfer is pollicization. A normal finger is sacrificed and transferred to the location of the absent thumb. This procedure is seldom used because it is not as aesthetically pleasing.

CORRECTION OF CONGENITAL DEFECTS

Hand deformities are often corrected on young children. Care of the pediatric patient requires special consideration and equipment. Keep this in mind when preparing to repair a variety of congenital problems.

Radial Dysplasia

Surgical correction of a clubbed hand is a complicated procedure and, depending on the extent of the deformity, may require the presence of an orthopedic surgeon as well as the plastic surgeon. A bone graft may be necessary, requiring a second operative site. According to the type and severity of the deformity, the correction may be accomplished in one operation or may require multiple surgeries. Five types of procedures have been developed to correct radial clubhand. They are:

1. Soft tissue release
2. Centralization
3. Replacement of the deficient radius

4. Tendon transfer
5. **Arthrodesis**

Procedures may be combined to achieve maximum function. Because Type III radial dysplasia is the most common type, this is the repair that will be described.

The patient experiencing positive results from physical therapy should undergo centralization within the first year of life. Stretching exercises and splinting should have advanced the wrist to the level of the distal ulna. The ulnar surface may be slightly remodeled so that the center of the wrist is directly over the distal ulna. Supportive structures may have to be remodeled and tendon rebalancing implemented in order to maintain the centralization and provide as much function to the hand and forearm as technically possible.

In addition to the centralization procedure, an osteotomy should be performed, if necessary, to correct a severe bow in the ulna. Stabilization at the osteotomy site may involve the placement of a K-wire or a bone graft (Figure 19-29).

A wedge of redundant tissue on the ulnar side of the wrist may be excised. The wound is irrigated and closed. The patient is placed in a restrictive dressing that may include a splint or cast. The patient is expected to be hospitalized overnight. A restrictive device may be placed on the unaffected arm to prevent accidental disruption of the dressing. Growth and function of the forearm and hand is not expected to be normal, although adequate function is anticipated.

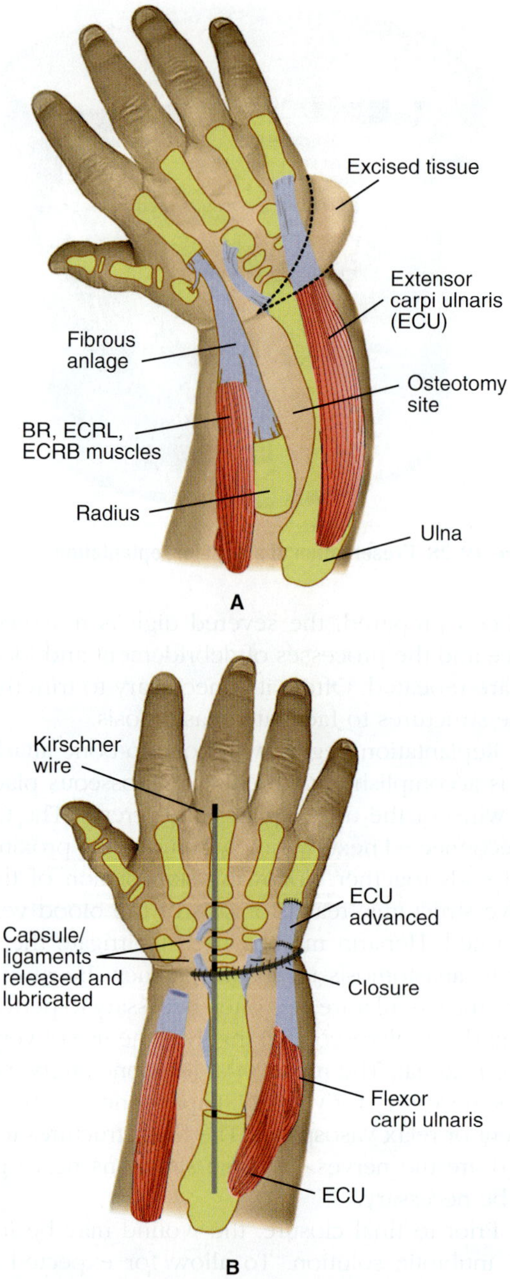

Figure 19-29 Centralization of a radial dysplasia: (A) Defect, (B) correction

Release of Syndactyly

Syndactyly repair may be quite simple, involving only soft tissue techniques, or it may be complicated and require bone and soft tissue grafts. Surgical intervention is recommended prior to the age of 8 and may be implemented at an even younger age. The type of incision used for the repair should be carefully considered to allow for growth and prevent later restriction of movement due to contractures. A simple web release will be described and is shown in Figure 19-30.

The intended incision lines on both the volar and dorsal surfaces of the hand are outlined with the surgical marking pen. Zigzag incisions are often used to allow for full-thickness coverage of the separated digits and diminish the future risk of developing contractures. Each flap of the Z is developed for later use in covering newly created interdigital space. If present, the fibrous band between the connected digits is cut, hemostasis achieved using cauterization, and the wounds closed using the full thickness tissue flaps developed following the initial incisions. A light dressing is applied. Immediate movement to the newly separated fingers is encouraged.

This is generally an out-patient procedure. A restrictive device may be recommended for a very young child to prevent wound disruption. The patient is expected to gain full use of all involved digits. Minimal postoperative physical therapy may be indicated.

Reduction of Polydactyly

Removal of an extra digit is usually a fairly simple procedure performed for cosmetic reasons only. Reductions of duplications of the thumb and small finger are generally the simplest. Central reductions attempting to create an aesthetically pleasing hand (or foot) are more involved.

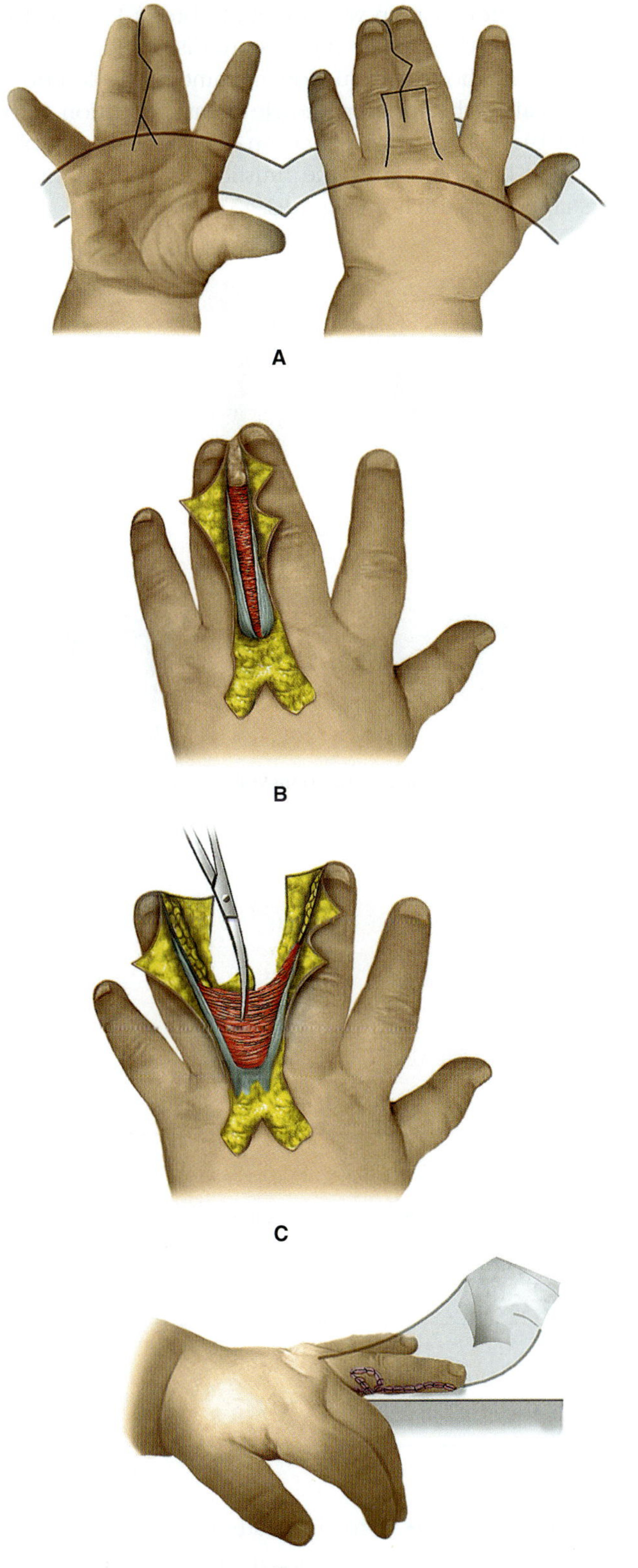

Figure 19-30 Release of syndactyly: (A) Planned incisions, (B) dissection, (C) separation, (D) closure

The simplest form of reduction is suture ligation to destroy the vascular pedicle at the base of the digit. This may be accomplished soon after birth without anesthesia. Often this leaves a small nubbin of tissue that may be excised later.

Simple excision may be performed on an infant under local anesthesia with the use of a body restraint. The extra digit is excised and the small wound closed.

More complex repairs may involve the patient being placed under general anesthesia and the excision of bone. A light dressing is applied. This is expected to be an outpatient procedure. A restrictive device may be used on the unaffected extremity to prevent wound disruption if the patient is a small child.

All types of duplication reduction should produce a good aesthetic result. The recovery period is short and no compromise of motion is expected.

MAMMOPLASTY

Mammoplasty is plastic reconstruction of the breast. The male and female breasts may be reconstructed for many reasons, some of them medical necessities and some aesthetic desires. The three most common types of breast surgery will be discussed: **augmentation** mammoplasty, reduction mammoplasty, and breast reconstruction following mastectomy. Preparation for all types of mammoplasty is similar; the following guide should be useful for the surgical technologist in assembling the necessary supplies for the basic procedure.

1. Prep tray
2. Basic surgical pack
3. Plastic instrumentation set
4. #15 scalpel blade
5. Local anesthetic with epinephrine, according to surgeon's preference
6. Syringes and needles for local
7. Fiberoptic retractor set
8. Electrosurgical pencil with needle tip and extension tip
9. Chest drapes
10. Suture material according to surgeon's preference
11. Dressings

A list of additional supplies necessary for the different types of mammoplasty will be provided in the description of the specific procedures.

REDUCTION MAMMOPLASTY

Hypertrophic male or female breasts may be reduced by means of liposuction or partial surgical removal. If major breast reduction is performed, liposuction may be used to contour nearby areas, such as the axilla, to provide an overall aesthetic result. Breast reduction may be desired because a person must restrict physical activities due to, or is self-conscious about, the size of the breasts. Most often, reduction mammoplasty performed on the female patient is a legitimate medical necessity done to relieve medical problems brought on by the weight of large breasts. These problems can include back, neck, and shoulder pain, skeletal deformities, skin irritations, and a decrease in respiratory function. A preoperative mammogram may be requested. This procedure is not recommended for women who intend to breast-feed, as the milk ducts leading to the nipples are disrupted.

The method of reduction mammoplasty described here is called the inferior pedicle breast reduction (Procedure 19-4). The primary incision lines resemble an old-fashioned keyhole, while the finished wound resembles the shape of an anchor (Figure 19-31).

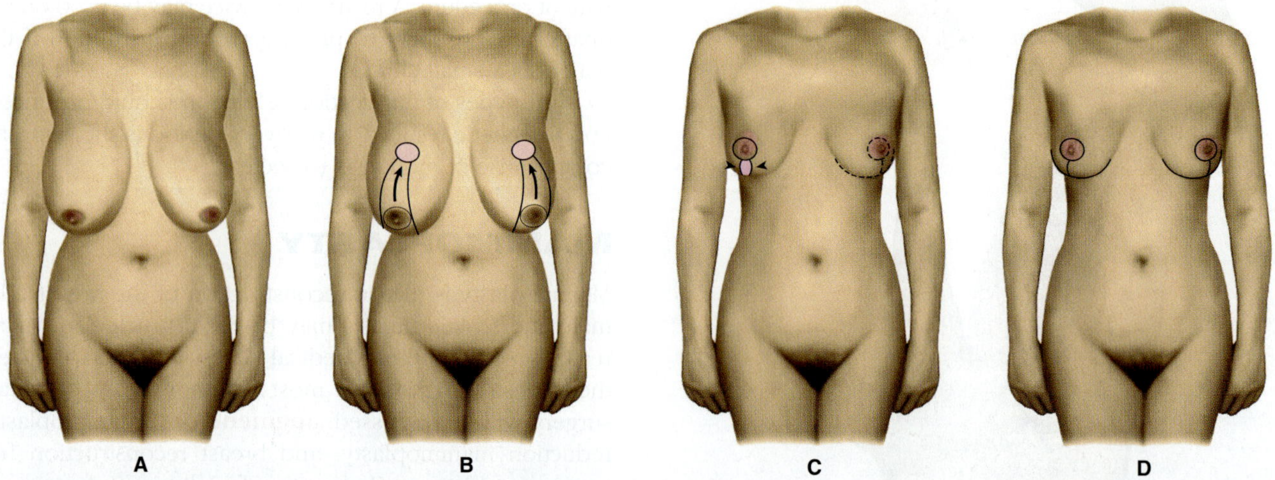

Figure 19-31 **Reduction mammoplasty: (A) Prior to surgery, (B) intended incision sites, (C) excess tissue removed, (D) final effect**

PROCEDURE 19-4 Reduction Mammoplasty

Equipment

- Padded footrest for modified sitting position
- Suction
- Fiberoptic headlight and light source
- Electrosurgical unit with needle tip and extension tip

Instruments

- Plastic instrumentation set
- Basic or minor procedures tray

Supplies

- Pack: basic pack
- Basin: basin set
- Gloves
- Blades: several #15 scalpel blades
- Drapes: folded towels and transverse sheet or folded towels and chest drape
- Suture: surgeon's preference
- Drains: none or surgeon's preference
- Dressings: surgeon's preference
- Drugs: local anesthetic of surgeon's choice, if used
- Miscellaneous:
  Sterile skin marking pen with ruler

PROCEDURE

19-4 Reduction Mammoplasty *(continued)*

Syringes: Luer-lock control with 25- or 27-gauge needles

Bulb syringe

Suction tubing

Elastic bandage

Skin staples and staple remover

Medical scale (for weighing breast tissue)

Laparotomy sponges

Areolar template

Liposuction supplies (if requested) (reduction only)

Banked blood if requested

Possible: autotransfusion system (available)

Operative Preparation

Anesthesia

- General

Position

- Supine, with each arm abducted 90° on a padded armboard

Prep

- Chest and breast: the area from the chin to the hips and the entire width of the patient, including the axillae

Draping

- The drapes (as described above) are applied to expose the entire chest and may be secured with skin staples

Practical Considerations

- The intended incision lines and landmarks are marked with indelible marker with the patient in Fowler's position. This is accomplished prior to the induction of the anesthesia, possibly before the patient is brought to the operating room
- Occasionally, the patient may require a transfusion and may be requested to donate a unit of blood in advance of the procedure to be stored for possible reinfusion

Operative Procedure	Technical Considerations
1. The initial incision is made around the existing areola.	**1.** Bleeding is controlled as it becomes evident with cauterization.
2. The surgeon must ensure a perfectly round incision for resizing.	**2.** The areolar template or "cookie cutter" is used to ensure a perfectly round incision.
3. The second incision is vertical, beginning at the bottom center of the areola continuing to the inframammary fold and then is extended laterally in each direction as needed.	**3.** Use original skin blade for this, then remove this blade from the Mayo stand and keep in a safe place, but do not reuse.
4. Deepithelization is the process that involves separating the skin from the underlying tissues. The dissection begins at the inverted T in the existing incision at the level of the inframammary fold and extends laterally in each direction until the circumference of the breast has been exposed.	**4.** Much of the dissection may be accomplished electrosurgically.
5. A pedicle is created that includes the nipple and areola, preserving the blood supply and innervation to that area.	**5.** The pedicle remains *in situ* and eventually a new opening in the skin is created to accommodate the existing tissue.

(continues)

PROCEDURE 19-4 Reduction Mammoplasty *(continued)*

6. The breast tissue is debulked—involving the removal of wedges of tissue radially.	**6.** The surgeon may desire the tissue removed from each side be weighed in the operating room by the circulator. The surgical technologist should exercise great care to keep the tissue specimens from the right and left breast isolated from one another.
7. Once the desired amount of tissue has been extracted, the new "keyhole" skin incision is made using the template.	**7.** Use a new #10 or #15 scalpel blade for this incision.
8. The wound is temporarily closed with staples. Any excess skin is removed.	**8.** The STSR should have several staplers on hand.
9. The process is repeated on the contralateral breast.	**9.** Due to a difference in breast size, the exact same amount (weight) of tissue may not be removed bilaterally. When temporary closure of the second breast has occurred, the patient may be placed in the Fowler's position to assess the breasts for size and symmetry.
10. It is common for the surgeon to reopen one or both wounds and make adjustments.	**10.** This may involve repositioning the patient several times.
11. Placement of the nipple-areolar pedicle begins the permanent closure.	**11.** Have suture ready in advance.
12. If desired, a drain is placed laterally.	**12.** Have drain available but open only upon surgeon's request.
13. The remaining wound edges are held in approximation with absorbable sutures. This process is repeated on the other side.	**13.** If liposuction is desired, it may be performed at this time.

Postoperative Considerations

Immediate Postoperative Care

- A fluff-type dressing is applied, followed by placement of a postsurgical support bra.
- The patient is expected to remain hospitalized for 1–3 days.
- Narcotic pain medication may be indicated for the first 24 hours.
- The patient should be educated in wound care and management of the drains prior to release from the hospital.

Prognosis

- The patient will have large permanent scars; however, the scars are under the breasts and should be hidden by the undergarment or bathing suit.
- The patient is expected to have full recovery. Resumption of normal activities is expected in about 2 weeks. However, the patient is instructed to refrain from vigorous exercise for 6–8 weeks.
- A repeat mammogram may be requested for comparison to the preoperative study in about 6 months.

Complications

- Hemorrhage
- Infection
- Scar tissue
- Patient dissatisfaction with appearance requiring further surgical intervention

PEARL OF WISDOM

For this procedure, the scales should be in the room to weigh breast tissue removed. These must be "zeroed out" prior to the start of surgery, to avoid incorrect readings.

AUGMENTATION MAMMOPLASTY

Augmentation mammoplasty is done to increase the size of the breast. Through the use of implants, breast size can be increased significantly. Until recently, silicone implants were the implant material of choice for most physicians and patients because of the close approximation to the look and feel of a natural breast. Today, however, concerns over potential health risks associated with the use of silicone have made its use almost nonexistent. While pharmaceutical companies continue to research other viable materials (for example, soybean oil), saline implants are currently the most widely used.

The breast implant itself is essentially just a bag or bladder composed of materials that are inert to the body—that is, materials that do not activate the body's defense mechanisms. The implants are available in various contours or shapes and sizes. The implants are usually introduced into the body empty and filled to a predetermined size by injecting saline (measured in cubic centimeters) through a port that the manufacturer has provided in the prosthesis.

The incisions may be placed in a variety of locations, all of which are designed to minimize or completely hide the surgical scar. Incision options include the periareolar line, the inframammary fold, an axillary crease, or in the umbilicus. Tunneling techniques may be used to place the implant with a variety of incisions. The surgeon and patient should discuss these options and together make the decision best suited to the individual situation.

Prior to surgery, the physician should collaborate with the patient in developing realistic expectations regarding the size of the implant to be used, and the planned outcomes.

In addition to the basic supplies previously listed, the surgical technologist will need to add the following items:

- Tunneling device (if necessary)
- Temporary implant sizers (if necessary)
- Permanent implants
- Syringes and solution to fill implants

The actual procedure for breast augmentation is a relatively simple one, performed most often in a physician's office under local anesthesia possibly enhanced with sedation. It usually takes less than an hour. The patient is placed in the supine position on the operating table, the skin prep is performed by the circulator, the drapes are applied, the local anesthetic is infiltrated, and the incision of choice is made. The pocket for the implant may be created either just under the existing breast tissue or beneath the pectoralis muscle. The subpectoral pocket may provide better long-term support of the prosthesis (Figure 19-32). This dissection process is repeated on the contralateral breast. At this point the trial implants or the permanent prostheses may be inserted. They are filled to the desired size. Often, the patient is raised to Fowler's position and the enhanced breasts are assessed for symmetry and size. Adjustments may be made at this time. Once satisfactory results are attained, the patient is returned to the supine position and the wounds are closed using a subcuticular running stitch. If necessary, temporary sizers are replaced with the permanent prostheses and then the wounds are closed. A light dressing is applied and a postsurgical bra provides support. Oral analgesics should be adequate for postoperative pain control. The patient is expected to return to normal activities within a few days.

The procedure itself should not prevent a woman desiring to breast-feed from doing so, although it should be kept in mind that there was minimal breast tissue present originally. It should be noted that implants may distort radiographic studies, such as mammography, making accurate diagnosis of breast cancer more difficult.

Pectoral implants are used to enhance the appearance of the male chest; the procedure for insertion closely follows that for breast implants in the female.

RECONSTRUCTION MAMMOPLASTY

Breast removal due to cancer or other disease may be one of the most psychologically devastating procedures that a woman may have to endure. Along with dealing with the diagnosis of cancer, many women feel that they have been stripped of their womanhood. Reconstruction mammoplasty can help to restore a woman's appearance, positive self-image, and quality of life.

For some patients, breast restoration may begin at the same time that the mastectomy is performed. The reconstructive process can involve more than one procedure. The nipple and areolar reconstruction is often the final stage. Some patients may choose to have surgery performed on the otherwise unaffected breast to gain symmetry. For patients with advanced malignancies, reconstruction may not be recommended.

A description of the different types of mastectomy can be found in Chapter 14. Several options for breast reconstruction exist, depending on the type of mastectomy that has been performed. These options include:

- *Implant reconstruction:* If the patient has enough remaining tissue, the surgeon may insert an implant similar to those used for augmentation mammoplasty under the existing muscle. Otherwise, a temporary device called a tissue expander is inserted in the same location that the final implant will be located.

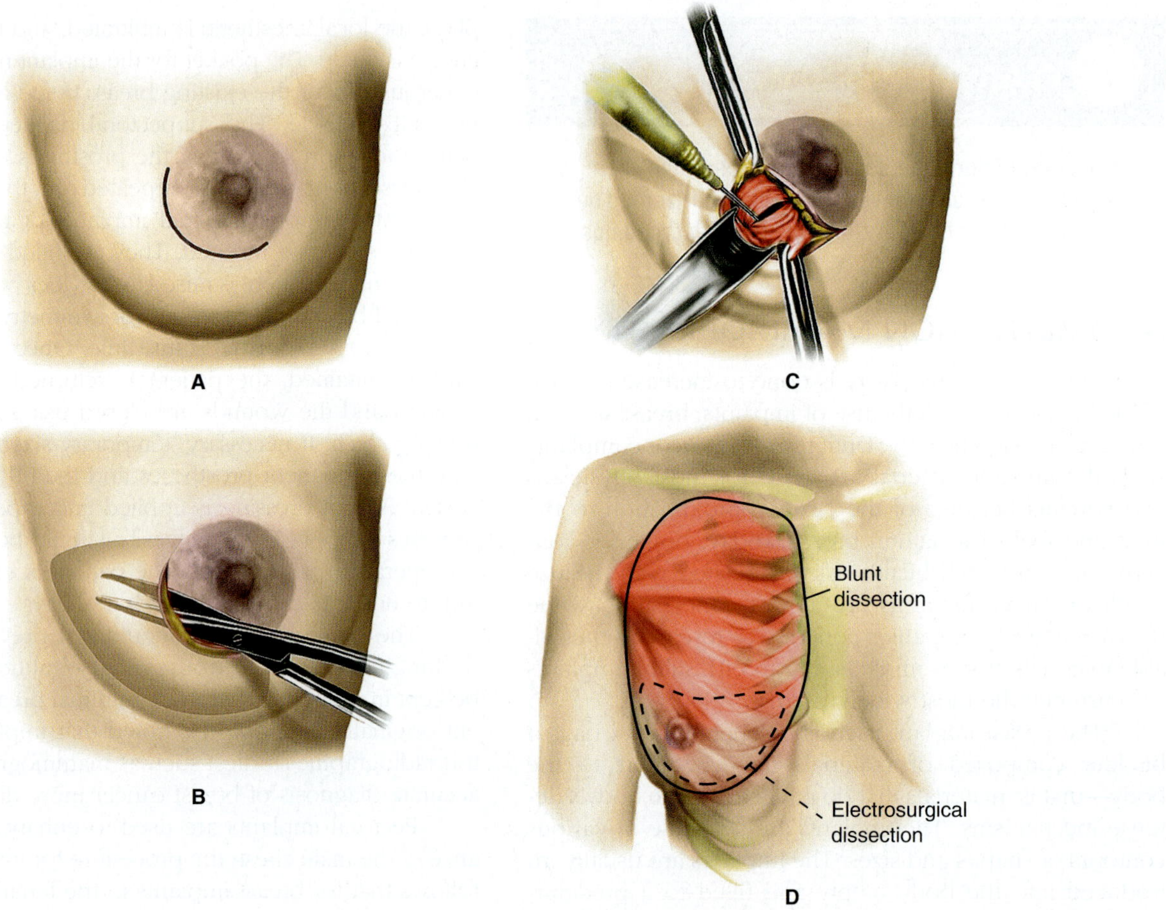

Figure 19-32 Augmentation mammoplasty: (A) Areolar incision, (B) creation of pocket, (C) pectoral muscle incision, (D) implant position

This temporary device allows for fluid to be gradually added at intervals to stretch the existing tissue. When the desired result is achieved, the permanent implant is substituted.

- *Flap reconstruction:* Flap reconstruction involves transferring tissue from one part of the body to another. The tissue may be taken from the abdomen, back, buttocks, or thigh. Two types of flap surgery exist.

1. *Free flap reconstruction* involves totally removing the tissue to be transferred from its original location and transplanting it to the chest. The blood vessels must be microscopically reconnected at the new site. The patient will not experience any sensation to the grafted area.
2. *Pedicle flap reconstruction* allows the tissue to be transferred to remain attached to its blood supply. It is relocated via a tunnel under the existing skin. The flap consists of the skin (if necessary), fat, and muscle. The flap may be used to create a pocket to accept an implant, or the tissue itself may create the new breast mound. The latissimus dorsi musculocutaneous flap and the transverse rectus abdominis musculocutaneous (TRAM) flap techniques are the two most commonly used pedicle flaps (Figure 19-33).

Pedicle flap reconstruction using a TRAM flap will be used to illustrate breast reconstruction. Patients who are excessively overweight or those who have previously undergone abdominal surgery may not be good candidates for this type of reconstruction. In addition to the items previously mentioned, the surgical technologist should consider the following:

- If the reconstruction is to be performed at the same time as the mastectomy, it may be necessary for the sterile surgical team members to use a new set of sterile supplies for the reconstructive portion of the procedure, to prevent the spread (seeding) of cancer cells.
- Tissue repair material such as synthetic mesh may be needed to reinforce the donor site.
- Closed wound drainage systems may be used at both surgical sites.
- A Doppler with a sterile probe should be available to identify the location of the major blood vessels serving the flap.

Breast reconstruction often immediately follows mastectomy and the patient remains under general anesthesia. The initial prep and draping should be done to accommodate the secondary procedure. Therefore, the entire chest and abdomen should be exposed. The ex-

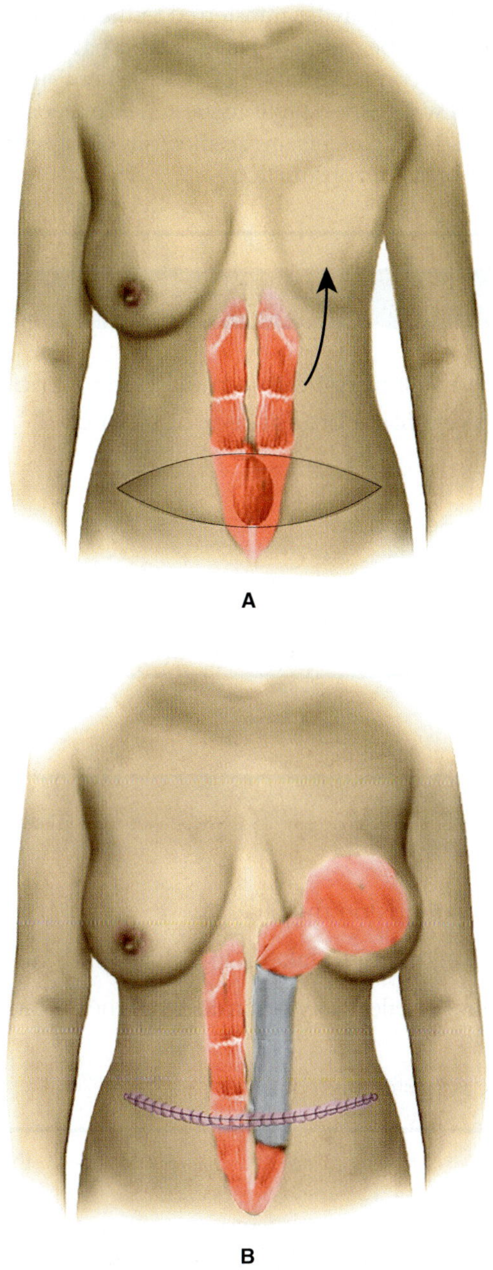

Figure 19-33 TRAM flap reconstruction: (A) Abdominal incision, (B) TRAM flap rotated into position

posed area should include the natural breast to use for comparison. The general surgeon and the plastic surgeon will have collaborated prior to the mastectomy regarding the type of mastectomy to be performed and the planned breast incision. Often, the general and plastic surgeons work together for the entire procedure, changing roles as primary surgeon and assistant as the case progresses. The general surgeon terminates the mastectomy portion of the procedure following removal of the breast and axillary contents, if necessary. Hemostasis is achieved and the wound is left open and covered with a sterile towel.

The plastic surgeon now becomes the primary surgeon, initiating the reconstructive portion of the procedure. The abdominal incision is a combination incision consisting of two transverse elliptical cuts above the umbilicus, one superiorly and one inferiorly creating an "island" of tissue. The surgeon dissects down to the anterior rectus sheath (fascia) achieving hemostasis as the need arises. The dissection may be accomplished with the use of electrosurgery. A transverse incision is made into the anterior rectus sheath and the inferior edge of the rectus abdominis muscle is transected. The epigastric vessels are located with the Doppler; the inferior vessels are ligated and the superior preserved to provide continued perfusion to the flap. Dissection continues superiorly developing the pedicle to the necessary length. The tissue remains attached to its pedicle and, once fully developed, is tunneled subcutaneously to the breast area and rotated into its new position in the existing mastectomy incision on the anterior chest wall. The rotational arc used is of extreme importance to preserve both the arterial and venous perfusion to the newly created breast. Any compromise in circulation could cause the flap to become ischemic and slough. The mound of tissue is left in position on the chest while the abdominal wound is closed. The vascular status of the flap is monitored visually for color and may be touched gently to check for warmth, or the Doppler may be reemployed.

If necessary, the abdominal wound may be reinforced with the use of a synthetic tissue repair material. The operating table may be flexed to facilitate tissue approximation and the abdominal wound is closed with the suture material of choice. A closed wound drainage system may be placed. Attention returns to the chest area. A final check of the integrity of the flap is made. Once the surgeon is satisfied that the flap is viable, the rectus muscle and adjacent tissue is shaped to create the breast mound and is then sutured into position. This maneuver will also close the existing mastectomy wound. A second closed wound drainage system may be placed at the lateral edge of this wound as well. This completes the first stage of the reconstruction. Nipple-areolar reconstruction is rarely planned as part of the first reconstructive procedure. If it is to be done, it will be performed at this time and may require accessing another surgical site. The abdominal wound is dressed and an abdominal binder or girdle may be applied. A loose fluff-style dressing is applied to the chest. Caution should be used not to place any unnecessary pressure on the wound that could compromise circulation. A postsurgical bra may be used for support.

The patient is expected to remain hospitalized for several days and will initially require the use of narcotics for pain relief. Ambulation will be painful, but should be encouraged immediately. The patient should be shown how to splint the abdominal wound for protection and comfort when coughing or ambulating. Wound and drain care should be explained to the patient prior to release from the hospital. Drains are normally extracted 10–14 days following the surgery. The patient is expected to return to her normal activities in 4–6 weeks. There will be permanent visible scars on both the abdomen and breast. If the nipple and areolar reconstruction was not done at the time of the original surgery, at least one more surgical procedure will be necessary for that purpose. This will most likely be performed in the plastic surgeon's office or in an ambulatory surgery center under local anesthesia. Tissue from another area of the body may be transferred to the area or a medical tattoo may be applied. Patients who have undergone TRAM flap reconstruction are at risk for herniation of the abdominal wall, especially if tissue repair material has not been used. Most patients are aesthetically satisfied with the results of breast reconstruction.

CASE STUDY

Selena had a modified radical mastectomy for breast cancer. She has completed her treatments and the wound is healed. It appears that she will survive this malignancy, and she has asked for a breast reconstruction.

1. What are the options for breast reconstruction for Selena?
2. Will implants or muscle be used?
3. What instruments will be required?

QUESTIONS FOR FURTHER STUDY

1. What are the steps in a "face-lift" procedure?
2. Why is the term *plastic* used to define this field of surgery?
3. What types of suture are typically used to close incisions or wounds on the face?
4. What are the reasons for the use of sterile mineral oil when preparing to take a split-thickness skin graft?
5. Describe the most commonly used technique for performing a cheiloplasty referred to as the "rotation advancement."
6. What are the purposes of using cocaine when a rhinoplasty is performed?

BIBLIOGRAPHY

Atkinson, L. J., & Fortunato, N. (1996). *Berry and Kohn's operating room technique* (8th ed.). St. Louis, MO: Mosby.

Borowitz, K. C., & Williams, C. (1998). *Children's medical center, University of Virginia* [Online]. Available from *http://avery.med.virginia.edu/medicine/clinical/pediatrics*

Burke, F., et al. (1990). *Principles of hand surgery*. New York: Churchill Livingstone.

Cohen, M. (1994). *Mastery of plastic and reconstructive surgery*. Boston: Little, Brown.

Georgiade, G. S., et al. (1992). *Textbook of plastic maxillofacial and reconstructive surgery* (2nd ed.). Baltimore: Williams and Wilkins.

Indiana Hand Center. (1997). *The Indiana Hand Center*. [Online]. Bloomington: MANUS. Available from *http://www.indianahandcenter.com*

McGuiness, A. M., et al. (2002). *Core curriculum for surgical technology* (5th ed.). Centennial, CO: Association of Surgical Technologists.

Meeker, M. H., & Rothrock, J. C. (1999). *Alexander's care of the patient in surgery* (11th ed.). St. Louis, MO: Mosby.

Neuman, J. F. (1997). Evaluation and treatment of gynecomastia [Online]. *American Family Physician 55*. Available from *http://www.aafp.org*

Smith, J. W., & Aston, S. J. (1991). *Grabb and Smith's plastic surgery* (4th ed.). Boston: Little, Brown.

Solomon, E., Schmidt, R., & Adragna, P. (Eds.). (1990). *Human anatomy & physiology* (2nd ed.). Ft. Worth: Saunders College Publishing.

Thomas, C. L. (1989). *Taber's cyclopedic medical dictionary* (16th ed.). Philadelphia: F. A. Davis.

CHAPTER 20

Genitourinary Surgery

Teri Junge

CASE STUDY

Homer is a 63-year-old male scheduled for a TURP.

1. What does TURP mean?
2. What is the most likely cause of Homer's bladder outlet obstruction?
3. What is the anesthetic of choice for Homer and why?
4. Homer and his wife are concerned about their marital relations following surgery. Can he expect his sexual function to be normal?

OBJECTIVES

After studying this chapter, the reader should be able to:

A 1. Discuss the relevant anatomy of the genitourinary system.

P 2. Describe the pathology that prompts genitourinary system surgical intervention and the related terminology.

3. Discuss any special preoperative genitourinary diagnostic procedures/tests.

O 4. Discuss any special preoperative genitourinary preparation procedures.

5. Identify the names and uses of genitourinary instruments, supplies, and drugs.
6. Identify the names and uses of special genitourinary equipment.
7. Discuss the intraoperative preparation of the patient undergoing the genitourinary procedure.
8. Define and give an overview of the genitourinary procedure.
9. Discuss the purpose and expected outcomes of the genitourinary procedure.

10. Discuss the immediate postoperative care and possible complications of the genitourinary procedure.

S 11. Discuss any specific variations related to the preoperative, intraoperative, and postoperative care of the genitourinary patient.

SELECT KEY TERMS

1. ACTH
2. afferent
3. calculi
4. conduit
5. cortex
6. ESWL
7. focal point
8. Gerota's fascia
9. Gibson incision
10. hilum
11. hirsutism
12. hypertrophy
13. hypospadias
14. incontinence
15. intravenous urogram (IVU)
16. medulla
17. prepuce
18. retroperitoneal
19. stoma
20. suprarenal glands
21. torsion
22. TURP
23. UTI
24. vesical trigone

ANATOMY

The anatomy covered in this chapter will include the urinary system and male reproductive anatomy. Female reproductive anatomy is covered in Chapter 15. Some comments on male and female differences will be noted when the difference concerns genitourinary surgery.

SUPRARENAL GLANDS

The **suprarenal** (adrenal) **glands** sit on the superior and medial portion of the kidneys (Figure 20-1). The suprarenal glands are endocrine glands with a **cortex** and **medulla**. The cortex secretes steroid-type hormones essential to the control of fluid and electrolyte balance in the body. The medulla secretes epinephrine and norepinephrine. These glands are essentially triangular in shape. They are 3–5 cm long, 2–3 cm wide, and approximately 1 cm thick. The glands are concave and the surface of the concavity sits on the kidney. They are enclosed within the renal fascia (**Gerota's fascia**) but separated from the kidney on the connecting side by a thin fascial sheet. The result is isolation in a fascial envelope. Small, separate accessory glands sometimes exist. These glands are highly vascular and receive multiple arteries from the inferior phrenic artery, abdominal aorta, and renal artery. The veins correspond to the arteries. The nerve supply comes via the celiac plexus and the greater thoracic splanchnic nerve.

Due to the anatomical proximity of the adrenal glands to the kidneys, a similar surgical approach is used; therefore the anatomy, pathology, and surgical procedures relating to this portion of the endocrine system are also included in this chapter, even though the general surgeon, rather than the genitourologist, usually performs adrenalectomy.

KIDNEYS

The two kidneys differ somewhat in location and size. The left kidney is normally larger than the right kidney. The right kidney is located slightly lower than the left. The kidneys are typically from 10–12 cm in length, 5–6 cm in width, and 3 cm in thickness. Nephrons are the functional unit of the kidney (refer to Plate 9A and B in Appendix A). There are more than 1 million nephrons, which are subdivided into two types: juxtamedullary and cortical nephrons. The juxtamedullary nephron extends deep into the medulla of the kidney, while the cortical nephron rarely does so. Each nephron itself is composed of two basic units: the renal corpuscle and the renal tubule.

Renal corpuscles consist of a network of capillaries, called the glomerulus, and Bowman's capsule, a double-layered cup of the renal tubule. The glomerulus and Bowman's capsule lie in the cortex of the kidney. The outer layer of a Bowman's capsule is the parietal layer; the inner

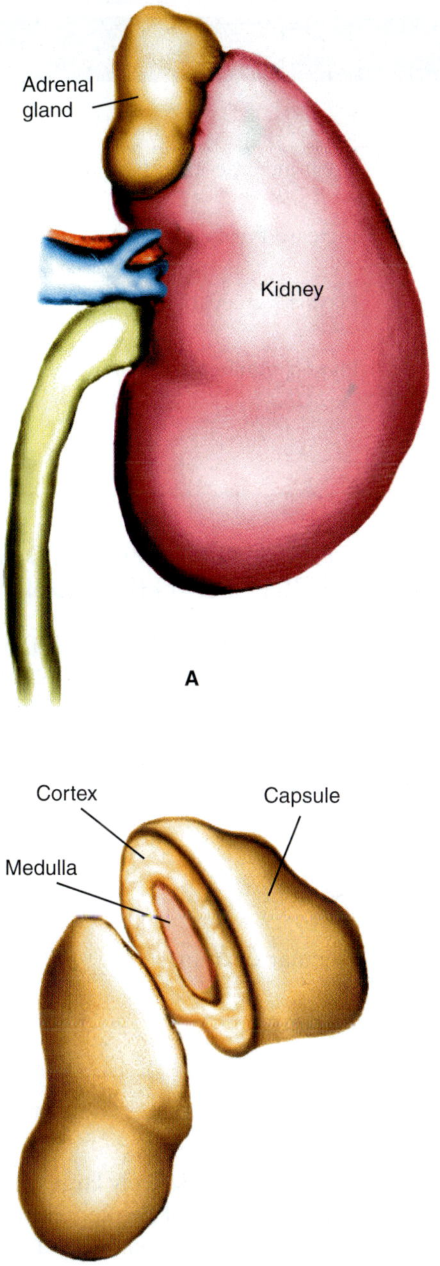

Figure 20-1 **Adrenal gland: (A) Location, (B) cross section**

is the visceral layer. The inner layer contains a special type of epithelial cells called podocytes. The podocytes send out multiple branches that adhere to the capillaries of the glomerulus. These grouped branches, along with the spaces between them, create a filter through which many substances must pass before entering a Bowman's capsule (Table 20-1). This filtration device helps separate blood in the glomerulus from the lumen of Bowman's capsule. It is one of a series of devices that collectively produce a filtration barrier.

Renal tubules make up the second component of the nephron (Table 20-2). The tubules consist of three units: the proximal convoluted tubule, the loop of Henle, and the distal convoluted tubule.

The kidneys are located in the **retroperitoneal** space in the lower thoracic and upper lumbar area (Figure 20-2). The kidneys are bilateral structures embedded in paravertebral gutters of fat and fibrous connective tissue formed by the relative positions of the vertebral column and psoas muscles. The kidneys are bounded by the psoas muscles on the medial side, the transverse abdominal muscles on the lateral, and the quadratus lumborum muscles posteriorly. Anteriorly, the kidneys relate to other abdominal organs. The suprarenal gland sits atop the superomedial surface of both kidneys. The medial border of the right kidney sits posterior to the second section of the duodenum. The superior portion of the right kidney lies in contact with the right lobe of the liver. The inferior one-third of the right kidney lies laterally to the right flexure of the colon and portions of the jejunum. On the other side, the pancreas lies across the **hilum** of the left kidney. The stomach touches the superior part of the left kidney. The spleen, also, makes contact. Inferior to these structures, the left flexure of the colon lies laterally and portions of jejunum medially.

The kidneys lie in a bed of fatty and fibrous connective tissue. The adipose and fibrous connective tissue form distinct layers around the kidney. A membranous sheet, the renal fascia, separates the fatty layers. The renal fascia sends out anterior and posterior laminae, both of which pass medially and unite. The laminae continue medially across the vertebral column. They pass anteriorly and posteriorly to the aorta and inferior vena cava. The

Table 20-1 Filtration System of the Kidney

STRUCTURE	COMPOSITION	ACTION
Glomerular capillary endothelium	Fenestrated endothelium	Restricts movement of blood, cells, and large molecules
Glomerular basement membrane	Glycoprotein matrix without pores	Allows passage of molecules smaller than plasma proteins
Bowman's capsule, visceral layer	Podocytes with filtration slits	Final barrier before slit pore and lumen of Bowman's capsule

Table 20-2 Renal Tubule Structure and Function

STRUCTURE	FEATURES	ACTION
Proximal convoluted tubule	Cortical Coiled Near renal corpuscle Cuboidal epithelium	Great increase in surface area Increased reabsorption and secretion
Loop of Henle	Descending: Thin wall of squamous cells Ascending: Thicker wall of cuboidal cells	Plays a significant role in urine concentration
Distal convoluted tubule	Cortical Thin walled Cuboidal cells Coiled structure	Plays a significant role in urine concentration

posterior fascia blends with the transversalis fascia over the vertebral column. On the inferior and medial side a portion of fascia continues along the ureter as periureteric fascia. The inferior pole of the kidney lies further from the medial line than the superior pole. The kidney is convex, and the medial border receives the renal blood vessels at an indention called the hilum. The renal pelvis exists in this area and becomes the descending ureter. A space is formed around the blood vessels and renal pelvis by the anterior and posterior surfaces of the kidney. The space is filled with fatty tissue.

Kidneys' smooth exterior results from investment by a fibrous capsule (Gerota's fascia). The kidney proper has two major zones. The outer zone has a high concentration of glomeruli, which makes it granular in appearance. This zone is called the cortex. The inner zone, the medulla, consists mostly of straight tubules and connecting ducts. It has a striated appearance. The innermost portion of the cortex begins to transition in appearance to more a medullary-like form. The tubules of this portion of cortex are called the pars radiata. Some cortical substance extends to the renal sinus and separates the straight tubules and collecting ducts of the medullary pyramids. This cortical substance is called the renal columns. A branch of the renal artery, the interlobar artery, crosses each renal column. The pyramidal shape of the medullary pyramids and the investing cortical substance effectively form a "lobe" of kidney.

The renal pyramids taper to form 8–12 renal papillae. These papillae enter the 4–13 minor calyces. The minor calyces are the initial portions of the system of extrarenal ducts. The minor calyces empty into two or three major calyces. Major calyces drain the superior, middle, and inferior portions of the kidney into a common renal pelvis. The renal pelvis passes inferiorly and medially beyond the hilum. As it nears the inferior border of the kidney, the extrarenal renal pelvis narrows and continues as the ureter. The ureter conducts urine from the renal pelvis to the bladder.

BLOOD VESSEL, LYMPHATIC, AND NERVE SUPPLY TO THE KIDNEY

As the abdominal aorta descends, it supplies branches that are classified as visceral, parietal, or terminal. In normal descending order, the arterial branches of the abdominal aorta are as follows:

- Inferior phrenic
- Celiac trunk
- Middle suprarenal
- First lumbar
- Superior mesenteric
- Renal
- Gonadal (testicular-ovarian)
- Second lumbar
- Inferior mesenteric
- Third lumbar
- Fourth lumbar
- Median sacral
- Common iliac

The renal arteries are relatively large and arise at the level of the upper boundary of the second lumbar vertebra. This point of origin is approximately 1 cm below the superior mesenteric artery. The renal arteries follow a transverse course from the aorta to the hilum of the kidney. They pass anterior to the crura of the diaphragm and the psoas muscles. The right renal artery is situated slightly lower than the left and is greater in length. The right renal artery passes posterior to the inferior vena cava, the head of the pancreas, and the second section of duodenum. The left renal artery passes posterior to the left renal vein, the pancreas, and the splenic vein. At the hilum of the kidney, the arteries form multiple branches that enter the kidney sinus both anterior and posterior to the renal pelvis. There they branch again into anterior and posterior interlobar branches and pass to the kidney substance of the renal columns. The renal arteries also form an inferior suprarenal branch that travels upward to the

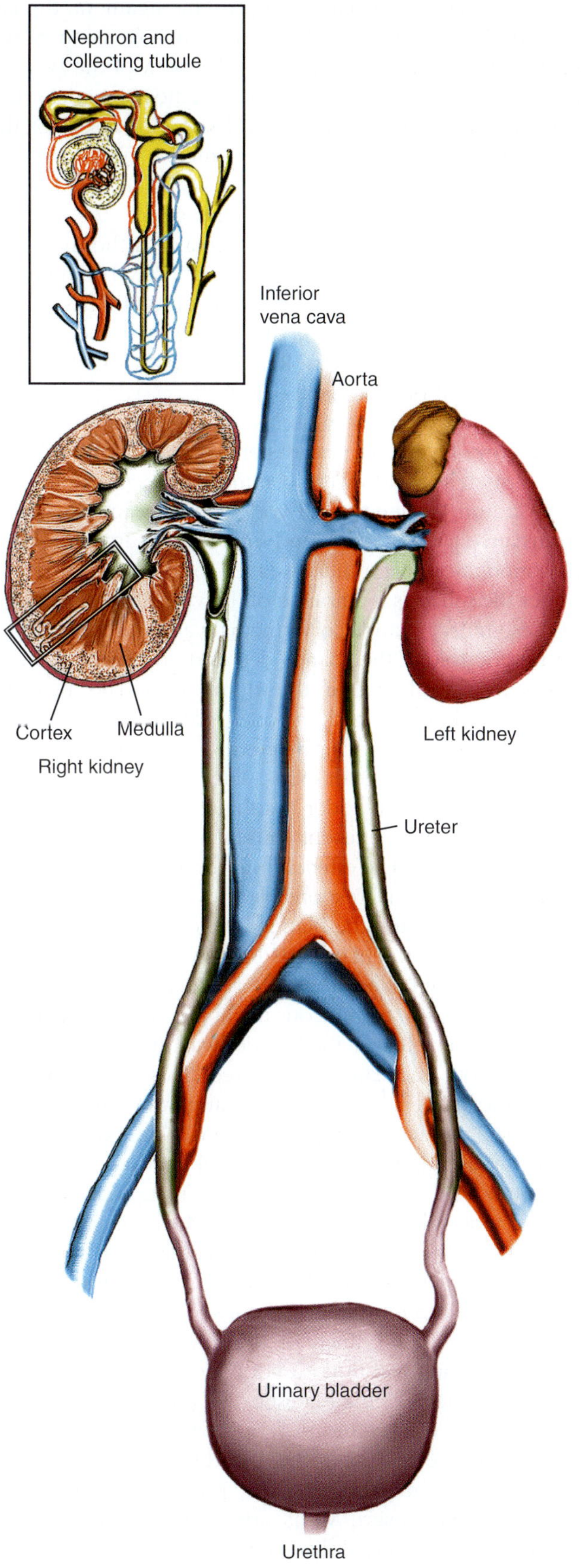

Figure 20-2 Kidneys, ureters, and bladder

lower portion of the suprarenal gland and ureteric branches to the ureter.

Almost one-fourth of the population has accessory renal arteries that arise from the aorta and pass directly to the kidney surface. These are more common on the left kidney and tend to arise below the renal artery itself.

The renal veins arise on both the anterior and posterior sides of the kidney sinus. They mostly lie anterior to the arteries. The left renal vein is longer than the right. The left renal vein passes anterior to the aorta below the superior mesenteric artery and terminates in the inferior vena cava. As it courses its way to the vena cava, the left renal vein accepts the left suprarenal and left testicular/ovarian veins and sometimes the left inferior phrenic and left second lumbar veins. The short right renal vein passes behind the second section of the duodenum and terminates on the right side of the inferior vena cava.

The kidney's lymphatic vessels form three plexuses. One plexus is formed in the substance of the kidney itself, one underneath the capsule, and one in the perirenal fat. The lymph trunks from the kidney substance and capsule join at the hilum and follow the course of the renal vein to the lumbar lymph nodes. The plexus of the perirenal fat drains directly to the lumbar lymph nodes.

The autonomic **afferent** innervation of the kidney comes from the renal plexus. The main efferent innervation is autonomic, vasomotor nerves. Neural activity does not affect kidney production or secretion directly. The effect on urine production is secondary to changes in blood supply.

URETERS

The ureters conduct urine from the kidney to the bladder. The ureters are thick-walled muscular tubes with a small lumen. They run their abdominal course in extraperitoneal connective tissue and the pelvic course in the retroperitoneal space. The ureters run their descending course on the psoas muscles until they cross the bifurcation of the common iliac arteries and enter the pelvis. The average length is 25 cm split evenly between the abdominal and pelvic sections. The ureters are crossed obliquely by the testicular/ovarian vessels and by their ipsilateral colic vessels. The abdominal portion's blood supply is from branches of the renal and testicular/ovarian arteries. Veins follow the arteries. Nerves of the abdominal portion come from the renal and testicular/ovarian plexuses. The pelvic section descends on the side of the pelvic wall. The course is curved forward and medially. As it nears the bladder, it is crossed by numerous other structures. The ureter terminates by running obliquely through the wall of the bladder for about 1.5 cm. The oblique course allows the bladder to prevent reflux through muscular contraction upon the ureter. The pelvic ureter in the female relates to other structures in such a way as to create several surgical problems. The vascular supply for the pelvic section of the ureter comes from branches of the superior and/or inferior vesical artery. Some branches may come directly from the internal iliac artery and, in the female, from the uterine artery. Veins correspond to the arteries.

URINARY BLADDER

Urine collects in the urinary bladder, which lies in the anterior half of the pelvis (Figure 20-3). The urinary bladder sits in a space bounded by the symphysis pubis on the front, the walls of the pelvis bilaterally, and the rectovesical septum posteriorly. Because the pelvis diverges as it ascends from the most inferior point, the space is roughly triangular in shape. The intimate space for the urinary bladder is created by structures of the pelvic walls, as follows:

Inferior—levator ani muscles

Superior—obturator internus muscles

Posterior—rectum (male: also the ductus deferens and seminal vesicles)

Anterior—abdominal wall

In the male, the bladder lies on and is attached to the base of the prostate gland. In the female, the bladder lies on the pelvic diaphragm. The bladder itself is invested in endopelvic fascia. The puboprostatic ligament, the lateral true ligament of the bladder, is an extension of the endopelvic fascia. It originates at the neck of the bladder and the base of the prostate and attaches to parietal fascia on the rear of the pubis and superior fascia of the pelvic diaphragm. This fixes the inferior portion of the bladder relatively well. Added stability of the bladder, in both sexes, results from the passage of the urethra through the structures of the perineum. In the male, additional stability is gained by the continuity between the neck of the bladder and the prostatic urethra. The median umbilical ligament connects the bladder with the connective tissue of the umbilicus. Relationships with other male structures will be discussed below.

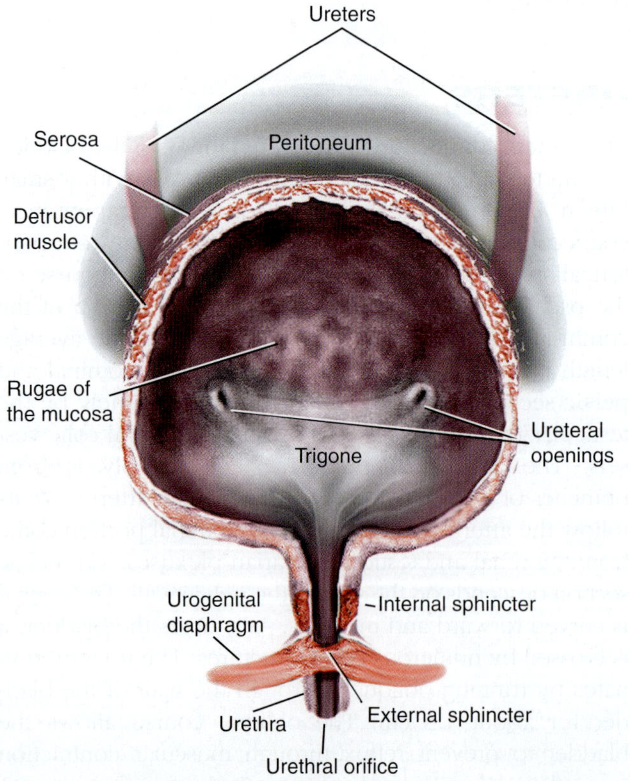

Figure 20-3 Bladder and urethra

The involuntary muscles of the bladder form a meshwork; layers are not existent. However, the orientation is such as to allow the common distinctions of external stratum (longitudinal orientation), middle layer (transverse to long axis), and internal stratum (longitudinal orientation). The muscle layers of the ureters extend under the mucous membrane of the vesical trigone. Some of these muscle bands curve medialward and form the interureteric fold. Other bands descend and crisscross in a thin submucosal sheet in the trigone area. The musculature of the bladder neck is somewhat difficult to understand. A vesical sphincter is referred to in most literature, but no annular sphincter exists. The action of the muscles of the neck of the bladder is sphincter-like, produced by the opposition of existent muscular arcades (structures made of arches). The effect of this arrangement is that the detrusor muscle is responsible for both emptying the bladder and closing the bladder orifice.

Internally, the bladder is lined with a mucous membrane that is wrinkled when the bladder is not distended. In the fundal area, the mucous membrane is firmly attached to the muscular coat of the bladder wall. It is, therefore, always smooth and can be visualized. This triangular area, called the **vesical trigone**, is an important clinical landmark. The ureteral openings are found at the posterolateral angles of the triangle and the urethral aperture at the inferior angle. The underlying muscular formation produces an interureteric fold between the two ureters. Normally, the openings to the ureters are approximately 3 cm apart.

Vascular supply to the bladder comes from the superior and inferior vesical arteries. These arteries arise from the anterior branch of the internal iliac artery. A plexus of veins within the endopelvic areolar tissue surrounds the neck of the bladder. The plexus extends over the seminal vesicles and ductus deferens to the point at which the ureters enter the bladder. In the male, the plexus communicates with the prostatic plexus, from which several vesical veins arise on each side. These empty into the internal iliac vein.

Innervation of the bladder is from the vesical plexus, which contains postganglionic sympathetic and preganglionic parasympathetic fibers. The vesical plexus of each side sits against the posterior-lateral portion of the bladder and terminal portion of the ureter. Nerve supply extends to the bladder, lower ureter, seminal vesicle, and ductus deferens. Parasympathetic actions serve the bladder-emptying reflex (contraction of the detrusor urinae muscle).

MALE REPRODUCTIVE SYSTEM

The male genital organs include the testes, ductus deferens, seminal vesicles, ejaculatory ducts, and the penis (refer to Plate 10). The prostate and bulbourethral glands are accessory structures.

PENIS AND MALE AND FEMALE URETHRA

The penis and scrotum are the superficial structures of the male urogenital triangle. The penis is a cylindrical structure composed of three cylindrical masses of cavernous tissue that are bound together by fibrous tissue and covered by skin. The cavernous structures of the penis, the two corpora cavernosa, are positioned on the dorsal side of the penis and lie side by side. The corpus spongiosum penis lies in the midline below these two structures. The corpus spongiosum penis expands distally forming a conical structure, the glans penis. The raised and backward-pointing margin of the glans penis is called the corona. The urethra passes through the corpus spongiosum penis and opens to the exterior via a slit-like opening, the external urethral orifice or meatus.

The skin covering the penis is thin, hairless, and somewhat dark. It is relatively loosely connected to the underlying structures. On the ventral surface, the skin exhibits a median raphe that is continuous with the raphe (seam or line of union) of the scrotum. At the distal base of the penis, the skin forms a free fold, the **prepuce** (foreskin), that resembles a mucous membrane and covers the glans penis.

The subcutaneous connective tissue of the penis is loose areolar tissue that contains no fat. This tissue is reinforced by smooth muscle fibers from the tunica dartos scroti. The superficial dorsal vein passes along the dorsal midline of the penis. The superficial dorsal vein joins the superficial external pudendal veins near the root of the penis. A layer of deep fascia encloses the cavernous bodies of the penis and the associated nerves and vessels.

The male and female urethras deserve special notice. The male urethra passes through the prostate gland, the urethral sphincter, the perineal membrane, and the penis. It is divided into three parts and totals about 20 cm in length. The three parts are called prostatic, membranous, and spongy. The prostatic section of the urethra passes through the prostate with a gentle forward curve and is 3–4 cm in length. The section receives most of the ducts of the prostate gland. The ejaculatory duct opens on each side of a urethral structure called the prostatic utricle. The membranous section crosses the annulus of the sphincter urethrae muscle and the perineal membrane. It is only about 2.5 cm in length. The bulbourethral glands perforate the perineal membrane and enter the spongy section of the urethra. The spongy section of the urethra is about 15 cm long. It enters the bulb of the penis just after the perineal membrane has been crossed and terminates at the external urethral orifice. The spongy urethra exists as a horizontal slit until near the external orifice where it becomes vertical.

The female urethra is only 4 cm long. It has sections that correspond to the prostatic and membranous portions of the male urethra. The lumen of the female urethra is about 5 mm in diameter. It is slightly concave in form, bending forward. The female urethra passes in front of the lower half of the vagina. Voluntary sphincter muscle surrounds the female urethra. Some of these muscle fibers help form the urethrovaginal sphincter. The urethra is separated from the vagina by loose areolar tissue. Skene's glands provide lubrication and enter the vestibule via the paraurethral ducts near the external urethral orifice. The blood supply comes via the inferior vesical and vaginal branches of the internal iliac artery.

TESTES

The testes are paired structures 4–5 cm long, 3 cm wide, and 2 cm thick that lie in the scrotum (Figure 20-4). The tunica vaginalis testis is an invaginated serous sac that covers most of the testis, epididymis, and lower end of the spermatic cord. The tunica vaginalis testis does not cover the posterior portion of the testis, and it is here that the blood vessels and nerves of the testis enter. The testes have a thick external covering of connective tissue called the tunica albuginea. The tunica albuginea turns into the testicular substance at its posterior border forming a mesh-like mediastinum testis. The mediastinum of the testis is crossed by the major ducts of the testis, the vessels, and lymphatics. A large number of convoluted seminiferous tubules lie between the septa of the testis. There are approximately 800 of these tubules. They unite to form the straight seminiferous tubules. These pass into the mediastinum and anastomose to become the rete testis. The channels of the rete testis unite to form 12–15 efferent ducts. These ducts pass through the tunica albuginea and form twisted masses called the coni epididymis. These form the head of the epididymis. The efferent ducts ultimately open into the single duct of the epididymis. The testicular arteries exit the abdominal aorta just below the renal arteries. These vessels are long and thin. They descend obliquely in the retroperitoneal space. The testicular arteries cross the psoas muscles, ureters, and external iliac arteries to enter the deep inguinal rings. The testicular arteries give off ureteral branches during their course. The testicular vein travels

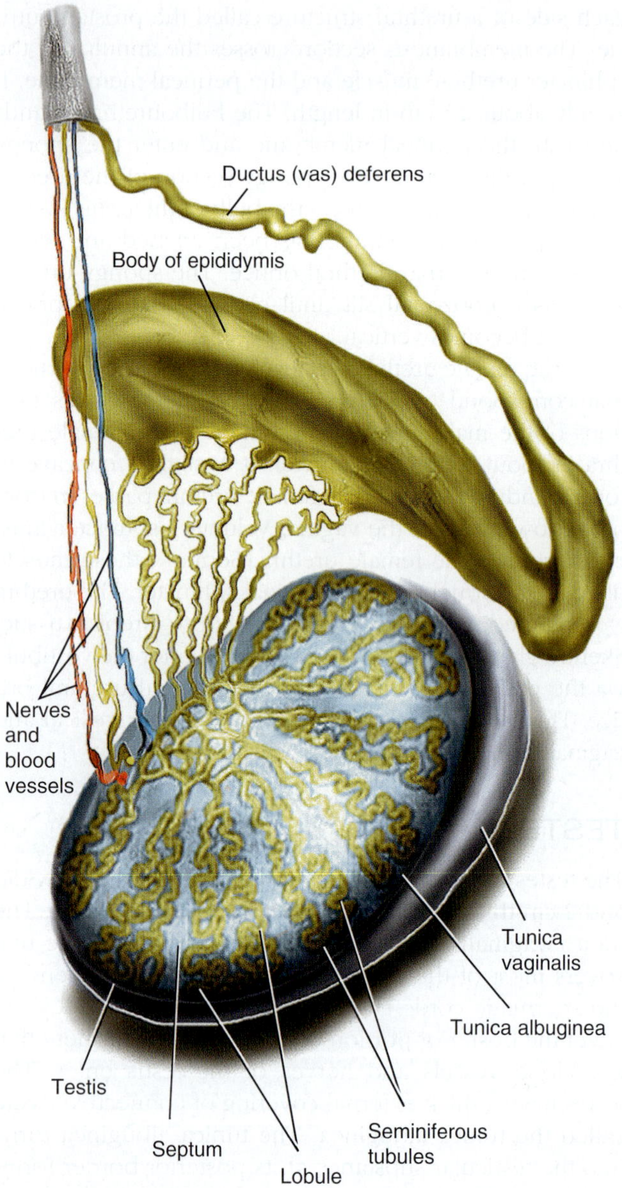

Figure 20-4 Testis

with the artery on the lateral side. The testicular artery exits the spermatic cord and forms several branches. Some of these branches travel with the ductus deferens to supply the epididymis, and others supply the substance of the testicle.

The testicular plexus contains parasympathetic fibers from the vagal system and sympathetic neurons from the 10th thoracic spinal cord segment.

DUCTUS DEFERENS

The ductus (vas) deferens arises from the duct of the epididymis and is about 45 cm long. The vas ascends through the inguinal canal as the center portion of the spermatic cord. It then runs backward and medially to descend on the fundus of the urinary bladder. It runs medial to the ureter and seminal vesicle. It narrows just above the base of the prostate and is joined by the duct of the seminal vesicle to form the ejaculatory duct. The ductus deferens has a thick muscular layer that delivers semen to the prostatic urethra by peristaltic action.

SEMINAL VESICLES

The seminal vesicles lie on the fundus of the bladder, enclosed by endopelvic fascia. They are about the size of a small finger and are blind pouches. The ductus deferens runs along their medial surface. The seminal vesicles narrow at the prostatic end and unite with the ductus deferens.

EJACULATORY DUCTS

About 2 cm long, these thin-walled ducts are formed by the unification of the ductus deferens and seminal vesicles. The ejaculatory ducts are contained within the prostate gland. They move downward and forward opening into the prostatic urethra at either side of the prostatic utricle.

PROSTATE GLAND

The prostate is a seminal tract accessory gland of conical shape that lies under the bladder. Its apex touches the perineal membrane. The rectovesical septum separates the prostate from the ampulla of the rectum on its posterior side. The lateral surfaces relate to the superior fascia of the pelvic diaphragm. The prostate is covered with endopelvic fascia. The fascial sheath is part of the puboprostatic ligaments. The urethra courses through the prostate, entering near the midbase and exiting on the anterior surface just above the apex. The ejaculatory ducts enter the posterior base and open at the prostatic utricle. The prostatic glandular elements are enclosed by a fibromuscular stroma and capsule. The gland is lobulated with about 50 lobules. Prostatic tubules lead to prostatic ducts that empty into prostatic sinuses on both sides of the urethral crest.

The arterial supply to the prostate consists of branches of the inferior vesical and middle rectal arteries. These are part of the internal iliac system. Veins form a prostatic plexus to the anterior and lateral portion of the gland. The deep dorsal vein of the penis joins this plexus. The prostatic plexus communicates with the vesical plexus. They empty into the sacral and internal iliac veins. The lymph vessels are part of the system of the seminal vesicles and bladder neck. They empty into the sacral and internal iliac nodes.

PATHOLOGY AFFECTING THE ADRENAL GLANDS

Pathological conditions affecting the adrenal gland typically produce signs and symptoms related to the gland's hormonal function.

CUSHING'S SYNDROME

Cushing's syndrome is a rare condition in which there is an overproduction of cortisol by the cortex of the adrenal gland. The hyperactivity of the adrenal gland may be stimulated by an overproduction of adrenocorticotropic hormone (**ACTH**) from the pituitary gland or may be from a tumor in the adrenal cortex itself.

Of those affected by Cushing's syndrome, 80% are considered to be of the ACTH, dependent type. The primary cause in this case is a pituitary tumor that causes an overproduction of ACTH, thereby causing the adrenal glands to overproduce cortisol. The cause in the remaining 20% of those with Cushing's syndrome is a tumor of the adrenal cortex. Adrenal cortex tumors may be benign (adenoma) or malignant (adrenal cell carcinoma).

The following are symptoms of overproduction of cortisol:

- Central body obesity
- Glucose intolerance
- Hypertension
- **Hirsutism**
- Osteoporosis
- Kidney stone formation
- Emotional instability
- Menstrual irregularity

Initial diagnosis of Cushing's syndrome is made with the use of blood and urine tests. If the syndrome is determined to originate in the pituitary, a CT or MRI scan of the brain will be performed. If the adrenal gland itself is suspected, an adrenal ultrasound, CT, or MRI will be used to confirm the location of the tumor.

Treatment will be determined according to the origin of the disease. Pituitary tumors will be surgically removed or treated with radiation therapy. Benign adrenal gland tumors may be removed endoscopically, while malignant tumors will require a more invasive traditional open procedure.

ADRENAL INSUFFICIENCY (ADDISON'S DISEASE)

The adrenal glands are essential in the secretion of hormones that maintain several body functions. When the adrenal glands fail to produce the hormones necessary to maintain fluid balance and blood pressure or they inhibit the response to stress, a critical situation may result.

Symptoms of adrenal insufficiency may develop gradually or appear suddenly (adrenal crisis). The symptoms include weight loss, weakness and fatigue, GI disturbances, low blood pressure, darkening of the skin, hair loss, and dramatic mood and behavior changes. An adrenal crisis may be triggered by stress to the body that includes infection, surgery, and trauma. Addison's disease may be a complication of certain illnesses such as TB and AIDS. It is critical that the health care team be aware of the patient's condition. Diagnosis is accomplished with biochemical laboratory tests and radiological examinations.

Treatment for Addison's disease is medical. Hormone replacement with corticosteroids is essential for life.

PHEOCHROMOCYTOMA

Pheochromocytoma is a tumor affecting the medulla of the adrenal gland causing an overproduction of adrenaline. The presence of excess adrenaline can prove deadly due to the severe hypertension that it causes.

The following are classic symptoms of pheochromocytoma:

- Severe headaches
- Excess sweating
- Tachycardia-palpitations
- Anxiety
- Tremor
- Pain in the epigastric region
- Weight loss
- Heat intolerance

Diagnosis for pheochromocytoma begins with 24-hour urine sampling and blood samples. Ultrasound, CT, and MRI may be used to locate a tumor of the adrenal medulla. One nuclear medicine study, called the MIBG scan, is available specifically for the detection and location of pheochromocytoma.

Treatment for pheochromocytoma is surgical. Most pheochromocytomas are small tumors that lend themselves easily to endoscopic removal.

PATHOLOGY AFFECTING THE URINARY SYSTEM

The urinary system is complex and important to the health of the body. It sometimes suffers from systemic diseases, neoplasms, and structural conditions.

BLADDER TUMORS

Bladder tumors usually present with hematuria, a symptom that is often ignored. Bladder tumors can be benign or malignant. They may appear as a single growth, but are often seen in multiples.

Benign tumors or papillomas occur only in young adults. **Intravenous urogram** (**IVU**) will likely be used to locate the tumor. Definitive diagnosis is made cystoscopically and the tumor is usually removed transurethrally. The tumors seldom recur and follow-up care is not usually indicated.

Malignant neoplasms arise from the epithelial lining of the bladder and usually affect individuals over the age of 50, most of them men. The tumor is mushroom shaped with a stalk-like attachment to the bladder wall. Intravenous urogram, cystoscopy, CT, and MRI may be used in diagnosis and determination of metastasis.

With early intervention, the malignancy may be removed transurethrally by cauterizing the stalk of the tumor and removing the remainder of the mass. If the tumor has invaded the bladder wall, partial cystectomy may be indicated. In advanced cases, a total cystectomy may be performed along with an additional procedure to divert the urine. Radiation and chemotherapy may be recommended. Bladder cancer has a tendency to recur and careful follow-up is necessary.

URINARY CALCULI

Calculi, or stones, are small solid particles that may form in one or both kidneys. It is possible for the stone to remain in its original location or travel through the urinary tract and become lodged at any point distal to the formation point. The presence of the stone will partially or totally obstruct the urinary tract. One or several stones may be present and they can vary in size from that of a grain of sand to a very large mass.

The size and location of the calculi will determine signs and symptoms, which can include:

- Painful urination
- Frequent urination
- Passage of small amounts of urine
- Flank pain (mild to severe with the exact site determined by the location of the stone)
- Nausea and vomiting
- Urinary tract infection
- Hematuria

Blood tests, urinalysis, and urine culture may be ordered to help determine the type of stone that may be present and to rule out the possibility of infection. Radiologic examinations such as X-ray, ultrasound, CT scan, and intravenous urography (formerly referred to as intravenous pyelogram or IVP) will provide information on the size and location of the obstruction.

The following four basic chemical types of urinary calculi exist:

- Calcium-based stones account for approximately 75% of urinary calculi. The causes of calcium-based stones vary. Dietary imbalances are blamed in most instances, but one type of calcium-based stone is associated with hyperparathyroidism. This type is treated with surgical removal of the parathyroid. Most recurrences of calcium-based stones can be avoided with diet modifications and pharmaceuticals.
- Another 15% of urinary calculi are determined to be struvite or magnesium ammonium phosphate stones that are traced to chronic urinary tract infections (**UTI**). Urinalysis will typically show a pH greater than 7.0 in these cases.
- Uric acid stones account for 6% of urinary tract stones. This condition is associated with gout. The urine pH will usually read less than 5.5.
- Cystine stones are caused by a metabolic defect in which renal tubular reabsorption of certain amino acids fails.

Uroliths (calculi) smaller than 4 mm have an 80% chance of spontaneous passage. Analgesics, anti-inflammatory medications, and muscle relaxants may aid this process. For calculi that do not pass spontaneously, several options for removal include:

- Extracorporeal shock wave lithotripsy (**ESWL**)
- Cystoscopicureteroscopicnephroscopic lithotomy
- Percutaneous lithotomy
- Open lithotomy

Urinary calculi recur in more than 50% of those affected. Diet and lifestyle changes can dramatically reduce the possibility of recurrence.

KIDNEY DISORDERS

Disorders of the kidney affect fluid and electrolyte balance, blood volume, and the ability to filter out waste products.

POLYCYSTIC KIDNEY DISEASE

Polycystic kidney disease (PKD) occurs when the parenchyma of the kidney is replaced by multiple fluid-filled benign cysts. The cysts begin their formation in the tubular portions of the nephrons and enlarge substantially. One kidney can contain thousands of cysts and may weigh up to 22 pounds. Polycystic kidney disease seems to affect both genders and all races equally. Approximately 500,000 people in the United States are affected by PKD. There are three types of polycystic kidney disease:

- Autosomal dominant PKD is one of the two inherited forms of the disease. The symptoms usually develop between the ages of 30 and 40. Ninety percent of all PKD falls into this category.
- Autosomal recessive PKD is the other inherited form, and is extremely rare. This type of PKD affects young children.
- Acquired cystic kidney disease develops in patients with long-term kidney problems. The symptoms occur later in life.

The symptoms of PKD include back and flank pain, headaches, hypertension, chronic urinary tract infections, hematuria, and the development of cysts in the kidneys and other organs such as the liver.

Family medical history is probably the most important factor in diagnosing polycystic kidney disease. The diagnosis may be verified with ultrasound. Treatment for PKD includes antibiotic therapy to resolve infection, and medication for pain. There is no cure. In the final stages of the disease, if both kidneys are affected, dialysis or transplantation will become necessary. Approximately 50% of persons affected by PKD progress to kidney failure or end-stage renal disease.

DIABETIC NEPHROPATHY

Diabetic nephropathy or sclerosis is also known by several alternate names such as Kimmelstiel-Wilson disease and diabetic glomerulosclerosis. Uncontrolled diabetes mellitus causes damage to many body systems, including the urinary system. The disease causes sclerosis to the glomerular apparatus of the kidney and may be accompanied by an excess of a connective tissue called hyaline. As the glomeruli are destroyed, so is the body's capability to filter the blood.

Some of the symptoms that the patient may experience are excessive thirst and edema. The clinical signs will include hypertension and proteinuria. Diabetic nephropathy is a progressive disease leading to chronic renal failure and continuing to end-stage renal disease within 2–6 years. Dialysis or kidney transplant will ultimately become a necessity.

END-STAGE RENAL DISEASE (ESRD)

End-stage renal disease (ESRD), or kidney failure, is a term that refers to the final stages of many types of kidney diseases, such as polycystic kidney disease or diabetic nephropathy, that occur when the filtration of the kidney is no longer effective. A person is considered to be in ESRD when the kidneys are functioning at less than 10% of their normal capacity. Almost half of the population suffering from ESRD is diabetic.

The patient should already be aware of the underlying condition leading to ESRD and be prepared for the eventual outcome. The main symptom is severely decreased or no urine output. This will probably be accompanied by malaise, fatigue, headache, hypertension, and decreased mental alertness. Laboratory findings will include increased creatinine and blood urea nitrogen (BUN) levels.

Death will occur from the accumulation of waste products and fluids if treatment is not started immediately. The only two treatments for ESRD are dialysis and kidney transplant.

Hemodialysis and peritoneal dialysis are the two types of dialysis that are available. Both methods of dialysis remove excess fluids and waste products from the body and require that an access port be established.

Hemodialysis

The first step in hemodialysis is establishing vascular access (Figure 20-5). Immediate access may be gained by

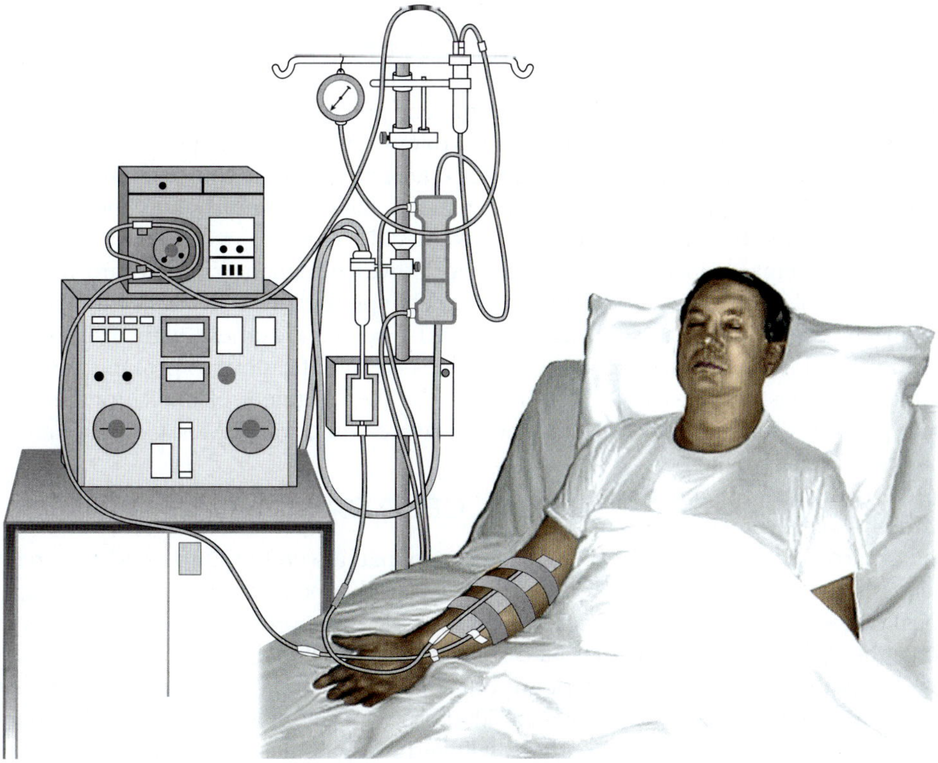

Figure 20-5 Hemodialysis

insertion of a temporary dual-lumen catheter. If dialysis is to be long term, a more permanent access site must be created. This is done surgically by inserting a polytetrafluoroethylene (PTFE) loop graft, sometimes referred to as a shunt, or creating an arteriovenous (AV) fistula, usually in the forearm on the nondominant side. The vessels of choice for a hemodialysis shunt or AV fistula are the cephalic vein and the radial artery. Both types of permanent vascular access need time to heal or mature prior to use.

Two dialysis cannulas (one for outflow and one for inflow) are connected, either percutaneously or to the exposed lumens of the catheter, and a portion of the patient's blood is pumped from the body to the dialysis machine. The dialysis machine has two compartments: one for the incoming blood and one for the necessary solution called dialysate. Between the two compartments is a semipermeable membrane much like the one found naturally in the kidney. As the blood passes over the membrane, the excess fluid and waste products are filtered into the dialysate while the vital substances such as blood cells and proteins that are too large to pass through the membrane are returned to the body. The dialysate, along with the waste and excess fluid, is discarded.

Hemodialysis may be accomplished at home or at a dialysis center. The standard schedule includes three treatments per week that may last from 2–4 hours each according to the individual situation.

Peritoneal Dialysis

Three options for peritoneal dialysis exist and require a different type of access (Figure 20-6).

The most common type of peritoneal dialysis is called continuous ambulatory peritoneal dialysis (CAPD). A permanent catheter (CAPD catheter) is placed in the lower peritoneal cavity. A small portion of the catheter remains outside the abdominal wall. Special tubing is connected to the catheter and dialysate is instilled by gravity into the peritoneal cavity. The dialysate remains in the peritoneal cavity for a specified amount of time (usually several hours). Instead of using a machine with a filter, the peritoneal membrane is the filter. Excess fluids and waste products from the abdominal blood vessels are drawn into the dialysate through the peritoneal membrane. When the prescribed amount of time has passed, the peritoneal fluid (dialysate and wastes) is drained by gravity into a bag, which is then discarded and the process begins again. The patient is usually capable of handling this type of dialysis at home without assistance.

Continuous cyclic peritoneal dialysis (CCPD) works by the same mechanism as CAPD; the difference is that a machine instead of gravity is used to pump and drain the dialysate. This is usually done at home while the patient sleeps.

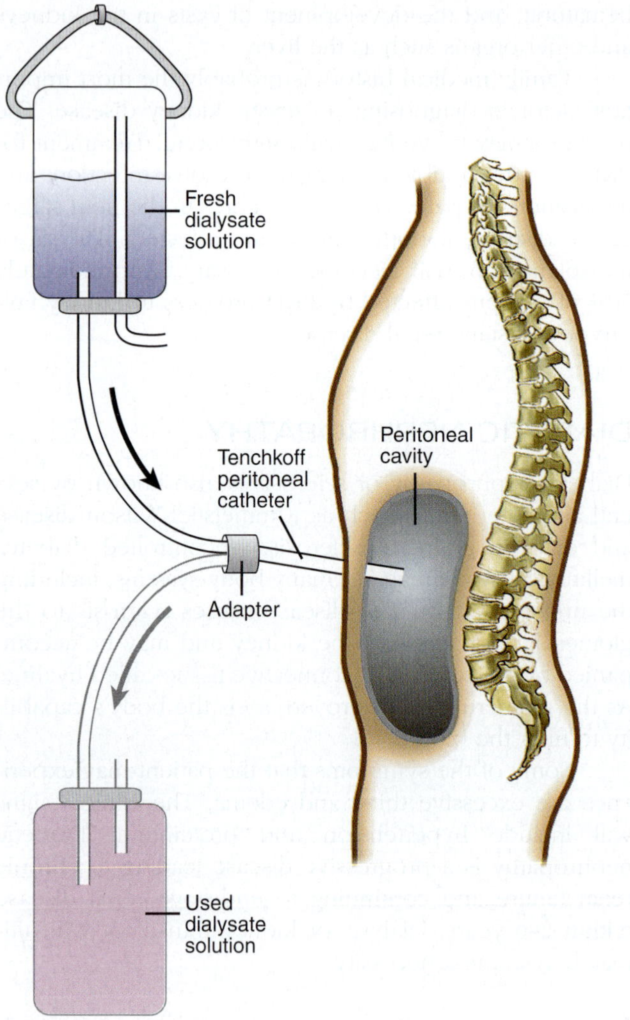

Figure 20-6 Peritoneal dialysis

Intermittent peritoneal dialysis (IPD) also involves the use of a pump. This is usually performed in a hospital setting and takes a greater amount of time than CCPD.

The patient, patient's family, and the health care team should decide together which approach is best suited to the individual situation. There are many pros and cons to each type of dialysis. Dialysis is not a cure for end-stage renal disease. Treatment with dialysis will require major lifestyle modifications to prolong the patient's life. This may be the treatment of choice or it may be a temporary measure while waiting for a kidney transplant.

RENAL CELL CARCINOMA

Renal cell carcinoma, also referred to as adenocarcinoma of the renal cells, is the most common type of kidney cancer. It is responsible for approximately 8,000 deaths in the United States each year. Renal cell carcinoma affects men twice as often as women and usually appears between the ages of 50 and 60. Development of renal cell carcinoma is directly linked to cigarette smoking and heredity and is often seen in patients with end-stage renal disease who are on dialysis.

Renal cell carcinoma causes a malignant change to cells lining the renal tubule, producing hematuria, flank pain, and the presence of a palpable mass. The patient may also suffer from hypertension, fatigue, and weight loss. The tumor easily invades the surrounding tissues and most commonly metastasizes to the lungs. It often has the opportunity to spread prior to detection.

Diagnosis of renal cell carcinoma is facilitated with abdominal ultrasound and CT scans. Additional information regarding local extension of the tumor or metastasis may be obtained with angiography or MRI.

Radical nephrectomy is the recommended treatment for renal cell carcinoma that has not spread. Early detection and surgery together produce the best results with the five-year survival rate around 75%. Attempts to treat this type of cancer with radiation, interferon, interleukin, hormones, and chemotherapy have not shown promise.

CONGENITAL NEPHROBLASTOMA

Congenital nephroblastoma, or Wilms' tumor, is a malignancy affecting the kidney that occurs in children primarily between the ages of 3 and 4. In 90% of the cases only one kidney is affected. The child is usually asymptomatic until the late stages of the disease when hypertension, hematuria, and abdominal enlargement are noted. The tumor is usually found incidentally on a routine exam.

Ultrasound, CT, and MRI will aid in diagnosing the extent of the tumor and any metastasis. Wilms' tumor is a mixed cell tumor that originates in the kidney and eventually replaces most of the involved kidney, causing hemorrhage and eventual necrosis. The tumor eventually affects the renal vein, causing thrombosis that can extend to the inferior vena cava. Nephroblastoma is spread through the blood, lymphatics, and extension of the tumor itself most commonly to the lungs and liver.

Surgical removal of the affected kidney is recommended and should be followed by radiation and chemotherapy. If treated prior to metastasis, the 5-year survival rate is 90%.

PATHOLOGY AFFECTING THE MALE REPRODUCTIVE SYSTEM

Much like the female reproductive system, the male reproductive system suffers pathological conditions unique to its hormonal, cellular, and structural character.

PHIMOSIS

Phimosis is a condition affecting the prepuce, or foreskin, that prevents it from retracting over the glans penis. The inability to retract the prepuce is attributed to a thin band of skin at the opening of the foreskin. Phimosis can be infantile or may occur in geriatric patients when the skin begins to lose elasticity. The inability to retract the foreskin for cleaning may lead to infection and may also cause pain during erection. The degree of phimosis can vary as well as the treatment options. Conservative treatments are available; circumcision is recommended for severe phimosis.

HYPOSPADIAS/EPISPADIAS

Hypospadias and epispadias are both congenital conditions of the urethra. Both conditions are more common in males, but can occur in females. Hypospadias is diagnosed when the urethral opening occurs on the underside of the penis or on the perineum of the male or in the vagina of the female. Epispadias is the developmental absence of the anterior wall of the urethra. The urethral orifice is located on the dorsum of the penis. Both conditions, if severe, may be surgically repaired.

BENIGN PROSTATIC HYPERTROPHY

Benign prostatic **hypertrophy** (BPH) is considered to be a normal part of aging affecting most men over the age of 50. As a man matures, the prostate increases is size; this is thought to be due to hormonal changes that occur throughout the life span. Eventually, the capsule surrounding the prostate prevents it from expanding outwardly, and it begins to exert pressure on the urethra, which it encircles. As the urethra narrows, the process of urination is disrupted leading to urgency, frequency, and urinary retention. Retained urine may lead to infection that may require systemic antibiotic treatment. Complete blockage of the urethra by the prostate is a urologic emergency requiring immediate intervention for drainage of the bladder.

Diagnosis of BPH usually begins with a digital rectal examination in the doctor's office. This will provide information about the size and condition of the gland. The next step in evaluation is to rule out the possibility of cancer. This is accomplished via a prostate specific antigen (PSA) blood test and possibly a biopsy.

BPH does not always require immediate treatment but some type of future intervention is inevitable. Pharmaceuticals are being developed to inhibit prostate growth and possibly even reduce the size of the prostate. Other medications act on the muscles of the prostate and bladder to improve urine flow. Options for minimally invasive procedures involve the transurethral introduction of microwaves or low-level radio-frequency energy to ablate the portion of the prostate causing the urethral obstruction. Transurethral resection of the prostate (**TURP**) is the surgical treatment of choice in 90% of surgeries performed to treat BPH. Open surgery is usually not necessary. Treatment for BPH usually does not involve removing the total gland; therefore continued growth of the remaining gland may cause the symptoms to recur in the future.

CANCER OF THE PROSTATE

Prostate cancer in the early stages is asymptomatic. As the tumor grows the patient will likely experience the same obstructive symptoms as those with BPH. Patients in the advanced stages of prostate cancer experience pelvic pain due to the tumor mass and bone pain from metastasis. Men over the age of 50 are most affected. It is not uncommon for a man to be diagnosed with both BPH and prostatic cancer.

The physician, on routine digital rectal examination (DRE), often detects early cancer of the prostate. Any abnormality noted should be followed up with a PSA blood test and a biopsy. If cancer is found to be present, further tests such as chest X-ray, CT, and bone scans may be performed to determine if any metastasis of the malignancy has occurred. Treatment will be based on the findings of these examinations.

Radical prostatectomy is performed either suprapubically or retropubically and is usually accompanied by pelvic lymph node dissection. Removal of the testicles (orchiectomy) may also be recommended. Radiation and/or hormone therapy may be the sole treatment or may be used as follow-up treatment after surgical removal of the prostate. Chemotherapy has not been found effective in treatment of prostate cancer.

CRYPTORCHIDISM

Cryptorchidism occurs when one or both testicles fail to descend to the final destination in the scrotum after the first year of life. The disorder is commonly associated with premature birth and is often accompanied by an inguinal hernia. The testicle may be found in the abdomen or, more commonly, in the groin. Location of the undescended testicle may be determined through the use of ultrasound. Human chorionic gonadotropin (HCG) may be used to induce testicular descent. If surgery is necessary, it should be performed at a young age to position (orchiopexy) the testicle in its normal location to prevent future infertility. If the testicle cannot be correctly positioned, removal (orchiectomy) may be necessary.

TESTICULAR TORSION

Torsion of the testicle is in actuality a twisting of the spermatic cord, which causes extreme pain (Figure 20-7). The spermatic cord contains the blood vessels that serve the testicle; twisting may reduce or obstruct the blood flow to the testicle producing ischemia or necrosis. Immediate reduction must occur or the testicle may be permanently compromised. Manual derotation is possible, but should be considered a temporary measure. Orchiopexy should be performed as soon as possible to prevent recurrence. The procedure may be done bilaterally because the gubernaculum that secures the testicle to the scrotum may be deficient on both sides.

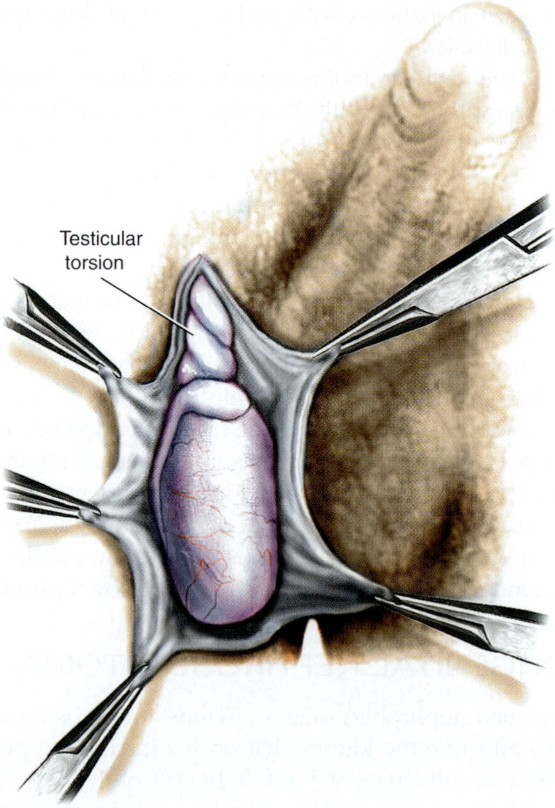

Figure 20-7 **Testicular torsion**

Every attempt should be made to determine the viability of the testis. Intravenous fluorescein in conjunction with a Wood's lamp or black light may aid in the diagnosis. Orchiectomy is necessary if the testis is necrotic.

TESTICULAR CANCER

Testicular cancer is usually first noticed during bathing or self-examination. Pain is not evident in the early stages of the disease. This aggressive type of malignancy usually strikes young men between the ages of 20 and 40. Infants with cryptorchidism are at higher risk than the general population for developing cancer of the testicle. Young men are often too embarrassed to report an abnormality in the groin area and unfortunately the disease is allowed to progress to an advanced stage.

Hematologic and ultrasonic studies may aid in diagnosis. CT scans, bone scan, and chest X-ray will help to determine if the malignancy has spread and will dictate treatment.

Orchiectomy is recommended and follow-up treatment with radiation or chemotherapy may be added to treat certain types of tumors. In some situations, if bilateral orchiectomy is to be performed, sperm can be preserved if future paternity is desired. Testicular implants are available to provide a better aesthetic postoperative appearance.

TRAUMA TO THE GENITOURINARY SYSTEM

Trauma can occur to any part of the male or female genitourinary tract and may result from a variety of causes. Motor vehicle accidents, abusive or forceful sexual activity, blunt physical combat (boxing or bicycle accident), and penetrating wounds (stab or gunshot) are a few examples of injuries that can occur. The patient may experience mild discomfort to intense pain; severe hemorrhage can lead to shock; or permanent impotence may result from an injury. A treatment plan will be developed according to the type and extent of the injury. Emergency care requiring immediate surgery may be necessary.

DIAGNOSTIC PROCEDURES/TESTS

Disorders of the genitourinary tract, whether congenital or acquired, are diagnosed through many of the standard procedures that apply to determining pathology in other body systems. Many of the usual methods of diagnosis have been thoroughly discussed in other chapters and will be only briefly mentioned as they apply to genitourinary conditions.

HISTORY AND PHYSICAL

A detailed history should be obtained from the patient or another reliable person if the patient is unable to provide the information. This step is time consuming; a patient, thorough clinician taking the family history and the patient's personal medical and social history will extract pertinent information. The person taking the history should also do visual and hands-on physical assessments of the patient. Occasionally, a clinician becomes dependent on laboratory and radiologic findings and skims over this part of the examination.

All men, as part of their health maintenance program, should perform routine testicular self-examination. Additionally, men over the age of 40 should have a yearly digital rectal examination to check for prostatic enlargement.

LABORATORY FINDINGS

Laboratory studies provide extremely accurate information about what is happening inside the body. Several types of studies are available to the genitourologist to help determine the etiology of the pathological process.

Microscopic examination is the most accurate method for determining blood and urine composition. Chemical reagent strips are available for fast general results for some tests. The chemical reagent strips are handy for a patient needing to monitor certain blood and urine levels several times per day. These home/office test strips are not highly accurate and occasional professional testing should be performed to verify the results.

HEMATOLOGY FINDINGS

Refer to the tables in Chapter 13 for normal hematology values and deviations that indicate the presence of a pathological process. It is important to realize that a great number of additional, more specific tests are available. The tables are intended to provide the reader with some basic information.

Specific hematologic examinations will require a patient to comply with certain prerequisites, such as remaining NPO for a specified period prior to the examination (Table 20-3).

Common chemistry findings are listed in Table 20-4.

One important blood value that has not been listed previously is the PSA test, which is useful in determining cancer of the prostate. Normal PSA is expected to be <4 ng/mL. An elevated PSA does not automatically indicate the presence of a malignant process, but should be followed up with a prostatic biopsy. Additionally, following prostatectomy for cancer, the PSA test is used as an indicator in determining the presence of metastatic processes. An increased phosphatase acid level is also an indicator for possible prostatic malignancy.

URINALYSIS

Urinalysis is the single most important laboratory examination used in diagnosing problems affecting the urinary tract. Several methods of collection are available. Ideally, the sample should be the first of the day and should be examined as soon after collection as possible. With the exception of samples requiring culture, the sample should be refrigerated if it cannot be examined immediately. Normal urinalysis findings are outlined in Chapter 13.

A simple voided specimen is commonly used. The patient simply urinates into a clean container. This method is ineffective if an infection is suspected; in that case, a clean-catch midstream sample or a catheterized specimen should be obtained.

Clean-catch sample requires patient cooperation, a moistened towelette, and a sterile specimen container. The patient is instructed to cleanse the area around the urinary meatus, start to void into the toilet, then begin to collect the sample partway through the excretion process, and allow the final portion of the urine to flow into the toilet again. The importance of keeping the inside of the specimen container and the lid sterile should be stressed to the patient. A child or bedridden patient may need assistance with this process. A bedpan or urinal may be substituted if the patient is immobile.

Catheterized specimens are obtained under completely sterile conditions and must be obtained with the assistance of a health care worker capable of maintaining sterile technique. The patient is awake during the procedure, and every possible measure to protect the patient's privacy and dignity should be taken. Patient education

Table 20-3 Hematology Findings

NORMAL RANGE	CONDITIONS IN WHICH VARIATIONS FROM NORMAL MAY OCCUR
Volume 7–9% of body weight (4000–6000 mL)	Decreased: hemorrhage, surgical shock, burns
Erythrocytes 4.5–5 million/mm^3	Increased: polycythemia, anoxia, chronic pulmonary disease, high altitudes, renal disease with increased secretion of erythropoietin, Cushing's syndrome
	Decreased: anemia, hemorrhage, leukemia
Reticulocytes 0.8–1% of RBC (red blood cells)	Increased: hemolytic jaundice, anemia with increased bone marrow activity
Leukocytes 5,000–10,000 mm^3	Increased: infections and tissue destruction, leukemia, metabolic disorders
	Decreased: irradiation, bone marrow aplasia
Neutrophils (PMN) 60–70% of WBC (white blood cells)	Increased: acute infections, gout, uremia, neoplastic diseases of the bone marrow, diabetic ketosis, massive necrosis, poisoning by mercury, lead, or digitalis
	Decreased: agranulocytosis, acute leukemia, measles, malaria, overwhelming bacterial infections
Lymphocytes 25–33% of WBC	Increased: whooping cough, chronic infections, infectious mononucleosis, chronic lymphatic leukemia, thyrotoxicosis
	Decreased: Hodgkin's disease, in response to adrenal cortical steroids, whole-body irradiation
Monocytes 2–6% of WBC	Increased: chronic bacterial diseases, tetrachloroethane poisoning, monocytic leukemia
Eosinophils 1–3% of WBC	Increased: hypersensitivity (hay fever, asthma, chronic skin diseases), helminthic infestations, leukemia
	Decreased: steroid therapy
Basophils 0.05–0.5% of PMN	Increased: acute severe infections, leukemia
Metamyelocytes 5% of PMN	Increased: acute severe infections, leukemia
Platelets 250,000–350,000	Increased: after trauma or surgery, after massive hemorrhage, polycythemia
	Decreased: thrombocytopenic purpura, lupus erythematosus, following massive blood transfusions
Hemoglobin 14–16 gm/100 mL	Increased: conditions in which there is an increase in erythrocytes
	Decreased: anemia, hemorrhage, leukemia
Hematocrit 42–47%	Increased: dehydration, plasma loss, burns, conditions in which there is an increase in erythrocytes
	Decreased: hemorrhage, anemia
Sedimentation rate Men 0–12 mm/hr Women 0–20 mm/hr	Increased: infection, coronary thrombosis, leukemia, anemia, hemorrhage, malignancy, hyperthyroidism, kidney disease Decreased: severe liver disease, malaria, erythema, sickle-cell anemia
Bleeding time 1–3 min	Increased: thrombocytopenia, acute leukemia, Hodgkin's disease, hemorrhagic disease of the newborn, hemophilia
Coagulation time 6–12 min	Increased: hemophilia, anticoagulant therapy
Clot retraction time Begins in 1 hr Completes in 24 hr	Increased: thrombocytopenia, acute leukemia, pernicious anemia, multiple myeloma, malignant granuloma, hemorrhagic disease of the newborn
Prothrombin time 10–15 sec	Increased: treatment with anticoagulants, hemorrhagic disease of the newborn, liver disease, hemophilia

Source: From *The Composition and Function of Body Fluids*, 2nd ed., by S. R. Burke, 1976, St. Louis, MO: C. V. Mosby.

prior to the procedure will lead to good cooperation and less tension. Commercially prepared sterile kits are available for catheterization. A nonretaining catheter, such as a Robinson, is used and may be referred to as a "straight cath." The same procedure is used to drain a patient's bladder prior to a short surgical procedure, such as a D&C, where bladder decompression is necessary.

The collection of a 24-hour urine sample is useful in determining some urinary and adrenal conditions. Blood urea nitrogen (BUN), creatinine, and catecholamine concentrations are studied. The first sample of the day is discarded. All urine excreted from that time to the same time the next day is collected and chilled.

(Text continues on page 750)

Table 20-4 Blood Chemistry Findings*

*Values depend to a certain extent on the technique used for the determination; therefore occasional discrepancies may occur when comparing different normal value charts.

NORMAL RANGE	CONDITIONS IN WHICH VARIATIONS FROM NORMAL MAY OCCUR
Albumin 3.5–5.5 g/dL	Increased: dehydration
	Decreased: renal disease, liver disease, malnutrition
Aldolase 3–8 units/mL	Increased: muscular atrophy, cancer, acute or chronic disease
Ammonia 20–160 μg/dL (diffusion)	Increased: liver disease
Amylase 60–160 Somogyi units/dL	Increased: pancreatitis, postgastrectomy, cholecystitis, salivary gland disease
	Decreased: hepatitis, thyrotoxicosis, severe burns, toxemia of pregnancy
Bicarbonate 21–28 mM/L	Increased: metabolic alkalosis
	Decreased: metabolic acidosis
Bilirubin Total 0.3–1.5 mg/dL Direct 0.1–0.3 mg/dL	Increased: biliary obstruction, impaired liver function, hemolytic disease
Blood gases	
pH arterial 7.35–7.45	Increased: alkalosis
pH venous 7.3–7.41	Decreased: acidosis
Po_2 arterial 95–100 mm Hg	Increased: administration of high concentrations of oxygen
	Decreased: hypovolemia, decreased cardiac output, chronic pulmonary diseases
Pco_2 arterial 36–44 mm Hg	Increased: respiratory acidosis, metabolic alkalosis
Pco_2 venous 40–45 mm Hg	Decreased: respiratory alkalosis, metabolic acidosis, hypothermia
Blood urea nitrogen (BUN) 8–18 mg/dL (adult)	Increased: fever, excess body protein catabolism, renal failure, congestive heart failure with decreased renal blood supply, obstructive uropathy
	Decreased: growing infant
Calcium Ionized 2.1–2.6 mEq/L Total 4.5–5.3 mEq/L Infants 11–13 mg/dL	Increased: hyperparathyroidism, vitamin D excess, multiple myeloma, thyrotoxicosis, sarcoidosis, bone cancer, fractures Decreased: hypoparathyroidism, acute pancreatitis, vitamin D deficiency, steatorrhea, nephrosis, rickets, Paget's disease, malabsorption, pregnancy, respiratory alkalosis
CO_2 combining power 45–70 vol% 21–28 mEq/L	Increased: emphysema, metabolic alkalosis Decreased: respiratory alkalosis, metabolic acidosis
CO_2 (measured as HCO_3) 25–35 mEq/L	Increased: respiratory acidosis, metabolic alkalosis Decreased: respiratory alkalosis, metabolic acidosis
Carboxyhemoglobin Suburban nonsmokers less than 1.5% saturation of hemoglobin Smokers 1.5–5.0% Heavy smokers 5.0–9.0%	Increased: industrial pollution, smoking
Chloride 95–105 mEq/L	Increased: dehydration, hyperchloremic acidosis, brain injury, steroid therapy, respiratory alkalosis, hyperparathyroidism
	Decreased: gastrointestinal loss, potassium depletion associated with alkalosis, diabetic ketosis, Addison's disease, respiratory acidosis, mercurial diuretic therapy
Cholesterol 150–250 mg/dL (varies with age and diet)	Increased: obstructive jaundice, renal disease, pancreatic disease, hypothyroidism, untreated diabetes mellitus, chronic pancreatitis, familial hypercholesterolemia
	Decreased: severe liver disease, starvation, terminal uremia, hyperthyroidism, cortisone therapy, anemia
Creatine phosphokinase Males 55–170 units/L Females 30–135 units/L	Increased: myocardial infarction, crush injury, hypothyroidism, tissue transplant rejection, cerebral vascular accident
Creatinine 0.6–1.2 mg/dL	Increased: acromegaly, renal failure
Fibrinogen 200–400 mg/dL	Increased: inflammatory processes
	Decreased: liver disease, hemorrhagic disease

(continues)

Table 20-4 *(continued)*

NORMAL RANGE	CONDITIONS IN WHICH VARIATIONS FROM NORMAL MAY OCCUR
Gastrin 40–150 pg/mL	Increased: peptic ulcers, gastric carcinoma, pernicious anemia
Globulin 2.5–3.0 g/dL	Increased: chronic infectious diseases, chronic hepatitis, sarcoidosis
Glucose 70–120 mg/dL (fasting)	Increased: diabetes mellitus, severe thyrotoxicosis, burns, shock, stress, after norepinephrine injection, pheochromocytoma (during attack), Cushing's syndrome, pancreatic insufficiency, diuretics
	Decreased: insulin overdosage, hyperplasia of islet cells, hypothalamic lesions, postgastrectomy dumping syndrome, liver disease, Addison's disease
Glutamic-oxaloacetic transaminase (SGOT) less than 40 units/mL	Increased: myocardial infarction, acute rheumatic carditis, cardiac surgery, cirrhosis, hepatitis, pulmonary infarction, acute pancreatitis, trauma, shock, skeletal muscle disease
Glutamic-pyruvic transaminase (SGPT) less than 30 units/mL	Increased: acute hepatitis, cirrhosis of liver, myocardial infarction, infectious mononucleosis
Glutathione reductase 10–70 units/mL	Increased: cancer, hepatitis
Hydroxybutyric dehydrogenase 140–350 units/mL	Increased: myocardial infarction, myocarditis, liver disease
Iodine (PBI) 4.0–8.0 μg/dL	Increased: hyperthyroidism, exogenous iodine intake, elevated serum protein
	Decreased: hypothyroidism, low serum protein
Iron, total 50–150 μg/dL	Decreased: hypochromic anemia, hemoglobinopathies
Isocitric dehydrogenase (ICD) 60–290 units/mL	Increased: hepatitis, pancreatic malignancy, preeclamptic toxemia, carcinomatosis of liver
Lactic acid Venous 5–20 mg/dL Arterial 3–7 mg/dL	Increased: lactic acidosis
Lactic dehydrogenase (LDH) 200–425 units/mL LDH_1 17–27% LDH_2 27–37% LDH_3 18–25% LDH_4 3–8% LDH_5 0–5%	Increased: myocardial infarction (LDH in heart muscle is stable so that when specimen is incubated, level remains elevated), hepatitis, skeletal muscle damage (LDH in liver and muscle is heat labile so that elevated levels return to normal after incubation), renal tissue destruction, pulmonary emboli, pneumonia, pernicious anemia, cerebral vascular accident
Lipids (values increase with age) Total 400–800 mg/dL	
Cholesterol 150–250 mg/dL (age 35 yr)	Increased: familial hypercholesterolemia, obstructive jaundice, renal disease, pancreatic disease, hypothyroidism, pancreatitis, untreated diabetes mellitus
	Decreased: severe liver disease, starvation, uremia, hyperthyroidism, cortisone therapy, anemia
Triglycerides 10–150 mg/dL (age 35 yr)	Increased: atherosclerosis, hyperlipemia, diabetes mellitus, lipid metabolism abnormality
	Decreased: deficient bile production, liver damage, poor intestinal absorption, lipid metabolism abnormality
Phospholipids 150–380 mg/dL (age 35 yr)	Increased: hyperlipidemia, atherosclerosis, lipid metabolism abnormality, diabetes mellitus
	Decreased: severe liver disease, malabsorption
Low-density lipoproteins (LDL) 45–50% of total lipids	Increased: hyperlipidemia, coronary artery disease
Magnesium 1.5–2.5 mEq/L	Increased: administration of magnesium compounds in presence of renal failure
	Decreased: severe malabsorption
Nonprotein nitrogen (NPN) 20–35 mg/dL	Increased: renal insufficiency

Table 20-4 *(continued)*

NORMAL RANGE	CONDITIONS IN WHICH VARIATIONS FROM NORMAL MAY OCCUR
Osmolality 280–295 mOsm/L	Increased: water loss, diabetes, azotemia, sepsis, lactic acidosis, liver failure, drug intoxication
	Decreased: water excess, sodium loss
Oxygen pressure Po_2 arterial 95–100 mm Hg	Increased: administration of high concentrations of oxygen
	Decreased: hypovolemia, decreased cardiac output, chronic pulmonary disease
pH	
Arterial 7.35–7.45	Increased: alkalosis
Venous 7.3–7.41	Decreased: acidosis
Phosphatase	
Acid 0.13–0.63 units/L (Bessey-Lowry)	Increased: prostatic malignancy
Alkaline	Increased: bone diseases and malignancies, liver disease, hyperparathyroidism, obstructive jaundice
Adults 0.8–2.3 units/L (Bessey-Lowry)	
Children 3.4–9.0 units/L (Bessey-Lowry)	
Phospholipids 150–380 mg/dL	Increased: hyperlipidemia, coronary artery disease, atherosclerosis, lipid metabolism abnormality
Phosphorus	
Adult 1.8–2.6 mEq/L	Increased: vitamin D excess, healing fractures, renal failure, hypoparathyroidism, diabetic ketosis, hyperthyroidism
Children 2.3–4.1 mEq/L	Decreased: hyperparathyroidism, rickets, osteomalacia
Potassium 3.0–4.5 mEq/L	Increased: shock, crush syndrome, anuria, Addison's disease, renal failure, diabetic ketosis
	Decreased: severe diarrhea, bowel fistula, diuretic therapy, Cushing's syndrome
Protein	
Total 6.0–7.8 g/dL	Increased: dehydration
	Decreased: renal disease, malnutrition, liver disease, severe burns
Albumin 3.5–5.5 g/dL	Increased: dehydration
	Decreased: renal disease, liver disease, malnutrition
Globulin 2.5–3.0 g/dL	Increased: chronic infectious diseases, sarcoidosis, Hodgkin's disease
Sodium 133–143 mEq/L	Increased: steroid therapy, hypothalamic lesions, head injury, hyperosmolar states
	Decreased: gastrointestinal loss, sweating, renal tubular damage, water intoxication, Addison's disease, diuretics, metabolic acidosis, inappropriate ADH syndrome, bronchogenic carcinoma, pulmonary infections
Thyroid hormone tests (expressed as thyroxin)	
T_4 (Murphy-Pattee) 6.0–11.8 μg/dL	Increased: hyperthyroidism
	Decreased: hypothyroidism
T_3 (resin uptake) 25–35% uptake	Increased: hyperthyroidism, thyrotoxicosis
	Decreased: hypothyroidism
Triglycerides (age 35 yr)	Increased: atherosclerosis, hyperlipemia, diabetes mellitus, lipid metabolism abnormality
	Decreased: deficient bile production, liver damage, poor intestinal absorption, lipid metabolism abnormality
Urea nitrogen (BUN) 8–18 mg/dL	Increased: renal failure, obstructive uropathy, congestive heart failure with decreased renal blood supply, fever, excess body protein catabolism
	Decreased: growing infant
Uric acid 1.5–4.5 mg/dL	Increased: gout, gross tissue destruction, renal failure, hypoparathyroidism
	Decreased: administration of uricosuric drugs (cortisone, salicylates)

Source: From *The Composition and Function of Body Fluids,* 2nd ed., by S. R. Burke, 1976, St. Louis, MO: C. V. Mosby.

The patient is provided with a collection device and one or more large storage containers for the urine. The sample is easily collected at home provided the patient is compliant. Often blood samples to measure plasma creatinine are ordered in conjunction with the 24-hour urine test.

Visual examination of the urine prior to microscopic study is often helpful. Preliminary diagnoses are often made based on the color and constancy of urine. Particular smells are also associated with certain pathological conditions.

Table 20-5 Composition of Urine

NORMAL RANGE	CONDITIONS IN WHICH VARIATIONS FROM NORMAL MAY OCCUR
Volume in 24-hr: 1200–1500 mL (varies greatly with fluid intake)	Increased: diabetes insipidus, absorption of large quantities of edema fluid, diabetes mellitus, certain types of chronic renal disease, tumors of brain and spinal cord, myxedema, acromegaly, tabes dorsalis
	Decreased: dehydration, diseases that interfere with circulation to kidney, acute renal failure, uremia, acute intestinal obstruction, portal cirrhosis, peritonitis, poisoning by agents that damage kidneys
pH 4.7–8.0	Increased: compensatory phase of alkalosis, vegetable diet
	Decreased: compensatory phase of acidosis, administration of ammonium chloride or calcium chloride, diet of prunes or cranberries
Specific gravity 1.010–1.020	Increased: dehydration, administration of vasopressin tannate, glycosuria, albuminuria
	Decreased: diabetes insipidus, chronic nephritis
Urea 20–30 gm	Increased: tissue catabolism, febrile and wasting diseases, absorption of exudates as in suppurative processes
	Decreased: impaired liver function, myxedema, severe kidney diseases, compensatory phase of acidosis
Uric acid 0.60–0.75 gm	Increased: leukemia, polycythemia vera, liver disease, febrile diseases, eclampsia, absorption of exudates, X-ray therapy
	Decreased: before attack of gout, but increased during attack
Ammonia 0.5–15.0 gm	Increased: diabetic acidosis, pernicious vomiting of pregnancy, liver damage
	Decreased: alkalosis, administration of alkalies
Creatinine 0.30–0.45 gm	Increased: typhoid fever, typhus, anemia, tetanus, debilitating diseases, renal insufficiency, leukemia, muscular atrophy
Calcium 30–150 mg	Increased: osteitis fibrosis cystica
	Decreased: tetany
Phosphates 0.9–1.3 gm	Increased: osteitis fibrosa, alkalosis, administration of parathormone
Chlorides 110–250 mEq	Increased: Addison's disease
	Decreased: starvation, excessive sweating, vomiting, pneumonia, heart failure, burns, kidney disease
Sodium 43–217 mEq	Increased: compensatory phase of alkalosis
	Decreased: compensatory phase of acidosis
17-Ketosteroids Men 5–27 mg Women 5–15 mg	Increased: Cushing's syndrome, adrenal malignancy, administration of cortisone, administration of ACTH, ovarian tumors
	Decreased: hypopituitarism, pituitary tumors, Addison's disease, myxedema, hepatic disease, chronic debilitating diseases
Aldosterone up to 15 μg	Increased: adrenal malignancy, conditions associated with excessive sodium loss, cardiac failure, nephrosis, hepatic cirrhosis
	Decreased: Addison's disease, eclampsia
Pressor amines Norepinephrine 5–100 μg Epinephrine 11.5 μg	Increased: essential hypertension, pheochromocytoma, severe stress, insulin-induced hypoglycemia
Amylase 8,000–30,000 Wohlgemuth units	Increased: early in acute pancreatitis, perforated duodenal ulcer, stone in common bile duct, carcinoma of the pancreas or bile duct, salivary gland disease
	Decreased: some liver diseases and some renal diseases

Source: From *The Composition and Function of Body Fluids,* 3rd ed., by S. R. Burke, 1980, St. Louis, MO: C. V. Mosby.

Table 20-6 Abnormal Constituents of Urine

CONSTITUENT	CONDITIONS IN WHICH VARIATIONS FROM NORMAL MAY OCCUR
Bence-Jones protein	Multiple myeloma, bone metastases of carcinoma, osteogenic sarcoma, osteomalacia
Albumin	Transient albuminuria may occur during pregnancy or prolonged exposure to cold, or following strenuous exercise; albuminuria present in nephritis, nephrosis, nephrosclerosis, pyelonephritis, amyloidosis, renal calculi, bichloride of mercury poisoning, and sometimes with blood transfusion reactions
Acetone	Diabetes mellitus, eclampsia, starvation, febrile diseases in which carbohydrate intake is limited, pernicious vomiting of pregnancy
Glucose	Unusually high carbohydrate intake, diabetes mellitus
Bilirubin	Obstructive jaundice, hemolytic jaundice, hepatitis, cholangitis
Urobilin and urobilinogen	Hemolytic jaundice, pernicious anemia, hepatitis, eclampsia, portal cirrhosis, lobar pneumonia, malaria
Erythrocytes	Glomerulonephritis, pyelonephritis, tuberculosis of kidneys, tumors of kidney, tumors of ureter and bladder, polycystic kidneys, calculi, hemorrhagic diseases, occasionally with anticoagulant therapy
Leukocytes	Increased in urethritis, prostatitis, cystitis, pyelitis, pyelonephritis (a few leukocytes are found in normal urine)
Casts	Glomerulonephritis, nephrosis, pyelonephritis, febrile diseases, eclampsia, amyloid disease, poisoning by heavy metals

Source: From *The Composition and Function of Body Fluids,* 3rd ed., by S. R. Burke, 1980, St. Louis, MO: C. V. Mosby.

The normal composition of urine is shown in Table 20-5; abnormal constituents are listed in Table 20-6.

RADIOLOGIC FINDINGS

Regular X-rays, ultrasound, CT scan, and MRI are important tools in diagnosing tumors and obstructions of the genitourinary tract.

KUB stands for kidney, ureters, and bladder. A KUB is an AP (anterior to posterior) radiographic view of the urinary system that provides basic information about the size, shape, and position of the organs. Certain types of calculi may be visible on a KUB.

IVU, previously called intravenous pyelogram (IVP), is an enhancement of the KUB that involves injection of a contrast medium into the patient's vein. The radiopaque material is filtered through the kidney and excreted. The procedure takes approximately an hour and provides an excellent outline of the entire urologic system. The patient should be NPO 8–12 hours prior to the test and may be asked to use a laxative or administer an enema in preparation for the IVU.

Retrograde urogram (previously called retrograde pyelogram) serves the same purpose as IVU. However, the contrast medium must be injected into the ureters with the use of a cystoscope because an obstruction is preventing the antegrade process from occurring. This may be performed in the physician's office, but is more commonly done in the more aseptic OR (cysto room) environment where anesthesia care is readily available if needed.

MIBG stands for metaiodobenzylguanidine and is a nuclear medicine study that is specifically designed to detect and locate pheochromocytoma.

BIOPSY

Biopsy is the only accurate way to determine the presence of malignancy and the exact cell type. Tissue samples are obtained using percutaneous, endoscopic, and open methods. According to the patient's needs, the procedure may be accomplished in the physician's office or a health care facility.

ENDOSCOPY

Endoscopy allows for visualization of the affected structures; tissue and fluid samples may be collected at the same time, and/or additional tests (such as retrograde urogram) performed. Transurethral endoscopy is commonly called cystoscopy, although enhanced instrumentation allows for viewing of all urinary tract structures and is not strictly limited to the bladder. Laparoscopic or retroperitoneoscopic procedures may also be performed to diagnose and treat conditions of the genitourinary system.

SPECIAL EQUIPMENT, INSTRUMENTS, SUPPLIES, AND DRUGS

The routine equipment for genitourinary surgery is very similar to that of general surgery. However, the items needed for transurethral procedures are highly specialized and many facilities have a specially equipped room set aside for just this purpose. Even though the procedures performed here are far more extensive than cystoscopy, the room is often still referred to as the "cysto" room. Some of the special features in the ideal "cysto" room include:

- Built-in table that will accommodate a patient in the lithotomy position and allow for fluoroscopy and regular X-ray
- Radiographic equipment that may be a permanent part of the operating table
- Radiation protective gear for team members and patient
- Adjacent darkroom for developing X-rays
- Back table that may be semicircular in shape
- Poles to support large, multiple bags or bottles of irrigation fluid
- Drainage system built into operating table or floor drain connected to sanitary sewer
- Adjustable sitting stool for the surgeon
- Multiple X-ray view boxes
- Built-in video, illumination, and electrosurgical equipment

In addition to the instrumentation and supplies used for general surgery procedures, the surgical technologist should consider adding several items to the major instrumentation set according to the type of procedure scheduled and the patient's individual situation. A list of suggestions follows.

General

- General surgery—major set
- Long instrumentation set
- Self-retaining abdominal retractor
- Mixter right angles
- Potts scissors
- Vascular instruments
- Bladder and prostate retractors

Kidney

- Pedicle clamps
- Stone/lithotomy forceps

Thoracic (Rib Resection)

- Self-retaining rib retractor (Finochietto)
- Alexander periosteotome
- Doyen rib elevator and raspatory
- Rib shears
- Sauerbruch rongeur
- Bailey rib contractor (approximator)

The instrumentation and supplies required for transurethral procedures are far more complex and unique to genitourinary surgery (Table 20-7).

A number of more common items are also used routinely in genitourinary surgery. They include:

- *Lubricant:* To facilitate entry of instrumentation into urethra; must be sterile
- *Foley catheter with drainage bag:* Size and style according to surgeon's preference
- *Alternate catheters:* For difficult catheterization; size and style according to surgeon's preference
- *Catheter guide:* Introduced into catheter lumen to facilitate insertion
- *Ureteral catheters:* According to surgeon's preference
- *Ureteral drainage bag:* Specially designed to accept unilateral or bilateral ureteral catheters and measure the drainage from each individually

PREOPERATIVE AND INTRAOPERATIVE PREPARATION

Many genitourinary (GU) procedures require that preoperative radiologic studies be available to the operative team. Be sure that any pictures/films and reports are requested in advance and are present in the OR for review. Additionally, intraoperative radiologic intervention may be necessary. The procedure should be scheduled in advance with the radiology department to be sure that the necessary equipment, technologist, and physician are available to the surgical patient at the appropriate time.

Choosing an anesthetic for genitourinary procedures takes many factors into consideration: type of surgery to be performed, anticipated position of the patient, age and physical condition of the patient, preference of the surgeon and the anesthesia provider and the patient's desire. Local, regional, or general anesthesia may be selected within these guidelines.

An indwelling urinary catheter, such as a Foley, is often used during genitourinary surgery. It is often necessary for the circulator to insert the catheter with the patient in the supine position prior to placing the patient in the operative position. In some situations the Foley is inserted as part of the operative procedure and is inserted from the main sterile field by the surgeon, assistant, or STSR.

Entry into the thoracic cavity may be planned according to the type of incision chosen or incidental due to pleural or diaphragmatic injury. The surgical technologist must plan ahead for the possibility of chest tube insertion in the event that pneumothorax occurs. Another option exists for evacuating air from the pleural space. A small amount of air may be allowed to escape the pleural space via a small flexible catheter such as a Robinson. The catheter is placed through the existing visible tear in the pleura or diaphragm and secured with a pursestring suture. The anesthesia provider performs a Valsalva maneuver to increase intrathoracic pressure, thereby expelling any air trapped in the pleural space through the catheter. While the pressure is maintained, the catheter is slipped out of the thoracic cavity as the pursestring suture is tight-

Table 20-7 Transurethral Instruments and Supplies

ITEM	DESCRIPTION
Urethral sounds (dilators)	Available in male, female, and pediatric designs and a variety of French sizes (8 Fr, or 2.6 mm, to 40 Fr, or 13.2 mm)
Lithotrite	Designed to crush bladder stones to allow for removal
Urethrotome	Cutting instrument designed for internal urethrotomy of the male or female urethra
Flexible endoscopic instruments	Adult and pediatric: cystoscope, ureteroscope, and nephroscope, each with a variety of accessories used for irrigation, biopsy, and stone extraction purposes (Figure 20-8)
Rigid endoscopic instrumentation	Adult and pediatric: components and accessories (Figure 20-9)
	Sheath: Hollow stainless steel tube available in a variety of sizes from 14–26 Fr. May have a port outfitted with stopcocks affixed to either side to allow for inflow and outflow of irrigation fluid
	Obturator: Blunt tip, fits inside sheath to facilitate introduction of the sheath into the urethra without traumatizing the mucosal lining. Size of obturator corresponds to the sheath
	Bridge: To accommodate added length of telescope. May have additional ports for introducing catheters, probes, electrodes, or forceps
	Deflecting mechanism: May be incorporated into the bridge or may be a separate instrument. A movable deflector that extends to the end of the sheath aids in placing accessories such as catheters or probes into the ureters
	Telescopic lens: Primary viewing component. Available with the lens angled at a variety of degrees. The surgeon will likely use the zero degree or straight lens first. A 120-degree lens is for retrograde viewing. Has a receptacle for attachment of the fiberoptic light cord
Resectoscope	Sheath: Range in size from 11–30 Fr. Resectoscope sheaths differ from cystoscope sheaths only in the fact that they have insulation to allow for use of electrosurgery
	Obturator: Same as above
	Telescopic lens: Same as above
	Bridge: Same as above
	Working element: Several styles available. Has receptacle for attachment of cautery cord. Receives an assortment of cautery loops, balls, and blades
Accessories	Luer-lock stopcocks to control the flow of irrigation fluid
	Light source with cable
	Electrosurgical unit with grounding pad, cable, and assortment of tips
	Video equipment: camera, monitor, VCR, etc.
	Tubing: Inflow for irrigation fluid. May have one or more entry sites. Outflow to collection unit or floor drain
Irrigation fluid	According to surgeon's preference. Water, saline, sorbitol, glycine, etc. Use of electrosurgical unit will affect the type of irrigant used; nonhemolytic and nonelectrolytic solutions are preferred
O'Connor shield	Disposable item that allows the surgeon to examine the prostatic urethra digitally through the rectum without contamination of the operative field
Pharmaceuticals	According to surgeon's preference. May include antibiotics, contrast media, etc. Fluorescein is an intravenous illuminating agent that shows orange when exposed to a Wood's lamp
Ellik evacuator or Toomey syringe	Forcefully removes tumor segments and blood clots from the bladder

ened and the negative pressure is restored, eliminating the need for a chest tube.

Patient position and the type of incision used are also influenced by many of the same factors that influence the type of anesthesia chosen. The three main positions used for surgery of the genitourinary system are lithotomy, supine, and lateral (and their variations). One of the most important criteria for choosing one incisional option over another is exposure. Optimum exposure is crucial to the identification of vital structures and the elimination of

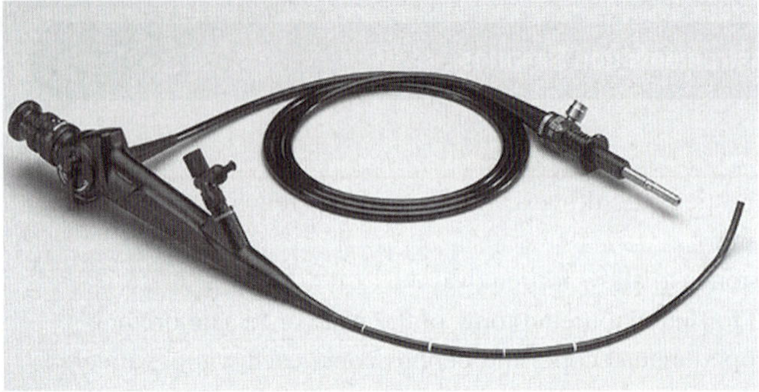

Figure 20-8 Flexible cystoscope ***(Courtesy of Olympus America)***

intraoperative and postoperative complications. Several operative approaches to the male reproductive system, peritoneal cavity (abdomen and pelvis), and retroperitoneum are available to the genitourologist.

INCISIONAL OPTIONS

Operative approaches include inguinal, scrotal, abdominal, Gibson, flank, and lumbar incisions.

INGUINAL INCISION

An inguinal incision is often used to access the scrotal contents of an adult or child. Cryptorchidism is often treated through an inguinal incision. This would also be the incision of choice for radical orchiectomy. A detailed description of the inguinal incision, prep, and draping can be found in Chapter 14.

SCROTAL INCISION

Scrotal incisions are performed to access the scrotal contents. This may be for the purpose of vasectomy, testicular biopsy, simple orchiectomy, or orchiopexy. Scrotal incisions are often carried out under local anesthesia with the patient in supine position. Shaving is usually not necessary, a minimal prep is performed, and limited drapes applied. Tension is applied to the scrotum and a transverse incision is made through the skin and dartos muscle. Hemostasis is achieved with the electrocautery. The tunica vaginalis is opened exposing the contents of the hemiscrotum. The wound is typically closed in two layers with interrupted absorbable sutures. Penrose drains are commonly used in this type of incision and postoperative edema is expected.

ABDOMINAL INCISIONS

Any abdominal incision may be used by the genitourologist. These are performed with the patient in the supine position and usually under general anesthesia. Most of the abdominal incisional information, along with recommendations for prepping and draping, can be found in Chapter 14. The low transverse incision or Pfannenstiel incision is covered in Chapter 15.

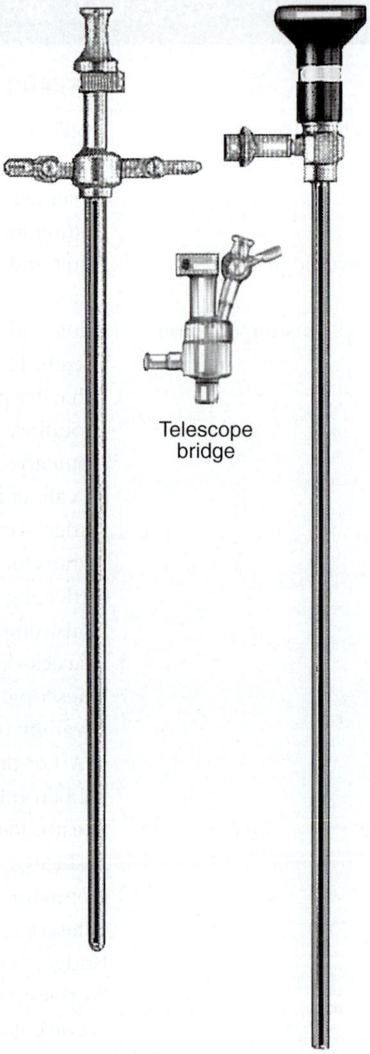

Figure 20-9 Rigid cystoscope, telescope bridge, and obturator

GIBSON INCISION

The **Gibson incision** is an extraperitoneal abdominal approach that is specifically designed for access to the lower portion of the ureter (Figure 20-10). It is sometimes used for implantation of a donor kidney. The patient is usually under general anesthesia and placed in a supine position on the operating table. If necessary, the Foley catheter should be inserted prior to final positioning. A bolster

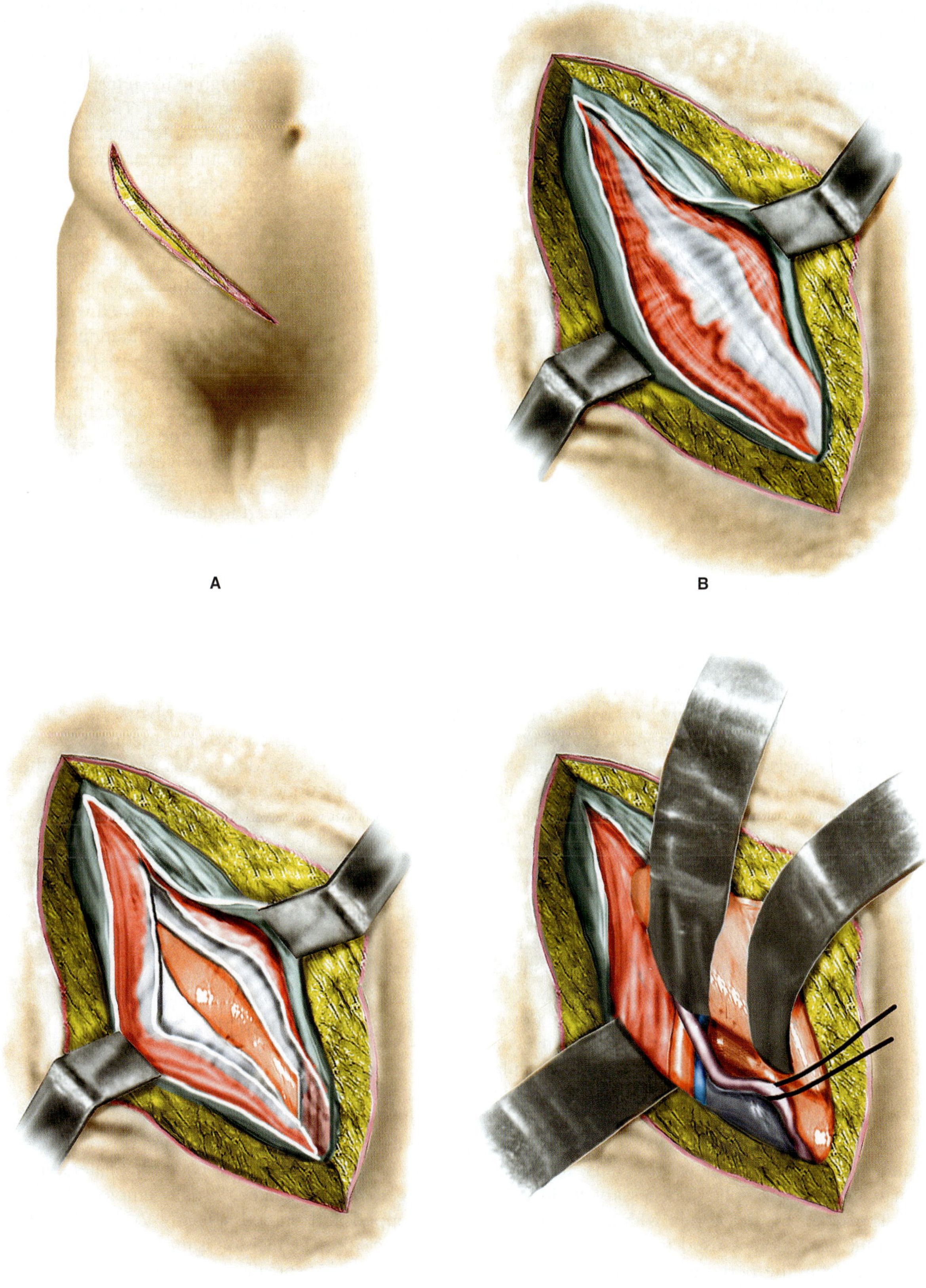

A B C D

Figure 20-10 Gibson incision: (A) Location of incision, (B) internal oblique exposed, (C) transversalis fascia opened, (D) ureter isolated may be placed under the hip on the operative side or the operating table may be hyperextended to enhance the surgeon's view anatomically. A pillow may be needed between the patient's legs. A shave is performed if necessary and the prep carried out from the mid-chest level to the mid-thigh and the entire width of the patient.

The incision begins medial to the anterosuperior iliac spine and curves downward and medially to slightly above the symphysis pubis. The external oblique muscle and the rectus sheath are incised, the rectus muscle is retracted toward the midline, and the internal oblique muscle and transversalis fascia are divided to expose the peritoneum. The peritoneum is retracted medially to expose the iliac vessels and the ureter. If additional exposure is needed, the inferior epigastric artery and vein can be ligated and the rectus muscle transected. Wound closure is systematic approximation of the fascias enclosing the internal and external oblique muscles and that of the anterior rectus.

FLANK INCISIONS

When the use of a flank incision is planned, general anesthesia is administered, and the patient placed in the lateral position with the affected side up. The area is shaved if necessary, a generous prep performed by the circulator, and drapes similar to those used for laparotomy are applied. Direct access is provided to the adrenal gland, kidney, and proximal ureter; the peritoneal cavity is not entered. The flank incision usually involves cutting the muscles. Only in a very limited approach to the mid-ureter can the muscle splitting flank incision be used. According to the exact surgical site, the flank incision may be subcostal, transcostal, or intercostal.

Subcostal flank incisions are appropriate if the preoperative radiographic studies show the kidney to be low lying or if the mid- to upper ureter is the intended target. The incision line extends from the rectus sheath around to the sacrospinalis muscle approximately 2 cm below the twelfth rib. The latissimus dorsi, external oblique, and internal oblique muscles are transected with the electrocautery. The subcostal neurovascular bundle is identified and gently retracted to prevent injury. The lumbodorsal fascia is opened exposing the perinephric fat and the Gerota's fascia surrounding the kidney and adrenal gland. The transversus abdominis muscle may be partially split if necessary to increase exposure. The wound is held open with a self-retaining retractor. Blunt dissection is used to free the retroperitoneal contents from the peritoneum and diaphragm allowing for anterior or posterior exposure of the renal pedicle. Wound closure is accomplished layer by layer with interrupted absorbable figure eight stitches. Skin may be stapled or sutured.

Transcostal incisions are used to expose the entire kidney, especially if it is high in the retroperitoneal space, and involves the resection of a rib. The incision is made directly over the rib selected for removal, usually the 11th or 12th. The muscles encountered are transected providing exposure of the periosteum. The periosteum is incised and dissected anteriorly with the Alexander periosteotome. This maneuver also separates the intercostal muscles from the rib. The undersurface of the rib is separated from the periosteum with a Doyen rib elevator. The segment of rib to be removed is grasped with a heavy instrument, and the anterior free or "floating" edge is freed from its fibrous attachments. The rib shears is used to sever the rib posteriorly and any rough edges are smoothed with a rongeur. The diaphragm and pleura should not be disturbed. Wound closure, in addition to that previously described, involves closure of the rib bed. This is accomplished in two layers with interrupted absorbable sutures placed in the muscle or fascia.

Intercostal incisions are usually planned between the 11th and 12th ribs and involve separation rather than resection. The dissection proceeds as described previously with the ribs to be separated stripped of their periosteum and the underlying pleura bluntly dissected away from both ribs. Care is taken to protect the intercostal neurovascular structures. A self-retaining rib retractor is placed between the ribs to be separated and opened far enough to provide adequate exposure. Rib fractures often occur during this process and this should not alarm the surgical team members. The closure of the intercostal incision will begin with the approximation of the ribs using the rib contractor. Three to four heavy absorbable sutures will be placed around the upper and lower ribs avoiding the intercostal vessels and nerves. Once the ribs have been secured, the contractor is removed and the closure proceeds as described for the subcostal incision.

LUMBAR INCISION

The lumbar incision provides limited exposure and is used for adrenalectomy, renal biopsy, or removal of a small low-lying kidney. This type of incision may be done with the patient in lateral or prone position; this is especially nice when there is a need for bilateral access. Use of a general anesthetic is usually employed and the area is prepped and draped similarly to that described for a flank incision. The incision is made below the 12th rib lateral to the sacrospinalis muscle and extends past the tip of the rib. The underlying muscles are divided with the electrocautery until the Gerota's fascia is exposed. Exposure of the retroperitoneal space can be enhanced by upward retraction of the 12th rib, which can be maintained with the use of a self-retaining retractor. The wound is closed like the subcostal flank incision.

SURGICAL PROCEDURES

Several procedures, both open and endoscopic, are used to treat conditions affecting the adrenal glands, urinary tract, and the male reproductive system.

ADRENALECTOMY

Adrenalectomy is surgical removal of one or both adrenal glands. Adrenalectomy is usually performed because of a tumor that causes Cushing's syndrome or pheochromocytoma. Adrenalectomy may also be considered in the treatment of certain types of reproductive malignancies (for example, breast or prostate cancer). Adrenalectomy may be accomplished endoscopically or via a traditional incision. Several factors will be used to determine the type of removal best suited to the patient's individual situation, including:

- Size of the tumor
- Type of tumor
- History of previous abdominal surgery

Endoscopic removal is best for small nonmalignant masses. Two approaches for endoscopic adrenalectomy are available: transabdominal laparoscopic or retroperitoneoscopic, either of which may be varied for surgery on the right or left adrenal gland.

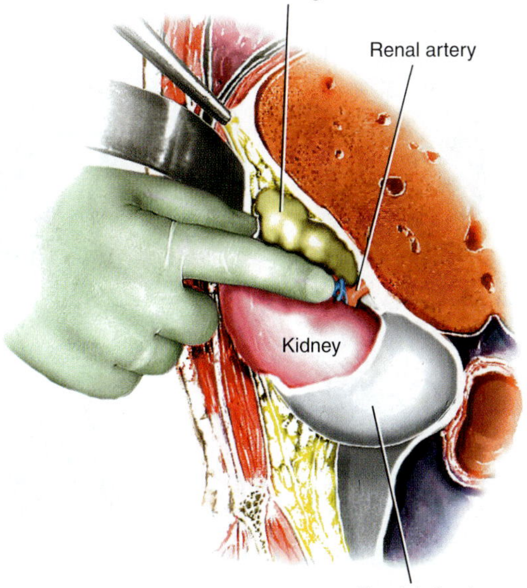

Figure 20-11 Open adrenalectomy

Large tumors and malignancies must be removed through a traditional incision (Figure 20-11). The approach to the adrenal gland is similar to that used for a nephrectomy, most likely a flank or lumbar incision.

The retroperitoneal space is exposed and Gerota's fascia opened. Dissection begins with the separation of superior perinephric fat; blood vessels are ligated as they are encountered. The kidney is retracted downward and the fibrous attachments to the adrenal surfaces are transected. Once mobilized, the adrenal gland is rotated to expose the major blood vessels. Ideally, the main adrenal artery is doubly clamped, transected, and ligated first, followed by similar steps on the vein. Any remaining fibrous attachments are freed and the specimen removed. The wound is irrigated and hemostasis achieved. A drain may be placed in the adrenal fossa and Gerota's fascia closed over the upper pole of the kidney. The remainder of the wound is closed in the usual fashion.

An adrenal mass that cannot be separated from the kidney may require an en bloc removal of both organs as would be performed in radical nephrectomy.

The patient is expected to remain hospitalized for 3–5 days and return to normal activities within 6–8 weeks. Follow-up care for the postadrenalectomy patient may include lifelong hormone replacement therapy. Chemotherapy may be recommended for those suffering from malignant adrenal tumors.

NEPHRECTOMY

Nephrectomy is total or subtotal removal of the kidney. The flank approach is the incision of choice in most situations. A midline incision will probably be used for radical nephrectomy due to malignancy.

Renal cooling is a technique used to preserve renal function during an episode of planned prolonged arterial occlusion (ischemia) of a kidney or portion of a kidney that is to remain in the patient, or a kidney scheduled for transplant. Renal cooling reduces the metabolic requirements of the kidney and lowers the possibility of tubular necrosis. The STSR will need sterile iced slush along with a sheet of sterile plastic or a Lahey intestinal bag to contain the iced slush. Preparation of the slush is a task that requires additional supplies and preparation time.

Subtotal nephrectomy may be accomplished at the upper or lower pole of the kidney only (Figure 20-12). Partial nephrectomy is performed to obtain a specimen for biopsy, remove small cancers, remove calculi that have caused damage to the surrounding parenchymal tissue, or to treat a traumatic injury. A generous flank incision is used, the Gerota's fascia entered, and the entire kidney mobilized to provide access to the renal artery, which must be isolated and controlled. Control of

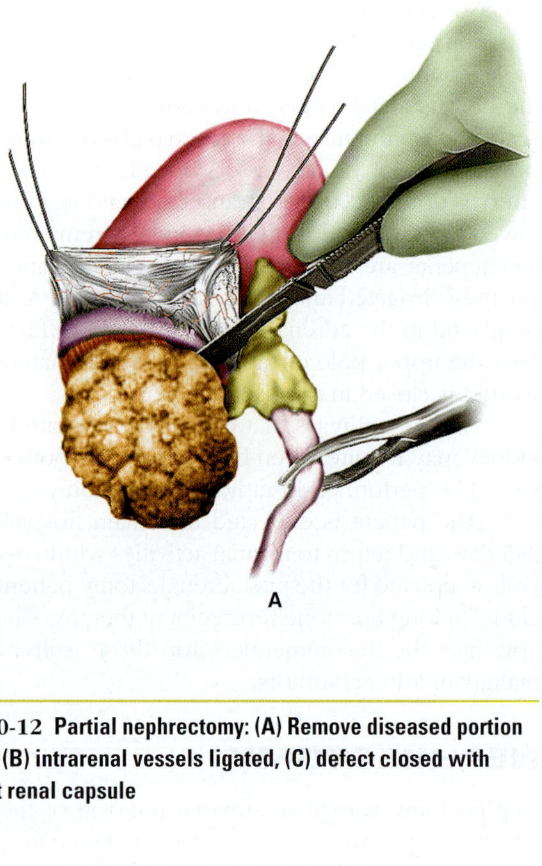

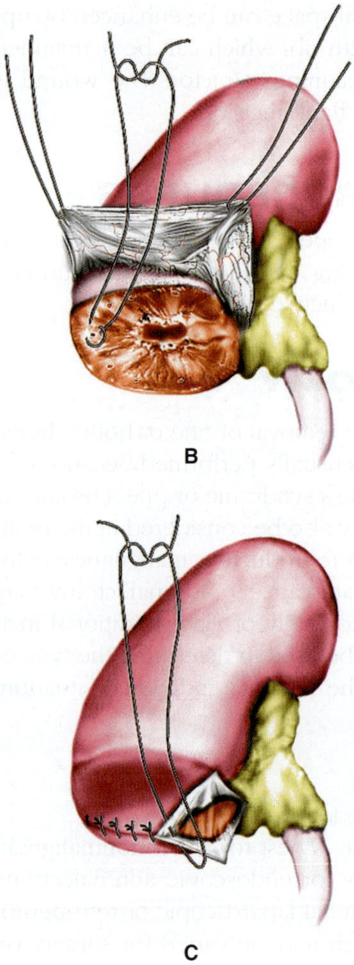

Figure 20-12 Partial nephrectomy: (A) Remove diseased portion of kidney, (B) intrarenal vessels ligated, (C) defect closed with redundant renal capsule

the artery may be accomplished with the use of a vessel loop or a small vascular clamp such as a spring bulldog. The renal capsule is incised and retracted from the operative site. The superior and inferior renal segments are clearly delineated and the appropriate segmental artery is isolated, secured, transected, and ligated. Following removal of the affected segment of the kidney, any visible intrarenal vessels should be ligated. Blood flow is slowly returned to the remaining portion of the kidney by releasing the tension on the vessel loop or clamp. The resulting defect is covered with a patch of peritoneum, omental fat, or the redundant renal capsule. A Penrose wound drain will likely be positioned adjacent to the renal closure, Gerota's fascia closed, and the remainder of the wound is closed. *Note:* The first closure count should clearly demonstrate that the constrictive device on the renal artery has been completely removed from the patient.

Simple nephrectomy is removal of the kidney (refer to Procedure 20-1 and Figure 20-13). The surrounding structures, including the adrenal gland, remain. Simple nephrectomy is performed for small malignancies, chronic obstructive disorders, benign tumors, or removal of a kidney to be used for transplant.

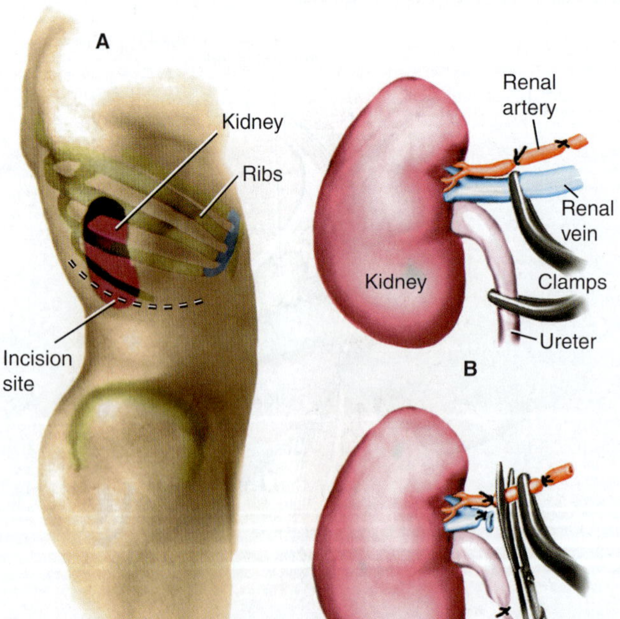

Figure 20-13 Simple nephrectomy: (A) Subcostal incision, (B) renal artery ligated first, (C) renal artery transected

PROCEDURE

20-1 Simple Nephrectomy

Equipment

- Electrosurgical unit
- Positioning aids

Instruments

- Major instrumentation set
- Long instrumentation set
- Self-retaining abdominal retractor
- Mixter right angles
- Potts scissors
- Vascular instruments
- Pedicle clamps
- Hemoclip appliers

Supplies

- Pack: basic
- Basin: double
- Gloves
- Blades: #10 × 2
- Drapes: laparotomy (transverse)
- Suture: according to surgeon's preference
- Drains: Penrose
- Dressings: three-layer
- Drugs: according to surgeon's preference
- Miscellaneous:
  - Electrocautery pencil
  - Extension for electrocautery
  - Irrigation fluid
  - Suction tubing
  - Gauze sponges
  - Laparotomy sponges
  - Peanut sponges
  - Hemoclips
  - Chest tubes, water-seal drainage system, and insertion tray (available)

Operative Preparation

Anesthesia

- General

Position

- Lateral, affected side up

Prep

- Insert Foley catheter (if ordered) prior to final patient positioning
- Shave if necessary
- Axilla to thigh and as far anterior and posterior as possible

Draping

- Foot sheet may be used
- Anticipated incision site is outlined with towels that are secured in place with adhesive, towel clips, staples, or suture
- Transverse laparotomy sheet
- Additional sheet may be necessary to cover the arm board

Practical Considerations

- Thoracic instruments are available if needed
- Preoperative radiographic films should be displayed in the OR

Operative Procedure	Technical Considerations
1. Subcostal flank incision is made approximately 2 cm below the 12th rib (Figure 20-13A).	**1.** A #10 blade on #3 knife handle will be used. Anticipate use of cautery and suction.

(continues)

PROCEDURE 20-1 Simple Nephrectomy *(continued)*

2. Latissimus dorsi, external oblique, and internal oblique muscles are transected.	**2.** Soft tissue retraction is initially achieved with Parker or Richardson retractors. Muscle segments may be doubly clamped, cut, and ligated or transected with the electrocautery.
3. Subcostal neurovascular bundle is identified and retracted.	**3.** Self-retaining retractor preceded by moist lap sponges is inserted. A vein retractor may be needed to retract the neurovascular bundle.
4. The lumbodorsal fascia is opened.	**4.** Provide new #10 blade (deep knife) followed by DeBakey tissue forceps and long Metzenbaum scissors.
5. If necessary, the transversus abdominus muscle is partially split.	**5.** Anticipate the use of a deeper retractor such as a Harrington at this point.
6. Gerota's fascia is opened.	**6.** Return scissors and tissue forceps to surgeon.
7. The renal pedicle is exposed anteriorly and posteriorly with the use of blunt dissection.	**7.** Surgeon may use fingers, peanut sponge on a long Mayo clamp, or a sponge on a stick for this step. Have all items prepared in advance.
8. Perinephric fat and the adrenal gland at the upper pole of the kidney are dissected.	**8.** Scissors and tissue forceps may be needed again or blunt dissection may continue. Unexpected bleeding may occur. Have hemoclips and suction available.
9. The ureter is isolated, doubly clamped, transected, and ligated.	**9.** Provide two Mayo clamps, Metzenbaum scissors, and suture of surgeon's preference. Automatically provide suture scissors of appropriate length after ligatures.
10. The kidney is retracted superiorly to expose the renal artery and vein.	**10.** Prepare pedicle clamps.
11. Renal artery is clamped first and then the vein (Figure 20-13B).	**11.** Prepare heavy nonabsorbable sutures. Surgeon may request that the suture be presented on a right angle to facilitate placement around artery and vein.
12. The vessels are doubly secured with heavy nonabsorbable sutures and transected (Figure 20-13C).	**12.** Prepare at least three sutures for each vessel.
13. Any remaining attachments are released and the kidney is removed.	**13.** Prepare to accept the specimen. Anticipate the use of body temperature irrigation fluid and obtain if necessary. Keep track of amount of irrigation fluid used and report to circulator or anesthesia provider at end of procedure.
14. Hemostasis is achieved.	**14.** Suction and cautery will be needed. Be prepared for the possibility that a suture ligature may be needed.
15. If necessary, a drain is placed and Gerota's fascia is closed.	**15.** Present moistened Penrose drain. Prepare and pass suture for closure.

PROCEDURE

20-1 Simple Nephrectomy *(continued)*

16. The wound is closed layer by layer with interrupted absorbable figure-eight stitches.
17. Skin is stapled and drain secured.

16. Several sutures will be needed for the figure-eight suturing technique. Count.
17. Provide stapling device and two Adson tissue forceps with teeth for skin closure. Prepare dressing material (additional absorbant layer material may be needed if drain has been placed).

Postoperative Considerations

Immediate Postoperative Care

- Patient is placed in the supine position for emergence from anesthesia and extubation.
- Intake and output is measured for 24–48 hours postoperatively.
- Respiratory effort may be decreased due to incisional pain, monitor oxygen saturation.

Prognosis

- Patient is expected to return to full activity in 6–8 weeks.
- Malignancy may need additional treatment (radiation or chemotherapy).
- Remaining kidney is expected to handle additional load without difficulty if not diseased.

Complications

- Hemorrhage
- Infection

PEARL OF WISDOM

If the pleural cavity is entered (intentionally or accidentally), chest tube insertion becomes necessary. The STSR should anticipate this possibility by obtaining the necessary equipment and supplies in advance. According to the patient's condition, chest tube insertion may be an urgent or emergent procedure.

If the kidney is intended for transplant, the living donor may be heparinized several minutes prior to removal. The artery, vein, and ureter are dissected in such a way that the maximum length is available for the implantation. The kidney is infused with cold Collins solution.

Radical nephrectomy is the removal of the kidney, adrenal gland, perirenal fat, upper ureter, and the Gerota's fascia, en bloc. Regional lymph nodes may be removed if the situation so dictates. Radical nephrectomy is usually accomplished through an abdominal incision with the patient in the supine position. The transperitoneal incision allows the abdominal organs to be inspected for metastases. The most direct approach to the renal vessels should be used. Keep in mind that minor anatomical variances are possible, and that the anatomy may be grossly distorted with certain types of tumors. Also, the STSR should be aware that slight differences will be noticed between right and left nephrectomy. A common approach for exposure of the renal vessels is through the posterior peritoneum medial to the inferior mesenteric vein (Figure 20-14).

The vein is typically isolated first, then retracted to expose the artery. Once the renal artery is isolated, three ligatures of strong nonabsorbable sutures are applied. Two ligatures are placed as close to the aorta as possible and the third approximately 1 cm distal to the aorta. The ligatures on the renal vein are placed similarly in relation to the vena cava. The vessels are transected between the second and third ties. If necessary, the vascular stumps can be further secured with stick ties of the same material used for the ligatures. The lower portions of Gerota's fascia are freed exposing the ureter, which is then doubly

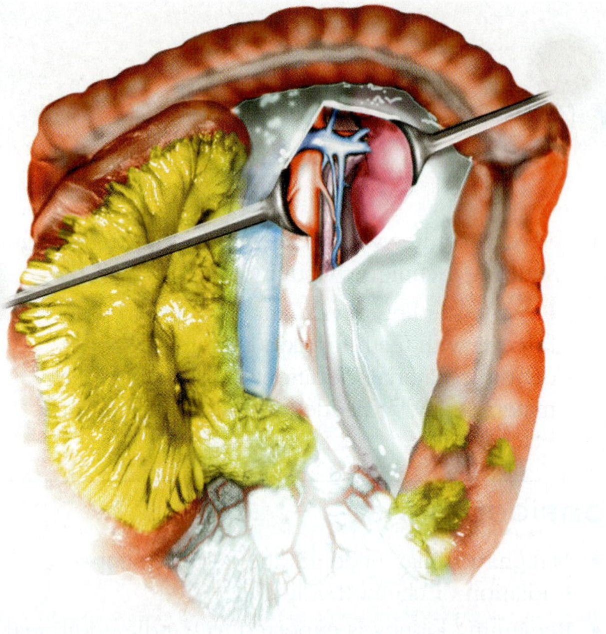

Figure 20-14 Transperitoneal exposure of renal vessels

clamped, transected, and ligated. If possible, the superior portion of Gerota's fascia is reserved until last, allowing for the best exposure and control of the adrenal vessels. Once all vessels are secured, all remaining attachments of Gerota's fascia are freed and the specimen is removed. The renal fossa is irrigated and inspected for any residual bleeding, which will be ligated or cauterized. If lymphadenectomy is planned, it is performed following nephrectomy. It is not usually necessary to drain the renal fossa. Usual wound closure methods are used.

RENAL TRANSPLANT

Organs for kidney transplant are obtained from three sources: cadavers, living relatives, or unrelated living donors. Compatibility is determined with serological studies.

Cadaveric donators are persons who have executed advanced directives requesting that their organs be used for transplant in the event that they become brain dead, but their circulatory function can be preserved until a recipient for their organs can be located. When an advance directive (formerly called a living will) is not available, the next of kin may authorize the procurement of the organs; of course, organ donation is not limited to kidneys.

The procurement (referred to in the past as "harvest") of cadaveric kidneys differs slightly from the operation performed on living donors. The brain dead patient is brought to the OR from the intensive care unit when all of the procurement teams have arrived and everything is prepared. An anesthesia provider is present even though the patient is technically dead. The anesthesia provider is responsible for maintaining the airway and cardiac status of the patient as long as is necessary. The patient is prepped and draped for laparotomy. A long vertical midline incision is used. If other organs are to be donated, they may be removed prior to the kidneys. Both kidneys are removed, preserving as much length as possible on the blood vessels (especially the right renal vein) and the ureters. The spleen and nearby lymph nodes may be removed to aid in tissue typing and cross-matching the donor with the recipient. The kidneys are flushed with Collins solution (a preservative) and packed in sterile iced slush for transport. It is common for procured organs to be transported to implantation centers all over the country.

Primitive wound closure techniques are generally employed when closing a cadaver. By the time of closure, just the basic OR team remains. Up to this point the case has been very exciting. Procurement teams from all over the country have been participating in the procedure. Suddenly the teams leave with their respective organs and there is no further use for the anesthesia provider. The operating room often gets very quiet and the fact that the patient is no longer being ventilated and the heart is not beating becomes apparent. The surgical team members should give some consideration in advance to their personal thoughts about organ donation and dealing with the body of the donor postoperatively. This can be an emotionally trying experience for the surgical team members.

Donations from living donors (related or unrelated) are handled in much the same way as a simple nephrectomy. Because the renal vein is longer on the left side, it is the preferred kidney for donation from a living donor.

Success of a kidney transplant is about 80% when the donation is from an unrelated donor. The success rate increases to 90% when the living donor is related, with the best results achieved when the donor is an identical twin.

RECIPIENT OPERATIONS

The kidney to be implanted is often referred to as the *graft*. The patient undergoes dialysis just prior to the transplant procedure to be sure that his or her fluid and electrolyte balance is optimal. Following dialysis, the patient is brought to the OR, receives a general anesthesia, and is positioned, prepped, and draped for surgery.

In an adult, the graft is usually placed in the right pelvis through a Gibson incision (Figure 20-15). The peritoneum and psoas muscles are separated to expose the iliac vessels. If the patient is male, the spermatic cord is mobilized and retracted. The internal iliac is the artery of choice for anastomosis of the renal artery. It is isolated; the branches are secured and then occluded with a vascular clamp. The distal portion is ligated and separated. If necessary, an embolectomy may be performed at this time. The arterial anastomosis is accomplished with 6–0 polypropylene sutures. The suturing technique will be according to the type of anastomosis performed; interrupted sutures will most likely be done with an end-to-end

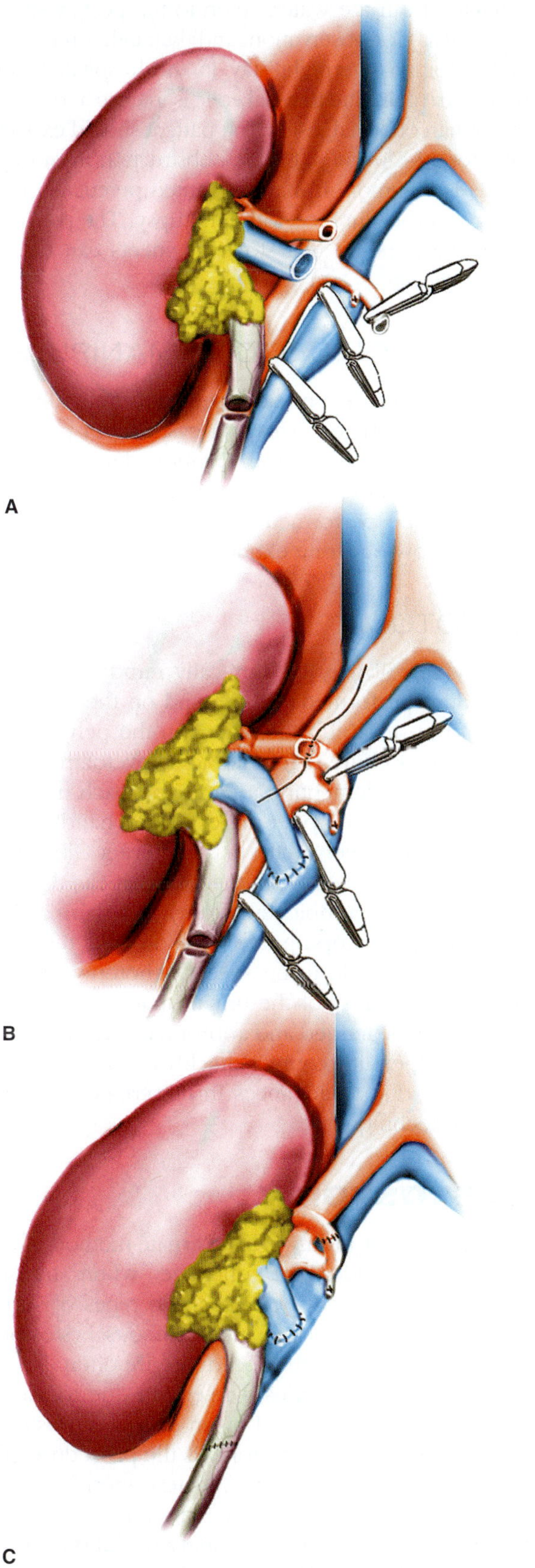

Figure 20-15 Renal transplantation (adult recipient): (A) Iliac vessels exposed, (B) renal artery and vein anastomosis, (C) donor kidney in place

anastomosis and continuous suturing techniques will be used with an end-to-side anastomosis. The renal vein is attached to the external iliac vein via an end-to-side anastomosis accomplished through a venotomy created between two vascular clamps. Perfusion is restored to the kidney and normal turgor and color should quickly return. Often urine is seen exiting the not-yet-attached ureter at this time. Any bleeding (anastomotic or otherwise) should be dealt with at this time. The patient's blood pressure should be maintained; mannitol may be given to increase urinary output. A ureteroneocystostomy is performed as the last step of the procedure. The use of a drain is not anticipated and normal wound closure techniques are implemented. A Foley catheter is placed for bladder decompression.

In children, the location of the graft is slightly different. A midline incision is used and the kidney is placed in the mid-retroperitoneum posterior to the right colon. The aorta and inferior vena cava are used for the vascular anastomoses. The rest of the procedure imitates the one previously described for the adult transplant.

STONE REMOVAL

Several methods are available to the genitourologist for removing urinary calculi. In many cases the stone will pass on its own with increased fluid intake, pain medication, and muscle relaxants. Some methods are minimally invasive and are performed percutaneously in the radiology department by the radiologist. Extracorporeal shock wave lithotripsy (ESWL) is a noninvasive treatment for urinary calculi, but it is very painful and often requires the use of sedation, regional, or general anesthesia. Endoscopy of the urinary tract may be performed to remove stones or an open procedure may be mandated.

EXTRACORPOREAL SHOCK WAVE LITHOTRIPSY

Extracorporeal shock wave lithotripsy is a noninvasive method of pulverizing urinary calculi so that the smaller fragments may be removed from the body with the urine (Figure 20-16). ESWL requires expensive, highly specialized equipment and many facilities have found it to be cost effective to share the expense with several other facilities. Often a mobile lithotriptor is purchased cooperatively or owned by a private corporation and leased to different sites. The mobile unit often arrives fully stocked and staffed; if not, this poses a complex situation for the operating team. Careful planning is needed to be sure that all necessary equipment and supplies are taken to the unit. If the procedure is to be done in the radiology department, the same equipment and supplies may need to be relocated.

A patient undergoing ESWL is positioned and secured in a semi-Fowler's position in a submergible chair following

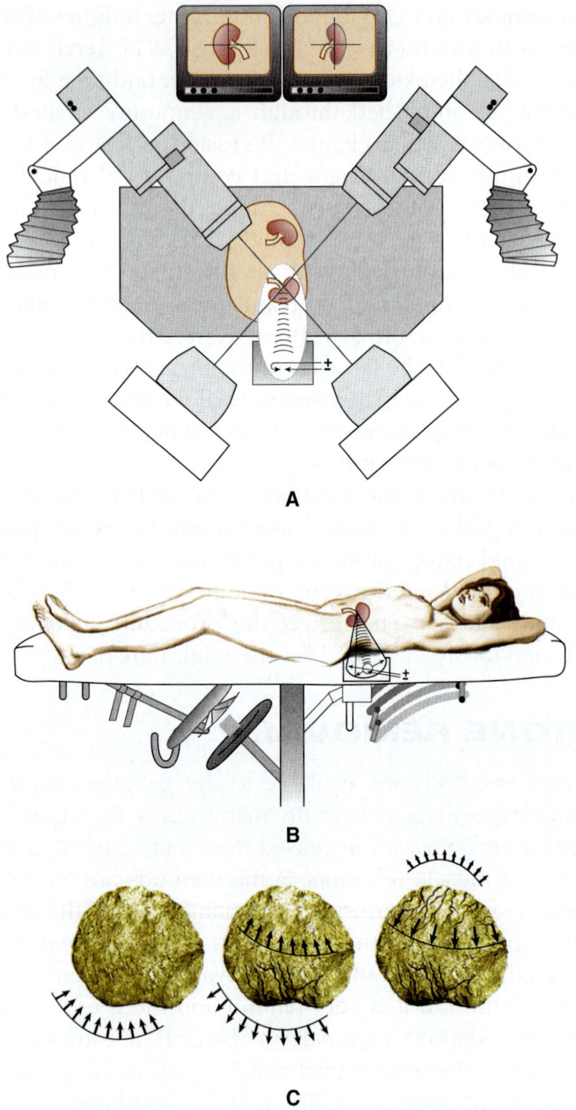

Figure 20-16 **ESWL: (A) Two X-ray beams crossing at focal point for proper positioning on stone, (B) focal point, (C) reflection of shock waves at first and second acoustical interfaces of the stone and surrounding fluid with fracture of the stone**

administration of general anesthesia. ESWL has been approved for treatment of kidney and upper ureteral stones. It has not been approved for bladder and lower ureteral stones and pregnancy is a contraindication. ESWL involves pinpointing the exact location of the stone with fluoroscopy or ultrasound and pulverizing the stone with shock waves generated by an electrical discharge through degassed deionized water in which the lower portion of the patient is submerged. Repetitive shocks are delivered to the calculi with reexamination of the stone by fluoroscopy after every 200 shocks. A 4-mm stone often requires more than 1,000 shocks to be pulverized. The maximum dose for one treatment is 2,400 shocks. Because of their size or composition, some stones may require multiple treatments. This may occur on consecutive days. Following treatment, the patient is extracted from the water, taken to the postanesthesia care unit (PACU) for observation, and then either released or admitted for an overnight stay in the hospital. Often postprocedure pain due to renal colic is intense and requires the use of narcotic analgesics. The patient should expect hematuria for 12–24 hours. Ureteral obstruction from stone fragments is common; it may be treated percutaneously, with an open procedure, or with lithotripsy. The patient should strain the urine so that stone fragments can be analyzed pathologically.

ENDOSCOPIC STONE MANIPULATION

Urinary stones may be accessed transurethrally, manipulated, and extracted. This is a cysto room procedure requiring specialized instrumentation that may include a stone basket, lithotrite, or lithotriptor. Retrograde urogram will likely be performed to demonstrate patency of the ureter following stone extraction.

LITHOTOMY

Urinary calculi may be surgically removed. The type of procedure performed will depend on the size and location of the stone. If the stone is in the pelvis of the kidney, the procedure is referred to as pyelolithotomy and a procedure implementing a flank approach may be used. Ureteroliths in the upper ureter will be handled similarly. Stones in the lower ureter may require a Gibson incision for access and stones in the bladder can be removed through a suprapubic cystotomy. The urinary tract is opened at the appropriate location and the stone extracted as a whole using special lithotomy or stone forceps. The integrity of the urinary tract must be restored. The wound is drained and appropriate closure techniques applied. Open lithotomy is quickly becoming an obsolete procedure due to advances in lithotripsy and minimally invasive techniques.

CYSTOSTOMY

Suprapubic cystostomy is an alternate method of catheterizing the bladder for drainage when transurethral catheterization is not possible. Two types of suprapubic cystostomy are available: percutaneous cystostomy and open cystostomy. Both procedures are often used in men experiencing acute urinary retention due to an obstruction of the urethra caused by an enlarged prostate.

Percutaneous cystostomy is the procedure of choice for bladder drainage when catheterization is not possible and following some operative procedures. Contraindications include previous abdominal surgical procedures and regional pathology. There is a risk of intraperitoneal damage. Commercially designed kits are available for percutaneous cystostomy. The procedure can be performed under local anesthesia. The pubic area is shaved and prepped. Then the local anesthetic is administered, superficially at first, and then down to the bladder using a longer (spinal) needle. The surgeon creates a small stab wound with a #11 blade and inserts the cystostomy tube medially just above the symphysis pubis. The bladder is likely distended due to an outlet obstruction and easily palpable. The cystostomy tube has a metal obturator to provide support for the tube. Once the catheter is advanced into the bladder, the obturator is removed. The tube is then secured (by inflating the balloon, if there is one, and suturing or taping it into position) and connected to a collection device. The patient should notice immediate relief. If the bladder is extremely distended, the amount of fluid allowed to exit may be regulated. Sudden decreases in intra-abdominal pressure can lead to a severe drop in the patient's blood pressure.

Open cystostomy is done when the simpler percutaneous cystostomy is contraindicated (Figure 20-17). Regional or general anesthesia is recommended. The area is shaved, prepped, and draped. A vertical or transverse incision is made in the midline superior to the symphysis pubis. The anterior rectus sheath is exposed, the fascia divided, and the muscle fibers split longitudinally. The transversalis fascia is then opened exposing the retropubic space. The peritoneum is displaced upwardly, two traction clamps or sutures are placed in the bladder wall, an opening into the bladder is created, and the catheter of choice (e.g., Malecot) is inserted. The STSR should have the suction apparatus ready at the moment the bladder is entered. The traction sutures are used to secure the catheter in position or a heavy pursestring suture is applied. The catheter may be brought to the outside of the body through the existing incision or through an additional stab wound. The small defect is closed and the catheter is fixed in position and attached to a drainage system. The small incision may be painful and require an

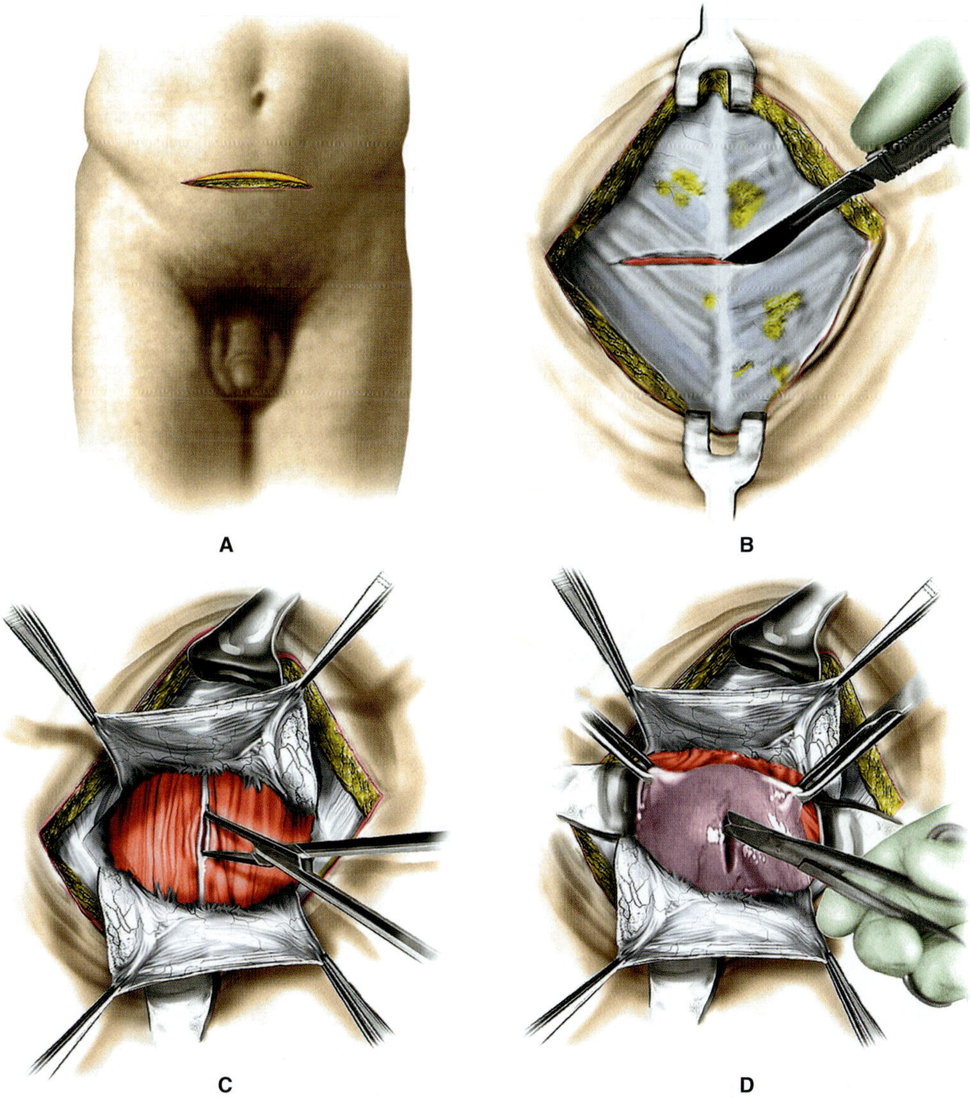

Figure 20-17 Open cystostomy: (A) Incision site, (B) fascia incised, (C) muscle split, (D) bladder incised

(continues)

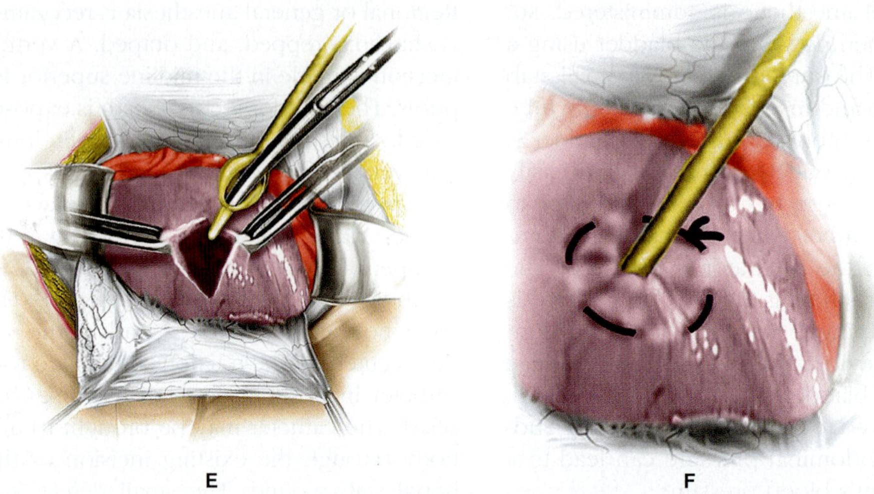

Figure 20-17 ***(continued):*** **(E) cystostomy tube inserted, (F) cystostomy tube secured with pursestring suture**

overnight hospitalization. If the patient is to be discharged with a catheter in place, management techniques should be taught or a visiting nurse schedule should be arranged.

CYSTECTOMY/ILEAL CONDUIT

Cystectomy is removal of the bladder. Partial or segmental cystectomy may be performed to remove a single invasive bladder tumor situated in the dome of the bladder. Occasionally, the need arises for a simple total cystectomy consisting of bladder removal only. Radical cystectomy differs slightly between male and female patients. In the male, the bladder, prostate, and seminal vesicles are removed; in the female, the dissection includes the bladder urethra, anterior vaginal wall, uterus, fallopian tubes, and ovaries. The radical procedure is for treatment of malignancies that have invaded the nearby tissues.

When the entire bladder is removed, a urinary diversion procedure must accompany cystectomy. Several surgical options are available for urinary diversion. Simple cutaneous ureterostomy is not a sound choice for long-term drainage, but may be temporarily implemented if the patient cannot tolerate a prolonged procedure. The ileal **conduit**, also called the ureteroileocutaneous diversion, is the standard procedure (Procedure 20-2). The patient wears an external appliance for collection of the urine. A final, more difficult to accomplish, option is the continent urinary reservoir (referred to as a Kock pouch) fashioned from reconfigured bowel to serve as the holding area for the urine. The reservoir has a capacity of 400–1200 mL and is emptied by periodic catheterization of an abdominal **stoma**. The stoma's continence is maintained by intussusception of the ileum just inside the stoma.

(Text continues on page 771)

PROCEDURE 20-2 Radical Cystectomy with Ileal Conduit—Male Patient

Equipment

- Electrosurgical unit

Instruments

- Major instrumentation set
- Long instrumentation set
- Self-retaining abdominal retractor
- Mixter right angles
- Hemoclip appliers
- Bowel instrumentation set

PROCEDURE 20-2 Radical Cystectomy with Ileal Conduit—Male Patient *(continued)*

Supplies

- Pack: basic
- Basin: double
- Gloves
- Blades: #10 (several)
- Drapes: laparotomy
- Suture: according to surgeon's preference
- Drains: according to surgeon's preference
- Dressings: three-layer and stoma bag
- Drugs: according to surgeon's preference
- Miscellaneous:
  - Electrocautery pencil
  - Extension for electrocautery
  - Irrigation fluid
  - Suction tubing
  - Gauze sponges
  - Laparotomy sponges
  - Peanut sponges
  - Hemoclips
  - Automatic stapling devices for bowel
  - Ureteral stents of surgeon's preference (available)

Operative Preparation

Anesthesia

- General

Position

- Supine, arms extended on arm boards

Prep

- Insert Foley catheter
- Shave if necessary
- Prep mid-chest to thigh and laterally as far as possible

Draping

- Foot sheet may be used
- Anticipated incision site outlined with towels secured in place with adhesive or towel clips
- Laparotomy sheet

Practical Considerations

- Patient will have full bowel prep (refer to Chapter 14)
- Ileostomy site may be predetermined and marked. (Be sure markings are not inadvertently removed during the skin prep.) Patient or caregiver is given instructions regarding stoma care
- Preoperative radiographic films should be displayed in the OR
- Variation (according to surgeon's preference): Patient may be placed in low lithotomy position (additional positioning aids and drapes will be necessary). The Foley catheter is inserted from the sterile field and the entire drainage system remains sterile throughout the procedure
- The genitourologist may request that a general surgeon and/or a gynecologist assist with the procedure
- Patient may have already undergone a series of radiation treatments that could negatively affect the tissue at the operative site
- Notify pathologist that frozen section specimens will be sent during procedure

Operative Procedure

1. A long vertical incision is used to enter the abdominal cavity.
2. The bladder is exposed and the intraperitoneal contents are palpated to be sure the area is free of unsuspected masses.

Technical Considerations

1. A #10 blade on #3 knife handle is used. Anticipate use of cautery and suction.
2. Warm, moist lap sponges are used to displace the bowel and a self-retaining retractor is placed. The procedure may be terminated at this point if it is determined that the tumor has progressed beyond resection.

(continues)

PROCEDURE 20-2 Radical Cystectomy with Ileal Conduit—Male Patient *(continued)*

3. The urachus is clamped and transected. The proximal end is ligated and the large clamp remains distally to be used for traction.	**3.** Large Mayo clamps are needed to clamp the urachus; one remains to provide bladder traction. Long, heavy nonabsorbable ties on a passer are needed for the proximal urachus.
4. If planned, a lymphadenectomy is performed at this time.	**4.** A combination of sharp and blunt dissection is used. Sharp dissection: Long scissors to surgeon's dominant hand and long DeBakey tissue forceps to the other hand. Blunt dissection: Surgeon may use fingers, peanut sponge on the end of a long Mayo clamp, or a sponge on a stick. Several specimens may be collected.
5. The bladder is freed from its attachments to the posterior symphysis down to the level of the puboprostatic ligaments.	**5.** Any bleeding is immediately controlled with the cautery, hemoclips, or ligatures (be prepared for any possibility).
6. Bladder is retracted medially, exposing the iliac blood vessels and obturator fossa on that side.	**6.** Sharp and blunt dissection continues. Suction will be used almost constantly.
7. 8–10 cm of vas is excised and the gonadal vessels are mobilized.	**7.** Sudden hemorrhage may occur. Long clamps are available at all times.
8. The dissection is repeated on the contralateral side.	**8.** Reorganize supplies and repeat procedural steps.
9. The pelvic peritoneum is incised and the dissection carried downward on each side of the bladder to free the superior and lateral aspects.	**9.** A #10 blade on long knife handle is needed. Follow with cautery.
10. The right paracolic gutter is incised to expose the ureter. The cecum, right colon, and small intestine are mobilized and retracted to the upper abdomen. Similarly, the peritoneum lateral to the sigmoid is opened and the ureter exposed.	**10.** Tools for dissection will be needed repeatedly. Observe progression of procedure and anticipate tools for use. More warm, moist packs are needed to retract intestine.
11. The ureters are isolated and dissected back as far as necessary. A segment of each proximal ureter is sent for frozen section to determine if the surgical margins are free of malignancy.	**11.** Prepare to accept two specimens for frozen section. Be sure that each is labeled anatomically.
12. The ureters are temporarily tucked into the upper abdomen until needed for the reconstruction.	**12.** Provide warm, moist lap sponges.
13. The bladder is pulled to one side with the traction clamp and the endopelvic fascia is opened and bluntly dissected inferiorly to its pedicle.	**13.** Reload peanut sponges and stick sponges as they become soiled. Provide clean lap sponges as needed throughout the procedure.
14. Dissection is repeated on the contralateral side and then both pedicles are doubly clamped, transected, and ligated. The process is repeated as many times as necessary for tissue in each pedicle.	**14.** Provide long Mayo clamps, long scissors, and ties preloaded on passers, followed by suture scissors of appropriate length.
15. The cul-de-sac of the male peritoneum is incised and the incision extended to the level of the existing lateral peritoneal incisions.	**15.** The incision may be initiated with a knife and extended with the long scissors. Tissue forceps are usually needed along with the scissors for dissection.

PROCEDURE

20-2 Radical Cystectomy with Ileal Conduit—Male Patient *(continued)*

16. The rectum and sigmoid are retracted, the bladder pulled forward, and the dissection carried toward the prostate and seminal vesicles.	**16.** Malleable retractor may be useful for rectal resection. Once retractors are set, dissection continues.
17. The hemorrhoidal vessels are encountered and are immediately clamped, transected, and ligated.	**17.** Continue clamp-clamp-cut-tie-cut-tie-cut routine. Suture is prepared in advance of need.
18. Mobilization continues toward the prostatic and membranous urethra. The structures affecting erectile function may be preserved with careful dissection, if this is a concern.	**18.** Blunt and sharp dissection continues. Provide suction and cautery as needed.
19. The Foley catheter is removed prior to securing the membranous urethra with two clamps. The urethra is transected and ligated with strong nonabsorbable sutures.	**19.** Syringe is needed to deflate Foley balloon. Provide clamps, scissors, and ligatures.
20. All remaining attachments are severed and the bladder removed. Hemorrhage is controlled. If pressure is needed to control bleeding, a Foley catheter with a 30-cc balloon may be inserted transurethrally, the balloon fully inflated, and external traction applied.	**20.** Prepare to accept bladder specimen. Suction and irrigation fluid may be used. Provide cautery or hemoclips as needed. Anticipate possible use of Foley catheter for hemorrhage control.
21. The area is packed with moist laparotomy sponges and the diversionary procedure begun.	**21.** Provide warm moist lap sponges. Prepare for intestinal portion of procedure. Keep in mind that entry to the GI tract will change the wound classification and that certain instruments used to create the conduit will require isolation on the sterile field.
22. The conduit is fashioned from a 20-cm length of terminal ileum. The designated segment of ileum is divided between two noncrushing intestinal clamps. Stapling devices may be used according to surgeon's preference.	**22.** Provide bowel clamps of surgeon's choice.
23. The corresponding mesentery is divided on both sides of the segment to be used for the conduit.	**23.** Stapling devices may be used to divide the mesentery or the routine clamp-cut-ligate system is employed.
24. The remaining ileum is positioned posteriorly, continuity restored with routine small bowel anastomosis, and the mesenteric defect closed.	**24.** Refer to Chapter 14 for technical considerations for small bowel anastomosis. Prepare stents if use is expected.
25. Both ureters are implanted into the ileal segment (Figure 20-18). Stents may be inserted if necessary.	**25.** Ileum is opened sharply and suture for anastomosis is provided. The procedure is repeated for the second ureter.
26. The proximal end of the conduit is closed.	**26.** Proximal ileum may be closed with suture or staples according to surgeon's preference.
27. The distal end is brought through the abdominal wall at a predetermined location through a separate incision.	**27.** Skin knife is needed, followed by cautery. Provide a pair of Army-Navy or small Richardson retractors.

(continues)

PROCEDURE 20-2 Radical Cystectomy with Ileal Conduit—Male Patient *(continued)*

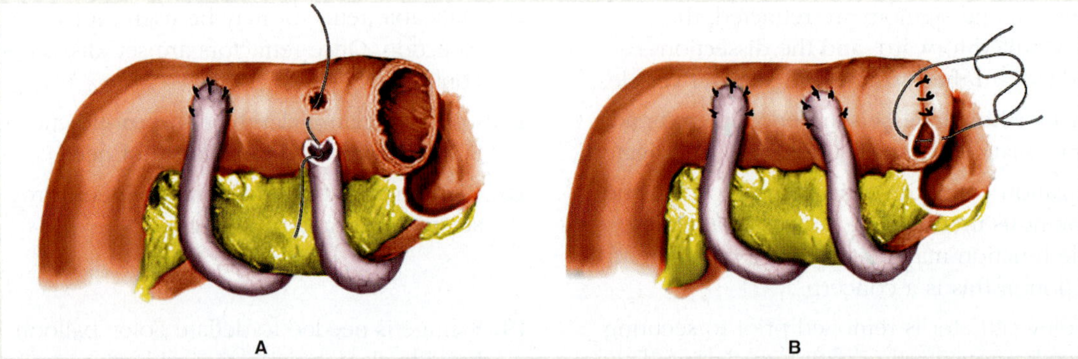

Figure 20-18 Ileal conduit: (A) Ureters implanted into ileal segment, (B) closure of proximal end of ileal conduit

28. The conduit is fixed into position and the stoma created by everting the ileal edge and affixing it to the skin (Figure 20-19).

28. Sutures are needed to secure the conduit to the abdominal wall. The stoma is affixed to the skin with sutures or staples.

29. The wound is inspected, hemostasis achieved, and wound drains inserted if necessary.

29. Provide warm irrigation fluid of surgeon's preference and suction. The Poole suction tip may be useful. Clamps, cautery, or hemoclips may be needed. Prepare wound drains.

30. The midline incision is closed in the usual manner.

30. Provide suture for closure. Count.

31. Dressings and a stoma bag are applied. Some surgeons prefer to catheterize the stoma to prevent urine contact with the external tissues until the stoma has matured.

31. Stoma bag may be customized. Provide heavy scissors. Provide catheter if requested.

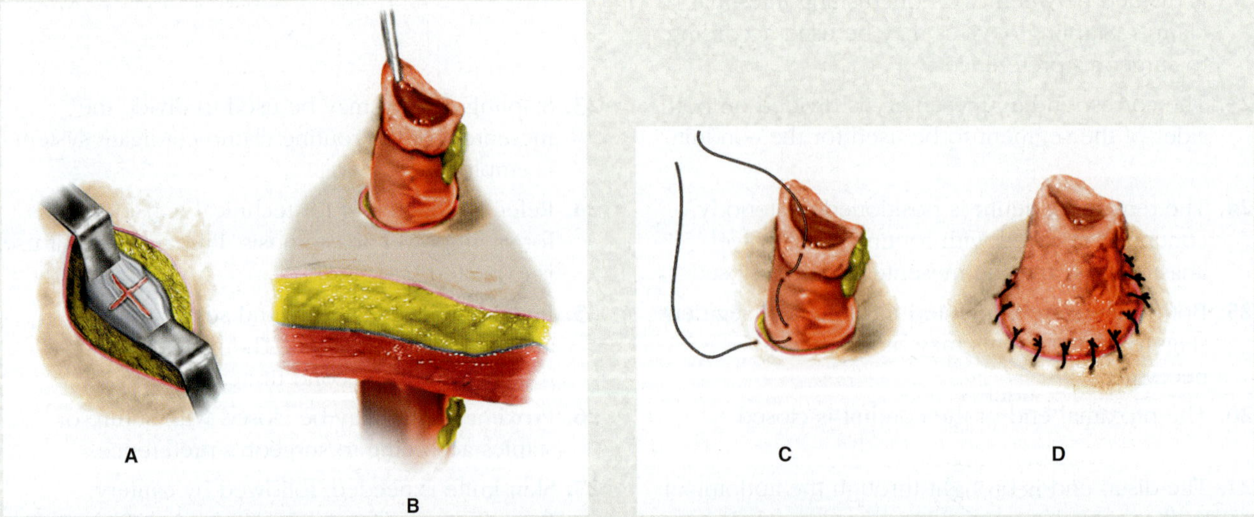

Figure 20-19 End ileostomy: (A) Abdominal incision for stoma, (B) ileum brought through abdominal wall, (C) ileal edge everted to create stoma, (D) end ileal stoma

PROCEDURE 20-2 Radical Cystectomy with Ileal Conduit—Male Patient *(continued)*

Postoperative Considerations

Immediate Postoperative Care

- Antibiotics and analgesics will be prescribed.
- Patient is expected to remain hospitalized for 5–7 days.
- Diet should be resumed slowly and patient should have a bowel movement prior to discharge.

Prognosis

- Patient or caregiver will be responsible for lifetime stoma care.
- Additional treatment for cancer may be necessary.
- Patient is expected to resume normal activities within 6–8 weeks.

Complications

- Hemorrhage
- Infection
- Leakage of the small bowel or ureteroileal anastomoses
- Irritation around the stoma
- Stenosis at the site of the stoma or the ureteroileal anastomoses

PEARL OF WISDOM

If seeding of malignant cells is of concern, the bladder may be filled with formalin solution prior to the urethral transection. The fluid should remain in the bladder and urethra for approximately 10 minutes to decrease the viability of potentially contaminating tumor cells. After the prescribed amount of time, the fluid is drained and the urethral dissection continues.

PROCEDURES FOR STRESS INCONTINENCE AFFECTING WOMEN

Several procedural options are available to women who experience stress **incontinence**. The objectives are to restore the posterior urethrovesical angle and elevate the base of the bladder, which may have been distorted during childbirth or as the natural result of aging.

Mild stress incontinence may be reduced following an anterior colporrhaphy. Colporrhaphy elevates the base of the bladder by eliminating redundant and weakened vaginal tissue. The gynecologist often performs this procedure in conjunction with vaginal hysterectomy (refer to Chapter 15).

Significant incontinent episodes may be eliminated with suprapubic vesicourethral suspension (Marshall-Marchetti-Krantz procedure) or endoscopic suspension of the bladder neck (Stamey procedure).

The Marshall-Marchetti-Krantz (MMK) procedure may be performed by the genitourologist or gynecologist in conjunction with abdominal hysterectomy or as a lone procedure (refer to Procedure 20-3 and Figure 20-20).

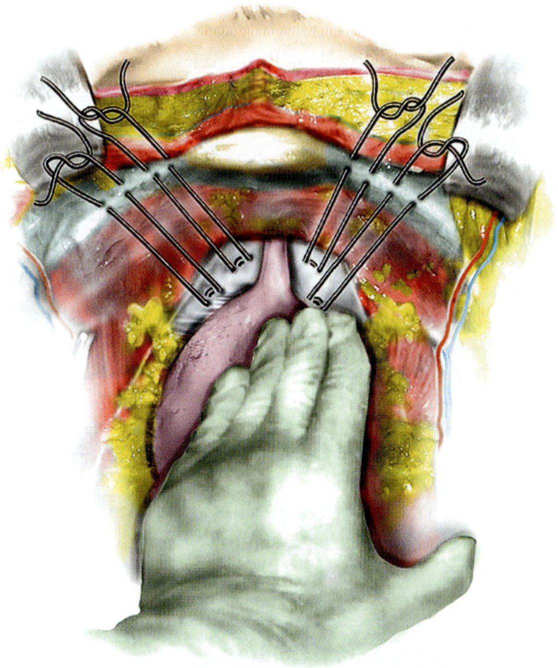

Figure 20-20 Marshall-Marchetti-Krantz procedure—suprapubic vesicourethral suspension with suture fixation to Cooper's ligament

PROCEDURE 20-3 Marshall-Marchetti-Krantz Procedure

Equipment

- Electrosurgical unit
- Positioning aids

Instruments

- Major instrumentation set
- Long instrumentation set
- Heaney needle holders × 2

Supplies

- Pack: basic
- Basin: double
- Gloves
- Blades: #10 × 2
- Drapes: laparotomy (transverse) plus an additional impervious ½ sheet
- Suture: according to surgeon's preference
- Drains: none
- Dressings: three-layer
- Drugs: according to surgeon's preference
- Miscellaneous:
  - Electrocautery pencil
  - Extension for electrocautery
  - Irrigation fluid
  - Suction tubing
  - Gauze sponges
  - Laparotomy sponges
  - Peanut sponges

Operative Preparation

Anesthesia

- General (preferred) or regional
- Lubricate and protect eyes

Position

- Supine with Trendelenburg's
- Frog-leg

Prep

- Remove anterior pubic hair
- Insert Foley catheter
- Prep mid-chest to thighs and laterally as far as possible
- Vulvar and internal vaginal prep also required

Draping

- Impervious sheet under buttocks
- Anticipated incision site is outlined with towels that are secured in place with adhesive or towel clips
- Transverse laparotomy sheet; disposable lap sheet may be cut to accommodate frog-leg position and provide vaginal access
- A towel may be used to temporarily cover the opening in the drape that will provide vaginal access

Practical Considerations

- Extra gloves and possibly an additional gown will be necessary for the assistant
- Foley catheter may be inserted by circulator preoperatively or from the sterile field by the surgeon, assistant, or STSR

Operative Procedure	Technical Considerations
1. A Pfannenstiel incision is used to approach the retropubic space.	1. A #10 blade on #3 handle is used for incision. Provide cautery and suction.

PROCEDURE

20-3 Marshall-Marchetti-Krantz Procedure *(continued)*

2. The bladder and urethra are freed from behind the symphysis pubis using blunt dissection techniques.	**2.** Surgeon may use fingers, peanut sponges on a long Mayo clamp, or a sponge on a stick for dissection. Prepare supplies in advance of need.
3. The endopelvic fascia is incised to allow for displacement of the bladder.	**3.** A #10 blade on a #3L handle may be needed, according to patient's size (depth).
4. The assistant will insert two gloved fingers into the vagina to elevate the base of the bladder (which is easily palpable due to the presence of the Foley catheter balloon) to facilitate suture placement and reduce tension.	**4.** Protect sterile field from contamination during this process.
5. Four heavy absorbable sutures are placed in strategic locations in the anterior vaginal wall bilaterally to the urethra and are secured in the posterior symphysis or Cooper's ligament.	**5.** Load sutures on Heaney needle holders for placement. Anticipate the use of all four sutures sequentially. A series of hemostats may be requested to "tag" the sutures until all have been placed and are ready for tying.
6. All sutures are positioned and then tied sequentially for optimum elevation of the bladder.	**6.** Provide suture scissors as needed. Assist circulator in changing assistant's gown and gloves as necessary. Provide towel to cover site following bladder elevation. Prepare drain, if requested. Anticipate wound closure and prepare suture.
7. A wound drain may be placed. The wound is closed and dressed in the usual fashion.	**7.** Count. Provide three-layer dressing material.
8. Vaginal packing may be inserted to temporarily reduce tension on the suture line.	**8.** Vaginal packing is inserted after abdominal dressing is in place.

Postoperative Considerations

Immediate Postoperative Care

- Blood-tinged urine may be noted in the Foley drainage bag.
- The Foley catheter may be removed in the PACU; the patient is expected to void normally.

Prognosis

- The patient may remain hospitalized overnight.

Complications

- Hemorrhage
- Infection
- Recurrence of urinary stress incontinence

PEARL OF WISDOM

The STSR should be cognizant that a potential for contamination of the field exists due to the vaginal and abdominal areas being incorporated in the same drape. The assistant will need to change gloves (and possibly gown) immediately after providing intravaginal urethral support during suturing.

Endoscopic suspension of the vesical neck (Stamey procedure) is accomplished by suspending the fascial attachments of the bladder to the rectus fascia with sutures that are placed with the use of a Stamey needle (Figure 20-21). The sutures are additionally supported with Dacron bolsters. Suture placement is verified cystoscopically at several intervals throughout the case. The patient is in lithotomy position under general anesthesia. Both the abdominal and perineal preps are carried out and a drape that exposes both areas must be used. A Foley catheter is inserted from the sterile field; it should remain sterile in its entirety throughout the procedure. The Foley will have to be extracted every time the endoscope is inserted and reinserted when the scope is removed. The procedure requires two small suprapubic incisions and a vaginal incision. When placement of all sutures is determined to be satisfactory, the sutures are tensioned and tied sequentially. The small wounds are closed and postoperative care parallels that described for the MMK procedure.

TRANSURETHRAL ENDOSCOPY OF THE GENITOURINARY TRACT

Transurethral endoscopy of the genitourinary tract provides an internal view of the structures. GU endoscopy is accomplished by introducing the scope through the male or female urethra with the patient in the lithotomy position. Anesthesia may be local, regional, or general. Viewing instruments are available in a variety of sizes and styles for several purposes.

Urinary tract endoscopy is commonly referred to as *cystoscopy,* although that limited term does not begin to identify all of the procedures that can be performed endoscopically. Often the procedure encompasses all of the structures of the genitourinary tract and is not limited strictly to "viewing." The main purpose of urinary tract endoscopy is diagnosis. In addition to viewing instruments, a variety of accessories are available to make cystoscopy an operative procedure as well. Current technological developments continue to expand the procedural capabilities of endoscopy. A brief listing of some of the procedures that are possible endoscopically follows:

- Retrograde urogram
- Visual diagnosis of a variety of genitourinary tract conditions
- Biopsy
- Bleeding tissue fulguration
- Prostate tissue removal (transurethral resection of the prostate, TURP)
- Removal of small bladder tumors (transurethral resection of bladder tumor, TURBT)
- Placement of ureteral stents in one or both ureters
- Calculi removal from any part of the GU tract
- Urethral enlargement

The role of the surgical technologist during the endoscopic procedure is minimal, but the responsibilities are of paramount importance.

The surgical technologist is responsible for assembling all of the necessary items according to the type of procedure scheduled and the surgeon's preference. If the health care facility does not have a designated cysto room, a major amount of equipment may need to be moved into the OR. Often the health care facility has designated a specific team of personnel that specializes in GU procedures

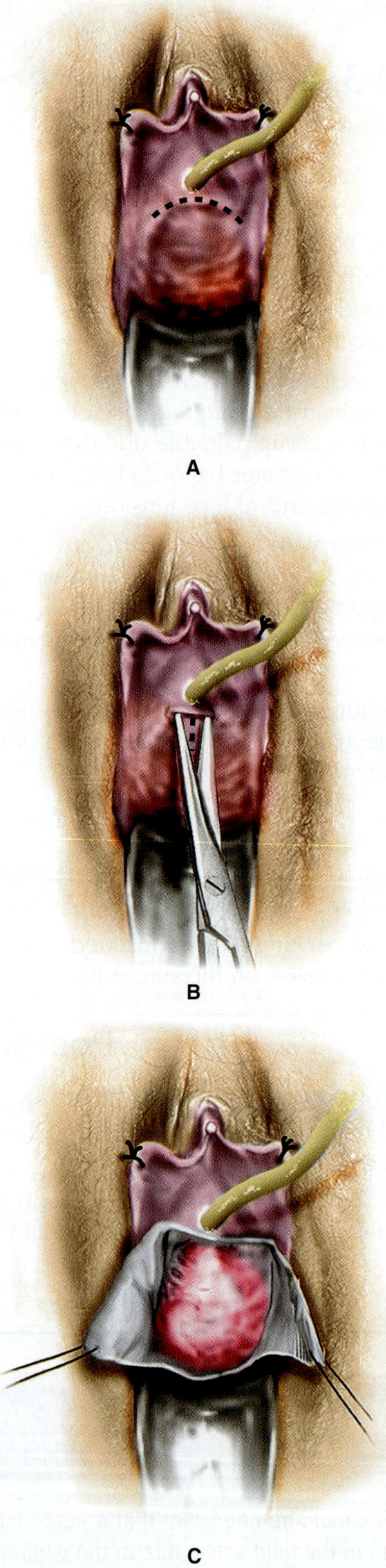

Figure 20-21 **Stamey procedure: (A) Vaginal incision site, (B) dissection to expose urethra, (C) urethra exposed**

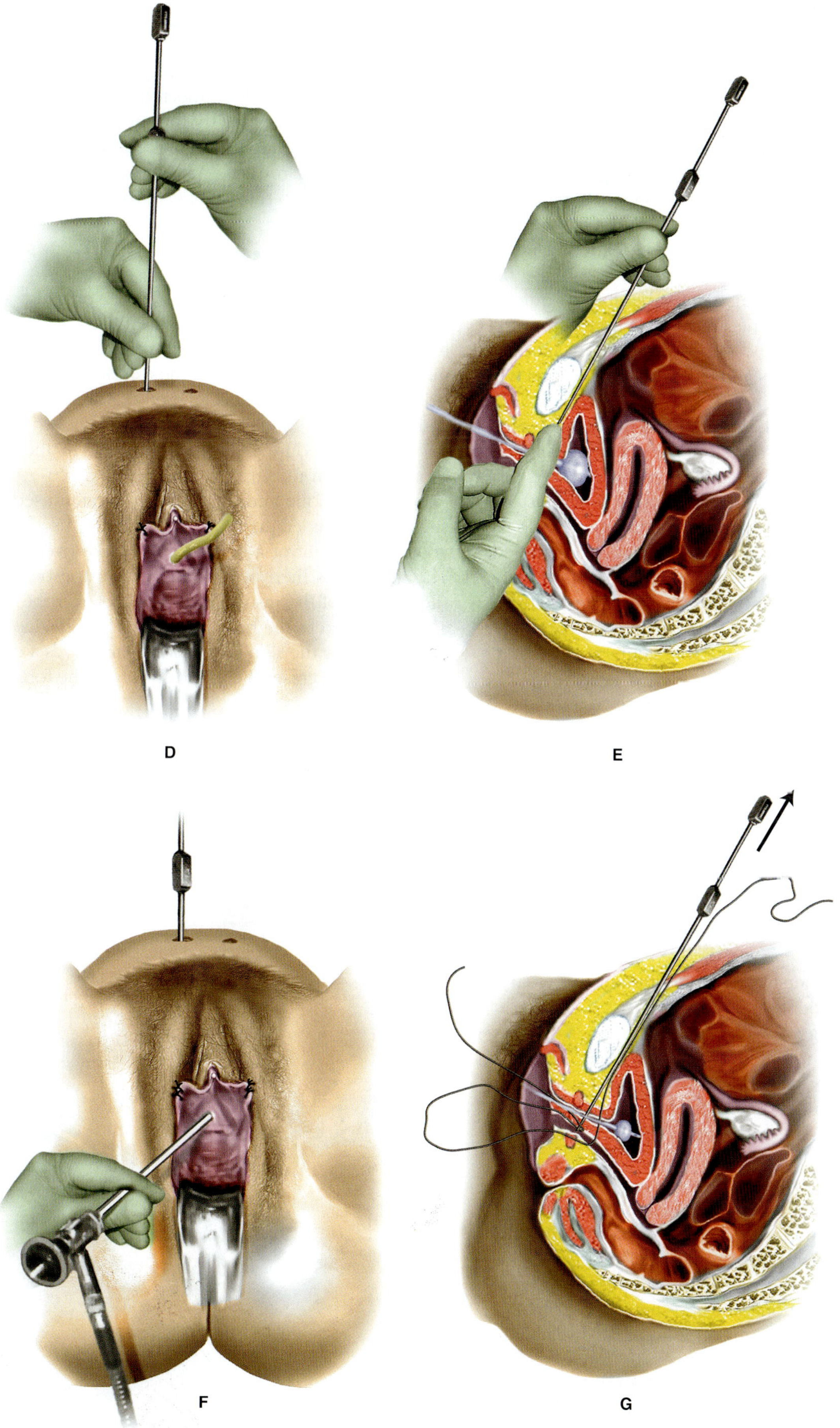

Figure 20-21 ***(continued):*** **(D) incisions for Stamey needle placement, (E) guiding Stamey needle into place, (F) verification of needle placement, (G) suture placement**

to work in the specialty area. This however, does not excuse the generalist from being responsible for knowledge of the equipment and procedures in case he or she is asked to fill in due to staff illness or other emergency.

Communication with the radiology department may be necessary to obtain preoperative films or arrange for intraoperative studies.

Because endoscopic equipment is extremely delicate, it is often stored in protective cases, in a nonsterile state. The surgical technologist must be able to quickly determine which instruments are suitable for steam sterilization and which must be sterilized using an alternate method. Items with lenses and electrical connections typically are not steam sterilized.

A sterile field must be created and maintained. Sterilized items must be transported to the operating suite using sterile technique. The surgical technologist is not required to "scrub in" for the endoscopy, but must organize the instruments and supplies on the sterile field for use by the surgeon. Some instruments must be assembled; all connections should be secure and fluid-tight. In many facilities it is permissible to don sterile gloves and perform the necessary tasks. Once the sterile field is prepared, the surgical technologist may leave the sterile area and deglove.

The surgical technologist may receive fluids and pharmaceuticals onto the sterile field from the circulator. These must be labeled for use by the surgeon. All irrigation fluids should be prepared in advance and placed for use.

The surgical technologist will assist the circulator with patient care once all of the components of the sterile field have been taken care of. Responsibilities may include:

- Positioning the patient for anesthesia and the procedure
- Applying the dispersive electrode if one is necessary
- Prepping the patient
- Assisting the surgeon with draping
- Receiving the nonsterile ends of the cables, cords, and tubings to be connected
- Connecting such devices as the cautery cords, light cable, video camera cord, irrigation (inflow and outflow) tubings, etc.
- Turning on and setting the devices as directed

The main role of the surgical technologist during the endoscopic procedure is to be certain that the irrigation fluid of choice is constantly available. The type of fluid used may change as the procedure progresses. Fluid inflow and outflow are monitored and should closely match.

A variety of urinary catheters should be available for insertion at the end of the procedure. The surgeon, circulator, or surgical technologist may perform this task.

Any specimens should be transferred from the sterile field to a properly labeled container for transport to the laboratory.

On completion of the procedure, several pieces of equipment must be disconnected and safely removed from the field. Drapes are then removed and discarded.

All urologic endoscopic procedures are expected to follow this basic routine. Any variances will be determined according to the patient's exact situation.

CIRCUMCISION

Circumcision is the removal of the prepuce (Figure 20-22). This is often performed on infants at the parent's request due to personal or religious reasons. Circumcision may also be done to treat phimosis. Circumcision is considered minor surgery; several methods are available (Procedure 20-4).

The procedure may be performed in the delivery room, newborn nursery, or physician's office. A minimal prep may be done and drapes are not often used. In this situation, a guided method is frequently used. This involves placement of a bell-shaped device over the glans. The foreskin is then pulled taught over the bell and the second part of the instrument is placed over the foreskin and connected to the base of the bell. The device is tightened, trapping the skin in position. This serves a dual purpose: it compromises the blood supply to the foreskin and

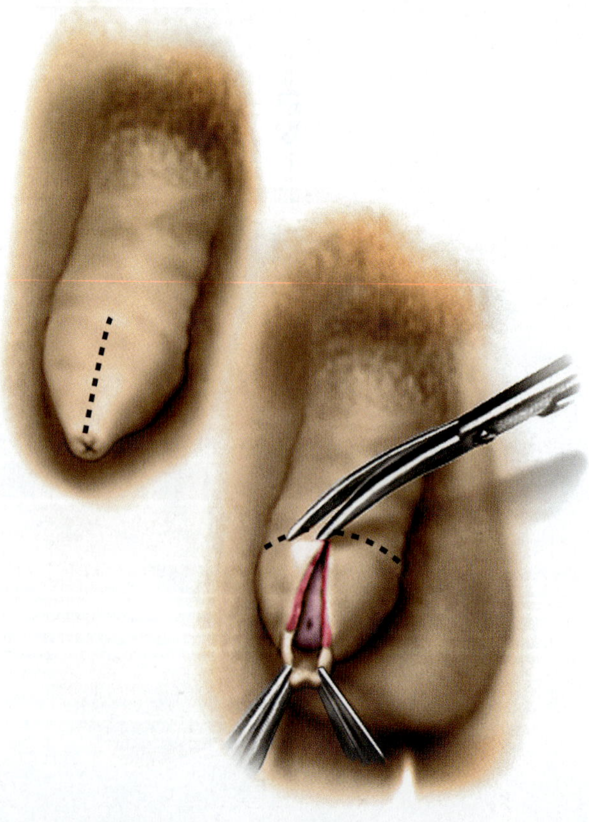

Figure 20-22 Circumcision

provides a protective surface for the surgeon to move the scalpel along as the foreskin is excised. The clamp is removed and sutures are placed if necessary. A frenulectomy may be performed at this time. A nonadherent dressing is loosely applied to the distal penis allowing for urination and preventing irritation by the diaper. The parents should be instructed on how to care for the wound. Pain medication if needed may be administered in the form of rectal suppository or oral liquid. Complete wound healing is expected within 7–10 days and no further care is necessary.

PROCEDURE 20-4 Circumcision

Equipment

- Electrocautery

Instruments

- Circumcision instrumentation tray

Supplies

- Pack: basic
- Basin: small
- Gloves
- Blades: #15
- Drapes: towels or small fenestrated sheet
- Suture: according to surgeon's preference
- Drains: none
- Dressings: adaptic
- Drugs: according to surgeon's preference
- Miscellaneous:
  Electrocautery pencil
  10-cc syringe and 25-gauge 1½-in. needle if use of local anesthetic is anticipated
  Gauze sponges
  Clean diaper, if applicable

Operative Prep

Anesthesia

- General preferred, local or regional may be used
- Local anesthesia may be used in addition to general anesthesia for postoperative pain control

Position

- Supine

Prep

- Shave not necessary
- Prep penis and small surrounding area
- Retract foreskin if patient's condition allows

Draping

- Three or four towels may be placed around the base of the penis or a small drape with a fenestration may be used

Practical Considerations

- Prep solution may be needed on sterile field if adequate preoperative prep was not carried out due to phimosis

Operative Procedure	Technical Considerations
1. Straight hemostat is applied to the posterior midline of the foreskin to provide hemostasis.	**1.** Provide straight hemostat. Clamp will likely remain in place several minutes.

(continues)

PROCEDURE

20-4 Circumcision *(continued)*

2. Clamp is removed and a dorsal slit is created.	**2.** A #15 knife blade or straight scissors is used to make the dorsal slit.
3. A circumferential freehand cut around the shaft is carried out as far back as the surgeon determines appropriate.	**3.** Knife or scissors is used to remove the foreskin. It may or may not be necessary to send foreskin as a specimen. Be familiar with facility policy. Gauze may be used to remove blood from field to enhance surgeon's visualization. Cautery may be used.
4. If frenulectomy is to be performed, it may be accomplished at this time.	**4.** Scissors or cautery may be necessary.
5. Raw edges of the small remainder of the foreskin are pulled together and sutured, leaving the glans and frenulum exposed.	**5.** Provide absorbable suture on short needle holder and Adson tissue forceps with teeth. Prepare to cut suture if requested. Count may not be required according to facility policy.
6. Nonadherent dressing is loosely applied to the distal penis.	**6.** Wrap adaptic around penis. Diaper, if applicable.

Postoperative Considerations

Immediate Postoperative Care

- Dressing is loosely applied to allow for urination.
- Oral analgesics should be adequate for pain control.
- Apply cold packs to minimize swelling.

Prognosis

- Circumcision is expected to be an out-patient procedure.
- Resume normal activities within 7–10 days.

Complications

- Hemorrhage
- Infection

PEARL OF WISDOM

Emotional needs of the male are considered. Provide privacy and protect patient's dignity as procedure allows.

ORCHIECTOMY

Orchiectomy is the removal of one or both testicles (Figure 20-23).

Radical orchiectomy is for the removal of a cancerous testicle. The entire contents of the hemiscrotum, the tunica vaginalis, and the spermatic cord are removed, usually through an inguinal incision.

Simple orchiectomy is the removal of only the testis and the epididymis. This is accomplished through a scrotal incision to remove an abscessed testicle or bilaterally in the treatment of prostate cancer to deprive the patient of androgens. The scrotum is opened, and the testis and spermatic cord are extruded through the wound. The cord above the testis is opened and the structures identified and separated. Each section is doubly clamped, transected, and ligated with nonabsorbable suture. If desired and the patient's condition allows, testicular prosthesis may be inserted at this time. A Penrose drain may be inserted and the wound is closed. A pressure dressing should be applied to reduce the risk of hematoma formation. This is considered minor surgery; the patient may remain hospitalized overnight and should be able to return to normal activities in 2–4 weeks.

ORCHIOPEXY

Orchiopexy is the surgical fixation of a testis in the scrotal sac (Figure 20-24). The procedure is most commonly performed to treat testicular torsion and to position a retracted testicle or one that has failed to descend (Procedure 20-5).

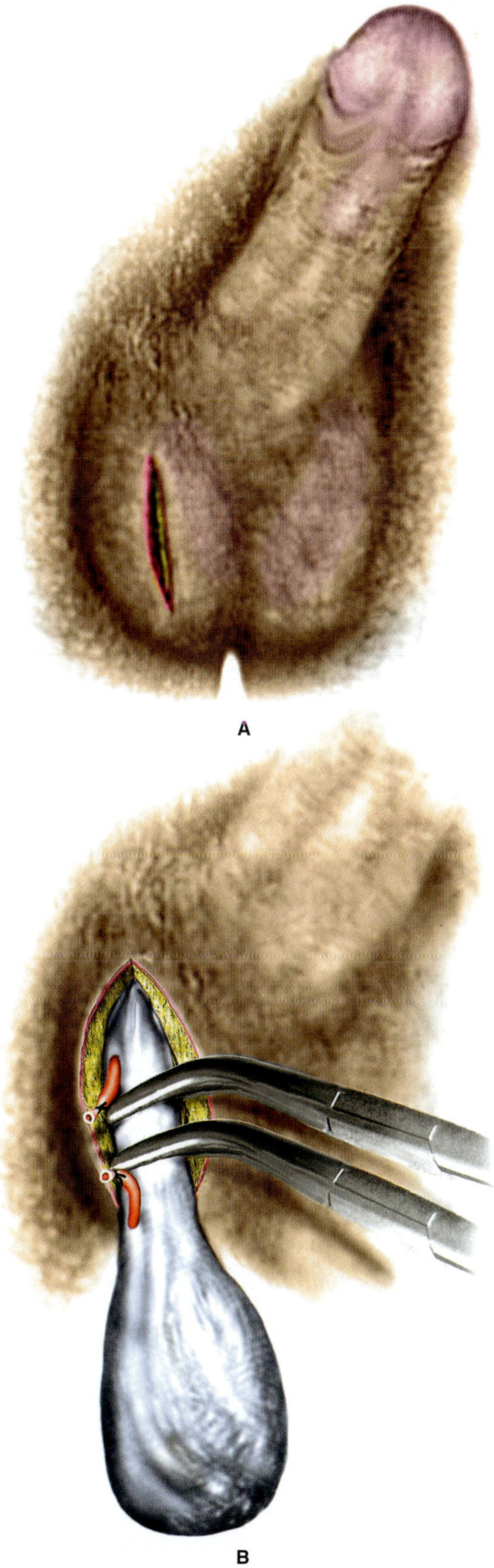

Figure 20-23 Simple orchiectomy: (A) Scrotal incision, (B) removal of testicle

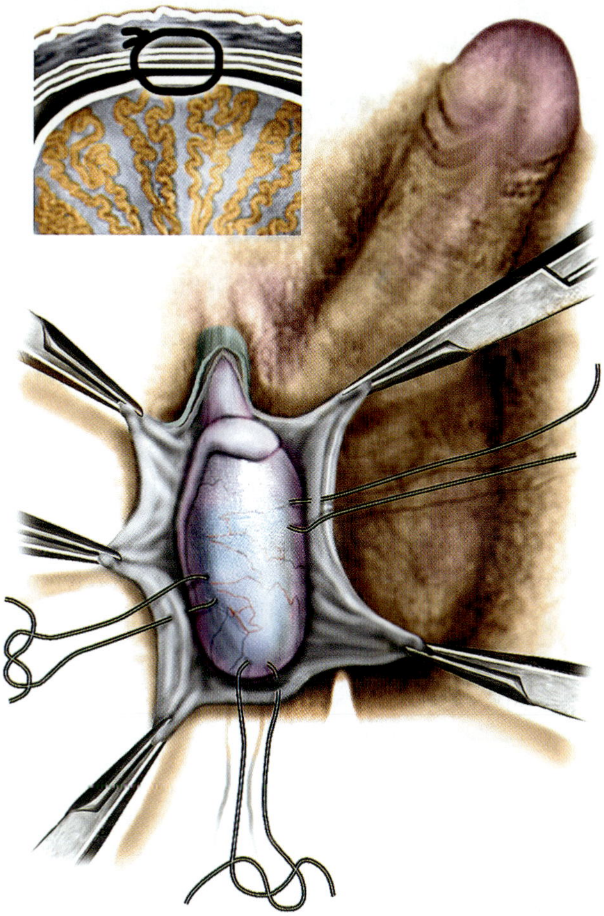

Figure 20-24 Orchiopexy

PROCEDURE 20-5 Orchiopexy

Equipment

- Electrosurgical unit

Instruments

- Minor instrumentation set

Supplies

- Pack: basic
- Basin: single
- Gloves
- Blades: #15 × 2
- Drapes: small fenestrated sheet
- Suture: according to surgeon's preference
- Drains: Penrose, if necessary
- Dressings: adaptic, gauze sponges, scrotal support
- Drugs: according to surgeon's preference
- Miscellaneous:
  Electrocautery pencil
  Gauze sponges

Operative Preparation

Anesthesia
- General preferred

Position
- Supine

Prep
- Shave may not be necessary
- External genitalia and small surrounding area are prepped

Draping
- Towel under external genitalia
- Area may be outlined with towels or a drape with a small fenestration may be used

Practical Considerations

- Orchiopexy is usually performed bilaterally, even if only one side is acutely affected

Operative Procedure	Technical Considerations
1. Tension is applied to the scrotum and an incision is made through the skin and dartos muscle.	**1.** A #15 blade is used for the scrotal incision. It may be necessary for the STSR to apply the scrotal tension.
2. Hemostasis is achieved.	**2.** Provide electrocautery pencil.
3. The tunica vaginalis is opened and the contents of the hemiscrotum exposed.	**3.** Dissection is often carried out with the electrocautery.
4. The testis is properly positioned in the scrotal sac.	**4.** Positioning is carried out manually.
5. The tunica albuginea is attached to the dartos muscle with three nonabsorbable stitches, one on each of the lateral aspects and one inferiorly.	**5.** Provide nonabsorbable suture of surgeon's preference. It may be necessary for the STSR to keep the testis in position while the surgeon sutures.
6. Drainage is usually not required and the wound is closed in two layers with interrupted absorbable sutures.	**6.** Provide suture of surgeon's preference. Count. Reorganize supplies for reuse on contralateral side.
7. Procedure is repeated on contralateral side.	**7.** Follow steps previously outlined.

PROCEDURE

20-5 Orchiopexy *(continued)*

Postoperative Considerations

Immediate Postoperative Care

- Postoperative edema is expected; advise patient to apply ice to minimize.

Prognosis

- Resume normal activities within 2 weeks.

Complications

- Hemorrhage
- Infection

PEARL OF WISDOM

In addition to the testicular incision, an inguinal incision may be required to mobilize the testis or repair any hernia that may coexist.

HYDROCELECTOMY

A hydrocele is an abnormal accumulation of fluid contained in the tunica vaginalis layer of the scrotum. The fluid buildup is often the result of trauma or infection. A hydrocelectomy is performed to remove the fluid-filled sac through a scrotal incision.

The patient is placed in the supine position and general anesthesia administered. An anterior incision is made over the location of the hydrocele with a #15 blade. Bleeding is controlled by clamping the vessels with a mosquito clamp and tying with 4–0 absorbable suture ties or cautery with a needle-point tip. The tunica vaginalis is exposed by incising the facial layers. With tenotomy scissors, Adson forceps, and blunt dissection, the hydrocele is dissected free. The contents of the sac may be aspirated with the use of a 20- or 22-gauge needle on a 10-cc syringe. The sac is opened with the scissors and inverted to surround the testis and epididymis. Excess tunica vaginalis may have to be excised using the scissors, and the edges of the tunica are sutured behind the testicle using a 4–0 or 5–0 absorbable suture. The testicle is resituated in the scrotal sac and a Penrose drain is placed within the scrotum and exteriorized through a stab incision. The scrotal incision is closed in layers with 4–0 or 5–0 absorbable sutures. A fluff dressing is applied and a scrotal support (jockstrap) placed to keep the dressing in place and to keep light pressure on the surgical site to aid in preventing postoperative scrotal edema.

VARICOCELECTOMY

Varicoceles are an abnormal dilation of the spermatic veins in the spermatic cord that drain the testicle, causing a slightly painful swelling of the scrotum. The condition usually occurs on the left side. Varicoceles cause a pooling of blood in the scrotum and consequently a rise in temperature. The rise in temperature affects the production of sperm and can kill sperm, resulting in infertility. A varicocelectomy, also referred to as varicocele ligation, is performed to prevent a decrease in the sperm count. The operation is performed by a variety of methods on an outpatient basis: (1) open inguinal incision, (2) microsurgery, (3) laparoscope, or (4) embolization.

For open procedures the patient is placed in the supine position and either general or spinal anesthesia administered. A transverse abdominal incision is made starting at the anterior superior iliac spine and extending to the lateral aspect of the rectus abdominis muscle. The scrotum and veins are emptied of blood to prevent postoperative varicocele. The veins are ligated with nonabsorbable ties and the wound closed in layers with absorbable suture.

The laparoscopic approach involves ligation of the spermatic vein. After insertion of the laparoscope, the internal inguinal ring, spermatic cord, and blood vessels are identified. The spermatic vein is dissected free from its attachments and ligated with two endoscopic clips. The vein is divided with endoscopic scissors between the two clips. The vein is ligated high up in the pelvis to avoid damaging the testicular artery.

HYPOSPADIAS REPAIR

Hypospadias is a congenital condition in the male in which the urethra ends on the ventral side of the glans penis, anywhere along the penile shaft, on the corona, or on the perineum. The degree of the chordee is determined by how proximal the urethral opening is located. Chordee is caused by fibrous bands that extend from the urethral opening to the tip of the glans. The goal of the procedure is to reposition the meatus at the center of the glans penis. The repair can be accomplished as a one-stage or two-stage procedure depending on the severity of the condition. The procedure is usually performed between the ages of 1 and 4. The following procedural discussion includes glanuplasty, chordee repair, urethroplasty describing the free skin graft technique, and skin cover. Each procedure is discussed separately.

For glanuloplasty, the patient is placed in the supine position with legs slightly apart; make sure the legs are properly supported and padded. General anesthesia is administered. Using a #15 knife blade, a circumferential incision is made just beneath the corona and slightly proximal to the meatus and corona. Using delicate scissors, the skin is stripped downward from the phallus by cutting the subcutaneous tissue. A transverse closure of the edge of the dorsal meatus to the distal glanular groove is completed with the use of small-diameter suture. The surgeon now places three traction sutures: (1) at the lateral region of the glans, (2) where the foreskin ends, and (3) at the top of the ventral meatus. The edges of the glans are sutured together on the ventral side in the shape of a V. Sutures placed in vertical mattress fashion approximate the glans below the meatus. The penile skin is brought back into position and reapproximated.

The chordee repair is the next procedure to be performed. The goal of the repair is to straighten the penis. A circumferential incision is made around the corona and distally to the urethral meatus. Dissection is carried down to the tunica albuginea of the corpora cavernosa. The fibrous bands are dissected free with delicate scissors and are freed along the entire penile shaft to the junction of the penis and scrotum. On completion of the release, the glans penis is closed with 4–0 or 5–0 absorbable sutures in a circumferential manner. If a urethroplasty is not indicated or will be performed at a later date, the dorsal incision is closed in interrupted fashion with 4–0 or 5–0 absorbable sutures.

Many different procedures are used for urethroplasty, including combinations of procedures. The free skin graft, which is usually used with a one-stage hypospadias repair, is described here. The surgeon makes a V-shaped incision on the glans. The penile skin is dissected free after the chordee repair is completed. The three points of the glans are dissected and held in a triangular-looking fashion by mosquito clamps. The ventral skin is used for the full-thickness graft. The skin is placed around a catheter that is used as a stent. The graft is proximally anastomosed to the urethra next to the corpora, and the middle glans dart is sutured to the corpora. A meatoplasty is performed and 4–0 or 5–0 absorbable sutures in interrupted fashion are placed around the meatus, glans, and down the dorsal penile shaft.

The last procedure to be performed as part of the repair is the skin cover. After the chordee repair and urethroplasty, the penis is resurfaced with skin. Excess dorsal foreskin is usually utilized. The excess skin is held upward with mosquito clamps. A small incision is made in the midline in order to deliver the glans penis through the hole. The skin flap is then sutured into place with 4–0 or 5–0 absorbable sutures placed in interrupted mattress fashion.

INSERTION OF INFLATABLE PENILE PROSTHESIS

A penile prosthesis is inserted for the treatment of male impotence. Impotence occurs for a variety of reasons including diabetes mellitus, pelvic trauma, damage to nerves, penile trauma, priapism, Peyronie's disease, and vascular disease. The goal is to enable the male to achieve an erection in order to have sexual intercourse. The following is a description of the procedure for the insertion of an inflatable penile prosthesis.

The patient is placed in the supine position and either general or spinal anesthesia is administered. A Foley catheter is placed to aid in identifying the intraoperative position of the urethra. The STSR should make sure the following instrumentation is available for the procedure: (1) Furlow inserter, (2) Hegar dilators, (3) assembly tool, (4) closing tool, and (5) various connectors. The most serious complication is infection. Aseptic technique must be strictly followed with careful draping of the patient. The anus must be well isolated from the operative field.

Using a #15 knife blade, the surgeon will make a midline incision from the penile base into the scrotum. A 14- or 16-Fr Foley catheter is inserted at this point in the procedure to aid in identifying the position of the urethra, and it is used to retract the urethra to the side. The tunica albuginea of both corpora is incised and traction sutures are placed. The corpora are dilated with the Hegar dilators, and the Furlow inserter is used to measure the corporal length. Then 1–0 or 2–0 absorbable sutures are placed along the incision of the tunica and tagged with mosquito clamps. The inflatable rods are packaged by the manufacturer with traction sutures attached at the distal end. The sutures are placed through a Keith needle and the needle is placed into the groove of the Furlow inserter. The Furlow inserter is placed through the corporal tunnel and the plunger at the end of the inserter is pushed to puncture the glans with the Keith needle. The needle is grasped with a heavy needle holder and pulled through the glans, allowing the inflatable rod to move into position. The Furlow inserter is removed and the inflatable rod is further placed into position. The procedure is repeated in the other corpora. The next step is the placement of the pump.

The external inguinal ring is located and a path bluntly formed with the fingers. Metzenbaum scissors are used to separate the transversalis fascia. Cooper's ligament is located and the fluid reservoir is positioned in the perivesical space. The fluid reservoir is filled and positioned against Hesselbach's triangle. The pump is placed in the scrotum, usually on the patient's dominant side, lateral to the testicle in a space bluntly dissected. The inflatable rods and fluid reservoir are connected to the pump with the appropriate connectors using the assembly tool to clamp in place. The pump and inflatable rods are tested.

The scrotal tunica albuginea is closed over the pump with a 3–0 or 4–0 absorbable suture in running fashion. To aid in preventing hemorrhage and healing, the penile prosthesis is partially inflated. The incision is closed with 3–0 or 4–0 absorbable suture, subcuticular fashion. The Foley catheter is left in place for approximately 24–48 hours. Dressing is applied.

VASECTOMY

Vasectomy is performed almost exclusively to obstruct the vas deferens in order to produce permanent sterility (Figure 20-25). This is an out-patient procedure usually done with a local anesthetic via bilateral scrotal incisions. The vas is grasped above the epididymis and manually separated from the adjacent cord structures, the local anesthetic administered, and a small incision made. The vas is delivered through the wound with the use of a clamp. The vas is clamped proximally and distally, ligatures are applied, and the midsection of the vas is removed. The remaining segments of the vas may be fulgurated to destroy the lumen. The wound is closed and the procedure repeated on the contralateral side. Mild pain and minimal swelling are expected. The patient should be able to return to normal activities within 2–5 days. The patient should realize that sterility is not immediate, because residual sperm may be contained in the GU tract. Ten to 15 ejaculations are usually necessary to evacuate the remaining sperm. Contraception should be practiced until sterility is verified with semen analysis. Although reanastomosis occurs in less than 1% of cases, the patient should be aware that there is a remote possibility of unexpected pregnancy.

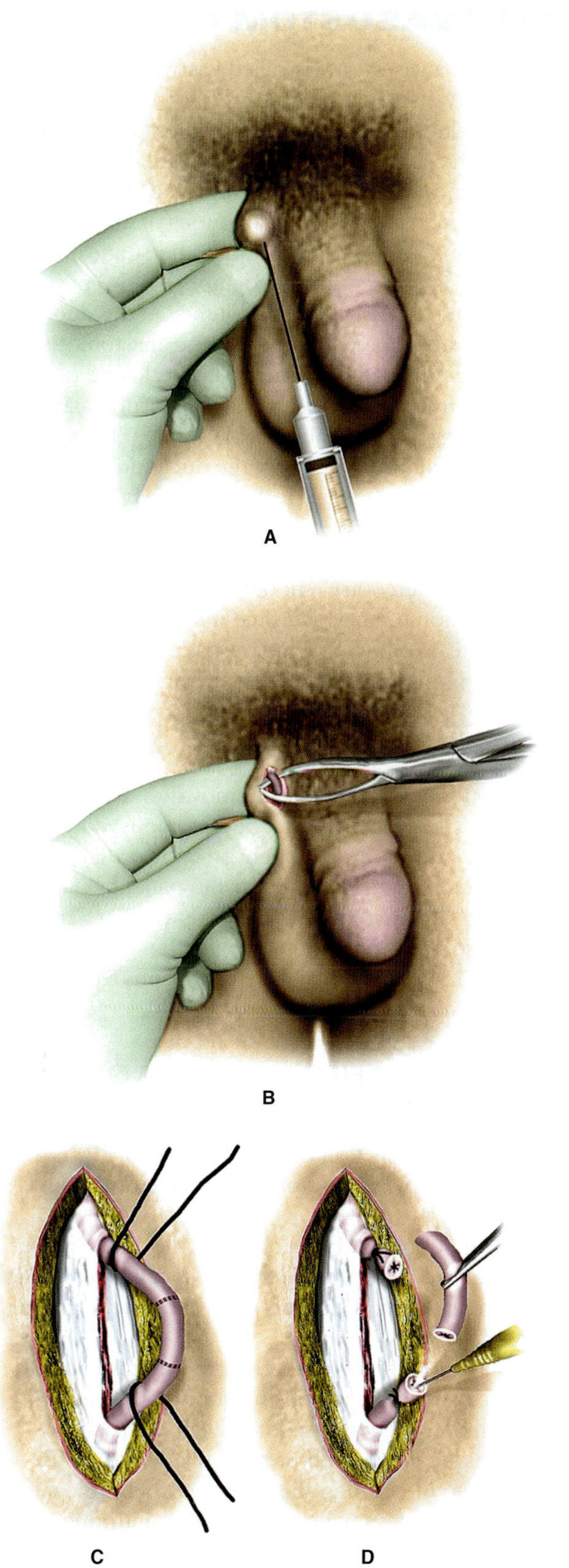

Figure 20-25 Vasectomy: (A) Anesthesia administration, (B) isolation of vas, (C) ligatures applied to proximal and distal vas, (D) midsection of vas removed and lumen of remaining vas fulgurated

VASOVASOSTOMY

Reversal of a vasectomy is called vasovasostomy. The procedure may also be done to correct obstructions of the vas deferens due to congenital anomalies, inflammation, or trauma. The severed ends of the vas are exposed through a scrotal incision and held in approximation with a specially designed clamp. Surgical loupes or an operating microscope may be used to enhance the surgical field. Any scar tissue is excised and vasography or the passage of a temporary stent demonstrates patency of the duct. The lumens may be dilated if necessary. The anastomosis may be accomplished simply with a one-layer closure of the vasal wall or a more complex two-layer closure may be performed using 10–0 nonabsorbable sutures. The vas may be stented to maintain patency of the duct during healing, but advanced microsurgical techniques may eliminate the need for the stent. The procedure is repeated on the contralateral side. The patient may remain hospitalized overnight. Intercourse should be avoided for approximately 1 month, at which time a semen analysis will be performed. Following vasovasostomy, conception is achieved approximately 50% of the time.

PROSTATECTOMY

Prostatectomy is the surgical removal of all or part of the prostate. The procedure can be accomplished transurethrally or may require an open procedure. The approach will be determined primarily by the patient's pathological condition. Removal of a cancerous prostate usually requires an open procedure, while the patient suffering from BPH (benign prostatic hypertrophy) is most often treated transurethrally.

TRANSURETHRAL RESECTION OF THE PROSTATE

Transurethral resection of the prostate (TURP) is a procedure that is typically performed in the cysto room (Figure 20-26).

The surgical technologist should be aware of several intraoperative complications specific to TURP that could negatively affect the outcome of the procedure. They include:

- It may be impossible to enter the urethra with the resectoscope due to obstruction. Conservative treatment, such as a modified catheterization technique along with urethral dilation, may be effective in opening the passage or a perineal urethrostomy may be performed to introduce the resectoscope.

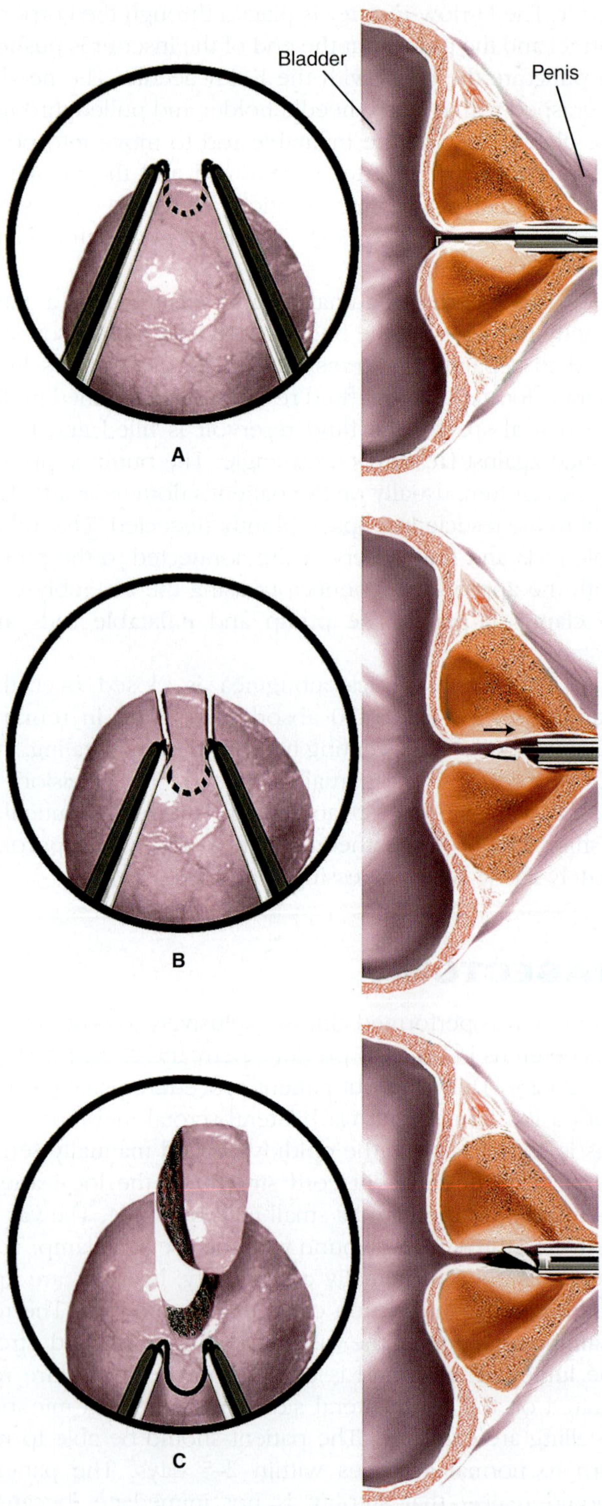

Figure 20-26 Transurethral prostatectomy: (A) Prostate gland visualized, (B) resectoscope used to remove hyperplastic tissue, (C) prostate chip separated

- Uncontrollable hemorrhage may obscure the visual field. The procedure may be terminated immediately and pressure applied to the area with a Foley catheter balloon under traction, or the procedure may be converted to an open procedure.
- Instrument malfunction is usually an easily correctable problem. Prompt troubleshooting techniques should be implemented to determine the source of the malfunction and to remedy the situation.
- A sudden jerking of one of the patient's legs is an indicator that the electrical stimulation from the cautery is irritating the obturator nerve and that perforation of the prostatic capsule may be imminent. Surgical team members should report any unexpected movement by the patient to the surgeon and anesthesia provider. Modification of the technique used by the surgeon can prevent nerve injury and prevent perforation of the capsule.
- Accidental perforation of the prostatic capsule leads to extravasation of the irrigating fluid onto the space surrounding the prostate. If noted immediately, the procedure is terminated once hemostasis is achieved and any remaining loose prostatic tissue is removed. The perforation should be documented with a urethrocystogram. If extravasation is extensive, a drain may be inserted to remove the fluid.

Systemic absorption of the irrigating fluid is a serious complication that stems from extensive extravasation. The irrigant is absorbed into venous circulation and puts a load on the circulatory system. This is referred to as TURP syndrome. Early signs include restlessness, confusion, nausea, and vomiting that are noted with the patient anesthetized regionally. The diagnosis is more difficult with a patient under general anesthesia. The patient's blood pressure is expected to rise. Late signs of systemic absorption of the irrigant affecting the neurological system are seizures, coma, and blindness; the respiratory and cardiovascular signs are pulmonary edema and congestive heart failure. Administration of furosemide by the anesthesia provider will help reduce the amount of intravascular fluid. The patient should be monitored for electrolyte and blood gas imbalances and have a central venous pressure (CVP) monitor inserted. Overnight observation in the intensive care unit is recommended. The procedure is terminated as soon as feasible following removal of any prostatic fragments and the attainment of hemostasis.

The patient is anesthetized regionally (preferred) or generally, then placed in the lithotomy position, prepped, and draped. The surgeon may place an O'Connor shield to allow for transrectal digital manipulation of the prostate during the procedure without fecal contamination.

If necessary, the urethra is dilated or a meatotomy is performed. A preliminary cystoscopy may be performed. Following removal of the cystoscope, the lubricated resectoscope is inserted. This may be done under direct vision, or a camera/video system can be used. A loop electrode for the electrocautery is used to resect or "scoop away" the enlarged prostate tissue. The resection requires multiple strokes or passes with the electrode. The loop may require frequent cleaning due to the adherence of biologic debris. A sterile brush is used for this purpose. The surgeon will intermittently remove tissue fragments with the Ellik evacuator. The bladder, prostatic fossa, and urethra are inspected for debris and any blood vessels that were not cauterized with the loop electrode will be coagulated with a blade or ball style electrode prior to final removal of the instrument.

A large Foley catheter (22–24 Fr) with a 30-cc balloon is inserted and the balloon inflated with water. (Some surgeons prefer the use of a three-way catheter to allow for continuous irrigation of the bladder postoperatively.) The catheter may be manually irrigated to assess hemostasis. Bladder drainage is expected to be clear or slightly tinged with blood. Grossly bloody drainage may be indicative of arterial bleeding. The surgeon will remove the catheter and reinsert the resectoscope, inspect the area for bleeding vessels, and fulgurate them. Traction may be applied to the Foley by taping the external portion to the patient's inner thigh. This maneuver applies moderate pressure to the operative site and may be helpful in reducing bleeding.

The amount of time required for TURP is directly related to the size of the prostate gland and can range from 30 minutes to 3 hours.

The patient remains hospitalized for several days until the urine draining from the catheter is clear, the catheter is removed, and the patient is able to void satisfactorily. Normal activity including sexual relations can be resumed in 4–6 weeks. Postoperative complications, although rare, include bleeding, infection, and urethral stricture. Urethral stricture may lead to urinary retention and retrograde ejaculation.

SUPRAPUBIC PROSTATECTOMY

Suprapubic prostatectomy is performed to treat adenomas that are too large to be removed endoscopically or to remove malignancy (Procedure 20-6 and Figure 20-27).

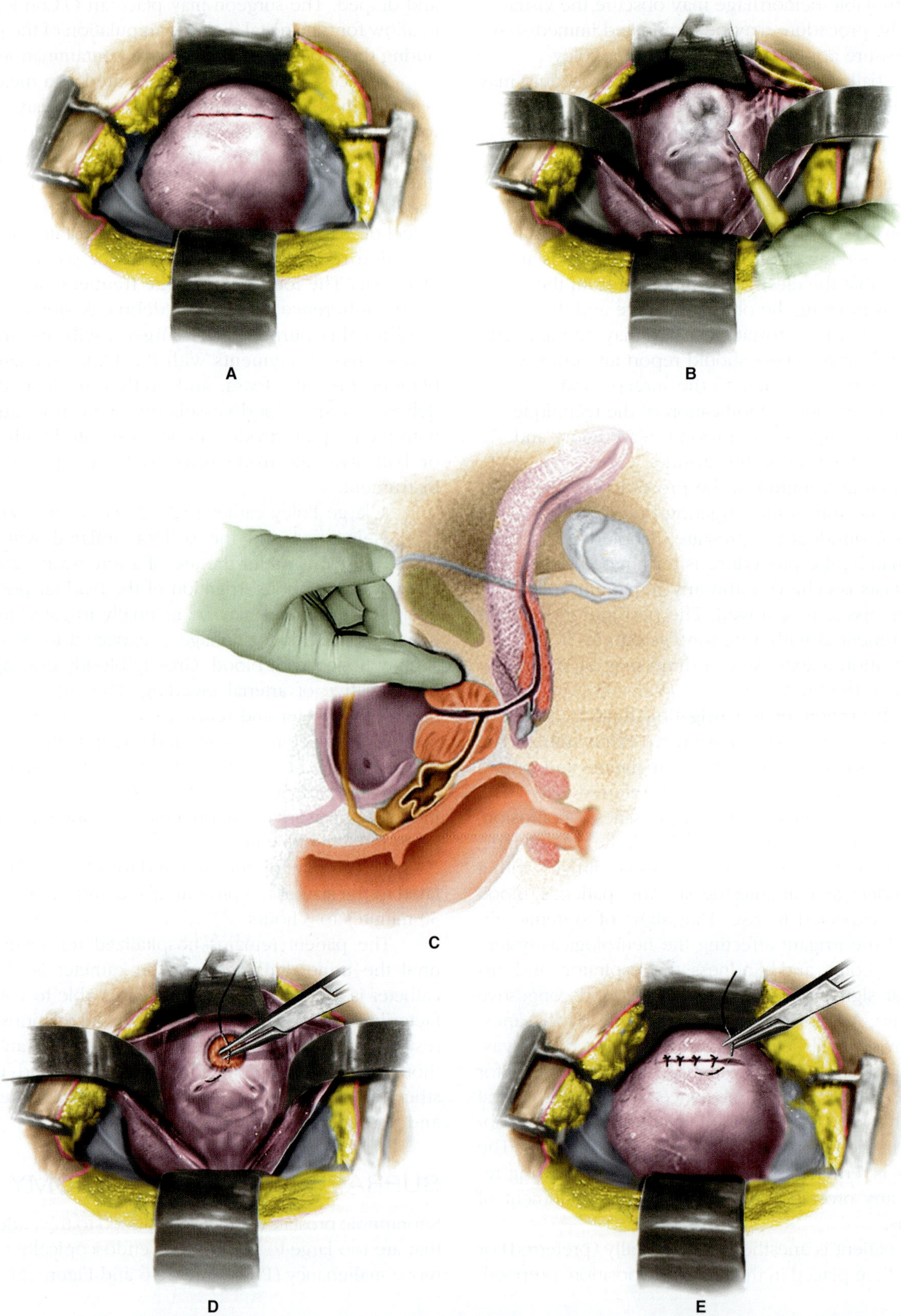

Figure 20-27 **Suppubic prostatectomy: (A) Bladder exposed through low transverse incision, (B) bladder entered, (C) blunt dissection of prostate, (D) prostate fossa sutured to bladder mucosa, (E) bladder closure**

PROCEDURE 20-6 Suprapubic Prostatectomy

Equipment

- Electrosurgical unit

Instruments

- Major instrumentation set
- Long instrumentation set
- Heaney needle holders
- Self-retaining abdominal retractor
- Hemoclip appliers
- Bladder retractor

Supplies

- Pack: basic
- Basin: double
- Gloves
- Blades: #10 (several)
- Drapes: laparotomy
- Suture: according to surgeon's preference
- Drains: Jackson-Pratt
- Dressings: three-layer
- Drugs: according to surgeon's preference
- Miscellaneous:
  - Electrocautery pencil
  - Extension for electrocautery
  - Irrigation fluid
  - Suction tubing
  - Gauze sponges
  - Laparotomy sponges
  - Peanut sponges
  - Hemoclips
  - 16-Fr Foley catheter with 5-cc balloon
  - Drainage bag
  - Lubricant
  - 22-Fr Foley catheter with 30-cc balloon

Operative Preparation

Anesthesia

- Regional or general

Position

- Supine

Prep

- Shave abdomen and pubic area
- Prep mid-chest to thighs and laterally as far as possible

Draping

- Foot drape may be used
- Towel under external genitalia
- Intended incision site is outlined with towels
- Laparotomy sheet is used; penis remains exposed

Practical Considerations

- Foley catheter is inserted and maintained within the sterile field
- Prior to bladder closure, a suprapubic catheter may be inserted to supplement bladder drainage or provide a means of bladder irrigation

Operative Procedure	Technical Considerations
1. A low transverse (Pfannenstiel) incision is made down to the level of the bladder (Figure 20-27A).	1. A #10 knife blade on #3 handle is used for the incision. Bleeding is controlled with electrocautery. Present retractors as necessary.
2. The peritoneum is reflected away from the dome of the bladder.	2. Blunt dissection by the surgeon's fingers or with a sponge stick is used.

(continues)

PROCEDURE 20-6 Suprapubic Prostatectomy *(continued)*

3. The bladder is entered suprapubically between two stay sutures and the ureters are visualized (Figure 20-27B).	**3.** The two stay sutures should be prepared in advance. Tags will be needed. "Deep" knife is used for cystotomy. Suction is used frequently.
4. Retraction is provided to expose the bladder outlet.	**4.** Provide retractors of choice. Moist lap sponges may be used to protect underlying tissue.
5. The Foley catheter is removed and the mucosa surrounding the base of the prostate is incised, avoiding the ureteral orifices.	**5.** Provide empty syringe to deflate Foley balloon. A #10 blade on a #3L handle is needed.
6. Retractors are removed and the prostate (or lobe) is dissected circumferentially with the surgeon's finger (Figure 20-27C).	**6.** Retrieve retractors; prepare for reuse.
7. The tumor is delivered into the bladder and removed. Specimen may be removed en bloc or dissection may continue if the prostatic lobes have been divided for removal.	**7.** Prepare to accept specimen.
8. Figure-eight sutures may be used in the prostatic fossa to control bleeding.	**8.** Sutures are prepared in advance. The Heaney needle holder may be useful.
9. The integrity of the bladder outlet is restored by suturing the mucosa of the bladder to the prostatic fossa (Figure 20-27D).	**9.** Six sutures are often used to reconnect the bladder to the prostatic fossa. Sutures are loaded in advance on the Heaney needle holders. All sutures may be placed and tagged, then tied sequentially.
10. A 22-Fr 30-cc Foley is inserted transurethrally and the balloon is inflated. If necessary to control hemorrhage, external traction may be applied to the Foley.	**10.** Prepare Foley for insertion by testing the integrity of the balloon and lubricating the tip. Prepare to connect collection device.
11. Bleeding may be difficult to control because the suprapubic approach does not provide good visualization of the prostatic fossa and it is difficult to maneuver a needle driver into the restricted space.	**11.** Electrocautery may be an effective choice.
12. Once hemostasis is achieved, the cystotomy is closed (Figure 20-27E).	**12.** Provide suture of surgeon's preference. Suture scissors will be necessary.
13. A Jackson-Pratt drain is placed in the retropubic space and the remainder of the wound is closed.	**13.** Provide drain and suture as needed. Count. Drain will likely be sutured in place.
14. A pressure dressing is applied.	**14.** Provide dressing materials.

Postoperative Considerations

Immediate Postoperative Care

- An epidural anesthetic may be useful in postoperative pain control.

Prognosis

- Patient is expected to remain hospitalized for several days until the urine is clear, the catheters are removed, and normal voiding occurs.

PROCEDURE

20-6 Suprapubic Prostatectomy *(continued)*

- The patient is expected to return to normal activities in 6–8 weeks.
- Sexual function and urinary continence should not be compromised.
- Additional treatment for malignancy may be indicated.
- Monitor PSA blood levels.

Complications

- Hemorrhage
- Infection

PEARL OF WISDOM

If the ureters are difficult to identify when the bladder is opened, intravenous indigo carmine may facilitate locating the orifices.

RETROPUBIC PROSTATECTOMY

Retropubic prostatectomy is accomplished in much the same manner as suprapubic prostatectomy. The advantage of the retropubic approach is that it provides better visualization of the prostatic fossa, allowing for better hemostatic control. The dissection is carried further retropubically, and instead of a cystotomy, a prostatic capsulotomy is performed between two stay sutures. Prior to the capsulotomy, the tissues overlying the prostate are moved laterally using blunt dissection techniques and the veins within the lateral pelvic fascia are secured with heavy sutures. The diseased prostate is separated from the capsule by sharp scissors dissection or bluntly with the surgeon's fingers. A tenaculum is applied to the prostate to aid in extraction and any remaining fibers are cut. The ureters are identified, hemostasis is achieved, a transurethral Foley catheter with a 30-cc balloon is inserted, and the capsulotomy is closed. A suprapubic catheter may be placed, along with a wound drain, and wound closure is carried out. Postoperative care and concerns are similar to those encountered with suprapubic prostatectomy.

PERINEAL PROSTATECTOMY

Perineal prostatectomy is rarely used. Although the incision provides excellent exposure to the prostatic fossa, there is a serious risk of injury to the rectum and a high incidence of impotence. The position and general anesthesia requirement also carry significant risk to the elderly patient. Exaggerated lithotomy position, which is enhanced with extreme Trendelenburg's position, is required to carry out the procedure.

CASE STUDY

Raymond is 35 years old. He lives in an area that has water with high mineral and salts content. He has been admitted to the emergency room with a diagnosis of kidney stones. This is his third admission for this condition.

1. What are kidney stones?
2. What are the treatment options for Raymond?
3. If he has surgery, what procedure will most likely be performed?

QUESTIONS FOR FURTHER STUDY

1. What is end-stage renal disease? Is it serious?
2. Which kidney is preferred for live donor transplantation, and why?
3. What types of incisions are most common to genitourinary surgery in the male?
4. When a simple nephrectomy is being performed, which is clamped first, the renal artery or vein and why?
5. What other purpose does the indwelling Foley catheter with balloon serve besides urinary drainage when a patient has undergone a TURP?
6. When a TURP is being performed, why should the surgical technologist report a sudden jerking of the patient's leg to the surgeon and anesthesia provider?

BIBLIOGRAPHY

Baker, L. A., & Gomez, R. A. (1998). Embryonic development of the ureter. *Semin. Nephrol. 18*(6), 569–584.

Burke, S. R. (1992). *Human anatomy and physiology in health and disease* (3rd ed.). Clifton Park, NY: Delmar Learning.

Carlson, B. M. (1999). *Human embryology and development biology* (2nd ed.). St. Louis, MO: Mosby.

Caruthers, B. L. (1999). Kidney development and function in the fetus. *The Surgical Technologist 31* (1), 16–19.

Clinical guideline—Varicocele management: Explanatory notes (2002, October 2). [Online]. Available from *http://freespace.virgin.net.cd.1/ech/Clinical%20Guidelines/varico.htm*

Culp, D. A., Fallon, B., & Loening, S. A. H. (1985). *Surgical urology* (5th ed.). Chicago: Year Book Medical Publishers.

Endocrine Web Inc. (1998). [Online]. Available from *http://www.endocrineseb.com*

Estes, M. E. Z. (1998). *Health assessment and physical examination.* Clifton Park, NY: Delmar Learning.

Fowler, J. E. (1990). *Manual of urologic surgery* (1st ed.). Boston: Little, Brown.

Gandy, A. (1995). *Pediatric database (PEDBASE).* [Online] Ontario: University of Western Ontario. Available from *http://www.icondata.com/health/pedbase*

Gilbert, B. R. (2003, February 21). *Microsurgical varicocele ligation—patient information* [Online]. Available from *http://www.ppol.com/services_varicocele.html*

Guyton, A. C. (1991). *Textbook of medical physiology* (8th ed.). Philadelphia: W. B. Saunders.

HealthAnswers.com, Inc. (1999). *Medical reference library* [Online]. Available from *http://www.healthanswers.com*

HealthGate Data Corporation. (1999). [Online]. Available from *http://www.healthgate.com*

McGuiness, A. M., et al. (2002). *Core curriculum for surgical technology* (5th ed.). Centennial, CO: Association of Surgical Technologists.

National Institutes of Diabetes and Digestive and Kidney Disease (NIDDK). (1998). [Online]. Available from *http://www.niddk.nih.gov/healthikidney.htm*

Quaintance, V. (1996). The principal methods of circumcision [Online]. Available from *http://www.users.dircon.co.uk/-vemon/ICIRC/circ methods.html*

Solomon, E. P., Schmidt, R. R., & Adragna, P. J. (1990). *Human anatomy and physiology* (2nd ed.). Ft. Worth, TX: Saunders College Publishing.

Stuart, R. O., & Nigam, S. K. (1995). Development of the tubular nephron. *Semin. Nephrol. 15* (4), 315–326.

Urology Page. (1995). *UROlog* [Online]. Available from *http://www.urolog.nl/uropage/engind_b.htm*

Wills, R. E., & Woodmansee, J. A. (1999). Radical nephrectomy in the treatment of renal cell carcinoma. *The Surgical Technologist 31* (1), 10–15.

Woodburne, R. T., & Burkel, W. E. (1988). *Essentials of human anatomy* (8th ed.). New York: Oxford University Press.

CHAPTER 21

Orthopedic Surgery

Kevin B. Frey

CASE STUDY

Marcella works evenings at a trauma center. She was just advised that a patient will be coming to the OR with a severe Colles' fracture. She is to be the STSR on the case.

1. What is a Colles' fracture?
2. What are the options for surgical intervention?
3. What equipment will Marcella need to secure?

OBJECTIVES

After studying this chapter, the reader should be able to:

A 1. Discuss the relevant anatomy and physiology of the musculoskeletal system.

P 2. Describe the pathology of the musculoskeletal system that prompts surgical intervention and the related terminology.

3. Discuss any special preoperative orthopedic diagnostic procedures/tests.

O 4. Discuss any special preoperative preparation related to orthopedic procedures.

5. Identify the names and uses of orthopedic instruments, supplies, and drugs.
6. Identify the names and uses of special equipment related to orthopedic procedures.
7. Discuss the intraoperative preparation of the patient undergoing an orthopedic procedure.
8. Define and give an overview of the orthopedic procedure.
9. Discuss the purpose and expected outcomes of the orthopedic procedure.
10. Discuss the immediate postoperative care and possible complications of the orthopedic procedure.

S 11. Discuss any specific variations related to the preoperative, intraoperative, and postoperative care of the orthopedic patient.

SELECT KEY TERMS

1. abduction
2. AC joint
3. adduction
4. amphiarthrosis
5. cancellous bone
6. cartilage
7. comminuted
8. compound fracture
9. cortical bone
10. diarthrosis
11. epiphysis
12. flexion
13. ligament
14. marrow
15. osteogenesis
16. pedicle
17. proximal
18. shoulder joint
19. splint
20. valgus

BONE AND BONE TISSUE

Bones are living tissue that provide form and structure to the human body and are actively involved in the maintenance of homeostasis. The skeletal system comprises the bones and other structures that make up the joints of the skeleton (refer to Plate 11 in Appendix A). Those other structures include the **cartilage**, tendons, and ligaments that hold the skeletal framework together (Figure 21-1).

The skeleton performs the following functions:

1. It provides a framework to support the body.
2. It serves as points of attachment for muscles, which in turn move the bones.
3. It protects some internal organs from injury; for example, the ribs protect the lungs.
4. It serves as a source of RBCs. Since it contains the red bone **marrow**, bone is one of the hematopoietic tissues of the body.
5. It serves as a storage site and source of calcium. Calcium is a necessary component of the blood clotting sequence and is needed for the normal functioning of the muscles and nerves.

BONE TISSUE

Bone is a specialized connective tissue that takes several basic forms (Figure 21-2). Bone cells are called osteocytes and the surrounding matrix is made up of calcium salts and collagen. The calcium salts give the bone the strength it needs to fulfill its supportive function. Osteocytes act as both bone-forming and bone-destroying cells. The osteocytes have the ability to not only synthesize, but also to resorb the matrix. The specific cells of bone will be discussed in more detail later.

Two types of bone tissue exist (Figure 21-3). Compact, or **cortical bone**, is the hard, dense tissue of bone that surrounds the marrow cavity. Found within compact bone are the haversian systems. A single haversian unit is made up of circular rings of bone matrix with implanted osteocytes that form a canal. Traversing each canal is a single venule and arteriole, which account for the rich vascularity of bone. The haversian units are connected to make up compact bone and are not found in **cancellous bone**. Each osteocyte is found in a space, or lacuna, of the matrix and extends filament-like processes through canaliculi (microscopic channels) called Volkmann's canals to contact adjacent osteocytes' processes and the blood vessels.

Cancellous, or spongy, bone is found at the ends of bone and lining the medullary marrow cavity. Cancellous bone gives the appearance of a sponge due to its porous matrix. The name *cancellous bone* is used to describe the appearance of the bone, but does not explain the structure. The end bone structure is composed of columns of bony substance called trabeculae with large spaces interspersed among the columns, hence giving it the appearance of a sponge. The columns are well suited for adapting to load bearing due to their formation along stress lines. Cancellous bone is composed of osteocytes and matrix.

Surrounding bone is a thin, fibrous layer of tissue called the periosteum. It is composed of two cell layers. The inner cambium layer is the area where new bone cells are formed. The collagen fibers of the periosteum serve as an anchor of attachment merging with those of the tendons and ligaments that are attached to bone. The periosteum is permeated with nerves and blood vessels that nourish the underlying bone, but by itself is not capable of providing enough nourishment to the bone cortex. The

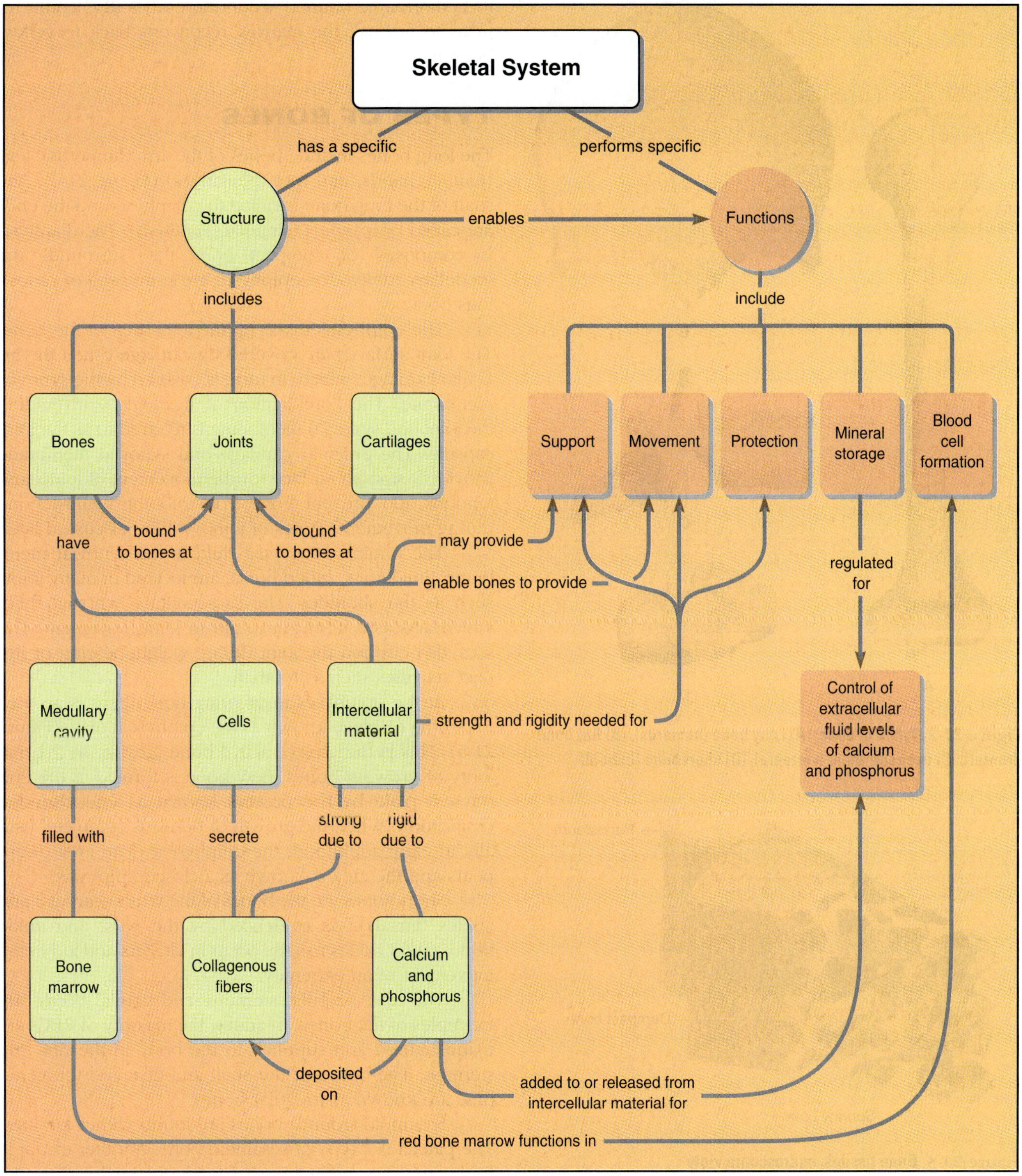

Figure 21-1 **Skeletal system concept map**

periosteum also serves as a layer of defense against infection of bone.

Bone marrow is a semisolid tissue that is found in the spaces of cancellous bone. In infants, adolescents, and young adults, red bone marrow is found in the cancellous bone at the ends of the long bones, sternum, ribs, and vertebrae. The red bone marrow is essential for the production of red blood cells (RBCs), platelets, and white blood cells (WBCs). In long bones, a medullary cavity extends through the shaft of the bone. A fibrous layer of

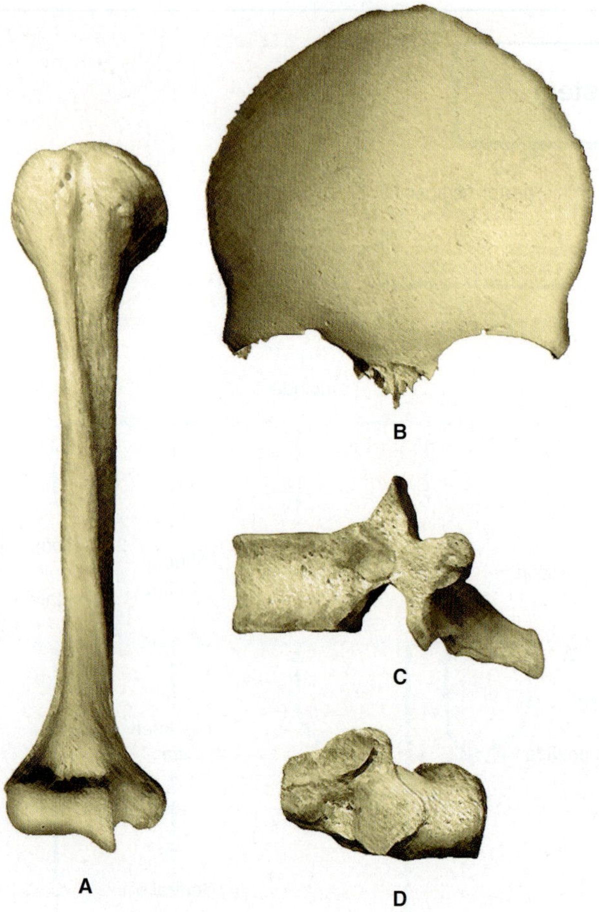

Figure 21-2 Types of bone: (A) Long bone (humerus), (B) flat bone (frontal), (C) irregular bone (vertebra), (D) short bone (cuboid)

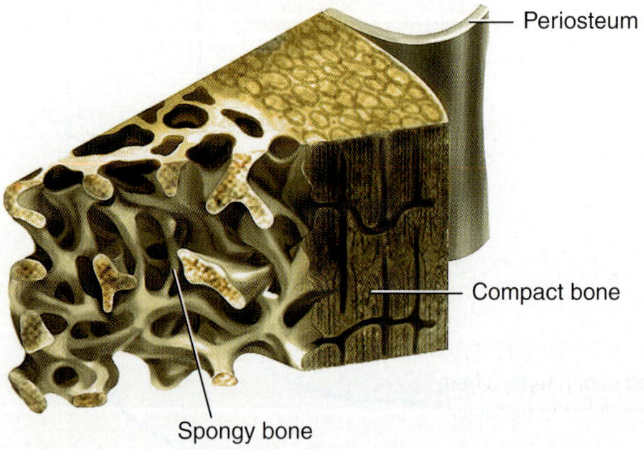

Figure 21-3 Bone tissues, microscopic view

tissue, similar to periosteum, lines the cavity and is called endosteum. In adults, the red bone marrow in the cavity is slowly replaced by yellow bone marrow that does not produce RBCs. The blood supply in yellow bone marrow is extensive and supplies the cortex of the bone. Interestingly, the yellow bone marrow in adults will convert back to RBC-producing red bone marrow in reaction to hemorrhagic trauma. When the body's RBC count returns to normal, the marrow reconverts back to yellow bone marrow.

TYPES OF BONES

The long bones include bones of the arm (humerus), legs (femur), hands, and feet (phalanges) (Figure 21-4). The shaft of the long bone is called the diaphysis and the ends are called **epiphyses** (singular, *epiphysis*). The diaphysis is composed of compact bone that surrounds the medullary cavity. The epiphyses are composed of cancellous bone.

The epiphyses make up the joint area of the bone. The joint surfaces are covered by cartilage called the articular cartilage, which, in turn, is covered by the synovial membrane. The combination of ligaments surrounding the joint and synovial membrane is referred to as the joint capsule. The articular cartilage and synovial membrane provide a smooth surface for the movement of joints and tendons and prevent bone from rubbing against bone during movement. Types of joints will be discussed later.

The origin of synovial fluid is the synovial membrane. Small sacs, called bursa, are located in many joints such as the shoulder. The sacs contain synovial fluid, which acts as a lubricant to aid in joint movement. The sacs also cushion the joint during weight-bearing or impact activities such as football.

At the epiphyses in growing bone there is an area under the cartilage known as the epiphyseal plate (Figure 21-5). This is the area of active bone growth. In the majority of growing bones, new bone is formed at the epiphyseal plate by the process known as endochondral ossification. When the growth of bones is complete, usually in early adulthood, the epiphyseal plate area disappears and the area is known as a closed epiphysis.

Short bones are the bones of the wrists (carpals) and ankles (tarsals). As evidenced by the wrist and ankle bones, short bones usually occur in clusters and aid in the movement of an extremity.

The ribs, scapula, sternum, and cranial bones are examples of flat bones. In adults, the majority of RBCs are manufactured and supplied to the body in the ribs and sternum. The bones of the skull and face and the vertebrae are known as irregular bones.

Sesamoid (round) bones are found within tendons. The patella is a type of sesamoid bone. Another example is the two sesamoid bones found on the head of the metatarsal in the foot forming what is referred to as the "ball" of the foot.

TYPES OF JOINTS

The area where two bones meet to form a joint is called the articulation; or, the bones articulate to form a joint. Joints are classified according to the movement that is

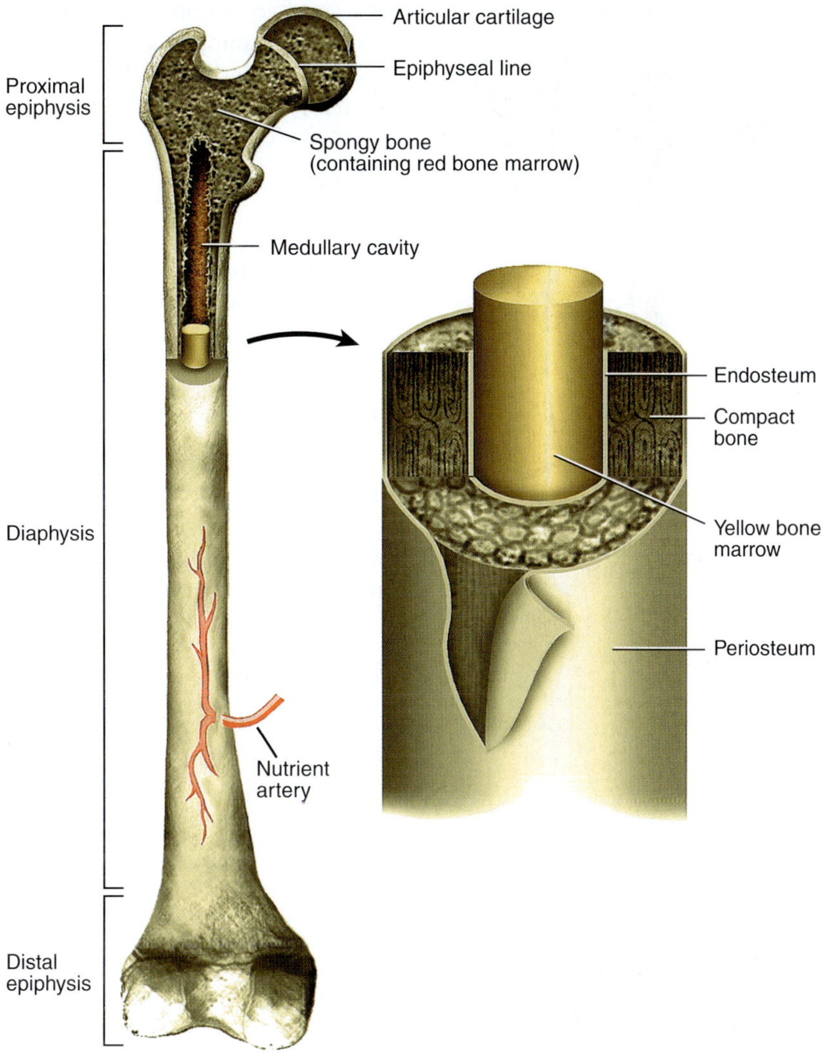

Figure 21-4 **Structure of long bones**

possible. The three general groups are called immovable, slightly movable, and freely movable joints.

IMMOVABLE JOINTS

A synarthrosis is an immovable joint. In synarthroses, the bones are in close contact with each other and separated by a thin layer of cartilage. An example is the suture lines of the cranial bones.

SLIGHTLY MOVABLE JOINTS

An **amphiarthrosis** is a joint that is slightly movable. Lying between the bones of the joint is a disk of fibrous cartilage that connects the bones. Examples of this type of joint include cartilage that connects the vertebrae and the disk of cartilage called the symphysis pubis that connects the pubic bones. This type of joint allows some movement due to the limited flexibility of the cartilage.

FREELY MOVABLE JOINTS

A **diarthrosis** joint is a freely movable joint (Figure 21-6). All diarthroses are also referred to as synovial joints because these joints all contain a synovial membrane that secretes synovial fluid. Diarthroses are further classified according to the movements they allow (Figure 21-7).

Ball-and-Socket Joints

This type of joint allows for the widest range of motion. It consists of a bone with a ball-shaped head that articulates with the cup-shaped socket in another bone. Movement in all planes is possible, including rotational. Examples include the shoulder and hip joints.

Condyloid Joints

The condyloid joint allows for movement in only one plane with some lateral movement. The joint is composed

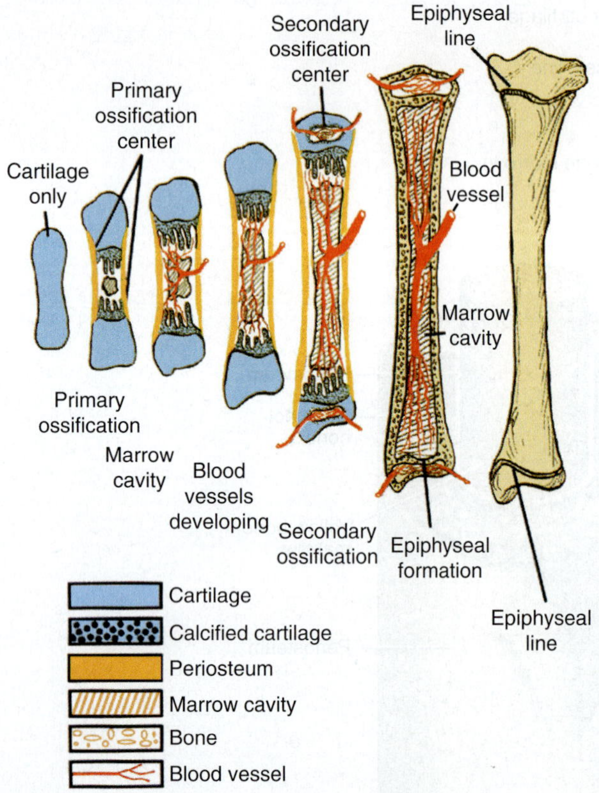

Figure 21-5 Long bone development

of a condyle of one bone fitting into the fossa of another bone. An example is the temporomandibular joint in which the condyle of the mandible fits into the fossa of the temporal bone.

Gliding Joints

Gliding joints allow side-to-side and twisting movements. The articulating surfaces of the bones in the gliding joint are either flat or slightly curved. An example of a gliding joint is the carpals of the wrist joint.

Hinge Joints

The elbow is a hinge joint. This type of joint allows movement in only one plane, much like the motion permitted by the hinge on a door. The hinge joint is formed by the convex surface of one bone fitting into the concave surface of the adjacent bone.

Pivot Joints

Pivot joints allow only a rotational movement around a central axis. The joint formed at the **proximal** end of the radius is a type of pivot joint.

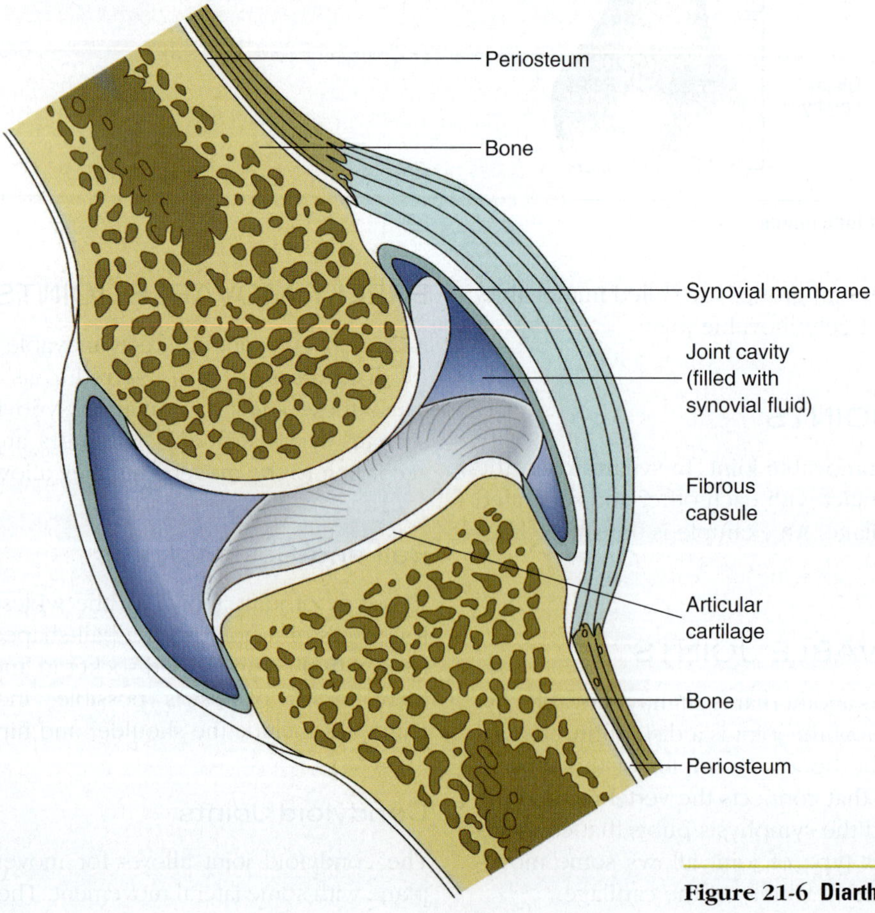

Figure 21-6 Diarthrosis (synovial) joint

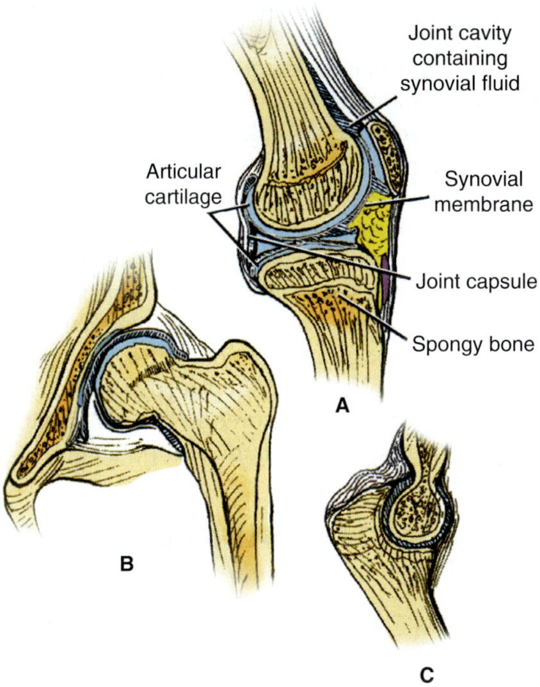

Figure 21-7 Joint types: (A) Hinge (knee), (B) ball and socket (hip), (C) hinge (elbow)

Saddle Joints

Saddle joints allow movement in a variety of planes. The articulating surfaces of the bones both have concave and convex regions. The surface of one bone fits into the equivalent surface of the other bone. An example is the joint formed by the trapezium of the wrist with the metacarpal of the thumb.

TERMS RELATED TO JOINT MOVEMENTS

The muscles attached to bone produce movements of diarthroses. Most often, one end of a muscle is attached to the immovable end of one bone of the joint; this is called the origin of the muscle. The other end of the muscle is attached to the movable end of the other bone; this is called the insertion of the muscle. When the muscle contracts, the muscle fibers pull the insertion toward the origin, causing the joint to move. The terms used to describe the various movements of joints are listed in Table 21-1.

BONE GROWTH AND BONE CELLS

During embryonic development, the skeleton begins to form within the first few weeks of life (Figure 21-8). At first the skeleton is made of cartilage and fibrous connective tissue that is gradually replaced by bone. The bones form by replacing the connective tissue in one of two

Table 21-1 Joint Movement Terminology

Term	Definition
Abduction	Moving a body part away from the midline of the body
Adduction	Moving a body part toward the midline of the body
Circumduction	Moving a particular body part in a circular path without moving the entire body part (e.g., moving a finger in a circular motion without moving the hand)
Rotation	Moving a body part around a central axis
Dorsiflexion	Bending the foot upward at the ankle joint
Plantar flexion	Bending the foot downward at the ankle joint
Eversion	Turning the foot outward or inside out at the ankle joint so the sole of the foot is shown outward
Inversion	Turning the foot outward at the ankle joint so the sole of the foot is pointing inward
Flexion	Bending a joint
Extension	Straightening a joint
Pronation	Pointing a body part downward (e.g., facing the palm of the hand downward)
Supination	Pointing a body part upward

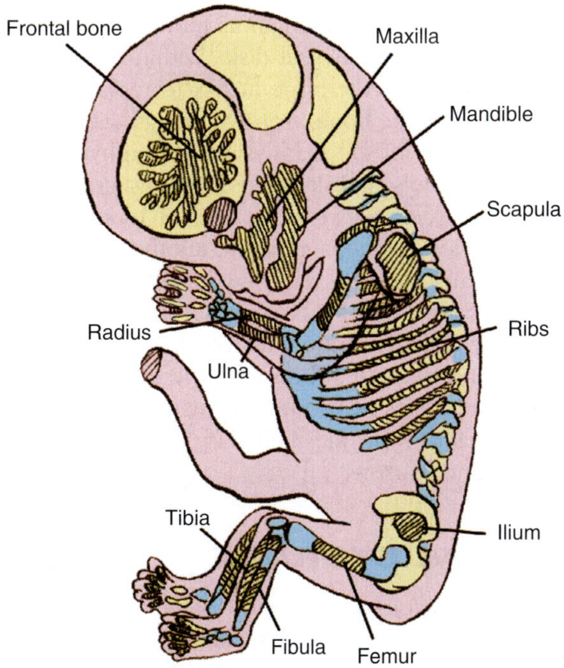

Figure 21-8 Embryonic skeleton

ways, creating some bones that are called intramembranous bones and others that are called endochondral bones.

INTRAMEMBRANOUS BONES

The cranial and facial bones first appear as fibrous connective tissue. Then some of the connective tissue cells called fibroblasts differentiate into osteoblasts, the bone-forming cells. The osteoblasts are active in producing the bone matrix, in a process called ossification. Bone growth continues in all directions with the deposit of calcium salts forming cancellous bone. Viable cells outside of the developing bone produce the periosteum. At the same time, the osteoblasts on the inner side of the periosteum form a layer of compact bone over the new cancellous bone. Eventually, the osteoblasts, when surrounded by the bone matrix, develop into osteocytes.

At birth, this process is not complete. The areas between the cranial bones are still composed of fibrous connective tissue called fontanels. These become ossified to form the suture lines by the age of 2 years.

ENDOCHONDRAL BONE

The rest of the bones of the embryonic skeleton are endochondral bone made of cartilage. Osteoblasts generate the bone matrix in the center of the diaphyses of the long bones, called the primary ossification center, and bone tissue develops from the center toward the ends of the bone. Later the band of cartilage called the epiphyseal disk is formed between the junction of the diaphysis with each epiphysis.

The bone grows in length as more cartilage is produced within the epiphyseal disk. Within the diaphysis, osteoblasts produce the bone matrix to replace the new cartilage causing the bone to grow in length. Once the ossification centers of the diaphysis and epiphysis join together, the epiphyseal disks are ossified and growth stops. This usually occurs between the ages of 16 and 25.

As the long bone is growing, another type of bone cell, called an osteoclast, is at work. Osteoclasts are the cells responsible for the breakdown and resorption of bone. They play an important role in the constant remodeling and shaping of bone. During embryonic development, osteoclasts reabsorb bone matrix in the center of the diaphysis to form the medullary canal that later fills with red bone marrow.

MINERAL STORAGE

Bone contains large quantities of calcium. Calcium is essential for many of the body's metabolic processes and calcium is constantly being removed from the bones to maintain normal blood calcium levels. This accounts for bone being an active tissue. When the body detects a low serum level of calcium, osteoclasts are stimulated by parathyroid hormone to break down bone tissue and increase the reabsorption of calcium from the bones into the blood, thereby increasing the circulating calcium level. Once the level is stabilized, the hormone calcitonin secreted by the thyroid gland acts on the osteoclasts to inhibit their activity and decrease the reabsorption of calcium from the bones. Osteoblasts are then activated to form new bone tissue. Due to the counteraction of osteoblasts and osteoclasts, the bone matrix is kept strong because the calcium in bone is replaced at a rate equal to its removal. Other minerals stored in bone tissue include phosphorus, magnesium, sodium, and potassium.

FACTORS THAT AFFECT BONE GROWTH

Besides the effect hormones have on bone, three other important factors affect the growth and maintenance of bone. They are heredity, nutrition, and exercise.

Heredity is not a well-understood mechanism in relation to bone growth. Individuals possess a potential for height that is most likely due to the genes inherited from both parents.

Nutrition is a key factor also, because the nutrients derived from food are the raw materials from which bone is produced. Without these nutrients, the bones cannot grow normally or be continually remodeled. Vitamin D is needed for the absorption of calcium and phosphorus to take place in the small intestine. Calcium, phosphorus, and protein are needed in the diet since these become a part of the bone matrix.

Weight-bearing exercise is also important. Bones are meant to bear normal weight and stress. Without this stress, bones lose calcium at a more rapid rate than it is replaced. Exercise such as walking is considered sufficient to maintain the density of bone.

CLINICAL AND BONE LANDMARK TERMS

Orthopedics is an area that uses specific language to identify anatomical landmarks, features, and relationships. Some of these terms are essential for a basic understanding of the specialty (Table 21-2).

PATHOLOGY

The musculoskeletal system is prone to numerous types of pathological conditions. A select number of these conditions is listed in Table 21-3.

(Text continues on page 805)

Table 21-2 Key Clinical and Landmark Orthopedic Terms

CLINICAL TERMS

Ankylosis	Abnormal stiffness or fixation of a joint usually resulting from the destruction of articular cartilage as occurs in rheumatoid arthritis.
Arthralgia	Pain in a joint.
Arthrocentesis	Puncture of a joint with a needle to withdraw synovial fluid for diagnostic purposes or to remove excess fluid due to trauma or infection.
Arthrodesis	Surgical fusion of a joint.
Arthroplasty	Surgical reconstruction and/or replacement of a joint to restore movement.
Arthroscopy	Surgical procedure in which the interior of a joint is visualized through the use of an endoscope inserted through a small incision.
Colles' fracture	Fracture of the epiphysis of the radius approximately 1 in. from the wrist joint causing the hand to be displaced in a dorsal and lateral position.
Laminectomy	Surgical removal of the posterior arch of the vertebra called the lamina to reduce pressure on a nerve root.
Osteochondritis	Inflammation of bone and cartilage.
Osteogenesis	Formation of bone.
Osteogenesis imperfecta	Genetic and congenital condition that involves the defective development of connective tissue resulting in deformed and abnormally brittle bones that are easily fractured.
Osteoma	Tumor of the bone.
Osteomalacia	Abnormal condition characterized by softening of the bone due to a loss of calcification of the bone matrix. The condition is a result of an inadequate amount of phosphorus and calcium in the blood for the mineralization of bone, caused by a deficiency of vitamin D.
Osteomyelitis	Inflammation and infection of bone and bone marrow usually caused by bacteria. Staphylococci are the most common causative bacteria.
Osteonecrosis	Destruction and death of bone tissue. Occurs frequently in the head of the femur due to a disease process or trauma that obstructs or destroys the blood supply to the femoral head.
Osteoporosis	Disorder characterized by the excessive loss of calcium from bone without replacement, causing a loss in bone density.
Osteotomy	Cutting or sawing of the bone.
Synovectomy	Surgical removal of the synovial membrane of a joint.

ANATOMICAL LANDMARKS AND TERMS FOR BONE

Appendicular skeleton	The 126 bones composing the upper and lower extremities of the body.
Axial skeleton	The 80 bones composing the cranium, vertebral column, sternum, and ribs.
Condyle	Rounded projection/process at the epiphysis of a bone that articulates with another bone and serves as the point of attachment for ligaments.
Crest	Narrow elongated ridge/elevation of bone, such as the iliac crest.
Distal	Away from the origin of the extremity.
Epicondyle	Projection on the surface of a bone located above a condyle.
Foramen	Opening in the bone for the passage of structures such as blood vessels, nerves, or ligaments. An example is the foramen magnum, a passage in the occipital bone through which the spinal cord passes into the spinal column.
Fossa	Hollow or depression on the surface end of a bone, such as the olecranon fossa.
Fovea	Another name for a depression on the bone but smaller than a fossa. An example is the fovea on the head of the femur, which serves as the point of attachment for the ligamentum teres.
Head	The enlarged, rounded, proximal portion of a bone, usually a long bone.
Process	Natural growth that projects from a bone. Condyles are an example of a process.
Proximal	Near the origin of the limb.
Trochanter	Large process on a bone. Examples are the lesser and greater trochanters of the femur that serve as points of attachment for various muscles.
Tubercle	Small knob-like nodule or eminence on a bone.
Tuberosity	Nodule or eminence on a bone that is larger than a tubercle.

Table 21-3 Orthopedic Conditions

CONDITION	DESCRIPTION
Arthropathies	
Arthritis	Inflammation of a joint.
	Note: The term *arthritis* is applied to rheumatoid as well as to osteoarthritis; however, it is only the rheumatoid type that shows all the signs of inflammation.
Rheumatoid arthritis (RA)	Rheumatoid arthritis involves connective tissue throughout the entire body, but mainly involves the synovium in the joint.
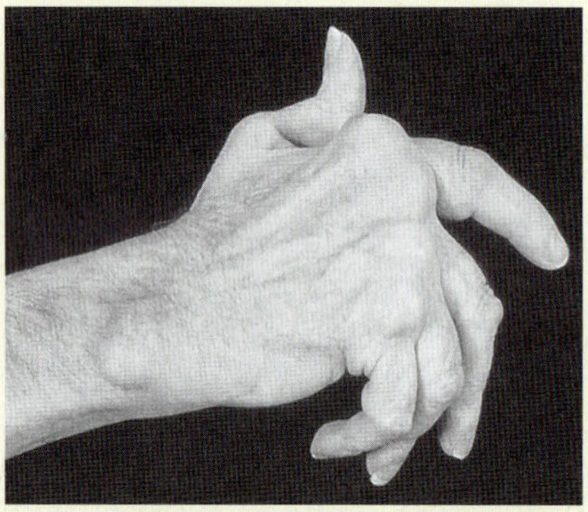	Rheumatoid arthritis is considered an autoimmune disease (abnormal response against one's own body). In the disease process, the body does not recognize its own natural antibodies as "self." Because the body thinks its own natural antibodies are foreign, it produces antibodies called rheumatoid factors (RF) that fight against its own natural antibodies. The disease starts with a simple synovitis and can progress through several stages, the last being joint immobility. Because of the role of RF antibodies, an RF test confirms RA.
	The inflammation is initiated by RF antibodies producing an inflammatory exudate called *pannus*. Movement is difficult and painful because the thick pannus adheres to the joint surfaces, producing *ankylosis*.
(Photo courtesy of SIU/Visuals Unlimited)	Diagnostic tests may include analysis of synovial fluid, antinuclear antibody, latex fixation tests, and rheumatoid factors. (For a detailed description of these and other tests, see Table 21-6.)
Osteoarthritis (OA)	Osteoarthritis is a degenerative disease of the joint and is a normal part of aging. Although the exact cause is unknown, the articular cartilage wears away, often because of overuse, exposing underlying bone. Pain is caused by the friction between the two bones as they glide across each other without the protection of the articular cartilage.
	The most effective treatment for both RA and OA is acetylsalicylic acids, such as aspirin, and nonsteroidal anti-inflammatory drugs (NSAIDs).
	Diagnosis is made by skeletal X-ray of arthritic joint.
Dislocations	A dislocation is the displacement of a bone from its socket, usually caused by trauma. The types of dislocations include compound or open, which is the complete displacement of the bone from its socket along with a break in the skin so that the joint communicates with the air; complete, which is the complete displacement of the bone from its socket with no break in the skin; and incomplete, subluxation, or partial, which is the slight displacement of the bone from its socket and does not involve communication with the air.
Internal derangement of the knee joint	Disruption in the arrangement of the structure, which therefore affects the function of the knee.
Bucket handle tear	A bucket handle tear includes abnormalities of the internal structures of the knee joint, such as C-shaped meniscus tears on the medial or lateral edge with the opposite side still attached. The torn edge resembles a bucket handle.
Joint mice	Joint mice, so called because of loose particles within the joint, are caused by repeated trauma to the knee. Joint mice often create a constant irritation within the joint cavity, which produces an excess of synovial fluid. When a particle becomes lodged between articulating surfaces, pain or a locking of the joint may occur.

Table 21-3 *(continued)*

CONDITION	DESCRIPTION
Tendons, Tendon Sheaths, and Bursa	
Bunion	A bony protuberance on the medial aspect of the first metatarsal. The condition is associated with hallux valgus deformity. A bony prominence projecting from a bone is called an exostosis. 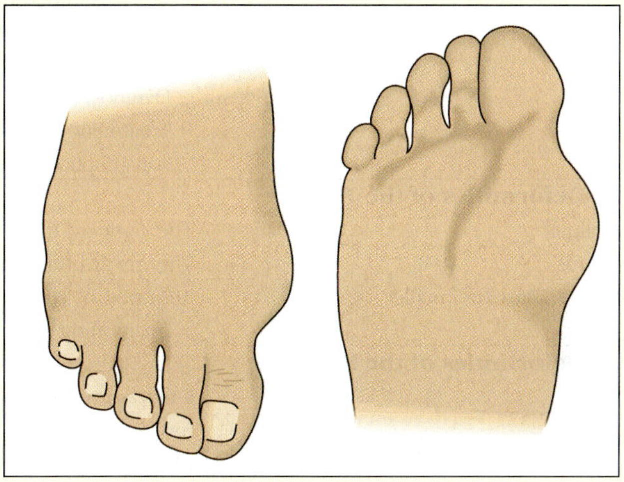
Ganglion of tendon sheath	A cystic growth commonly occurring on the dorsum of the wrist. 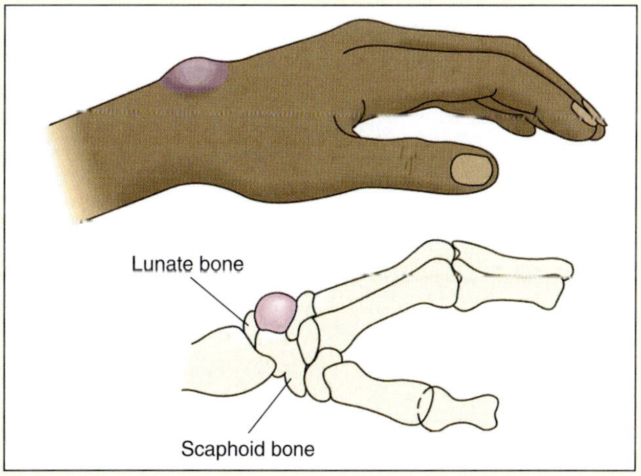
Osteopathies and Chondropathies	
Osteomalacia	A softening of bone caused by abnormal calcium deposits. *Note:* It can be caused by a lack of vitamin D or by malabsorption of calcium and is called rickets in children.
Osteomyelitis	Inflammation of the bone and sometimes of the bone marrow *Note:* Osteomyelitis is caused by the presence of pyogenic bacteria, usually *Staphylococcus*. The infection can spread to the bone through the blood from a previously injured site, or the microorganism can infiltrate the bone directly following open fractures, surgical reductions, or other exposures to the air.
Osteoporosis	Condition of decreased bone density due to a loss of bony substance and diminished osteogenesis—the bone becomes porous and fragile, and fractures are common.

(continues)

Table 21-3 *(continued)*

CONDITION	DESCRIPTION
Osteopathies and Chondropathies *(continued)*	
Primary osteoporosis	Primary osteoporosis is idiopathic; however, contributing factors include reduction in calcium intake and hormonal imbalance. It is most commonly seen in postmenopausal women.
Secondary osteoporosis	Secondary osteoporosis is caused by extended drug use, particularly steroids, or by extended periods of inactivity. In general, osteoporosis is usually seen in elderly women who first come to a health care facility complaining of back pain, because the vertebral column is most commonly affected. Diagnosis is mainly through X-rays of the thoracic and lumbar vertebrae. Treatment is preventive by increasing bone mass through proper dietary consumption of calcium and vitamin D and through exercise.
Acquired Deformities of the Toe	
Hallux valgus	The outward turning of the great toe away from the midline.
Hallux varus	The inward turning of the great toe toward the midline.
Hammer toe, claw toe, mallet toe	Acquired or congenital deformities of the toes as a result of abnormal positioning of the interphalangeal joints.
Acquired Deformities of the Hip	
Coxa valga	Outward turning of the hip joint.
Coxa vara	Inward turning of the hip joint.
Genu valgum	Knock-kneed; the knees are in close position and the space between the ankles is increased. 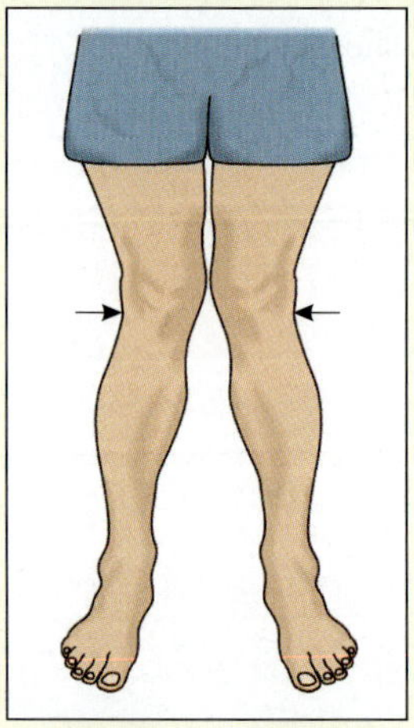
Genu varum	Bowlegged; the space between the knees is abnormally increased and the lower leg bows inwardly. 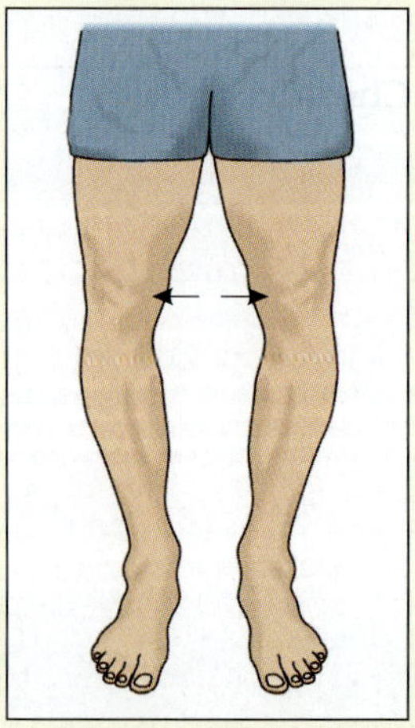

Table 21-3 ***(continued)***

CONDITION	DESCRIPTION
Congenital Anomalies	
Talipes valgus	Outward turning of the foot away from the midline. 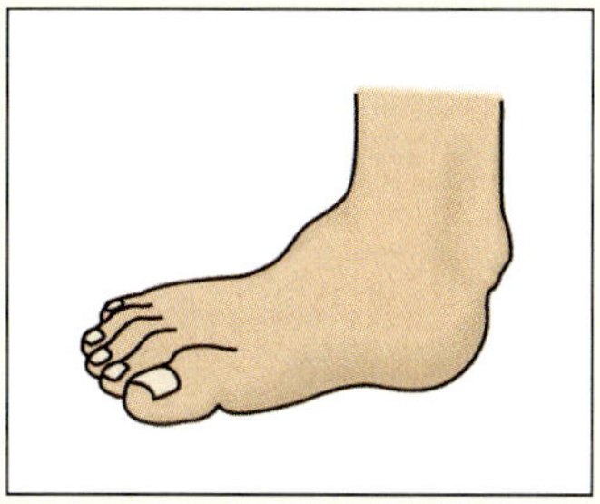
Talipes varus	Inward turning of the foot toward the midline. 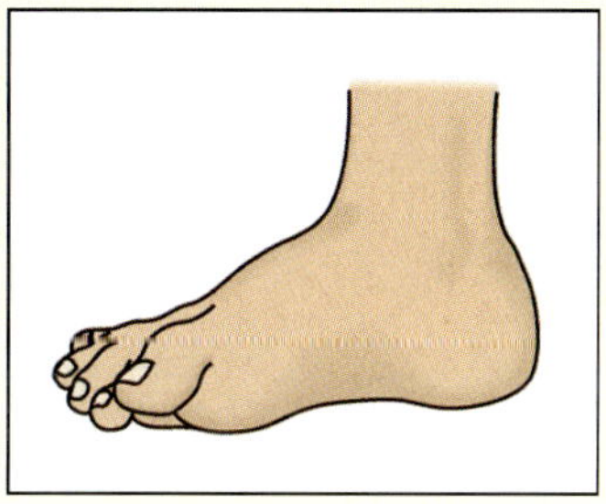
Note: All varieties of talipes can be acquired.	
Injuries	
Fractures	Discontinuity of the normal alignment of bone. *Note:* Most fractures are caused by accidents, although some are pathological (fractures caused by diseased bones).
Classification of fractures	Fractures can be grouped according to the following list: • *Whether or not the bone pierces the skin* If the bone pierces the skin, it is called a compound or open fracture. If the fracture does not pierce the skin, it is called a simple or closed fracture. • *Type of fracture line through the bone* If the fracture line is continuous through the bone, it is called complete. If the fracture line is not continuous through the bone, it is called incomplete or partial. A type of partial fracture is a greenstick fracture, which like a green stick or twig from a tree will bend on one side and break on the other. • *Direction of the fracture line* In a linear fracture, the line of the fracture runs parallel to the axis of the bone. A spiral fracture is where the fracture line curves around the bone. A transverse fracture is where the fracture line is across the bone. In an intra-articular fracture, the fracture line is on the joint surfaces of bone. • *Miscellaneous fractures* Pott's fracture, a break of the lower fibula, is an outdated term. Colles' fracture is a break of the distal radius.

(continues)

Table 21-3 *(continued)*

CONDITION	DESCRIPTION
Injuries *(continued)*	
Classification of fractures *(continued)*	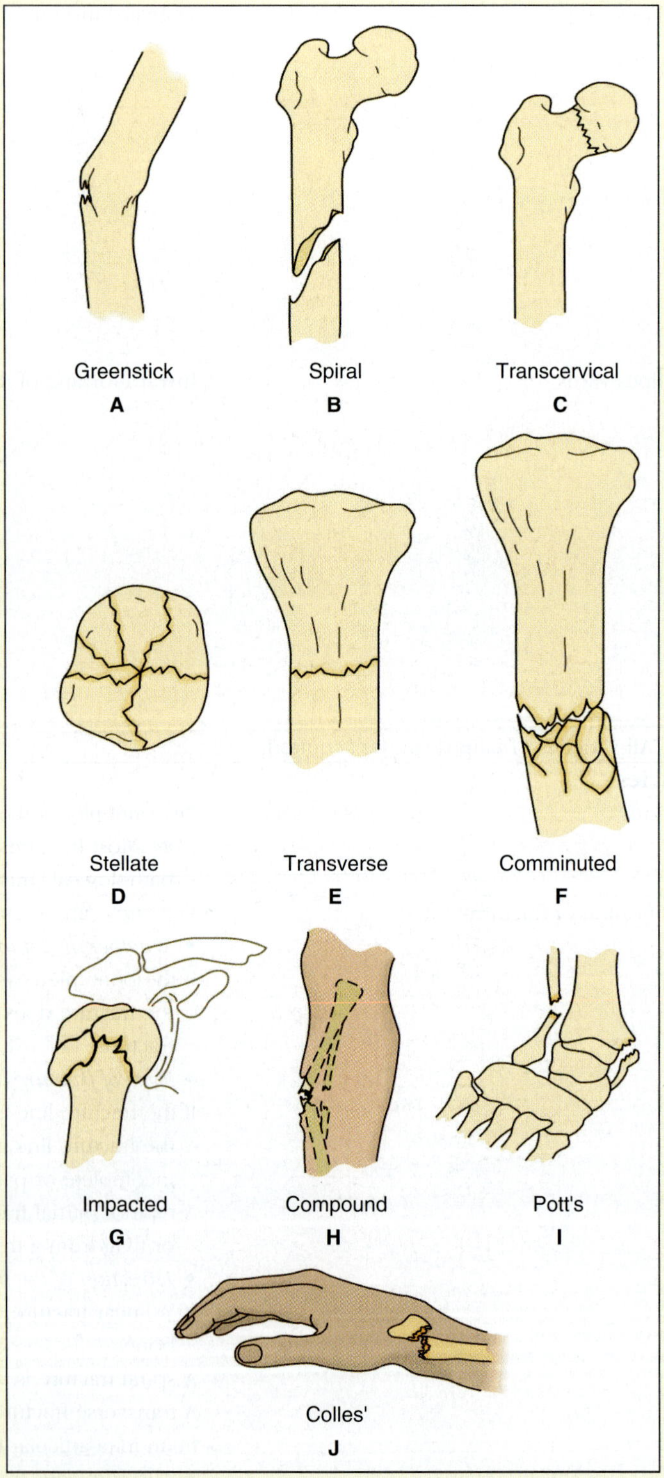
Sprains	Injury to the joint characterized by the rupture of some or all fibers of the supporting ligament.

Table 21-3 *(continued)*

CONDITION	DESCRIPTION
Malignant Neoplasms	
Ewing's tumor	Malignant tumor of bone affecting mostly boys between 5 and 15 years of age; the cure rate is currently greater than 60% with proper treatment such as chemotherapy, radiation therapy, and surgery.
Multiple myeloma; plasma cell myeloma	Malignant neoplasm of the marrow plasma cells resulting in bone destruction and overproduction of immunoglobulins and Bence Jones protein (see Table 21-6).
	Note: Treatment is chemotherapy.
Osteogenic sarcoma; osteosarcoma	Malignant tumor of the long bones, particularly the femur, commonly metastasizing to the lungs.
	Note: Treatment is chemotherapy and surgery.
Benign Neoplasms	
Chondroma	Benign tumor of cartilage.
Giant cell tumor	Tumor of the epiphysis of long bones, particularly the distal femur at the knee; commonly seen in the 20–40 age group.
	Note: Treatment is removal of the tumor followed by bone grafting.
Osteoma	Benign tumor of bone.

Source: From *Modern Medical Language* by C. E. Collins, 1996, St. Paul, MN: West Publishing Co. Reprinted with permission.

TYPES OF FRACTURES

Fractures are classified according to the type of fracture and extent of damage (Table 21-4). Fractures are either complete, in which the fracture completely interrupts the continuity of bone, or incomplete, in which the fracture is partial and some of the bone is still intact.

A term discussed in conjunction with fractures, but which is not a fracture in itself, is subluxation. A subluxation is an incomplete dislocation—the abnormal, incomplete separation of two articulating bones. A complete separation of a joint is called luxation.

NORMAL BONE HEALING

When a bone fracture occurs, complete bone healing is expected in 8–12 weeks under the right circumstances. For complete union of a fracture, the site of injury should be completely immobilized (internal or external fixation) and in proper alignment, the patient should be in good general health, well nourished, and infection free, and all physiological mechanisms to facilitate the normal process of bone healing should be intact.

The normal process of bone healing (**osteogenesis**) involves the following five stages:

1. Inflammation
2. Cellular proliferation
3. Callus formation
4. Ossification
5. Remodeling

The inflammatory stage begins at the time of injury and lasts approximately 2 days. The fracture hematoma, which is a result of the extravasation of blood caused by the injury, is formed during this time. The blood clot serves as a foundation for the subsequent cellular proliferation stage.

The cellular proliferation stage begins approximately on the second day following the traumatic event. Macrophages debride the area and allow for the formation of a fibrin mesh that seals the approximated edges of the fracture site. The fibrin mesh serves as the foundation for capillary and fibroblastic ingrowth. A soft tissue or periosteal callus is formed on the outer surface or cortex of the fractured bone by the collagen-producing fibroblasts and osteoblasts.

The callus formation stage lasts 3–4 weeks. The soft tissue growth continues and the bone fragments grow toward one another, bridging the gap. Osteoblasts form a matrix of collagen that invades the periosteal callus bridging the fracture site and uniting the two ends of the bone. Fibrous tissue, cartilage, and immature bone stabilize the fracture site.

The ossification stage begins 2 or 3 weeks following the injury and can last 3 to 4 months. The matrix of osteoblasts, now called the osteoid, calcifies, firmly uniting the bone. The bone is now able to accept mineral deposits.

The remodeling stage is the maintenance state of normal bone. Following a fracture, any devitalized tissue is removed and the new bone is organized to provide maximum support and function. Osteoblastic and osteoclastic activity should be equal, constantly resorbing and

Table 21-4 Types of Fractures and Causes

TYPE	DESCRIPTION	CAUSE
Avulsion	Bone and other tissues are pulled from normal attachments.	Direct force; most often extremity is bent in abnormal manner.
Bucket handle	Dual vertical fractures on the same side of the pelvis.	Direct force or anterior compression of the pelvis.
Butterfly	Associated with comminuted type of fracture; butterfly-shaped piece of fractured bone.	Direct or rotational force.
Comminuted (segmental)	Fracture with more than two pieces of bone fragment; may have notable amount of associated soft tissue trauma.	Direct crushing force.
Compound (open)	Broken end of bone has penetrated skin exposing the bone. Significant damage may be present to surrounding blood vessels, nerves, and muscles.	Moderate to severe energy that is continuous until bone reaches level of tolerance. Usually produced by direct force.
Depressed	Fracture occurs when bone is driven inward, frequently seen with cranial fracture.	Moderate to severe direct force.
Displaced	Fracture in which bone ends are out of alignment.	Direct force to area.
Greenstick	The fracture occurs in only one cortex of the bone. The bone splits longitudinally and is not a complete break; sometimes referred to as an incomplete or stress fracture.	Minor direct energy. Repetitive direct force such as jogging on a hard surface every day or jumping (basketball).
Impacted	The broken ends of each bone are forced into each other, usually creating many bone fragments.	Compressive force.
Intra-articular	Bones inside a joint are fractured.	Direct force to the joint area.
Oblique (type of linear fracture)	Fracture occurs at an oblique angle across both cortices.	Direct force possibly with some compression.
Simple (closed)	Fracture is in normal anatomical position and the skin is not broken.	Moderate energy that continues until bone reaches level of tolerance. Usually direct force.
Spiral	Fracture that curves around bone.	Direct twisting force or distal part of bone unable to move.
Spontaneous (pathological)	Fracture occurs without trauma; usually associated with bone weakened by a tumor or other disease process.	Minor force can cause fracture, such as leaning on the arm for support.
Stellate	Fracture occurs at central point in which additional breaks in bone radiate from the central point.	Direct force of moderate energy.
Transverse	Horizontal fracture through the bone.	Direct force toward the bone.

reforming the bone. The process of remodeling continues throughout the life cycle and is affected by local stress on the individual bone, circulation, nutrition, and hormones. Any disruption of the homeostasis will result in a pathological condition.

PATHOLOGICAL BONE HEALING

A disruption at any stage of bone healing or maintenance can be responsible for a variety of abnormal conditions. Fracture healing is a process that goes through stages to reach the end result. If the process is interrupted, the final result may be devastating for the individual. Interruptions of the normal path of bone healing include poor immobilization of the fracture, distraction of the bone fragments, deficient or nonexistent blood supply to the bone, infection, and interposition of soft tissue.

The majority of fractures must be immobilized to hold the bones in place in order for healing to take place. Movement of the fractured bones can cause disruption of the hematoma, thus prolonging the healing process and causing additional bleeding at the fracture site. Excellent immobilization must be achieved to assure a stable union.

Distraction is a term used to describe bone fragments that are separated so that bone contact does not occur. Distraction can be caused by too much weight applied to skeletal traction. The gap between the bone fragments created by distraction is filled with granulation tissue, which delays the healing. The excessive tension placed by distraction on the blood vessels may decrease the blood supply to the fracture site, which also increases healing time.

Distraction is linked with the complication known as interposition of soft tissues. The gap formed by distraction can allow soft tissue to grow over the ends of one or both fracture fragments. The soft tissue seals off the surface of the fractured bones disallowing the hematoma to form and inhibiting callus formation. The result is a poor union of the fracture.

A vascular necrosis occurs when the capillary network or collateral circulation cannot be reestablished following a traumatic injury or when the vascular system is disrupted by other means. This can be pharmacological (e.g., steroid use), pathological (e.g., diabetes), or idiopathic. Decreased blood supply to the bone may lead to irreversible necrosis.

Compound fractures compromise the integrity of the skin and allow for the possible entry of microorganisms to cause infection of the bone and injury to surrounding soft tissues. Infection can delay healing and lead to serious consequences such as a generalized infection of the bone and bone marrow. Osteomyelitis, a serious infection of bone, starts as a local infection and can lead to chronic osteomyelitis.

Individuals heal at different rates, but the average time required for a fracture to heal does not ordinarily vary much from person to person. *Delayed union* is a term used to describe an increase in the healing time of fractures. The reasons for delayed healing are pathological (e.g., osteoporosis), mechanical (e.g., distraction of the fracture site or inadequate immobilization), or traumatic, referring to the type of injury sustained (e.g., **comminuted** fractures).

Nonunion is when the fractured bone ends do not unite. The presence of infection and movement of the fracture site are what usually cause nonunion. Infection and movement cause continual bleeding at the fracture site and a continual breakdown of the fragile hematoma. The fracture gap may increase to a point where the fracture ends have no chance of healing and a permanent nonunion exists.

Malunion occurs when the fracture heals in a position that does not resemble the original anatomical form of the bone and alters the mechanical function of the bone.

Compartmental syndrome is an increase in pressure within a closed space that usually occurs in the forearm and tibia. The fractured ends of the bone cause excess pressure that leads to neurovascular compromise. Tissue viability may be affected, increasing the risk for infection, and permanent nerve damage can occur. Other causes of compartmental syndrome are from a cast that is placed too tight or intracompartmental bleeding.

The forearm and leg are divided into compartments composed of bones, muscles, and nerves. Fascia and skin create the compartments that surround these structures. When a fracture occurs, pressure within the compartment increases due to the bleeding and swelling of tissues. The fascia can expand only so far to accommodate the swelling. When the fascia reaches its limit, the pressure is directed inward and compresses the blood vessels and nerves. Eventually the capillary circulation to the muscle stops. When the circulation is compromised the muscles become ischemic; necrosis begins in 2–4 hours and becomes irreversible in 12 hours. Nerve damage starts within 30 minutes and after 12 hours, if the swelling is not stopped, there will be irreversible loss of muscle function.

Other soft tissues can be damaged by fractures. Tendons and ligaments are involved in avulsions. When the fracture occurs, the tendon or ligament avulses a small piece of bone to which it was attached. If left untreated, a dysfunction in the movement of the extremity may occur. Avulsions are commonly associated with fractures of the phalanges. Visceral damage may also occur from fractures. Examples of serious damage include a fracture of the pelvis in which the bladder is ruptured and the female internal reproductive organs are damaged, and a rib fracture that punctures a lung causing it to collapse.

CASTS

A cast is one of the more common methods utilized to immobilize a fracture. The complications of distraction and malalignment can be avoided with the application of a cast to the extremity. A common option is a closed reduction of the fracture with the subsequent application of a cast.

Fiberglass is a popular type of casting material. Fiberglass is inexpensive and lightweight compared to other casting materials and is used in a clinic when immobilizing a fracture. Plaster has been used for years as the standard material for applying casts. Usually a plaster cast is applied after a surgical procedure and later replaced with the lighter fiberglass cast to aid the patient in mobility.

The majority of surgery departments have a cast cart that contains all the necessary supplies for application of a cast in the OR. The supplies include a disposable bucket for lukewarm water, Webril and stockinette of various sizes, plaster casting material of various widths and lengths, and heavy-duty scissors. The surgeon will first apply Webril or a stockinette to the extremity to protect the patient's skin from the cast (Figure 21-9). The casting

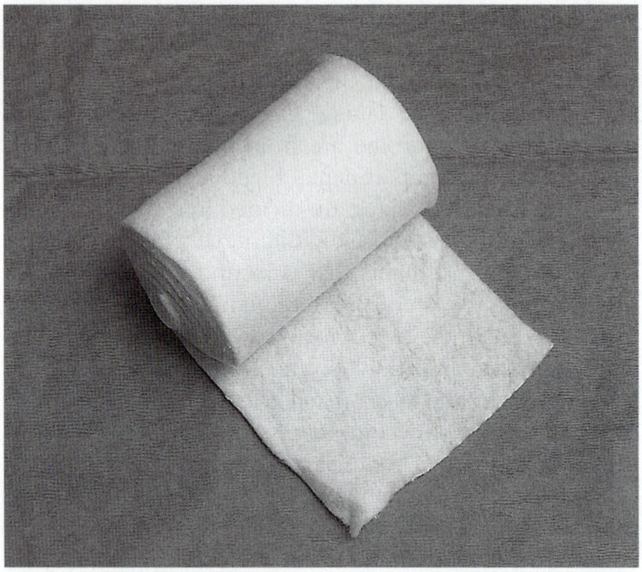

Figure 21-9 Under-casting material—cast padding

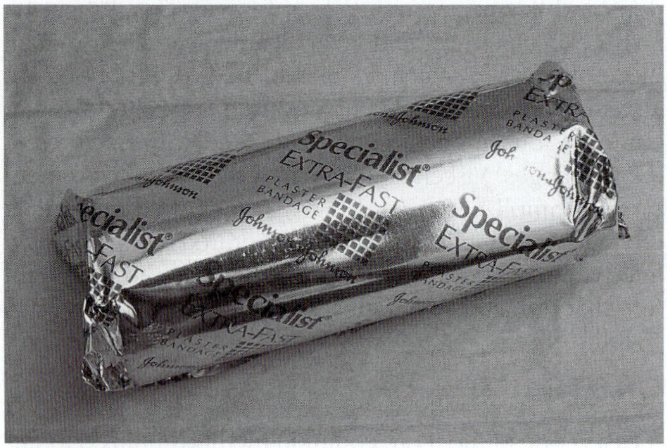

Figure 21-10 Casting material—plaster

material quickly begins to harden once wet, requiring that all the necessary materials for casting be ready.

If a **splint** is being applied, flat sheets of the casting material will be used. The surgeon will indicate how many layers thick the splint should be and the length of the splint. If necessary, the heavy-duty scissors is used to cut the material. The circulator wets the cast material and the surgeon applies it to the extremity and holds it in place until it hardens.

When applying a cast, rolls of casting material are used (Figure 21-10). These rolls are available in a variety of widths; the correct width is chosen according to the extremity or body part that requires casting. The circulator submerges the roll and holds it under the water until the bubbles stop rising to the surface, which indicates that the roll is adequately wet. Numerous types of casts can be made (Table 21-5).

Table 21-5 Types of Casts

TYPE	DESCRIPTION
Short arm cast	Applied from below the elbow to the metacarpal heads; wrist fracture
Long arm cast	Applied from axilla to metacarpal heads; fracture of forearm or elbow
Short leg cast	Applied from tibial tuberosity to metatarsal heads; ankle and foot fractures
Long leg cast	Applied from hip to metatarsal heads; fracture of femur, tibia, fibula, ankle
Cylinder cast	Applied from the groin to the ankle; required when complete knee immobilization is desired
Hip spica cast	Applied to trunk, complete leg of affected side, one-half of unaffected leg
Body jacket cast	Applied to trunk of body to immobilize the spine

DIAGNOSTIC TERMS AND PROCEDURES

Select common orthopedic terminology and procedures used for diagnostic activity are presented in Table 21-6.

THE SKELETON

The skeleton consists of 206 bones (refer to Plates 7 and 11). These bones are divided into what are called the axial and appendicular skeletons. The axial skeleton consists of the skull, vertebral column, ribs, and sternum. The appendicular skeleton consists of the arms, legs, shoulders, and pelvis.

THE SKULL

The human skull is divided into the cranium and facial bones. The entire skull consists of 22 bones; 8 of them make up the cranium and 14 form the facial skeleton. The only movable bone of the skull is the mandible.

CRANIUM

The primary purpose of the cranium is to enclose and protect the brain. The bones of the cranium also provide points of attachment for the muscles that permit chewing and head movement. A few of the cranial bones contain paranasal sinuses, air-filled cavities lined with mucous membrane that are connected by passages to the nasal cavity. The sinuses aid in reducing the weight of the skull.

Table 21-6 Diagnostic Terms and Procedures

TERM	DESCRIPTION
Range of motion (ROM)	Degree to which a joint can be moved in any range, including abduction, flexion, extension, dorsiflexion.
	Note: Range is measured in degrees. For example, limited joint movement may be 55 degrees; full-range movement, 360 degrees.
Lachman and Drawer	Tests ligament stability of the knee.
Sulcus test	Tests ligament stability of the shoulder.
Laboratory Tests	
Analysis of synovial fluid	Synovial fluid is aspirated (withdrawn) and then examined. This test is used to distinguish between osteoarthritis, rheumatoid arthritis, and gout. In rheumatoid arthritis, rheumatoid factors are present in the synovial fluid.
Antinuclear antibody (ANA)	ANAs are antibodies the body produces against its own nuclear material; their presence indicates autoimmune diseases such as systemic lupus erythematosus.
Bence Jones protein	Bence Jones protein is produced by malignant plasma cells and secreted by the bone marrow in multiple myeloma. Initially, this protein is catabolized by the kidneys; however, as the disease progresses, the protein is produced in such large amounts that the kidneys are unable to cope. The excess spills over into the urine where it can be detected by laboratory examination.
Cultures	Cultures are used to isolate and identify microorganisms causing disease. These tests are used in diagnosing infectious diseases such as osteomyelitis and septic arthritis.
Erythrocyte sedimentation rate (ESR)	This test measures the rate at which red blood cells fall or settle to the bottom of a test tube. Red blood cells fall faster during inflammations, elevating the ESR above its normal value. This test, in conjunction with other tests, helps diagnose inflammatory conditions such as ankylosing spondylitis and rheumatoid arthritis.
Human leukocyte antigen B27 (HLA)	HLAs are proteins found on white blood cells. The occurrence of HLA-B27 is seen in ankylosing spondylitis.
Latex fixation tests (agglutination tests)	This test is used to diagnose rheumatoid arthritis because it detects rheumatoid factors.
Rheumatoid factors (RF)	This test measures the quantity of RF in the blood. Rheumatoid factors are proteins present in the blood and synovial fluid of patients with rheumatoid arthritis.
Serum alkaline phosphatase (SAP)	Alkaline phosphatase is important in the building of new bone. However, increased levels indicate bone disease such as multiple myeloma, osteomalacia, osteogenic sarcoma, and rheumatoid disease.
Serum and urinary calcium and phosphorus	Calcium and phosphorus are important constituents of bone. Abnormal values are present in osteoporosis and osteomalacia.
Serum urate	Elevated amounts of serum urate are present in patients with gout.
Urinary uric acid	Elevated amounts of urinary uric acid are found in patients with gout.
Radiology and Diagnostic Imaging	
Arthrography	X-ray of a joint after injection of a contrast medium.
Bone scans	A visual image of bone is displayed following injection of technetium (^{99m}Tc), a radioactive substance. This substance is picked up by bone undergoing abnormal metabolic activity and shows up as dark areas on the image. Bone scans are useful in detecting tumors and are used to distinguish between osteomyelitis and cellulitis.
Computed tomography (CT)	A CT scan is an X-ray of an organ or body detailing that structure at various depths. Multiple radiographs are taken at multiple angles, and the computer reconstructs these images to represent a cross-section or "slice" of the structure.

(continues)

Table 21-6 *(continued)*

TERM	DESCRIPTION
Radiology and Diagnostic Imaging (*continued*)	
Magnetic resonance imaging (MRI); nuclear magnetic resonance (NMR)	This is a noninvasive imaging technique that relies on the body's responses to a strong magnetic field.
Skeletal X-rays	This simple X-ray of bone is often used to initially evaluate patient's complaints. No contrast media or radioactive substances are used.
Clinical Procedures	
Arthrocentesis (aspiration of synovial fluid)	Removal of synovial fluid for analysis in such conditions as gout, rheumatoid arthritis, hematoma, and infection.
Arthroscopy	Diagnostic and therapeutic procedure used to inspect certain joint cavities. The instrument used is an arthroscope. The scope houses a video camera, and the image is projected onto a television monitor. Arthroscopy is most commonly used on the knee joint. The advantages of this procedure include the use of local anesthetic, a quick recovery time, and a reduced hospital stay.

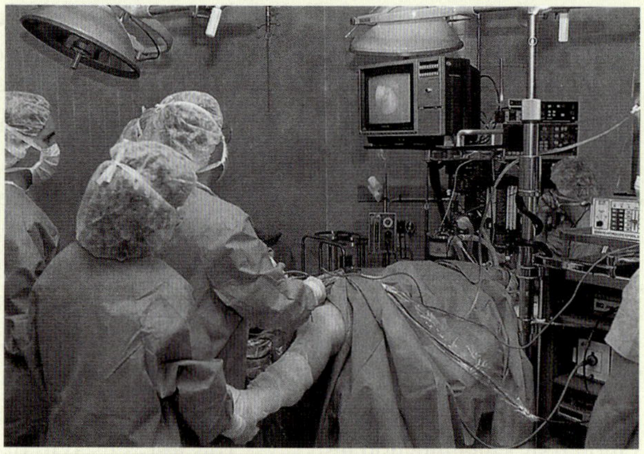

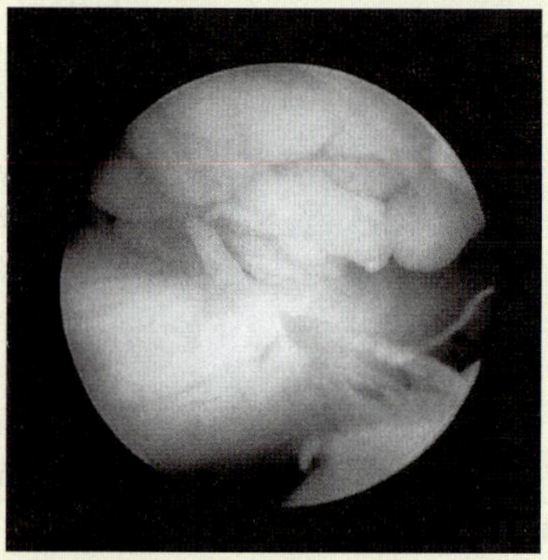

(Photo courtesy of SIU/Visuals Unlimited)

TERM	DESCRIPTION
Aspiration of bone marrow	Withdrawal of bone marrow for the evaluation of bone marrow disease, such as blood dyscrasias (abnormalities) and multiple myeloma.
Biopsy	Removal of a piece of bone that is to be examined by a pathologist for diagnostic purposes. *Note:* This test is used to diagnose tumors and chronic infections such as osteomyelitis.

Source: From *Modern Medical Language* by C. E. Collins, 1996, St. Paul, MN: West Publishing Co. Reprinted with permission.

The eight bones of the cranium are as follows:

- *Frontal bone:* Found above the eyes forming the anterior or forehead portion of the cranium. The supraorbital foramen, through which blood vessels and nerves pass to supply the tissues of the forehead, is found in the frontal bone. Above each eye in the frontal bone is a pair of frontal sinuses.
- *Parietal bones (2):* A pair of bones, one located on each side of the skull, forms the roof and sides of the cranium. The two parietal bones meet in the midline of the cranium at the sagittal suture and join the frontal bone at the coronal suture.
- *Occipital bone:* Forms the back and base of the cranium. The occipital bone joins the parietal bones along the lambdoidal suture. The foramen magnum, through which the spinal cord exits the brain to travel through the vertebral column, is located in the occipital bone.
- *Temporal bones (2):* A pair of bones found on each side of the cranium join the parietal bone along the squamosal suture. The temporal bones form parts of the sides and base of the cranium. The external auditory meatus is located in the temporal bones. Within each bone is a depression called the mandibular fossa that articulates with the processes of the mandible to form the temporomandibular joint (TMJ). Slightly below each external auditory meatus are two processes, the mastoid and styloid process. The mastoid process serves as a point of attachment for particular muscles of the neck; the styloid process serves as a point of attachment for muscles of the tongue and pharynx.
- *Sphenoid bone:* Lodged between several other bones in the anterior portion of the cranium. The sphenoid bone aids in forming the base and sides of the cranium, and the floors and sides of the orbits. A depression, called the sella turcica, in which the pituitary gland rests, is found in the sphenoid. The sphenoid also contains the two sphenoid sinuses.
- *Ethmoid bone:* Located in front of the sphenoid bone. The ethmoid bone consists of two areas, one on each side of the nasal cavity, that are joined by thin horizontal plates called the cribriform plates. Projecting superiorly between the two plates is a triangular process of ethmoid bone called the crista galli. This process serves as a point of attachment for the meninges. Another plate, the perpendicular plate, projects inferiorly in the midline from the cribriform plates to form the majority of the nasal septum. Four scroll-shaped plates called the nasal conchae project inward from the lateral side of the ethmoid bone. The conchae increase the surface area of the nasal mucosa. The small air spaces found in the lateral ethmoid bone are called ethmoid sinuses.

FACIAL BONES

The 14 facial bones form the basic shape of the face. They also serve as sites of attachment for muscles that move the jaw and control facial expressions. The following are the facial bones:

- *Maxillae (2):* The maxillae form the upper jaw, floors of the orbits, and sides and floor of the nasal cavity. Each maxilla contains a maxillary sinus, the largest of the paranasal sinuses. The palatine processes of the maxillae form the anterior portion of the hard palate. The maxillae contain the sockets for the upper teeth.
- *Palatine bones (2):* The palatine bones are located behind the maxillae. They serve a dual role by forming the posterior section of the hard palate and floor of the nasal cavity.
- *Zygomatic bones (2):* The zygomatic bones form the prominences of the cheeks and also help form the lateral walls and floors of the orbits.
- *Lacrimal bones (2):* The lacrimal bones are located between the ethmoid and maxillae in the medial wall of each orbit. An opening in each lacrimal bone allows for the passage of the nasolacrimal duct to drain tears to the nasal cavity.
- *Nasal bones (2):* The long, thin nasal bones are fused at the midline to form the bridge of the nose.
- *Vomer:* The flat vomer bone is located along the midline within the nasal cavity. Posteriorly it joins the perpendicular plate of the ethmoid bone to form the nasal septum.
- *Mandible:* The mandible is a horseshoe-shaped bone with a flat portion projecting upward called the mandibular angle. As previously mentioned, the mandibular condyle articulates with the temporal bone to form a condyloid joint. The mandible serves as attachment for muscles used during chewing, such as the large masseter muscle. The superior border of the mandible contains sockets for the lower teeth.
- *Inferior nasal conchae (2):* Extend horizontally along the lateral walls of the nasal cavity.

In addition to the cranial and facial bones, the three ossicles are contained within the middle ear. The hyoid bone is just below the mandible anterior to the trachea.

VERTEBRAL COLUMN

The vertebral column travels from the skull to the pelvis and is composed of the bony vertebrae. Between each vertebra are disks of fibrous cartilage called intervertebral disks. The vertebrae are connected to each other by supporting ligaments. The functions of the column are to support the head and trunk of the body and protect the spinal cord. The spinal cord travels through the vertebral canal.

ANATOMICAL STRUCTURE OF THE VERTEBRAE

The vertebrae differ in structure according to the region of the vertebral column in which they are located, but they do share common characteristics.

The anterior portion of the vertebra is called the body. The body is thick and round in shape. A vertical row of these bodies is what supports the head and trunk. The intervertebral disks, which separate the vertebral bodies, serve as cushioning devices to prevent damage to the vertebral column due to forces produced by walking, jumping, and falling.

Projecting posteriorly from each vertebral body are two short extensions called **pedicles**. Two bony plates, called laminae, arise from the pedicles and fuse in the back to become the spinous process. Together the pedicles, laminae, and spinous process complete the vertebral arch to form the vertebral foramen, through which the spinal cord travels.

Located between the pedicles and laminae is the transverse process, which extends laterally and inferiorly toward the back. Various ligaments and muscles are attached to the transverse processes. Projecting superiorly and inferiorly from each vertebral arch are the superior and inferior articulating processes. These processes serve as the point of attachment for the ligaments that connect each vertebra to the one above and the one below it.

BONES OF THE THORACIC REGION

The bones of the thoracic region include the ribs, sternum, and costal cartilage. The function of the thoracic cage is to protect the visceral organs of the thoracic cavity and play a role in breathing.

RIBS

Most individuals have 12 pairs of ribs with one pair attached to each of the 12 thoracic vertebrae. The first 7 rib pairs are called the true ribs and join the sternum directly by their costal cartilages. The remaining 5 pairs are called false ribs because their cartilages do not connect directly to the sternum. Instead, the cartilages of the false ribs connect and their cartilages join the seventh costal cartilage. The last 2 pairs of ribs are called floating ribs since they have no cartilaginous attachments to either the sternum or each other.

STERNUM

The sternum, commonly called the breastbone, is located along the midline in the anterior portion of the thoracic cage. It is a flat, elongated bone that is divided into three sections: the upper manubrium, the middle body, and the lower small xiphoid process. The manubrium communicates with the clavicles by facets on its superior border. The true ribs attach to the body.

CLAVICLES

The clavicle, referred to as the collarbone, is a long, slender, doubly curved bone that acts as a brace for the scapula and aids in keeping the shoulder in place. It articulates medially with the manubrium and laterally with the acromion process of the scapula. It is attached to the underlying coracoid process of the scapula by the coracoclavicular ligaments.

SCAPULA

The scapula or shoulder blade is a broad, flat, triangular-shaped bone located on either side of the upper back forming the posterior portion of the shoulder girdle. The posterior surface of each scapula is divided into unequal portions by a spine. This spine, or ridge of bone, leads to the acromion process and the coracoid process. The acromion process articulates with the clavicle and provides attachments for muscles of the arm and chest.

Between the processes on the lateral side of the scapula is a fossa called the glenoid cavity that serves as the socket for the head of the humerus. This forms the ball-and-socket **shoulder joint**.

PECTORAL GIRDLE

The pectoral or shoulder girdle consists of the glenohumeral, sternoclavicular, and acromioclavicular (AC) joints. Of the three joints, the glenohumeral has the widest range of motion. The **AC joint**, located at the top of the shoulder, is an articulation between the lateral end of the clavicle and the flattened, small process located on the border of the acromion (Figure 21-11). Surrounding the shoulder joint are four muscles collectively referred to as the rotator cuff. The four muscles are the infraspinatus, teres minor, subscapularis, and supraspinatus. The tendons of the four muscles insert onto the capsule of the humeral head allowing the muscles to provide a variety of movements of the shoulder joint. The main function of the rotator cuff is to provide stability and strength to the shoulder joint.

HUMERUS

The humerus is the longest and largest bone of the upper extremity. It extends from the scapula to the elbow (Figure 21-12). Its upper end is the smooth and rounded ball that fits into the glenoid fossa of the scapula. Just below the head of the humerus are two processes called the

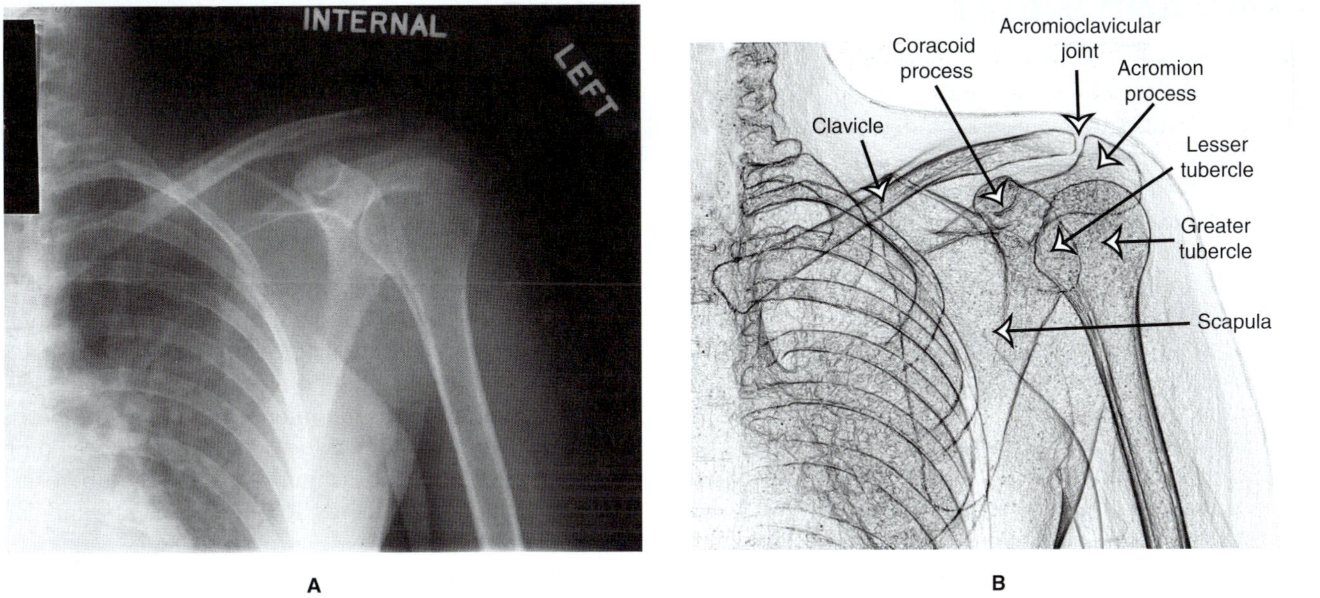

Figure 21-11 Shoulder: (A) X-ray, (B) schematic

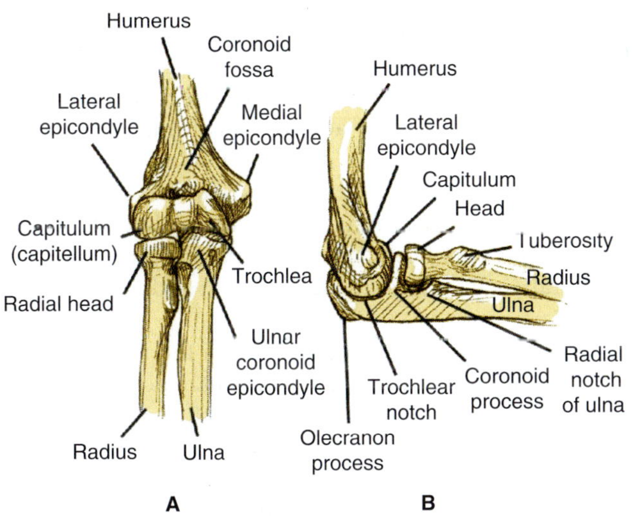

Figure 21-12 Elbow: (A) Anterior, (B) lateral

greater and lesser tuberosities. A narrow circumferential depression along the lower margin of the articular surface of the humerus separating the head from the tubercles is called the anatomical neck. Just below the tubercles is a region called the surgical neck, so named because it is a common site for fractures.

The greater tubercle is located on the lateral side of the humeral head. The supraspinatus, infraspinatus, and teres minor tendons insert on the greater tubercle. The lesser tubercle is located on the anterior side and serves as the site of insertion of the subscapular tendon. Lying in a deep groove between the tuberosities called the bicipital groove is the tendon of the biceps muscle. Near the middle of the humeral shaft is the deltoid tuberosity. It provides an attachment for the deltoid muscle that raises the arm horizontally and laterally.

At the distal end of the humerus there are two condyles. The lateral condyle is called the capitulum; it articulates with the head of the radius. The articular surface of the medial condyle, called the trochlea, articulates with the ulna.

RADIUS AND ULNA

The radius extends from the elbow to the wrist and rotates around the ulna. An easy way to remember on which side of the arm the radius lies, is to recall that it is on the "thumb" side of the arm and hand. The proximal end articulates with the capitulum of the humerus and the radial notch of the ulna. This allows the radius to rotate around the ulna during movement. Just below the head of the radius is a process called the radial tuberosity, which serves as an attachment for the tendon of the biceps muscle. The distal end is divided into two articular surfaces. The lateral surface articulates with the carpal bones of the wrist. Located on the lateral surface is the styloid process, which provides attachments for the ligaments of the wrist. The medial surface articulates with the distal end of the ulna.

The proximal portion of the ulna, the trochlea, articulates with the humerus. Two processes, called the olecranon and coronoid processes, are located on each side of this articulation. Both processes provide attachments for muscles.

The somewhat rounded head on the distal end of the ulna articulates with a notch of the radius called the ulnar notch. The ulna also has a styloid process that provides attachments for ligaments of the wrist.

HAND AND WRIST

The skeletal bones of the wrist and hand consist of the carpals, or wrist bones; metacarpals, or bones of the palm; and the phalanges, or bones of the digits (Figure 21-13). The distal row articulates with the metacarpal bones. The proximal row articulates with the radius and fibrous cartilage of the ulna.

The eight carpal bones are arranged in two rows. The distal row, from the radial to the ulnar side, is arranged as follows: trapezium, trapezoid, capitate, and hamate. The proximal row consists of the scaphoid (also called navicular), lunate, triquetrum, and pisiform. The scaphoid is the main link of the carpal bones; it stabilizes and coordinates the movement of the two rows. Each carpal bone has smooth articular surfaces for contact with other carpals and rough surfaces for the attachment of ligaments.

The five metacarpal bones are located in the palm. The metacarpals articulate proximally with the distal row of carpal bones; distally, the head of each metacarpal articulates with a phalanx. The bones are cylindrical in shape and the heads are rounded, forming the knuckles. There are 14 phalangeal bones in each hand: three bones in each finger and two in the thumb.

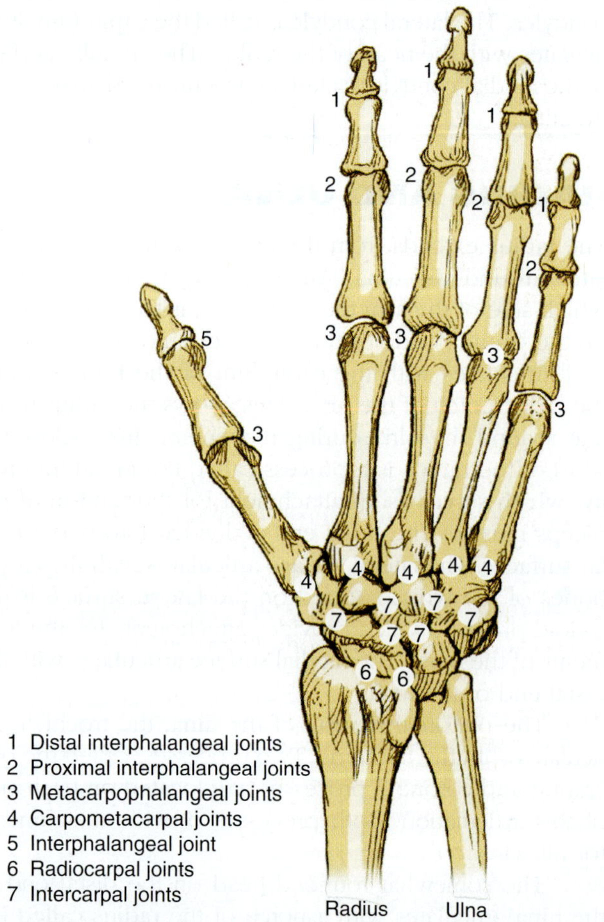

Figure 21-13 Hand and wrist joints

PELVIS

The sacrum, coccyx, and pelvic girdle form the circular pelvis. (Refer to Chapter 15 for more details on the pelvis.) The pelvis provides support for the trunk and attachments for the femur. The pelvis is created from the fusion of three bones called the ilium, ischium, and pubis. Together they are referred to as the ox coxae or innominate bone.

The ilium forms the superior portion of the pelvis and is the largest of the three bones. The ilium flares outward in a ridge called the iliac crest. This crest serves as a primary site for obtaining bone for bone grafts.

The ischium forms the inferior portion of the pelvis and is the strongest of the three pelvic bones. Located on the lower portion of the ischium is the ischial tuberosity, which provides attachments for the ligaments and leg muscles.

The pubis is the anterior portion of the pelvis. The two pubic bones join at the midline to form the symphysis pubis. The symphysis pubis is actually a disk of fibrous cartilage that serves to connect the two pubic bones.

HIP AND FEMUR

The hip is a ball-and-socket joint formed by the deep, round fossa, called the acetabulum, located in the innominate bone and the head of the femur (Figure 21-14). A capsule, ligaments, and muscles stabilize the hip. The iliofemoral ligament connects the ilium with the femur anteriorly and superiorly, and the ischiofemoral and pubofemoral ligaments join the ischium and pubis to the femur.

The femur is the largest bone in the body, extending from hip to the knee. The proximal end of the femur consists of the femoral head and neck, and the greater and lesser trochanters (Figure 21-15).

The greater trochanter is located on the upper, lateral part of the upper shaft of the femur. It serves as the point of insertion for the gluteus medius and gluteus minimus. The iliopsoas muscle inserts into the lesser trochanter. Located at the distal end of the femur are the lateral and medial condyles that articulate with the condyles of the tibia to form the knee joint. The femoral condyles are separated by a depression called the patellar surface (groove) forming the articulating surface for the patella.

TIBIA AND FIBULA

The patella is a sesamoid bone contained within the quadriceps tendon. The patellar tendon travels across the anterior surface of the patella as the tendon originates and inserts above and below the knee joint. The posterior surface of the patella articulates with the femur.

The capsule of the knee joint is attached as follows (Figure 21-16):

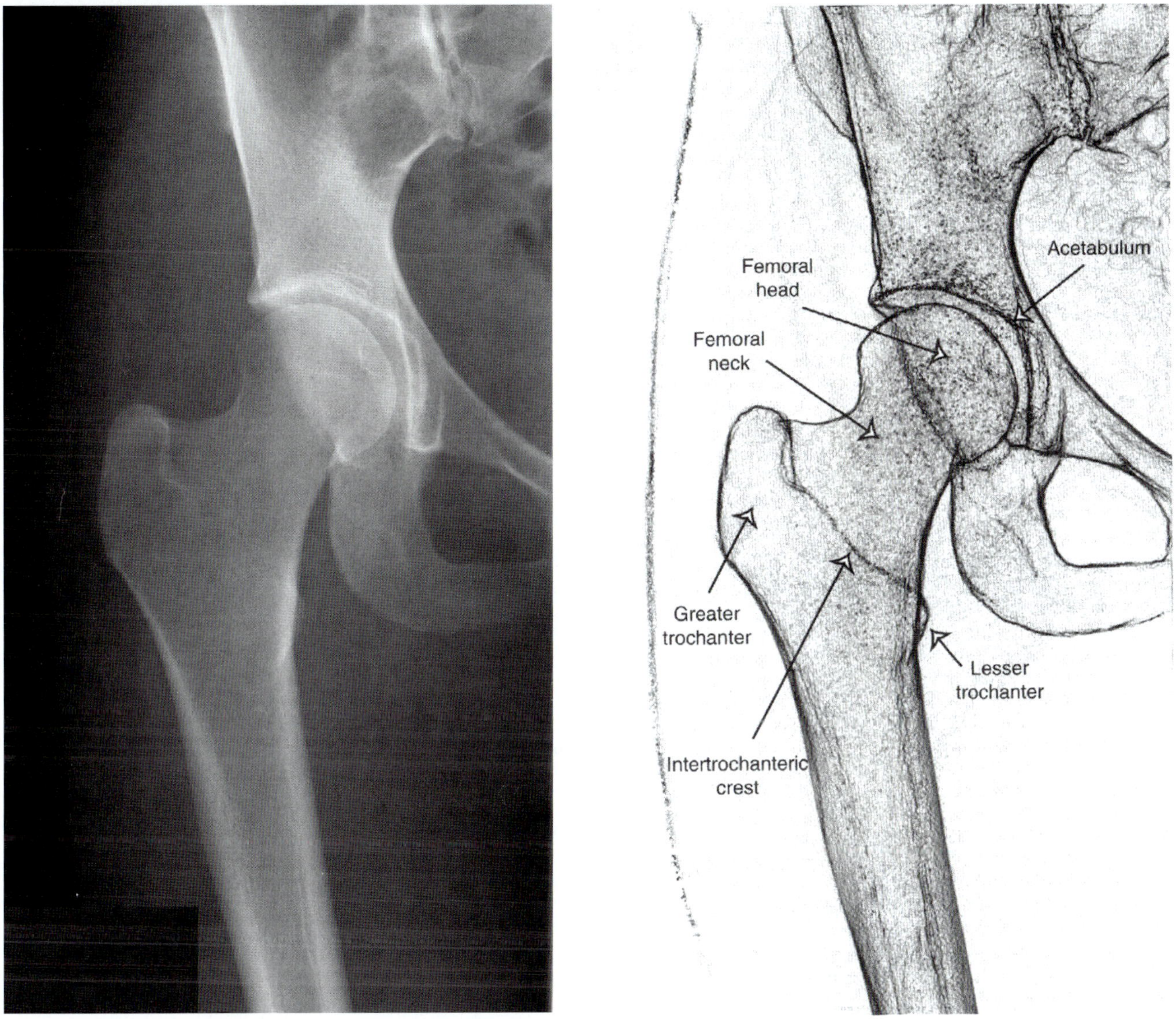

A B

Figure 21-14 Hip: (A) AP X-ray, (B) schematic

1. Proximally to the lateral and medial condyles of the femur
2. Distally to the lateral and medial condyles of the tibia
3. Superior end of the fibula

The capsule is stabilized as follows:

1. Anteriorly by the patellar and quadriceps tendons
2. Laterally and medially by the medial and lateral collateral ligaments
3. Posteriorly by the popliteus and gastrocnemius muscles

Two large **ligaments** located in the knee joint help stabilize the movement of the joint. The ligaments are called the anterior and posterior cruciate ligaments and are located in the intercondylar region of the knee joint. The posterior cruciate ligament (PCL) is attached to the posterior midline surface of the tibia and passes anteriorly, attaching to the medial condyle of the femur. The PCL prevents the femur from sliding anteriorly on the tibia, especially when the knee is bent.

The anterior cruciate ligament (ACL) is attached to the posterior lateral condyle of the femur and to a notch in the midline of the tibia between the tibial condyles. The ACL prevents the femur from sliding posteriorly on the tibia, prevents hyperextension of the knee, and limits the medial rotation of the femur when the leg is in a fixed position with the foot planted. A common injury of the knee is a torn ACL, which requires surgery to either repair or replace the ACL.

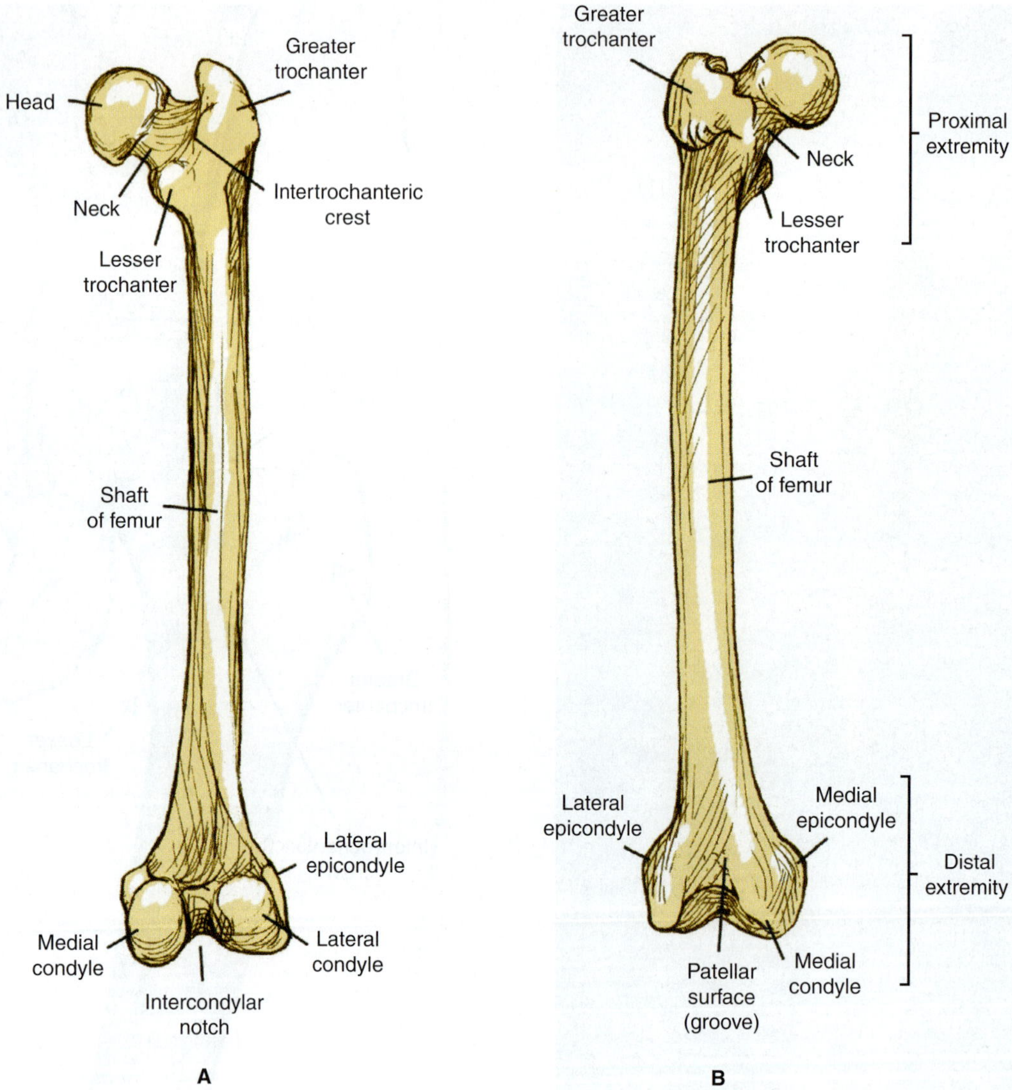

Figure 21-15 **Femur: (A) Posterior, (B) anterior**

The knee joint is cushioned to withstand activities such as walking, jumping, and running by a pair of menisci called the lateral and medial meniscus. The menisci are thick, crescent-shaped pads of cartilage that rest on the upper articular surface of the tibia. Injuries to the menisci, particularly athletic injuries, are common and result in various types of tears in the cartilage, such as the bucket handle tear.

The tibia, or shinbone, is the larger, thus stronger, bone of the lower leg. It is located on the medial side. Located at the proximal end of the tibia are the medial and lateral condyles that articulate with the condyles of the femur to form the knee joint. Distally, the tibia articulates with the talus bone forming part of the ankle joint. Laterally, it articulates with the fibula. The medial prominence is called the medial malleolus.

The fibula is located on the lateral side of the lower leg. It is a nonweight-bearing bone that serves as a site for attachment of ligaments and muscles of the lower leg. A prominence called the lateral malleolus articulates with the talus bone to form the other portion of the ankle joint.

ANKLE AND FOOT

The ankle joint consists of seven tarsal bones whose names are as follows: calcaneus, navicular, cuboid, medial cuneiform, middle cuneiform, and lateral cuneiform (Figure 21-17). The largest of the anklebones is the calcaneus, which is located inferiorly to the talus and forms the heel. The calcaneus aids in supporting the weight of the body and provides an attachment for the muscles of the foot.

The five metatarsals are equivalent to the metacarpals of the hand (Figure 21-18). The distal ends of the metatarsals articulate with the first phalanges of the

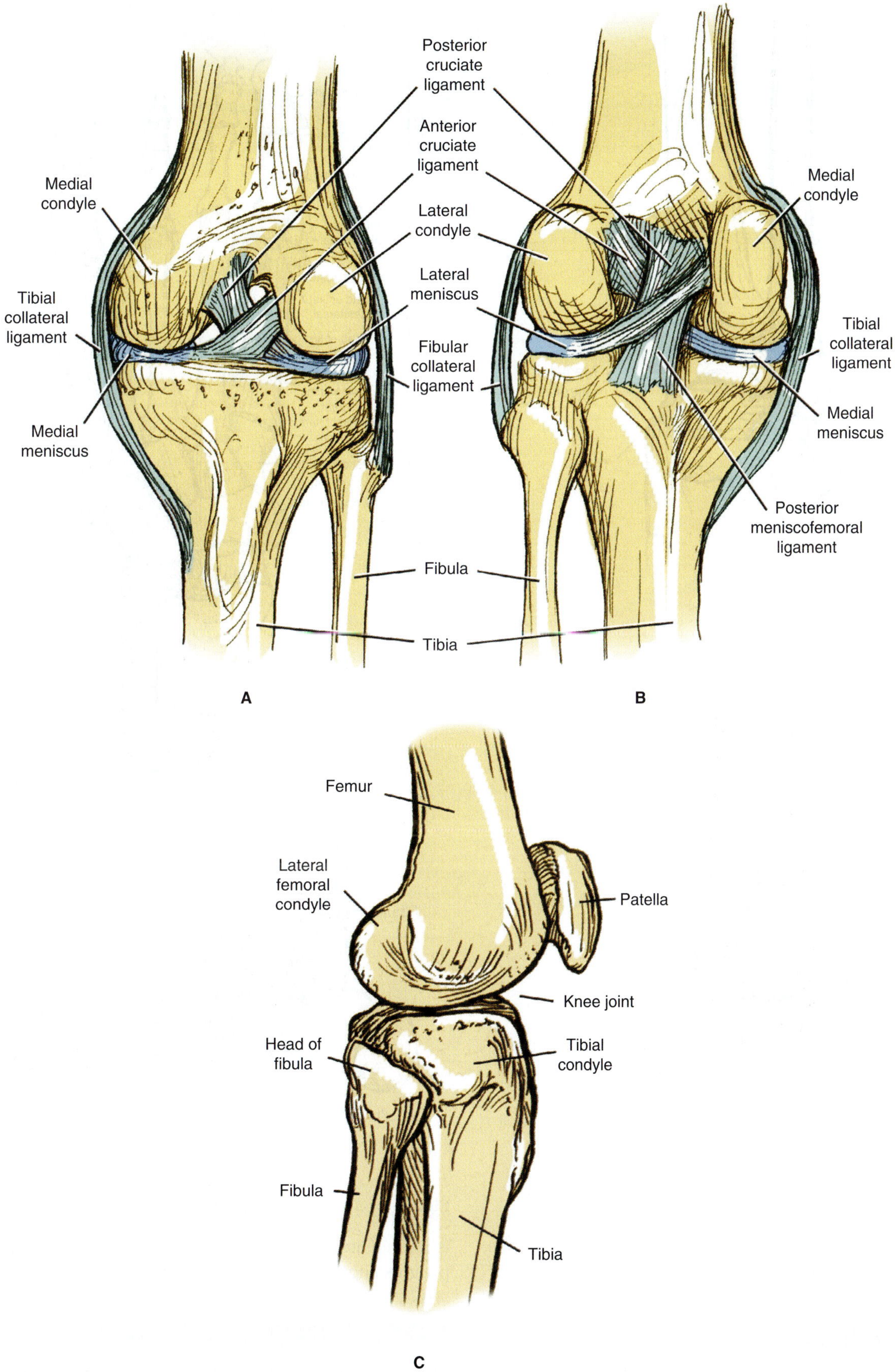

Figure 21-16 **Knee: (A) Anterior, (B) posterior, (C) lateral**

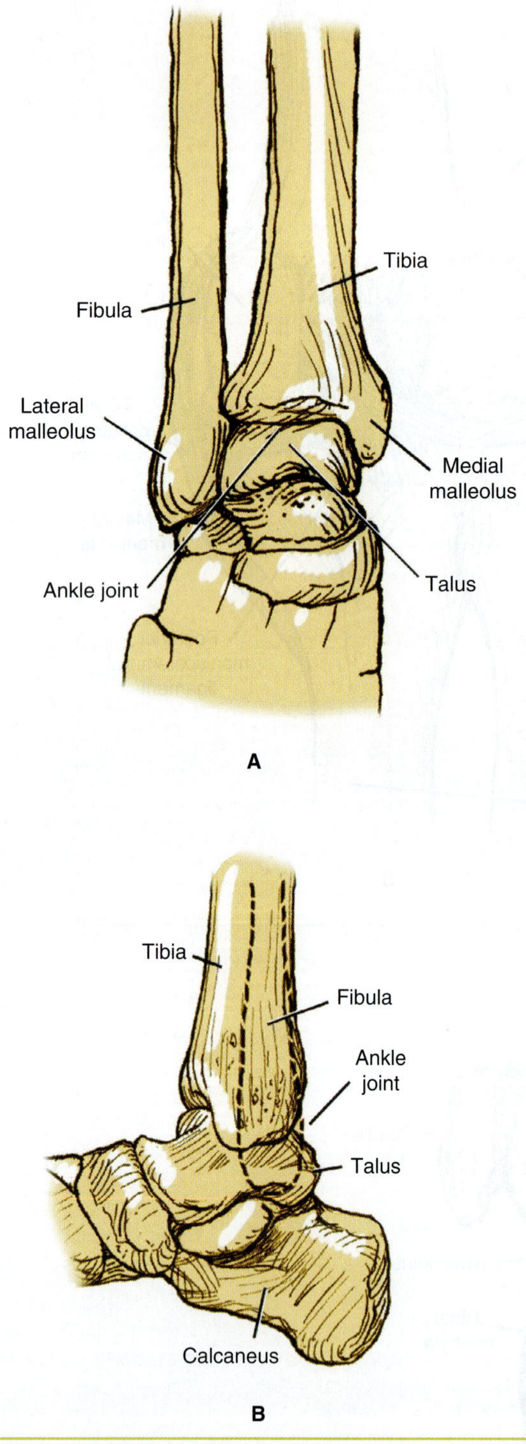

Figure 21-17 **Ankle: (A) Anterior, (B) lateral**

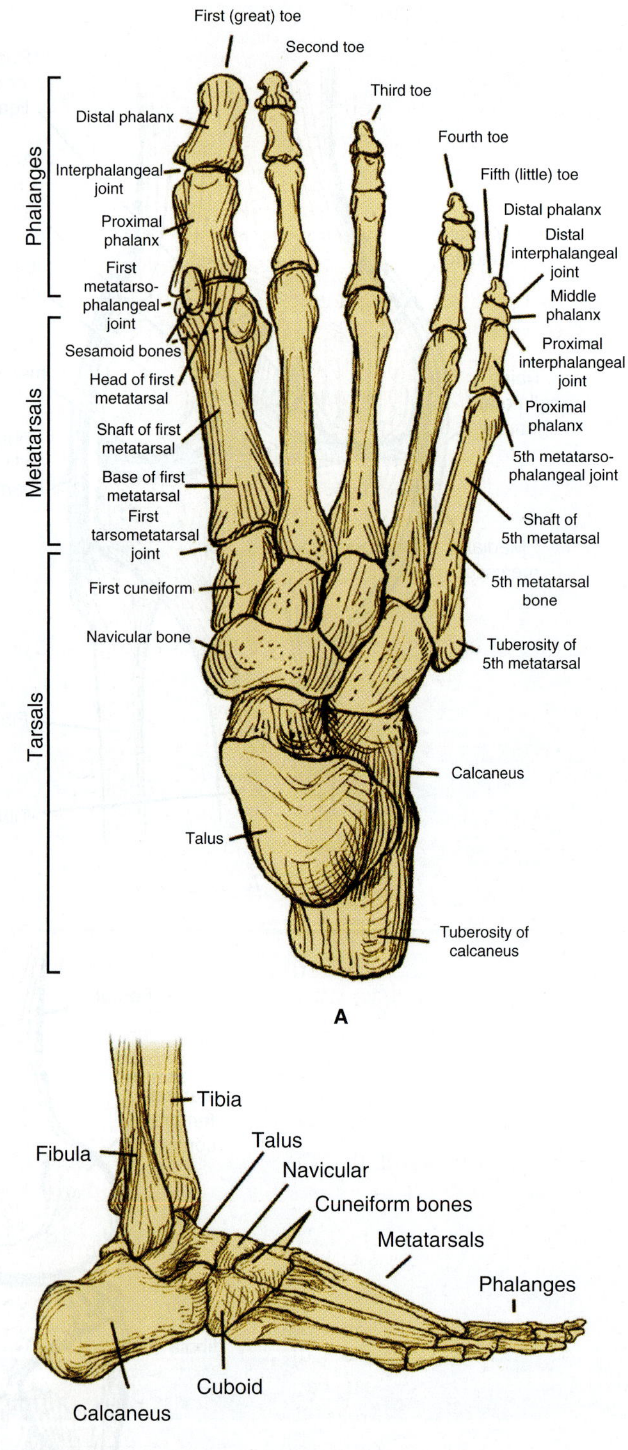

Figure 21-18 **Foot: (A) Superior, (B) lateral**

toes. The phalanges consist of three per toe except for the great toe, which only has two.

EQUIPMENT

Orthopedic surgery is known for its special requirements in terms of equipment and instrumentation. The following is a brief introduction to the complex and continuously progressing world of orthopedic equipment.

POSITIONING DEVICES

The positioning of the orthopedic surgical patient can be quite involved, particularly when the patient has sustained a severe fracture. The selected position should provide adequate exposure of the operative site (while maintaining body alignment and possibly alignment of the fractured bones), prevent pressure on the muscles and nerves, and prevent compression of blood vessels.

The choice of position is based on the type of procedure, location of the injury, and the surgeon's preference. Often, the OR table safety strap is not sufficient to stabilize the patient and other positioning devices are required to secure the patient. When positioning the patient, the OR team must know the meaning of common orthopedic directional terms such as **flexion**, extension, lateral, medial, **abduction**, and **adduction**.

Many positioning devices are commercially available to hold an extremity in place during surgery. Some of the positioning devices can be sterilized in order to be utilized intraoperatively at the sterile field. Two popular types of devices are the foot holder utilized during total knee arthroplasty procedures and the shoulder positioner, which allows for distraction of the joint to aid in visualization. The advantage of using sterile positioning devices is the ability to reposition the extremity during the surgical procedure.

The lateral position is frequently used for operations on the hip and shoulder. The vacuum beanbag is often used to stabilize the patient in the lateral position, eliminating the need for roll towels and tape over the hips. The beanbag can be contoured to the body shape of the patient by adjusting the beanbag while the air is suctioned out.

The prone position is used for procedures on the back, posterior portion of the shoulder, and Achilles tendon. The prone position is often facilitated with the use of the Wilson frame, Andrews frame, and OR table. The Andrews frame maintains the patient in a modified knee-chest position. The Wilson and Andrews frames are placed on top of the OR table and the patient is rolled onto the frame after being anesthetized on the gurney.

A fracture table is commonly used for surgery on a hip fracture and for femoral nailing. The fracture table must be well understood by the personnel using it in order for it to be properly set up. Fracture tables have several moving parts and can cause injury to the patient and OR personnel if not correctly handled. The patient can be placed in the supine or lateral position using a fracture table. The following description is for placing the patient in the supine position on the fracture table.

The pelvis is stabilized against a perineal post that must be well padded, usually with Webril, to prevent damage to the external genital structures and perineal nerve. The foot of the injured extremity is placed in a "boot" that is also well padded. The boot is attached to a traction bar that can rotate the leg or applies traction to it. The foot can be secured in the boot with the use of Velcro straps or by wrapping an Ace or Coban bandage around the foot. The unaffected leg is placed in a boot that is abducted to allow for the C-arm fluoroscope to be positioned over the injured site.

PNEUMATIC TOURNIQUETS

Pneumatic tourniquets are frequently used for surgical procedures on extremities. The use of the tourniquet provides a bloodless surgical site, which aids visualization. The surgeon will exsanguinate the extremity by elevating it and wrapping, distally to proximally, with an Ace or Esmarch bandage. After exsanguination is accomplished, the tourniquet is inflated. A popular tourniquet is the double-cuffed pneumatic tourniquet. If one cuff fails to inflate, the second cuff provides the needed pressure. In addition, the cuffs can be inflated alternately to reduce constant pressure on one site of the extremity. To avoid a pressure-induced injury to the nerves and blood vessels, continuous tourniquet pressure should not be applied for more than 1 hour on an upper extremity or for more than 1½ hours on the thigh. After 1 hour of pressure, the surgeon should be notified, and again every 15 minutes thereafter.

TRACTION

Traction alignment can be used preoperatively, intraoperatively, and postoperatively. Traction is used to immobilize a joint, reduce a fracture, and align a body part. The three types of traction are manual, skin, and skeletal. Skeletal traction is frequently applied in the operating room.

Application of skeletal traction is a sterile procedure. The sterile instruments used for the insertion of skeletal traction include knife handle with #15 knife blade, hand or power drill, Steinmann pins, traction bow, and pin cutter. Traction frames are placed on the patient's postoperative bed and weights are used to apply the traction.

LASERS

The use of lasers in orthopedic surgery has been slowly increasing. With the development of new techniques and improved instrumentation, the laser may become even more attractive in the future.

The CO_2 and contact Nd:YAG lasers have seen limited use during knee arthroscopy. The same two lasers have been successfully used on the soft tissues during a total joint arthroplasty and lumbar laminectomy. CO_2 is used to aid in the removal of methyl methacrylate (MMA) during a revision arthroplasty. The laser changes the consistency of the MMA, allowing for its easy removal.

RADIOGRAPHY

Radiography is frequently used during orthopedic surgery, particularly during the repair and/or reduction of fractures. The two most popular types of radiography are standard X-rays, in which the cassette is draped with a sterile cassette cover by the STSR, and fluoroscopy.

Fluoroscopy provides the surgical team with the ability to view the procedure as it progresses, allowing confirmation of the fracture reduction or placement of pins, screws, and/or plates. The C-arm is a convenient fluoroscopy machine that can be directly positioned over the operative site. A sterile C-arm drape is commercially available, which allows the surgeon to adjust the C-arm's position during the procedure.

AIR FLOW

The prevention of infection is critical during orthopedic procedures, especially those involving open bone from a fracture or during a total joint arthroplasty. The invasion of the interior of bone by microorganisms can have devastating effects for the patient. Body exhaust suits are frequently worn by the members of the sterile surgical team during repair of severe fractures and total joint replacement. Laminar air flow systems provide highly filtered air, one-direction flow of air, and continuous air exchanges that reduce the microbial count.

CONTINUOUS PASSIVE RANGE-OF-MOTION MACHINES

Surgeons frequently order the use of the Continuous Passive Range-of-Motion Machines (CPMs) for the patient after major knee, elbow, shoulder, and femoral surgical procedures. The CPM provides the following advantages:

1. Aids in decreasing pain and swelling at the operative site
2. Reduces joint stiffness resulting from the patient being bedridden
3. Inhibits the formation of adhesions
4. Provides early mobility
5. Decreases the effects of immobilization, such as muscle wasting

TRANSCUTANEOUS ELECTRIC NERVE STIMULATION

The transcutaneous electric nerve stimulation (TENS) unit can be used to suppress postoperative pain by stimulating large sensory nerve fibers. It is a portable, battery-operated unit with electrodes that are placed on the skin near the source of the pain. Because the overstimulation of the large-diameter sensory neurons blocks the perception of pain sensations carried by unmyelinated fibers, TENS is effective after total joint replacements and repair of severe fractures.

ELECTRICAL STIMULATION OF BONE

Osteogenesis is influenced by artificially applied electrical stimulation. Due to the low level of current generated by the device, electrical stimulation can be used in the presence of implants, both internal and external. The types of stimulators available include implantable, percutaneous, and external. The disadvantage of using electrical stimulation is that it requires immobilization of the extremity for a long period of time, which can slow the rehabilitation.

The electrical stimulator is used in the treatment of nonunion or delayed union of bone fractures to speed the healing process. Infected nonunions that have undergone debridement also benefit from electrical stimulation that inhibits bacterial growth.

SAWS, DRILLS, AND REAMERS

Instruments powered by air, nitrogen, or electricity have virtually eliminated the need for hand-operated saws and drills. The use of power instruments reduces operative time and improves both surgical technique and postoperative results. The manufacturer's instructions must be followed for cleaning, sterilizing, and lubricating power instruments.

The surgical technologist must be familiar with the assembly of the power instruments, including safety factors. The majority of power instruments include a safety device that prevents the inadvertent activation of the instrument. Power instruments can be heavy and should not be placed on the patient when not in use.

Two directional terms must be understood in relation to the use of power saws. An oscillating saw is one in which the saw blade moves from side to side, or oscillates. In a reciprocating saw, the saw blade moves back and forth, or reciprocates. Various bone cuts can be achieved using the two types of motion. The operative procedure or particular step in the procedure will dictate which will be needed.

ARTHROSCOPIC EQUIPMENT

Arthroscopic surgery is frequently performed for diagnostic purposes, for repair of tissues within a joint, and as an adjunct to surgical procedures such as anterior cruciate ligament repair. Arthroscopy is usually performed on the knee, ankle, elbow, and wrist joints. To perform the arthroscopy the surgeon requires well-functioning equipment that allows clear visualization of the interior of the joint.

The required equipment includes:

1. Video monitor
2. Light source box
3. Arthroscopy pump and tubing for fluids
4. Powered shaving system
5. Camera system

6. Video recording system
7. Photograph system

SUPPLIES

The field of orthopedics requires sophisticated equipment and instrumentation. A large number of supplies are required. Casting materials were discussed above. Other commonly used supplies are discussed in this section.

IMPLANTS

Implants are a routine part of many orthopedic surgical procedures. Implants include screws, plates, wires, pins, intramedullary nails and rods, and total joint components. An adequate inventory of implants is required in order to meet the needs of surgery. The inventory can be based on surgeon's preference, number of procedures performed per year requiring the use of implants, and cost.

The Food and Drug Administration requires proper documentation and tracking of implants. The majority of implants, particularly total joint implants, nails, and rods, include a manufacturer's label with the required information that can be attached to the patient's operative record and filed in the patient's permanent record. The STSR assists the circulator by supplying the information if a label is not available. The information should include:

1. Number of implants used
2. Type of implant(s)
3. Size of implant(s)
4. Manufacturer's serial number(s)

A variety of alloys are used to manufacture implants. The most frequently used alloys include titanium, stainless steel, and cobalt-chromium. It is very important that implants of the same alloy are used when surgery is performed. If implants composed of different alloys are placed in the patient, they will corrode, causing a breakdown of the implant. This will delay healing and may possibly cause an infection.

Implants should never be reused. Scratches that can occur on the surface of an implant can cause complications if the implant is reused. These complications may include corrosion of the implant, irritation, and infection of the bone due to the imperfection's "digging" into the bone. If an implant, particularly a total joint implant, is dropped, it should not be used since it may have become marred or scratched.

SUTURE

Orthopedic surgeons use a wide range of suture (Table 21-7). Ligaments and tendons are made of tough collagen tissue that has a poor vascular supply and, compared to vascular tissues, they heal more slowly. Generally, nonabsorbable suture is used to repair ligaments, tendons, muscles, and bone. Absorbable suture is preferred to close the periosteum.

METHYL METHACRYLATE

Methyl methacrylate (MMA), also referred to as bone cement, is routinely used during total joint arthroplasty. Bone cement stabilizes and keeps the implants in the correct anatomical position. The cement fills the cavity and spaces of the bone to form a bond between the implant and bone. The STSR is responsible for mixing the sterile powder and liquid to create the cement. The majority of ORs have incorporated the use of a closed mixing system that is attached to suction to exhaust the fumes created during the process of mixing the cement. The fumes are irritating to the mucous membranes and possibly toxic to the liver.

PHARMACOLOGY

Routine pharmacological supplies used in orthopedics include antibiotics, hemostatic agents, and steroids.

Table 21-7 Suture Used in Orthopedic Surgery

SUTURE MATERIAL	DESCRIPTION	USE
Surgical steel	Most inert and strongest of all suture material; lacks elasticity	Tendons; bone to bone, such as sternum closure
Polyester (Ethibond)	Braided suture that is superior to any other braided suture in decreasing drag through tissue	Tendon to bone
Polypropylene (Prolene)	Monofilament strand almost as inert as stainless steel; acceptable substitute for steel, but easier to handle	Tendon to bone
Nylon (Nurolon)	Multifilament with minimal tissue reaction	Tendon to bone
Chromic	Moderate tissue reaction; chemically treated to slow absorption	Periosteum
Polyglactin (Vicryl)	Coated multifilament; slow absorption	Periosteum

ANTIBIOTICS

Antibiotics are used intravenously and mixed with irrigation solutions. A common practice is for the surgeon to have the individual managing anesthesia inject an antibiotic through the patient's IV just before the skin incision is made. First-generation cephalosporins (Ancef, Keflex, and Cefadyl) are the antibiotic of choice. The second-generation cephalosporin Mefoxin is also frequently used. Polymixin, bacitracin, and Cefadyl are common antibiotics mixed with irrigation solutions or injected into the bags of solution to be used with the pulse lavage system.

HEMOSTATIC AGENTS

Hemostatic agents that are frequently used include Gelfoam, Avitene, thrombin, and bone wax. Gelfoam is used in its pad form and placed on the bone where the capillary bleeding is taking place. The Gelfoam must be moistened in warm saline and the excess is squeezed out before it is applied. Gelfoam may also be dipped in thrombin or epinephrine.

Avitene is an absorbable hemostatic agent that is applied dry using some type of smooth forceps. Avitene is applied directly to the oozing surface of bone; pressure must be immediately applied with a dry 4 × 4 sponge to ensure the Avitene adheres to the wound surface.

Thrombin is a hemostatic agent of bovine source. Thrombin must be used only as a topical agent and never injected. The STSR must keep the thrombin separate from other solutions and make sure it is labeled. Orthopedic surgeons tend to prefer to use thrombin in liquid solution rather than powder form. Thrombin kits can be purchased that include a spray bottle for applying the thrombin to the oozing surface.

Bone wax is a sterile mixture of beeswax that aids in stopping oozing from cut surfaces of bone. The STSR can roll small pieces of the bone wax into balls that are then applied to the wound site by the surgeon.

STEROIDS

Steroids are used for their anti-inflammatory action. Patients may receive shots of cortisone, a short-acting steroid, or betamethasone, a long-acting steroid, to reduce inflammation in a joint area caused by trauma. The steroid may be given therapeutically to treat the inflammation and preoperatively and postoperatively to aid in reducing tissue inflammation caused by surgery.

PROCEDURES

There are many orthopedic procedures and most have several variations. The procedures in this chapter illustrate common types of procedures with their unique problems and techniques.

BONE GRAFTING

The iliac crest is the optimal source for obtaining autogenous cancellous and cortical bone for use in bone grafting for many purposes. These purposes include filling in a cavity after the removal of a large amount of bone, filling in areas that have experienced loss of bone due to trauma or disease process, and promoting the fusion of a joint.

The site for taking the graft is separately draped and a separate instrument setup is used. Instruments for taking the graft include various sizes of gouges, osteotomes, and curettes, and a mallet. A power saw may be used to shape the graft(s) if necessary.

The most abundant source of cancellous bone is found in the posterior portion of the iliac spine, just below the iliac crest (Procedure 21-1). When the anterior portion of the ilium is used as the bone graft donor site, the patient experiences less postoperative discomfort than if the bone is taken from the medial aspect of the ilium. The following description is for taking bone from the posterior ilium; the method is basically the same as for taking bone from the anterior ilium.

PROCEDURE

21-1 Bone Graft Procedure, Donor Site

Equipment

- Positioning devices may be required
- Electrosurgical unit
- Power equipment available

Instruments

- Basic orthopedic set
- Straight and curved osteotomes
- Gouge set
- Curettes

PROCEDURE

21-1 Bone Graft Procedure, Donor Site *(continued)*

Supplies

- Orthopedic pack
- Special drapes as needed
- Basin set
- Gloves
- Blades
- Suture of choice

Operative Preparation

Anesthesia
- General

Position
- Lateral (or as needed)

Prep
- Donor site
- Recipient site

Draping
- Donor site
- Recipient site

Practical Considerations

- Have X-rays or MRIs in OR
- Notify radiology of possible intraoperative X-ray
- Have C-arm near OR
- Follow radiology safety procedures
- Notify orthopedic technician if external stabilization methods needed postoperatively

Operative Procedure	Technical Considerations
1. An oblique incision is made from the highest point of the iliac crest going downward and medially.	**1.** A second Mayo stand may be useful for graft procurement.
2. Iliac crest is exposed using sharp dissection.	**2.** Blunt rakes are used for retracting.
3. Gluteal fascia is incised with scalpel and the gluteal muscles bluntly separated in the direction of their fibers. Muscles are retracted to provide exposure.	**3.** Deeper retractors may be employed.
4. Using a curved osteotome, a cut is made around the periphery of the ilium just below the crest outlining the total area of the graft.	**4.** Always accompany an osteotome with a mallet.
5. Additional cuts are then made outlining longitudinal strips that will be taken as the graft.	**5.** All of the cuts may be made with the osteotome or a power saw may be used.
6. Using a gouge, the strips of cancellous grafts are removed.	**6.** Blood is suctioned with an Asepto syringe and saved in a basin. Graft material is placed in the blood until ready for use.
7. Bone wax is packed into the area denuded of bone.	**7.** Roll pieces of bone wax into small balls to hand to the surgeon.
8. Closure: gluteal muscle and fascia are sutured to the iliac crest. The gluteal fascia along with periosteum is sutured to the bone using interrupted sutures. The remainder of the wound is closed in routine fashion.	**8.** A perforating towel clip is used to create a small hole in the medial crest of the ilium. Drains may be placed. A pressure dressing is applied to aid in protecting the wound and hemostasis.

(continues)

Postoperative Considerations

Immediate Postoperative Care
- Transport to Postanesthesia Care Unit (PACU)
- Observe for local hemorrhage
- Careful movement to avoid dislodging graft

Prognosis
- Return to normal activities
- May have some restrictions on types of activities

Complications
- Hemorrhage
- Wound infection
- Bone infection
- Failure of graft

PEARL OF WISDOM

Be sure graft is stored in a safe location until time of use. Be sure to transfer graft over sterile field.

KNEE ARTHROSCOPY

Knee pathology is usually diagnosed by physical examination, with radiography (Figure 21-19A), and with MRI (Figure 21-19B). Arthroscopy of the knee is performed for diagnostic purposes, for removal of loose bodies that can cause the knee joint to lock in place, for shaving the patella and torn meniscus, and for insertion of instruments to perform a meniscectomy or repair (Procedure 21-2).

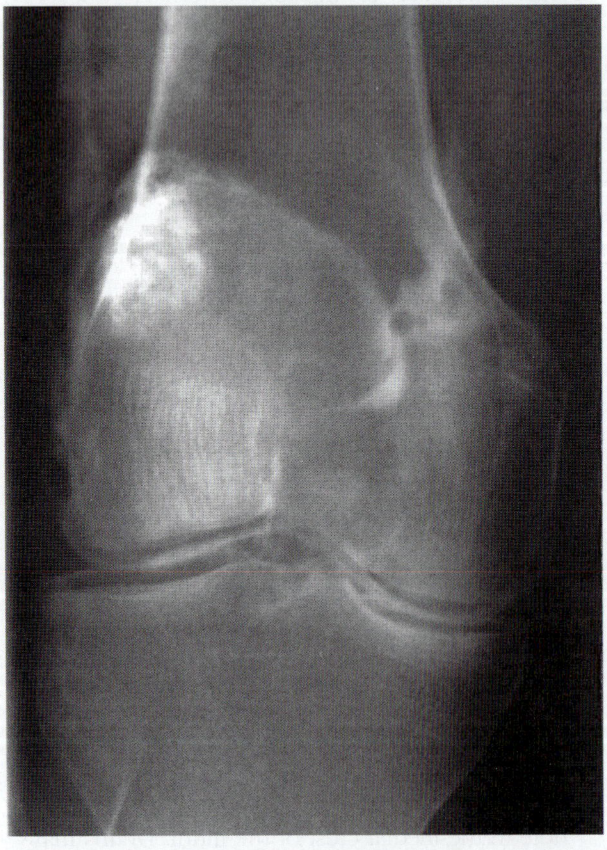

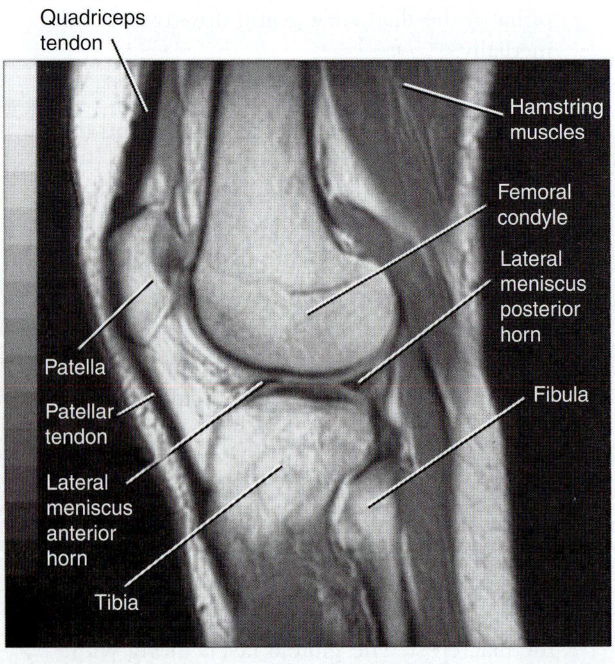

Figure 21-19 **Knee diagnostics: (A) X-ray, (B) MRI**

PROCEDURE

21-2 Knee Arthroscopy

Equipment

- Positioning devices (as needed)
- Electrosurgical unit
- Video equipment
- Light source
- Tourniquet
- Fluid pump
- Power source for arthroscopic shaver

Instruments

- Arthroscopy set
- 30-degree arthroscope; have 70-degree available
- Nerve hooks: small and large
- Arthroscopic powered shaver
- Various arthroscopic graspers

Supplies

- Orthopedic pack
- Special drapes if needed
- Basin set
- Gloves
- Blades
- Suture of choice (4–0 or 5–0 nylon or undyed synthetic nonabsorbable is often used)
- Dressing: 4 × 4 sponges, Webril or Kerlix wrapped around knee joint, 6-in. Ace bandage

Operative Preparation

Anesthesia

- General, spinal, or local anesthesia can be used depending on the extent of the operative procedure

Position

- Supine
- The end of the OR table may be lowered according to surgeon's preference
- A padded lateral post is attached to the side of the OR table approximately at the level of the mid-thigh to facilitate placing countertraction on the knee joint to open the medial side

Prep

- Affected leg—circumferential

Draping

- Lower extremity draping method

Practical Considerations

- Prior to prep, surgeon will perform an examination under anesthesia (EUA) to confirm diagnostic findings
- Have X-rays or MRIs in OR
- Notify radiology of possible intraoperative X-ray
- Have C-arm near OR
- Follow radiology safety procedures
- Notify orthopedic technician if external stabilization methods needed postoperatively
- Check monitors and photographic equipment
- Apply tourniquet preoperatively but do not inflate until surgeon requests

Operative Procedure

1. A #11 knife blade is used to make an incision that is lateral to the patellar tendon and just above the joint line.

Technical Considerations

1. Arthroscopy pump tubing must be primed prior to use.

(continues)

PROCEDURE 21-2 **Knee Arthroscopy** *(continued)*

2. Irrigation/inflow cannula is inserted using the sharp trocar and/or blunt trocar according to surgeon's preference.	**2.** Tubing leading from a bag of lactated Ringer's or saline solution is connected to the opening on the side of the cannula.
3. The joint is distended either by fluids entering the joint by gravity or with the use of the arthroscopy pump.	**3.** Finish passing equipment to circulator to connect.
4. Second stab incision is made anterolaterally allowing for insertion of the sharp trocar and sheath just inside the capsule of the knee.	**4.** Employ necessary sharps precautions for #11 blade and trocars.
5. Sharp trocar is removed and replaced with the blunt. The sheath is now advanced into the knee joint. The blunt trocar is removed and the 30-degree scope is inserted.	**5.** The camera is attached to the top of the scope and the light source to the side. Tubing attached to the inflow trocar is usually switched to the inlet valve/port on the side of the arthroscope sheath. The inflow trocar is now the outflow trocar.
6. For additional incisions, the surgeon inserts the spinal needle under direct vision as a guide to make an anteromedial stab incision.	**6.** This incision serves at the entry for inserting probes and instruments.
7. Beginning in the suprapatellar pouch, the patellofemoral joint is visualized. Next the medial and lateral aspects of the knee are viewed to examine the menisci and ACL.	**7.** Assist with leg stabilization as needed. Remote control may be used to document procedure with still photos.
8. The probe or nerve hook is inserted. It is used to determine if the menisci and ACL are intact or have suffered a tear.	**8.** The shaver may be used to shave the posterior surface of the patella that displays a frayed appearance due to osteoarthritis. Gently pressing down on the patella will aid the surgeon in shaving the movable patella.
9. The scope is inserted in the opposite portal (medial side of knee joint) to complete the examination by looking at the medial femoral condyle, medial meniscus, and posterior cruciate ligament.	**9.** A common tear of meniscus is the "bucket handle" tear.
10. At the end of the procedure, the fluid is allowed to freely flow through the knee joint, thoroughly irrigating the site.	**10.** Small pieces of tissue that are not irrigated out can get wedged in the joint causing the knee to lock into place.
11. The sheaths are removed. Wounds are closed.	**11.** Adson tissue forceps and needle holder with suture is used to close the portals; ½-in. Steri-Strips are applied over the incision sites. It is a routine practice for the surgeon to inject a local anesthetic, usually 0.25% Marcaine, within the joint to aid in postoperative pain management.

PROCEDURE

21-2 Knee Arthroscopy *(continued)*

Postoperative Considerations

Immediate Postoperative Care
- Transport to PACU
- Observe for local hemorrhage

Prognosis
- Return to normal activities

Complications
- Hemorrhage
- Wound infection

PEARL OF WISDOM

Be sure all videoscopic equipment is in working order prior to use.

- Prime fluid pump.
- Balance camera color field.
- Be sure cable/electrical connections are secure.
- Be sure camera remote has charged batteries.

ARTHROSCOPIC REPAIR OF MENISCAL TEAR

Injury to the menisci is one of the most common knee injuries (Figure 21-20). Various types of tears can occur in the meniscus, the most common being what is called the *bucket handle*. The bucket handle consists of an incomplete longitudinal tear with displacement of the inner portion of the meniscus. When a tear of this type is encountered, an arthroscopic partial meniscectomy, or repair, can be completed (Procedure 21-3).

The aim of meniscal surgery is preservation of as much of the cartilage as possible. The goal of the surgeon is to leave the rim of meniscus intact to aid in cushioning and stabilizing the knee joint. Extensive tears require a total meniscectomy, but this leaves the knee somewhat unstable.

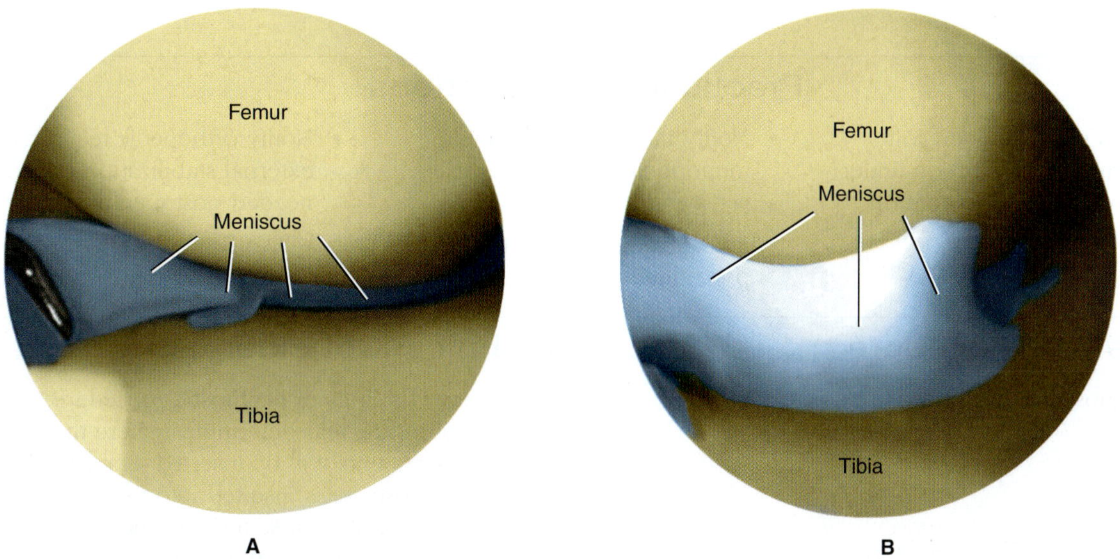

Figure 21-20 **Torn meniscus: (A) Medial meniscus tear with fragment, (B) fragment dislocated into knee joint**

PROCEDURE

21-3 Arthroscopic Repair of a Torn Meniscus

Equipment

- Tourniquet
- Fluid pump
- Power source for arthroscopic shaver
- Video equipment
- Light source
- Positioning devices as needed
- Electrosurgical unit
- Appropriate extremity holder

Instruments

- Arthroscopy set
- Meniscal repair instrument set
- Meniscus suture
- Pituitary rongeur
- Small scissors
- Long Beaver knife handle with blade
- Arthroscopic shaver

Supplies

- Orthopedic pack
- Special drapes if needed
- Basin set
- Gloves
- Blades
- Suture of choice (4–0 or 5–0 nylon or undyed synthetic nonabsorbable is often used)
- Dressing: 4 × 4 sponges, Webril or Kerlix wrapped around knee joint, 6-in. Ace bandage

Operative Preparation

Anesthesia

- General, spinal, or local anesthesia can be used depending on the extent of the operative procedure

Position

- Supine
- The end of the OR table may be lowered according to surgeon's preference
- A padded lateral post is attached to the side of the OR table approximately at the level of the mid-thigh to facilitate placing countertraction on the knee joint to open the medial side

Prep

- Affected leg—circumferential
- Donor site (if graft procedure)

Draping

- Lower extremity draping method

Practical Considerations

- Prior to prep, surgeon will perform an examination under anesthesia (EUA) to confirm diagnostic findings
- Have X-rays or MRIs in OR
- Notify radiology of possible intraoperative X-ray
- Have C-arm near OR
- Follow radiology safety procedures
- Notify orthopedic technician if external stabilization methods needed postoperatively
- Check monitors and photographic equipment

Operative Procedure	Technical Considerations
1. Diagnostic arthroscopy is performed.	**1.** Observe findings of diagnostic procedure: location of the tear determines where the scope and instruments will be inserted. For a medial tear, arthroscope is inserted into the medial portal and the cannula is inserted into the lateral portal site. Vice versa for a lateral tear.

PROCEDURE

21-3 Arthroscopic Repair of a Torn Meniscus *(continued)*

2. A probe is inserted to identify and free up the torn section of the meniscus.
3. A clamp is inserted to grasp the torn meniscus. A cutting instrument such as the Beaver knife or scissors is used to resect the meniscus (Figure 21-21).

2. An 18-gauge spinal needle may be used to identify a fourth incision site.
3. The surgical options are to resect or repair. Adjust instrumentation according to surgeon's decision.

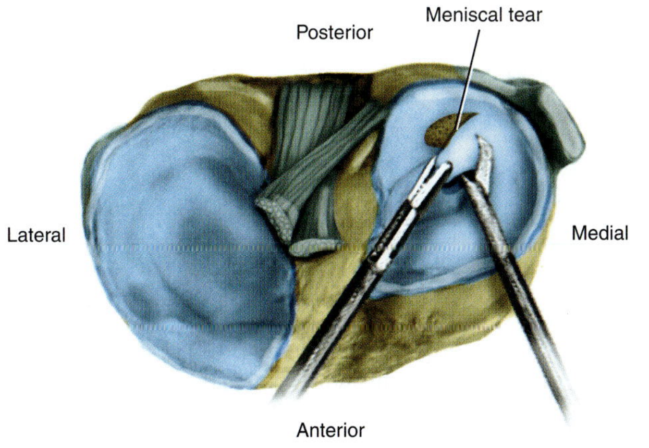

Figure 21-21 Arthroscopic meniscal resection

4. Pituitary rongeur or arthroscopic shaver with side cutting blade can be used to smooth the edge of the torn area and create an even line of tissue.

4. If the meniscal tear is going to be repaired, the instrumentation from the meniscal repair set will be used. The instrument set will contain various cannulas that are straight or curved; the type of cannula required is determined by the location of the tear.

5. The cannula is positioned and each needle with suture is inserted into the cannula, through the meniscus, and across the tear, forming a loop of suture over the tear.
6. The needle is passed through the anterolateral portal so the sutures pass through the medial meniscus.
7. The needle tips are palpated under the skin and the surgeon, using a #15 knife blade, makes a small incision in order to pull the suture out of the knee joint.

5. Meniscal repair kits are commercially available that contain two long Keith needles attached by suture. The suture of preference is usually 0 or 2–0 Vicryl, PDS, or Prolene.
6. The STSR may be asked to operate the camera while the surgeon performs the repair.
7. After the sutures are placed, the knee is flexed and extended to ensure that the range of movement is not constricted. Watch sterile field carefully during manipulation. A needle holder may be used to initially grasp and deliver the needle from the wound.

8. The needles are cut off and the suture tied to bring the torn edges of the meniscus together.

8. The sutures are usually tied with the knee extended. Prepare for closing while sutures are tied.

(continues)

PROCEDURE 21-3 Arthroscopic Repair of a Torn Meniscus *(continued)*

9. After the repair is completed, the knee joint is thoroughly irrigated. The closure and dressing are the same as for a diagnostic arthroscopy.	**9.** Prepare dressing material. Local anesthetic may be injected to aid in postoperative pain control.

Postoperative Considerations

Immediate Postoperative Care

- Transport to PACU
- Observe for local hemorrhage

Prognosis

- Return to normal activities
- May require postoperative rehabilitation (physical therapy)

Complications

- Hemorrhage
- Wound infection
- Joint infection

PEARL OF WISDOM

If the STSR is required to operate the camera or stabilize the extremity during the repair, be sure all necessary items are within the surgeon's reach.

ARTHROSCOPIC ANTERIOR CRUCIATE LIGAMENT REPAIR

The anterior cruciate ligament (ACL) averages a length of 38 mm and width of 10 mm that is made up of collagen fibers. The blood supply to the ACL is from the middle genicular artery, and the ACL receives its innervation from the tibial nerve.

The femoral attachment is the medial aspect of the lateral femoral condyle in the intercondylar notch. The ACL inserts into the interspinous area of the tibia. It is an important stabilizing structure and the most frequently injured ligament of the knee. ACL tears often occur in younger athletic patients who play basketball and football; in older patients, the tears are most often from skiing injuries. The tear is usually due to noncontact deceleration that produces a **valgus** twisting injury. An example is an athlete who places the foot and pivots in a quick manner in the opposite direction.

MRI is used as an aid to diagnose and confirm an ACL tear. Several clinical diagnostic tests can also be used as aids in diagnosing a tear. A popular test is the Lachman test, and the following is a description for a tear of the right knee. The knee is placed in 15 degrees of flexion and slight external rotation to relax the iliotibial band. The surgeon will place the right hand on the medial side of the calf while the left hand grabs the lateral aspect of the thigh. The right hand pulls the lower leg slightly in an anterior direction, while the left hand pushes the upper part of the leg slightly posteriorly. In this way, the surgeon can determine if a tear has occurred and the millimeters of displacement.

If the patient does not respond to rehabilitation, exercises, and other nonoperative treatment, arthroscopic repair has become the standard for surgical treatment. ACL repair involves replacement of the ligament with autograft, synthetic ligament, or allograft. Autografts are most often used and include patellar tendon graft (the most frequently used), iliotibial band, or semitendinosus tendon.

Instrumentation and equipment include the basic orthopedic instrument set, knee arthroscopic instruments, video equipment, ACL guide system, bone tunnel plugs, fixation device such as bone screws, staples, or spiked washers (surgeon's preference), power drill, microsagittal saw, and tourniquet.

The surgeon will perform an examination under anesthesia (EUA) before the skin prep and draping are performed. A diagnostic arthroscopy will be carried out to confirm the diagnosis and perform any preliminary procedures such as repairing a meniscal tear. Refer to Procedure 21-2, Knee Arthroscopy, on pages 825–827. The rest of this discussion concentrates on the ACL repair.

NOTCHPLASTY

The portion of the ACL that remains is debrided using a full-radius resector attached to the arthroscopic shaver. A notchplasty is performed using a 4.5-mm arthroplasty bur, osteotome, and rasp. Notchplasty widens the anterior portion of the intercondylar notch by removing 3–5 mm of bone and recessing the roof of the intercondylar notch to prevent impingement on the ACL graft.

PATELLAR TENDON HARVEST AND PREPARATION

A small incision is made on the distal lateral portion of the femur downward to the lateral aspect of the femoral condyle. The femoral aiming device is positioned and the guide pin inserted at the femoral site into the posterior and superior area of the intercondylar notch. A second anterior incision is made below the knee that is medial to the tibial tubercle. The tibial aiming device is positioned and the guide pin inserted at the anterior tibial incision into the intercondylar notch just medial to the site of ACL attachment to the tibia. The pins are now replaced with #1 or #2 suture that is passed through the pin sites. The surgeon then moves the knee through a series of motions to confirm that the measurements of the aiming devices are correct.

A longitudinal midline incision is made near the patellar tendon. Small retractors are placed to expose the tendon. The surgeon inserts a Joker underneath the tendon and moves it proximally and distally to loosen the tendon from its attachments. The surgeon uses either a marking pen or the cautery to outline 1-in.-long patellar and tibial bone plugs. Two 2 mm holes are drilled in the patellar and tibial bone plugs. Using the microsagittal saw, the surgeon begins the removal of the central one-third portion of the patellar tendon with the 2.5-cm tibial and patellar bone plugs. The bone saw is initially used for the harvest, and the task is completed with a ¼-in. curved osteotome.

The STSR should clear a small area on the back table for the surgeon to prepare the graft for insertion. A green towel should be laid down to reinforce the area and prevent a tear in the sterile table cover. The surgeon uses a tendon-sizing device to stretch the tendon to full length to aid in preparation. The surgeon then uses curved Mayo scissors to debride the graft and size it to the appropriate width, usually 10–12 mm. The sharp edges of the bone plugs may be gently crushed and formed with pliers. The surgeon will place heavy nonabsorbable synthetic sutures (usually #2 and #5 Ethibond) through the drill holes for the tibial and femoral tunnels.

FEMORAL AND TIBIAL TUNNEL

The two-incision approach is the established standard for arthroscopic ACL reconstruction as opposed to the one-incision technique that presents obstacles to proper placement of the graft. The lateral condyle is exposed in the second incision and Hohmann retractors placed to protect the soft tissues and the vastus lateralis.

An angled curette is used to create the starting point for the femoral tunnel. The guide pin is reinserted and overdrilled with the cannula to create a 10-mm tunnel. The tibial tunnel is created in the same fashion. The tunnels are smoothed using a curette or abrader (egg-shaped bur) placed on the arthroscopic shaver.

GRAFT INSERTION AND FIXATION

Prior to placing the graft, each end of the graft is marked with a skin marker. The inflow should be turned off since the saline will cause the graft to expand. As one last step prior to graft insertion, the surgeon may use a pituitary rongeur to remove soft tissue that surrounds the outer portion of the femoral tunnel to facilitate in passage of the graft. The smaller of the bone plugs is placed into the tunnel first, ensuring that the cortical side of the proximal bone plug is facing posteriorly. Under arthroscopic visualization, a Schnidt clamp is passed up the tibial tunnel to grab the stay sutures to pull them out of the tibial tunnel and help in passing the graft. The surgeon also confirms that the bone plugs are in place by viewing the blue marks that were made on the edge of each bone plug. Both ends of the graft are fixed with either staples, bone screws with spiked washers, or the more commonly used interference screws or bioabsorbable screws. The graft is fixed with the knee in 20–30 degrees of flexion to maintain the physiological tension. Under arthrosopic exam, the surgeon will confirm there is no impingement of the graft with the knee in full extension.

WOUND CLOSURE AND POSTOPERATIVE REHABILITATION

Prior to wound closure, the joint is thoroughly irrigated. During the procedure the STSR should have collected as much as possible of the bone chips created during the reaming of the femoral and tibial tunnels. The surgeon may place the chips in the defect caused by the harvesting of the patellar tendon as an aid in healing. A bone tamp may be used to keep the chips in place. Other options from which surgeons can choose are either not repairing the tendon at all or repairing the tendon with a 0 Vicryl, simple or horizontal mattress suture technique. Regardless of the choice of the surgeon, the paratenon must be repaired. The rest of the wound closure is accomplished in the usual fashion for knee surgery procedures.

A bulky dressing is placed and a hinged knee brace may be placed. Current studies are showing that there is no difference in the surgical outcome between patients who wear a brace and those who do not. During the postoperative period up to the eighth week, the patient will use crutches or a cane for assisted ambulation in combination with rehabilitation that includes range-of-motion exercises, straight leg raises, TENS unit, toe raises, and minisquats. By 2 weeks postoperative, the patient should be able to obtain 0 degrees of extension and 90 degrees of flexion by 4 weeks.

ABOVE-THE-KNEE AMPUTATION

Amputations are most often performed because of trauma or disease that inhibits a good vascular supply to the extremity. Diabetic patients, who are prone to nonhealing ulcers and poor vascularity to the extremities, are at risk for amputation, in particular the foot and leg. The goal of the surgery is to preserve as much of the movement of the proximal leg as possible and to allow the patient to eventually ambulate with a prosthesis. However, the health of the patient often determines if he or she will be a good candidate for a prosthesis.

Amputations are performed quickly in order to control hemorrhaging; consequently, the STSR must be prepared to keep up with the surgeon during the procedure. The patient receives either general or spinal anesthesia. The skin prep and draping are done in the normal fashion for an extremity with application of the tourniquet prior to the skin prep. The level of the bone resection will be approximately 4–6 inches proximal to the knee joint line. The surgeon will use a #10 knife blade to make an incision that is in the shape of the mouth of a fish. The STSR must have several lap sponges available to soak up blood to aid in exposure. The surgeon will also control bleeding with the cautery.

Using sharp and blunt dissection, the surgeon creates two skin flaps: an anterior flap so the scar will be in the posterior, and a long adductor muscle flap that will be used to suture across the end of the resected femur. The anterior muscles are transected with a #10 knife blade or Liston amputating knife (Figure 21-22). The femur can now be transected. The femoral periosteum is elevated with a Key elevator or #10 knife blade. The surgeon may use either a power saw, Gigli saw (Figure 21-23), or Satterlee bone saw (Figure 21-24). The posterior muscles are identified and transected. The STSR must be prepared with several clamps and nonabsorbable suture ties for the surgeon to doubly clamp, ligate, and cut the major blood vessels. The end of the sciatic nerve is clamped with a Schnidt clamp and ligated with cautery.

The posterior muscles are freed from their attachments to the femur with a Key elevator and the periosteum is cut circumferentially with the knife blade at the level of the femoral bone transection. The surgeon uses a 7/64 drill bit to drill holes into the cortex of the transected end of the femur. The adductor flap is sutured across the femoral end, utilizing the drill holes, while the STSR keeps the femur in adduction as the surgeon ties down the adductors. The surgeon will either suture the quadriceps to

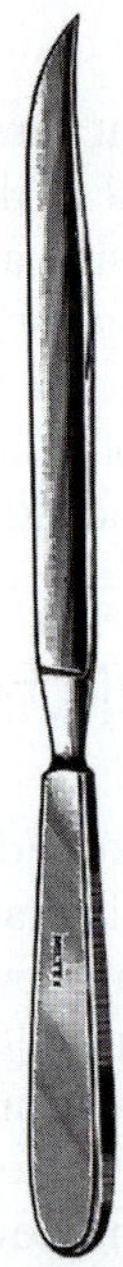

Figure 21-22 Liston amputating knife *(Photo courtesy of Miltex, Inc.)*

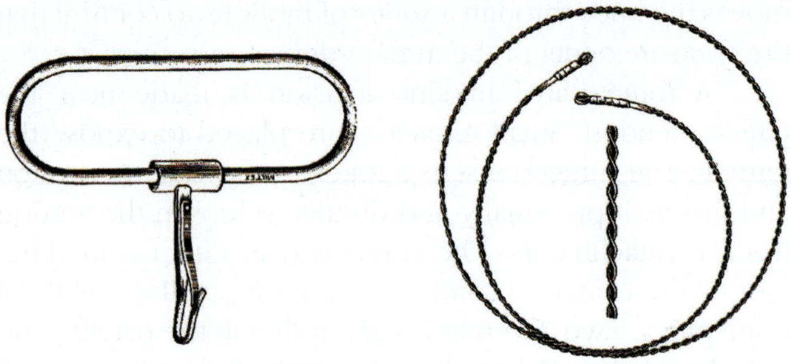

Figure 21-23 Gigli-Strully saw handle and Gigli 12-in. saw *(Photo courtesy of Miltex, Inc.)*

the posterior femur or adductor flap. While the surgeon is suturing the quadriceps in place, the STSR will keep the femur in extension position to avoid hip flexion contracture. A bulky dressing will be placed and often the patient is transported to the ICU for an overnight stay and then moved back to the ward.

ENDOSCOPIC CARPAL TUNNEL RELEASE

Carpal tunnel syndrome (CTS) is a common entrapment syndrome of the upper extremity that is frequently work related and possibly due to repeated motions. To relieve the symptoms of CTS, the transverse carpal ligament (TCL) is surgically released to relieve the pressure on the median nerve.

The median nerve innervates the forearm and long finger flexors. It also provides the palm of the hand, index finger, and thumb their sensory ability.

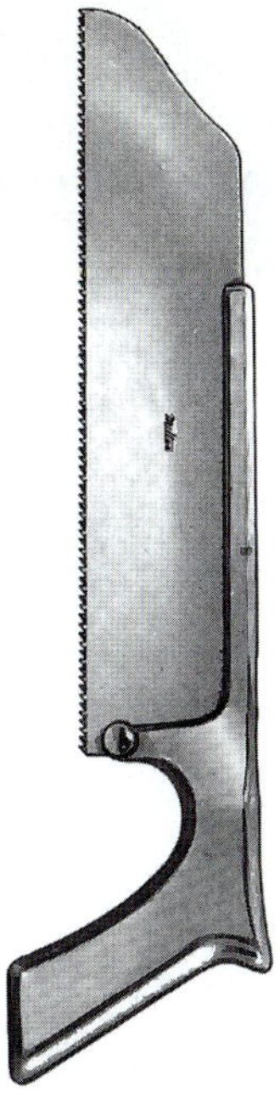

Figure 21-24 **Satterlee bone saw** ***(Photo courtesy of Miltex, Inc.)***

The roof of the carpal tunnel is the TCL. The carpals are arranged in two rows of four forming a concavity on their anterior or palmar surface. The TCL transversely covers this concavity through which the long flexor tendons and the median nerve pass. The TCL is attached ulnarly to the hamulus, or hook, of the hamate bone and radially to the tuberosity of the scaphoid and trapezium bones.

The median nerve enters the carpal tunnel on the palmar side of the wrist in proximity to the radial side of the palmaris longus tendon. Anteriorly the median nerve is covered by the TCL and posteriorly on the radial side by the flexor tendons.

Patients with CTS present with the following clinical signs and symptoms:

1. Tingling of the fingers
2. Numbness in the fingers, often nocturnally waking the individual
3. Loss of sensation in the fingers
4. Decrease in motor control

The endoscopic release of the TCL can be accomplished with one of two operative methods (Procedure 21-4). The first is the single-incision approach and the second is the two-incision approach developed by Dr. James Chow.

Contraindications for performing an endoscopic CTR are the presence of infection, recurrent CTS, and previous surgery of the wrist that may have caused scarring and adhesions at the operative site.

The advantages of performing an endoscopic CTR include rapid return of strength, less scarring and fewer adhesions, less pain, and ability to return to normal activity sooner than if an open procedure were performed. The disadvantages include limited ability to visualize other anatomical structures, possible inability to control a bleeding vessel, and possibility of causing injury to the structures of the carpal tunnel such as the flexor tendons and median nerve.

PROCEDURE 21-4 Endoscopic Carpal Tunnel Release

Equipment

- Videoscopic equipment
- Tourniquet
- Fluid pump
- Light source

Instruments

- Endoscopic set
- Plastic or minor set
- Tenotomy scissors
- Camera
- Light cord
- 4-mm, 30-degree scope
- Ragnell retractors
- Blunt trocar and sheath
- Probe knife
- Triangle knife
- Retrograde reverse cutting blade

(continues)

PROCEDURE 21-4 Endoscopic Carpal Tunnel Release *(continued)*

Supplies

- Minor pack
- Special drapes if needed
- Basin set
- Gloves
- Blades
- Suture of choice
- Dressing of choice
- Extra towels

Operative Preparation

Anesthesia
- Regional block with the use of the tourniquet and sedation

Position
- Supine
- Operative hand/arm table

Prep
- Upper extremity—circumferential

Draping
- Upper extremity draping method

Practical Considerations

- Notify orthopedic technician if external stabilization methods needed postoperatively.
- Check monitors and photographic equipment.
- Chairs (for surgeon and STSR) opposite each other.

Operative Procedure (Chow)	Technical Considerations
1. A marking pen is used to identify the entry portal. A 1-cm transverse incision is made with a #15 knife blade through the fascia exposing the flexor tendon.	**1.** Aid the surgeon's view by slight manual retraction of the fingers away from the incision area.
2. The flexor tendon is retracted radially with two Ragnell retractors; the space between the flexor tendon and ulnar neurovascular bundle is identified.	**2.** Hand retractors and prepare trocar assembly.
3. A blunt trocar sheath assembly is inserted distally into the identified space underneath the TCL. The wrist is now placed in dorsiflexion with the use of a stack of hand towels. Simultaneously, the trocar is slightly lifted up along the arch of the hook of hamate and advanced distally to the base of the carpal ligament, staying outside of the flexor tendon sheath.	**3.** A "lead hand" may also be used in conjunction with stacked towels to retract fingers and thumb.
4. Near the predetermined exit portal, the trocar is advanced into the subcutaneous tissue. A second small incision is made and the trocar sheath assembly is pushed through the opening.	**4.** Secure knife for second incision.
5. The blunt trocar is removed, leaving the sheath in place. The endoscope is inserted proximally into the sheath.	**5.** Place lens of the endoscope in warm water prior to insertion, to prevent fogging. Have antifog solution available. Q-tips inserted distally can be used to wipe the lens.

PROCEDURE

21-4 Endoscopic Carpal Tunnel Release *(continued)*

6. The blunt probe is inserted distally and is used to dissect the bursal membranes covering the opening of the sheath.	**6.** Often the STSR is responsible for operating the scope and camera to follow the surgeon as cuts are made.
7. The carpal ligament can now be identified. The sheath is dissected proximal to distal until the TCL is clearly visualized.	**7.** Concentrate on maintenance of camera position.
8. The probe knife is introduced to begin the release of the distal to proximal edge of the TCL.	**8.** The probe knife only allows forward cutting action.
9. A triangle knife is now introduced to cut the midsection of the TCL.	**9.** Hand triangle knife.
10. A retrograde reverse cutting blade is inserted into the incision made by the triangle knife and is drawn distally, joining the first two cuts together and completely releasing the distal aspect of the TCL.	**10.** Maintain continuous flow of irrigation fluid.
11. The endoscope is now removed and placed in the distal end of the sheath.	**11.** Have Q-tips ready to wipe the lens.
12. The probe knife is used to cut the proximal edge of the TCL and the retrograde reverse cutting knife is used to complete the proximal dissection.	**12.** Follow facility protocol for sharps handling.
13. The scope is removed, trocar reinserted, and the sheath removed. The two entry portals are sutured with 4–0 or 5–0 nylon. Dressing usually consists of fluffs kept in place with Coban.	**13.** A volar plaster splint may be indicated. A small amount of antiseptic or antibiotic solution may be used to irrigate the entry portals before closure is begun.

Postoperative Considerations

Immediate Postoperative Care

- Transport to PACU
- Observe for local hemorrhage
- Check for neural function

Prognosis

- Return to normal activities
- May require postoperative rehabilitation

Complications

- Hemorrhage
- Wound infection
- Median nerve damage

PEARL OF WISDOM

Good visualization is the key to endoscopic procedures. Know how to troubleshoot all aspects of visualization problems. Be prepared to clean the endoscopes immediately.

COLLES' FRACTURE

Colles' fracture is an angulated fracture of the distal radius at the epiphysis approximately 1 in. from the wrist joint. The fracture causes the hand to assume a dorsal and lateral position until treated. Colles' fractures are treated either through closed reduction and application of a cast, external fixation, or, for a comminuted fracture, internal fixation with Kirschner wires (K-wires).

EXTERNAL FIXATION OF COLLES' FRACTURE

External fixation of a fracture provides optimal reduction and immobilization of a fractured bone. The advantages of using an external fixating device include decreased interference with the joint, early mobilization for the patient, and elimination of the need for casting.

Many types of external fixators are commercially available, varying in design depending on the area of the body for which they are intended.

Common features of external fixation devices include:

- Threaded or smooth Steinmann pins and/or Kirschner wires
- Clamps and rings to connect and hold the device together
- Long smooth rods that serve as the supporting device for the clamps and rings

The placement of an external fixation device is a sterile procedure (Procedure 21-5). The external fixator is usually available from the manufacturer in its own sterile package and does not require any type of processing by the central sterile supply department.

PROCEDURE 21-5 External Fixation of a Colles' Fracture

Equipment

- Fluoroscopy machine

Instruments

- Basic orthopedic instrument set
- Power drill
- Pin cutter

Supplies

- Orthopedic pack
- Special drapes if needed
- Basin set
- Gloves
- Blades
- Fixation device and accessories
- Dressing: 4 × 4 sponges dipped in povidone-iodine solution and wrapped around the sites of the entry of the pins

Operative Preparation

Anesthesia

- General or regional

Position

- Supine

Prep

- Upper extremity

Draping

- Upper extremity draping method

Practical Considerations

- Have X-rays or CT scans in OR
- Notify radiology of possible intraoperative X-ray
- Have C-arm in OR
- Follow radiology safety procedures

Operative Procedure	Technical Considerations
1. Fracture is reduced under fluoroscopy. An external frame may be placed to stabilize the fracture.	1. Assist with positioning and stabilize the extremity as needed.

PROCEDURE

21-5 External Fixation of a Colles' Fracture *(continued)*

2. A small longitudinal incision is made from the base of the second metacarpal to the middle of the shaft. The soft tissue is bluntly dissected down to the bone. Small Hohmann retractors may be used.

2. A #15 knife blade is used. The metacarpal incision is performed first to ensure proper length of the fixator.

3. A drill guide is used as a directional aid and to protect the surrounding soft tissues from the drill bit.

3. Be sure that the size of the drill guide coordinates with the selected drill bit. The size is usually imprinted on the guide.

4. Pins are inserted with the use of a power drill.

4. Pins will be placed above and below the fracture site.

5. The distal (metacarpal) pins are inserted at a 45- to 60-degree angle with the tips imbedded in, but not penetrating, the far cortex.

5. A marking pen may be used to mark the sites of insertion.

6. A longitudinal incision is made in the forearm and tissues are bluntly dissected down to the bone. The sensory branch of the radial nerve must be preserved.

6. Blunt rakes are used to provide gentle retraction.

7. Fluoroscopy is used throughout the procedure to confirm the placement of the pins and that the reduction of the fracture is maintained.

7. Wear lead gloves if necessary.

8. Proximal (radial) pins are inserted in the fashion described for the distal pins.

8. The surgeon may place pins so that a slight protrusion is achieved through the far cortex for osteopenic bone.

9. Clamps and/or joints are slipped over the pins and the longitudinal supportive rod is put in place.

9. Be sure the securing screws on the frame are facing laterally to facilitate tightening.

10. A frame is placed over the pins and the clamps are secured. Tightening the clamps holds the fracture in reduction.

10. Wrenches are used to tighten the frame (Figure 21-25).

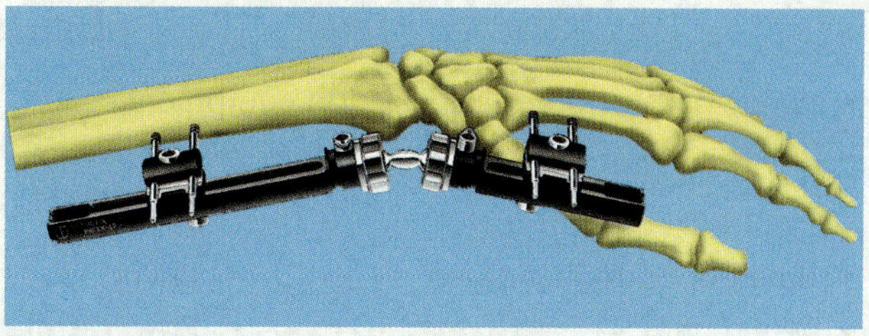

Figure 21-25 External fixation—Colles' fracture

11. Any flexion/extension, radial/ulnar, length, and supination/pronation deviations are corrected by adjusting the frame.

11. More than one wrench may be useful.

12. A final X-ray is taken to confirm pin placement and fracture reduction.

12. Be sure patient and all team members are protected from radiation.

13. Dressing is applied.

13. Sutures are generally not needed.

(continues)

PROCEDURE

21-5

External Fixation of a Colles' Fracture *(continued)*

Postoperative Considerations

Immediate Postoperative Care

- Transport to PACU
- Observe for local hemorrhage
- Pain management

Prognosis

- Return to normal activities
- May require postoperative rehabilitation

Complications

- Hemorrhage
- Wound infection
- Nerve damage

PEARL OF WISDOM

Anticipate the use of fluoroscopy and X-ray machines. Follow all radiation safety procedures.

INTERNAL K-WIRE FIXATION OF A COLLES' FRACTURE

Colles' fractures may be stabilized by internal as well as external methods. The internal approach is represented by K-wire fixation (Procedure 21-6).

PROCEDURE

21-6

Internal K-wire Fixation of a Colles' Fracture

Equipment

- Armboards or other stabilization equipment

Instruments

- Small open reduction set
- Wire cutter
- Pliers
- Power drill
- K-wire set

Supplies

- Orthopedic pack
- Special drapes if needed
- Basin set
- Gloves
- Blades
- Suture of choice
- Dressing

PROCEDURE 21-6

Internal K-wire Fixation of a Colles' Fracture *(continued)*

Operative Preparation

Anesthesia
- General

Position
- Supine with the affected arm laid on the hand table

Prep
- Upper extremity

Draping
- Extremity draping method

Practical Considerations

- Have X-rays or MRIs in OR
- Notify radiology of possible intraoperative X-ray
- Have C-arm near OR
- Follow radiology safety procedures
- Notify orthopedic technician if external stabilization methods needed postoperatively

Operative Procedure	Technical Concíderations
1. Fracture is reduced under fluoroscopy.	1. Be sure patient and staff are protected from radiation. STSR may be asked to stabilize extremity during closed reduction.
2. A small stab incision is made.	2. A #15 or #11 blade is used.
3. Pins are inserted with the use of a power drill.	3. The number of pins inserted depends on the location of the fracture.
4. Fluoroscopy is used throughout the procedure to confirm pin placement.	4. Wear lead gloves if necessary.
5. Pins are cut close to the skin surface. Ends may be angled to reduce risk of injury due to protrusion of the pin.	5. Provide pin cutter and pliers.
6. Final radiographic verification is achieved and dressings are applied.	6. Antibiotic ointment may be applied and if gauze is used it may be cut with a bandage scissors to facilitate placement around the pin. External stabilization (cast or splint) may be applied.

Postoperative Considerations

Immediate Postoperative Care
- Transport to PACU
- Observe for local hemorrhage
- Postoperative X-rays

Prognosis
- Return to normal activities
- May require postoperative rehabilitation

Complications
- Hemorrhage
- Wound infection
- Nerve damage

PEARL OF WISDOM

Be sure that when the pin is cut, the free end does not become airborne and cause injury.

METACARPAL PHALANGEAL JOINT ARTHROPLASTY

Metacarpal phalangeal joint (MPJ) arthroplasty is indicated in patients for the following reasons: severe dislocation, volar subluxation, or disabling deformity with articular cartilage damage due to rheumatoid or degenerative arthritis. The goals of the surgery are to restore function to the finger through joint alignment and stability and to relieve chronic pain. However, the patient should not expect to have the same amount of grasping strength as previous to developing the disabling condition.

In addition to a hand set and the instrumentation for implants, other items that will be needed are properly sized implants, small Hohmann retractors, skin hooks, powered bur, and several #15 knife blades. A Bier block with tourniquet will most likely be the anesthesia of choice.

The patient is placed in the supine position and the operative arm and hand placed on the hand table. After the tourniquet is in place and the Bier block administered, the arm is prepped from fingers to mid-biceps and the extremity drape placed. The initial transverse incision is made over the metacarpal to expose the extensor tendons. The veins and nerves located between the metacarpal are preserved. The surgeon continues the dissection by releasing the intrinsic tendons and joint capsule. The STSR should remember to change the knife blade frequently during the surgical procedure; the blades will quickly dull when the surgeon is dissecting tendon and bone.

Next the surgeon accomplishes the metacarpal neck resection. Using the knife blade, the collateral ligaments are released from the metacarpal neck. Two Hohmann retractors are placed underneath the metacarpal neck to elevate it, and a small saw is used to transect the metacarpal head at the neck. A small rasp is used to smooth the bone ends. The proximal phalanx is prepared first. The bur is used to make the initial entry into the medullary canal and next the broaches are used. The same process is then completed for the metacarpal.

Various sizes of prosthesis are used to facilitate the correct fit. STSRs should wipe their gloves off to remove any talc before handling the prosthesis, even though this should have been done before the beginning of the case. Once the appropriate size of implant is chosen, the ends are positioned within the medullary canals. The surgeon then irrigates the surgical wound and begins closure. The capsular flaps are secured with a horizontal mattress suture to cover the implant to aid in decreasing the risk of infection, and the extensor tendon is realigned with suture. Dressing and a forearm splint are placed.

TRIPLE ARTHRODESIS

The result of a triple arthrodesis is the fusion of the subtalar, calcaneocuboid, and talonavicular joints. The procedure is most effective for individuals suffering from a forefoot or hindfoot deformity. Such deformities are the result of clubfoot, rheumatoid arthritis, or poliomyelitis. The procedure is contraindicated in children younger than 10–12 years of age since the procedure limits the foot growth and has a high failure rate. Postoperatively the procedure only allows plantar flexion and dorsiflexion motions.

The instrumentation and equipment include a basic orthopedic instrument set, power saw and drill, rasp, bone graft instruments, AO compression plates and screws, Kirschner wires, Hohmann retractors, Crego retractors, and small lamina spreader.

The patient receives either general or spinal anesthesia and is placed in the supine position with a sandbag bump placed under the hip on the operative side. The skin prep involves the foot to the midcalf circumferentially. The iliac crest is also prepped to obtain bone for the bone grafting portion of the procedure. Extremity draping is in usual fashion except to ensure that the iliac crest is exposed.

Depending on the surgeon's preference, the incision will be oblique, which parallels the subtalar joint, or anterolateral, which is a longitudinal incision between the tip of the lateral malleolus and the base of the fourth metatarsal. The extensor digitorum brevis is resected from its point of insertion, and soft tissue dissection is continued with a #15 knife blade and rongeur.

The first resection is the subtalar joint. A Crego elevator (Figure 21-26) is placed around the calcaneus at the level of the joint. The joint capsule is incised and the lamina spreader (Figure 21-27) placed. The articular surface of the subtalar joint is removed and smoothed using the power saw, osteotome, curette, and rasp. Next the articular surface of the calcaneocuboid joint is removed by the same method. Last, the articular surface of the talonavicular joint is removed. The head of the joint is manually brought into the wound to facilitate the resection. If the head of the joint cannot be exposed well enough, the surgeon will use a #15 knife blade to release the joint to attain as much mobility as possible. The STSR must ensure that as much of the resected bone as possible is saved for the bone graft, which might enable the surgeon to avoid having to obtain bone from the iliac crest.

The correction of the hindfoot valgus is achieved by fixation of the subtalar joint. The surgeon places a screw,

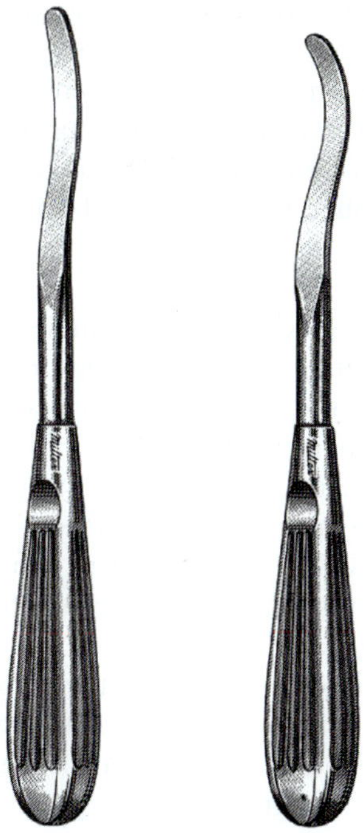

Figure 21-26 **Crego periosteal elevators** ***(Photo courtesy of Miltex, Inc.)***

the usual length being 65 mm, anterior to posterior or posterior to anterior. The forefoot rotation is corrected with fixation of the talonavicular joint. A smooth Steinman pin is inserted toward the center of the head of the talus. Third fixation involves the calcaneocuboid joint, which corrects the forefoot abduction and adduction. Two 4.5-mm cannulated screws will be crossed placed from the anterior process of the calcaneus to the cuboid.

After fixation is achieved, the bone graft is placed. A rongeur is used to cut the bone into small pieces. The bone is placed around the talonavicular joint, in the gap at the calcaneocuboid joint, and in the sinus tarsi. Bone tamps with a mallet may be used to tap the bone graft into place.

The surgeon will thoroughly irrigate the surgical wound site, check the foot and heel for alignment, place a Jackson-Pratt suction drain, and close the wound in layers. A short leg cast or splint will be applied. The pins remain for approximately 6 weeks and the patient may begin weight bearing 10–12 weeks postoperatively.

ACHILLES TENDON REPAIR

The Achilles tendon is most often ruptured, either partially or totally, by a traumatic incident such as avulsion or laceration. Athletes are a common group of individuals at risk for an Achilles tendon rupture, in particular, "weekend athletes." The treatment is surgical repair of the rupture, which must be performed as soon as possible before the tendon atrophies. When the tendon is still of adequate length, the torn ends of the tendon are sutured together. Occasionally the rupture will occur near the calcaneus, necessitating the reinsertion of the proximal end of the tendon into the bone.

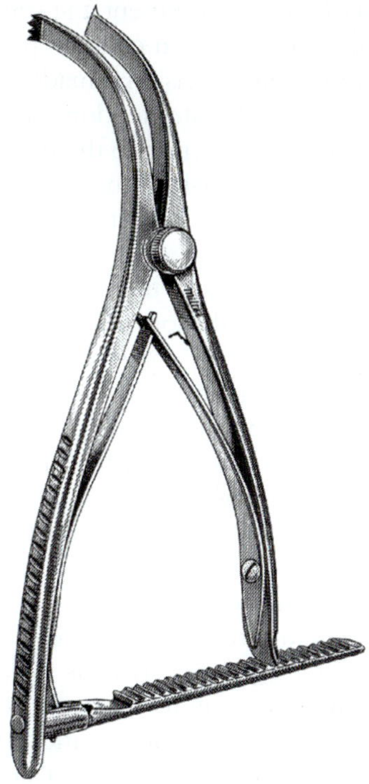

Figure 21-27 **Inge lamina spreader, 6 in.** ***(Photo courtesy of Miltex, Inc.)***

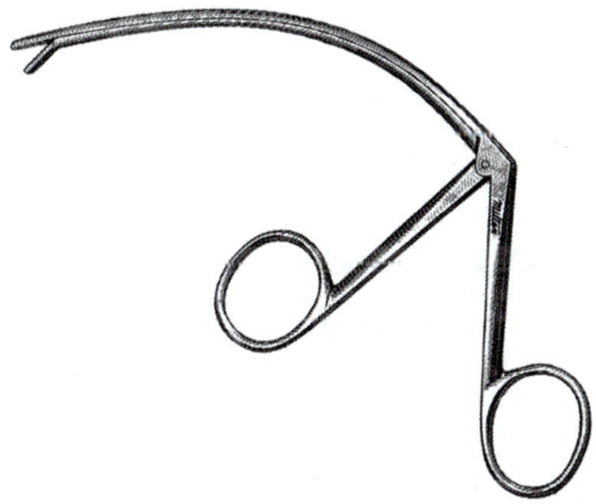

Figure 21-28 **Miltex tendon-pulling forceps** ***(Photo courtesy of Miltex, Inc.)***

A basic orthopedic instrument set will be needed and the surgeon may want a flexible or rigid tendon-pulling forceps (Figure 21-28) available to grasp the proximal portion of the tendon to bring into place for the repair. The patient receives either general or spinal anesthesia; either way, a tourniquet will be needed.

Place the tourniquet while the patient is in the supine position, before turning him or her to the prone position; it is difficult to apply the tourniquet in the prone position. The leg is prepped from mid-thigh to the toes and draped with an extremity drape. Blood is exsanguinated from the leg and the tourniquet inflated.

If an assistant is not present, the surgeon will ask the STSR to maintain the foot in equinus position during the surgery. A longitudinal incision is made with the #10 knife blade medial to the Achilles tendon and carried down to the paratenon. In comparison to the flexor tendons in the hand, which have an outside synovial sheath covering the tendon, the Achilles tendon has no such sheath and is covered by the paratenon.

The ruptured ends of the Achilles tendon are identified. Exploration of the proximal end may occur. The Achilles tendon is always under some degree of constant tension, even when an individual is at rest. Consequently, on rupture, the proximal end may retract upward along the gastrocnemius muscle and require retrieval with the tendon-pulling forceps or other atraumatic clamp. Another atraumatic clamp is placed on the other ruptured end of the tendon and the ends are brought together to achieve the original tendon length.

Several suture repair techniques can be utilized by the surgeon. One popular type is called the Krachow whip stitch, in which suture is placed along each tendon edge to accomplish the approximation. The suture often used is #5 Tycron or Ethibond on a noncutting needle. The surgeon next closes the paratenon over the site of the tendon repair to aid in healing and preventing adhesions from forming. The rest of the wound is closed in layers and a splint dressing applied with the foot maintained in equinus position. After 10 days the splint is removed and approximately 6 weeks postoperative the patient will be able to perform gradual weight bearing.

BUNIONECTOMY

A bunion, medically referred to as hallux valgus, is described as a bony exostosis located on the medial side of the first metatarsal head of the great toe. Bunions are common in females due to the common shoe styles worn by women, including pointed toes and high heels. Other dispositions to developing a bunion include flatfeet, imbalance due to muscle difficulties, and foot pronation. The patient experiences pain and swelling of the great toe.

Various types of surgical procedures are used to treat the condition such as the Aken, Chevron, McKeever, and Keller techniques. All of these procedures have the same outcome of removing the exostosis and realigning the great toe. The goals of surgery are to correct the deformity by removing the exostosis, restore the normal range of motion, and remove the abnormal bony portions to prevent reoccurrence. The Keller technique is described here.

In addition to a basic orthopedic instrument set, Kirschner wires, a power wire-driver, and a microsagittal saw will be needed. Several #15 knife blades will be needed and they will need to be changed often during the procedure.

The patient is placed in the supine position. It is important to confirm which foot will be operated on because patients often have bunions on both feet. A tourniquet is applied to the proximal portion of the thigh. The foot up to the level of the midcalf is circumferentially prepped. Draping for an extremity is accomplished in the usual fashion. A foot drape with a single opening may be used or, if the patient will be having both feet operated upon, a drape with dual openings is available.

A medical incision is made beginning at the neck of the proximal phalanx and extended through the subcutaneous tissue. The joint capsule is opened by making a flap incision to expose the exostosis. The capsular tissue and other soft tissue attachments are stripped from the base of the proximal phalanx of the great toe and metatarsal head. Using the microsagittal saw, the proximal one-third of the proximal phalanx is excised. Using the #15 knife blade, the periosteum and capsular tissues are dissected from the proximal fragment.

Alignment of the joint is maintained by placing two smooth 5⁄64 Steinmann pins across the metatarsal joint. The Steinmann pins hold the bony surfaces apart and are left in place for approximately 4 weeks. The wound is thoroughly irrigated and closed. The dressing is applied so as to maintain toe alignment.

OPEN REDUCTION-INTERNAL FIXATION OF THE HUMERUS

Most fractures involving the shaft of the humerus are best treated with closed reduction and immobilization. Indications for treatment by ORIF include:

- Closed reduction will not produce optimal alignment of the fracture and could contribute to healing disorders such as malunion.
- Soft tissue injuries caused by the fracture are present and require treatment.
- The fracture is spontaneous (pathological) due to an osteoma.

Patients who benefit the most from an ORIF of the humerus are those who sustained a fracture with no comminution (Procedure 21-7).

Due to the large rotational forces placed on the humerus, it is recommended that a broad 4.5 dynamic compression plate (DCP) be used. The length of the plate should be at least five times the diameter of the bone. Depending on the surgeon's preference, an anterior or posterior approach for plating can be used for mid-shaft fractures of the humerus. Some surgeons favor the anterior approach to avoid injury to the radial nerve, which lies posteriorly in the spiral groove of the shaft.

PROCEDURE

21-7 ORIF of the Humerus

Equipment

- Tourniquet
- Power source for instruments

Instruments

- Basic orthopedic instrument set
- Power drill
- ORIF instrument set
- Drill bits
- Tap
- Depth gauge
- Drill and tap guides
- K-wires of various sizes
- Countersink
- Screws and plates of various sizes
- Bone-holding and reduction forceps
- Handle for tap
- Hexagonal screwdriver

Supplies

- Orthopedic pack
- Special drapes if needed
- Basin set
- Gloves
- Blades
- Suture of choice
- Dressing

Operative Preparation

Anesthesia

- General

Position

- Supine, with a roll towel used as a bump under the scapula of the affected side. The arm is positioned on a hand table

Prep

- Includes the hand, entire arm, and past the shoulder up to the border of the neck in case the incision has to be extended

Draping

- Upper extremity draping method

Practical Considerations

- Have X-rays or MRIs in OR
- Notify radiology of possible intraoperative X-ray
- Have C-arm near OR
- Follow radiology safety procedures
- Notify orthopedic technician if external stabilization methods needed postoperatively

Operative Procedure	Technical Considerations
1. The incision for an anterolateral approach to the shaft of the humerus is centered at the level of the fracture. In the upper portion of the arm the skin incision follows the anterior border of the deltoid muscle and continues distally along the lateral border of the biceps muscle.	**1.** A #10 knife blade and electrocautery are used.

(continues)

PROCEDURE

21-7 ORIF of the Humerus *(continued)*

2. Proximal exposure is further achieved by extending the incision, along with deep dissection, along the deltopectoral groove. The cephalic vein is encountered in the groove and is retracted medially or laterally along with the deltoid muscle.

   2. Provide retractors according to patient size and surgeon's preference.

3. The radial nerve is identified. It lies just below and behind the deltoid insertion, on the posterior surface of the humerus in the spiral groove, and twists around the humeral shaft. The entire length of the nerve should be identified so the placement of retractors does not injure the nerve.

   3. Blunt retractors are used without much force applied to avoid injury to the vein and nerve.

4. Distal to the insertion of the deltoid, the biceps muscle is separated from the underlying brachialis muscle and retracted medially. Rake retractors are most likely used throughout the entire procedure.

   4. Blunt, not sharp, dissection is used.

5. At the distal edge of the incision, the origin of the brachialis is identified. At this level, the brachialis muscle blends in with the insertion of the deltoid muscle. The muscle fibers of the brachialis muscle are split down its middle in a longitudinal fashion in such a manner that the lateral third of the brachialis muscle can now be easily retracted.

   5. Deeper retractors may be substituted as procedure progresses.

6. Splitting the brachialis down the middle allows distal exposure of the humerus and prevents damage to the radial nerve, which, at this point, is winding around the humerus laterally and is protected by the musculospiral groove. This also allows exposure as far as the elbow joint.

   6. Have all instruments ready on the Mayo. You may be required to help with postioning and stabilizing the arm.

7. The elbow is flexed to 90 degrees, which allows for easier retraction of the brachialis muscle both laterally and medially, plus it facilitates exposure of the operative site.

   7. The STSR may hold the arm to maintain the position.

8. The brachialis muscle is split down the middle lateral portion to finish the exposure of the humeral shaft and begin the ORIF.

   8. Continue with blunt dissection technique.

9. The fracture is reduced and the bone ends are kept in place with reduction forceps or clamps.

   9. Reduction instruments used include Lohman clamp, bone reduction forceps (similar to perforating towel clamps), and self-retaining bone clamp. The Lohman provides the dual advantage of keeping the fracture reduced and holding the plate in place.

PROCEDURE 21-7 ORIF of the Humerus *(continued)*

10. The correct size plate is chosen and held in place over the fracture site on the bone. Using a drill the surgeon may place one or two K-wires to also aid in holding the fracture together. The first hole is drilled through the opening in the plate and into the bone. The depth of drill hole is measured. The tap is used to prepare the drill hole for the screw. The screw is placed.

10. Instrumentation for the placement of screws follows the same sequence for each screw. Screws are placed above and below the fracture. The correct size drill bit is selected, loaded on the power drill, and handed to the surgeon. A drill guide may be used. Prepare and hand depth gauge. Prepare and hand tap. (Screws that are self-tapping can be identified by an angled notch near the tip of the screw.) Select, load, and hand screw on a driver. (The screw is loaded on the hexagonal screwdriver and kept in place with the holding sleeve. As the surgical technologist hands the screwdriver with screw to the surgeon, the size of the screw is restated as confirmation.) Repeat for all holes in the plate.

11. The incision is closed in layers with 0 and 2–0 Vicryl suture. Skin staples are used and dressing applied.

11. Confirm the size of the plate and screws with the circulator, including the number of each sized screw that was implanted.

Postoperative Considerations

Immediate Postoperative Care

- Patient's arm placed in a sling
- Transport to PACU
- Observe for local hemorrhage

Prognosis

- Return to normal activities
- May require postoperative rehabilitation

Complications

- Hemorrhage
- Wound infection
- Joint infection

PEARL OF WISDOM

There are two main categories of screws available: self-tapping and nontapping. You must be able to identify them on sight. Nontapping screws require that the drill hole be tapped with a tapping device prior to placement of the screw.

SHOULDER JOINT ARTHROSCOPY

Arthroscopy of the shoulder joint, just as with knee arthroscopy, has seen several advancements in relation to surgical instrumentation that allows many procedures to be performed. It is highly beneficial as a diagnostic tool for evaluating patients with chronic shoulder problems and for repairing some types of defects. Procedures that can be performed include the removal of loose bodies, bursectomy, rotator cuff repairs, and repair of impingement syndrome. The following describes an arthroscopy for diagnostic reasons.

The patient is placed either in the lateral or semi-Fowler's position, depending on surgeon's preference. If the patient is placed in lateral position, a vaccum beanbag is used to maintain the position. The operative arm is placed in suspension with 5–15 pounds of weights placed on the pulley system to achieve distraction of the glenohumeral joint. Once the procedure begins, the surgeon may ask for additional weight to be added.

The skin prep involves base of neck, shoulder, scapula, chest to midline, and circumference of the arm up to the level of the elbow. Draping varies according to surgeon's preference, but involves draping the arm free as to permit a full range of shoulder motion during the surgical procedure. Instruments and equipment that are used for a knee arthroscopy are used for a shoulder arthroscopy.

The surgeon will begin by establishing the posterior portal that affords the best visualization of the shoulder joint. The surgeon positions his or her index finger at the point of the coracoid process and inserts an 18-gauge spinal needle just lateral to the process. The STSR hands the surgeon a 20-cc Luer-Lok syringe filled with normal saline for injection through the spinal needle into the shoulder joint to distend the joint and facilitate placement of the trocar and arthroscope. The surgeon may or may not inject up to 5 mL of Marcaine with epinephrine to aid in controlling bleeding.

The spinal needle is removed and the surgeon uses a #11 knife blade to make the stab incision at the point of the spinal needle insertion. The sharp trocar with sleeve is inserted through the joint capsule. The sharp trocar is removed and replaced with the blunt trocar, which is used to enter the shoulder capsule. The blunt trocar is removed and the 30-degree arthroscope is placed. The camera and light source are attached to the arthroscope as are the inflow and outflow tubing to facilitate the distention of the joint.

After the surgeon has examined the shoulder joint and if an operative procedure is warranted, an anterior portal is established. The surgeon establishes the portal using the spinal needle and a #15 knife blade. The site of the portal is lateral to the coracoid process, in the interval between the subscapularis and supraspinatus. Surgical instruments are placed through the anterior portal. The arm is placed through a series of movements and rotations for the surgeon to visualize the various anatomical structures of the shoulder joint.

At the conclusion of the procedure, the surgeon allows plenty of fluid to flow through the joint for irrigation purposes and removal of any loose bodies. Marcaine will be injected into the joint to minimize postoperative pain. The stab wounds are dressed with 4 × 4 sponges and the arm placed in a sling.

ACROMIOPLASTY

Candidates for an acromioplasty are afflicted by impingement syndrome, which limits the range of motion of the shoulder. Often the patient will have completed a rehabilitation program for up to 6 months to attempt to relieve the symptoms and if no improvement is noted, the patient is a candidate for acromioplasty surgery.

The equipment, instruments, supplies, and operative preparation are identical to those for the repair of a rotator cuff. The surgeon makes an incision with the #10 knife blade in an anteroposterior direction between the tip of the acromion and the AC joint. The incision is carried down to the fascia and two Gelpi retractors are placed for exposure. The fascia is freed from its attachments to the deltoid, but left in place for closure at the end of the procedure. Surgeons have two options concerning the deltoid muscle: (1) Dissect through the muscle fibers or (2) dissect off of the deltoid for later reattachment. This description involves dissecting through the muscle fibers.

The deltoid is split anterolateral by blunt and sharp dissection and with the use of cautery. The deltoid is dissected from the anterior acromion and the coracoacromial ligament is excised to expose the undersurface of the acromion. Blunt retractors are placed for exposure. The acromioplasty described here is the Rockwood technique. First, the portion of the anterior acromion that extends beyond the anterior edge of the acromion is resected using a power saw or osteotome. The undersurface of the acromion is beveled with the power saw. A bone rongeur and bone rasp are used to smooth the bone surfaces and remove any sharp edges. The wound is closed in layers and dressing placed similar to that for a rotator cuff repair.

REPAIR OF ROTATOR CUFF

The rotator cuff of the shoulder is composed of four muscles that form a cuff around the shoulder joint. The muscles stabilize the joint and allow it to perform a variety of movements. The four muscles are the infraspinatus, subscapularis, supraspinatus, and teres minor. The four muscles originate in the scapula and their tendons insert onto the tuberosities of the humerus. The acromion is the lateral extension of the spine of the scapula, forming the highest point of the shoulder and articulating with the clavicle. The acromion, also called the acromion process, provides attachment for the deltoid and trapezium muscles. (Refer to the beginning of the chapter for additional anatomical information.)

Injuries to the rotator cuff, specifically tears, will vary in their severity. The need for surgery is based on clinical findings and the degree to which the injury affects the patient's ability to function normally. Surgery, if indicated, should be performed as soon as possible to avoid atrophy and loss of tissue due to a delay in performing the repair. Surgical repair of a previously uninjured shoulder should provide the patient with an optimal result.

In addition to rotator cuff injuries, dislocation and ligament damage commonly occur in the shoulder. Repair of the rotator cuff illustrates the issues and procedures of ligament repair (Figure 21-29) (Procedure 21-8). The

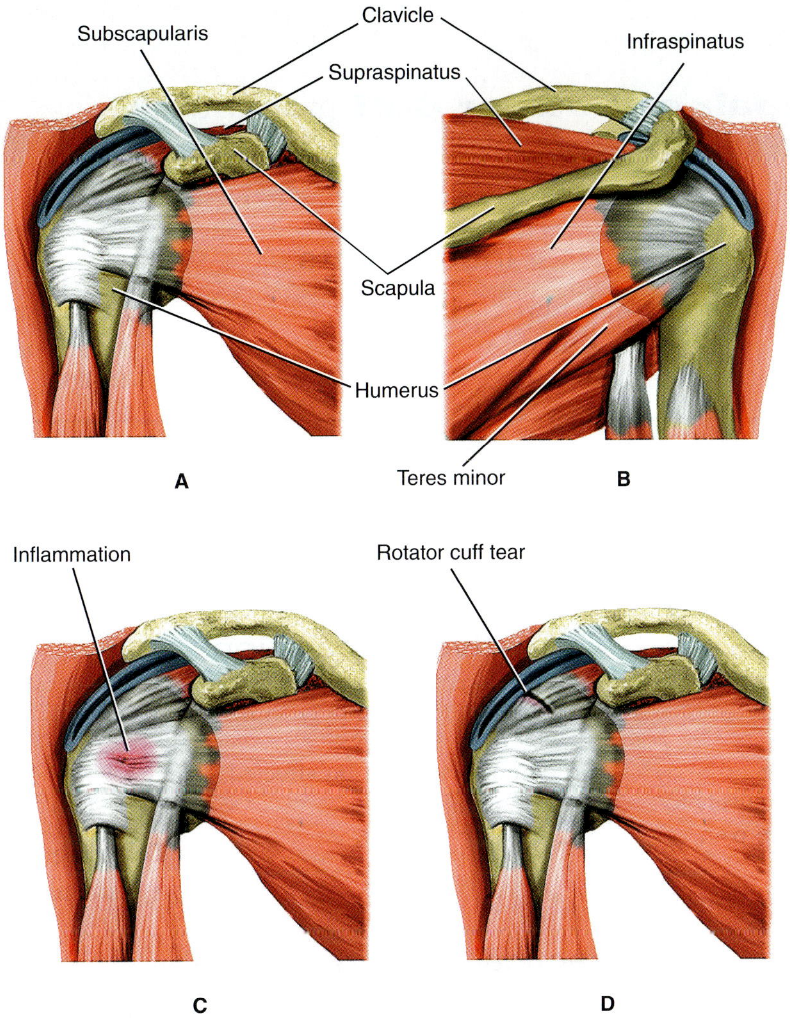

Figure 21-29 **Rotator cuff: (A) Anterior, (B) posterior, (C) inflamed tendon, (D) tear**

semi-Fowler's position, also known as the beach chair position, is often selected for the procedure. The patient is situated close to the edge of the table so the affected arm can be manipulated during surgery. The opposite arm is tucked at the patient's side. The midsection of the table is slightly flexed and the foot is dropped. The back of the OR table is brought forward and a rolled towel is placed under the scapula to slightly elevate the operative site. Some surgeons use an arm-holding device to hold the operative arm in place, eliminating the need for an extra person to hold the arm during the surgical procedure.

(Text continues on page 851)

PROCEDURE 21-8 Repair of Rotator Cuff

Equipment

- Power sources for instruments

(continues)

PROCEDURE 21-8 Repair of Rotator Cuff *(continued)*

Instruments

- Basic orthopedic instrument tray
- Power drill
- Saw
- Bur
- Bankart shoulder retractors
- Arthrex or Mitek rotator cuff anchors

Supplies

- Orthopedic pack
- Special drapes if needed
- Basin set
- Gloves
- Blades
- Suture of choice
- Dressing

Operative Preparation

Anesthesia

- General
- Scalene block may be administered preoperatively to aid with postoperative pain

Position

- Supine or semi-Fowler's
- Roll under scapula on affected side

Prep

- Wrist, arm, shoulder region, and a portion of the anterior chest

Draping

- Extremity draping method

Practical Considerations

- Have X-rays or MRIs in OR
- Notify radiology of possible intraoperative X-ray
- Have C-arm near OR
- Follow radiology safety procedures

Operative Procedure	Technical Considerations
1. The oblique skin incision is made along the anterolateral border of the acromion, ending about 5 cm inferior to the acromion process (Figure 21-30).	**1.** Scalpel, electrocautery, and retractors will be used in that order.
2. The incision is carried through the subcutaneous tissue down to the fascia. Next, large medial and lateral full-thickness flaps are mobilized and retracted medially and laterally.	**2.** Two techniques can be used for the dissection of the deltoid muscle. One technique leaves the deltoid origin attached to the acromion. The other technique calls for the origin to be dissected from the acromion and reattached at the end of the case.
3. The muscle fibers of the deltoid are split a short distance, no more than 5 cm distal to the acromion process, between the anterior and central origins.	**3.** Curved Mayo scissors are used to dissect the thick muscle fibers.
4. The incision is then deepened to expose the subacromial bursa, which is opened, using scissors. This incision allows a limited view of the underlying structures.	**4.** Long curved Mayo or Metzenbaum scissors are used.

PROCEDURE

21-8 Repair of Rotator Cuff *(continued)*

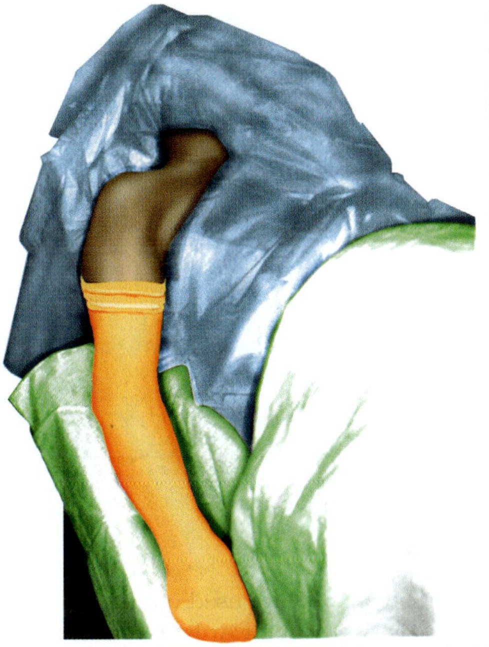

Figure 21-30 Position and draping

5. The exposure of the surgical site is improved with the use of the Bankart shoulder retractors. The surgeon can now clearly identify the coracoacromial ligament, which is resected with the use of cautery.	**5.** The surgeon may use a mallet to lightly tap the Bankart retractors into place.
6. The acromion is resected using a curved osteotome and mallet or saw and rongeur.	**6.** A rasp may be used to smooth the bone edges.
7. The exposure is now complete. The tear in the tendon can be identified and the quality of the tissue available for the repair can be assessed.	**7.** Retention suture may be passed through the tendon to keep it out of harm's way when the trough is created.
8. The repair is begun creating a bony trough near the tuberosity. The trough is created with a rongeur, curette, curved osteotome, or powered bur. A 4- to 5-mm-wide and 25-mm-long trough is made in the space between the greater tuberosity and the articular surface.	**8.** Have irrigation available to cool the tissue and remove debris if power is used to create the trough. Place power equipment in "safe" mode when not in use.
9. The suture of choice to repair the cuff is usually nonabsorbable #2. When suturing the edge of the tendon to the bone, the surgeon should elevate the arm while the sutures are tied. The elevation keeps the soft tissue from experiencing undue tension from the sutures and permits the tissue to be easily approximated (Figure 21-31).	**9.** Communicate with surgeon regarding suture preference in specific situation.

(continues)

PROCEDURE 21-8 Repair of Rotator Cuff *(continued)*

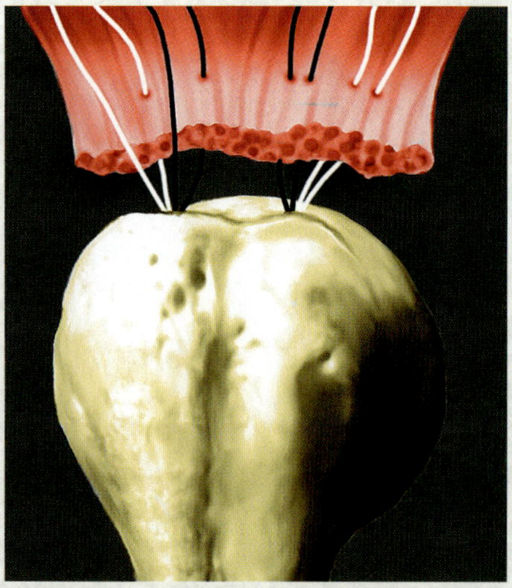

Figure 21-31 Sutures placed for repair

10. The surgeon uses the power drill to make holes in the trough to allow passage of the suture through the trough. Often a surgeon uses a suture passer to draw the suture out through the drill holes. The suture is tied down and the torn tendon of the rotator cuff is secured to the bone.

10. An alternative to suture used quite often by surgeons is the Mitek or Arthrex rotator cuff anchor. After the anchor is placed in the bone, the suture is passed through the torn tendon and tied (Figure 21-32).

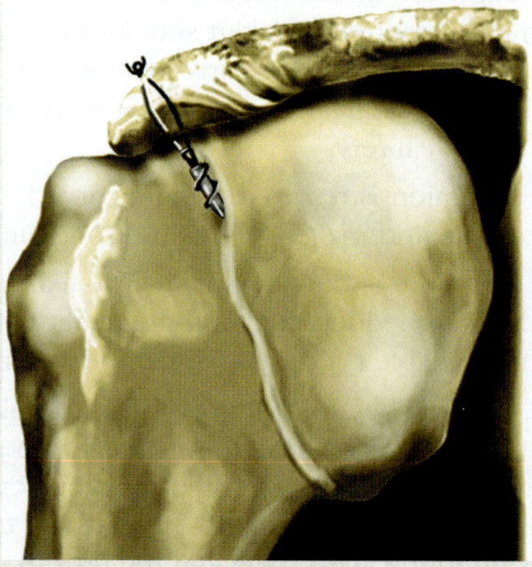

Figure 21-32 Use of an anchor

11. The closure of the wound can now be completed. The deltoid is closed with absorbable or nonabsorbable suture, depending on the surgeon's preference. The subcutaneous layer is closed with 2–0 or 3–0 absorbable sutures, and the skin with either 4–0 nylon or staples.

11. Wound will likely be irrigated with antibiotic solution. Prepare suture for closure. Initiate count.

PROCEDURE 21-8 Repair of Rotator Cuff *(continued)*

12. Bulky dressing is applied with a strip of Xeroform over the skin closure, 4 × 4 sponges or fluffs, and ABD pad that is held in place by tape. A sling or shoulder immobilizer is used.	**12.** Assist with dressing application and immobilization as needed.

Postoperative Considerations

Immediate Postoperative Care

- Transport to PACU
- Observe for local hemorrhage

Prognosis

- Return to normal activities
- May require postoperative rehabilitation

Complications

- Hemorrhage
- Wound infection
- Joint infection

> **PEARL OF WISDOM**
>
> Small amounts of irrigation fluid are dropped onto the bits of power drives that are used to create the trough. The water prevents overheating and damage to the bone. Be sure all team members are wearing appropriate PPE. Fluid will splatter.

A procedural variation to this technique, involving the detachment and reattachment of the deltoid muscle, is as follows:

- The cautery is used to start a full-thickness dissection of the deltoid muscle. The initial cautery incision is extended in a medial to lateral direction.
- A #15 knife blade is then used to sharply dissect the deltoid from its attachments on the anterolateral portion of the acromion.
- At the end of the surgical procedure it is essential that a strong deltoid repair be performed. The full thickness of the deltoid is reapproximated to the acromion by passing #2 Ethibond sutures through two or three drill holes made in the acromion.

INTERNAL FIXATION OF FEMORAL SHAFT FRACTURE

Fractures of the femoral shaft are due to either to trauma or pathological disease. Femoral fractures require attention and repair as soon as possible after the injury occurs. A delay of 12 hours or more can lead to difficulties in reducing the fracture. If surgery must be delayed, it is recommended that the leg be put in traction. Ipsilateral trochanteric or condylar fractures often occur in conjunction with a femoral shaft fracture.

The choices for treatment of a femoral fracture include closed reduction, skeletal traction, and surgical repair. Surgical repairs that have been used in the past, but have fallen out of favor include external fixation and plates and screws. The complications associated with plates and screws have been infections and broken or bent screws and plates, which have contributed to femoral refracture. The standard method of treatment is the use of intramedullary fixation nails, which in this instance are referred to as femoral nails.

The advantages of the femoral nail are:

1. Increase and evenly spread the load sharing of the bone. When bone heals it requires a load across the site of the fracture to promote osteosynthesis, which prevents femoral refracture.
2. Scarring is reduced.
3. Intraoperative blood loss is minimal.
4. Infection rate is low.
5. The fracture hematoma is preserved at the fracture site.

The type of nail to be used depends on the type and location of the fracture, whether ipsilateral trochanteric or condylar fractures are present, and whether bone fragments are present. Types of nails include flexible nails such as the Enders type, interlocking nails such as the

Russell-Taylor rod, and standards nails such as the AO nail. The following description is for the use of the AO titanium femoral nail system using a standard nail.

In addition to a basic orthopedic instrument set, the AO femoral nail instrumentation is needed and well as a power reamer and drill with long guide wires. Fluoroscopy is used during the procedure. The patient is placed in the supine position on the fracture table with traction to reduce the fracture. The entire leg and hip region is prepped and draped.

The instruments required for opening the femur include power drill, calibrated wire guide, 13-mm cannulated drill bit, large reverse awl, tissue protector, radiographic ruler, and, for cannulated nails, a guide rod.

The surgeon first confirms the nail length with the use of fluoroscopy. An AP view of the proximal femur is established. The ruler is held along the lateral side of the thigh and placed until the top is level with the tip of the greater trochanter. The skin is marked at this level. An AP of the distal femur is next taken. The proximal end of the ruler is placed at the skin mark and the nail length is read from the ruler.

The surgeon makes a longitudinal incision proximal to the greater trochanter through the gluteus medius and maximus. Using the power drill the 3.2 calibrated guidewire is placed in the medullary canal to a depth of 100 mm at the entry point where the nail will be placed. The 13-mm cannulated drill bit with tissue protector is placed over the guidewire and drilled to a depth of 100 mm. The opening that is created will allow the insertion of 9- to 12-mm nails. For 13- to 15-mm nails, the broach is used instead to enlarge the opening. The drill bit is removed after the opening has been created.

The STSR now assembles the insertion instruments. Here we describe the use of cannulated nails. The correct connecting screw is placed into the insertion handle and secured to the nail with the ball hexagonal screwdriver. The driving cap is screwed onto the insertion handle. This serves as the striking point when the hammer is used.

The STSR hands the assembly to the surgeon, who manually inserts the nail into the femoral opening as far as possible. For cannulated nails the nail is inserted over the guidewire, which passes through an opening in the side of the insertion handle. Next the surgeon is given the hammer to drive the nail into the distal metaphysis. The guidewire is now removed.

The proximal locking bolts are placed next. The standard aiming arm is attached to the insertion handle. The STSR assembles the triple trocar assembly, 11.0/8.0-mm protection sleeve, 8.0/4.0-mm drill sleeve, and 4.00-mm trocar. The assembly is inserted into the handle through a stab incision to the bone and the 4.0-mm trocar is removed. The STSR loads the 4.0-mm calibrated drill bit onto the power drill and hands it to the surgeon, who drills through both cortices until the drill sleeve presses against the cortex. The locking bolt length is read from the calibrated drill and communicated by the surgeon to the STSR. The locking bolt, protection sleeve, and screwdriver are handed to the surgeon for insertion of the locking bolt. The procedure is repeated for the second proximal locking bolt.

The distal locking bolt is now placed with the use of fluoroscopy. The C-arm is placed to show the most distal hole in the femoral nail. Using the #10 knife blade, a stab incision is made over the site of the distal hole. The STSR will hand the surgeon the power drill with the 4.0-mm drill bit, which is placed in the distal hole and drilled through both cortices. Using the depth gauge, the length of the locking bolt is obtained. However, the STSR should help the surgeon in remembering to add 2–4 mm to the reading to make sure the thread of the bolt engages the far cortex. The STSR hands the surgeon the correct size bolt, holding sleeve, and screwdriver for insertion of the bolt.

The insertion instruments are removed. The STSR hands the surgeon the hexagonal screwdriver and end cap to be threaded onto the proximal end of the nail. The STSR should be prepared to hand the surgeon the ratchet wrench to tighten the end cap. The surgeon closes the stab incisions, places the dressings, and the patient is taken to the PACU.

REPAIR OF HIP FRACTURE

There are several categories of hip fractures and hip fractures with an associated dislocation. The type of fracture determines the treatment, including whether the treatment is nonoperative or operative. The operative fractures that require ORIF are intertrochanteric, subtrochanteric, femoral neck, and basilar neck fractures. Fractures are common in the elderly and females who have osteoporosis. The fracture can disrupt the blood supply to the femoral head resulting in bone necrosis; consequently, fractures should be treated as soon as possible.

The following discussion is for repair of intertrochanteric fractures with the use of the AO Dynamic Hip Screw/Dynamic Condylar Screw (DHS/DCS) system. Intertrochanteric fractures most often reduce without complications; however, ORIF is indicated to prevent malunion due to the rotation of the lower extremity.

A fracture table is used with the patient in the supine position to reduce the fracture. Fluoroscopy is also used to confirm the reduction and throughout the procedure to confirm the placement of the hip screw with plate. Instrumentation and equipment include a basic orthopedic instrument set, DHS specialty instruments and implants, bone reduction clamps, power drill, and reamer.

The standard 38-mm barrel length for the plate and 135-degree barrel angle is most commonly used. After the patient is prepped and draped, the surgeon makes an incision distally from the greater trochanter downward the approximate length of the implant. The dissection is carried downward with the #10 knife blade through the fascia lata and vastus lateralis to expose the fracture site.

The DHS/DCS guide pin is handed to the surgeon by the STSR for placement in the femoral head. The guide pin that comes with the DHS/DCS instrument set is designed for use with the set, so no other guide pin should be substituted. The appropriate angle guide is placed along the axis of the femoral shaft, and the guide pin is inserted with the power drill into the center of the femoral head. The guide pin remains in place for the rest of the procedure. If the guide pin is accidentally removed during the procedure it must be immediately reinserted. The guide pin often comes out when the triple reamer is removed. To reinsert, insert a lag screw backward into the short centering sleeve. This is placed partway into the femoral head for use as a guide to reinsert the guide pin. The surgeon uses a hammer to reseat the guide pin.

The surgeon now determines the reaming and tapping depth and screw length. The direct measuring device is slid over the guide pin to measure the depth of the guide pin insertion. The measurement is a direct reading. The surgeon communicates the reading to the STSR who then subtracts 10 mm from the reading. For example, if the direct reading is 100 mm, the reamer setting, tapping depth, and screw length will be 90 mm. For the rest of this description, 90 mm will be used.

The appropriate triple reamer is assembled. Extra care must be taken while assembling the triple reamer since it is very sharp. The triple reamer can be assembled by the STSR during setup and the depth established intraoperatively. To assemble, select the reaming head that goes with the DHS plate and barrel length. The set screw on the reaming head is aligned with the flat side of the drill bit. Slide the cutting end of the reaming head over the coupling end of the drill bit, and continue sliding the reaming head until the noncutting end of the reaming head is level with the calculated depth, which in this instance is 90 mm. The reaming head is secured into the notch and locked into place with the locking nut.

The triple reamer assembly is placed on the power drill using the large quick coupling device. The reamer is placed over the guide pin and drilled into the femoral head. This accomplishes three things: (1) drills for the lag screw, (2) countersinks for the plate/barrel junction, and (3) reams in preparation for the plate barrel. While the surgeon is drilling, the STSR should frequently irrigate the area with small amounts of normal saline to prevent thermal necrosis of the bone.

If necessary the surgeon will use the calibrated tap. The tap is assembled by sliding the short centering sleeve over the tap, and the tap is inserted into the T-handle quick-coupling device. Release the collar of the T-handle and tug on the tap to make sure it is fully seated in the T-handle quick coupler. The surgeon now inserts the tap over the guide pin and taps to the correct depth, again 90 mm.

At this point the STSR puts the lag screw insertion assembly together with the correct size lag screw. To assemble, the coupling screw is inserted into the guide shaft. The coupling screw is screwed into place on the end of the lag screw. The tabs on the guide shaft should fit into the slots located on the lag screw. The long centering sleeve is placed over the wrench. Last, the guide shaft/lag screw assembly is inserted into the wrench until it stops.

The assembly is placed over the guide pin and the lag screw inserted. The wrench, long centering sleeve, coupling screw, guide shaft, and guide pin are removed. Removal of the guide pin requires the use of the power drill in reverse. The surgeon next needs the impactor and hammer to seat the plate. The last step of the procedure involves placing 4.5-mm cortex screws using the standard AO screw insertion technique to fix the plate against the femur.

The surgeon irrigates the wound, traction is released, one or two Jackson-Pratt drains placed, the wound closed in layers, and dressing placed. The patient should begin weight bearing as soon as possible, often the first postoperative day.

TOTAL HIP ARTHROPLASTY

Patients with a degenerative joint disease (DJD) such as osteoarthritis benefit from total hip arthroplasty, the surgical procedure also called total hip replacement (Procedure 21-9). The total hip prosthesis consists of a femoral and an acetabular component (Figure 21-33). The femoral component replaces the femoral head and neck after they have been resected. The shaft of the femoral prosthesis fits down the middle of the femur shaft. The femoral prosthesis is available in different sizes, types, and length of neck to accommodate the size of the patient. The stem of the prosthesis is either collarless or has a collar that rests on the rim of the resected femur.

The development of modular components has greatly increased the efficiency of the acetabular component and decreased the amount of surgery required in the event of a total hip revision. Metal acetabular cups that are used when cementing is indicated have a slightly rough, textured posterior surface and a polyethylene cup that snaps into the metal shell. Cups not requiring cement have a porous surface on the posterior side.

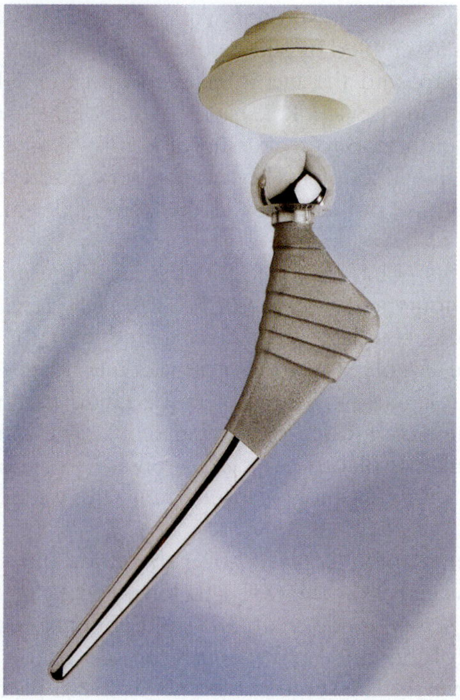

Figure 21-33 Hi-Nek total hip prosthesis: (A) Acetabular component, (B) femoral component ***(Courtesy of Corin Medical, Cirencester, Gloucestershire, United Kingdom)***

Methyl methacrylate (MMA) is used for cementing a hip prosthesis that requires the use of bone cement. The MMA adheres to the metal but not to the bone. Rather, it fills the cavity and spaces of the bone to form a bond between the prosthesis and the bone to keep the prosthesis in place. MMA is available as a sterile mixture of liquid and powder that is mixed by the STSR on the back table. A closed mixing system that exhausts the fumes is recommended for mixing the liquid and powder. The cement hardens in approximately 12–15 minutes.

Several total hip replacement systems are offered by the various orthopedic medical companies. The surgeon's preference usually dictates which company's system will be used. Since each system requires specific instrumentation, there is no "universal" set of hip instruments.

Active individuals with healthy bones and no previous bone diseases or complications are ideal candidates for a noncemented total hip replacement. Conversely, a cemented prosthesis is usually best for patients with osteoporosis, particularly older individuals.

Table 21-8 lists instrumentation that is required for a total hip arthroplasty. The list is generalized; specifics will vary according to the hip system being used and the surgeon's expectations. The list of instruments to place on the large Mayo stand or Mayfield overhead table does not include the specialty hip instruments.

(Text continues on page 859)

Table 21-8 Instrument Trays and Equipment for Total Hip Arthroplasty

INSTRUMENT TRAYS AND EQUIPMENT	
Basic orthopedic set	Hohmann retractors
Meyerding retractors	Self-retaining retractors
Curettes	Cobb elevators
Serrated rongeur	Osteotomes
Long Bovie tip	Large mallet
Pulse lavage	Regular tip and brush tip for lavage
Power saw and drill	4 × 4s soaked in thrombin
Cement	Cement gun
Closed cement mixing system	

INSTRUMENTS ON LARGE MAYO STAND	
Suture scissors	Curved Mayo scissors
#3 knife handles with #10 blades	Long tissue forceps
Sharp and blunt Hohmann retractors	Self-retaining hip retractor
Small and medium Meyerding retractors	Medium Cobb elevator
Medium curved and straight Lambotte osteotome	Serrated rongeur
Two Kocher clamps	Long Bovie tip
Power saw and drill	Two curved Crile clamps
Two Mayo-Hegar needle holders	Bone hook
Medium curette	Freer elevator
Large Key periosteal elevator	Pliers
Large mallet	

PROCEDURE

21-9 Total Hip Arthroplasty

Equipment

- Power sources for instruments
- Special operative table of choice
- Positioning equipment

Instruments

- See Table 21-8
- Total hip replacement system of choice

Supplies

- Orthopedic pack
- Special drapes if needed
- Basin set
- Gloves
- Blades
- Suture of choice
- Dressing

Operative Preparation

Anesthesia

- General or spinal

Position

- Lateral, with the affected hip exposed

Prep

- From the umbilicus, over the hip region, to the entire leg and foot

Draping Special Sequence:

- Four towels are used to square off the operative site and are kept in place with four towel clips
- Next a plastic U-drape is placed under the leg and the tails are placed using the lateral edge of the buttock and iliac crest as guides
- A stockinette is rolled up to the mid-thigh
- Coban is wrapped around the stockinette
- Two three-quarter sheets are used. One is laid transversely at the level of the umbilicus; the other is also laid transversely at the mid-thigh
- An impervious U-drape is placed last with the tails going toward the feet

Practical Considerations

- Have X-rays or MRIs in OR
- Notify radiology of possible intraoperative X-ray
- Follow radiology safety procedures

Operative Procedure	Technical Considerations
1. Watson-Jones incision is used. Incision is made with the midpoint over the lateral aspect of the greater trochanter and extended approximately 5–6 cm proximally and distally to the base of the trochanter, curving anteriorly at both ends.	**1.** The Watson-Jones incision is large. Electrocautery and appropriate retractors will be needed.
2. The subcutaneous tissues are divided. The fascia lata overlying the vastus lateralis is incised. The incision is carried distally the length of the incision.	**2.** The assistant will need laparotomy sponges for soaking up blood and as an aid in manually retracting tissues.

(continues)

PROCEDURE

21-9 Total Hip Arthroplasty *(continued)*

3. The interval between the gluteus medius and fascia lata muscles is located and dissection is continued between the two structures.	**3.** The self-retaining Charnley hip retractor with blades is placed into position.
4. The origin of the vastus lateralis is located in the distal portion of the incision. A longitudinal incision is made through the structure to expose the proximal femoral shaft.	**4.** The surgeon will most likely need a #7 or long #3 knife handle with a #10 blade.
5. The hip capsule is now incised, allowing the hip joint to be dislocated delivering the femoral head into the surgical wound.	**5.** Provide manual traction if necessary to dislocate joint.
6. The femoral osteotomy guide is placed over the lateral femur and neck. The point is marked where the reciprocating saw will be used to remove the head of the femur. The mark and cut are made approximately 1 cm proximal to the lesser trochanter.	**6.** Hand the femoral osteotomy Hohmann guide. Prepare reciprocating saw. Blunt Hohmann retractors are placed around the femoral neck; one large Hohmann is placed under the neck and one sharp Hohmann is placed distal to the lesser trochanter to deliver the femur into the wound. The STSR may be asked to hold the leg in place to keep it flexed, internally rotated, and horizontal.
7. Attention is now turned to the acetabular cup. The rim of the acetabulum is inspected for osteophytes. If present, they are removed with the rongeur to create a smooth acetabular rim. Care is taken to remove the rest of the posterior capsule.	**7.** The STSR should have a laparotomy sponge ready to remove/clean dissected bits of osteophytes from the jaws of the rongeur.
8. Acetabular reamers are used to ream the acetabular cup to remove the articular cartilage. The acetabulum is reamed until osteochondral bone is exposed.	**8.** The acetabular reamers are hemispheric in shape with several small, sharp blades on their surface for cutting the cartilage. The smallest reamer is used first and progression to larger sized reamers is 2 mm at a time. The STSR must make sure to keep the reamers in a proper size order until the surgeon is finished reaming the acetabulum. The STSR should also verbalize the size of the reamer when handing it to the surgeon.
9. Several holes are drilled approximately 1 cm in depth into the floor of the acetabulum in the ilium, ischium, and pubis. Each hole is then undercut with a curette to act as a seating hole for the bone cement.	**9.** A small drill bit, such as $\frac{5}{32}$ in., is used.
10. Trial acetabular components are now positioned in the reamed-out cavity. The cup is examined to determine bony coverage, size, and position within the acetabulum. The cup must be covered with bone, especially along the superior, posterior, and lateral margins. The trial is removed. The acetabulum is irrigated with the pulse lavage to remove any debris.	**10.** During pulse lavage, the STSR is mixing the first batch of cement and loading it into the cement gun (the cement gun looks like a specialized caulking gun).

PROCEDURE 21-9 Total Hip Arthroplasty *(continued)*

11. The acetabulum is thoroughly dried with laparotomy sponges. Then the acetabulum is filled with the cement.	**11.** A curette may be used to force cement into the previously drilled seating holes.
12. The acetabular metal shell component is manually guided into place. The acetabular impactor with mallet is used to gently seat the component in the cavity. Excess cement is removed from around the cup both manually and with a small curette.	**12.** The STSR should keep track of the time to help the surgeon estimate when the bone cement will be sufficiently hardened. The polyethylene insert is put into place later.
13. The foot is now lowered toward the floor and internally rotated to expose the proximal end of the femur.	**13.** Prepare femoral canal reamer on T-handle.
14. The femoral canal reamer on the T-handle is inserted manually down the shaft of the femur.	**14.** Rasps should be placed in order from the smallest rasp to the largest. The rasp is locked into place on the rasp handle.
15. The femoral rasps are used next. Care is taken not to penetrate the femur and in the process break the femur into pieces.	**15.** The surgeon is given the smallest rasp, also called a broach, and utilizes a back and forth motion to remove the cancellous bone. The surgeon will use the rasp manually and/or with a mallet. Larger rasps are successively used until cortical bone is exposed.
16. The final broach is left seated and serves as the femoral trial component. The femoral neck is first prepared with the round calcar reamer. Next, the trial head and neck are placed on the broach to confirm the size that is correct.	**16.** An X-ray may be taken to ensure correct fit of the prosthesis prior to cement application.
17. The rasp/trial is removed. The pulse lavage is used to clean out the femoral canal. The brush tip is used to aid in cleaning out the canal.	**17.** While the canal is being lavaged, the surgical technologist is mixing the second batch of cement and loading it into the cement gun.
18. The cement restrictor is placed into the femoral canal.	**18.** Notify the surgeon when cement is ready to use. The cement restrictor is used to prevent cement from entering the medullary canal.
19. The cement is injected down the femoral canal.	**19.** Prepare permanent prosthesis for insertion.
20. The femoral component is placed in the canal using the femoral impactor. (Great care is taken to introduce the prosthesis in such a way as to obtain the valgus position.)	**20.** The STSR keeps track of the time from when the cement is injected down the femoral canal. Keep a small piece of cement rolled into a ball on the back table to help in determining when the cement is hardened.
21. Once the cement hardens, the femoral head is positioned onto the stem. The femoral head impactor and mallet are used to seat the head on the stem.	**21.** The component is small and round. Be sure that it is passed securely.
22. The polyethylene insert is snapped into the acetabular shell.	**22.** Assist with manual reduction of the joint if necessary.

(continues)

23. The hip is reduced and moved through a range of motions to check for stability and positioning (Figure 21-34).

23. Sharp towel clips are used to hold the skin edges together.

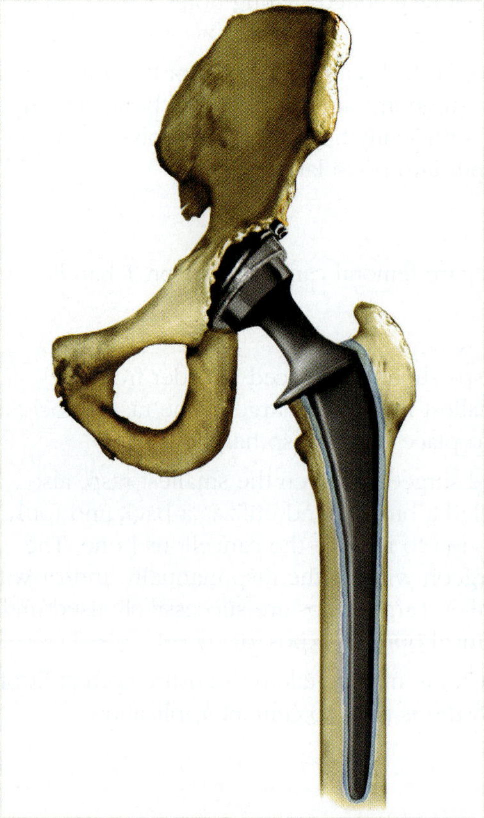

Figure 21-34 **Total hip arthroplasty (prosthesis in place)**

24. One or two hemovac drains will be placed. The first is placed deep in the hip joint and the second is placed in the subcutaneous area.

24. Prepare drains for insertion. Anticipate closure.

25. The fascia is closed with interrupted sutures and the skin is closed with staples.

25. Routine closure. Initiate count. Anticipate application of dressings.

Postoperative Considerations

Immediate Postoperative Care

- Abduction splint placed between patient's legs to immobilize the joint
- Transport to PACU
- Observe for local hemorrhage

Prognosis

- Return to normal activities
- May require postoperative rehabilitation

Complications

- Hemorrhage
- Wound infection
- Joint infection
- Intraoperative femoral fracture

PEARL OF WISDOM

The STSR should verbalize the size of the rasp when handing it to the surgeon. In fact, all items that are sized should be verbally identified when used.

TOTAL KNEE ARTHROPLASTY

Total knee arthroplasty is performed to place components that substitute for the surfaces of the knee joint. The normal surfaces are damaged due to disease such as degenerative joint disease or years of wear and tear, in athletes in particular who are involved in impact sports. The goal of the procedure is to restore normal function of the joint and relieve chronic pain.

The knee is one of the more difficult, challenging joints for which an implant system has been developed. The reason is because knee motion occurs in three planes: (1) abduction and adduction, (2) rotation, and (3) extension and flexion. In addition, the system should serve to preserve the normal ligaments while replacing the worn bone surfaces. Total knee replacement systems are based on the tricompartmental implants that replace the opposing femorotibial joint and the patellofemoral joint, but preserve the posterior cruciate ligament. The surgeon also has the choice of using either a cemented or noncemented prosthesis. The noncemented prosthesis is further categorized into porous design to allow bony ingrowth or press-fit design.

The instrumentation and equipment needed for the procedure include tourniquet, basic orthopedic instrument set, total knee specialty instruments, trials and implants, power drill and oscillating saw, MMA (if used), cement gun, and pulse lavage. The sterile members of the surgery team will wear the body exhaust suit ("space suit") for infection control purposes.

General anesthesia is administered, and the patient is placed in the supine position with a hip bump being preferred by some surgeons. The tourniquet is applied and the leg and hip prepped. Prior to the skin prep being performed, a foot bump will have been placed on the OR table. A sheet or towel is rolled and wrapped with tape to maintain the roll and then taped to the table. The operative foot is placed against the bump to maintain the knee in a hyperflexed position during the procedure.

INCISION

The foot is placed against the foot bump to flex the knee. An anterior midline straight longitudinal incision is made starting approximately 6–12 cm proximal to the superior pole of the patella, extending over the patella and ending at the medial border of the tubial tuberosity. The initial incision is made through the skin and subcutaneous layers with a #10 knife blade. Curved Mayo scissors are placed underneath the exposed superficial retinaculum to spread the layer proximally and distally, and the Mayo scissors are then used to incise the layer.

Next the surgeon excises the infrapatellar fat pad. The back end of the scalpel handle or flat end of forceps is used to bluntly separate the space between the fat pad and the patellar tendon. The #10 knife blade is used to complete the excision of the fat pad.

The medial and lateral knee capsular exposure is now accomplished. The capsule is medially and laterally reflected from the upper portion of the proximal tibia. The capsulotomy is performed in a circumferential manner using an osteotome. To fully expose the medial tibial plateau and complete the deep capsular exposure, the surgeon first uses the knife blade and completes the capsular elevation with a curved ½-in. osteotome. Osteophytes on the rim of the femur and tibia are removed with a rongeur.

To evert the patella, the surgeon performs the following incisions. Using the knife blade, the anterior attachments of the lateral meniscus of the tibia are incised. A Kocher clamp is attached to the retinaculum of the medial side of the patella and tension is placed on the patellofemoral ligament by slightly pulling on the Kocher. Curved Mayo scissors are used to spread the patellofemoral ligament and to incise the ligament off of the femur.

The articular exposure is completed when the surgeon incises the tibial insertion of the ACL, allowing the tibia to be subluxated forward for complete visualization of the plateau surfaces. A rongeur is used to remove any remaining osteophytes from the femoral condyles, intercondylar space, and articular margins of the tibia and patella.

PROXIMAL TIBIAL RESECTION

The knee is hyperflexed using the bump, and curved retractors are placed to protect the medial collateral ligament, patellar tendon, and capsule during resection of the proximal tibia. A blunt-tipped Hohmann retractor may be placed behind the posterior tibia to bring it forward into an anterior position. The remaining menisci are excised using a #10 knife blade. A Kocher clamp is used to grasp the menisci, pull them into the joint, and transect with the knife blade.

The tibial cutting jig is positioned by placing the spike into the proximal tibial spines. The ankle clamp is placed by wrapping the spring around the ankle and attaching it to the other side of the clamp. The alignment rod is positioned in the clamp slightly medial to the tibial tubercle and the second spike is gently hammered into the proximal end of the tibia.

The stylus is attached to the tibial cutting block and both are lowered until the tip of the stylus rests on the tibial plateau. A ⅛-in. drill bit is used to drill approximately 3 in. deep in preparation for the tibial fixation pins, which are placed in the holes marked on the tibial cutting block. The alignment rod and stylus are removed and alignment of the cutting block is confirmed. The oscillating saw is used to resect the proximal tibia. The STSR should frequently irrigate the area with small amounts of normal saline during resection to prevent thermal bone necrosis.

FEMORAL PREPARATION AND RESECTION

A rongeur is used to remove osteophytes from the intercondylar notch of the femur. The 8-mm intercondylar drill bit is used to drill a hole in the center of the distal end of the femur. The femoral intramedullary (IM) alignment guide with IM rod is inserted into the drill hole and seated in place.

The AP femoral cutting guide is attached to the femoral IM alignment guide by gently tapping two pins into place through the cutting guide into the holes in the alignment guide. Two more pins are used to pin the AP cutting guide into place. The femoral alignment guide and IM rod are then removed. Retractors are kept in place to protect the patellar tendon and MCL, and the AP cuts are made with the oscillating saw. On completion of the resection of the posterior femur, small portions of uncut bone may still be present. The surgeon will use a straight 1-in. osteotome placed through the saw cut and gently tap it with the hammer to remove the uncut bone.

The distal femoral cutting block is attached to the distal femoral cutting guide. The block is chosen based on the height of the patient. The IM rod is reinserted into the distal femoral cutting guide assembly and placed into the femoral canal. The cutting guide should be in contact with the intercondylar notch. Two pins are tapped into place to position the cutting block, the IM rod and cutting guide assembly are removed, and the distal femoral cut is made. The AP measuring guide is placed on the flat cut surface of the femur and the size of the femoral component is confirmed.

The last set of femoral cuts to be made are the chamfer cuts. The femoral finishing guide or chamfer cutting guide is centered between the epicondyles and gently hammered into place with the use of the impactor. Two fixation pins are placed anteriorly to secure the guide to the femur. A ¼-in. drill bit is used to make two holes into the distal end of the femur. The anterior and posterior chamfer cuts are accomplished with the oscillating saw.

TIBIAL STEM PREPARATION

The tibial size is reexamined for accuracy using the tibial trial plate. The tibial trial plate is also used as a jig to prepare seating holes for the pegs or stem that will be on the undersurface of the permanent tibial prosthesis.

PATELLAR RESECTION

The center of the patella is determined by aligning the center of the prosthetic patellar implant with the center of the patella bone. Cautery is used to slightly burn the patellar bone, marking the medial and lateral articular borders of the patellar facet. The surgeon will also use a caliper to measure the thickness of the patella. The correct patella cutting jig is held in place with a clamp and through the clamp the surface of the patella is resected.

TRIAL REDUCTION AND PLACEMENT OF PROSTHESES

A final trial reduction is performed using the trial components. The tibial tray is placed first followed by the tibial insert, femoral component, and patellar component. The surgeon puts the knee through a series of motions to confirm normal joint movement.

The trial components are removed and pulse lavage used to thoroughly irrigate the bone surfaces. Often an antibiotic is mixed with the irrigation solution. If bone cement is to be used, while the surgeon is irrigating, the STSR is responsible for mixing the cement and receiving the permanent prostheses from the circulator. The size of the prostheses are confirmed with the surgeon one last time before opening. If a prosthesis is dropped on the floor, it cannot be resterilized and used. Scratches on the surface of the prosthesis may have occurred when dropped and could cause complications if the prosthesis were placed in the knee. The STSR should replace any used lap sponges on the sterile field with clean unused sponges.

The STSR loads the cement into the cement gun and hands it to the surgeon. The surgeon places the cement on the cut bone surfaces and the prostheses are placed. The STSR should keep a small piece of bone cement on the back table and let the surgeon know when it has hardened. The surgeon will use a Freer elevator, smooth forceps, and/or knife blade to trim excess cement from around the prostheses.

WOUND CLOSURE AND DRESSING

The tourniquet is released and hemostasis achieved with cautery before wound closure is started. The knee is placed in 35 degrees of flexion during wound closure. The surgeon's preference will determine if a closed-suction drainage device will be put into place. A bulky compressive dressing is placed and, if no postoperative complications are experienced, the patient will be discharged 3–4 days postoperatively.

CASE STUDY

Cheryl is a downhill skier. She fell while cutting through deep powder. She said that she heard a "pop" while she was twisting and falling. Cheryl was diagnosed with a tear of the anterior cruciate ligament. She is in the OR for an arthroscopic repair.

1. What equipment is necessary for all arthroscopic procedures?
2. Can ligaments be repaired? How? Give another example.

QUESTIONS FOR FURTHER STUDY

1. What safety steps should be followed when using cement in orthopedic procedures?
2. What is the difference between a Steinmann pin and a K-wire?
3. What is the difference in structure between a self-tapping and a nontapping screw?
4. What is the purpose of placing a cement restrictor within the femur during a total hip arthroplasty?
5. When a carpal tunnel release is being performed, what is the reason for incising the transverse carpal ligament for the purpose of releasing it?
6. Place the following in their order of use during a knee arthroscopy: blunt trocar, irrigation/inflow cannula, sharp trocar, #11 knife blade.

BIBLIOGRAPHY

Agur, A. M. (1999). *Grant's atlas of anatomy* (9th ed.). Baltimore: Lippincott Williams & Wilkins.

Allen, G. (1998). The diagnosis and treatment of carpal tunnel syndrome. *The Surgical Technologist 30,* 9–18.

Anderson, K. (Ed.). (1998). *Mosby's medical, nursing, & allied health dictionary* (5th ed.). St. Louis, MO: Mosby.

Ball, K. A. (1990). *Lasers: The perioperative challenge.* St. Louis, MO: Mosby.

Bullock, B. L. (1996). *Pathophysiology: Adaptations and alterations in function.* Philadelphia: J. B. Lippincott.

Chow, J. C. Y. (No date). *Endoscopic release of carpal tunnel ligament* [Film]. Available: Smith & Nephew Dyonics, Inc., 160 Descomb Road, Anodver, MD 01810.

Collins, C. E., & Davies, J. J. (1996). *Modern medical language.* St. Paul, MN: West Publishing Co.

Ethicon, Inc. (1994). *Ethicon wound closure manual.* Author.

FDA. (2000). Medscout. *U.S. Food and Drug Administration* [Online]. Available from *http://www.medscout.com*

Gilmer, P. (No date). Repair of supraspinatus/infraspinatus tear. In *Wheeless' textbook of orthopaedics* [Online]. Available from *http://www.medmedia.com*

Goldstein, L. A., & Dickerson, R. C. (1981). *Atlas of orthopaedic surgery* (2nd ed.). St. Louis, MO: Mosby.

Gray, H. (1989). *Anatomy: Descriptive and surgical.* St. Louis, MO: Mosby.

Hitner, H., & Nagle, B. T. (1994). *Basic pharmacology for health occupations* (3rd ed.). New York: Glencoe.

Hole, J. W., Jr. (1995). *Essentials of human anatomy & physiology* (5th ed.). Dubuque, IA: Wm. C. Brown.

Junge, T. (1999, Summer). *Bone healing: Normal and disrupted.* SFA Newsletter, AST. Englewood, CO: Publisher.

Marks, S. C., Jr., & Hermey, D. C. (1996). The structure and development of bone. In J. P. Bilezikian, L. G. Raisz, & G. A. Rodan (Eds.), *Principles of bone biology.* San Diego: Academic Press.

Martin, J. T., & Warner, M. A. (1997). *Positioning in anesthesia and surgery* (3rd ed.). Philadelphia: W. B. Saunders.

Medmedia. (No date). Above the knee amputation. In *Wheeless' textbook of orthopaedics* [Online]. Available from *http://www.medmedia.com*

Medmedia. (No date). Achilles tendon rupture. In *Wheeless' textbook of orthopaedics* [Online]. Available from *http://www.medmedia.com*

Medmedia. (No date). Anterior cruciate ligament. In *Wheeless' textbook of orthopaedics* [Online]. Available from *http://www.medmedia.com*

Medmedia. (No date). Application of external fixators for distal radius fracture. In *Wheeless' textbook of orthopaedics* [Online]. Available from *http://www.medmedia.com*

Medmedia. (No date). Arthroscopy of the shoulder joint. In *Wheeless' textbook of orthopaedics* [Online]. Available from *http://www.medmedia.com*

Medmedia. (No date). Keller procedure. In *Wheeless' textbook of orthopaedics* [Online]. Available from *http://www.medmedia.com*

Medmedia. (No date). MP joint arthroplasty. In *Wheeless' textbook of orthopaedics* [Online]. Available from *http://www.medmedia.com*

Medmedia. (No date). Open acromioplasty. In *Wheeless' textbook of orthopaedics* [Online]. Available from *http://www.medmedia.com*

Medmedia. (No date). Plate fixation of humeral shaft fracture. In *Wheeless' textbook of orthopaedics* [Online]. Available from *http://www.medmedia.com*

Medmedia. (No date). Repairs of the medial meniscus. In *Wheeless' textbook of orthopaedics* [Online]. Available from *http://www.medmedia.com*

Medmedia. (No date). Total knee arthroplasty. In *Wheeless' textbook of orthopaedics* [Online]. Available from *http://www.medmedia.com*

Medmedia. (No date). Triple arthrodesis. In *Wheeless' textbook of orthopaedics* [Online]. Available from *http://www.medmedia.com*

Peacock, E. E., Jr. (1984). *Wound repair* (3rd ed.). Philadelphia: W. B. Saunders.

Salerno, E. (1999). *Pharmacology for health professionals*. St. Louis, MO: Mosby.

Scanlon, V. C., & Sander, T. (1997). *Essentials of anatomy and physiology* (2nd ed.). Philadelphia: F. A. Davis.

Schauwecker, F. (1982). *Practice of osteosynthesis* (2nd ed.). New York: Thieme-Stratton, Inc.

Synthes. (1995). DHS®/DCS® dynamic hip and condylar screw system: Technique guide [Brochure]. Paoli, PA: Autuor.

Welling, K. R. (No date). Rotator cuff surgery. *The Surgical Technologist 31,* 11–18.

CHAPTER 22

Cardiothoracic Surgery

Paul Price

CASE STUDY

Robert, a 54-year-old mechanic, arrives in the emergency room complaining of severe chest pain that radiates to his back and difficulty taking a deep breath. He has smoked two packs of cigarettes a day for 20 years and is grossly overweight. His father and brother both died of heart disease.

1. What does the physician suspect is wrong?
2. What tests should the physician order?
3. Will surgical intervention be necessary, and if so, what kind?
4. What procedure is typically attempted before surgery, and where is this procedure performed? What specialist performs this procedure?

OBJECTIVES

After studying this chapter, the reader should be able to:

A 1. Discuss the relevant anatomy of the cardiovascular and respiratory systems.

P 2. Describe the pathology that prompts cardiac or thoracic surgical intervention and the related terminology.

3. Discuss any special preoperative diagnostic procedures/tests for the patient undergoing cardiac or thoracic surgery.

O 4. Discuss any special preoperative preparation procedures.

5. Identify the names and uses of cardiovascular and thoracic instruments, supplies, and drugs.
6. Identify the names and uses of special equipment for the cardiac or thoracic procedure.
7. Discuss the intraoperative preparation of the patient undergoing a cardiac or thoracic procedure.

8. Define and give an overview of the cardiac or thoracic procedure.
9. Discuss the purpose and expected outcomes of the cardiac or thoracic procedure.
10. Discuss the immediate postoperative care and possible complications of the cardiac or thoracic procedure.
11. **S** Discuss any specific variations related to the preoperative, intraoperative, and postoperative care of the patient undergoing a cardiac or thoracic procedure.

SELECT KEY TERMS

1. alveoli	7. ductus arteriosus	13. oxygenated	19. stent
2. aneurysm	8. hyaline cartilage	14. pericardium	20. systole
3. arrhythmia	9. infarction	15. pleura	21. tachycardia
4. atria	10. infiltrate	16. prolapse	22. tamponade
5. bradycardia	11. mediastinum	17. PVC	23. ventricles
6. cardiac cycle	12. myocardium	18. regurgitation	

ANATOMY OF THE CHEST

The anatomical structures described below include the thorax, trachea, bronchial tree, and lungs. Anatomy of the heart is discussed in a separate section.

THE THORAX

The thoracic cavity is formed by the sternum and costal cartilages anteriorly, the thoracic vertebrae posteriorly, the ribs laterally, and the diaphragm inferiorly. The sternum consists of the inferior xiphoid process, the middle body, and the superior manubrium. The junction of the manubrium and body forms the sternal angle. The 12 ribs are attached to the thoracic vertebrae posteriorly. The seven true ribs articulate directly with the sternum anteriorly by a strip of costal cartilage, and the next three false ribs articulate with the sternum indirectly by attachment to costal cartilage. The last two false, or floating, ribs lack any cartilaginous attachment to the sternum.

The three divisions of the thoracic cavity are separated by a serous membrane called the **pleura**, and consist of a right and left pleural cavity on either side of the **mediastinum**. Within the right pleural cavity is the right lung, consisting of three lobes, and within the left pleural cavity is the smaller left lung, consisting of two lobes. The third division of the thorax is called the mediastinum. It contains the esophagus, trachea, thymus, lymph nodes, and the heart and its great vessels. Divided into anterior, middle, posterior, and superior regions, the mediastinum is bounded superiorly by the thoracic inlet, inferiorly by the diaphragm, anteriorly by the sternum, and posteriorly by the vertebral column.

The thoracic cavity is lined by the parietal pleura, which adheres to the inner surface of the ribs, the **pericardium** of the heart, and the superior surface of the diaphragm. The outer surface of each lung is covered by the visceral pleura that lies against the parietal pleura, separated by a potential space called the pleural space. This space contains a lubricating serous fluid that prevents friction between the lungs and pleura during respiration.

The thorax plays a major role in respiration due to its elliptical design. As the diaphragm and external intercostal muscles contract, the ribs and sternum are elevated and the size of the thoracic cavity increases significantly (Figure 22-1). Thoracic volume increases as pulmonary pressure decreases, forcing air into the lungs.

The principal muscles of the thorax associated with inspiration are the diaphragm (the most important muscle of inspiration) and external intercostals. Accessory muscles for inspiration include the sternocleidomastoid and scalenes (Figure 22-2). The muscles associated with expiration are the internal intercostals, external oblique, internal oblique, transversus abdominis, and rectus abdominis muscles.

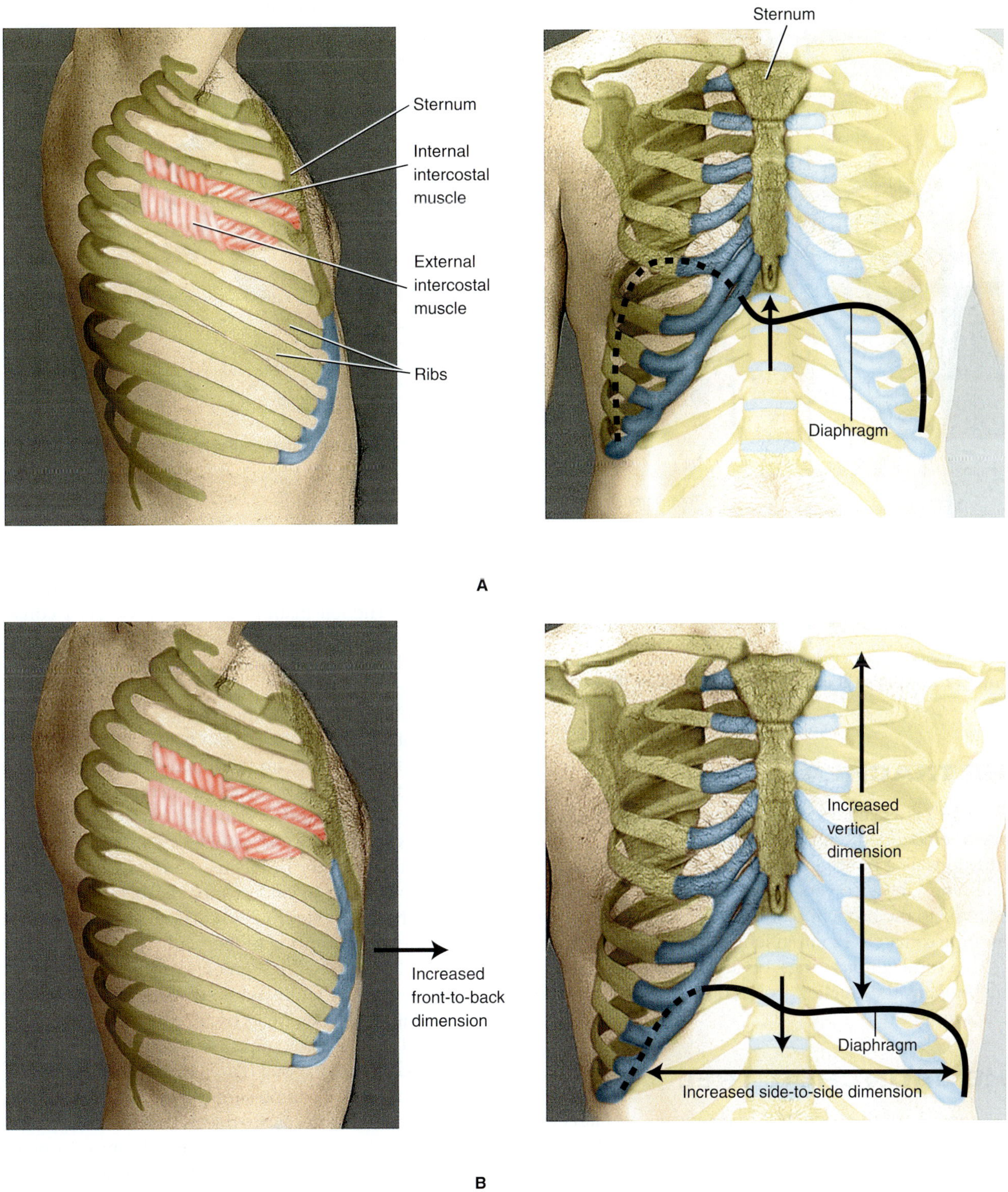

Figure 22-1 Thoracic changes during respiration: (A) Expiration, (B) inspiration

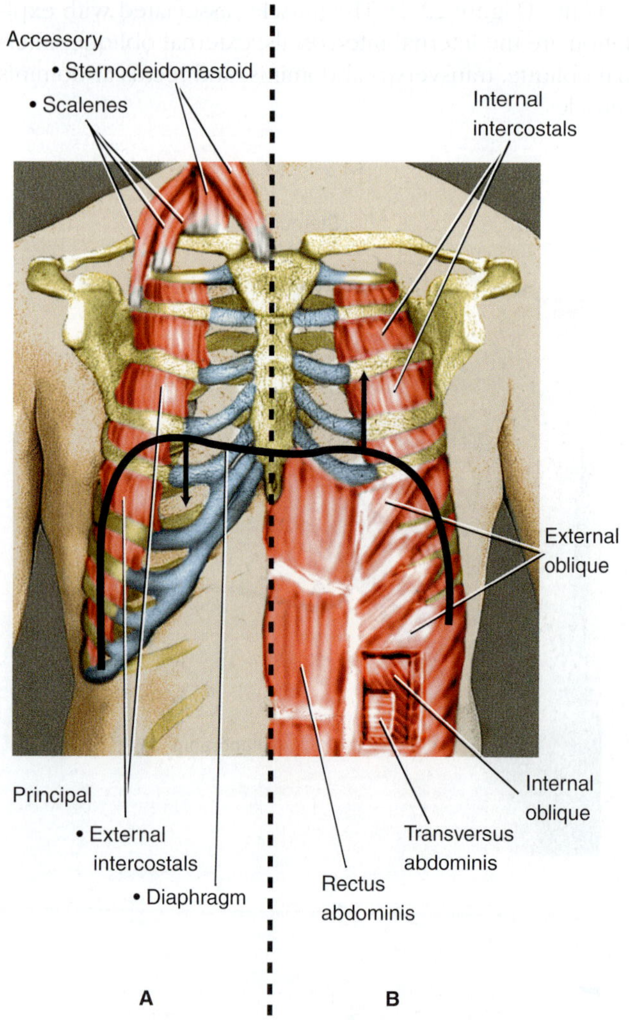

Figure 22-2 Muscles of respiration: (A) Inspiration, (B) expiration

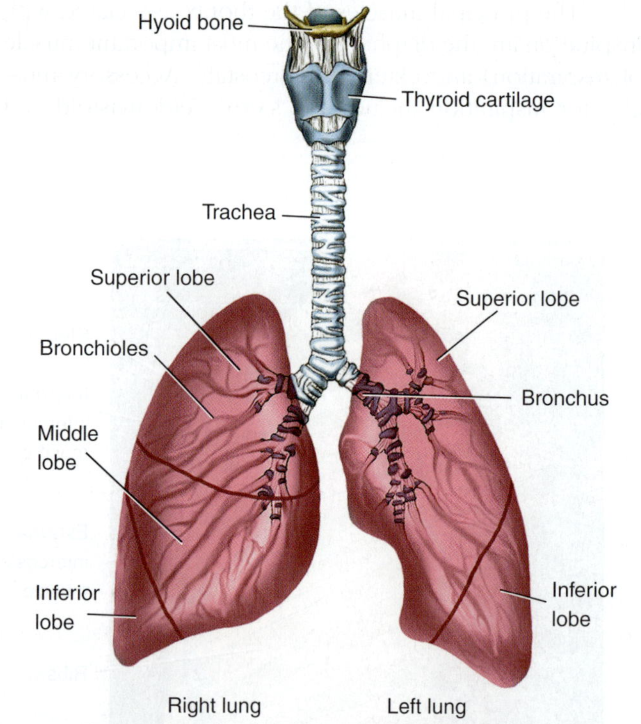

Figure 22-3 Trachea, lungs, and related structures

THE TRACHEA

The trachea is a cylindrical pipe composed of smooth muscle with embedded C-shaped rings of **hyaline cartilage**. It functions as a passageway for air from the atmosphere to the lungs and vice versa (Figure 22-3). It extends from the larynx to the bronchi of the thoracic cavity, and measures approximately 12 cm in length and 2.5 cm in diameter. The cartilaginous rings on the anterior and lateral walls prevent the trachea from collapsing and blocking the flow of air.

THE BRONCHIAL TREE

The branches of the bronchial tree serve as air filters and passageways for the distribution of air to the **alveoli** of the lungs.

At the level of the fifth thoracic vertebra, the trachea divides into the right and left primary bronchi at a point referred to as the carina. The right primary bronchus is slightly larger than the left, with a more pronounced vertical slant. The left main bronchus, however, is considerably longer than the right. These tubes are also composed of smooth muscle embedded with incomplete cartilaginous rings.

The inner walls of the primary bronchus are lined with ciliated mucosa, as are the walls of the trachea. The goblet cells that make up the mucosa secrete a substance that entraps foreign particles in incoming air. The cilia then pass the entrapped particles out of the respiratory tract, preventing possible respiratory tract infection.

As the primary bronchus enters the lung, it subdivides into smaller, secondary lobar branches, one for each lobe of the lung (Figure 22-4). These secondary bronchi subdivide even further to become tertiary (segmental) bronchi that supply the segments of the lung.

The bronchopulmonary segments function as individual units, each having its own bronchus, pulmonary artery, and pulmonary vein. They are held together by delicate connective tissue. Disease may be limited to specific segments that can be surgically removed without disturbing the function of other segments.

The segmental bronchi subdivide into bronchioles that enter small compartments of the bronchopulmonary segments, called lobules (the basic units of the lungs). The bronchioles subdivide into smaller, terminal bronchi-

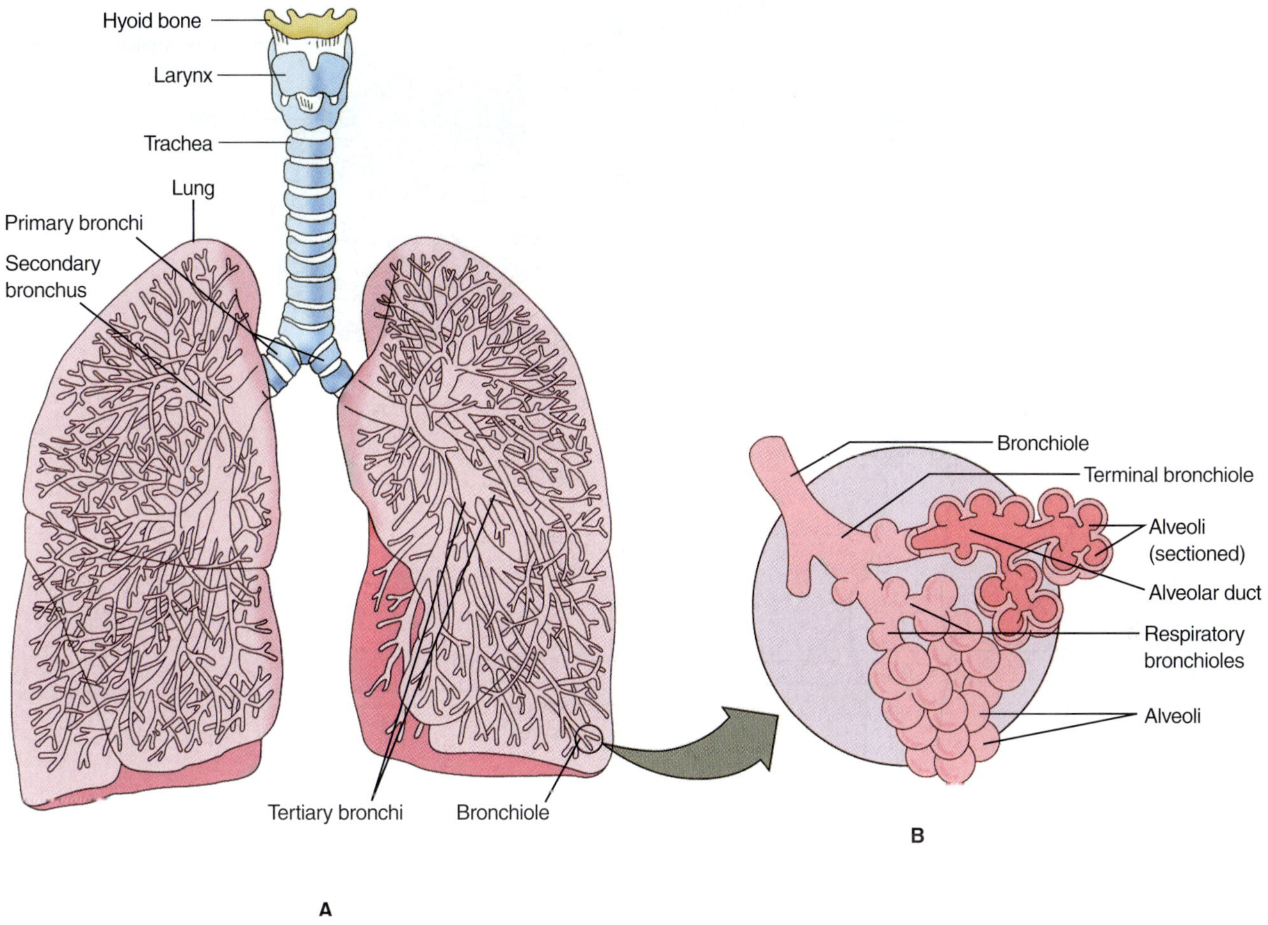

Figure 22-4 Bronchial tree: (A) Bronchial divisions, (B) bronchiole

oles, and then continue to subdivide into respiratory bronchioles (the first structures in the sequence that deals with the exchange of gases), terminating in microscopic branches that divide into alveolar ducts. Around each alveolar duct are round structures called alveoli (Figure 22-5). The alveoli are constructed of simple squamous epithelium and provide a large surface area for the exchange of oxygen from the alveolar sacs into blood and carbon dioxide from blood into the alveolar sacs.

THE LUNGS

The lungs are large, spongy organs shaped somewhat like a cone, that extend from the diaphragm to an area slightly above the clavicle. Each is designed to exchange carbon dioxide for oxygen (Figure 22-6). Each lung is suspended in its respective pleural cavity by an attached main bronchus and its corresponding pulmonary artery, superior pulmonary vein, inferior pulmonary vein, and lymphatic vessels. Pulmonary plexuses run anteriorly to these structures, and the vagus nerve runs posteriorly alongside the bronchial arteries. These structures enter the lung on its medial surface through a region called the hilum.

The lobes of the left lung are referred to as inferior and superior lobes and are separated by an oblique fissure. The lobes of the right lung are referred to as inferior, middle, and superior, and they are separated by an oblique and horizontal fissure.

Blood that is low in oxygen is delivered from the right ventricle of the heart to the left lung for oxygen infusion by way of the left branch of the pulmonary artery. The right lung receives blood from the right branch of the pulmonary artery. Blood that has been infused with oxygen enters the left atrium of the heart by way of the four pulmonary veins (Figure 22-7).

Oxygenated blood for nourishment of the bronchi and bronchioles is delivered by bronchial arteries that typically arise from the aorta just beyond the arch. However, these arteries may arise from aortic arch, subclavian, or innominate arteries or from any of the upper intercostal arteries.

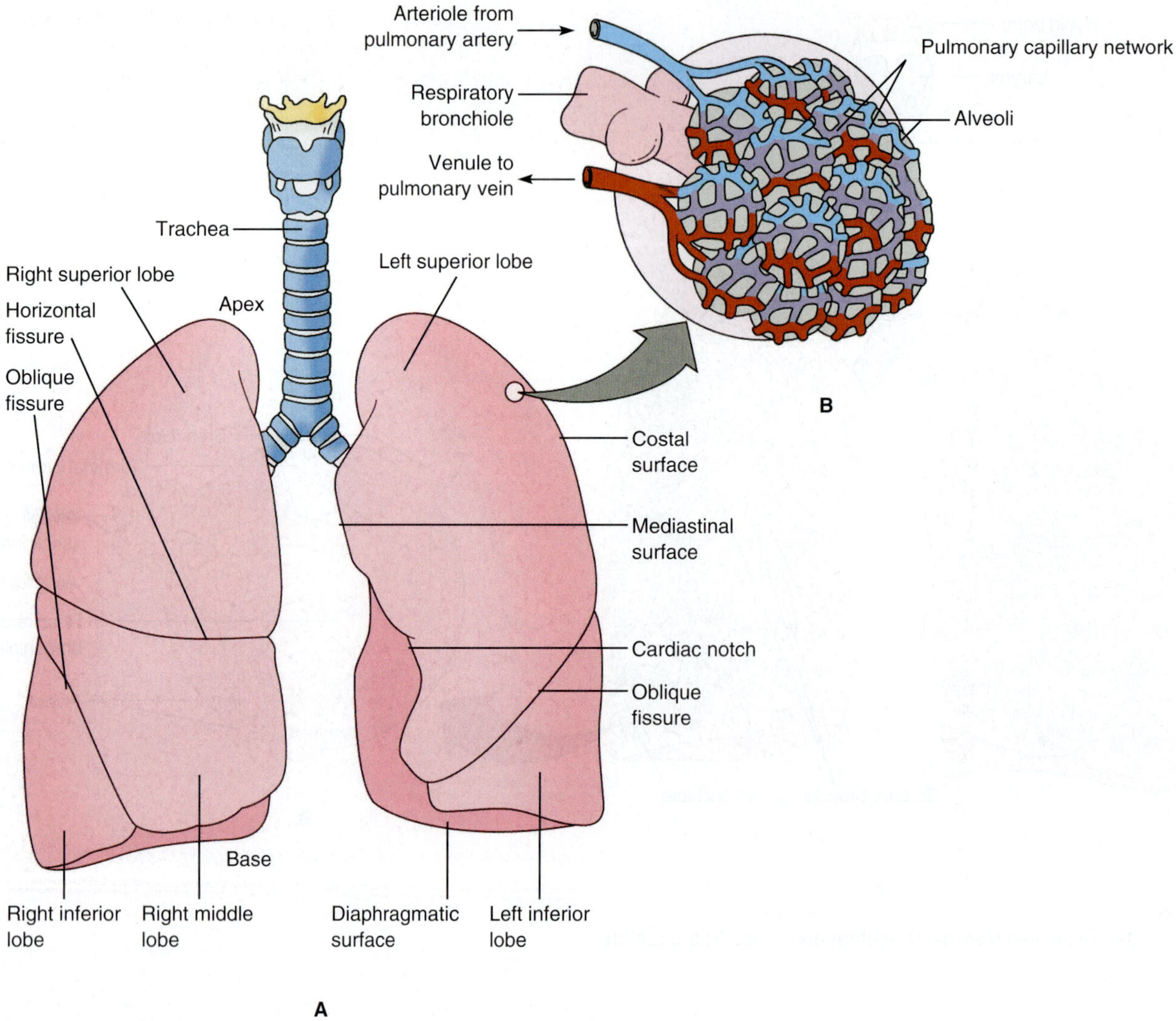

Figure 22-5 Lung structure: (A) Lobes and fissures, (B) alveoli and exchange of gases

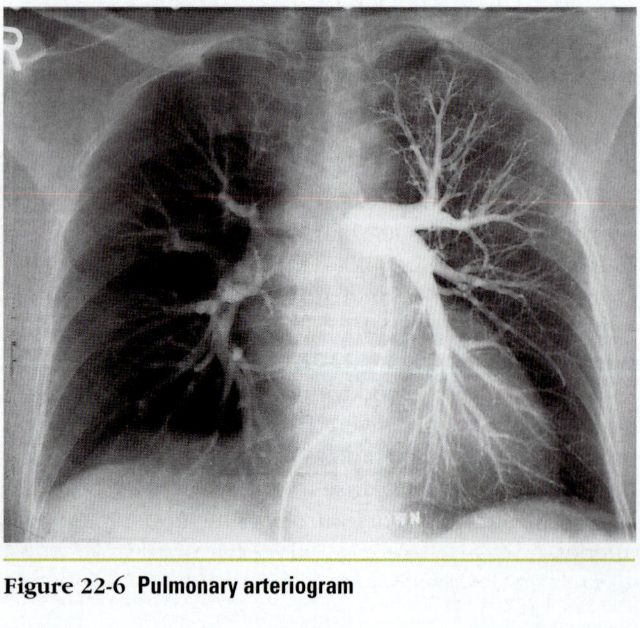

Figure 22-6 Pulmonary arteriogram

ANATOMY AND PHYSIOLOGY OF THE HEART

The human heart is a marvelous design of nature. The role it plays within the cardiovascular system is essential for the circulation of blood, which carries waste substances away from cells to excretory organs for elimination, and vital nutrients and oxygen from the respiratory and digestive organs to cells throughout the body. The circulatory system is also responsible for the transportation of hormones, enzymes, and other important biochemical substances necessary for the proper maintenance and health of the body.

LOCATION OF THE HEART

The heart is a hollow, muscular organ, and is the approximate size of a man's clenched fist. It is located within the mediastinum, slightly off center of the midline of the

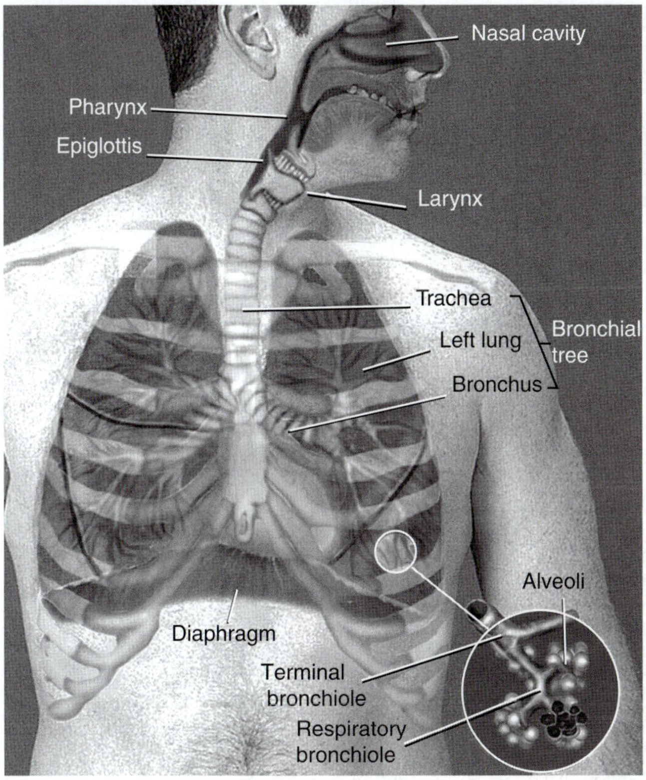

Figure 22-7 Pathway of respiration

thorax, with approximately two-thirds of the organ on the left side (Figure 22-8). It sits just behind the body of the sternum, between the attachments of the second through sixth ribs, and rests on the diaphragm. Posteriorly, the heart sits against the bodies of the fifth through eighth thoracic vertebrae. Within the thorax, the heart lies diagonally, with the distal apex tapering to the left of the midline and the broad, proximal portion lying to the right of the midline.

COVERINGS OF THE HEART

The entire heart is enclosed in a loose sac called the pericardium, which protects the heart and keeps it from rubbing against the thoracic wall. The pericardium consists of two parts:

- *Fibrous pericardium:* a tough, loose-fitting sac that attaches to the large vessels arising from the superior aspect of the heart, the posterior aspect of the sternum, the vertebral column, and the central portion of the diaphragm. It is not, however, attached to the heart itself. The fibrous pericardium is composed largely of white fibrous connective tissue (Figure 22-9).
- *Serous pericardium:* consists of a parietal layer that lines the inside of the fibrous pericardium, and a visceral layer (epicardium) that consists of a thin, serous covering attached to the surface of the heart. Between these two membranes is a potential space called the pericardial cavity, which contains a few drops of serous fluid designed to reduce the friction between the membranes as the heart moves.

THE HEART WALL

The wall of the heart is composed of three layers:

- The epicardium, which is the outer layer of the heart, provides protection and is composed of the visceral pericardium.
- The **myocardium**, which makes up the bulk of the heart wall, is composed of specially constructed cardiac muscle cells that contract and force blood from the heart's chambers.
- The endocardium, which is the inner lining of the heart wall, lines all of the heart's chambers and valves. The endocardium is composed of endothelial tissue, which consists of a single layer of flattened cells.

THE HEART CHAMBERS

The heart is divided internally by four chambers, two on the upper half of the heart and two on the lower half. The upper chambers are called **atria** (singular, atrium) and are designed to receive blood from the veins of the body. The lower chambers are called **ventricles** and are designed to pump blood into arteries leading away from the heart.

The walls of the atria are relatively thin compared to those of the ventricles, which have a thicker myocardium for pumping blood. The right ventricle has a thinner myocardium than does the left ventricle. The right ventricle pumps blood a short distance to the lungs against moderately low resistance to flow. The left ventricle pumps blood to all other portions of the body against great resistance to flow, and therefore needs the extra muscle for increased contractile force.

The chambers of the heart are divided into right and left portions by the septum. The septum between the atria is referred to as the interatrial septum; the interventricular septum separates the ventricles.

THE HEART VALVES

The atrium on each side of the heart communicates with its corresponding ventricle through an opening called the atrioventricular orifice, which is guarded by an atrioventricular valve (AV valve). The atrioventricular orifice between the right atrium and the right ventricle is guarded by the tricuspid valve, named for its three leaf-like appendages, or cusps.

Fibrous cords called chordae tendineae are attached to the cusps on the ventricular side. These cords originate from papillary muscles that project outward from the walls of the muscle. The chordae tendineae prevent the cusps of the valve from folding back into the atrium, causing

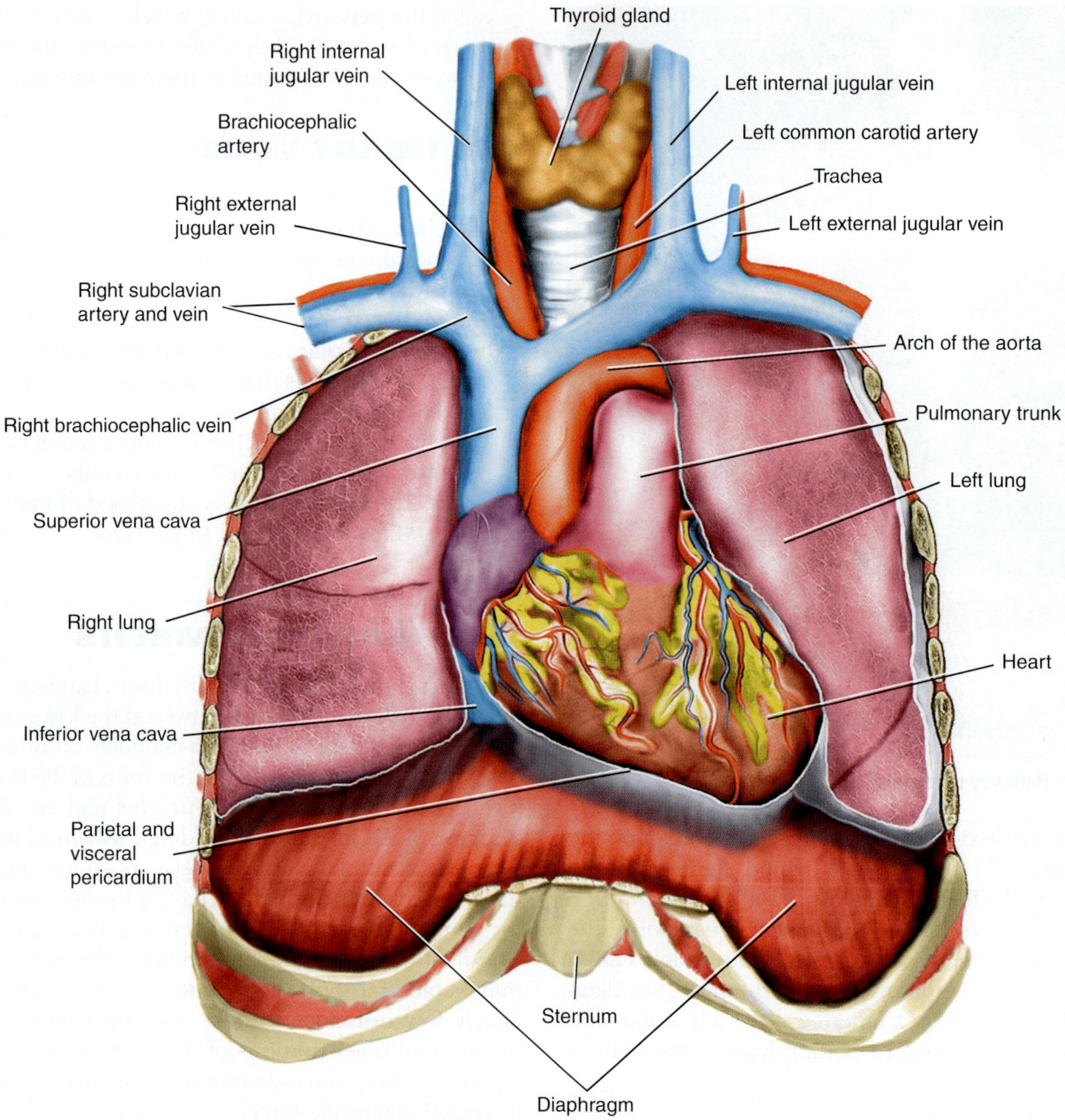

Figure 22-8 Structures within the thorax

incomplete closure of the valve and allowing blood back into the atrium.

The cusps fold open when blood pressure is greater on the atrial side, allowing blood to flow passively into the ventricle. When ventricular pressure is greater, the cusps close shut, and the only exit for the blood is across the pulmonary semilunar valve (so called for its three half-moon-shaped flaps), and into the pulmonary trunk. This valve opens as the right ventricle contracts; back flow is prevented when blood backs up against the valve in the pulmonary trunk after the ventricles relax, causing the semilunar valve to close.

Blood from the lungs enters the left atrium and crosses through the atrioventricular orifice across the atrioventricular valve referred to as the mitral valve. This valve has two cusps, and is appropriately named the bicuspid valve. It prevents blood in the left ventricle from backing up into the left atrium, a condition referred to as mitral **regurgitation**.

When the thick walls of the left ventricle contract, the mitral valve closes against the pressure of the blood within the chamber, and blood is ejected into the large artery known as the aorta. At the base of the aorta is another semilunar valve called the aortic semilunar valve, also consisting of three cusps. This valve prevents blood from flowing back into the left ventricle during ventricular relaxation.

BLOOD FLOW THROUGH THE HEART

The right atrium receives blood that is low in oxygen and high in carbon dioxide from two large veins: the superior

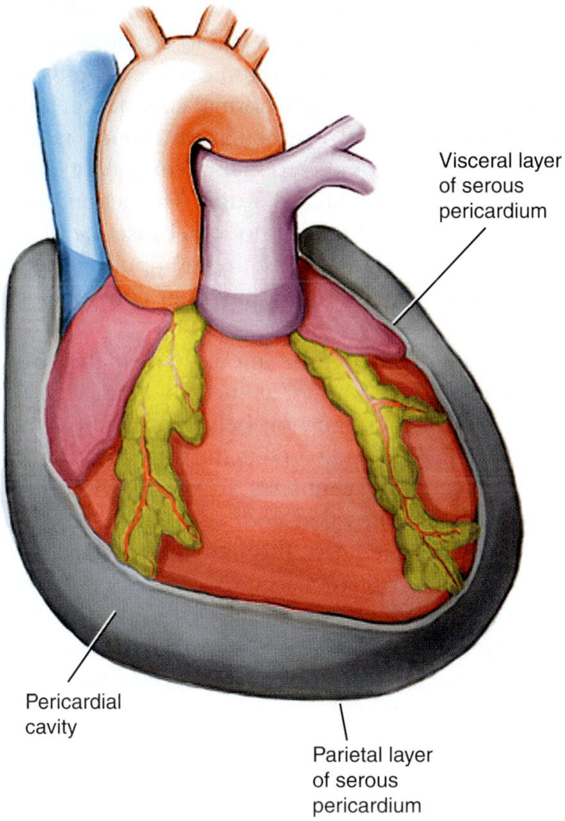

Figure 22-9 Pericardium

vena cava brings in venous blood from the upper portion of the body, and the inferior vena cava brings in venous blood from the lower portions of the body. A smaller vein, the coronary sinus, also empties into the right atrium, draining blood from the wall of the heart. Increased blood pressure in the right atrium causes the tricuspid valve to open, allowing blood to flow somewhat passively into the right ventricle. As blood pressure increases in the right ventricle, the valve closes. Increased pressure within the right ventricle causes the pulmonary semilunar valve to open, and blood is pumped under pressure into the pulmonary artery and on to the lungs for oxygenation. When the right ventricle relaxes, the blood in the pulmonary trunk pushes against the pulmonary semilunar valve and closes it, preventing regurgitation back into the right ventricle.

From the branches of the pulmonary artery, blood enters the capillaries of the alveoli of the lungs. Oxygen and carbon dioxide are exchanged between the blood in the capillaries and the air in the alveoli. The freshly oxygenated blood, which is now low in carbon dioxide, returns to the heart by way of four pulmonary veins and empties into the left atrium. As pressure increases in the left atrium, the atrial wall contracts and the mitral valve opens, moving blood through the left atrioventricular orifice and into the left ventricle. As the left ventricle contracts, the mitral valve closes, and blood enters the aorta through the aortic semilunar valve, where it is propelled to the body.

BLOOD SUPPLY FOR THE HEART

The myocardium of the heart receives oxygenated blood for nourishment from two arteries, both of which originate in the ascending aorta, just above the aortic semilunar valve. The right coronary artery divides into two main branches: the posterior descending artery, which sends branches to both ventricles; and the marginal artery, which sends branches to the right ventricle and right atrium. The left coronary artery divides into two main branches: the anterior descending artery, which supplies blood to both ventricles; and the circumflex artery, which supplies blood to the left ventricle and left atrium.

Both ventricles receive their blood supply from branches of both the right and left coronary arteries. Each atrium receives blood from only a small branch of the corresponding coronary artery. The left ventricle's myocardium receives the most blood, and therefore the most oxygen and nutrients, because of its larger myocardium and increased capacity for pumping.

After blood has nourished the myocardium with oxygen and nutrients and picked up its carbon dioxide wastes, it is delivered back to the right atrium by way of the coronary sinus. The coronary veins that lead into the coronary sinus closely parallel the path of their corresponding arteries.

THE CARDIAC CYCLE

A single **cardiac cycle** includes everything that occurs within the heart during a single heartbeat. In each cardiac cycle, pressure changes occur as the atria and ventricles alternately contract and relax, and blood flows from areas of higher pressure to those of lower pressure. As the atria of the heart relax, the ventricles contract and vice versa. The term **systole** refers to the phase of contraction, and the term diastole refers to the phase of relaxation. For a resting heart rate of 75 beats/minute, each cardiac cycle lasts about 0.8 seconds.

After three-fourths of the blood within the atria has passively drained into the ventricles through the atrioventricular orifice, the walls of the atria contract, forcing the remainder of blood into the ventricles. This contraction is called atrial systole. Contraction of the heart's chambers increases the pressure of the fluid within it. After atrial systole, the walls of the atria relax. This is referred to as atrial diastole.

The contraction of the ventricular wall is referred to as ventricular systole, and the relaxation phase of the ventricles is referred to as ventricular diastole. During ventricular systole, pressure within the ventricles rises sharply.

Once blood pressure within the ventricles exceeds the pressure within the atria, the atrioventricular valves close, allowing pressure within the atria to build. When ventricular pressure exceeds the pressure within the pulmonary artery and the aorta, the semilunar valves open and blood is pumped into those arteries (ventricular ejection). As blood leaves the ventricles, pressure falls below that of the arteries, and the semilunar valves are closed by the pressure of blood within the arteries. The lower pressure within the ventricles during ventricular diastole allows the atrioventricular valves to open once again, and blood begins to flow from the atria into the ventricles.

During ventricular systole, the pressure within the left ventricle rises to about 120 mm Hg, while the pressure within the right ventricle rises to approximately 30 mm Hg. This is a reflection of the left ventricle's thicker myocardium, which is necessary for the left ventricle to pump oxygenated blood to the rest of the body.

CARDIAC OUTPUT

Cardiac output is the amount of blood ejected from the left ventricle into the aorta or from the right ventricle into the pulmonary artery. Cardiac output (CO) equals the stroke volume (the volume of blood ejected by the ventricle with each contraction) times the number of heartbeats per minute. In a typical adult at rest, stroke volume (SV) averages about 70 mL/beat and a heart rate (HR) of 72 beats/min. Therefore, CO = SV × HR or 70 mL/beat × 72 beats/min. The result of 5040 mL/min or 5.04 L/min is approximately the total amount of blood volume within the typical adult male.

CARDIAC CONDUCTION

The cardiac conduction system coordinates the events of the cardiac cycle. Located throughout the heart are specialized areas of tissue that transmit electrical impulses throughout the myocardium for the rhythmical activity of the heart.

The conduction system's key component is the sinoatrial node (SA node), which is located in the right atrial wall just inferior to the opening of the superior vena cava. The SA node acts as a natural electrical pacemaker, and so is referred to as the heart's pacemaker. In other words, the cells of this specialized tissue have the ability to excite themselves. The SA node fires an electrical impulse that spreads into the myocardium and stimulates cardiac muscle fibers to contract in a rhythmic manner. On their own, the autorhythmic fibers in the SA node initiate action potentials 90–100 times per minute, but specific neurotransmitters and hormones can stimulate the autonomic nervous system's parasympathetic division to slow the rate to approximately 75 beats per minute.

The impulse fired by the sinoatrial node spreads throughout atrial tissue and down to the atrioventricular (AV) node, located in the septum between the two atria. This node provides the only normal conduction pathway between the atrial and ventricular syncytium, which are fibers that are interconnected in branching networks that, when stimulated, contract as a unit. The action potential slows considerably at the AV node because the fibers are much smaller, causing a delay in the impulse. This delay allows time for the atria to empty their contents into the ventricles.

From the AV node, the impulse enters the atrioventricular bundle, also known as the bundle of His. This is the only electrical connection between the atria and the ventricles. The AV bundle enters the upper portion of the septum between the ventricles and divides into left and right bundle branches that course along the septum toward the apex of the heart. It is here that the electrical impulse enters larger diameter conduction fibers known as Purkinje fibers, which spread the action potential to the apex of the left ventricle and upward to the remainder of the ventricular myocardium, resulting in a twisting ventricular contraction.

Parasympathetic and sympathetic nerve fibers for the heart originate within the medulla oblongata of the brain stem, becoming part of the right and left vagus nerves and terminating in the SA node and AV node. The parasympathetic division of the autonomic nervous system is responsible for slowing the heart rate, utilizing a neurotransmitter called acetylcholine to dampen SA and AV nodal activity.

Sympathetic fibers from the brain stem travel to the thoracic region of the spinal cord and reach out to the SA and AV nodes by way of cardiac accelerator nerves, which secrete the neurotransmitter norepinephrine to accelerate heart rate and myocardial contraction.

The body, in its quest for homeostasis, seeks a balance between parasympathetic and sympathetic stimulation of the heart. When the body is at rest and the heart rate is at its average 72 beats/min, the parasympathetic division is in control. The SA node typically fires at 90–100 beats/min, so acetylcholine is dampening the node's action through the parasympathetic fibers of the autonomic nervous system.

ANATOMICAL DEVELOPMENT OF THE HEART

The human heart begins its development just before the end of the third week of gestation. Development begins with the formation of two separate tubes that originate from mesodermal cells called endocardial tubes. One end of each tube represents the eventual arterial component of the heart and the other represents the venous component. Eventually, these two endocardial tubes fuse at specific regions in the center, forming one tube called the primitive heart tube. The primitive heart tube has the following five specific regions:

- Ventricle
- Sinus venosus
- Atrium
- Bulbus cordis
- Truncus arteriosus

The bulbus cordis and truncus arteriosus eventually become the pulmonary trunk and aortic arch, while the sinus venosus and atrium become the inferior and superior vena cava and atrial chambers. The ventricle becomes, of course, the ventricular chambers. Myocardial contraction begins by the beginning of the fourth week.

By the seventh week, a partition develops to form separate ventricular chambers, as does a wall that separates the right and left atrium. An opening between the two atrial chambers, referred to as the foramen ovale, remains until birth. At birth, the foramen ovale closes, leaving a depression in the interatrial septum called the fossa ovalis.

Fetal blood secures its oxygen and vital nutrients from maternal blood, bypassing the digestive and respiratory organs. The placenta assumes the function of these organs, interchanging gases, nutrients, and wastes between the fetal and maternal blood.

Two umbilical arteries carry fetal blood to the placenta, and the umbilical vein returns blood with high levels of oxygen and nutrients from the placenta, entering the fetus through the umbilicus and extending branches into the liver. Together, the two umbilical arteries and the one umbilical vein constitute the umbilical cord.

The ductus venosus is a continuation of the umbilical vein. Only small amounts of blood are shunted to the fetal liver by way of the branches of the umbilical vein. Most of the blood from the placenta is moved through the ductus venosus and into the inferior vena cava.

The **ductus arteriosus** connects the pulmonary artery with the descending thoracic aorta, allowing blood to enter into the fetal circulation without going through the lungs. This structure closes at birth.

The foramen ovale is an opening in the interatrial septum. The foramen ovale is a passageway for blood from the right atrium into the left atrium, diverting blood from the fetal lungs (Figure 22-10).

As soon as the umbilical cord is severed, the umbilical arteries and umbilical vein no longer function, and the placenta is expelled shortly after birth. The ductus venosus becomes the ligamentum venosum of the liver, the umbilical vein becomes the round ligament of the liver, and the ductus arteriosus becomes a fibrous cord that helps to stabilize the aorta and pulmonary artery within the thoracic cavity.

After birth, with the elimination of placental circulation, closure of the ductus arteriosus, and a decrease in pulmonary vascular resistance, the right ventricle ejects all of its blood into the pulmonary circulation, and the normal cardiopulmonary circuit is established.

OPERATIVE PATHOLOGY

Operative pathology of the following is described below: chest wall, mediastinum, lungs, thoracic trauma, thoracic outlet syndrome, thoracic aortic **aneurysm**, coronary artery disease, valvular disease, cardiomyopathy, cardiac dysrhythmias, and acyanotic and cyanotic congenital heart defects.

THE CHEST WALL

The most common congenital deformity of the chest is a funnel-shaped, asymmetrical depression due to a posterior displacement of the sternal body, referred to as pectus excavatum (Figure 22-11). In extreme cases, the sternum may even reach the vertebral column. Symptoms include bronchospasm, exercise intolerance, dysrhythmias, chest pain, and dyspnea. Surgical repair before the age of 5 produces the best results.

Pectus carinatum refers to a deformity of the chest wall that results in a prominent sternum, most often caused by an upward curve of the lower costal cartilages. In some cases, the manubrium and upper ribs are pushed outward with a posteriorly angulated body that suddenly projects anteriorly. The patient is often asymptomatic, but dysrhythmia and dyspnea on exertion may be present. Surgical repair is often performed for cosmetic reasons.

Sternal fissures may be classified as superior sternal cleft, inferior sternal cleft, and complete cleft of the sternum. A complete cleft of the sternum is rare, and involves a protrusion of exposed mediastinal structures through a thin covering of skin and fascia. There is also a free communication between the peritoneal and pericardial cavities. Surgical repair involves the suturing of a synthetic mesh over the sternal defect, primary closure of the pericardium, and closure of the abdominal wall defects with rectus sheaths.

Inferior sternal clefts are often one of many other related defects, such as free communication between the pericardial and peritoneal cavities, omphalocele defect, and crescentic deficiency of the diaphragm; and heart defects, such as tetralogy of Fallot or ventricular septal defect.

Superior sternal clefts extend from the clavicular heads to the fourth costal cartilage. The heart and great vessels are exposed through the cleft, and are only covered by skin and fascia. Repair can be achieved with bilateral oblique chondrotomies that are rotated to the midline and wired or sutured in place.

THE MEDIASTINUM

Typical of the lesions found within the mediastinum are thymomas, lymphomas, and germ cell tumors. Mass lesions

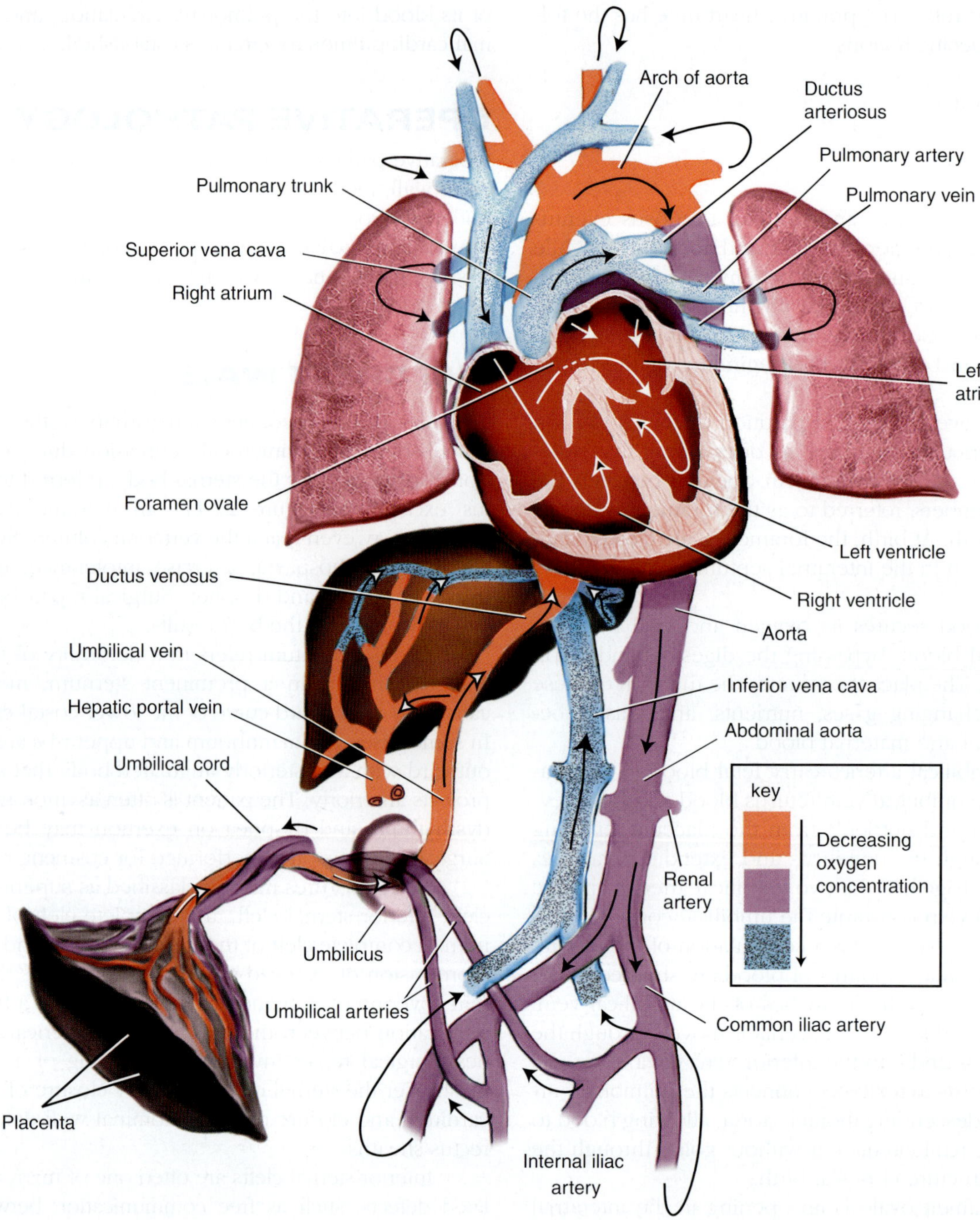

Figure 22-10 Fetal circulation

tend to be enterogenous cysts, lymphomas, neurogenic tumors, and pleuropericardial cysts. The most common tumors found within the mediastinum of children are neurogenic tumors; in adults, thymomas and lymphomas appear most frequently. Of the patients with mediastinal lesions, 40% are asymptomatic, and the remaining 60% have symptoms that are nonspecific. Complaints typically include cough, dyspnea, and chest pain. Symptomatic lesions are malignant in 60% of all patients.

THE LUNGS

Carcinoma of the lung is the leading cause of death due to cancer in the United States. Approximately 150,000 people die from the disease each year. Most of the affected are male, but as more females take up cigarette smoking and workplace trends change, the numbers are evening out. In most cases, lung cancer is the result of cigarette smoking. In fact, 90% of all patients with carcinoma

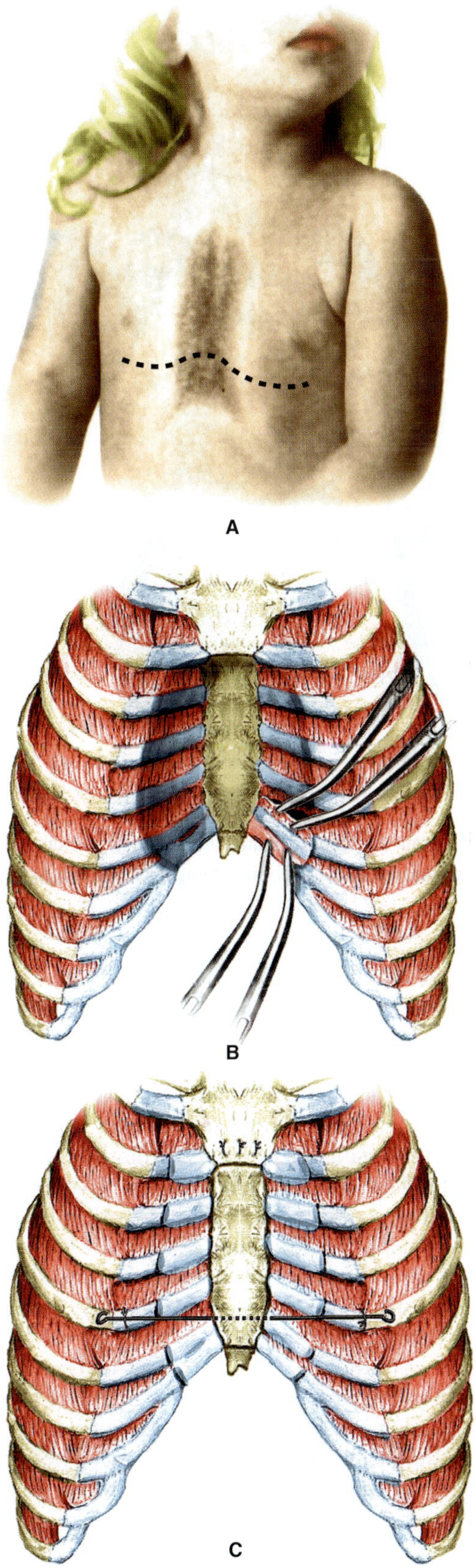

Figure 22-11 **Pectus excavatum repair: (A) Defect and incision outline, (B) pectoralis muscles elevated from chest wall, (C) chest wall stabilized (K-wire) following repair**

of the lung are cigarette smokers. Cigarette smoke contains a number of known carcinogens, the worst of which are the polycyclic hydrocarbons. These substances promote malignant transformation of bronchial cells (most new lung growths begin in the bronchi) through the activation of oncogenes and tumor suppression gene inhibition. Cigarette smoke also contains irritants that, in combination with the carcinogens, create preneoplastic lesions that eventually become cancerous.

Lung tumors are divided into four major subgroups: small cell carcinoma, squamous cell carcinoma, adenocarcinoma, and large cell carcinoma. Tumors may also be of a mixed pattern. Tumors of the lung are usually metastases from other sites, most commonly the kidney or the colon, although primary lung tumors are not uncommon. Primary lung tumors are highly invasive, and may metastasize locally to the prescalene lymph nodes, esophagus, and pericardium. Distant metastatic sites include the brain, adrenal glands, liver, or skeleton.

A small percentage of patients are asymptomatic, with detection of tumor made by routine chest X-ray. Most patients, however, present with persistent cough, hemoptysis, and shortness of breath. Intrathoracic extrapulmonary symptoms, such as pleural effusion, pain on inspiration, or clubbing of fingers, are present if lesions permeate the pleural space.

The prognosis for those afflicted with the disease is poor, as only 13% live 5 years or more after diagnosis. Mortality is related to tumor type and size on diagnosis. Initial diagnosis is made by chest X-ray and sputum cytology test, but definitive diagnosis is made with a biopsy from fiberoptic bronchoscopy. Early detection of bronchial tumors cannot be made with X ray, only with bronchoscopy. Mediastinoscopy is useful for the evaluation of nodal involvement of lung carcinoma.

THORACIC TRAUMA

Injuries to the chest wall and its underlying structures may be caused by blunt or penetrating force. Blunt chest injuries are usually the result of deceleration in motor vehicle accidents and falls, whereas firearms and knives are often the culprits in penetrating chest injuries. Penetrating wounds have only a site of entry, while perforating wounds have both an entry site and an exit site. Trauma to the chest wall alerts the physician to possible internal injury. For instance, fracture of the first or second rib may indicate thoracic aorta, innominate (brachiocephalic) artery, or subclavian artery injury.

In the emergency room, the physician should look for respiratory disturbances and hemodynamic instability related to the thorax. Cardiac contusion should be considered in rapid deceleration injuries. A chest X-ray is essential for the detection of fractures, hemothorax, pneumothorax, and lung contusion. Computerized axial tomography, MRI, angiography, and echocardiography

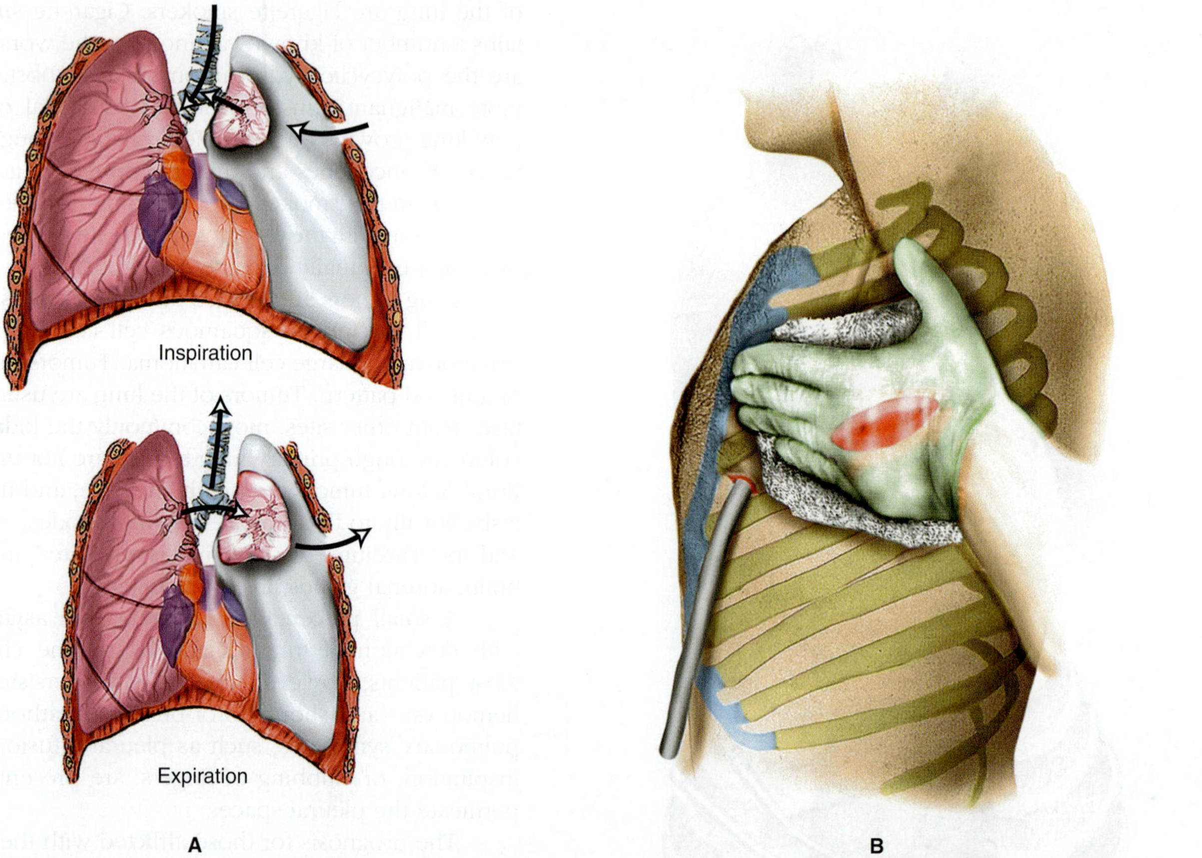

Figure 22-12 Penetrating chest trauma and treatment: (A) Open pneumothorax: Air from the outside rushes into the pleural cavity, compromising the function of the lungs. (Arrows indicate air movement during respiration.) (B) Tube thoracostomy: The open wound is occluded and a chest tube is inserted, permitting lung reexpansion

are all useful for diagnosing internal thoracic organ injuries.

Although sternal fracture is uncommon, minor rib fractures occur frequently with trauma to the chest. In fact, the number of rib fractures is a good indicator of the severity of chest trauma. Multiple rib fractures resulting in the loss of bony support of the chest wall may result in a chest wall motion that is opposite of the normal movement of the chest wall, a condition known as flail chest. Fractures of the first or second ribs are accompanied by multisystem trauma approximately 50% of the time. The neurovascular bundle is especially susceptible to injury with first and second rib fractures; diagnosis is confirmed by selective angiography.

Blunt or penetrating chest trauma may result in an accumulation of air and alveolar gas in the pleural cavity that takes up space normally occupied by the lung. The lung is unable to expand and so partially collapses. This condition is known as a pneumothorax, and is treated with tube thoracostomy (chest tube).

An open pneumothorax results from a large penetrating wound to the chest that exposes the pleural space to atmospheric pressure (Figure 22-12). As the diaphragm contracts, air is sucked into the wound, competing with normal ventilation. This type of wound should be completely covered with a dressing and a chest tube should be placed away from the wound.

A dangerous condition known as tension pneumothorax occurs when air escapes from a bronchus into the pleural cavity, but cannot regain entry back into the bronchus. Increasing air pressure within the pleural cavity causes collapse of the lung, decreased venous return due to mediastinal shift, and eventual cardiovascular collapse. Treatment should be immediate, and includes the placement of a large-gauge needle into the second or third intercostal space for pleural space decompression and tube thoracostomy.

Trauma to the chest may result in hemorrhage into the pleural cavity. Posterior placement of one or two chest tubes will effect drainage, but massive amounts of blood should be surgically removed because such a hemothorax may be providing hemostasis for a large vessel injury that will need to be repaired.

Trauma to the mediastinum may result in cardiac **tamponade** and contusion, aortic injury, esophageal injury, and air embolism. Cardiac tamponade is the compression of the heart due to a collection of blood or fluid within the pericardium, usually as a result of penetrating

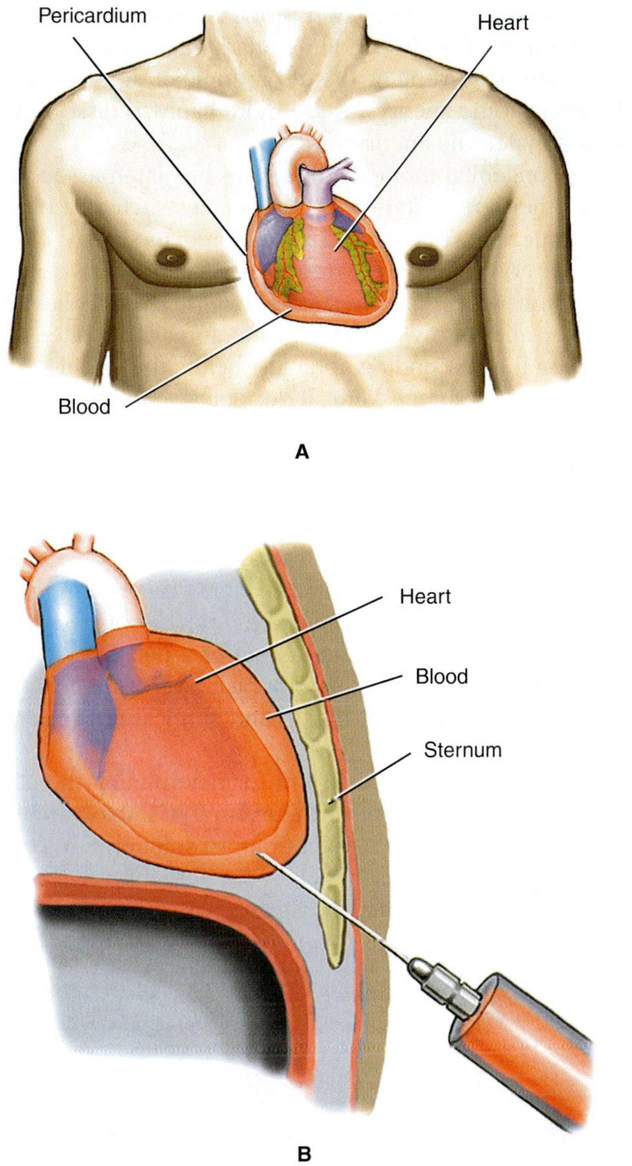

Figure 22-13 Cardiac tamponade: (A) Fluid within pericardial cavity, (B) pericardial aspiration with needle and syringe

trauma (Figure 22-13). The mass of fluid or blood interferes with atrial and ventricular filling, compromising the flow of blood to the myocardium from the coronary arteries. Contractility is slowed and cardiac output is reduced. This condition is often present with tension pneumothorax. The patient typically presents with hypotension, distended neck veins, **tachycardia**, and muffled heart sounds. Central venous pressure is increased as arterial blood pressure falls.

Treatment for cardiac tamponade must be immediate. Pericardial aspiration through a small subxiphoid incision is the first step in treatment, but the surgeon must be ready for median sternotomy or thoracotomy in case the pericardiocentesis results in massive blood loss.

Cardiac contusion usually affects the more anterior right ventricle and is often the result of blunt trauma by deceleration-type injuries. Collision with the steering wheel of a car is typical.

Injury to the thoracic aorta as a result of blunt or penetrating trauma is associated with a high mortality rate and requires immediate surgical treatment. Aortography confirms the location and extent of the tear.

THORACIC OUTLET SYNDROME

Thoracic outlet syndrome refers to a variety of symptoms associated with compression of the brachial plexus nerve complex and subclavian vessels at the superior aperture of the thorax. These structures follow a path to the upper extremity through the cervicoaxillary canal. Compression of the neurovascular bundle generally occurs in the proximal portion of the canal. Symptoms include arm pain, vasomotor symptoms, paresthesia of fingers, and atrophy of the muscles of the hand. Thoracic outlet syndrome may be caused by a drooping shoulder girdle, an adventitious fibrous band, cervical rib, continual hyperabduction of the arm, or, most commonly, an abnormal first rib.

Classification of thoracic outlet syndrome may be arterial thoracic, neurological, or venous thoracic. Arterial thoracic outlet syndrome is a result of subclavian artery compression and results in severe ischemia of the arm. Neurological thoracic outlet syndrome is generally a result of hyperextension of the neck or upper back and causes symptoms of throbbing pain in the extremity and paraesthesia of the neck and arms. Venous thoracic outlet syndrome involves the external compression of the axillosubclavian vein. Symptoms include pain, cyanosis, and arm swelling.

THORACIC AORTIC ANEURYSM

An aneurysm is a sac formed by localized dilatation of the walls of an artery due to structural weakening. The strength of an arterial wall is in the elastic tissue of the tunica media. Destruction of this layer by any disease diminishes the strength of the vessel wall.

Arterial aneurysms may be classified according to cause, shape, location, or structure. There are two types of aneurysm: true aneurysm, in which the wall of the sac consists of one or more of the layers that make up the wall of the blood vessel; and false, or pseudoaneurysms, which are pulsatile hematomas that are not contained by the vessel layers but are confined by a fibrous capsule. False aneurysms are caused by disruption of the vessel wall or of the anastomotic site between graft and vessel, with blood contained by surrounding tissue. Atherosclerotic aneurysms are classified as true aneurysms.

Dilatation of the aorta may occur as a consequence of aging, atherosclerosis, infection, inflammation, trauma, congenital malformation, or medial degeneration. The principal consequences of atherosclerosis of the aorta are aneurysm formation or obstruction. The atherosclerotic aorta cannot adapt to changes of blood pressure that occur during the normal cardiac cycle. The aorta is unable to expand during systole, and blood pressure must increase to force blood through a smaller arterial lumen. The increased pressure from inside forces dilatation of the inelastic aorta, and an aneurysm forms on the weakened arterial wall.

Aneurysms of the aorta may occur in several forms (Figure 22-14). They may be spindle shaped (fusiform), which involve the entire circumference of the artery, or they may appear as eccentric bubble formations (saccular), which only involve part of the circumference of the artery. A dissecting aneurysm involves hemorrhage into the arterial wall, which widens and splits due to a defect in the tunica media and tunica intima caused by the great hemodynamic forces associated with aneurysm formation and atherosclerosis. Classifications of the dissecting aortic aneurysm are:

Type I: Dissection of the ascending aorta and aortic pouch extending to the iliac bifurcation.

Type II: Dissection of the ascending aorta only.

Type III: Dissection originates at or distal to the left subclavian artery and extends distally for some distance. This dissection does not involve the thoracic aorta proximal to the left subclavian artery.

Aneurysm formation may occur at any point along the length of the aorta, while obstruction is usually confined to the abdominal aorta. Thoracic aneurysms may occur in the ascending, arch, or descending aorta. When the aortic arch or descending aorta are aneurysmal, there is usually involvement of the abdominal aorta as well. Thoracic aortic aneurysms are more likely to dissect than abdominal aortic aneurysms.

Congenital thoracic aneurysms are often associated with other congenital cardiac anomalies such as a bicuspid aortic valve or coarctation. Acquired aneurysms of the thoracic aorta occur most frequently in males between the ages of 40 and 70 as a result of hypertension. Following trauma, aneurysms of the thoracic aorta most often develop in the descending aorta just below the origin of the left subclavian artery. Vertical deceleration injuries are often responsible for aneurysm formation of the ascending thoracic aorta.

The patient with thoracic aorta aneurysm may be asymptomatic, but advanced dilatation may impinge on surrounding intrathoracic structures. Chest pain is the most common complaint, but may only be present in the supine position. Many aneurysms are discovered accidentally during routine chest X-ray or a detailed medical examination. Rupture of the thoracic aortic aneurysm is associated with high mortality, and surgical repair is imperative.

Ultrasonography is useful for determining the size, shape, and location of the aneurysm, but angiography is the defining diagnostic study. Contrast solution is injected through a catheter inserted into the femoral artery, and the aneurysm is outlined by X-ray.

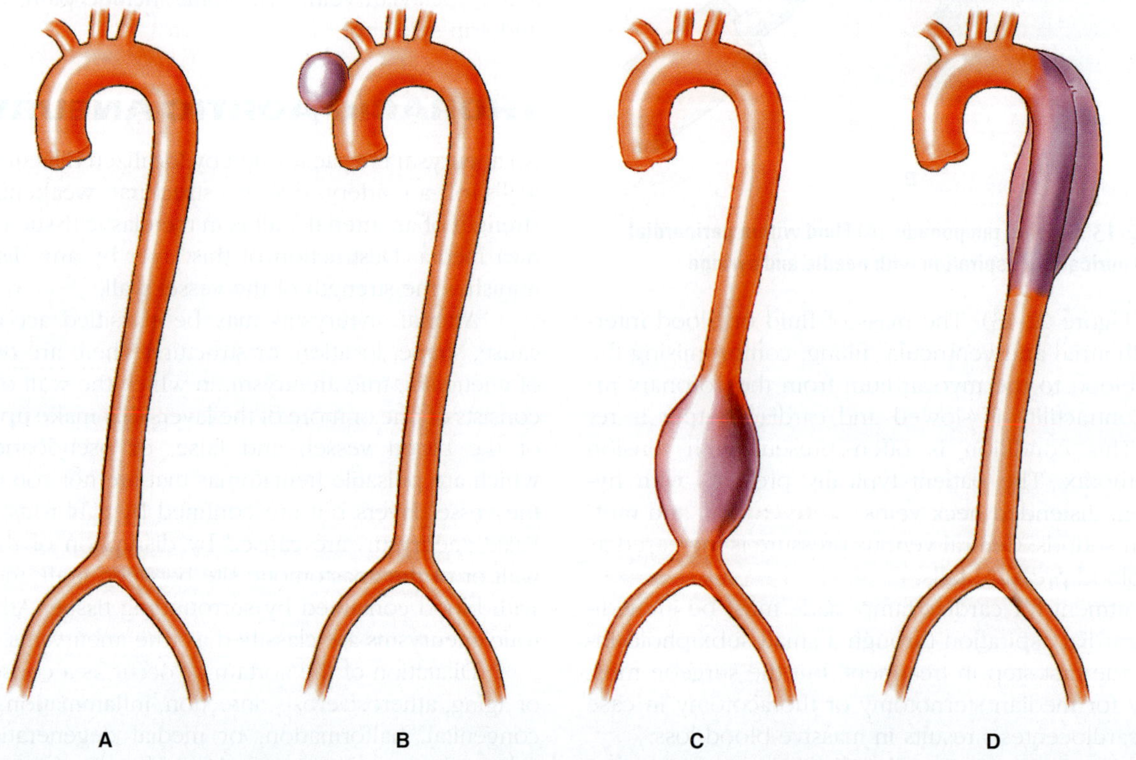

Figure 22-14 Various forms of aneurysms: (A) Normal aorta, (B) saccular aneurysm, (C) fusiform aneurysm, (D) dissecting aneurysm

CORONARY ARTERY DISEASE

Coronary atherosclerotic heart disease is the most common type of coronary artery disease, and is recognized as the leading cause of death in the industrialized Western world. Each year approximately 1 million Americans die from the disease, and the annual economic costs are staggering, averaging in the tens of billions of dollars.

Risk factors for coronary atherosclerosis include:

- *Age:* Older people are far more likely to be affected.
- *Sex:* The disease affects more males than females. Female sex hormones are thought to play a role, and estrogen therapy for postmenopausal women is currently being studied.
- *Race:* There is a higher mortality rate among nonwhites.
- *Genetics:* A familial disposition is thought to have both genetic and environmental origins.
- *Hypertension:* High blood pressure will accelerate the development of atherosclerosis, particularly if it develops at an early age.
- *Cigarette smoking:* This is one of the most important risk factors associated with the disease. The negative effects on the cardiovascular system are partially related to nicotine, tar, carbon monoxide, and other harmful components of cigarette smoke.
- *Diet:* A diet rich in saturated fats (especially animal fats) contributes to the development of the disease.
- *Obesity:* Overall, obese people develop atherosclerosis at an earlier age and have more significant lesions than do those who weigh less. Elevated serum levels of lipids, such as cholesterol, lipoproteins, and triglycerides, directly correlate with the extent and severity of the atherosclerosis. Obese individuals are also more prone to hypertension, diabetes, and glucose intolerance; it is these associated factors that may be the link between obesity and atherosclerosis.
- *Clotting factors:* Soluble clotting factors, such as thrombin, fibrin, and platelets, play a role in the formation of atherosclerotic lesions.
- *Psychosocial influences:* Individuals in lower socioeconomic positions are more likely to smoke, are more obese, and have higher rates of hypertension than those in positions of higher economic status. Individuals who are under constant pressure to perform, or who can be labeled "overachievers," are more likely to develop atherosclerosis.

The term *atherosclerosis,* from the Greek *athere,* meaning "gruel" or "porridge," and *scleros,* meaning "hard," describes a condition that involves the formation of an atheroma in the intima of medium and large arteries. Atheromas are the prototypical lesions of atherosclerosis, and consist of a soft central region composed of lipids and cellular debris covered by a tough layer of fibrous tissue. Calcium salts are eventually deposited into the arterial walls and the atheromas, resulting in a hardening of the artery. The result of the atherosclerotic process is a reduction of blood flow to the target tissues.

The atheroma is also highly thrombogenic, launching small pieces, or thrombi, into the bloodstream. These pieces can become lodged in smaller vessels such as cerebral or coronary arteries and may completely occlude the lumen of the vessel with subsequent infarction.

The first step in the formation of the atheroma (Figure 22-15) is believed to be an injury to the endothelial lining of the arterial wall. Blood platelets and lipoproteins are deposited into the injury as a repair mechanism, and growth factors released from the platelets stimulate the growth of new smooth muscle tissue in the arterial wall. Changes in the metabolism of the smooth muscle cells promote the accumulation of cholesterol and other lipids within the cells' cytoplasm, which, when leaked across the cell membrane into the interstitial spaces, attract scavenger macrophages. The macrophages secrete biologically active substances that cause further damage to the arterial wall. Eventually, collagen is deposited into the lesion and scar tissue begins to form, narrowing the lumen of the artery.

Progressive, chronic, myocardial ischemia, the underlying pathogenic mechanism of coronary atherosclerosis, develops as a result of the progression of narrowing of the lumen of the coronary artery due to atheroma formation. It is ischemia that is responsible for the clinical manifestations of coronary atherosclerosis: angina pectoris, which occurs when myocardial oxygen demand exceeds supply, and is characterized by substernal or retrosternal "crushing" pain that often radiates to the throat, back, or left arm; acute myocardial **infarction**, which results in the death of heart muscle tissue; and sudden cardiac death.

Sudden occlusion of the vessel results in acute myocardial infarction and treatment must be immediate. The area of damage by myocardial infarction depends on the coronary artery affected and the amount of myocardial tissue served by the artery. For example, an occlusion of the proximal right coronary artery will result in infarction of the right ventricle and posterior wall of the left ventricle; an occlusion of the proximal circumflex branch of the left coronary system will result in infarction of the lateral wall of the left ventricle; and an anterior ventricular wall infarction is typically caused by occlusion of the proximal left anterior descending artery. Smaller areas of damage occur in the myocardium when occlusion occurs in one or more distal branches of the coronary arteries.

Coronary artery lesions usually occur near the origin and bifurcation of the main coronary vessels, but diffuse involvement throughout the branches is seen in advanced cases. Most lesions occur in the left anterior

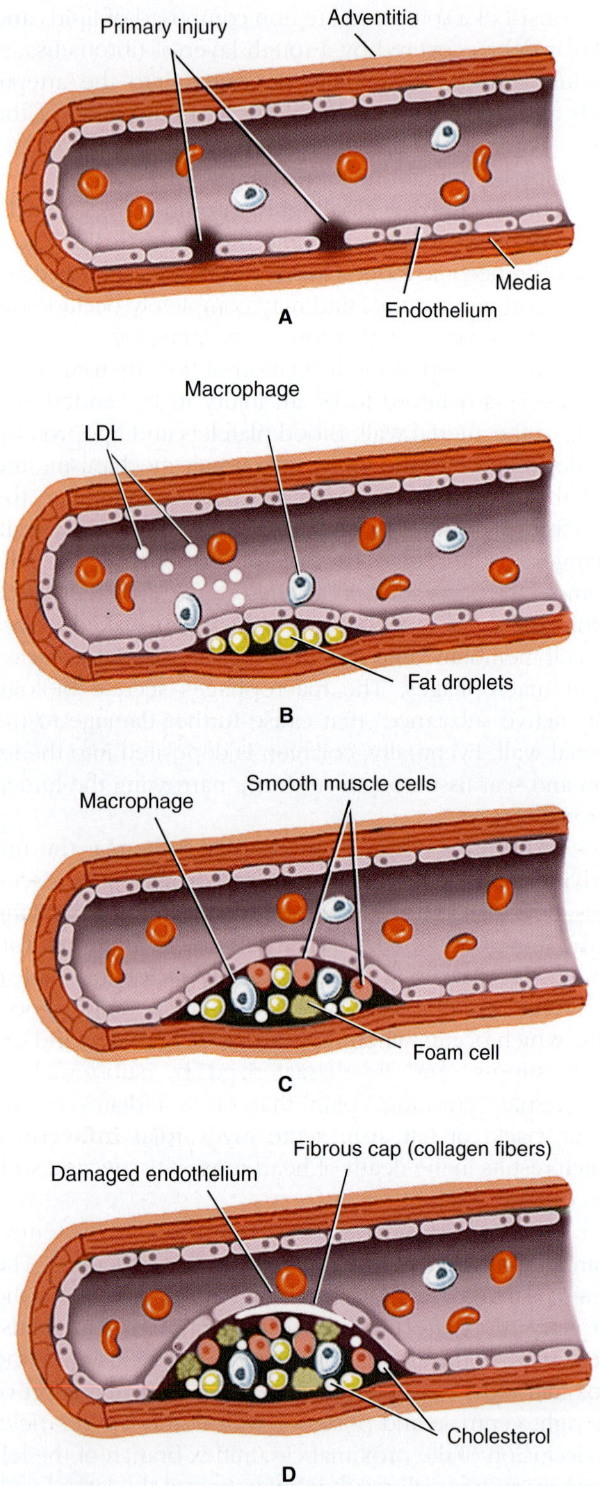

Figure 22-15 Atheroma formation: (A) Endothelial injury, (B) influx of lipids, (C) accumulation of lipids, proliferation of smooth muscle cells, and accumulation of macrophages, (D) atheroma

descending artery, or LAD. The LAD accounts for 50% of all atherosclerotic lesions of the coronary system, the right coronary artery accounts for 30–40%, and the circumflex branch of the left coronary system accounts for 15–20% of the lesions.

Within 24 hours of a myocardial infarction, temperature is elevated and white cell count is increased due to myocardial necrosis. Death of the myocardial cells also brings about the release of certain enzymes that enter the bloodstream. The following enzymes can be detected in the blood work:

- Creatine kinase (CK) levels increase and peak in 24–36 hours.
- The level of serum aspartate aminotransferase (AST) increases rapidly in 4–6 hours and peaks in 24–48 hours.
- Lactate dehydrogenase (LD) levels begin to increase the first day after attack and persist at high levels for 10–20 days.

Sudden death from myocardial infarction (MI) occurs in approximately 25% of cases, usually as a result of ventricular fibrillation (a major dysrhythmia in which the walls of the ventricle flutter without coordinated contraction, and blood is not pumped away from the heart), heart block, and asystole (cardiac arrest).

Diagnosis of MI is based on the presenting symptoms and evidence of impaired heart function that is found by physical examination, electrocardiography, and abnormal serum enzyme levels.

Drug therapy is aimed at reducing myocardial oxygen demand, and includes vasodilators such as nitroglycerin, beta-adrenergic blocking agents, and calcium channel blockers, which inhibit the movement of calcium ions across the cell membranes via the calcium channel.

The cardiac catheterization laboratory, or "cath lab," is often the next stop after the emergency room for the patient suffering an acute MI. The cardiologist can insert a temporary pacemaker wire into the right ventricle of the heart to stabilize heart rhythm, and can also insert catheters into the coronary arteries for the injection of contrast solutions, which, under fluoroscopy, can outline the coronary artery lesion and the extent of the blockage. Contrast solution injected into the left ventricle can clearly outline the damage to the left ventricular wall.

If necessary, the cardiologist can insert balloon-tipped catheters into the affected coronary artery and compress the atheroma against the artery wall. This is known as percutaneous transluminal coronary angioplasty (PTCA), and is discussed in detail later. Placement of a prosthetic intravascular **stent** (Figure 22-16) to maintain the cylindrical lumen produced by the balloon is also an option.

The cardiologist can also perform intracoronary thrombolysis, which involves the injection of an enzyme called streptokinase that can break down thrombi and thereby enlarge the lumen of the artery.

Surgical intervention in the form of coronary artery bypass grafting (CABG) may be necessary. The procedure may not necessarily prolong life or reduce the occurrence

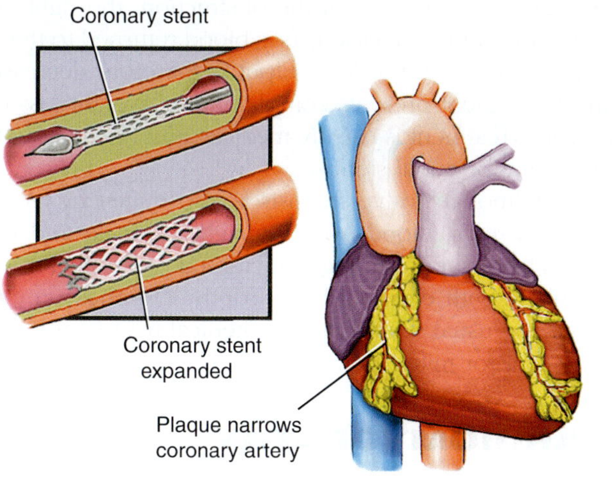

Figure 22-16 Intracoronary stent

of myocardial infarction, but it does reduce angina and improve activity tolerance, thereby improving the quality of life. Once damaged, however, the myocardium cannot be repaired.

Complications of myocardial infarction include:

- Myocardial rupture, which may occur as a result of a softening of the necrotic ventricular myocardium and an increased ventricular pressure. As blood escapes from the ventricle into the pericardial sac, the heart is compressed, interrupting normal rhythm. This potentially lethal condition is known as cardiac tamponade and is usually treated by pericardiocentesis.
- Cardiac aneurysm, or a ballooning of the ventricular wall, can be a result of increased ventricular pressure and scar tissue in the ventricular wall formed by massive myocardial infarctions.
- Heart failure and cardiogenic shock. As a result of inadequate perfusion of tissues by a failing heart, multisystem organ failure may develop. The most dangerous of these is cerebral ischemia, which may lead to irreversible brain damage. But it is the kidneys that are most often damaged. Typical signs of renal failure, such as oliguria and anuria, are common.

VALVULAR DISEASE

Disease of the semilunar or atrioventricular valves of the heart can lead to stenosis of the valves, a condition that can obstruct the normal flow of blood from one region of the heart to another, or to valvular insufficiency, which can cause a reflux of blood into the area from which the blood was ejected during systole. This reverse flow, usually involving the mitral and tricuspid valves, is known as regurgitation. As the valvular disease progresses, the myocardium enlarges to compensate for insufficient flow, and, unless treated surgically with prosthetic valve replacements, congestive heart failure is bound to ensue.

Rheumatic fever may cause calcium deposition and fibrous tissue formation on the leaflets of the mitral valve. This results in an immobile valve, and the atrioventricular orifice between the left atrium and left ventricle becomes progressively narrower. Half of the patients with the disease will develop atrial fibrillation, and blood flow from the atria to the ventricles is not ejected normally because the contraction is eliminated. Blood stagnated in the atria may form thromboses that could result in arterial embolization.

Diagnosis of mitral valve stenosis is established by clinical symptoms: dyspnea on exertion as a result of pulmonary hypertension; dysphagia or bronchitis as a result of left atrial hypertrophy; and excessive fatigue and weakness due to a decreased cardiac output. On auscultation, an opening snap may be heard, which is the result of a forceful opening of the valve, followed by a diastolic rumbling (murmur).

Mitral valve stenosis can also be diagnosed by cardiac catheterization, which, with the placement of catheters, can provide information on cardiac output from the left ventricle as well as pulmonary artery pressures. A comparison of pressures within the atrium and ventricle can provide a pressure gradient across the valve. Noninvasive diagnosis can be achieved with an echocardiogram, which can outline left atrial enlargement, fusion of the mitral leaflets, and obstruction of flow from the left atrium to the left ventricle.

Surgical interventions include mitral valve replacement, which will be described in detail later, and commissurotomy, which is the separation of the fused leaflets at their borders (known as the valve's commissures), and reattachment to the chordae tendineae.

Mitral regurgitation can also be caused by mitral valve **prolapse** (MVP). This form of mitral insufficiency is a condition in which some portion of the mitral valve is pushed back too far during ventricular contraction, usually due to redundant tissue on one or both leaflets or papillary muscle dysfunction. The valve leaflets are pushed in the direction of the left atrium during systole, and blood flows backward. MVP, in the vast majority of patients, is a benign condition requiring no treatment.

Medical treatment is similar to that for mitral stenosis. Surgical intervention involves mitral valve replacement or a valvuloplasty, which involves direct suturing of the torn leaflets. Occasionally, an annuloplasty is performed, which involves the suturing of a prosthetic ring into the circumference of the mitral annulus. As the sutures are pulled together, the size of the atrioventricular orifice is reduced and proper valve function is restored.

Aortic valve stenosis is less common than mitral valve disease and usually affects males. It can be caused by rheumatic fever, but atherosclerosis can be responsible for the condition in the elderly. Congenital valvular malformation is the predominant factor in aortic stenosis, causing the patient to become more susceptible to endocarditis or rheumatic fever.

Aortic stenosis impedes the flow from the left ventricle into the aorta, resulting in hypertrophy of the left ventricle as the ventricle struggles to overcome the increased resistance of its outflow tract. As the hypertrophied ventricle becomes dysfunctional, cardiac output is decreased; back flow to the left atrium and pulmonary circulation result in left atrial and pulmonary hypertension. The enlarged ventricle may also compress the coronary arteries at a pressure exceeding coronary perfusion pressure, resulting in myocardial ischemia and angina, exacerbated by the increased oxygen demands of the hypertrophied ventricle's myocardium. Eventually, heart failure will ensue.

The true extent of stenosis and cor pulmonale (overload of the right ventricle due to pulmonary hypertension) can be attained with cardiac catheterization. Echocardiography will show a thickened aortic valve and ventricular wall, with abnormal movement of the aortic leaflets.

Medical management is the first line of treatment, with the use of digitalis glycosides, sodium restriction, and diuretics for congestive heart failure. Nitroglycerine can be used to treat angina. Surgical intervention involves the replacement of the aortic valve with a prosthetic, which will be discussed in detail later.

Aortic regurgitation, like aortic stenosis, is frequently caused by rheumatic fever, which damages the leaflets of the valve and results in an incomplete closure. Marfan syndrome is another etiologic factor. This disease, which affects connective tissue systemically, results in necrosis and aneurysm formation of the ascending aorta. The dilation of the aortic annulus pulls the leaflets apart, resulting in valvular insufficiency. Congenital malformation of the valve results in susceptibility to bacterial endocarditis and rheumatic fever; aortic regurgitation is therefore imminent.

When the leaflets of the aortic valve close improperly, the outlet between the left ventricle and the aorta remains open to a degree, and blood that has been expelled into the aorta across the aortic valve flows back into the left ventricle during diastole. The ventricle hypertrophies and must contract more forcefully to expel this increased volume of blood.

Diagnosis is made on auscultation with a blowing diastolic murmur over the ascending aorta. Cardiac catheterization reveals the extent of the valvular insufficiency, the degree of ventricular overload, the stroke volume, and ejection fraction.

Tricuspid stenosis is uncommon and usually occurs in conjunction with mitral or aortic stenosis. Blood returning to the heart from systemic circulation is backed up because the valve is not allowing proper flow from the right atrium into the right ventricle, thereby increasing systemic venous pressure. As blood backs up into the right atrium as a result of the obstruction, the right ventricle's output is decreased, as is blood returned to the left side of the heart. Cardiac output is therefore decreased, and the patient presents complaining of weight loss and fatigue. Treatment is usually medical, and is similar to the treatment for mitral stenosis.

Pulmonary valve stenosis is also quite rare. As the valve narrows, blood from the right ventricle and right atrium backs up, resulting in increased pressures for both chambers with eventual hypertrophy. Dyspnea on exertion is the usual symptom, and medical treatment is similar to that for mitral stenosis.

CARDIOMYOPATHY

Cardiomyopathy is a general term designating primary disease of the myocardium, often of obscure and unknown etiology. In response to injury, the heart often enlarges, restricting its normal function. Cardiomyopathy can appear in many forms, including alcoholic, congestive, hypertrophic, infiltrative, and restrictive cardiomyopathies.

Alcoholic cardiomyopathy may occur in the individual who consumes large amounts of ethanol over a long period. Ethanol has a toxic effect on cardiac tissue, and eventually results in cardiac enlargement and low cardiac output. The onset of alcoholic cardiomyopathy is gradual, with fatigue and dyspnea on exertion as the first symptoms. Physical examination usually reveals a cardiac murmur, edema, hypertension, and an increasing central venous pressure.

Congestive cardiomyopathy is characterized by cardiac enlargement, especially of the left ventricle, myocardial dysfunction, and congestive heart failure.

Hypertrophic cardiomyopathy is characterized by an extensive thickening of the left ventricular myocardium and septum. Blood flow from the atria to the ventricles may be affected as well. Young males are most often affected, but the disease can also occur in a familial form that affects males and females equally.

Infiltrative cardiomyopathy results in the deposition of abnormal substances in the myocardium, as may occur in amyloidosis. The foreign material results in restrictive cardiomyopathy because the heart cannot expand adequately to receive the inflowing blood. The ventricular walls become excessively rigid, impeding ventricular filling. Restrictive cardiomyopathy is marked by normal systolic function of the heart but abnormal diastolic function.

Cardiomyopathies are incurable. Currently, the best treatment is heart transplantation, but new treatments are being tested with promising preliminary results.

CARDIAC DYSRHYTHMIAS

Individuals with heart disease often experience disturbances in normal heart rhythm, which can decrease cardiac output, damage the myocardium, and lead to eventual cardiac arrest. These cardiac dysrhythmias can be caused by many factors, including hypoxia, acidosis, electrolyte imbalances, myocardial infarction, drugs, hypotension, hemorrhage, hypovolemia, or pneumothorax. Most dysrhythmias are caused by abnormalities in impulse formation or abnormalities in conduction due to a blockage somewhere along the neural pathway.

Sinus dysrhythmia is the most common dysrhythmia, and is typically found in young adults and the elderly. This dysrhythmia is the physiological cyclic variation in heart rate related to vagal nerve impulses to the sinoatrial node. It is a benign rhythm that usually requires no treatment.

Sinus tachycardia, characterized by an atrial and ventricular rate of 100 beats per minute or more, is associated with the ingestion of nicotine, alcohol, or caffeine. It is a normal response to fear, excitement, or physical exertion. It is also associated with hyperthyroidism, hypovolemia, or hypotension. Sinus tachycardia is generally benign, but can cause a decrease in cardiac output if there is an underlying myocardial impairment.

Sinus **bradycardia**, characterized by an atrial and ventricular rate of 60 beats per minute or less, is considered beneficial because it reduces myocardial oxygen demands. It is often seen in well-conditioned athletes. It can become so slow, however, that cardiac output is reduced, resulting in eventual heart failure if left untreated. Atropine works well in the treatment of bradycardia.

Dysrhythmias originating in the atria include premature atrial beat, atrial tachycardia, atrial flutter, and atrial fibrillation.

The premature atrial beat arises from an ectopic focus somewhere within the atria. It is often associated with stress or the consumption of caffeine or nicotine, but may also accompany inflammation or myocardial infarction. It is considered benign, and treatment usually consists of the omission of tobacco or caffeine from the individual's lifestyle.

Atrial tachycardia is characterized by an atrial rate of 150–250 beats per minute. Sudden occurrence of atrial tachycardia is referred to as paroxysmal atrial tachycardia, and transient episodes are not uncommon in children and young adults. Symptoms usually involve palpitations and anxiety, but no treatment is necessary unless the atrial rate exceeds 200 beats per minute or the episode continues for an extended length of time.

Treatment for extended episodes of atrial tachycardia include carotid sinus stimulation or the intravenous administration of beta blockers or verapamil. Valsalva's maneuver may also be helpful in restoring normal rhythm, as will stimulation of the vagus nerve.

Atrial flutter involves rapid atrial activity at a rate of 250–350 beats per minute. Generally, as a prevention mechanism, the conduction of each impulse from the atria to the ventricles is blocked by the AV node. Despite this safety control, the ventricular rate may still exceed 150 beats per minute and could result in a decrease in cardiac output.

Direct current stimulation (cardioversion) is the treatment of choice for conversion to normal sinus rhythm, but digitalis will usually slow the ventricular rate in recurrent episodes. Patients who do not respond to either treatment may be candidates for atrial pacing.

Atrial fibrillation is another common dysrhythmia encountered in clinical practice, and involves a rapid and disordered beating of the atria, usually at a rate of 350–600 beats per minute. As in atrial flutter, the atrial impulse to the ventricles is increased, and the ventricular rate is usually 100–180 beats per minute. Without the propulsion of blood from the atria to the ventricles ("atrial kick"), cardiac output is reduced. Cardiac output is also affected by the irregular ventricular rhythm caused by the irregular atrial impulses.

Atrial fibrillation may be a chronic or transient condition. If chronic, heart disease may be an underlying problem. Morbidity associated with atrial fibrillation is the result of the following three detrimental conditions:

- An irregular heartbeat, which causes patient discomfort and anxiety
- Loss of synchronous atrioventricular contraction, which comprises cardiac hemodynamics resulting in varying levels of congestive heart failure
- Stasis of blood flow in the left atrium, which increases the vulnerability to thromboembolism

Ventricular dysrhythmias can be classified as benign premature ventricular contractions, complex PVCs, or malignant (lethal).

A premature ventricular contraction (**PVC**) is a contraction of the ventricle that occurs before it is expected in a normal series of cardiac cycles. PVCs that are benign usually are five or less per hour, and are often seen in normal persons in the absence of heart disease. These may be caused by a stretching of the anterior papillary muscle of the right ventricle during mechanical activity.

Complex PVCs (greater than 10–30 per hour) may occur in patients with or without heart disease. Those that occur in patients without heart disease may possibly be due to biochemical abnormalities or patches of myocarditis. Those that occur with left ventricular dysfunction are potentially lethal and should be treated with antiarrhythmic drugs.

Many are not aware of benign PVCs, and it may be wiser with some individuals not to direct their attention to the ectopic beats if they have no evidence of heart disease because of the anxiety that may be induced. The frequency of PVCs may be reduced by the elimination of caffeine, tobacco, and alcohol. The avoidance of stress factors and frequent exercise are also encouraged. If all general measures fail, and symptoms interfere with the quality of life, antiarrhythmic drugs may be utilized.

Ventricular tachycardia is present when three or more PVCs occur in succession, usually at a rate of

140–250 beats per minute. It is referred to as sustained if it lasts longer than 30 seconds or requires termination because of hemodynamic instability. The nonsustained types last less than 30 seconds and stop spontaneously. The sustained PVCs or nonsustained PVCs with hemodynamic instability are referred to as malignant dysrhythmias, and are usually seen in patients with cardiac disease.

A ventricle is said to flutter when it is contracting regularly, but at a very rapid rate (250–350 contractions per minute). Ventricular flutter presents as regular oscillations on electrocardiogram and is likely to be due to damage to the myocardium.

Ventricular fibrillation is also characterized by rapid ventricular contractions, but in an uncoordinated fashion. During this dysrhythmia, small regions of the myocardium contract and relax independently of all other areas. As a result, the myocardium fails to contract as a whole and the walls of the fibrillating ventricle are completely ineffective at pumping blood. Unless this dangerous dysrhythmia is converted by electric shock (defibrillation), death will most certainly ensue.

The ventricles can be stimulated to fibrillate by a variety of factors, including ischemia associated with coronary artery obstruction, electric shock, or trauma to the heart.

Dysrhythmias may also be caused by an interference in normal cardiac impulse conduction. These "heart blocks" are impairments of conduction in heart excitation and are influenced by the fact that certain cardiac tissues other than the SA node may act as pacemakers. For instance, damage to the SA node may cause the AV node to take over the functions of cardiac pacing, in essence functioning as a secondary pacemaker.

Atrioventricular blocks occur in the atrioventricular junction tissue (atrioventricular node, bundle of His, or its bundle branches). The block is often characterized as first-, second-, or third-degree AV block.

First-degree AV block occurs when conduction time is prolonged but all atrial beats are followed by ventricular beats. This delay could be in the AV node, bundle of His, or any of the bundle branches. Second-degree AV block occurs when some, but not all, atrial beats are conducted to the ventricles. Third-degree AV block can occur in the AV node, bundle of His, or any of the bundle branches. In this type of block, no impulses whatsoever are conducted by the junctional tissues, owing to pathological factors. This condition may be permanent or paroxysmal, and if syncopal attacks occur in conjunction with bradycardia, it is known as Adams-Stokes disease. This disease is the main indication for use of a permanent cardiac pacemaker.

CONGENITAL HEART DEFECTS

Congenital heart defects are usually divided into two types based on alteration in circulation: (1) acyanotic, in which there is no mixing of unoxygenated blood in the systemic circulation, and (2) cyanotic, in which unoxygenated blood enters the systemic circulation. Cyanosis is present because of a failure of delivery of pulmonary venous return to the systemic circulation or a reduction in the volume in pulmonary blood flow.

ACYANOTIC DEFECTS

Acyanotic defects are generally obstructive lesions that can lead to heart failure because of the burden placed on the ventricle, or shunt lesions that increase pulmonary flow. These defects include ventricular septal defect (VSD), atrial septal defect (ASD), patent ductus arteriosus (PDA), coarctation of the aorta, and pulmonary stenosis.

Ventricular Septal Defect

A ventricular septal defect (VSD) is an abnormal opening in the wall between the right and left ventricle. The size of the defect may vary from the size of a pinhole to a complete absence of the septum, resulting in a common ventricle. This opening allows a certain amount of oxygenated blood from the left ventricle to be shunted through the defect to the right ventricle. From the right ventricle, the blood is pumped back to the lungs, even though it has already been refreshed with oxygen. This inefficient shunting of oxygenated blood displaces blood that needs oxygenation. The heart must pump an increased amount of blood, resulting in an enlargement of the heart.

Symptoms associated with VSD may not occur until several weeks after birth. An infant with a large VSD will not grow normally and may appear undernourished. Pulmonary hypertension is often present because of the increased amount of blood within the pulmonary artery and its branches. If the defect is small, the only clinical finding is a heart murmur. These smaller defects often close spontaneously, but if the defect is large, surgical repair with either a synthetic prosthetic patch or a pericardial patch is recommended to prevent serious problems. Surgical repair of the VSD usually restores the blood circulation to normal, with a good long-term prognosis.

Atrial Septal Defect

An atrial septal defect (ASD) is an abnormal opening in the wall between the two atria. There are three types of ASD: ostium secundum, sinus venosus, and ostium primum. The ostium secundum type is in the midatrial septum and is the most common. The sinus venosus type of defect occurs high in the septum near the entrance of the superior vena cava in the right atrium. This type of defect is usually associated with anomalous pulmonary venous drainage, in which one or more pulmonary veins drain into the right atrium rather than the left. The ostium primum is located low in the anterior portion of the septum and is associated with other defects in the atrioventricular canal, usually with a cleft of the mitral valve.

The ASD results in a shunting of oxygenated blood from the left atrium across the defect into the right atrium. If the defect is large or of the ostium primum type with marked shunting of flow, the work load of the right side of the heart is increased. Pulmonary hypertension, enlargement of the pulmonary artery and its branches, and enlargement of the heart's right side may be a result of this increased workload. In later stages, right-sided heart failure and a reversal of the shunt with subsequent cyanosis may ensue.

The atrial septal defect is closed under direct vision with a pericardial or synthetic prosthetic patch. Small openings can be closed with suture only.

Patent Ductus Arteriosus

Patent ductus arteriosus (PDA) is a failure of that fetal structure to completely close after birth. In fetal life, the ductus arteriosus connects the pulmonary artery to the aorta in order to shunt oxygenated blood directly into the systemic circulation by bypassing the lungs. It usually extends from the origin of the left pulmonary artery to just distal to the origin of the left subclavian artery. It may coexist with other anomalies such as ventricular septal defect, coarctation of the aorta, and pulmonary stenosis.

Surgery is recommended for PDA and the ductus should be divided after 1 year of age or earlier if there is congestive heart failure. Since the defect is outside the heart chamber, a cardiopulmonary bypass is not required. If a ductus is found late in life and there is a small shunt, surgery is usually not recommended. Surgery in the adult can present problems because the ductus is usually calcified, brittle, and aneurysmal.

Coarctation of the Aorta

Coarctation of the aorta is a localized narrowing of the aorta in an otherwise normal vessel. In the adult form, the narrowing is usually distal to the left subclavian artery or just distal to the ligamentum arteriosum. In infantile aortic coarctation, the obstruction is proximal to the ductus arteriosus. Heart catheterization and aortography should be done to demonstrate the exact site of the narrowing and to evaluate or detect any associated lesions. Elective surgery is often recommended at 3–6 months of age because, if performed earlier, obstruction may recur. However, some surgeons prefer to wait until the third or fourth year. Surgery is necessary because of the high incidence of complications, including stroke, hypertension, a ruptured aorta, and congestive heart failure. Because the defect is outside the heart chambers, only the thoracic cavity is entered.

Pulmonary Stenosis

Pulmonary stenosis is a narrowing at the entrance to the pulmonary artery. This lesion can be in the pulmonary valve, in the pulmonary artery itself (infundibular), or in the peripheral pulmonary arteries. Peripheral pulmonary artery stenosis is usually associated with pulmonary valvular stenosis, supravalvular aortic stenosis, coarctation of the aorta, ventricular septal defect, or tetralogy of Fallot. Surgery or percutaneous balloon valvuloplasty is indicated if the patient is symptomatic. However, in asymptomatic patients with moderate or severe stenosis there is no full agreement as to when to intervene. Those with significant subvalvular stenosis require surgical resection. Entry into the right ventricle is usually required to gain access to the stenotic area, necessitating open-heart surgery.

CYANOTIC DEFECTS

Cyanotic defects include tetralogy of Fallot, transposition of the great vessels, tricuspid atresia, and truncus arteriosus.

Tetralogy of Fallot

Tetralogy of Fallot is the most common cyanotic heart defect in children. The classic form (of which there are several variations) includes the following four defects:

1. Ventricular septal defect
2. Infundibular or pulmonary valve stenosis
3. An aorta that overrides the ventricular septal defect
4. Right ventricular hypertrophy

The first three defects are congenital and the fourth is acquired as a result of the increased pressure within the right ventricle. Older children with this disease often give a history of squatting after exercise and are subject to hypoxic spells. Squatting relieves the symptoms of dyspnea and faintness that can occur after exertion by causing a rise in the common ventricular pressure. Pulmonary artery flow is enhanced as a result of the increased ventricular pressure, and more oxygenated blood enters the left side of the heart.

Tetralogy of Fallot results in cyanosis, which may appear soon after birth, in infancy, or later in childhood. These "blue babies" may have sudden episodes of severe cyanosis with rapid breathing and may even lose consciousness. Other complications of the disease include infective endocarditis, blood-clotting problems, cerebral infarction or embolism, cerebral abscess, and, rarely, right ventricular failure. Therefore, early total surgical correction should be done for all cases to avoid these complications.

Infants with severe tetralogy of Fallot may require a shunt between the aorta or subclavian artery and the pulmonary artery to increase blood flow to the lungs. This shunt allows for more blood flow to the lungs for increased oxygen saturation, which reduces cyanosis and allows the child to grow and develop until a total repair can be done when the child is older.

Most children with tetralogy of Fallot have the defects repaired before school age. The procedure involves closing the ventricular septal defect and removing the obstructing muscle. If the pulmonary valve is narrow, it is opened; if it is small, a synthetic graft or pericardial patch may be needed to finish the repair. Postoperative prognosis varies a great deal. Usually it is good, but it depends largely on the severity of the defects, especially the severity of pulmonary stenosis.

Transposition of the Great Vessels

Transposition of the great vessels generally refers to a condition in which the pulmonary artery leaves the left ventricle and the aorta exits from the right ventricle, although other transpositions may occur. Obviously, this type of circulation is incompatible with extrauterine life. A shunt between the systemic and pulmonary circuits must exist for such patients to survive. The shunt may be at the atrial, ventricular, or pulmonary artery level. For example, septal defects or patent ductus arteriosus will permit blood to enter the systemic circulation and/or pulmonary circulation for mixing of unoxygenated and oxygenated blood. Cyanosis and dyspnea are usually present from birth and may be followed by congestive heart failure.

Echocardiography can identify the great vessel and their reversed origin and may also identify any associated defects. Heart catheterization and angiographic studies confirm the diagnosis. The aorta is seen arising anteriorly from the right ventricle with its valve more superior than normal, and the pulmonary artery is seen arising from the left ventricle.

During heart catheterization, a small interatrial communication can be enlarged by pulling a balloon catheter through the defect for increased shunting (balloon atrial septostomy). A direct surgical creation of a large atrial septal defect is seldom necessary. After 3–9 months of age, total repair should be considered. Procedures for correction include the atrial switch, the Senning atrial switch, and the Rastelli procedures. The Mustard procedure redirects the venous blood within the atria by excision of the septum and creates a new septum with a pericardial patch or prosthetic material. The pericardial patch or synthetic material is positioned so that blood within the pulmonary vein flows across the tricuspid valve to the right ventricle and then out the aorta, and the caval blood flows across the mitral valve to the left ventricle and then into the pulmonary artery.

Tricuspid Atresia

Tricuspid atresia is the absence of the tricuspid valve and orifice. No opening exists between the right atrium and the right ventricle. The defect is usually associated with atrial and ventricular septal defects with underdevelopment of the right ventricle. This defect can be subdivided into those with normally related great vessels or those with transposition of the great vessels. The most common type of tricuspid atresia is one with normally related great vessels, an atrial septal defect, a small ventricular septal defect, a small right ventricle, and pulmonic stenosis. The circulation from the vena cavae passes across the atrial septal defect, mixes with the blood from the pulmonary veins, and then passes to the left ventricle, where some goes out to the pulmonary arteries via the ventricular septal defect and the rest goes out through the aorta.

Cyanosis appears early, and an early death is not uncommon. Those rare patients who survive to a second decade are usually those with transposition and pulmonary stenosis, or transposition without pulmonary stenosis.

Shunt procedures recommended have been vena caval to right pulmonary artery anastomosis (Glenn procedure), and systemic artery to pulmonary artery anastomosis (Blalock-Taussig procedure, Potts or Waterston procedure). Other palliative procedures include balloon atrial septostomy (described earlier), and pulmonary arterial banding in those with excessive pulmonary blood flow. Later, a corrective procedure described by Fontan can be performed that completely separates the two circulations and physiologically corrects the anomaly. In this procedure, the right atrium is connected to the pulmonary artery by using a conduit with a valve, with another valve inserted into the orifice of the inferior vena cava.

Truncus Arteriosus

Truncus arteriosus is characterized by having a single artery arising from both ventricles. The pulmonary arteries usually arise from one of several positions on a truncal (main part, or stem) vessel. In type 1, the pulmonary arteries arise at the base of the truncal vessel from a single main pulmonary trunk; in type 2, the pulmonary arteries arise posteriorly from the ascending truncal vessel; in type 3, the pulmonary arteries arise laterally from the ascending truncus; and in type 4, there is no true pulmonary arterial system, and the lungs are supplied by the bronchial arteries.

Patients with truncus arteriosus must have a ventricular septal defect to survive. Cyanosis is usually noted, but if pulmonary blood flow is good, cyanosis is less severe.

Echocardiography reveals the large truncal vessel overriding the ventricular septum, only one semilunar valve, and an enlarged left atrium. The diagnosis is established by cardiac catheterization and angiocardiograms. All patients should be considered for surgical correction unless there is severe pulmonary vascular disease. Early in life, total correction should be attempted using the conduit procedure. In this procedure, the pulmonary arteries are disconnected from the aorta, and the resultant defect in the aorta is repaired. The right ventricle is opened, and the ventricular septal defect is patched. A valve-containing prosthetic conduit is placed from the right ventricle to the pulmonary arteries. Surgery should be performed soon after birth, since pulmonary vascular obstructive disease can develop and cause early fatality.

DIAGNOSTIC PROCEDURES: THORAX

Diagnostic procedures of the structures of the thorax include bronchoscopy, mediastinoscopy, anterior mediastinotomy, thoracoscopy, and thoracentesis.

BRONCHOSCOPY

Bronchoscopy (Figure 22-17) is an invasive diagnostic and/or therapeutic procedure for the evaluation of hemoptysis, infection, carcinoma of the lung, and damage to the lungs due to smoke inhalation. It is also useful for retrieving foreign objects lodged in an airway and for laser treatment of endobronchial tumors. Bronchoscopy is also useful for postoperative evaluation of the transplanted lung.

Bronchoscopes may be rigid or flexible. The rigid scope is equipped with a fiberoptic light carrier for illumination of the trachea and primary bronchi and side channels for anesthetic gas and oxygen administration. Rigid bronchoscopy is typically used for the removal of foreign objects in children, although it may occasionally be used for biopsy of a large central mass or for evaluating hemoptysis. Equipment for rigid bronchoscopy includes a rigid bronchoscope, straight and up-biting biopsy forceps, suction cannula, specimen cup (Lukens tubes), grasping forceps, sponge carriers, fiberoptic telescope, light source, and fiberoptic light cord.

The smaller flexible fiberoptic bronchoscope allows for visualization of the upper, middle, and lower lobe bronchi, and may have a video camera attached for viewing on a screen. Transbronchial lung biopsy for the examination of pulmonary **infiltrate** is also performed through the flexible scope.

Cytologic specimens from bronchial washings delivered through the flexible bronchoscope are essential for the diagnosis of lung disease. Bronchial brushings and needle aspirations may also be performed through the flexible bronchoscope, and specimens taken with a flexible biting tip forceps may be sent to the laboratory for tissue identification.

Because the scope is introduced through the mouth and into the bronchial tubes, the procedure is not treated as a sterile one. Generally, the patient is not draped, but personnel should wear gowns, gloves, masks, and eye goggles for personal protection from body fluids. Ideally, the scope should be sterilized, but high-level disinfection is adequate for most hospitals. Flexible bronchoscopy is generally performed under a local anesthetic in the endoscopy department, but for the evaluation of intrabronchial tumors before thoracotomy, the procedure is performed in the OR under general anesthesia.

MEDIASTINOSCOPY

For the evaluation of nodal involvement or mediastinal masses in patients with carcinoma of the lung, a scope may be introduced through the pretracheal fascia and into the superior mediastinum (Figure 22-18). Mediastinoscopy is generally performed after CT scan has demonstrated hilar or paratracheal adenopathy. Because an incision is made, the procedure is a sterile one and is performed under general anesthesia.

An extrapleural mediastinotomy through the anterior second intercostal space may be performed to evaluate lymph nodes around the aortic arch on the left side that cannot be reached by mediastinoscopy. Mediastinotomy provides an approach for the examination of the anterior hilum and the aortopulmonary window area.

THORACOSCOPY

Thoracoscopy (Figure 22-19) is a minimally invasive endoscopic approach to the thoracic cavity for examination of the pleura and entire pulmonary mantle, mediastinum, thoracic wall, sympathetic chain, diaphragm, and pericardium. Biopsies of lung, mediastinal nodes, or pleura

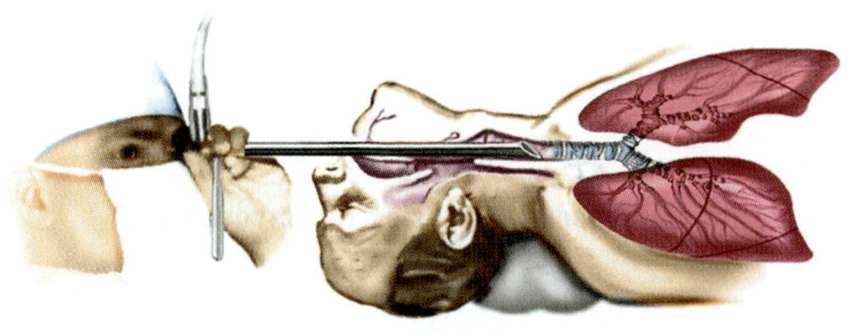

Figure 22-17 Rigid bronchoscopy

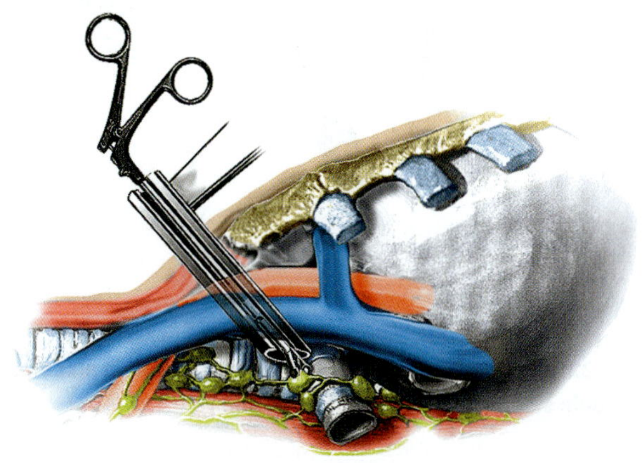

Figure 22-18 Mediastinoscopy

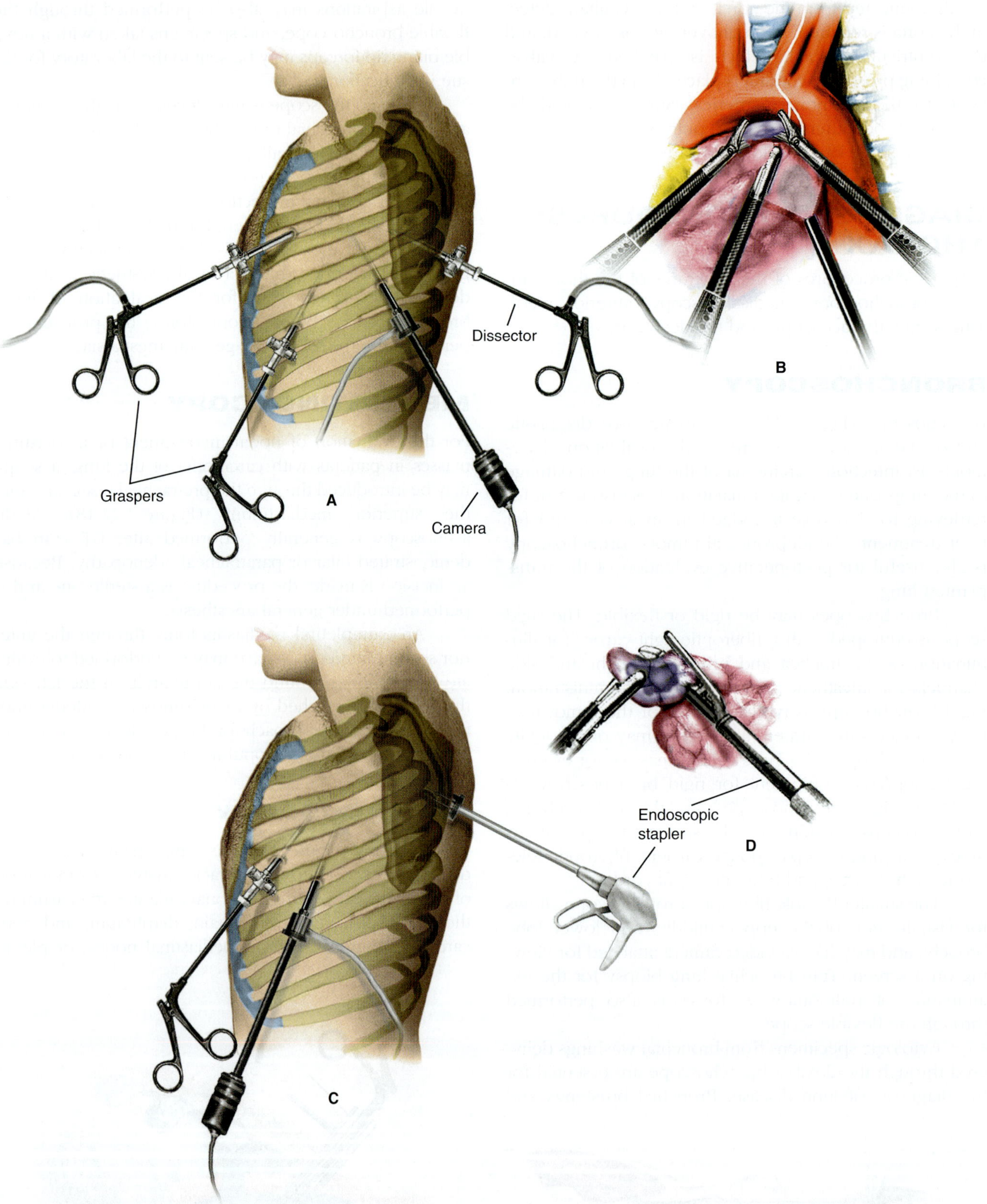

Figure 22-19 **Thoracoscopy: (A) Trocar and instrument placement, (B) exposure and dissection of lung lesion, (C) introduction of endoscopic stapler, (D) stapling of lung lesion**

may be taken through the scope for diagnosis of peripheral lesions. The procedure is performed in the OR under general endotracheal anesthesia so that the lung can be deflated for visualization.

THORACENTESIS

Thoracocentesis involves the placement of a needle into a posterior portion of the pleural space for the analysis of pleural effusion. The procedure is generally performed as an aid in the diagnosis of inflammatory or neoplastic diseases of the pleura or the lung. Therapeutic applications for thoracentesis include the removal of fluid accumulations from within the thoracic cavity. CT scan or ultrasonography may be necessary for proper needle placement.

DIAGNOSTIC PROCEDURES: CARDIAC

Diagnostic procedures of the heart include plain X-ray films, computed axial tomography (CAT scan), magnetic resonance imaging (MRI), electrocardiography, echocardiography, and cardiac catheterization.

RADIOLOGIC STUDIES

Anteroposterior (AP) and lateral X-rays of the chest can determine the overall size of the heart and great vessel configuration, as well as any valvular or intracoronary calcification. Asymptomatic pericardial cysts and cardiac tumors may also be detected on plain films.

CT scan and MRI are useful for the evaluation of pericardial and intracardiac and extracardiac masses. CT scan is especially useful for the detection and evaluation of thoracic aorta dissection. MRI can detect abnormal positioning of intracardiac structures.

Electrocardiography, echocardiography, and cardiac catheterization are also useful diagnostic procedures for the evaluation of cardiac disease. For a detailed description of these procedures, refer to Chapter 13.

SURGICAL INTERVENTION: THORACIC

Surgical procedures for the treatment of lung disorders require thoracotomy or thoracoscopy, a less invasive procedure performed primarily for lung biopsy.

SPECIAL PREOPERATIVE CONSIDERATIONS

For the patient undergoing surgery of the thoracic cavity, special considerations should be given pertaining to respiratory function. Often the patient is anxious because of the impending procedure and breathing difficulties related to his or her condition. The patient with carcinoma of the lung or traumatic injury to the chest is fearful of the possibility of death either intraoperatively or postoperatively.

The patient's chart should be reviewed by surgical team members for history, physical, consent, diagnostic findings, and laboratory results. Diagnostic tests for review include routine chest X-ray, CT scan or MRI, arterial blood gases, bronchoscopy and sputum analysis, mediastinoscopy, and pulmonary function. The chest X-ray should accompany the patient to the operating room. The patient should be typed and cross-matched for blood replacement because of the possibility of injury to major vessels within the thorax or mediastinum.

The surgical team should ensure that all necessary equipment for positioning and for the procedure is in the room and in proper working order well before the patient arrives. The surgeon's preference card should be checked for any supplies or instruments that may be lacking, especially if the case supplies were gathered by someone other than the person who will be scrubbing the procedure.

It is always a good idea to speak with the surgeon before setup begins to gain insight into any possible procedural deviations.

SPECIAL INSTRUMENTATION, SUPPLIES, DRUGS, AND EQUIPMENT

For intrathoracic procedures, the surgical technologist should be prepared for possible preoperative flexible bronchoscopy or mediastinoscopy. Preoperative bronchoscopy is important for appreciation of important structural features and intrabronchial tumor margins. Mediastinoscopy is useful for biopsy of lymph nodes before thoracotomy for lung resection.

Equipment for preoperative flexible bronchoscopy includes a flexible bronchoscope, endotracheal adaptor, flexible biopsy forceps, light source, and fiberoptic light cable. Supplies include gown, gloves, suction tubing, small basin with saline, gauze sponges, and water-soluble lubricant. Typically, a bronchoscopy cart with all necessary supplies and equipment is available for the surgical technologist and need only be checked for completeness. Because this procedure is for viewing of intrabronchial structures only, additional specimens may not be taken.

Equipment for mediastinoscopy includes a light source and fiberoptic light cord, mediastinoscope, suction tips, biopsy forceps, hemoclip applicator, grasping forceps, and electrosurgical unit. Instrumentation for mediastinoscopy includes a minor instrumentation set. Sterile supplies include gowns, gloves, suction tubing, electrosurgical pencil, Ray-Tec sponges, Telfa, 20-gauge needle, and towels and thyroid sheet for draping.

The patient is positioned supine, and the head is extended by placing a roll under the shoulders. A small,

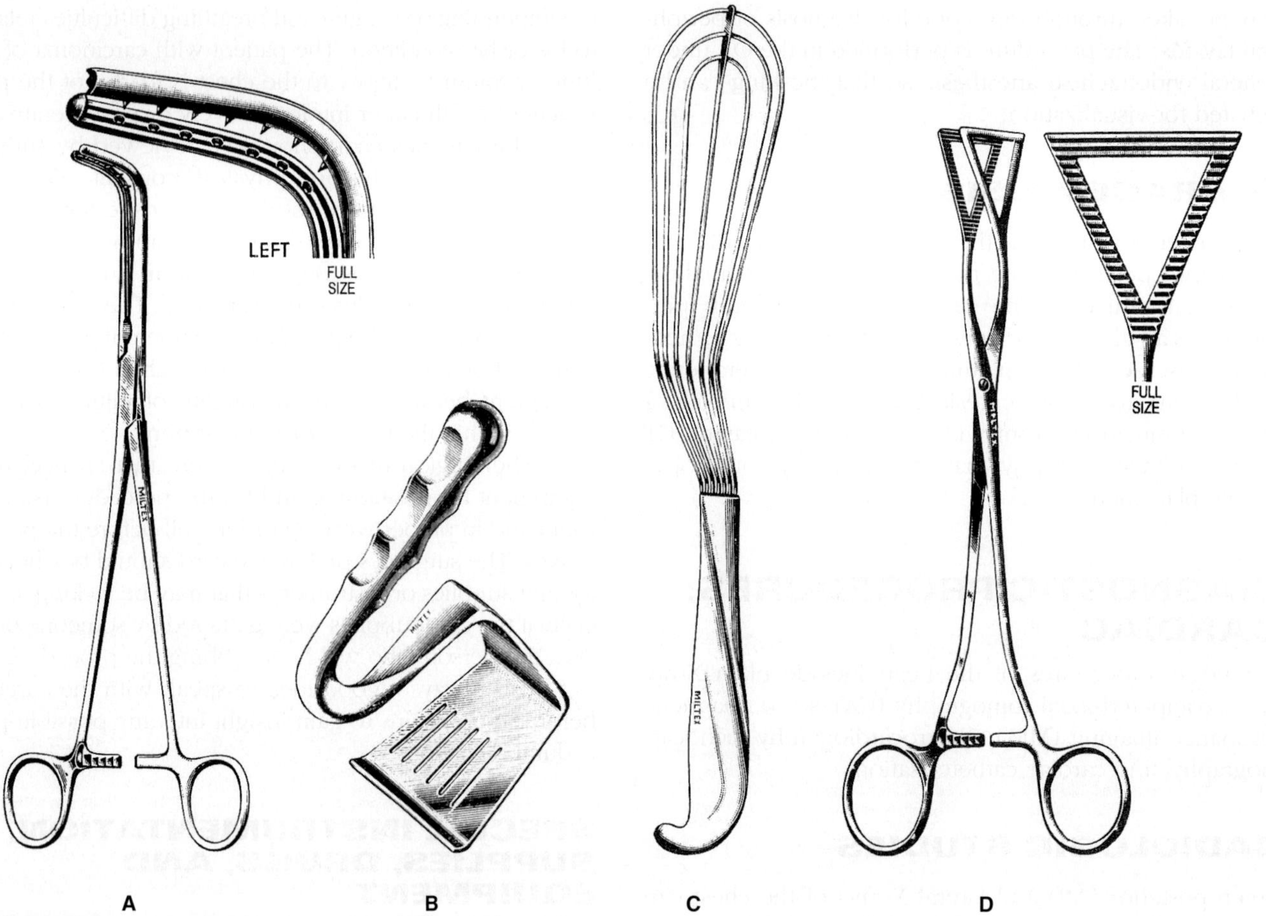

Figure 22-20 Thoracic instrumentation: (A) Sarot bronchus clamp, (B) Davidson scapula retractor, (C) Allison lung retractor, (D) Lovelace lung grasping forceps *(Courtesy of Miltex Instrument Co., Inc.)*

transverse incision is made 1–2 cm above the suprasternal notch and carried down to the platysma muscle. Dissection is continued through the pretracheal fascia until the trachea is exposed and freed by finger dissection from surrounding structures. The mediastinoscope is introduced, and lymph node biopsies are taken. The platysma muscle is closed with interrupted absorbable sutures after removal of the scope, and skin closure is achieved with a subcuticular stitch.

Equipment for thoracotomy includes electrosurgical unit, Cell Saver, and fiberoptic light source and headlight. A defibrillation unit should also be available.

Instrumentation for thoracotomy (Figure 22-20) includes a major set and chest (thoracotomy) set. A major vascular set may also be necessary, although some thoracotomy sets contain any necessary vascular instrumentation. Hemoclip applicators of all sizes are essential. Median sternotomy will require a sternal saw and sternal retractor.

Specialty supplies include hemoclips of all sizes, transverse laparotomy sheet, magnetic mat, peanut dissectors, Cell Saver suction tubing, chest tubes and closed seal drainage system, straight or Y-type connector for chest tubes, vessel loops, and automatic stapling devices for lobectomy, wedge resection, or pneumonectomy. For every thoracotomy, 2–0 and 3–0 silk suture ties (24–32 in. length) on carriers and Prolene or silk ligature sutures (stick-ties) are essential. Laparotomy sponges are used in all thoracotomy procedures.

Intraoperative drugs for thoracic procedures include Marcaine 0.25% or Xylocaine 1% for postoperative anesthesia, heparin for intra-arterial irrigation, papaverine for vasoconstriction control, and antibiotic irrigation of the surgeon's choice.

PATIENT PREPARATION

After the patient has been transported to the OR from the holding area, he or she is assisted in moving from the transport stretcher to the OR table and a strap is placed 2 inches above the patient's knees. Anesthesia personnel prepare and apply or insert monitoring equipment that may include a Swan-Ganz catheter for pulmonary wedge pressure and central venous pressure (CVP) readings, an arterial catheter for the monitoring of arterial blood pressure and blood gases (ABGs), and ECG, oxygen saturation, temperature, and blood pressure equipment. For intrathoracic procedures, the anesthesia provider may prefer to use a double-lumen endotracheal tube so that the affected lung can be collapsed during the surgical procedure without interfering with the unaffected lung's ventilation. The use of the double-lumen endotracheal tube (Figure 22-21) requires careful monitoring of ABGs and O_2 saturation because of the increased possibility of right-to-left shunt through the nonventilated lung.

After induction and intubation, the patient is repositioned if necessary. Approaches for intrathoracic procedures are typically anterolateral, posterolateral, or median sternotomy in the supine position. Other less common approaches include transaxillary for lower lobe wedge resection or biopsy, and supraclavicular for resection of the phrenic nerve or surgical treatment of thoracic outlet syndrome. Posterolateral positions provide access to the entire hemithorax and are typically utilized for lung resection or access to the diaphragm, descending aorta, or thoracic esophagus. Anterolateral approaches are utilized for lung biopsy or removal of a localized lesion. Median sternotomy provides access to both lungs and structures within the mediastinum. Thoracoabdominal approaches in the lateral position provide access to upper abdominal viscera through a low thoracotomy incision and opening of the diaphragm. An upper abdominal incision may be joined with a low thoracotomy incision for increased exposure.

For posterolateral positioning, OR personnel should have available 4-in. adhesive tape, the bean bag (placed flat on the OR table before the patient's arrival with a sheet on top and suction tubing and suction device nearby), surgical towels, sheets, sandbags, and pillows.

The patient is pulled to the edge of the OR table, then rolled and lifted to the unaffected side. Care must be taken to prevent tension on CVP and arterial lines, Foley catheter, and the endotracheal tube. Typically, at least four people are necessary to move a patient of average weight: one on each side, utilizing the draw sheet; one at the foot of the OR table, controlling the patient's feet; and the anesthesia provider at the head of the table, controlling the patient's head and neck and preventing tension on the IV, arterial and CVP lines, Foley, and endotracheal tube. Heavier patients may require more assistants for positioning.

The bean bag is molded to the patient and suction is applied for hardening and stabilization. Adhesive tape is placed across the pelvic girdle and the shoulders and fastened to the OR table for increased stabilization (some surgeons may prefer to use bolsters and adhesive tape alone, without the use of the bean bag). Surgical towels are placed under the adhesive tape to protect superficial structures. The lower leg is flexed to establish a base, and the upper leg is bent only slightly to prevent hyperextension. Pillows are placed between the legs to protect the peroneal nerve, and a soft roll is placed under the axillary region to prevent damage to the brachial plexus. The upper arm is flexed slightly and raised above the head to retract the scapula, and it is supported by pillows or an elevated, padded armboard attached to the OR table. The

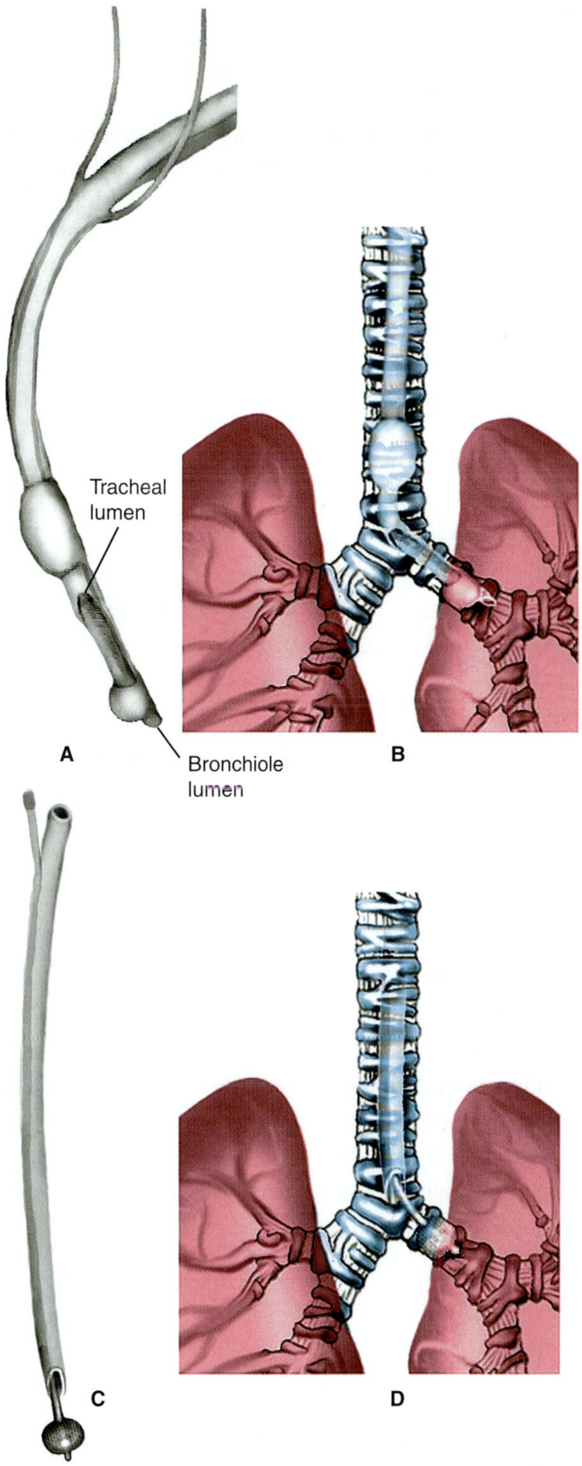

Figure 22-21 Specialized endotracheal tubes: (A) Double-lumen endotracheal tube with separate bronchial and tracheal balloons, (B) tubes are most often placed with the tip (bronchial lumen) in the left mainstem bronchus, (C) a single-lumen endotracheal tube with an endobronchial balloon, (D) balloon positioned to occlude the left mainstem bronchus

lower arm is extended slightly less than 90 degrees on a padded armboard and secured. Bony prominences are identified and padded as necessary, and the head of the table is lowered slightly.

For an anterolateral approach, the patient is left in the supine position after intubation and rolls are placed under the shoulder and hip of the affected side for an elevation of approximately 40 degrees. The arm on the affected side is moved away from the body and placed on a pad; an axillary roll may be placed under the unaffected axilla for brachial plexus protection. Bony prominences are identified and padded.

After positioning, the patient is prepped to the proper perimeters and draping begins. For lateral positions, a fenestrated transverse drape sheet over towels and an incision drape is the best choice. For median sternotomy, a nonfenestrated, reinforced heart sheet or fenestrated laparotomy sheet over towels secured by incision drape is effective.

THORACOSCOPY

Endoscopic examination of the thoracic cavity is achieved through a thoracoscope (Procedure 22-1). Peripheral lesions may be diagnosed through the thoracoscope; the diaphragm, pericardium, sympathetic chain, and mediastinal lymph nodes are also accessible for biopsy or treatment.

PROCEDURE 22-1 Thoracoscopy

Equipment

- Video monitors for viewing
- Videocassette recorder
- Light source
- Electrosurgical unit
- Nd:YAG laser (optional)
- Suction/irrigation unit
- A defibrillation unit should be available in case ventricular fibrillation occurs

Instruments

- 10-mm 0° and 30° lens
- Camera and cord
- Fiberoptic light cord
- Endoscopic graspers (toothed, serrated, and blunt)
- Suture ligators and carriers
- Endoscopic Pennington
- Endoscopic lung retractors
- Endoscopic clip applicators
- Scissors (hooked, micro, and straight)
- Dissectors and probes (electrosurgical unit may be hooked up to scissors or probe)
- Soft tissue instruments for incision and closure (hemostats, retractors, suture scissors, knife handles, and small needle holders)
- Major set, vascular set, and chest set available for emergencies

Supplies

- Pack: basic or laparoscopy
- Basin set
- Gloves
- Blades (#15)
- Drapes: transverse laparotomy sheet or laparoscopy sheet
- Suture: 4–0 Vicryl on a small cutting needle for subcuticular closures; ¼-in. Steri-Strips
- Drains: chest tube 28 Fr
- Dressings: 4 × 4 gauze
- Drugs: Marcaine 0.25% or lidocaine 1% with epinephrine (1:100,000) for hemostasis and postoperative anesthesia
- Miscellaneous:
  - Ray-Tec sponges
  - Endoscopic electrosurgical cord
  - Lens defogger
  - Magnetic pad
  - Camera cord cover
  - Various syringes and hypodermic needles
  - Electrosurgical pencil
  - Irrigation/suction assembly
  - Suction tubing
  - 10–12 mm trocars (blunt and sharp)
  - Reducers
  - Endoscopic linear stapling device
  - Pleur-evac closed water-seal drainage system

PROCEDURE 22-1 Thoracoscopy *(continued)*

Operative Preparation

Anesthesia

- General with double-lumen endotracheal tube intubation

Position

- Lateral (partial or full), with the affected side up
- The arm on the unaffected side is secured to an armboard
- An axillary roll is placed, and the arm on the affected side is placed onto a Mayo tray and padded with pillows and secured

Prep

- Prep extends from the shoulder and axilla to the iliac crest, to just above the level of the table on both sides

Draping

- The incision site is square-draped with folded towels and covered with a transverse laparotomy or laparoscopy sheet

Practical Considerations

- Make sure that the patient's X-rays are in the room
- Check with the surgeon about Foley catheter placement
- The STSR should be prepared for an open thoracotomy
- The lens should be cleaned and defogged periodically
- The STSR should pass off the light cord, irrigation tubing, suction tubing, camera cord, and electrosurgical cord
- The STSR should not allow the lens with light cord attached to touch the drape as it may ignite the drape

Operative Procedure	Technical Considerations
1. A 1.5-cm skin incision is made over the intercostal space after injection of the incision site with lidocaine 1%.	**1.** Dissection is carried through the intercostal space with electrocautery to prevent blood from obscuring the optical system.
2. A 10-mm trocar is placed into the pleural space after deflation of the lung, and the thoracoscope is introduced through the trocar and into the pleural cavity (Figure 22-22).	**2.** The initial port is typically established at the midaxillary line between the fourth and seventh intercostal space.
3. Sites for second and third incisions are chosen and made for accessory endoscopic and conventional instrumentation.	**3.** No trocar is necessary for insertion of these instruments. Accessory instrumentation is necessary for dissection, retraction, ligation, suction/irrigation, and excision.
4. Diagnosis may be made visually or the procedure of choice is carried out.	**4.** Be vigilant of any condition (e.g., hemorrhage) that may require immediate thoracotomy.
5. After removal of the scope, a chest tube is inserted and hooked up to a closed water-seal drainage system. Incisions are closed with subcuticular stitches.	**5.** Incisions are closed in a subcuticular fashion with 4–0 Vicryl on a small cutting needle. Argyle chest tubes between 28 and 32 Fr are used for drainage.

(continues)

PROCEDURE

22-1 Thoracoscopy *(continued)*

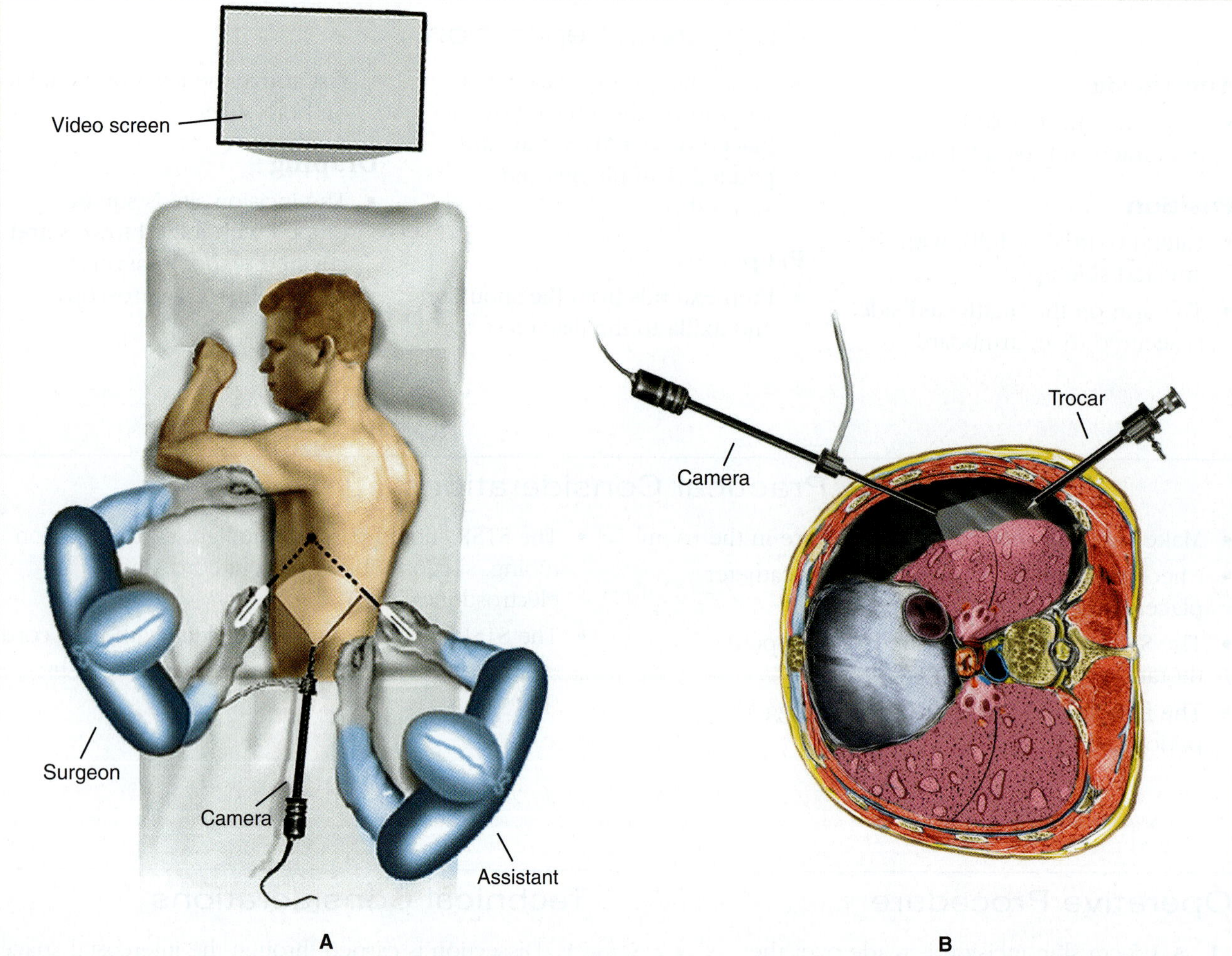

Figure 22-22 Thoracoscopy: (A) Trocar placement, (B) intrathoracic view

Postoperative Considerations

Immediate Postoperative Care

- The chest tube should be attached immediately to the closed water-seal drainage system to prevent clot formation within the tube.

Prognosis

- Depends on the pathological condition. Recovery time for these less invasive procedures is much shorter than for open thoracotomy.

Complications

- Atelectasis
- Pneumonia
- Respiratory insufficiency
- Pneumothorax
- Hemorrhage
- Pulmonary embolus
- Subcutaneous emphysema
- Mediastinal shift
- Acute pulmonary edema
- Infection

PEARL OF WISDOM

As with any endoscopic procedure, proper camera positioning is essential. But unlike laparoscopic procedures, the thorax cannot be insufflated for expansion; therefore, double-lumen endotracheal tubes that allow single-lung ventilation and collapse of the lung on the affected side are essential.

SCALENE/SUPRACLAVICULAR NODE BIOPSY

Palpable nodes in the scalene fat pads are prime sites for metastasis from lungs via the mediastinal lymphatics. Biopsy of these nodes is essential before thoracotomy, because these nodes represent the last of the lymphatic drainage chain. Positive nodes after biopsy indicate metastatic malignancy, and thoracotomy is not advised.

Equipment for this procedure includes electrosurgical unit and suction unit. A minor set includes any necessary instrumentation, and supplies include sterile specimen cup, Telfa, electrosurgical pencil, suction tubing and tip, and Ray-Tec sponges.

Patients for scalene node biopsy are positioned supine with the head extended and turned toward the unaffected side. After prepping, the patient is square-draped with folded towels and a thyroid sheet. A small incision is made 2 in. above the clavicle to the posterior border of the sternocleidomastoid muscle. Dissection is carried through the platysma muscle, retractors are inserted, and the scalene fat pad is identified and biopsied. The incision is closed.

THORACOTOMY FOR UPPER LOBECTOMY

If a neoplasm is confined to a particular lobe of the lung and hilar nodes are not involved, a lobe of the lung can be removed without disturbing other portions of the lung (Procedure 22-2). Most conditions requiring lobectomy, however, are inflammatory in nature, making lobectomy more difficult to perform than pneumonectomy because of increased adhesions. Secondary hilar structures are also difficult to dissect and anomalies occur frequently.

(Text continues on page 899)

PROCEDURE 22-2 Thoracotomy for Upper Lobectomy

Equipment

- Cell Saver
- Fiberoptic light source
- Fiberoptic headlight
- Defibrillation unit should also be available
- Electrosurgical unit
- Suction system

Instrumentation

- Major set
- Chest set
- Major vascular set necessary if chest set does not contain proper vascular instrumentation
- Hemoclip applicators of various lengths and sizes
- Sternal saw and sternal retractor if median sternotomy necessary

Supplies

- Pack: basic
- Basin set
- Gloves
- Blades (#20, #10, #15)
- Drapes: towels, plastic adhesive drape, transverse laparotomy sheet
- Suture: 2–0 and 3–0 silk suture ties (24–32 in. length) on carriers

(continues)

PROCEDURE 22-2 **Thoracotomy for Upper Lobectomy** *(continued)*

- Prolene or silk ligature sutures (stick-ties)
- Closure suture of surgeon's preference
- Drains: chest tubes (Argyle)
- Dressings: inner contact layer, 4 × 4s, ABD
- Drugs:
  - Antibiotic irrigation
  - Xylocaine 1% without epinephrine for postoperative pain control
- Miscellaneous:
  - Hemoclips of all sizes
  - Magnetic mat
  - Electrosurgical pencil
  - Electrosurgical extension blade
  - Suction tubing
  - Asepto syringes
  - Kitner dissectors
  - Cell Saver suction tubing
  - Chest tubes
  - Pleur-evac closed seal drainage system
  - Straight or Y-type connector for chest tubes
  - Vessel loops or umbilical tapes
  - Stapling devices

Operative Preparation

Anesthesia

- General

Position

- A posterolateral approach is generally utilized for lobectomy because it gives the surgeon more maneuverability. The supine position is required for median sternotomy
- The arm on the unaffected side is placed onto an armboard, and the arm on the affected side is placed onto a padded Mayo or double armboard supported by pillows
- The torso is supported with pillows or kidney rest, and the lower leg is flexed as a base while the upper leg is extended
- A pillow is placed between the legs and the feet and ankles are padded
- Tape is placed across the shoulder and hip and secured to the OR table

Prep

- The skin is prepped for a posterolateral incision with prep perimeters from the shoulder and arm to the iliac crest, and to just above the level of the table

Draping

- The incision site is square-draped with towels, and covered with plastic adhesive drape and transverse laparotomy sheet
- For median sternotomy, a nonfenestrated, reinforced heart sheet or fenestrated laparotomy sheet over towels secured by incision drape is effective

Practical Considerations

- A well-trained surgical technologist should have extensive knowledge of anatomy and physiology of the thorax. Procedures of the chest should be studied extensively
- The surgical technologist should know the steps of the thoracic procedure so that he or she can anticipate the moves of the surgeon. Knowing what the thoracic surgeon is doing is a huge benefit, because it allows the surgical technologist to understand the meaning behind a particular step, rather than simply to follow orders or repeat memorized steps
- The surgical technologist should understand that the patient is at a high risk for injury due to the lateral positioning necessary for most thoracic procedures. Skin integrity and joint conditions should be assessed preoperatively, pressure points must be identified and properly padded, and

PROCEDURE

22-2 Thoracotomy for Upper Lobectomy *(continued)*

peripheral nerves and vessels must be protected. Hyperextension of limbs must be prevented, and proper stabilization of the patient in the lateral position is mandatory. The surgical technologist should use stabilizing devices and pads liberally. Tension on arterial, IV, CVP, ET tube, and urinary lines must be prevented during positioning

- When opening sterile supplies, smaller items, such as blades and sutures, should be opened into the large basin. Larger items opened onto the back table should be opened in proximity to the area where they will eventually end up when setting up for the procedure. This reduces unnecessary movements and allows for a quicker setup during an emergency. If another team member opens sterile supplies while the surgical technologist scrubs, the surgical technologist should remind that person of this opening procedure. Haphazard opening of numerous sterile supplies will add precious minutes to a procedure setup
- Thoracic surgery can be challenging for even the most experienced surgical technologist, especially during emergency procedures. Proximity to major vessels should alert the surgical technologist to be prepared for vessel injury at any moment. Pledgeted double-armed polypropylene sutures should be always at the ready, as should silk or polypropylene suture ligatures. 2–0 or 3–0 silk ties of 24–32 in. length loaded on carriers should be available at all times.

Operative Procedure	Technical Considerations
1. After the patient has been prepped and draped, an incision is made into the fourth intercostal space (fifth or sixth interspace incision is made for the right middle lobe and lower lobe dissections).	**1.** Incision is made with a #10 blade on a No. 3 handle, or a #20 blade on a No. 4 handle.
2. A rib spreader is placed, and the pleura is incised. The anterosuperior portion of the hilar pleura is incised and separated.	**2.** Once the thorax is opened it is unlikely that the rib instruments will be reused. Remove them from the Mayo stand.
3. The fissure between the upper and lower lobes is opened, and dissection of the pulmonary artery is begun.	**3.** During the thoracic procedure, the STSR should keep a calculation of the amount of irrigation used because of the potential for blood replacement. If sponges are to be weighed, throw off sponges only after they are completely soaked with blood.
4. Pulmonary artery and pulmonary vein lobar branches are identified, isolated, doubly ligated, and divided.	**4.** Thoracic procedures require the STSR to always think a few steps ahead of the surgeon so that the surgeon never has to wait for a loaded suture or instrument. Time is of the essence during an injury to a major vessel of the thorax, and it requires the STSR to move quickly and think clearly.
5. The upper lobe bronchus is freed by blunt dissection, and a bronchus clamp or staple gun is placed at least 1.5–2 cm from the main bronchial trunk.	**5.** Have stapler loaded and sutures prepared. The bronchus is divided quickly. Entry of the bronchial tree will change the wound classification and may result in contaminated instruments. Be prepared to isolate any contaminated instruments or supplies.

(continues)

PROCEDURE 22-2 Thoracotomy for Upper Lobectomy *(continued)*

6. The bronchus is divided and closed with nonabsorbable sutures or staples fired from the auto-suture device.

6. Be aware of the surgeon's and surgical assistant's moves at all times. Closely listening and watching during the procedure allows for anticipation. During an emergency this is vital because the procedure may quickly deviate from normal.

7. A pleural flap is placed over the bronchial stump and secured with sutures. The remaining lobes are checked for air leaks, and the wound is closed after placement of chest tubes.

7. Body temperature irrigation will be needed to fill the thorax to check for leaks. The anesthetist will perform the Valsalva's maneuver. Prepare for chest tube placement, wound closure, and appropriate counts.

Postoperative Considerations

Immediate Postoperative Care

- The STSR should be prepared for an injection of Marcaine 0.25% during skin closure for postoperative pain control.
- The lines from the chest tubes must be hooked up to the closed suction unit and suction should be turned on immediately to prevent clotting within the chest tubes.
- Transfer from the OR table to the recovery room stretcher should be made with care so that arterial, IV and CVP lines, Foley catheter, and ET tube are not accidentally removed.
- The STSR should remain sterile, as should the Mayo and back table, until the patient has safely left the OR.
- After the thoracic procedure, the patient may be transferred to the recovery room with the endotracheal tube in place to ensure adequate postoperative ventilation and air exchange, the two most important factors for postoperative consideration in thoracic procedures.

Prognosis

- Depends on the pathological condition and the patient's preoperative status.

Complications

- Atelectasis
- Pneumonia
- Respiratory insufficiency
- Pneumothorax
- Hemorrhage
- Pulmonary embolus
- Subcutaneous emphysema
- Mediastinal shift
- Acute pulmonary edema
- Infection

PEARL OF WISDOM

Emergency chest procedures allow little time for a proper setup. Find out what approach the surgeon will be taking (usually posterolateral or median sternotomy) and prepare the items first that will allow you access to the injury. If approach is through median sternotomy, a scalpel followed by an electrosurgical pencil will be the first items the surgeon will want. While the surgeon is making the incision, prepare the sternal saw and pass off the Cell Saver suction line. After the sternotomy, a sternal retractor will be required. At this point, laparotomy sponges and the suction from the Cell Saver will be necessary. Once hemorrhage is controlled, the STSR can properly set up for the remainder of the procedure.

THORACOTOMY FOR RIGHT PNEUMONECTOMY

Pneumonectomy is the removal of an entire lung. Wedge resection, segmental resection, and lobectomy are resections that involve the removal of a portion of the lung. The chief indication for pneumonectomy is bronchogenic carcinoma. Less common indications include multiple lung abscesses, bronchiectasis, and extensive unilateral tuberculosis.

The approach for pneumonectomy is posterolateral because it offers the best overall access to hilar structures. After prepping, the patient is prepped and draped with folded towels, incision drape, and transverse laparotomy sheet, a posterolateral incision is made through the fifth intercostal space and the rib is resected. The ribs and soft tissue are protected with moist laparotomy sponges, and a rib spreader is placed between the ribs for retraction of the chest wall. The lung is mobilized by dividing adhesions between parietal and visceral pleura, and the pulmonary ligament is divided. The pulmonary artery is dissected, and its branches are occluded with vascular clamps, double-ligated with Prolene suture ligatures, and divided. The superior and inferior pulmonary veins are dissected, clamped, double-ligated, and divided, as well. The bronchus is exposed with blunt dissection, and connective tissue surrounding the bronchus is ligated and excised. A Sarot bronchus clamp is applied to the bronchus near the tracheal bifurcation, and the bronchus is divided with a knife. Nonabsorbable mattress sutures are applied in a mattress fashion, and the clamp is removed. If a stapling device is applied to the bronchus instead of the bronchus clamp, staples are fired and the bronchus is divided with a knife. The azygos vein is isolated, ligated, and divided, and the bronchial stump is covered with a pleural flap secured by sutures. Chest tubes are placed into the pleural space, brought out through stab incisions in the chest wall, and connected to a closed drainage system (e.g., Pleur-evac). A Bailey rib approximator is placed and heavy chromic sutures are placed around the ribs bordering the incision for closure. The chest tubes are secured to the skin with a heavy silk, and the wound is closed in the usual manner.

THORACOTOMY FOR WEDGE RESECTION OR SEGMENTECTOMY

Relatively small lesions of the lung can be removed for biopsy through a thoracotomy approach. A wedge resection involves the removal of a triangular-shaped piece of parenchyma after staples have been applied with an automatic stapling device or the tissue has been clamped and sewn. Approach depends on location of the lesion, and no ribs need be excised. If the specimen removed is

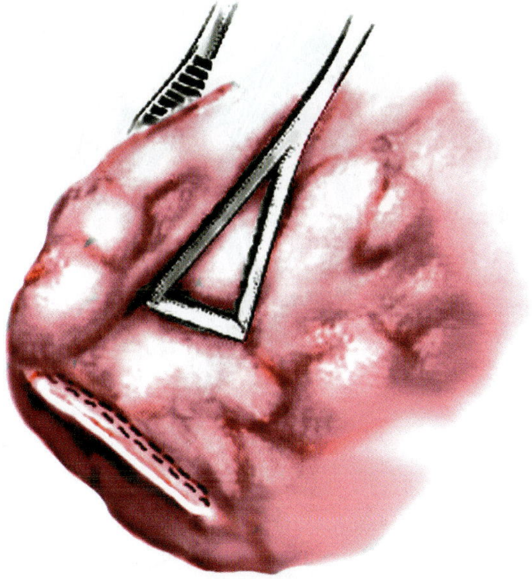

Figure 22-23 Segmental resection

confirmed by frozen section as malignant, a lobectomy may be necessary. If benign, a chest tube is placed into the pleural space and attached to a closed drainage system. The wound is closed in the usual manner.

Segmentectomy (Figure 22-23) involves the removal of an individual bronchovascular segment of a lung due to bronchiectasis, cysts, blebs, or benign lesions. The segments' arteries, veins, and bronchus are isolated, ligated, and divided, and the segment is removed and examined. A chest tube is placed and attached to a closed drainage system, and the wound is closed in the usual manner.

DECORTICATION OF LUNG

If blood or pus from a chest injury is not properly drained from the pleural cavity, it coagulates and forms a fibrin layer over the visceral and parietal pleura that interferes with the proper expansion of the lung (Figure 22-24). The condition is called empyema.

With the patient in the posterolateral position, the fifth intercostal space is entered, and a rib spreader is placed. Clotted blood or pus is removed, and adhesions between the parietal and visceral pleura are excised. The lung is inflated to demonstrate the extent of entrapment, and the fibrin layer is incised with a scalpel. A plane of cleavage is established with healthy lung bulging through the fibrin from underneath. Separation continues with blunt dissection (a finger and/or peanut dissector). After the entire visceral membrane has been removed, the lung is expanded and proper inflation is established. The retractor is removed, chest tubes are placed, and the wound is closed in the usual manner.

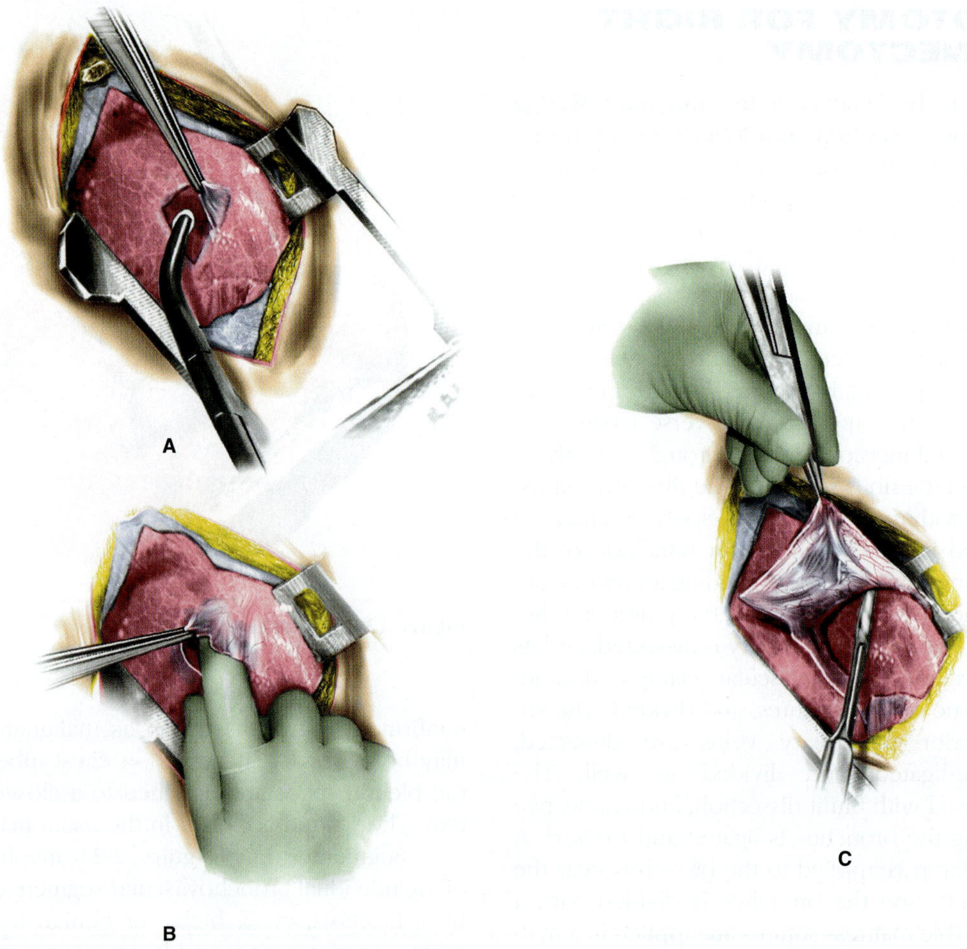

Figure 22-24 **Decortication of the lung: (A) An incision is made in the fibrous membrane, (B) begins with blunt dissection, (C) sharp dissection may be required if membrane is adhered to visceral pleura**

SURGICAL INTERVENTION: CARDIAC (ADULT)

The surgical procedures of the adult heart described in this section include pericardectomy, aortocoronary bypass, aortic and mitral valve replacements, heart transplants, percutaneous transluminal coronary angioplasty, and pacemaker implantations.

PREOPERATIVE CONSIDERATIONS

The patient who is to undergo cardiac surgery is often apprehensive about his or her condition and fearful of intraoperative or postoperative death. Surgical personnel should take the time to ensure the patient that all is well, and that he or she is in good and capable hands.

Cardiac surgery is typically performed in the largest room of the OR suite to accommodate a larger number of OR personnel and necessary equipment such as the cardiopulmonary pump, Cell Saver, hypothermia unit, defibrillator unit, and electrosurgical and suction units.

The cardiac patient may come from the cardiac care unit on an ICU bed with monitoring lines in place. Occasionally, the patient will be brought over from the cardiac catheterization lab, usually for an emergency procedure. Percutaneous transluminal coronary angioplasty (PTCA) procedures are performed in the "cath lab," and the OR's cardiac team is typically asked to stand by in case the patient requires an emergency open-heart procedure. Coronary angioplasty balloons can dissect a coronary artery during inflation, and this will require immediate surgical repair. These emergencies require the team to open sterile supplies and to set up for the procedure very quickly, often as the patient is being moved to the OR table. The patient brought over from the cardiac catheterization lab will generally have sheaths inserted into the femoral vein and artery.

Because so many supplies are necessary for cardiac procedures, the surgical technologist should take the time to check them against the preference card and obtain any missing items. Because there are so many sterile items to be opened, smaller items should be opened into the basin, and larger items should be opened onto strategic locations that minimize motion during setup. This process is especially important for emergency cardiac procedures because setup time is limited.

Anesthesia for cardiac procedures should be administered by physicians who are specially trained in cardiac anesthesia. The patient will require a high degree of monitoring intraoperatively and postoperatively. Intraoperative invasive monitoring includes:

- An arterial line within the radial or femoral artery for measurement of direct arterial blood pressures and arterial blood gas studies.
- A Swan-Ganz pulmonary artery catheter that indirectly measures left atrial and left ventricular pressures by assessing right atrial, right ventricular, and pulmonary artery wedge pressures. The Swan-Ganz may also be used to monitor central venous pressures.
- Other lines may be inserted directly into the aorta or left atrium by the surgeon for direct pressure readings.
- Urinary drainage catheter with temperature sensor for the measurement of urinary output and core temperature.
- Transesophageal echocardiography.

Noninvasive intraoperative monitoring includes:

- BP cuff for the indirect measurement of arterial blood pressure
- Pulse oximeter for the measurement of oxygen saturation of hemoglobin
- ECG

On arrival, the patient's chart should be reviewed for history, physical, consent, diagnostic findings, and laboratory results. Diagnostic studies for review include:

- Resting ECG
- Stress test ECG
- Chest X-ray
- Echocardiography
- Cardiac catheterization studies that include ventricular, atrial, and pulmonary pressures, and cardiac output with ejection fraction recordings
- Digital subtraction cine-arteriograms of the left ventricle and coronary arteries (Often a drawing is made by the cardiologist of the coronary arteries and coronary artery stenoses.)
- Radionuclide imaging
- Thoracic aorta arteriograms and MRI studies (if the patient is to have a ventricular aneurysm repaired)
- Electrophysiology studies

In addition to diagnostic findings, the anesthesia provider should examine preoperative pulmonary function, coagulation studies, and arterial blood gas studies. The patient will have been typed and cross-matched for blood replacement, and OR personnel should check with the blood bank to ensure that the proper blood is available.

PATIENT PREPARATION

The median sternotomy with the patient in the supine position offers the best approach to the heart and great vessels for surgical repair and cannulae placement for cardiopulmonary bypass. Posterolateral thoracotomy may be utilized for access to the descending aorta.

Pressure points should be identified and padded, and arms should be placed at the patient's side and properly padded.

Typically, three Mayo stands are utilized for coronary bypass procedures, and two for aneurysm repair or valve replacement procedures. Coronary bypass procedures that will utilize a saphenous vein graft will require a third Mayo stand for saphenous vein harvesting. Some surgical technologists can manage the case with only one Mayo stand for all cardiac procedures.

TECHNIQUES OF CARDIOPULMONARY BYPASS

The pump oxygenator, or "heart-lung machine," is the apparatus used in cardiac surgery to remove unoxygenated blood from the venous system, oxygenate and filter it, and return it to the arterial system. By assuming the roles of the heart and lungs, the pump oxygenator (Figure 22-25) allows the heart to be stopped so that delicate cardiac procedures may by performed. It also allows the lungs to be deflated for better exposure of the heart and major vessels.

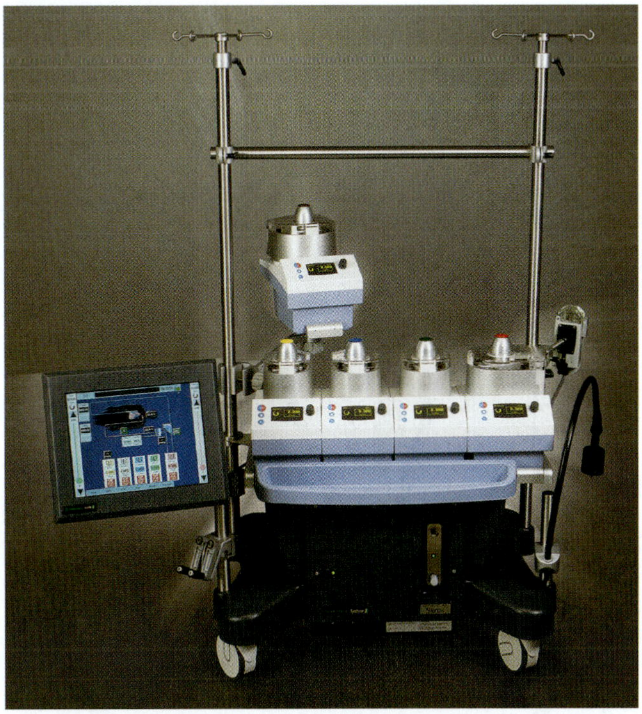

Figure 22-25 Terumo® Advanced Perfusion System 1 *(Courtesy of Terumo Cardiovascular Systems Corporation)*

The name "heart-lung machine" indicates what is required to produce extracorporeal circulation: the oxygenation of blood (replacing the function of the lungs) and the pumping of blood (replacing the function of the heart).

The pump oxygenator is relatively simple in design. Venous blood is removed from the body by way of a sterile plastic tube (cannula) that is placed into the right atrium or venae cavae and shunted through an oxygenator. The oxygenator may be a bubble or microporous-membrane type, and it is equipped with a reservoir and heat exchanger that allows the temperature of the blood to be manipulated as needed. After blood has been oxygenated, a roller pump moves the blood from the reservoir back to the arterial system. Additional pumps are used for removing blood from the operative site (using "cardiotomy suckers" on the operative field) and vented blood from the left ventricle (Figure 22-26). This blood is added to a reservoir for oxygenation and sent back into the arterial system, preventing blood loss.

The placement of cannulas into the right atrium or venae cavae for draining venous blood to the pump oxygenator and the ascending aorta for the return of arterial blood from the pump oxygenator is referred to as *cannulation* (Figure 22-27). Before cannulation, heparin (300 U/kg) must be administered to prevent clotting.

Note: If the right atrium is to be opened (for tricuspid valve replacement or repair of ASD), a venous cannula is placed into the superior vena cava and another in the inferior vena cava. For most cardiac procedures, however, a two-stage venous cannula is sufficient.

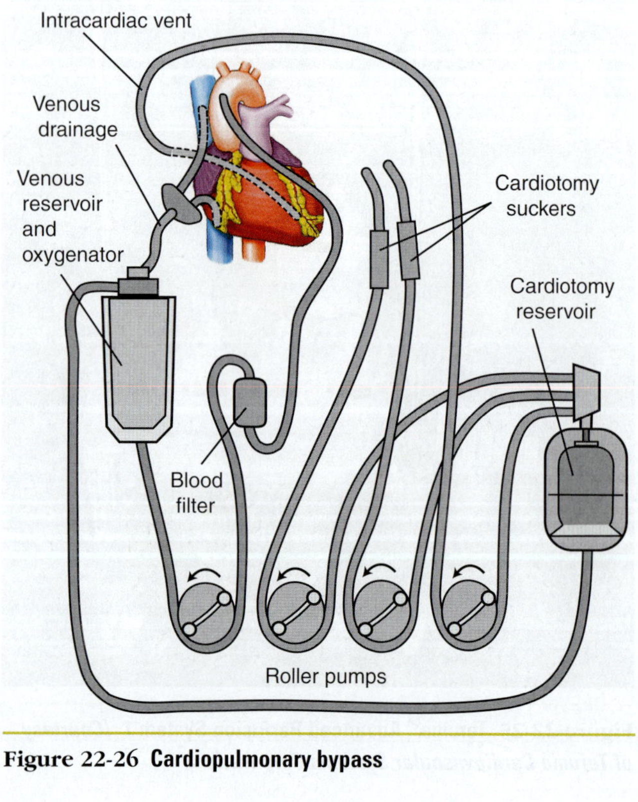

Figure 22-26 Cardiopulmonary bypass

After venous and arterial cannulation, saline-filled polyvinyl chloride tubing from the pump oxygenator is attached to each cannula and secured. As the connections between the pump lines and the arterial and caval cannulas are made, great care is taken to prevent air bubbles from forming within the bypass circuit.

Because left ventricular pressures are elevated in a motionless heart, causing lung damage or ventricular distension, a vent is placed into the left ventricle (Figure 22-28). In addition to lowering left ventricular pressure, venting also removes air from the heart.

For optimal visualization during coronary artery bypass procedures, left ventricular venting is accomplished with a cannula placed through the ascending aorta and into the left ventricle. The cannula is attached to a small, needle-vented suction line from the pump oxygenator.

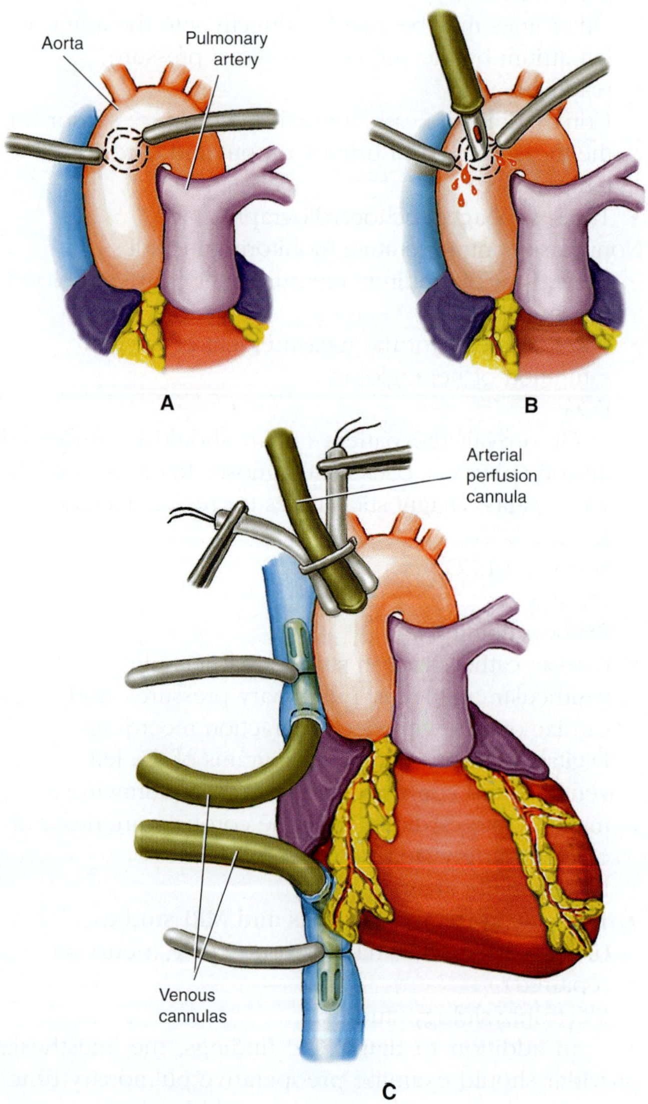

Figure 22-27 Arterial and venous cannulation: (A) Pursestring sutures are placed in the ascending aorta. (B) Aortic cannula is secured by tightening the pursestring sutures over the rubber catheters. (C) Completed arterial and venous cannulation

TECHNIQUE Aortic Cannulation

1. After median sternotomy, a self-retaining retractor is placed and an incision is made into the pericardium. Traction sutures are placed into the pericardium and secured to the retractor or chest wall.
2. The aorta is exposed, and two pursestring sutures are placed high on the ascending aorta, to allow room for proximal vein grafts and the cardioplegia/venting cannula.
3. Large red rubber catheters that have been cut into 4-in. pieces are placed over each pursestring suture and the needles are cut off of the suture ends. A Rochester-Pean or Crile hemostat clamp is placed on the ends of each pursestring. A Satinsky partial-occlusion clamp may be placed onto the aorta if the aorta is not calcified.
4. An incision is made into the aorta between the pursestring sutures with a #11 knife blade, and the metal, bevel-ended tip of the aortic cannula is placed into the arteriotomy. The cannula is allowed to fill with arterial blood that is held in check by a stopper on the proximal end.
5. The cannula is held in place by the rubber catheter tourniquets (keeper) that are cinched tightly over the pursestring sutures and clamped with a hemostat. A heavy silk suture is tied around the cannula and rubber keepers.

TECHNIQUE Venous Cannulation

1. A single pursestring suture is placed into the right atrial appendage, and a red rubber catheter is placed over the pursestring suture. The needles are removed from the suture and either a Rochester-Pean hemostat clamp or a Crile hemostat clamp is placed on the suture ends.
2. A Satinsky partial-occlusion clamp is secured over the incision site.
3. The incision is made into the right atrial appendage with a #15 blade or Metzenbaum scissors.
4. A two-stage venous cannula that drains blood from the right atrium, inferior vena cava, and coronary sinus is inserted, and the red rubber catheter is cinched tightly over the pursestring suture, securing the cannula. The hemostat is clamped to the rubber catheter tourniquet.
5. A heavy silk suture is placed around the cannula and the rubber keepers.

Utilizing a Y-shaped cannula, the cardioplegia solution can be administered through the same aortic puncture site as the venting line.

Myocardial protection during cardiopulmonary bypass is accomplished with systemic hypothermia, topical myocardial hypothermia, and the administration of cold potassium cardioplegia solution into the coronary arteries via the aortic root and/or the coronary sinus via the right atrium. Hypothermia reduces the oxygen demands of the myocardium, and so is the technique utilized most often for cardiac procedures.

After cannulation and the initiation of cardiopulmonary bypass, a Fogarty cross-clamp is placed across the ascending aorta. A needle/cannula assembly for the administration of cold (4°C) potassium cardioplegia solution that inhibits myocardial contraction is inserted into the aortic root, and the paralyzing solution is infused into the coronary arteries at frequent intervals. Retrograde administration of cardioplegia is useful for second operations for coronary

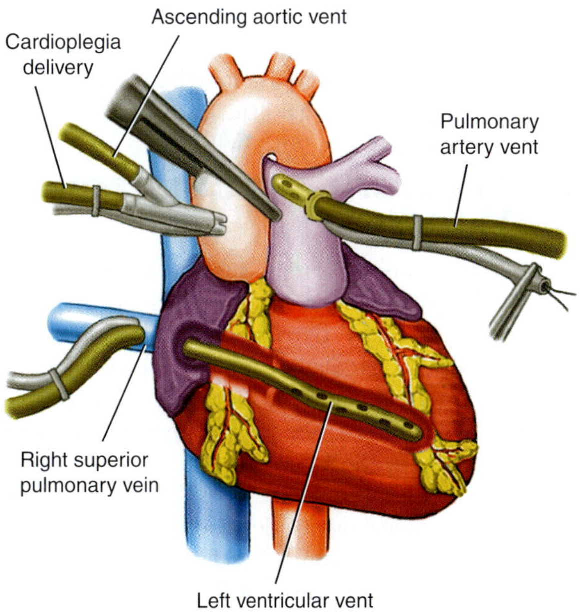

Figure 22-28 **Left ventricular venting**

TECHNIQUE Left Ventricular Vent Placement via the Left Atrium

1. A single pursestring suture is placed into the anterior surface of the right superior pulmonary vein.
2. A small incision is made in the pulmonary vein and dilated.
3. A 20-Fr left heart venting catheter is inserted and guided into the left ventricle.
4. The venting catheter is attached to a suction line from the pump oxygenator.

artery stenosis and valvular procedures and can be accomplished via a catheter placed into the coronary sinus via the right atrium that is held in place with a pursestring/tourniquet combination.

After cardioplegia infusion, ice slush, or ice cold saline (4°C) is placed around the heart. A myocardial insulating pad may also be placed behind the heart. After hypothermic techniques have been employed, the systemic temperature of the patient often falls to 32°C. Utilizing the heat exchanger on the pump oxygenator, the temperature can be taken down even further. A moderate temperature of approximately 28°C reduces oxygen demand on the myocardium by half.

Continuous warm blood cardioplegia is an alternative to hypothermic techniques for myocardial preservation, but is not widely used because of visualization problems during the coronary artery anastomoses.

If the patient has an inadequate ascending aorta due to short length, or if scarring from a previous procedure prevents quick access through a sternotomy, then cannulas for cardiopulmonary bypass may be inserted into the common femoral or external iliac artery.

MECHANICAL CIRCULATORY ASSISTANCE

For patients who need cardiac support because they are waiting for cardiac transplantation or cannot be weaned from cardiopulmonary bypass, mechanical devices designed to assist in circulatory functions may be utilized. Procedures on the descending thoracic aorta may also require mechanical assistance for left heart bypass to provide blood flow to the lower portion of the body while the aorta is occluded.

The mechanical device designed for circulatory support after cardiac procedures is called an intra-aortic balloon pump (IABP). Insertion of the balloon pump may increase cardiac output to a level that would permit separation from the pump oxygenator and allow time for the heart to recover (Figure 22-29).

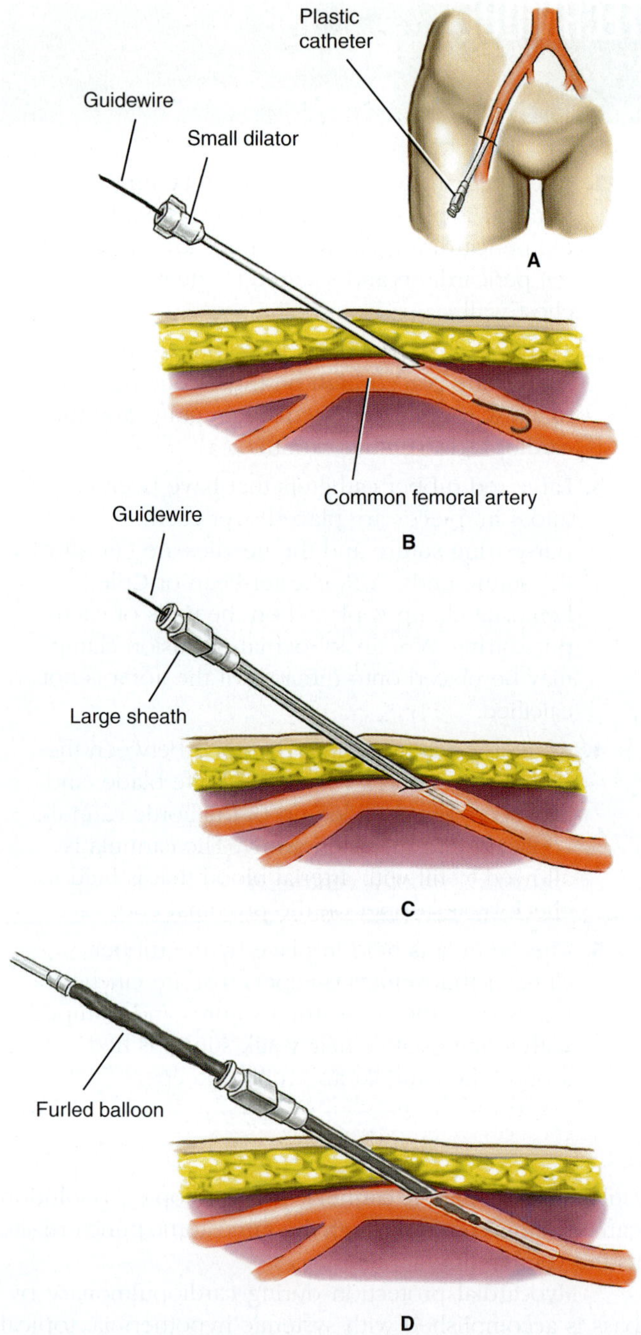

Figure 22-29 **Intra-aortic balloon pump insertion: (A) Needle cannula assembly is inserted into femoral artery. (B) Small dilator is threaded over guidewire. (C) Large sheath is inserted over guidewire. (D) Balloon is inserted into sheath**

To be completely effective, the IABP must lower left ventricular pressure during systole (when the balloon is deflated) and increase coronary artery circulation during diastole (when the balloon is inflated) (Figure 22-30).

TECHNIQUE Insertion of the IABP

1. After percutaneous needle/cannula assembly placement into the femoral artery, a guidewire is threaded through the arterial cannula and the cannula is removed.
2. The artery is dilated to a 12-Fr diameter with plastic, graduated dilators threaded over the guidewire.
3. A balloon sheath/dilator assembly is inserted over the guidewire, and the dilator is removed.
4. The IABP catheter with a large balloon wound tightly around the distal end is inserted through the sheath and advanced slowly to a position just distal to the left subclavian artery.
5. The balloon is unwound and the catheter is attached to the pump. The pump is then activated.

Patients who cannot be separated from cardiopulmonary bypass by conventional methods or IABP may benefit from the use of a ventricular assist device (VAD). The VAD is designed to boost cardiac output and rest an ailing left ventricle by diverting blood away from the left ventricle, through an artificial pump, and into the aorta for systemic circulation.

For procedures on the descending thoracic aorta, blood flow must be maintained to distal tissues. The use of a heparin-coated impeller flow pump for left ventricular bypass permits work to be done on the descending thoracic aorta and also supplements cardiac output for an ailing left ventricle. Through cannulas inserted into the common femoral artery and left atrium, the pump pulls blood away from the left ventricle and propels it into the aorta.

CORONARY ARTERY BYPASS GRAFTING

Surgery for coronary artery stenosis has become the most commonly performed cardiac procedure during the past 20 years. It involves the revascularization of myocardium that has become ischemic due to stenotic or occluded coronary vessels. A saphenous vein or the internal mammary artery (IMA) is sewn to the affected coronary artery at a point distal to the stenosis (Figure 22-31).

Coronary artery bypass grafting (CABG) (Procedure 22-3) generally involves cardiopulmonary bypass (CPB), although coronary artery grafting can be done without

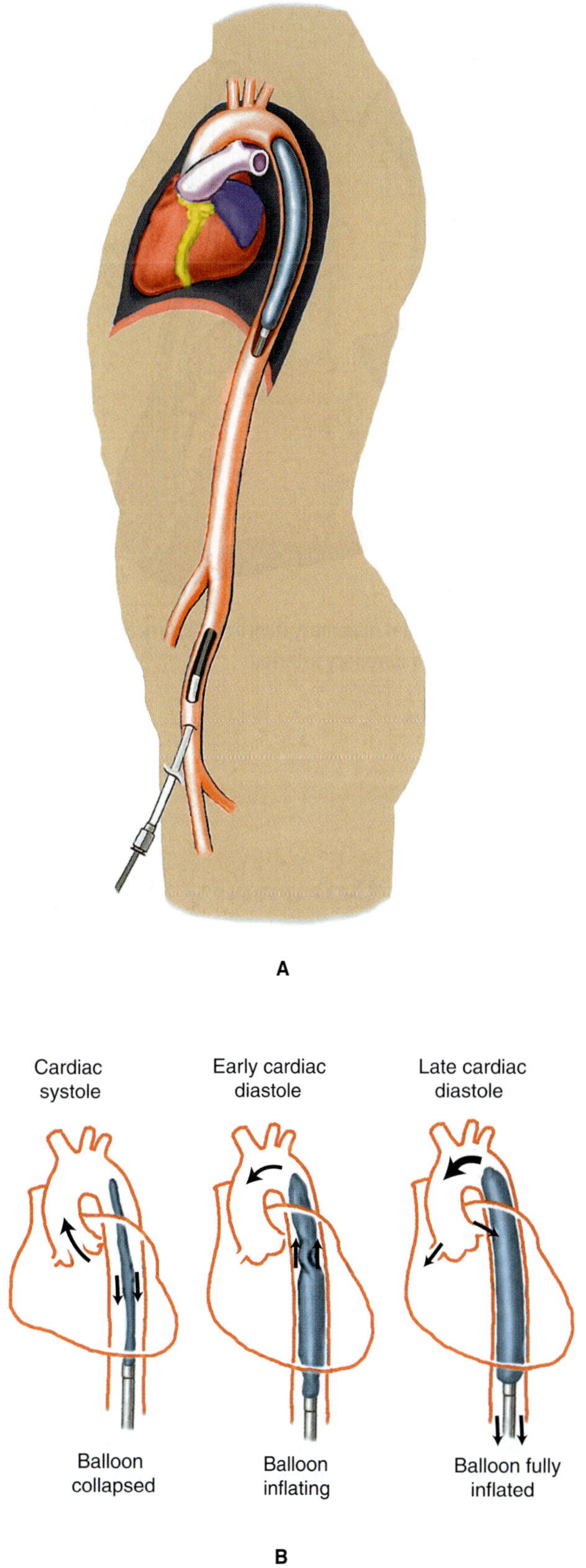

Figure 22-30 **IABP mechanics: (A) The balloon is situated in the descending aorta. (B) The balloon is deflated during cardiac systole and inflated during diastole**

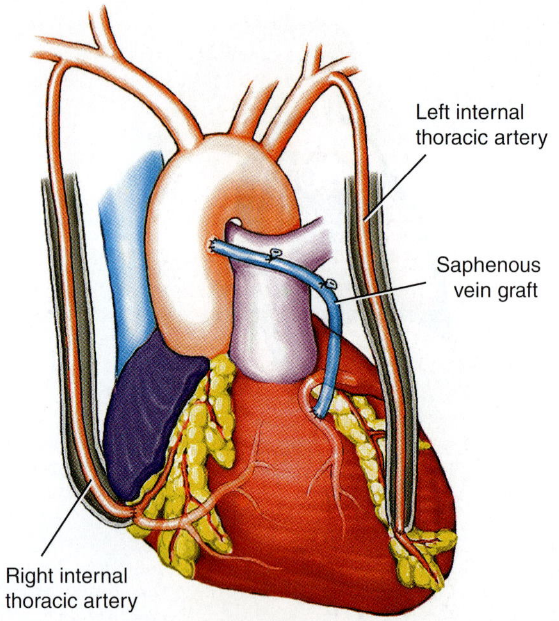

Figure 22-31 **Internal mammary (thoracic) artery and saphenous vein anastomosed to coronary arteries**

CPB under certain conditions. New, less invasive procedures have also been developed for coronary artery bypass grafting. The minimally invasive direct coronary artery bypass procedure (mid-cab) is useful for certain coronary artery lesions, and follows the trend in medicine for less invasive surgery in general. The heart is not stopped for the procedure, and only a 4-in. incision is required for access to the coronary vessels. The new "limited bypass" surgery will not replace conventional coronary bypass procedures because many patients are not viable candidates for this type of procedure. For those patients who are eligible, the mid-cab procedure offers shorter hospital stays for less cost than conventional bypass surgery.

Conventional coronary bypass procedures are performed routinely in this country, however, and this discussion will concern the technique for coronary artery grafting with either IMA and/or saphenous vein under cardiopulmonary bypass.

(Text continues on page 911)

PROCEDURE 22-3 Coronary Artery Bypass Grafting

Equipment

- Cardiopulmonary bypass machine
- Hypothermia and temperature unit
- Hypothermia mattress
- Cell Saver
- External pacemaker
- Defibrillator unit
- Electrosurgical unit
- Suction system
- Ice (slush) machine
- Argon laser for sternal coagulation (optional)

Instruments

- Open heart sets (Typically, one open heart set contains all necessary instrumentation to place the patient on cardiopulmonary bypass, and the other contains instrumentation for saphenous vein dissection and the cardiac procedure.)
- Self-retaining mammary artery retractor
- Sternal saw
- Oscillating saw may be necessary for repeat heart procedures
- Delicate coronary artery instruments, such as those designed by Diethrich, include various sizes of coronary scissors, dilators, bulldogs, heparin needles, Castroviejo needle holders, and vascular forceps
- An endoscope may be used for saphenous vein removal

PROCEDURE

22-3 Coronary Artery Bypass Grafting *(continued)*

Supplies

- Pack: heart
- Basin set
- Gloves
- Blades (#10, #11, #15, #20, Beaver)
- Drapes: nonfenestrated heart sheet
- Suture:
  - Cannulation sutures of the surgeon's choice (e.g., Prolene or Ethibond)
  - 5–0, 6–0 Prolene
  - 0, 2–0, 3–0, 4–0 silk for pericardial stays, chest tube suture, and ties
  - Stainless steel sternal wires
  - Closure sutures of the surgeon's choice
- Drains: chest tubes (Argyle)
- Dressings: surgeon's preference
- Drugs:
  - Sodium heparin mixed with sodium chloride for intra-arterial irrigation and for soaking the saphenous vein before anastomosis
- Topical papaverine for the prevention of vasospasm, especially involving the internal mammary artery
- Antibiotic solution of surgeon's choice mixed with saline for irrigation
- Various topical coagulants
- Miscellaneous:
  - Internal defibrillator paddles and cord
  - Venous and arterial cannulae
  - Cardioplegia needle and administration set
  - Cell Saver suction tubing
  - Alligator pacing cables
  - IV tubing and needles for intrachamber pressure readings
  - Bone wax
  - Gelfoam
  - Surgicel
  - Electrosurgical pencils (one for saphenous vein retrieval and the other for the chest)
  - Teflon felt pledgets
  - Aortic punch
  - Left ventricular sump catheter
  - Coronary artery direct perfusion cannula
  - Pacemaker wires
  - Closed seal drainage unit (e.g., Pleur-evac)
  - Hemoclips of various sizes
  - Teflon or Dacron patch material
  - Red rubber catheters for tourniquets and rubber shods
  - Umbilical tape
  - Vessel loops
  - Disposable bulldog vascular clamps
  - Y-connector for chest tubes
  - Fogarty inserts for aortic cross-clamp
  - Saphenous vein cannula
  - Various size syringes and needles

Operative Preparation

Anesthesia

- General

Position

- Supine, with legs externally rotated (frog-leg position)

Prep

- One person preps as an assistant holds both legs. This allows the legs to be prepped circumferentially
- The patient is prepped from the jaw line to the toes, and the chest and abdomen are prepped to the edge of the OR table

Draping

- The assistant holds the legs as the STSR places a three-quarter sheet underneath both legs
- Impervious stockinettes are placed over both feet, and the STSR takes the legs from the assistant
- The legs are externally rotated and flexed at the knees for access to the saphenous vein. The chest and abdomen are square-draped, and the genitals are covered with a folded towel and secured
- The drape is placed for access to the anterior chest, abdomen, inguinal area, and leg
- After draping, the STSR will bring up the pump lines, electrosurgical cords, Cell Saver suction line, defibrillator cable, and regular suction line and secure to the drape

(continues)

PROCEDURE 22-3 Coronary Artery Bypass Grafting *(continued)*

Practical Considerations

- Generally, only those surgical technologists who have been properly trained in open-heart surgery are allowed to scrub cardiac procedures
- The STSR must have good anticipatory skills, and should understand cardiovascular anatomy and physiology, as well as cardiac procedural sequence
- The STSR should be thinking five steps ahead of the surgeon throughout the procedure, and should pay attention at all times
- It is important that the STSR understand cardiac dysrhythmias and their relationship to the cardiac procedure, and be able to understand all pressure readings
- Room-temperature saline should be used up to the point of aortic cross-clamping; thereafter, cold saline is to be used until the rewarming period. Warm saline should be used after rewarming begins
- There should never be water on the back table. It would be too easy to accidentally use water instead of saline when filling the cannulae. Water will cause lysing of RBCs
- Be ready to go back on the pump at a moment's notice. Do not discard cannulae after removal, and keep cannulation sutures ready after the patient is removed from CPB. Keep wire cutters and sternal retractor sterile until the patient is safely out of the OR
- For repeat cardiac procedures, be prepared to cannulate femorally. The oscillating saw may be used for sternotomy to prevent cutting into ventricular adhesions to the sternal wall
- Pass off defibrillation cables at the same time as electrosurgical cords. The surgeon will not want to wait for the defibrillation paddles if they are suddenly needed
- Wet the surgeon's hands with saline when tying polypropylene sutures to prevent breaking them
- Remind the circulator to turn on the suction to the closed-seal drainage unit as soon as the chest tubes are connected to it. This prevents clots from forming in the chest tubes
- Keep your Mayo stand and back tables as neat as possible
- Check polypropylene sutures for knots or kinks before passing to the surgeon. If one is found, do not try to untie it. Load another as quickly as possible
- Laying a light-colored paper towel over the Mayo stand during anastomoses helps make the polypropylene sutures visible
- Watch polypropylene sutures for dragging when passing them to the surgeon. They can be easily snagged on items between the Mayo stand and the surgeon. Keep tension off the suture as well
- Keep the field clear of instruments, blood-soaked sponges, etc. Wring out blood from laparotomy sponges into a bowl and suction with the pump sucker
- Do not confuse the terms "atrial" and "arterial" when passing cannulation stitches. One is for the right atrium, and the other is for the aorta. Typically, the arterial cannulation stitch is placed first, but if aortic pressure is high, the right atrium will be cannulated first
- Remember that the key to doing a good job is knowing *why* you are doing things. Don't just memorize the steps

Operative Procedure	Technical Considerations
1. An incision is made extending from the sternal notch to the xiphoid process and vessels are coagulated.	**1.** Prepare the sternal saw and the sternal retractor. For repeat sternotomies, an oscillating saw is used so that a ventricle that may be adhered to the chest wall is not cut.
2. The sternum is opened with a sternal saw, and a self-retaining sternal retractor is inserted.	**2.** If the internal mammary artery (IMA) is dissected for coronary artery anastomosis, a mammary retractor is placed instead of the sternal retractor.

PROCEDURE

22-3 Coronary Artery Bypass Grafting *(continued)*

3. The pericardium is incised and retracted with sutures.

3. Retraction sutures are prepared in advance as their use is anticipated.

4. If the left IMA is to be used for left anterior descending artery anastomosis, the IMA is dissected as a pedicle graft proximally from the level of the subclavian artery and distally to the costal margin. Side branches are occluded with small clips.

4. The pedicle graft is soaked in a papaverine solution to prevent vasospasm. A papaverine-soaked 4 × 4 is usually wrapped around the graft.

5. The saphenous vein is harvested from one or both legs by a separate team at the same time that the chest is opened. Tributaries are ligated during dissection with small hemoclips and 4–0 silk ties (Figure 22-32).

5. If the saphenous vein is not taken endoscopically, then dissection is carried out with a #10 blade on a No. 3 handle, Metzenbaum scissors, and DeBakey forceps. Hemoclip appliers must be reloaded for immediate reuse.

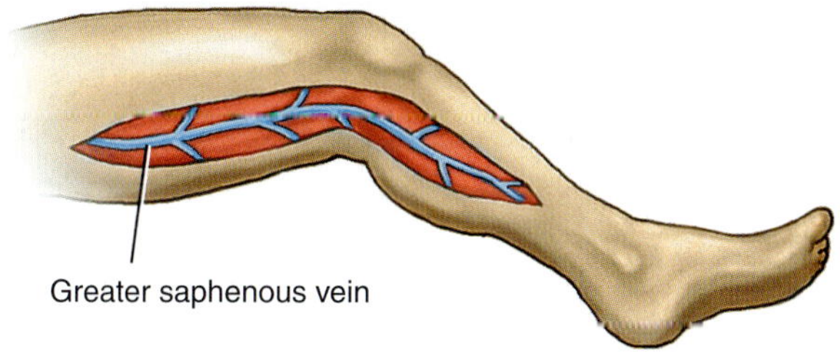

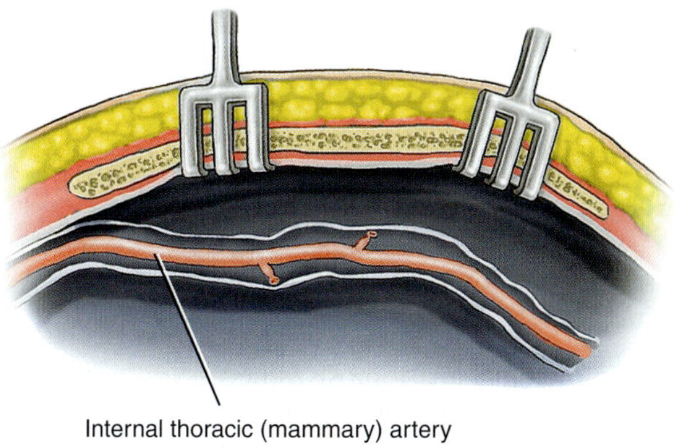

Figure 22-32 Graft options for CABG: (A) Saphenous vein dissection, (B) internal mammary artery dissection

6. The vein is flushed with heparinized saline to identify any branches that may have been missed, and the vein is stored in a heparin/saline solution until needed.

6. Flushing is facilitated by a saphenous vein cannula inserted into the vein and secured with a silk tie. Tributaries are tied off with a 4–0 silk tie.

(continues)

PROCEDURE 22-3 Coronary Artery Bypass Grafting *(continued)*

7. Cardiopulmonary bypass is initiated utilizing techniques discussed previously.

8. Coronary artery stenoses are identified, and an arteriotomy is made just distal to the stenosis.

9. The internal mammary artery or saphenous vein is anastomosed to the affected coronary artery with 6–0 or 7–0 gauge polypropylene sutures.

10. A Satinsky partial-occlusion clamp is applied to the ascending aorta, and a 4.5-mm hole is made in the isolated section of the aorta with an aortic punch (Figure 22-33).

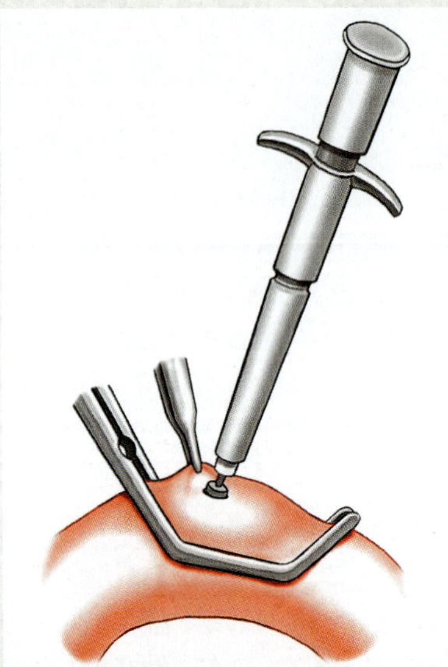

Figure 22-33 Aortic punch

7. The pump lines should be easily accessible and ready to hook up to the cannulae. An Asepto filled with warm saline should be ready to displace air bubbles during hookup.

8. A #64 Beaver blade and handle are useful for the arteriotomy. Tenotomy scissors and Diethrich angled coronary scissors should be available.

9. A disposable bulldog vascular clamp is used to occlude the distal end of the IMA.

10. Pass vascular clamp of appropriate size as needed. Prepare aortic punch and sutures if saphenous vein graft is used.

11. The proximal saphenous vein is anastomosed to the aorta in an end-to-side fashion with size 6–0 polypropylene sutures.

12. The Satinsky partial-occlusion clamp is removed, and needle aspiration of the graft is performed to remove air.

13. Cardiopulmonary bypass is discontinued, chest tubes are placed for the evacuation of fluid and air, and the sternum is closed with heavy-gauged stainless steel wire. The chest is closed in the usual manner.

11. No proximal anastomosis is necessary for the IMA because only the distal end of the artery is transected. The proximal portion remains intact at its origin of the subclavian artery.

12. Needle aspiration is carried out with a 25-gauge ⅝-in. needle on a 10-cc syringe.

13. Use caution when passing wire to avoid puncture of gloves. Have wire twisters, cutters, and closing suture ready. Count as necessary. Chest tubes are secured to the skin with 0 silk on a cutting needle.

PROCEDURE 22-3 **Coronary Artery Bypass Grafting** *(continued)*

Postoperative Considerations

Immediate Postoperative Care

- As usual, the STSR and the back table should remain sterile until the patient has safely left the OR. Wire cutters, sternal retractor, cannulation stitches loaded on needle holders, and cannulae should be available in case the patient must be placed back on cardiopulmonary bypass.
- Care must be taken when transferring the patient from the OR table to the CCU bed. The patient will have monitoring lines, an ET tube, and urinary and chest drainage tubes in place. These can be easily disturbed if tension is placed on them during the move.

Prognosis

- Depends on the condition of the myocardium, especially the left ventricle, and the degree of atherosclerosis. Time spent on cardiopulmonary bypass is also a factor.

Complications

- Complications that may occur postoperatively include clotting problems related to systemic heparinization and cardiopulmonary bypass, which can damage platelets as they pass through the machine. Electrolyte imbalances, hypervolemia, pulmonary edema, atelectasis, and metabolic acidosis may occur if CPB time is extended. Transient cerebral ischemia and cerebral edema may also result from prolonged CPB. Precautions against embolism and hypothermia during the cardiac procedure are essential.
- Postoperative bleeding is monitored closely by CCU personnel through chest tube drainage. Excessive bleeding may be caused by clotting mechanism deficiencies related to CPB, and can lead to cardiac tamponade if left untreated. If bleeding is deemed excessive, the patient is returned to the OR and the chest is reopened for hemorrhage control. So-called "bring-back hearts" require the use of wire cutters to cut through sternal wires, sternal retractor, suction, laparotomy sponges, electrosurgical unit, and polypropylene sutures with and without pledgets loaded on needle holders.

PEARL OF WISDOM

In emergencies, think about what you will be doing first, and prepare the items necessary to do those things. Think about what you need to get into the chest and cannulate (scalpel, electrosurgical pencil, sternal saw, sternal retractor, Cell Saver suction, pump lines, cannulation stitches). Anything else can wait.

AORTIC VALVE REPLACEMENT

Aortic valves are the most frequently replaced valves in cardiac surgery (Procedure 22-4). Aortic valve dysfunction, as discussed previously, may result from rheumatic disease, acute infection, atherosclerotic heart disease, or congenital defects. Stenotic valves are often a natural effect of aging. Whatever the etiology, almost all patients with either aortic valve stenosis or a leaky aortic valve will require surgical valve replacement. A few, however, will do well with a simple repair.

There are basically two types of valve for replacement: biologic (tissue) and mechanical. A valve that combines synthetic material with animal tissue is also frequently used. The tissue valves may be harvested from a pig or a human cadaver, and may also be constructed from the pericardium of a cow. Unlike mechanical valves that have a tendency to form blood clots, placement of a tissue valve does not require anticoagulant therapy for the recipient. Porcine (pig) and human donor valves usually wear out after a period of 10–15 years, and so are not suitable for implantation in younger patients.

Mechanical valves are constructed from modern ceramics, and are usually implanted into patients under the age of 65 because of their longer life span. These valves require the use of anticoagulant therapy because of their tendency to form blood clots. Other risks associated with the use of the mechanical valves are hemorrhage and endocarditis.

A valve that combines bovine pericardium with polyester and plastic, such as the Carpentier-Edwards bioprosthesis valve, lasts approximately 14 years and is another option for patients over the age of 65. The leaflets of the valve are constructed from pericardial tissue, while the supporting structure is made from polyester and plastic.

In certain instances, a diseased aortic valve can be replaced with the patient's own healthy pulmonary semilunar valve. The pulmonary valve is then replaced with a human donor valve. The benefit to this type of valve replacement is that no foreign synthetic substance or animal tissue is introduced into the body, so there is little risk of rejection or clot formation.

(Text continues on page 916)

PROCEDURE 22-4 Aortic Valve Replacement

Equipment

- Cardiopulmonary bypass machine
- Hypothermia and temperature unit
- Hypothermia mattress
- Cell Saver
- External pacemaker
- Defibrillator unit
- Electrosurgical unit
- Suction system
- Ice (slush) machine
- Argon laser for sternal coagulation (optional)

Instruments

- Open heart sets (Typically, one open heart set contains all necessary instrumentation to place the patient on cardiopulmonary bypass, and the other contains instrumentation for the cardiac procedure.)
- Sternal saw
- An oscillating saw may be necessary for repeat heart procedures
- Valve sizers, handle, and rings will be necessary to size the annulus
- Valve retractors will be necessary for leaflet and annulus retraction
- Valve scissors will be needed to cut away the diseased valve

Supplies

- Pack: heart
- Basin set
- Gloves
- Blades: (#10, #11, #15, #20)
- Drapes: nonfenestrated heart sheet
- Suture:
  - Cannulation sutures of the surgeon's choice (e.g., Prolene or Ethibond)
  - Valve suture (typically, Ethibond)
  - 0, 2–0, 3–0, 4–0 silk for pericardial stays, chest tube suture, and ties
  - Stainless steel sternal wires
  - Closure sutures of the surgeon's choice
- Drains: chest tubes (Argyle)
- Dressings: surgeon's preference
- Drugs:
  - Sodium heparin mixed with sodium chloride
  - Antibiotic solution of surgeon's choice mixed with saline for irrigation
  - Various topical coagulants
- Miscellaneous:
  - Internal defibrillator paddles and cord
  - Venous and arterial cannulae
  - Cardioplegia needle and administration set
  - Cell Saver suction tubing
  - Alligator pacing cables
  - IV tubing and needles for intra-chamber pressure readings
  - Bone wax
  - Gelfoam or Surgicel
  - Electrosurgical pencil
  - Teflon felt pledgets
  - Aortic punch
  - Left ventricular sump catheter

PROCEDURE 22-4 Aortic Valve Replacement *(continued)*

Pacemaker wires

Closed seal drainage unit (e.g., Pleur-evac)

Red rubber catheters for tourniquets and rubber shods

Umbilical tape

Y-connector for chest tubes

Fogarty inserts for aortic cross-clamp

Various size syringes and needles

Operative Preparation

Anesthesia

- General

Position

- Supine

Prep

- From jaw line to mid-thigh, to just above the level of the table on both sides

Draping

- A folded towel is secured to the groin with towel clips or skin staples. The chest is square-draped with towels. Plastic adhesive drapes are placed over the towels, and a nonfenestrated heart sheet is placed over the patient

Practical Considerations

- Generally, only those surgical technologists who have been properly trained in open-heart surgery are allowed to scrub cardiac procedures
- The STSR must have good anticipatory skills, and should understand cardiovascular anatomy and physiology, as well as cardiac procedural sequence
- The STSR should be thinking five steps ahead of the surgeon throughout the procedure, and should pay attention at all times
- It is important that the STSR understand cardiac dysrhythmias and their relationship to the cardiac procedure, and be able to understand all pressure readings
- Room-temperature saline should be used up to the point of aortic cross-clamping; thereafter, cold saline is to be used until the rewarming period. Warm saline should be used after rewarming begins
- There should never be water on the back table. It would be too easy to accidentally use water instead of saline when filling the cannulae. Water will cause lysing of RBCs
- Be ready to go back on the pump at a moment's notice. Do not discard cannulae after removal, and keep cannulation sutures ready after the patient is removed from CPB. Keep wire cutters and sternal retractor sterile until the patient is safely out of the room
- Pass off defibrillation cables at the same time as electrosurgical cords. The surgeon will not want to wait for the defibrillation paddles if he suddenly needs them
- Keep the field clear of instruments, blood-soaked sponges, etc. Wring out blood from laparotomy pads into a bowl and suction with the pump sucker
- Do not confuse the terms "atrial" and "arterial" when passing cannulation stitches. One is for the right atrium, and the other is for the aorta. Typically, the arterial cannulation stitch is placed first, but if aortic pressure is high, the right atrium will be cannulated first
- Remember that the key to doing a good job is knowing *why* you are doing things. Don't just memorize the steps
- The STSR should ensure that the valve sizers are for the valve being replaced. Don't use aortic valve sizers for mitral valves and vice versa
- Do not open the valve prosthesis until you and the surgeon have checked to make sure it is the one you need

(continues)

PROCEDURE 22-4 **Aortic Valve Replacement** *(continued)*

Operative Procedure	Technical Considerations
1. A median sternotomy is performed and cardiopulmonary bypass is initiated.	**1.** Bone wax is used to seal off bleeders from the sternal walls. 2–0 silk pericardial stays retract the pericardium and are often secured to the sternal retractor.
2. For the maintenance of a bloodless field, a left ventricular vent is placed through the right superior pulmonary vein and into the left ventricle.	**2.** Follow sequence for cannulation previously outlined. Cardioplegia solution is prepared in advance of need.
3. The aorta is cross-clamped, and cardioplegia is infused in a retrograde fashion through the coronary sinus. If the aortic valve is incompetent, cardioplegia may be infused through the ascending aorta.	**3.** A large Fogarty aortic cross-clamp with plastic, atraumatic inserts is frequently used to occlude the aorta.
4. An incision is made into the aorta, the edges are retracted with sutures, and the exposed aortic valve is inspected.	**4.** Retraction sutures are ready. Prepare valve retractors and scissors for use.
5. Leaflets are resected and calcium deposits are carefully removed from the annulus for eventual placement of sutures.	**5.** The STSR should ready the valve sizers at this point, and the circulator should be ready to open the proper valve. Be sure the prosthesis holder is readily available.
6. The annulus is sized and the prosthesis is selected. The prosthesis is delivered to the annulus on a prosthesis holder.	**6.** Tissue prosthetics must be rinsed in saline according to protocol. Follow the manufacturer's instructions for rinsing porcine valves, typically, 2–3 minutes in three different bowls.
7. Interrupted, nonabsorbable, multifilament sutures of alternating colors are placed into the annulus and through the skirt of the valve, and the valve is carefully pushed down into place.	**7.** The STSR should keep close track of the sutures to be loaded and of the needles that are returned by the surgeon. Wet valve and sutures with saline when placing valve into annulus.
8. The sutures are tied and the motion of the prosthetic leaflets is tested.	**8.** The STSR should have a French-eyed needle available in case the surgeon needs to place another suture through the annulus after the needles have been cut off.
9. The aortic incision is closed with nonabsorbable sutures and the cross-clamp is removed.	**9.** Ethibond is the suture of choice for aortic incision closure.
10. Air is removed from the left ventricle, the cross-clamp is removed, and CPB is discontinued. Chest tubes are placed for the evacuation of fluid and air, and the chest is closed in the usual manner (Figure 22-34).	**10.** Patient is warmed, the heart restarted, and the cannulas removed. Prepare chest tubes and closing suture. Count as needed.

PROCEDURE

22-4 **Aortic Valve Replacement** *(continued)*

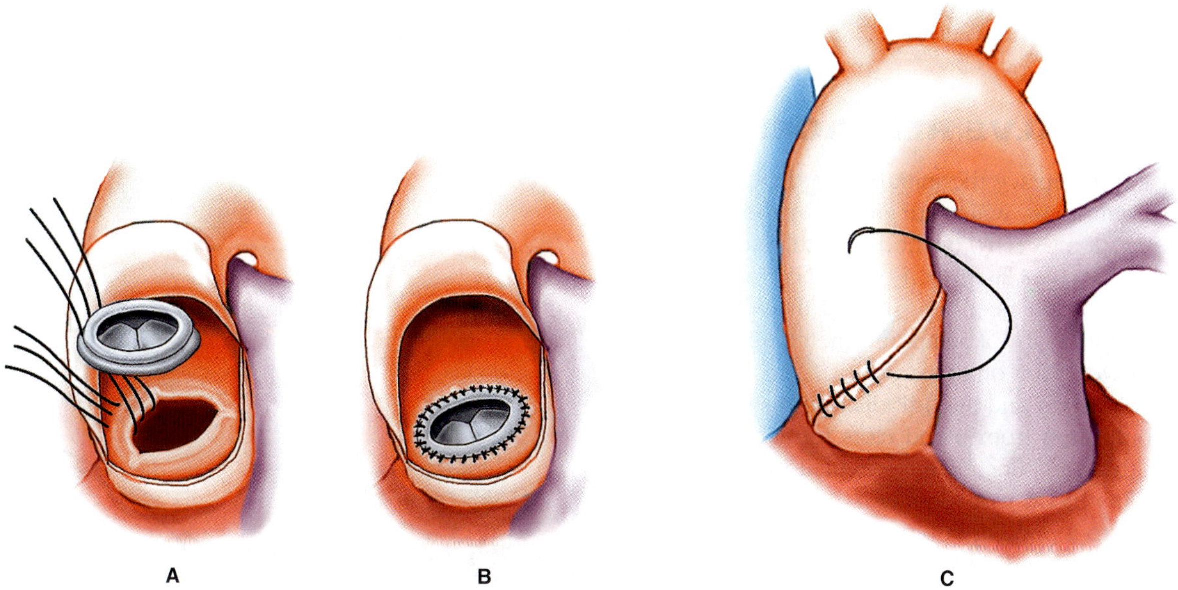

Figure 22-34 **Prosthetic valve placement: (A) Sutures are placed through the annulus and the skirt of the valve prosthesis. (B) The valve is positioned and the sutures are tied. (C) The aortic incision is closed**

Postoperative Considerations

Immediate Postoperative Care

- As usual, the STSR and the back table should remain sterile until the patient has safely left the OR. Wire cutters, sternal retractor, cannulation stitches loaded on needle holders, and cannulae should be available in case the patient must be placed back on cardiopulmonary bypass.
- Care must be taken when transferring the patient from the OR table to the CCU bed. The patient will have monitoring lines, IV, ET tube, and urinary and chest drainage tubes in place. These can be easily disturbed if tension is placed on them during the move.

Prognosis

- Good to excellent

Complications

- Postoperative infections can be potentially fatal. Implanted cardiac prosthetics increase the risk for infection and should be handled with strict attention to sterile technique. An infection of a valve prosthetic can cause embolism, endocarditis, or mechanical failure, any of which is potentially fatal. Infections of the sternum generally require debridement.

PEARL OF WISDOM

For repeat cardiac procedures, be prepared to cannulate femorally. The oscillating saw may be used for sternotomy to prevent cutting into ventricular adhesions to the sternal wall.

MITRAL VALVE REPLACEMENT

The decision to replace the mitral valve depends on the severity of symptoms, which are graded by the New York Heart Association (NYHA) method. Breathlessness on exertion is graded as a class 3 or 4 on the NYHA scale, and generally indicates a need for surgery. If uncontrollable atrial fibrillation is also a symptom, then surgery is indicated at a lower point on the scale.

Mitral stenosis and atrial fibrillation may cause systemic embolization from blood clots formed within the left atrium that are launched into circulation from the left ventricle. This blood clot formation, as discussed previously, is due to a pooling of blood within the left atrium. Surgery is usually indicated for the patient with mitral stenosis and atrial fibrillation because of this tendency for clot formation.

The mitral valve can be either repaired or replaced. Procedures for surgical repair include closed mitral commissurotomy (CMC), open mitral valvotomy for mitral stenosis, or mitral annuloplasty or valvuloplasty for mitral regurgitation. As with the aortic valve, a mitral valve prosthesis requires a lifetime of anticoagulant therapy, so mitral valve repair, if possible, is preferable over replacement.

CMC is performed infrequently in this country, but certain developing nations still depend on the procedure for the treatment of mitral stenosis because CPB is not necessary to perform closed mitral commissurotomy (Figure 22-35). Through an anterior lateral thoracotomy incision, the left ventricle is incised and a Tubb's dilator is placed through the wall of the ventricle and across the left atrioventricular orifice (a finger in the left atrium serves as a guide for the dilator). The blades of the dilator are spread, and the stenotic mitral valve is widened.

Open mitral commissurotomy for mitral stenosis requires a median sternotomy and CPB. An incision is made into the left atrium and the mitral valve is visualized. If the valve leaflets are fused together at the line of closure (commissure), an incision is made into the leaflets and they are separated. Areas of calcification are removed, and the atrium is closed.

Mitral valve annuloplasty (Figure 22-36) is done to correct an annular dilatation of the posterior leaflet of the mitral valve due to a contraction of the papillary muscle that shortens the chordae tendineae. The leaflet edges of the valve do not come together properly, and mitral regurgitation results. A prosthetic ring is selected and interrupted sutures are placed through the annulus and into the prosthetic ring. The sutures are tied and the annulus is drawn snugly against the ring, thus creating a competent valve.

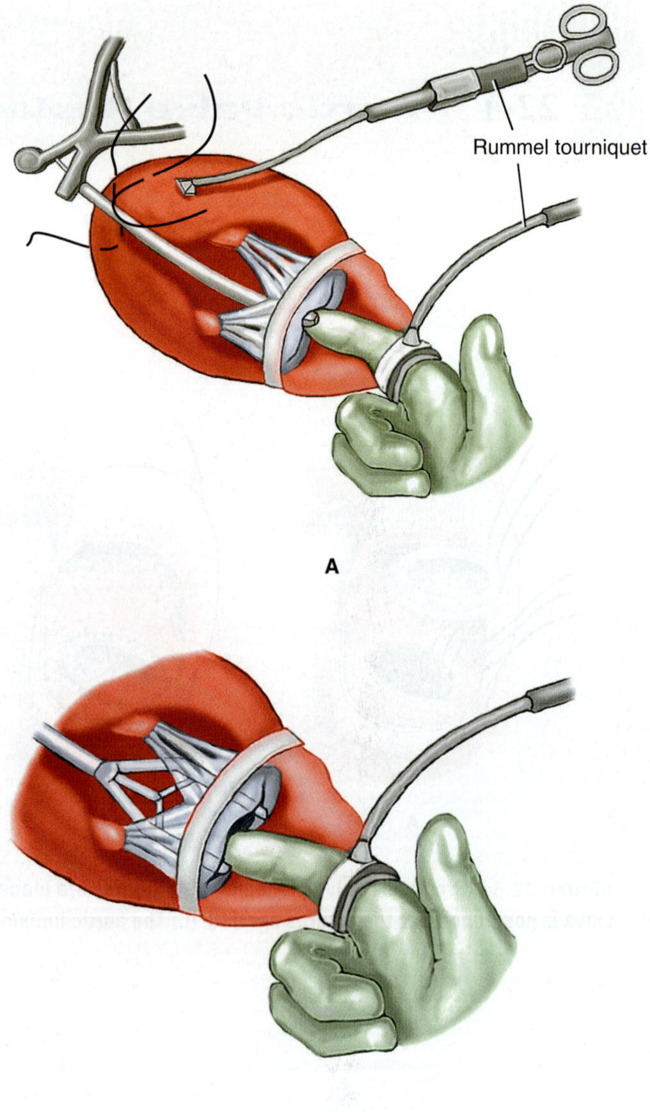

Figure 22-35 **Closed mitral commissurotomy: (A) A mitral valve dilator is inserted through the left ventricle and into the mitral valve after the valve is explored with the index finger. (B) The dilator is opened**

Mitral valvuloplasty for mitral regurgitation is done to repair the valve's leaflets or to shorten or repair the chordae tendineae associated with the leaflets.

Mitral valve replacement (Figure 22-37) is performed when damage is too extensive for repair. Many types of prosthetic valves are available for this procedure (bovine pericardial, porcine, bileaflet, or disk). The surgeon chooses the prosthesis after assessing factors asso-

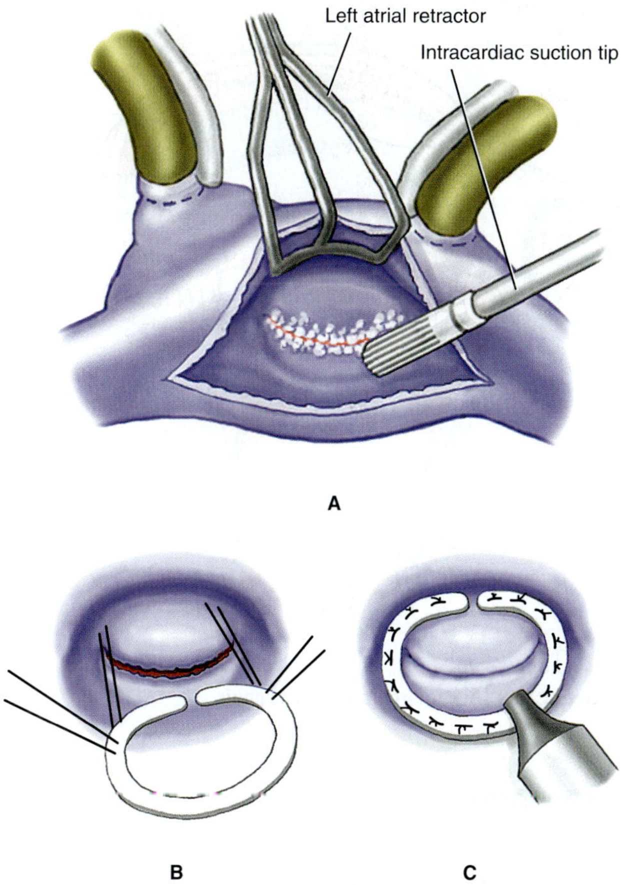

Figure 22-36 Mitral valve annuloplasty: (A) The left atrium is opened and retracted to expose the mitral valve. (B) Sutures are placed through the annulus and the ring. (C) The ring is positioned, the sutures are tied, and an Asepto syringe filled with saline is used to check valve competency

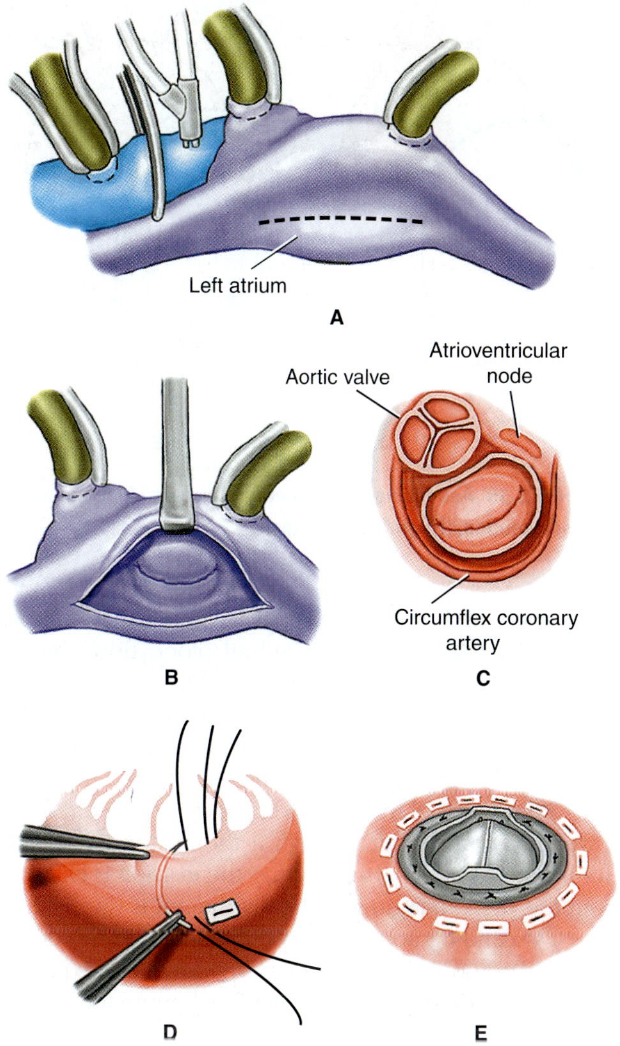

Figure 22-37 Mitral valve replacement: (A) Atrial incision site, (B) mitral valve exposed, (C) cross section showing related anatomical structures, (D) sutures are placed in the annulus, (E) prosthesis in place

ciated with each patient. As with the aortic valve prosthesis, risks include thromoembolism, hemorrhage, and endocarditis. Patients with a mitral valve prosthesis must receive anticoagulant medication for the remainder of their lives.

Preservation of as much valve tissue as possible is preferable, especially the posterior leaflet and its supporting structures.

Occasionally, the tricuspid valve will become leaky, resulting in tricuspid regurgitation. If the condition is severe, a De Vega annuloplasty may be performed. This type of repair involves the placement of a pursestring suture around the circumference of the annulus. The pursestring is drawn tightly enough to reduce the back flow of blood from the right ventricle into the right atrium.

THORACIC AORTIC ANEURYSMECTOMY

Aneurysms of the thoracic aorta may be defined as a localized or diffuse dilation of the vessel diameter to more than 5 or 6 cm. Aneurysms may occur in the ascending, arch, descending, or thoracoabdominal aorta, but the ascending aorta is exposed to the greatest velocity of blood exiting the heart and is the site of 40% of all TAAs.

Treatment of the TAA involves segmental resection of the aneurysm with synthetic graft replacement. Grafts placed within the aneurysmal wall are generally preferable over complete excision of the aneurysm because they spare adjacent structures (Figure 22-38).

Aneurysms of the ascending aorta may also involve a diseased aortic valve, as in patients with Marfan's syndrome. Therefore, repair of the ascending aorta with a woven Dacron graft should also include aortic valve replacement with right and left coronary ostia reimplantation into the synthetic graft. If the aneurysm extends to the proximal aortic arch, the common femoral artery is cannulated; otherwise, cannulation is in the ascending aorta.

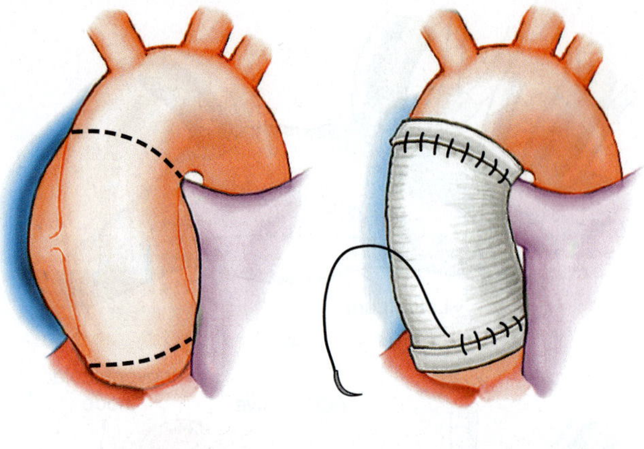

Figure 22-38 **Ascending aortic aneurysm repair: (A) Ascending aortic dissection, (B) graft anastomosis**

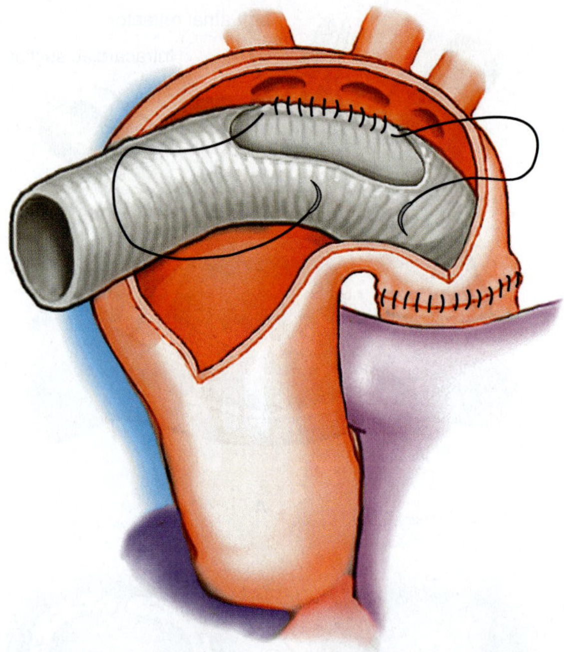

Figure 22-39 **Aortic arch aneurysm repair**

Aortic arch aneurysm repair (Figure 22-39) is complicated by interruption of cerebral blood flow. To preserve cerebral function during repair, the patient's head is packed in ice and the core temperature is dropped to 15°C. The bypass pump is then turned off, and the aneurysmal arch is replaced with synthetic graft.

Aneurysms of the descending aorta are repaired with a woven Dacron graft through a thoracotomy approach (for thoracoabdominal aneurysms, the incision is extended from the costal margin and the diaphragm is divided).

Descending aortic aneurysms (Figure 22-40) do not require cardiopulmonary bypass, but generally require an atrial-to-femoral bypass with centrifugal pump for continuation of blood flow to all vessels distal to the thoracic aorta.

PERICARDIECTOMY/ PERICARDIAL WINDOW

Dense fibrous scarring of the heart as a result of constrictive pericarditis often obliterates the pericardial space and can decrease myocardial contractility. Diastolic filling of the ventricles, however, is the most serious consequence of pericarditis, which is believed to be primarily viral in origin.

TECHNIQUE

Replacement of the Mitral Valve with a Prosthesis

1. The chest is opened in the usual manner, and CPB is initiated. Generally, superior and inferior vena caval cannulation is utilized.
2. Venting catheters are placed for the removal of air, and the aorta is cross-clamped.
3. Cardioplegia is generally infused in a retrograde fashion through the coronary sinus.
4. An incision is made into the left atrium, and the mitral valve is exposed and inspected.
5. The valve is sized, and the correct prosthesis is selected.
6. Sutures of alternating colors are placed through the annulus in an interrupted fashion. (*Note:* The sutures are pledgeted if the annulus is not stable.)
7. Sutures are placed through the ring of the prosthesis, and the prosthetic is lowered into position. The sutures are tied and cut.
8. The valve is inspected for proper function, and a venting catheter is placed through the valve and into the left ventricle for the removal of air while the left atrium is closed.
9. Air removal techniques are employed, the cross-clamp is removed, and CPB is discontinued. Chest tubes are placed for the evacuation of fluid and air, and the chest is closed in the usual manner.

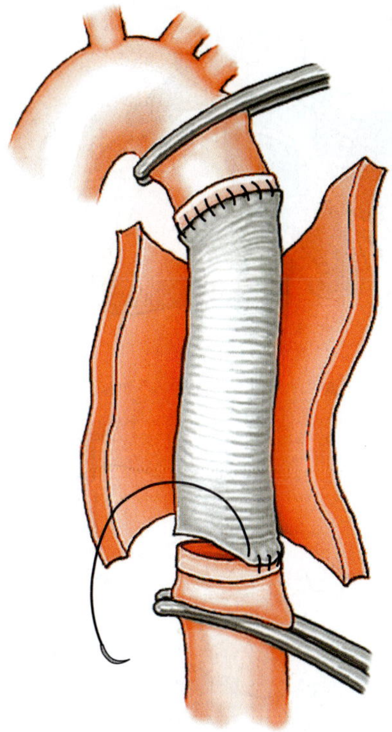

Figure 22-40 Descending aortic aneurysm repair

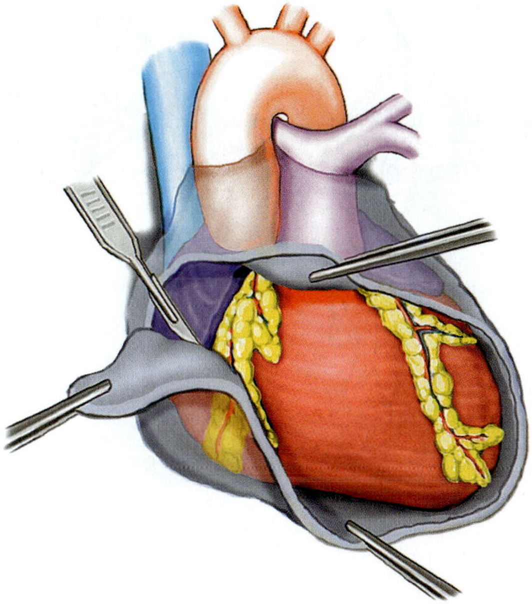

Figure 22-41 Pericardial window: approach through median sternotomy—decortication begins with left ventricle

Pericardiectomy (Figure 22-41) is typically performed with cardiopulmonary bypass on standby, and the approach is typically through median sternotomy. Sternal saw and sternal retractor are necessary, and the STSR should have all bypass supplies handy and ready to open.

After sternotomy, the phrenic nerves are identified and protected, and the pericardium is incised. Decortication begins with the left ventricle to prevent the development of pulmonary edema and right heart failure, which could occur as a result of beginning with the right ventricle. A plane is developed between parietal and visceral pericardium. Caution must be taken to prevent calcified portions of the parietal pericardium from penetrating the heart's chambers, especially the atria. If perforations do occur, the STSR should be prepared with loaded 4–0 or 5–0 pledgeted Prolene sutures. Decortication continues until the atria, ventricles, and both cavae are freed. Chest tubes are placed and connected to closed system drainage. The sternum is closed with stainless steel wire, and the remainder of the wound is closed in the usual manner.

HEART TRANSPLANTATION

Heart transplants are the third most common transplant operations performed in the United States (after corneal and kidney transplants). Heart transplants are indicated for patients with severe myocardial damage caused by coronary artery disease, cardiomyopathy, heart valve disease with congestive heart failure, and severe congenital heart disease.

Heart/lung transplants are performed on patients who will die from end-stage lung disease (usually pulmonary hypertension) that also involves the heart.

Rejection of the new heart is an ongoing battle for the heart transplant patient. The body's immune system treats the new organ as foreign tissue and immediately sets out to attack it. But with the discovery of the immunosuppressive agent cyclosporine A that is used in conjunction with the drugs azathioprine and prednisone, the chances for organ rejection have been greatly diminished. Approximately 80% of all heart transplant patients are alive 2 years after receiving the donor heart.

The biggest problem facing the patient who is to undergo the procedure is organ procurement. At any given time, approximately 2,000 patients are waiting for a heart or heart/lung transplant, and 25% of these will not survive the wait. Donors must be individuals who are brain dead but are kept alive by a respirator. Efforts by hospitals and organizations nationwide are addressing the organ shortage, and results are beginning to be noticed.

Heart procurement (Figure 22-42) is usually performed in tandem with other transplant teams who remove corneas, liver, pancreas, kidneys, and lungs from a fresh cadaver. The heart team exposes the heart through a median sternotomy, and the pulmonary artery, aorta, and venae cavae are dissected free for adequate length. The superior vena cava is ligated, followed rapidly by the ligation of the inferior vena cava at the level of the diaphragm. The aorta is cross-clamped and cold cardioplegia is infused through the aortic root. An incision is made into the pulmonary vein to vent the left atrium, and cold saline is poured over the heart. The pulmonary veins, pulmonary artery, and aorta are divided, and the heart is

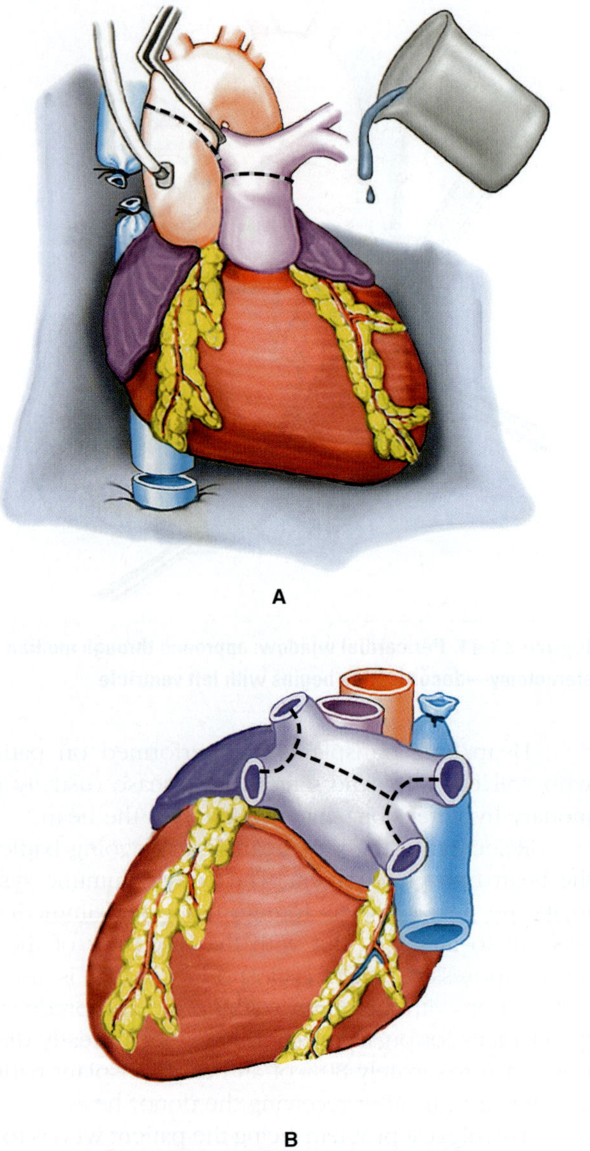

Figure 22-42 **Donor heart: (A) Procurement (anterior view), (B) great vessel anastomosis sites (posterior view)**

placed into ice cold saline for inspection. After inspection, the heart is packed in ice for transport and eventual transplantation.

The heart recipient (Figure 22-43) is placed on cardiopulmonary bypass and cooled. The aorta is cross-clamped high on the ascending aorta, and the atria are excised. The pulmonary artery is excised distal to the pulmonary valve, and the aorta is excised distal to the aortic valve. The donor left atrium is anastomosed to the recipient left atrium, and vents are placed into the left ventricle and ascending aorta for the eventual removal of air. The donor right atrium is then anastomosed to the recipient right atrium, and the patient is warmed. The aortic anastomosis is completed, and air is removed from the heart and aorta through the vents. The cross-clamp is removed from the aorta, the heart is defibrillated, and CPB is discontinued.

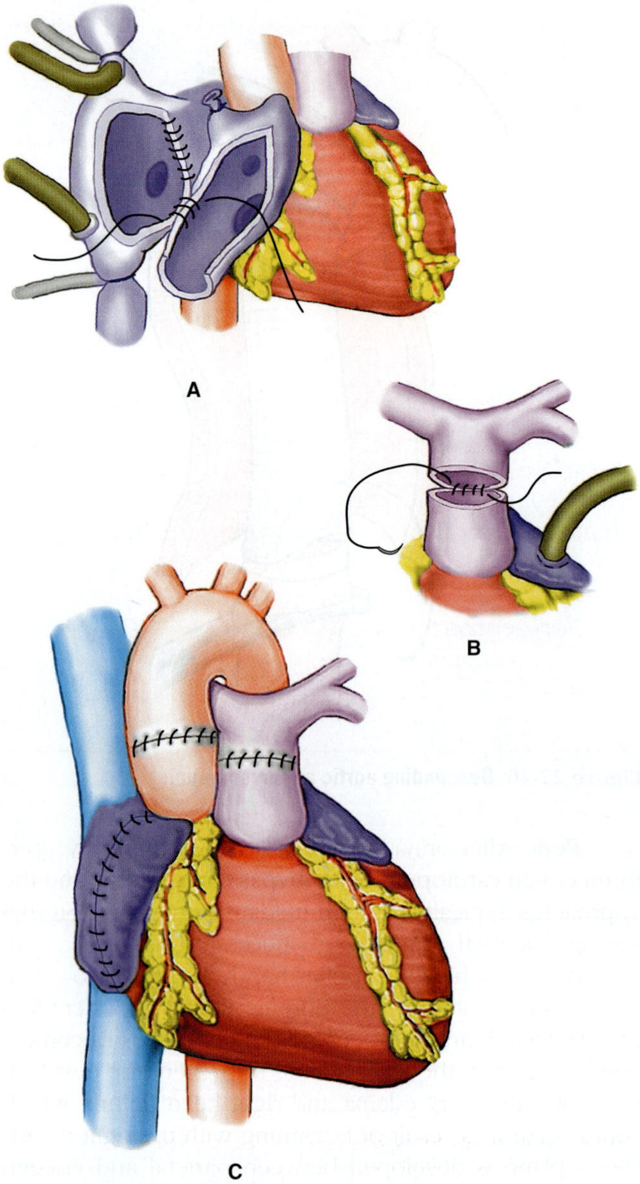

Figure 22-43 **Transplanted heart: (A) Atrial anastomosis, (B) pulmonary trunk anastomosis, (C) completed anastomoses**

Chest tubes are placed for the evacuation of fluid and air, and the chest is closed in the usual manner.

PERMANENT PACEMAKER INSERTION

Cardiac pacing is used to manage various dysrhythmias, most commonly heart block and bradycardia. The permanent pacemaker consists of a pulse generator and electrodes. Two types of electrodes are available for implantation: endocardial leads that are generally placed through the subclavian vein into the right ventricle or atrium; and epicardial leads that are attached directly to the myocardium during cardiac surgery or through a subxiphoid approach.

The pulse generator is powered by a lithium source, and generally lasts 6–10 years before requiring surgical replacement. Future energy sources for the pulse generator include plutonium-238 for nuclear power and an indefinite battery life. The pulse generator controls energy output, heart rate, and pacing modes. Pacing modes include a fixed rate (asynchronous) mode that fires at a preset rate, and a demand (standby) mode that senses the patient's heart beats and is stimulated to fire when the rate drops below a preset standard. The fixed-rate mode is rarely used because it competes with the heart's own rhythm, and could result in ventricular fibrillation.

The endocardial electrode can be placed into the right ventricle or the right atrium. If the patient has problems with pacing from the SA node, the lead can be placed into the right atrium, where pacing more closely resembles the normal electrical activity of the heart. Electrode placement into the right ventricle causes retrograde depolarization.

For permanent pacemaker placement (Figure 22-44), the right upper chest is injected with lidocaine 1% in preparation for generator placement. A transverse incision is made for the creation of the generator pocket, taking care not to place the generator too close to the clavicle or too close to the axilla. The patient is then placed into the Trendelenburg position and the head is turned to the opposite side. A large-gauged needle with a syringe attached is introduced into the right subclavian vein and venous blood is aspirated into the syringe, indicating proper placement. The syringe is removed, and a J-tipped guidewire is threaded through the needle and guided under continuous fluoroscopy into the right atrium. The needle is removed over the J-wire, and a dilator-sheath assembly is placed over the wire and into the subclavian vein. An electrode is inserted into the sheath and advanced under fluoroscopy into the right ventricular apex, where it is stabilized. If a dual-chamber pacemaker is used, the second lead is stabilized in the right atrial appendage. Once lead placement is verified, the sheath is removed. The electrodes are then attached to an external generator for testing, and, once proper pacing is established, attached to the pulse generator. The pulse generator is then inserted into the chest pocket, and the pocket is closed.

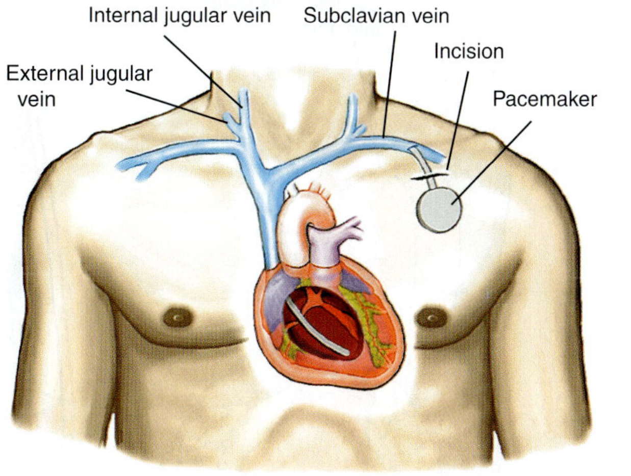

Figure 22-44 Pacemaker

PERCUTANEOUS TRANSLUMINAL CORONARY ANGIOPLASTY

Since the development by Grüntzig of a double-lumen catheter with a cylindrical polyvinyl balloon, percutaneous transluminal coronary angioplasty (PTCA) has become one of the major tools for treatment of certain coronary artery lesions. The polyvinyl balloon will not expand beyond a predetermined circumference, allowing compression of an atheroma against the wall of the coronary artery with minimal risk of arterial dissection. The procedure is performed in the cardiac catheterization laboratory; OR standby is necessary in case problems arise that require surgical correction.

To perform coronary angioplasty (Figure 22-45), temporary pacing electrodes are introduced into the femoral vein and guided into the right ventricle for the control of **arrhythmias** during the procedure. An arterial needle is then inserted into the common femoral artery, and a guiding J-wire is introduced through the arterial needle and into the abdominal aorta. The needle is removed, and a large dilator-sheath assembly is threaded over the J-wire. The dilator is removed, and a guiding catheter is inserted into the sheath and pushed over the aortic arch, with the tip of the catheter in the coronary orifice. Contrast solution is injected under fluoroscopy to identify the location of the coronary lesion. The angioplasty balloon and guiding wire are inserted into the guiding catheter, and the guiding wire is carefully manipulated to slide through and past the coronary lesion, creating leverage for the passage of the angioplasty balloon. The balloon is then pushed over the guiding wire and is seated at the center of the lesion. The balloon is inflated slowly with a saline/contrast mixture so that it can be observed under fluoroscopy. After deflation, contrast solution is injected into the coronary artery and films are made of the results. An intracoronary stent can be placed at the site of the lesion after balloon repair.

SURGICAL INTERVENTION: CARDIAC (PEDIATRIC)

Surgical procedures for repair of congenital heart defects include correction of atrial and ventricular septal defect, patent ductus arteriosus, aortic coarctation, tetralogy of Fallot, and transposition of the great arteries.

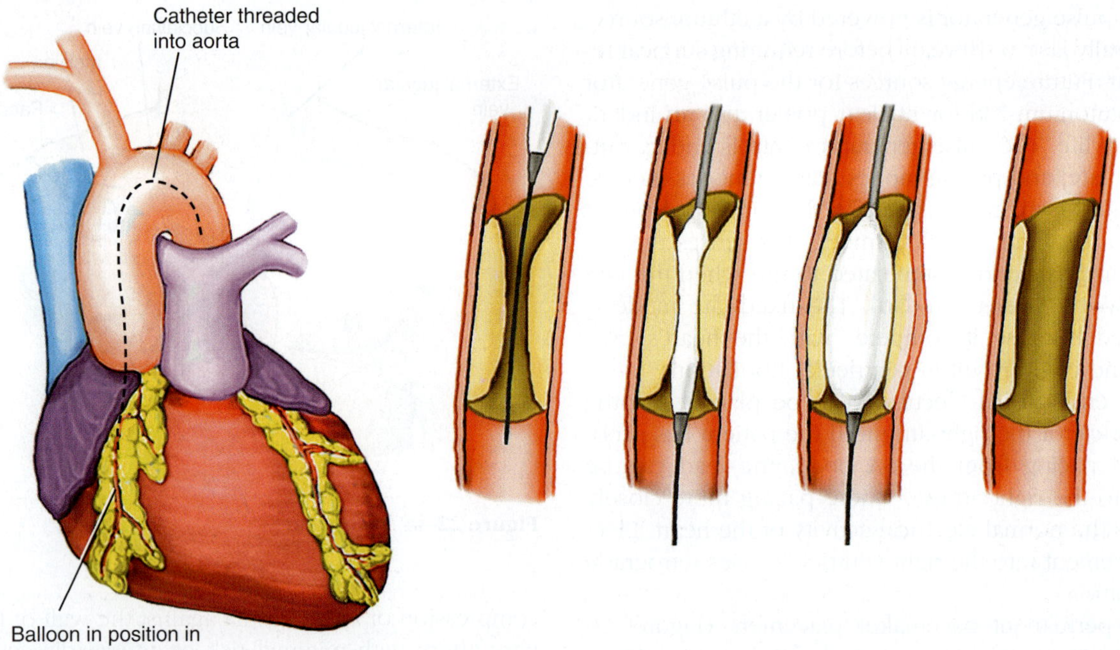

Figure 22-45 Percutaneous transluminal coronary angioplasty

SPECIAL PREOPERATIVE PREPARATION

Most adult cardiac procedures are coronary bypasses or valve replacements. Pediatric heart procedures are typically congenital heart defect repairs of acyanotic or cyanotic classification.

The pediatric patient is at greater risk of hypothermia than the adult patient, so the OR temperature is generally raised well before the patient arrives. Warming blankets are utilized during the procedure, and the patient's temperature is closely monitored with temperature probes.

Blood loss should be closely monitored by the surgical team because of the pediatric patient's low blood volume. Sponges should be weighed by circulating personnel, and irrigation amounts should be measured accurately by the STSR.

Pediatric cardiac instruments are smaller and more delicate than adult cardiac instruments, but are basically the same in type. A sternal saw is not necessary for infants. The sternum is typically cut with Mayo scissors.

Prosthetic patch materials or pericardial pieces are frequently used in pediatric cardiac procedures for repair of congenital defects. Small-gauged polypropylene sutures with and without pledgets are also frequently used.

ATRIAL SEPTAL DEFECT

The primary indication for surgical repair of the atrial septal defect is the presence of symptoms. Surgery may also be indicated in the infant who is asymptomatic but has clear echocardiographic evidence of right ventricular volume overload. The child who is asymptomatic for the defect should undergo surgical repair around the age of 4 or 5. If symptoms are present, intervention should come at any age without hesitation.

Atrial septal defects were the first repairs attempted on the pediatric heart because of their relative simplicity, but were done without the benefit of cardiopulmonary bypass to stop the heart. Today, virtually all septal defect repairs are done with the aid of CPB.

The heart is approached through median sternotomy, and CBP is initiated with a hypothermic core temperature established at 32°C. The aorta is cross-clamped, and cardioplegia is administered. The right atrium is incised, the defect is inspected, and a decision is made as to whether primary closure or patch closure is to be performed. If significant tension will be the result of a primary closure, then a patch should be utilized. A patch of pericardium should be sufficient, especially in the presence of tricuspid regurgitation. Closure with or without a patch is with a running polypropylene, and before the suture line is completed, the atrium is filled with cold saline to remove air. After completion of the suture line, the right atrium is closed and CBP discontinued.

VENTRICULAR SEPTAL DEFECT

A ventricular septal defect (VSD) is repaired in a fashion similar to the atrial septal defect; that is, with a small Dacron patch sewn over the defect (primary closure is rare for the VSD). Smaller VSDs are generally left alone, especially if the patient is asymptomatic. Asymptomatic patients should undergo cardiac catheterization at the age of 1, and if pulmonary pressures are elevated, the VSD should be repaired at that time to prevent irreversible pulmonary vascular disease later in life. Large VSDs should be repaired surgically, especially if the patient has a significant left-to-right shunt or an elevated right ventricular pressure.

Septal defects of the ventricle may occur as conoventricular septal defects (the most common of the VSDs), with an outer rim composed of membranous tissue; as muscular ventricular septal defects, with an outer rim composed of muscle only and occurring anywhere in the trabecular portion of the septum; as atrioventricular canal type ventricular septal defects that lie beneath the tricuspid valve with all or part of the septum of the AV canal missing; and as conal septal defects that result from a defect within the infundibular septum.

Our discussion will concern the conoventricular septal defect. The challenge for this procedure is to close the VSD completely without damaging the conduction system of the heart. The heart is approached through median sternotomy, and the patient is placed on CPB and cooled. (*Note:* For patients weighing less than 8 kg, deep hypothermia to a temperature of 18°C with total circulatory arrest is also an option.) If a patent ductus arteriosus is present, it is ligated and divided before the right atrium is opened to prevent air from entering the systemic circulation. After antegrade cardioplegia delivery, the right atrium is opened and the leaflets of the tricuspid valve are retracted. If a patch closure is chosen for repair, then pledgeted, interrupted, nonabsorbable sutures of 6–0 gauge are utilized to hold a Dacron patch in place over the VSD. The atrium is closed, and CPB is discontinued.

PATENT DUCTUS ARTERIOSUS

Once the diagnosis of patent ductus arteriosus is established, surgical intervention should be planned because it is highly unlikely that spontaneous closure will occur in the few weeks after birth, especially if the patent ductus arteriosus is large (Figure 22-46). If the patient is asymptomatic, an elective procedure should be performed within 3 months of diagnosis. If symptoms are present, the procedure should be performed immediately. CPB is not necessary for the procedure.

For closure of the patent ductus arteriosus, the patient is placed in the right lateral position, and the left chest is entered through the third or fourth intercostal space. The pleura is opened and retracted with sutures. Great care must be taken when retracting the left lung to expose the ductus because of its friability and noncompliance. After identification of the left recurrent laryngeal nerve, the parietal pleura is dissected away from the ductus. A small right-angle clamp is passed underneath the lower margin of the ductus, and a silk ligature is passed

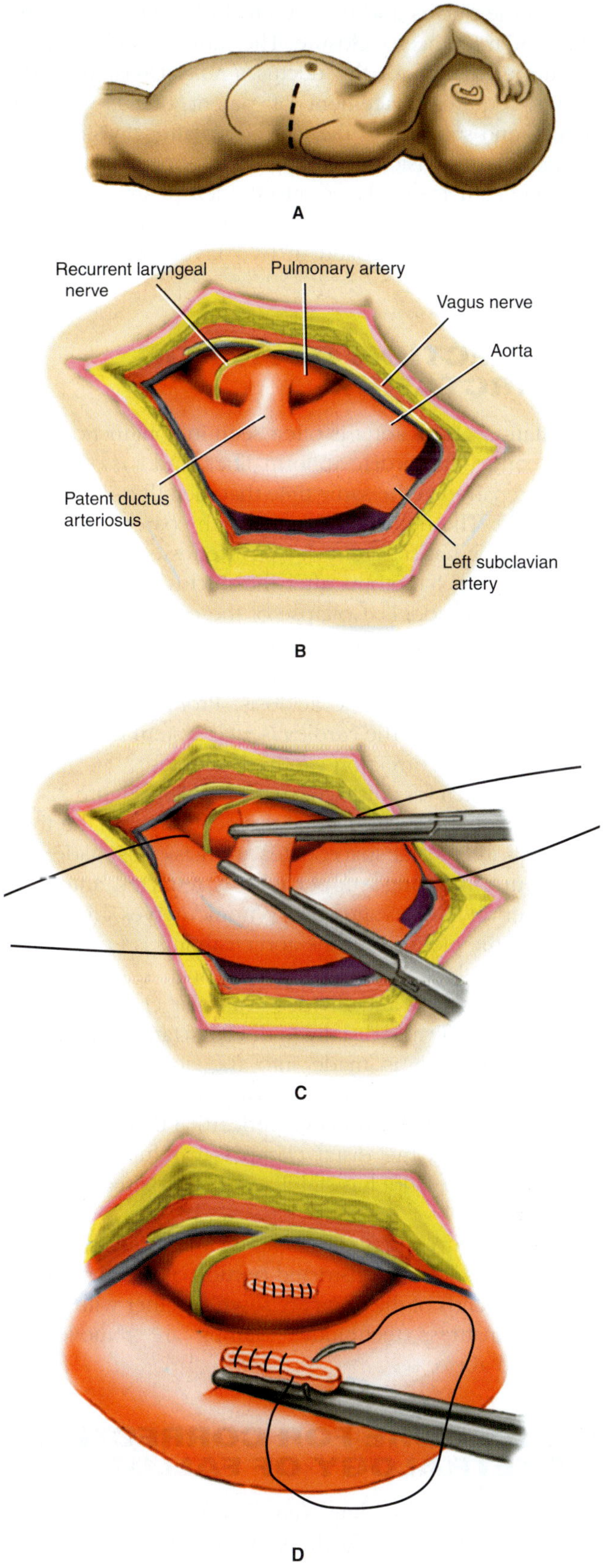

Figure 22-46 Repair of patent ductus arteriosus: (A) Planned incision site, (B) exposure of patent ductus arteriosus, (C) clamp application, (D) suturing of free edges

around the ductus and tied. A small hemoclip is also applied for assurance of closure. The same is performed for the upper margin of the ductus. (*Note:* Division of the ductus requires placement of patent ductus vascular clamps and suturing of the free edges after division.) After ligation or division, the pleura is left open, and a small drainage catheter is placed into the left pleural space for the drainage of fluid and air. The ribs are approximated and the wound is closed in two layers with running sutures.

CORRECTION OF AORTIC COARCTATION

Coarctation of the aorta is often seen in conjunction with other congenital cardiac abnormalities, and it is often surgically repaired at the same time that the other defects are addressed. The neonate or infant with coarctation of the aorta usually has a patent ductus arteriosus and presents with dramatic symptoms after the ductus closes and the coarctation remodels. Collapse of the cardiovascular system ensues rapidly, with hypotension, tachycardia, and tachypnea as the initial symptoms, followed within hours by anuria and metabolic acidosis. Prompt resuscitation and stabilization of the cardiovascular system is necessary before surgical correction can be attempted.

Approach for aortic coarctation repair (Figure 22-47) is through a left posterolateral thoracotomy into the third or fourth intercostal space. After an incision is made into the pleura, the lung's upper lobe is retracted anteriorly and inferiorly. The vagus and phrenic nerves are identified, and the pleura over the aortic isthmus is excised and retracted with sutures. The patent ductus arteriosus is identified, ligated, and divided. Vascular clamps are applied proximally and distally to the coarctation, and a longitudinal incision is made into the aorta. A piece of Dacron or Gore-Tex graft is sewn into the aortotomy to widen the aorta (occasionally, pericardial tissue is utilized as a graft), and the distal clamp is carefully removed. Once blood pressure has stabilized, the proximal clamp is removed.

For end-to-end, tissue-to-tissue anastomosis, clamps are applied and the constricted portion of the aorta is excised. The ends of the aorta are sewn together with a continuous mattress technique. Clamps are removed as described above.

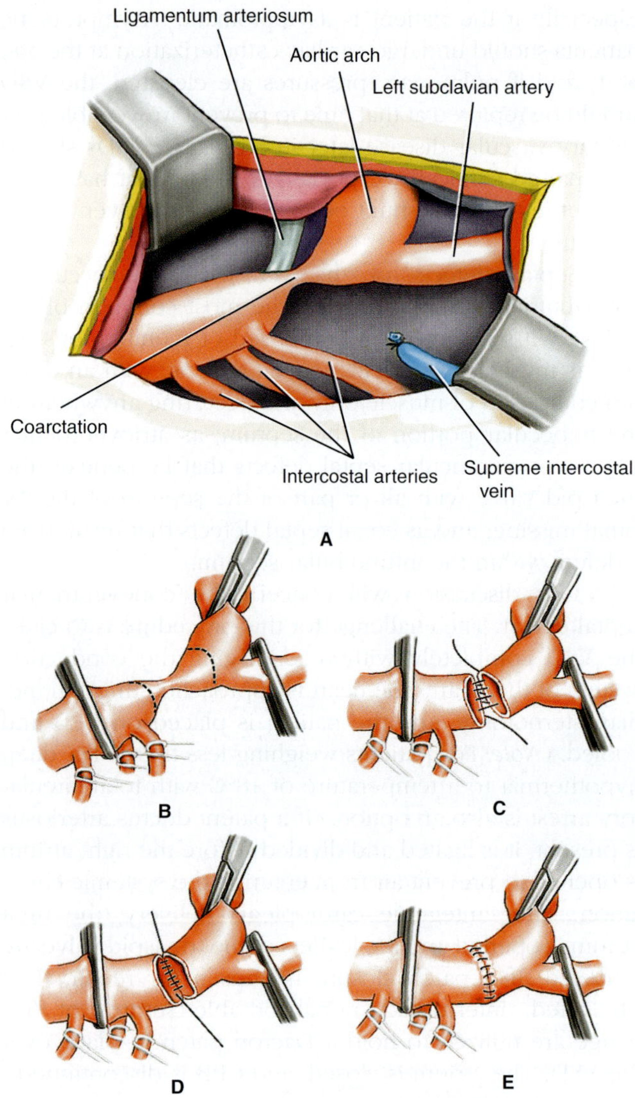

Figure 22-47 End-to-end anastomosis for repair of aortic coarctation: (A) Exposure of coarctation, (B) incision sites, (C) anastomosis of free edges, (D) advance of closure, (E) anastomosis complete

PROCEDURE FOR CORRECTION OF TETRALOGY OF FALLOT

Due to symptoms of hypoxemia and hypoxia, approximately 70% of patients with tetralogy of Fallot (TOF) and pulmonary stenosis will require surgical correction during the first year of life. Approximately 30% will die within the first year if left untreated. Early repair minimizes secondary damage to the heart, brain, and lungs.

Approach for repair of TOF is through median sternotomy. A small pericardial patch is excised for subsequent reconstruction of the right ventricular outflow tract. CPB and cooling are initiated in the usual manner. The pulmonary trunk is dissected away from the right and left pulmonary branches and the ascending aorta, and the aorta is cross-clamped for cardioplegia infusion at 18°C. Circulation is stopped, and the right atrial cannula is removed for exposure. A vertical incision is made into the infundibulum, and the VSD is identified. The VSD is closed with a Dacron patch and interrupted horizontal mattress sutures reinforced with Teflon pledgets, taking care not to suture any conduction tissue in proximity. The ventricular septum is searched for any additional defects. If the pulmonary annulus is hypoplastic, it is patched. If the pulmonary valve leaflets are calcified, they are incised. The right ventricular outflow tract patch is molded, and the right heart is filled with saline. Cardiopulmonary bypass is reinstated with a single cannula placed into the right atrium, just below the opening of the superior vena cava. While the patient is warming, the pericardial patch is sewn to the right ventricular outflow tract with a continuous 5–0 Prolene suture, and a 19-gauge catheter is pushed through a pursestring suture into the epicardium of the right ventricle for postoperative monitoring. Air in the heart is removed through a needle placed into the ascending aorta, and the lungs are inflated to remove air from the pulmonary veins. CPB is discontinued, and the chest is closed in the usual manner.

PROCEDURE FOR CORRECTION OF TRANSPOSITION OF THE GREAT ARTERIES

Various procedures are utilized for surgical correction of transposition of the great arteries. The Senning and Mustard techniques recruit the right ventricle as the systemic pump, while the arterial switch recruits the left. The arterial switch is the preferred method because of late complications associated with the Senning and Mustard techniques, specifically atrial dysrhythmias and right ventricular dysfunction. Also, the left ventricle is the better chamber for systemic propulsion of blood because of its thicker myocardium and concentric contraction pattern.

For the arterial switch, approach is through median sternotomy. CPB can be initiated in a number of ways, depending on the surgeon's preference or length of procedure. A single venous cannula is placed into the right atrium and the aorta is cannulated distally for subsequent aortic anastomosis. A segment of pericardium is harvested, and hypothermia is initiated. The ductus arteriosus and left and right pulmonary branches are dissected free, and the pump oxygenator is turned on. The patent ductus arteriosus is then doubly ligated and divided. The ascending aorta is dissected away from the main pulmonary artery and clamped when the patient's core temperature reaches 18°C. Cold cardioplegia is delivered through an ascending aorta cannula. The aorta is divided just distal to the coronary arteries, and the left and right coronary ostia are excised with a large portion of the surrounding aortic wall. The pulmonary artery is transected just distal to the pulmonary valve and just proximal to the pulmonary bifurcation. The distal pulmonary artery is brought anterior to the aorta and is held in position by rubber loops. The coronary implantation sites are prepared by excising the anterior portion of the native proximal pulmonary artery, and the coronary ostia are sewn to the implantation sites with a continuous 7–0 Prolene suture. A small piece of pericardium is sewn to the coronary-neoaortic anastomosis to prevent kinking of the coronary arteries. The distal aorta is then anastomosed to the proximal pulmonary artery with a continuous polydioxanone suture. The atrial communication is closed through a right atriotomy. After air is removed from the left side of the heart through a vent in the ascending aorta, the aortic cross-clamp is removed. The coronary ostia in the neopulmonary artery are patched with pericardium, and the patient is warmed. The patient is slowly weaned from CPB, and heart rate, systemic blood pressure, and left atrial pressures are closely monitored. The patient's incision is closed in the usual manner.

CASE STUDY

Jim, a 50-year-old diabetic, is taken to the cardiac cath unit for a coronary angiogram and left ventriculogram after arriving in the ER with severe chest pains. The cardiologist discovers a lesion in the left main coronary branch and immediately orders an emergency CABG.

1. Why is a lesion in this location more dangerous than any other coronary lesion?
2. Could an angioplasty be performed to repair the lesion?

QUESTIONS FOR FURTHER STUDY

1. What is the proximal saphenous vein sutured to during CABG?
2. What is the purpose of the left ventricular vent?
3. What is the purpose of the IABP, and where is it positioned?
4. During cannulation, where are the cannulas of the pump oxygenator machine placed for cardiopulmonary bypass surgery?
5. Describe what occurs when a patient experiences a mediastinal shift.
6. During a pericardiectomy what should the CST be prepared to give to the surgeon if calcified portions of the parietal pericardium penetrate the heart's chambers?

BIBLIOGRAPHY

Anthony, C. P., & Thibodeau, G. A. (1979). *Textbook of anatomy and physiology* (10th ed.). St. Louis, MO: Mosby.

Bianchi, S., Duran, C. M., Gometza, B., Kumar, N., & Prabhakar, G. (1993). Vanishing De Vega annuloplasty for functional tricuspid regurgitation. *J. Thorac. Cardiovasc. Surg.* [Online]. Available from *http://www.hsforum.com/HeartSurgery/References/TVR.hsf*

Campbell, D. B., Pierce, W. S., & Waldhausen, J. A. (Eds.). (1996). *Surgery of the chest* (6th ed.). St. Louis, MO: Mosby-Year Book.

Cassmeyer, V. L., Long, B. C., Phipps, W. J., & Woods, N. F. (Eds.). (1991). *Medical-surgical nursing concepts and clinical practice* (4th ed.). St. Louis, MO: Mosby-Year Book.

Castañeda, A. R., Jonas, R. A., Mayer, J. E., & Hanley, F. L. (1994). *Cardiac surgery of the neonate and infant*. Philadelphia: W. B. Saunders.

Damjanov, I. (1996). *Pathology for the health-related professions* (1st ed.). Philadelphia: W. B. Saunders.

Davis, J. H., & Sheldon, G. F. (Eds.). (1995). *Surgery: A problem-solving approach* (2nd ed.). St. Louis, MO: Mosby-Year Book.

Gazes, P. C. (1990). *Clinical cardiology* (3rd ed.). Philadelphia: Lea and Febiger.

Grabowski, S. R., & Tortora, G. J. (1996). *Principles of anatomy and physiology* (8th ed.). New York: Harper-Collins.

Harvey, A. M., Johns, R. J., McKusick, V. A., Owens, A. H., & Ross, R. S. (Eds.). (1988). *The principles and practices of medicine* (22nd ed.). East Norwalk, CT: Appleton & Lange.

Healthanswers.com. (1997). Heart transplant [Online]. Available from *http://www.healthanswers.com/database/ami/converted/003003.html*

Heartdisease.com. (1997). Mitral stenosis: Surgical options [Online]. Available from *http://heartdisease.tqn.com/library/weekly/aa050497.htm*

Heartsource Publications. (1997). Aortic arch repair expertise yields multiple benefits for Heart Institute patients. *Rush Cardiac News* [Online]. Available from *http://www.rpslmc.edu/Med/Heart/Newsletter/Win97/p4.html*

Hole, J. W. (1987). *Human anatomy and physiology* (4th ed.). Dubuque, IA: Wm. C. Brown.

Mid-Atlantic Surgical Associates. (1998). Double valve replacement (Text version) [Online]. Available from *http://www.heartsurgeons.com/valvetext.htm*

News Channel 9 at ABC, WTVC. (1998). Heart valve switch [Online]. Available from *http://www.wtvc.com/healthwatch/hw059.html*

O'Connor, R. (1998). Thoracic aneurysms [Online]. Available from *http://www.emedicine.com/EMERG/topic28.htm*

O'Toole, M. (Ed.). (1997). *Miller-Keane encyclopedia & dictionary of medicine, nursing, and allied health* (5th ed.). Philadelphia: W. B. Saunders.

Sabiston, D. C., Jr. (1997). *Textbook of surgery. The biological basis of modern surgical practice* (15th ed.). Philadelphia: W. B. Saunders.

Sanders, T., & Scanlon, V. C. (1995). *Essentials of anatomy and physiology* (2nd ed.). Philadelphia: F. A. Davis.

CHAPTER 23

Peripheral Vascular Surgery

Paul Price

CASE STUDY

Gregory is a 67-year-old man who has come to the emergency room complaining of bouts of weakness in his right leg that have been progressively getting worse. His wife has noted that he appears confused during these bouts and often has trouble speaking. The speech difficulties and confusion last only about a day, and then he is back to normal. The right extremity weakness, however, improves only slightly after each bout, leaving Gregory a bit weaker each time. Gregory put off seeing a doctor because of the transient nature of his attacks. His wife, however, is worried that he is having a stroke. Gregory has been a pack-a-day smoker for 40 years.

1. What tests may be ordered?
2. What is the possible diagnosis?
3. What surgical procedure will be scheduled?

OBJECTIVES

After studying this chapter, the reader should be able to:

A 1. Discuss the relevant anatomy of the peripheral vascular system.

P 2. Describe the pathology that prompts surgical intervention of the peripheral vascular system and the related terminology.

3. Discuss any special preoperative peripheral vascular diagnostic procedures.

4. Discuss any special preoperative preparation procedures.

O

5. Identify the names and uses of peripheral vascular instruments, supplies, and drugs.
6. Identify the names and uses of special equipment.
7. Discuss the intraoperative preparation of the patient undergoing the peripheral vascular procedure.
8. Define and give an overview of the peripheral vascular procedure.
9. Discuss the purpose and expected outcomes of the peripheral vascular procedure.
10. Discuss the immediate postoperative care and possible complications of the peripheral vascular procedure.

S

11. Discuss any specific variations related to the preoperative, intraoperative, and postoperative care of the patient undergoing peripheral vascular surgery.

SELECT KEY TERMS

1. adventitia	7. embolus	13. mitigate	19. phrenic
2. bifurcation	8. Fogarty catheter	14. morbidity	20. pledget
3. capillary	9. in situ	15. mortality	21. plethysmography
4. claudication	10. innominate	16. occlusion	22. sinus
5. contralateral	11. intima	17. papaverine	23. thrombus
6. diastole	12. ischemia	18. patency	24. valve

PERIPHERAL VASCULAR SURGERY

Peripheral vessel procedures are often performed on patients with advanced atherosclerosis that affects the extremities, abdominal and thoracic viscera, and the brain. The surgical technologist should be aware of this, and should take proper precautions during patient preparation. The surgical technologist should have a good understanding of the pathology and the anatomy and physiology involved in peripheral vascular procedures. Knowledge of any preoperative procedures that may have been used for diagnosis is essential, as well. The outcome of each peripheral vascular procedure performed depends on the ability of OR personnel to function as a team, trusting that each member will perform with utmost skill and professionalism.

SURGICAL ANATOMY

The peripheral vascular system refers to a closed system of blood vessels that transports blood away from the heart to the body's tissues, and then back again to the heart.

BLOOD VESSELS

Arterial blood is pumped by the heart through a large system of blood vessels called arteries; therefore, arterial blood refers to blood that is transported away from the heart to the tissues of the body. The arteries are large in size as they leave the heart, but begin subdividing into progressively smaller arteries as they move into various regions of the body. These arteries grow progressively smaller until they become arterioles, which in turn become **capillaries**. Capillaries are microscopic vessels designed to exchange nutrients and wastes between the blood and tissue fluid around the cells in specialized areas called capillary beds. After this exchange, capillaries unite to form venules, the smallest of veins (Figure 23-1). These venules, in turn, unite to form progressively larger blood vessels called veins, which eventually become the superior and inferior vena cava, the largest of veins. Veins, then, are designed to transport blood back to the heart.

Arterial blood pumped away from the left ventricle of the heart enters the aorta, the largest of the arteries, and begins its trip through the progressively smaller arteries toward the arterioles, which become capillaries (Figure 23-2).

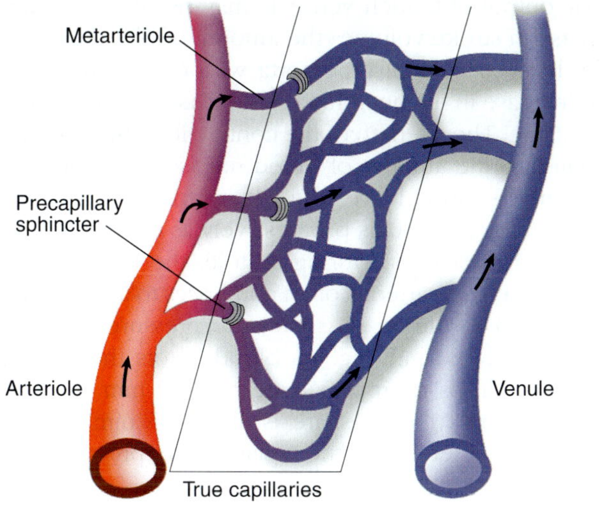

Figure 23-1 Capillary bed connecting an arteriole to a venule

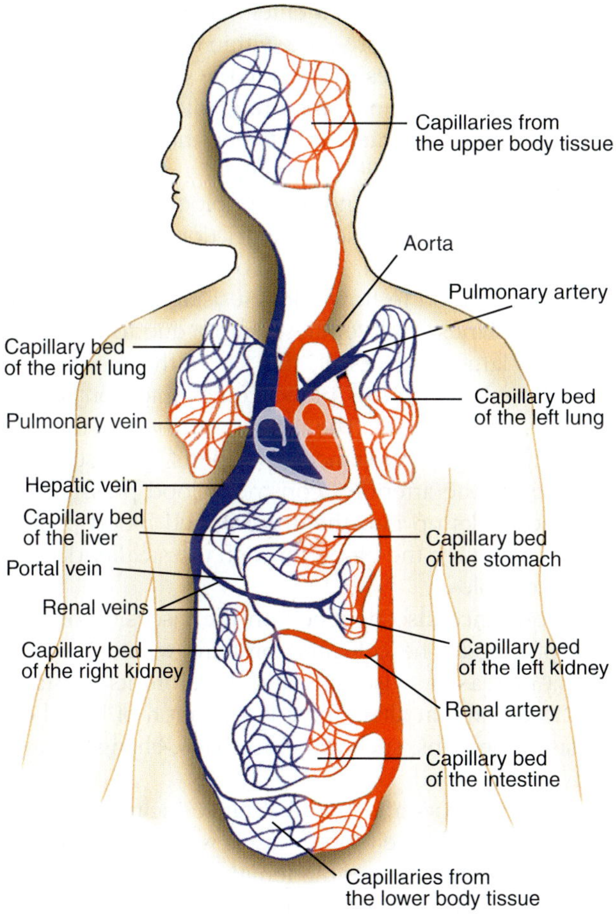

Figure 23-2 Systemic, pulmonary, renal, and portal blood circuits

Wastes, nutrients, O_2, and CO_2 are exchanged, and then venous blood begins its trip back to the heart in the venules, which grow progressively larger to become veins. Venous blood is then emptied into the inferior and superior vena cava, and deposited into the right atrium of the heart.

STRUCTURE OF THE ARTERY AND THE VEIN

The wall of an artery consists of three layers called tunics. The outer layer is called the tunica **adventitia** and consists of connective tissue. This layer attaches the artery to the surrounding tissues and also contains tiny vessels called vasa vasorum that nourish the cells of the arterial wall.

The middle tunic is called the tunica media and is the thickest of the three layers of the arterial wall. This layer includes elastic fibers and smooth muscle fibers that completely encircle the artery. The smooth muscles in this layer are innervated by sympathetic branches of the autonomic nervous system. Impulses from these nerves can cause the smooth muscles to contract, resulting in a narrowing of the lumen, which is the channel for blood flow within the vessel. This process is referred to as vasoconstriction. The inhibition of the impulses from the autonomic nervous system allows the smooth muscles to relax, resulting in an increase of the diameter of the lumen. This is referred to as vasodilation. Vasoconstriction results in a rise in blood pressure, while vasodilation results in decrease in blood pressure.

The inner tunic is called the tunica **intima** and is composed of a lining of endothelium. This layer is in contact with the blood; the lining of this layer must be smooth so that platelets can flow without being damaged.

The walls of arterioles are very thin, and consist of only a layer of simple squamous epithelium surrounded by a small amount of smooth muscle and connective tissue.

The epithelial layer of the capillaries is very thin as well, and contains openings or pores where two adjacent epithelial cells overlap. These pores vary in size, depending on their location. Within the endocrine and digestive systems, the pores are very large, with increased permeability due to their larger diameter. The pores of the capillaries of the muscular system, however, are very small. Within the nervous system, the brain has capillaries with tightly packed endothelial cells, comprising a system of protection for delicate neurons called the blood–brain barrier.

Veins are composed of the same three layers as arteries, but there are differences in their relative thickness. The middle layer of the venous wall is poorly developed, with far less smooth muscle tissue. The tunica adventitia is the thickest layer of the vessel, consisting of collagen and elastic fibers, while the tunica intima is much thinner than that of the artery. The lumen of a vein, however, is larger than that of an artery (Figure 23-3).

Blood pressure within a vein is low and venous blood must work against gravity in most regions of the body on its trip back to the heart. Therefore, the veins are equipped with flap-like **valves** made of thin layers of tunica intima that close if blood begins to back up in a vein. Veins pass between groups of skeletal muscles, and when these muscles contract, blood is pushed upward in the

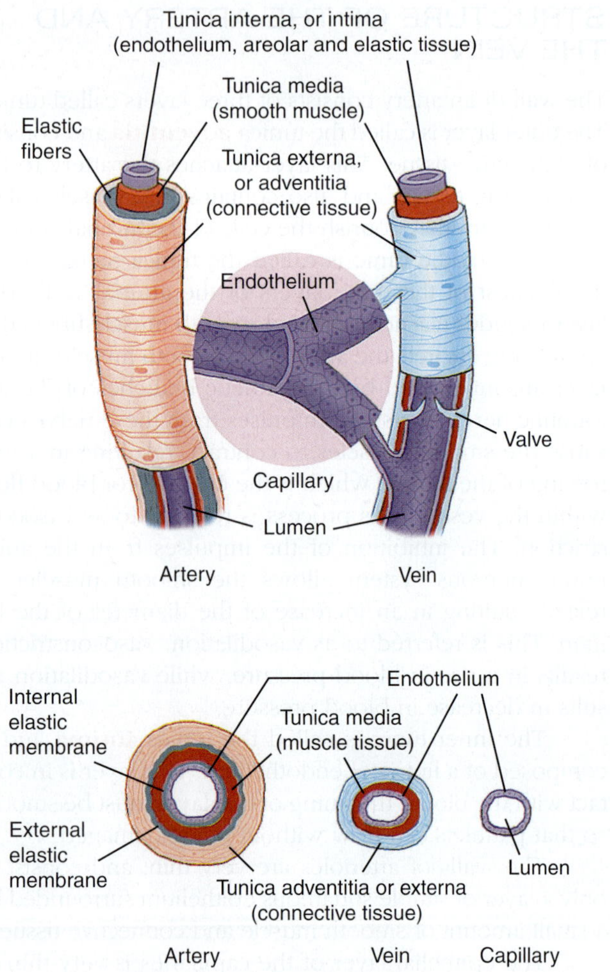

Figure 23-3 Blood vessel types and structure

vein toward the heart. When the skeletal muscles relax, the vein's valves prevent the blood from moving back away from the heart.

BLOOD PRESSURE

Blood pressure is the force that blood exerts against the internal walls of blood vessels. Arterial blood pressure is dependent on many factors, including blood volume, the strength of a ventricular contraction, resistance, blood viscosity, and heart rate.

Blood pressure is dependent on the volume of blood within the cardiovascular system. The average adult has approximately 5 liters of blood. If a large amount of blood is lost due to hemorrhage, the blood pressure falls; in fact, a true indication of hemorrhage is a rapidly falling blood pressure. If volume is added to the cardiovascular system by blood transfusion or if water is retained in the body, blood pressure rises because there is more fluid, and therefore more pressure, against the walls of the arteries.

Arterial blood pressure also depends on the strength of the heart's ventricular contraction. The cardiac output of the left ventricle may rise if there is an increase in stroke volume (the amount of blood ejected by the left ventricle into the aorta with one contraction) or an increase in the heart rate, as long as resistance remains the same. The strength of the contraction, then, is directly related to the amount of blood released into the arterial system. As blood leaves the left ventricle and enters the aorta, its pressure falls progressively as the distance from the heart increases. During systole, the blood pressure within the large arteries of an adult rises to approximately 120 mm Hg; during **diastole**, the pressure falls to approximately 80 mm Hg. As blood enters the arterioles, pressure drops to approximately 35–40 mm Hg, and in the capillaries the pressure is about 15 mm Hg. Once blood has entered into the venae cavae, pressure is very near zero.

The blood pressure gradient for the entire systemic circulation is the difference between the mean blood pressure within the aorta and the mean blood pressure within the venae cavae as it enters the right atrium of the heart. For example, if pressure within the ascending aorta is 120 mm Hg, and pressure within the superior vena cava is 2 mm Hg, the systemic pressure gradient is 118 mm Hg. Without a pressure gradient between the arterial and venous system, blood will not circulate.

Resistance is the hindrance of blood flow within the cardiovascular system due to the friction of blood against the walls of the vessel. It must be overcome by blood pressure for blood to flow. Most resistance is in the arterioles, capillaries, and venules, simply due to their small size. The larger the vessel, the lower the resistance to blood flow because less blood comes into contact with the walls of the vessel. The vasoconstriction of arterioles increases vascular resistance, and therefore raises blood pressure. As the arterioles constrict, blood pressure rises as blood backs up into the arteries, and blood pressure increases to force the blood through the smaller diameter of the arterioles.

Resistance also depends on the viscosity, or thickness, of blood. The cells and proteins within the blood plasma increase its viscosity, and therefore its resistance. Any condition that alters the concentration of blood cells or plasma proteins, such as hemorrhage, changes the viscosity of the blood.

Other factors affecting resistance include the diameter and length of the blood vessels within the cardiovascular system. The greater the length of the vessel and the smaller its diameter, the greater the resistance to flow. Heart rate also affects blood pressure. As the heart beats faster, each contraction of the left ventricle leaves less time for the ventricle to refill, and so less blood is pumped into the aorta for systemic circulation. With a decreased cardiac output, arterial blood volume is decreased, and blood pressure is lowered. A change in heart rate will affect the blood pressure only if that change corresponds to an increase or decrease in the cardiac output.

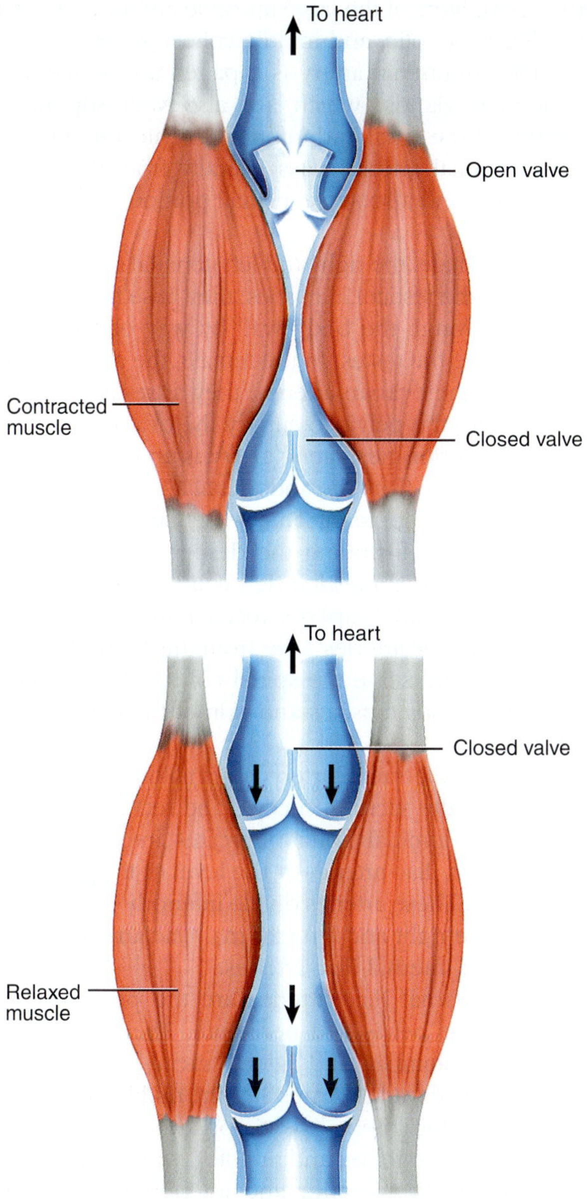

Figure 23-4 Skeletal muscle moves venous blood

Venous blood pressure, as mentioned previously, is much lower than arterial pressure. As blood approaches the right atrium of the heart, its pressure is near zero. Venous return to the heart does not rely, then, on cardiac output, but rather on other factors. As skeletal muscles contract, they squeeze the blood inside the veins upward against gravity (Figure 23-4). Many veins, especially those in the arms and legs, have semilunar valves that catch the blood moving toward the heart, preventing back flow (Figure 23-5).

In addition, respiratory inspiration squeezes blood from the abdominal veins upward toward the heart by pushing the diaphragm against the abdominal organs, which creates a decrease in thoracic cavity pressure and an increase in the pressure within the abdomen. As a result, a large volume of blood moves from the compressed abdominal veins into the veins of the thoracic cavity.

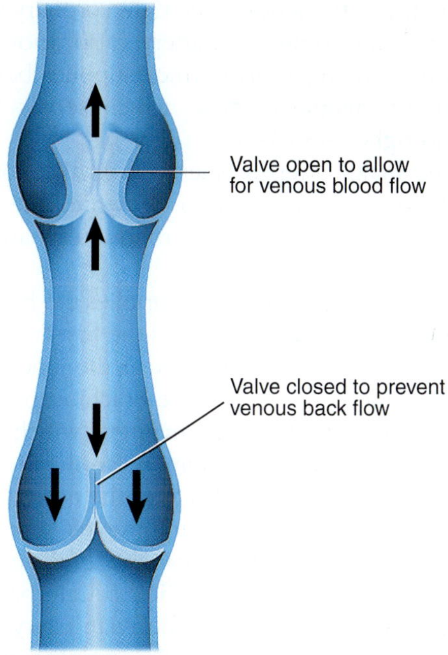

Figure 23-5 Venous valves

Venous blood pressure within the right atrium is referred to as central venous pressure (CVP). CVP is of importance because of the effect it has on the pressure within the large peripheral veins. If the heart is beating weakly, CVP increases, and blood backs up into the venous system, causing the pressure within the system to rise. If the heart beats strongly, CVP is low as blood enters and leaves the heart efficiently. Other factors that lead to an increase in CVP are tricuspid regurgitation or an increase in systemic blood volume.

THE ARTERIAL SYSTEM

The aorta, which is the largest artery in the body, begins as the ascending aorta, ascending from the left ventricle of the heart. Just beyond the aortic semilunar valve are the left and right aortic **sinuses**, which are small dilatations of the aorta that precede the only branches of the ascending aorta, the left and right coronary arteries. The aortic sinuses contain the aortic bodies, which are specialized receptors within the epithelial lining that function to control blood pressure and oxygen and carbon dioxide concentrations.

The coronary arteries, as explained previously, supply the myocardium with oxygenated blood. They lie within a groove that encircles the heart called the atrioventricular sulcus. Branches of the left coronary artery are the anterior interventricular artery (also known as the anterior descending artery), which supply both ventricles, and the circumflex artery, which serves the left atrium and the left ventricle. Branches of the right coronary artery are the posterior interventricular artery (also known as the posterior descending artery), which supplies both ventricles, and the marginal artery, which serves the right atrium and right ventricle.

Three major arteries emerge from the aortic arch: the brachiocephalic artery (also known as the **innominate** artery), the left common carotid artery, and the left subclavian artery.

The brachiocephalic artery supplies the blood to the tissues of the arm and head, and is the first branch of the aortic arch, veering to the right. Near the junction of the sternum and the right clavicle, the brachiocephalic artery bifurcates into the right subclavian artery, which leads into the right arm, and the right common carotid artery, which serves the brain and the right side of the neck and head.

The left common carotid and the left subclavian arteries are the second and third branches of the aortic arch, and serve the same function as their counterparts on the right side. Just beyond the left subclavian artery, the aorta becomes the descending aorta. The portion of the descending aorta that lies above the diaphragm is known as the thoracic aorta, which passes downward from the 4th through 12th thoracic vertebrae; that portion below the diaphragm is known as the abdominal aorta.

Branches of the descending aorta supplying the thoracic wall are the superior **phrenic** arteries and the posterior intercostal arteries. Branches supplying the viscera of the thorax are the bronchial, pericardial, mediastinal, and esophageal arteries.

In the abdominal aorta, branches serve the abdominal wall and the abdominal viscera. The visceral branches include the celiac artery, which is a thick, short artery that immediately divides into three arteries: the left gastric, splenic, and common hepatic arteries.

The common hepatic artery has three main branches: the hepatic artery proper (left and right hepatic branches), which serve the liver and gallbladder; the gastroduodenal artery, which serves the stomach, the body of the pancreas, and the duodenum; and the right gastric artery, which serves the stomach.

The splenic artery has three main branches: the left gastroepiploic artery, which serves the stomach; the pancreatic artery, which serves the tail of the pancreas; and the polar arteries, serving the spleen.

The left gastric artery serves the lesser curvature of the stomach and the esophagus.

The inferior phrenic arteries supply blood to the inferior surface of the diaphragm and adrenal glands.

The superior mesenteric artery is an unpaired vessel arising anteriorly from the abdominal aorta, just below the celiac trunk. This vessel branches to supply numerous abdominal organs: the pancreas and duodenum are served by the inferior pancreaticoduodenal artery; the small intestine is served by the ileal and jejunal intestinal arteries; and the cecum, appendix, and ascending and transverse colons of the large intestine are supplied by the ileocolic, right colic, and middle colic arteries.

The suprarenal artery is a paired artery that serves the adrenal glands, which are also well supplied by branches of the renal and inferior phrenic arteries.

The renal arteries pass laterally from the aorta to each kidney and also serve a small portion of the adrenal glands.

In the male, the right and left gonadal arteries are referred to as the testicular arteries; they arise from the aorta and pass through the body wall by way of the inguinal canal to serve the testes. In the female, the arteries are referred to as the ovarian arteries; they arise from the aorta and pass into the pelvis to supply the ovaries.

The inferior mesenteric artery is an unpaired vessel arising anteriorly from the abdominal aorta, just above the **bifurcation** of the aorta. This vessel supplies lower abdominal organs, including the descending and sigmoid colons of the large intestine (left colic and sigmoid arteries) and the rectum (superior rectal artery).

The lumbar arteries arise from the posterior surface of the aorta and serve the spinal cord and its meninges, as well as various muscles and skin of the lumbar region of the back.

The middle sacral artery is a small, unpaired vessel that supplies the sacrum, coccyx, and rectum.

The abdominal aorta bifurcates into the left and right common iliac arteries at the level of the fourth lumbar vertebra. These arteries divide inferiorly into two main branches: the right and left external iliac arteries, and the right and left internal iliac arteries.

The internal iliac arteries are the principal blood supply for the pelvis and perineum. Their branches include the iliolumbar and lateral sacral arteries, which serve the pelvic wall and muscles; the middle rectal artery, which serves the internal pelvic organs; the vesicular arteries (superior, inferior, and middle), which serve the urinary bladder; the superior and inferior gluteal arteries, which supply the buttocks; the obturator artery, which supplies the upper medial thigh muscles; and the internal pudendal artery, which supplies the external genitalia and is responsible for blood engorgement of the female genitalia and penile erections in men.

The external iliac arteries become the femoral arteries as they exit the pelvic cavity and cross the inguinal ligament. Two branches arise from the external iliac arteries: the inferior epigastric artery, which serves the skin and abdominal wall muscles; and the deep iliac circumflex artery, which supplies the muscles of the iliac fossa.

The femoral arteries, which pass fairly close to the anterior surface of the upper thigh, send branches back into the pelvic region to supply the genitals and lower abdominal wall. Branches include the medial and lateral femoral circumflex arteries, which supply muscles in the proximal thigh and encircle the femur; and the deep femoral artery (profundus femoris), which is the largest branch of the femoral artery and serves the hip joint and hamstring muscles of the thigh.

The femoral artery continues down the medial and posterior side of the thigh at the back of the knee joint, where it becomes the popliteal artery. The popliteal artery supplies a few small branches to the knee joint, then divides into two branches. The first branch, the anterior tibial artery, serves the anterior aspect of the leg, and, at the ankle, becomes the dorsalis pedis artery, which serves the ankle and dorsum of the foot. The second branch, the posterior tibial artery, continues down the posterior side of the leg between the knee and the ankle. The posterior tibial artery sends off a large branch called the peroneal artery, which supplies the peroneal leg muscles. At the ankle, it bifurcates into the lateral and medial plantar arteries, which supply the bottom of the foot. The lateral plantar artery joins with the dorsal pedis artery to form the plantar arch.

Arterial blood supply for the left upper extremity begins at the aortic arch, where the left subclavian artery originates. The right subclavian artery branches from the brachiocephalic artery. The subclavian arteries pass laterally deep to the clavicle, and as they enter the axillary region, they become the axillary arteries. As the axillary arteries enter the brachial region of the arm, they become the brachial arteries, which continue along the medial side of the humerus. The major branch of the brachial artery is the deep brachial artery, which serves the triceps muscle. At the end of the elbow, the brachial artery divides into the medial ulnar and lateral radial arteries. The largest branch of the radial artery is the radial recurrent artery, which supplies the elbow. The branches of the ulnar artery are the anterior and posterior ulnar recurrent arteries. The ulnar and radial arteries pass inferiorly to the palm, where branches fuse to form palmar arches. From these arise palmar digital arteries, which supply the fingers and thumb.

Blood for the head and neck originates from the two common carotid arteries that pass along either side of the trachea in the neck. The right common carotid originates from the brachiocephalic artery, and the left common carotid arises directly from the aortic arch. Small branches of the common carotid artery supply the larynx, thyroid gland, anterior neck muscles, and lymph glands.

The common carotid artery bifurcates into the internal and external carotid arteries at the superior border of the larynx. The external carotid artery supplies structures in the neck and head area external to the skull. The main branches include the superior thyroid artery, which serves the hyoid muscles, larynx and vocal cords, and the thyroid gland; the ascending pharyngeal artery; the lingual artery, which supplies the tongue and sublingual salivary gland; the facial artery, which supplies the palate, chin, lips, and nose; the occipital artery, which serves the posterior scalp, the meninges of the brain, and the posterior neck muscles; and the posterior auricular artery, which supplies the ear.

Near the mandibular condyle, the external carotid divides into the superficial temporal artery, which serves the parotid salivary gland; and the maxillary artery, which supplies the teeth and gums, muscles of mastication, nasal cavity, eyelids, and meninges of the brain.

The internal carotid and the vertebral arteries supply blood to the brain. The internal carotid artery enters the base of the skull through the carotid canal of the temporal bone. After arising from the subclavian arteries, the paired vertebral arteries enter the skull through the foramen magnum. Once inside the skull these two arteries unite to form the single basilar artery. The two internal carotid arteries and the basilar artery unite in a circular arrangement at the base of the brain near the sella turcica called the circle of Willis. This circle is formed by the union of the anterior cerebral arteries, which branch from the internal carotid arteries, and the posterior cerebral arteries, which branch from the basilar artery. The posterior communicating arteries connect the posterior cerebral arteries and the internal carotid arteries. The anterior cerebral arteries are connected by the anterior communicating artery (refer to Plate 15A in Appendix A).

THE VENOUS SYSTEM

The dural sinuses are blood channels that receive blood from the cerebral, ophthalmic, cerebellar, and meningeal veins of the brain. These include the superior sagittal sinus, inferior sagittal sinus, straight sinus, and basilar plexus, which are all unpaired sinuses of the brain. The paired sinuses include the cavernous, superior petrosal, inferior petrosal, occipital, transverse/lateral, and sigmoid sinuses.

The veins of the brain include the superior cerebral vein, inferior and medial veins, the great cerebral vein of Galen, and the superior and inferior ophthalmic veins. The veins that receive blood from these numerous sinuses and veins within the brain are the right and left internal jugular veins. Therefore, the internal jugular veins drain the brain and the meninges, as well as the deep regions of the face and neck. These veins course downward, beneath the sternocleidomastoid muscle and alongside the common carotid artery in the neck, and eventually empty into the right and left subclavian veins. The union of the internal jugular and the subclavian veins creates the brachiocephalic, or innominate veins. The brachiocephalic veins then merge into a single superior vena cava, which enters into the right atrium of the heart.

The right and left external jugular veins course downward laterally alongside the internal jugular vein and superficial to the sternocleidomastoid muscle. These veins drain the parotid glands and superficial structures of the face and scalp, eventually emptying into the right and left subclavian veins.

The right and left vertebral veins descend through the transverse foramina of the cervical vertebra alongside the vertebral arteries. These veins drain deep structures of the neck, including the vertebrae, and eventually empty into the subclavian veins.

The superficial tissues of the upper extremities are drained by the cephalic and basilic veins. The cephalic vein courses along the lateral side of the arm from the hand to the shoulder, eventually emptying into the axillary vein. Just beyond the axilla, the axillary vein becomes the subclavian vein.

The basilic vein passes upward along the medial side of the arm and merges with the brachial vein just below the head of the humerus to form the axillary vein. The deep tissues of the upper extremity are drained by the radial, ulnar, and brachial veins, which course upward within the same regions as their counterpart arteries. The radial veins receive blood from the dorsal metacarpal veins; the ulnar veins receive blood from the palmar venous arch; and the brachial veins join into the axillary veins.

The abdominal and thoracic walls are drained by tributaries of the brachiocephalic and azygos veins. The right and left brachiocephalic, as mentioned earlier, are formed by the union of the subclavian and internal jugular veins. The brachiocephalic vein drains the head, neck, arms, and upper thorax. The left brachiocephalic vein is the entry point for the thoracic duct of the lymphatic system. The thoracic duct enters the right brachiocephalic vein at the junction of the right internal jugular and subclavian veins. The azygos vein receives the ascending lumbar, hemiazygos, accessory azygos, and bronchial veins in the thorax, as well as certain intercostal and subcostal veins that drain the muscles of the thoracic wall. The azygos originates in the dorsal abdominal wall and courses superiorly to the right side of the vertebral column to join the superior vena cava. Blood from the abdomen and pelvis enters the inferior vena cava for return to the right atrium of the heart. The inferior vena cava, however, does not drain the veins of the spleen, pancreas, gastrointestinal tract, or gallbladder. The blood from these organs is drained into the hepatic portal vein, which is formed by the union of the superior mesenteric vein and the splenic vein. The superior mesenteric vein drains blood from the small intestine and the splenic vein drains blood from the spleen. The hepatic portal vein transports the blood to the liver. In the liver, the blood, which contains absorbed nutrients of digestion, enters capillaries called hepatic sinusoids, which filter the blood through the hepatic liver cells. This venous pathway is called the hepatic portal system.

Bacteria that is present in the portal vein is filtered by the phagocytic action of the Kupffer cells within the hepatic sinusoids. After passing through the hepatic sinusoids, blood is carried through a series of merging vessels into the hepatic veins, and eventually makes its way back to the inferior vena cava.

As the inferior vena cava ascends through the abdomen, it picks up other tributaries from the abdomen. These include the left and right renal veins from the kidney, the suprarenal veins from the adrenal glands, the inferior phrenic veins, and the gonadal veins from the ovaries or testicles.

The veins of the lower extremities are divided into two groups: the superficial group and the deep group. The deep veins of the lower extremities have the names of their corresponding arteries. The anterior and posterior tibial veins drain blood from the deep veins of the foot. At the knee, these veins unite to form the popliteal vein, which continues upward into the thigh and becomes the femoral vein, which drains blood from the deep femoral vein and lateral-medial circumflex veins in the upper thigh. As the femoral vein approaches the inguinal ligament, it receives blood from the great saphenous vein, the longest vein in the body. Near its junction with the femoral vein, the great saphenous vein receives blood from the upper thigh, groin, and lower abdominal wall.

At the level of the sacroiliac joint, the external iliac vein merges with the internal iliac vein, which carries blood away from the reproductive, urinary, and digestive organs, and becomes the common iliac vein. The left and right common iliac veins merge at the level of the fifth lumbar vertebra to form the inferior vena cava (refer to Plate 15B).

OPERATIVE PATHOLOGY AND DIAGNOSIS

Vascular abnormalities involving the extremities increase in frequency with age and are a major cause of disability in the United States. Although peripheral manifestations are frequently symptoms of a generalized, systemic disease, the peripheral problem itself demands solution for the well-being of the patient. Reconstructing an occluded peripheral artery will not cure the patient of atherosclerosis, but it will **mitigate** a major problem for the patient.

The signs and symptoms of peripheral arterial disease are determined by the location and degree of vascular obstruction, the rapidity with which this obstruction develops, and the presence or absence of collateral channels. The initial symptom of arterial disease is the pain of muscle ischemia and **claudication**, usually felt as a cramping pain or dull ache.

Claudication is the primary indicator of occlusive vascular disease. Claudication means "to cramp" and is brought on only by exercise and relieved by rest. Patients may describe this subjective feeling as cramping, aching, weakness, or stiffness brought on by exercise. Its etiology is probably related to a product of ischemic muscle metabolism.

The location of ischemic pain is determined by the sites of arterial obstruction. If pain is felt in the calf muscles, the major obstruction is probably in the superficial femoral artery. Obstruction of the common femoral artery or the external iliac artery usually translates into pain in the thigh. Pain in the buttock may be caused by an obstruction in the common iliac artery or distal aorta. Impotence may represent distal aortic disease.

Acute arterial **occlusion** often causes constant pain in an extremity at rest. Excruciating pain is an early prominent feature after complete occlusion of a large, normal artery, and is usually an indication of embolism. The signs and symptoms of acute occlusion are described by the four Ps: painful, paresthetic, pale, and pulseless. Generally, the site of the occlusion can be deduced from the level of change in skin temperature: inguinal ligament, aortic occlusion; mid-thigh, iliac artery occlusion; lower leg, superficial femoral occlusion; ankle and foot, popliteal occlusion.

Palpation of brachial, radial, carotid, aortic, femoral, popliteal, and pedal pulses provides important information for diagnosis. These pulses are graded from 0 to 4+, with a score of 0 indicating complete absence of pulse. Of the special diagnostic aids, the Doppler flow probe has assumed the most important role in the evaluation of patients with peripheral vascular disease. These extraordinarily sensitive devices can detect flow in pedal vessels in cases of severe **ischemia**.

Diagnostic procedures and tests for the evaluation of peripheral vascular disease include (discussed in detail in Chapter 13):

- **Plethysmography** for patients with diffuse small vessel arterial disease
- Doppler probe for the measurement of blood flow to a particular artery
- Phleborheography for diagnosis of deep vein thrombosis
- Computed axial tomography, magnetic resonance imaging, and ultrasonography for the detection and evaluation of carotid artery atherosclerosis or thoracic or abdominal aortic aneurysm
- Angiography, the gold standard for the diagnosis and evaluation of vascular disease

ARTERIAL EMBOLISM

A sudden loss of circulation to an extremity is usually an indication of arterial embolism. In addition to blood clots, emboli may consist of fat, air, or even portions of tumor that circulate through the cardiovascular system until they eventually become lodged in smaller vessels, blocking blood flow to an extremity or organ. **Morbidity** associated with embolism remains high and consistent at 15–30%, not necessarily because of the ischemic limb but because of the underlying disease that led to the formation of the **embolus**.

Major emboli lodge at bifurcations or the origin of large branches, at sites of anatomical narrowing, and at sites of pathological narrowing, such as an atherosclerotic superficial femoral artery. Approximately 80% of peripheral emboli affect the lower limb with the common femoral bifurcation accounting for almost half the cases.

Emboli may originate from the left atrium in patients with atrial fibrillation or from the left ventricle when the endocardium is damaged and the ventricle contracts poorly. Recent studies suggest that 90% of all patients with arterial emboli have an underlying heart disorder, although emboli may also be shed from the aorta to the extremities.

Obviously, the underlying source for arterial embolism must be established for proper treatment and to prevent recurrence. The first practical decision in the treatment of the patient with arterial embolism is whether or not the patient can tolerate angiography and general anesthesia. Treatment of recent myocardial infarction or ventricular dysrhythmia assumes priority. However, simultaneous attempts should be made to restore peripheral circulation.

For the unstable patient, nonoperative therapy is the best option. High dosages of anticoagulants such as heparin allows the patient's own fibrinolytic system to lyse the occluding clot. More recently, enzymatic lysis of the embolus has been advocated. The enzyme (urokinase or streptokinase) is delivered through an intra-arterial catheter placed at the proximal extent of the clot. If enzyme therapy is not successful, surgery for the direct removal of the embolus or **thrombus** is the next option.

For the patient with no acute complicating cardiovascular condition, evaluation should be thorough but delay in treatment should be avoided. Electrocardiogram and echocardiogram should be obtained, and enzymatic therapy during angiography should be attempted. If unsuccessful, surgery is the next option.

Surgical intervention for the removal of emboli (arterial embolectomy) involves an incision made into the affected artery for the removal of thromboembolitic material and the restoration of flow to the extremity. The insertion of a balloon-tipped **Fogarty** (embolectomy) **catheter** into the arteriotomy facilitates the removal of the embolus (Figure 23-6).

ARTERIOSCLEROSIS OBLITERANS

Arteriosclerosis obliterans is a generalized disease affecting the arterial system, and, as discussed previously, involves

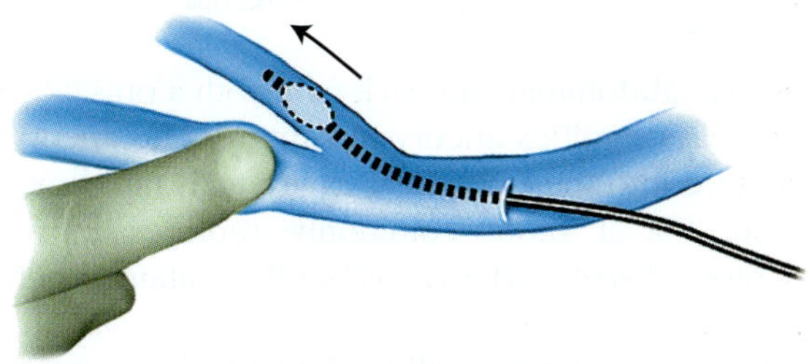

Figure 23-6 Insertion of Fogarty catheter

the formation of an atheroma within the lumen of an artery that restricts blood flow to target tissues. It has a remarkably consistent pattern of involvement that is segmental in nature. The segmental nature of involvement makes vascular reconstruction to relatively normal vessels distal to the disease possible in most instances.

The two main areas of early peripheral involvement are the aortic bifurcation and the distal superficial femoral artery at the adductor canal. The process may then progress to involve other portions of the arterial system.

The physical examination of patients with vascular insufficiency reveals severely thickened, deformed nails, shiny skin, and decreased hair growth. Significant pallor on examination and exercise of the extremity is an important sign.

Medical management for nondisabling claudication is preferable over surgical management, and involves the following:

- Cessation of smoking
- Control of hypertension
- Weight reduction
- Dietary management of hyperlipidemia
- Exercise (walking to the point of claudication three times a day)
- Proper care of the feet

Collateral blood flow will usually form in a period of 6 months. As a general rule, surgery for the relief of claudication alone should not be performed until therapy has been attempted for a period of 6 months, unless the condition is worsening rapidly.

ANEURYSMS OF THE ABDOMINAL AORTA

Aortic disease may have a profound effect on an individual's overall health because of all the important arteries that originate from this large vessel; however, almost all patients with abdominal aortic aneurysm are diagnosed while the patient is still asymptomatic.

Aneurysms of the abdominal aorta are generally fusiform. The majority arise below the origin of the renal arteries and terminate at the bifurcation of the aorta or common iliac arteries. Occasionally, one or both renal arteries may arise from an abdominal aneurysm, without involvement of the superior mesenteric artery. Aneurysms may also extend beyond the bifurcation of the common iliac arteries into the external or internal iliac arteries (Figure 23-7).

Severe abdominal and back pain with a pulsatile abdominal mass signifies aneurysm rupture. The aneurysm may rupture into the peritoneal cavity with rapid exsanguination, but it more commonly ruptures into the retroperitoneal space where it is briefly contained before fatal hemorrhage occurs.

The risk of rupture is difficult to predict on an individual basis, although patients with large aneurysms are at greater risk. Hypertension increases the likelihood of rupture for any given size of aneurysm. Operative **mortality** is very low (2–3%) for the elective procedure, but once rupture has occurred, operative mortality rises steeply and may exceed 80% for the patient in shock. Therefore, elective surgical correction is highly advisable.

The recommended treatment for aneurysms of the abdominal aorta is resection with synthetic graft replacement, although percutaneous stent reinforcement is rapidly gaining popularity. For grafting, the Y-shaped, bifurcated Dacron material is used if the common iliac arteries are involved; if not, a straight Dacron graft is used (Figure 23-8).

CT scan is useful in the diagnosis of abdominal aortic aneurysm. It can provide information about the extent of the aneurysm, the location of thromboembolytic material, and whether or not leakage has occurred. Ultrasound is also useful for initial detection, but cannot provide much more information. Once the aneurysm is detected, the patient should undergo aortic angiography so that surgery may be planned in detail. An aortogram can reveal important factors such as renal artery involvement, renal artery stenosis, visceral arterial disease, and additional occlusive or aneurysmal disease in the internal iliac and runoff vessels. Intimal degeneration in the juxtarenal aorta that would preclude safe infrarenal clamping may also be revealed by aortogram.

The patient with abdominal aortic aneurysm should be assessed for coronary artery disease before undergoing aneurysmal repair because atherosclerosis of the coronary arteries is a major determinant of mortality after arterial reconstruction. If the patient is asymptomatic for aneurysmal disease but has symptomatic coronary artery disease, coronary artery bypass grafting or percutaneous transluminal coronary angioplasty should be attempted before the aneurysm repair. If the patient is symptomatic for both diseases, simultaneous repair for both the aneurysm and the coronary stenoses is advisable.

Aneurysms may also occur in the smaller peripheral arteries. Atherosclerotic aneurysms of the femoral and popliteal arteries are likely to shed emboli and finally thrombose rather than rupture. The patient typically complains of foot or calf pain. Examination reveals a pulsating mass in the groin or behind the knee and irregular red-blue patches of skin on the foot. Continued embolization and loss of the extremity are inevitable in the untreated patient.

Iliac artery aneurysm rupture is more likely than aneurysms of the popliteal and femoral arteries. These aneurysms are generally not detected on physical examination or routine X-ray, and so are allowed to progress to rupture.

In an otherwise healthy patient, surgery is the best option for femoral, popliteal, and iliac artery aneurysms. The procedure involves resection of the aneurysm and arterial reconstruction with a synthetic Dacron graft.

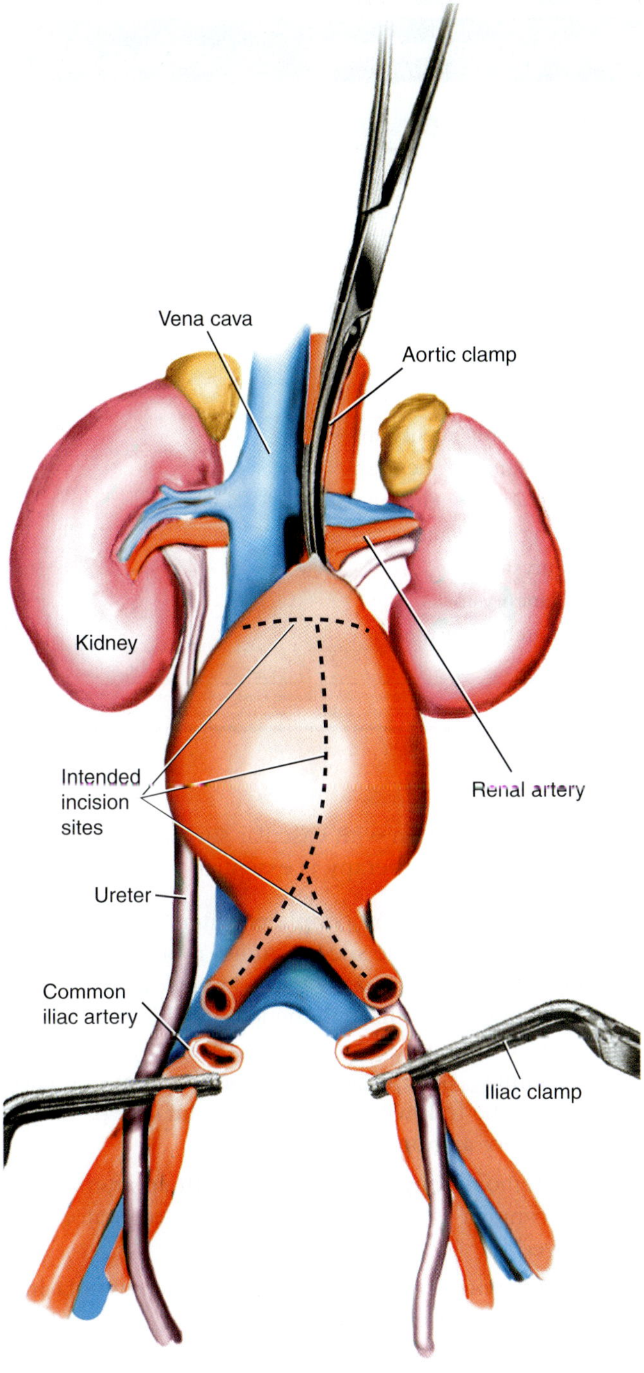

Figure 23-7 **Abdominal aortic aneurysm**

SURGICAL INTERVENTIONS

Peripheral vascular surgery may involve any part of the body; however, there are several basic approaches and some common features for peripheral vascular surgery. Common approaches used in peripheral vascular surgery include:

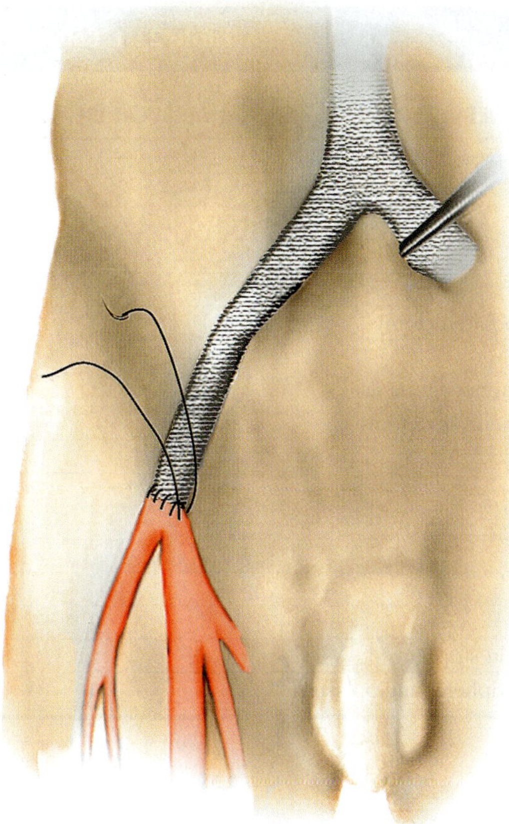

Figure 23-8 **Bifurcated aortic graft sutured in place**

- Median sternotomy
- Thoracotomy
- Thoracoabdominal incisions
- Anterior abdominal incisions
- Localized incisions for peripheral vascular procedures

Common procedures are found in Table 23-1.

PERIPHERAL VESSEL ANGIOPLASTY

Balloon dilatation of the peripheral artery (percutaneous transluminal angioplasty) is an option for patients with symptomatic atherosclerotic disease. The procedure has been demonstrated to be effective in both initial reports and long-term follow-up. Initial theories of the mechanism of angioplasty advocated compression of plaque against the arterial wall as the most significant factor in recanalization, but more recent, extensive evaluation has demonstrated that a "cracking" of the plaque with subsequent healing and neointima production as the predominant factor.

Short areas of iliac artery stenosis can be dilated with approximately a 90% success rate. Femoral artery angioplasty results depend largely on popliteal artery runoff. In general, excellent symptomatic relief can be achieved

Table 23-1 Common Procedures in Peripheral Vascular Surgery

GENERAL TYPE FOR PERIPHERAL VASCULATURE	SPECIFIC PROCEDURES
Bypass	Aortofemoral bypass
	Femoropopliteal bypass
	Femorofemoral bypass
	Axillofemoral bypass
	Popliteal to post-tibial bypass (*in situ*)
Endarterectomy	Carotid endarterectomy
	Aortic endarterectomy
Arteriovenous fistula	AV fistula formation (shunt)
Aneurysmectomy	Abdominal aortic aneurysm
	Thoracoabdominal aneurysm
	Ascending aortic aneurysm
	Descending aortic aneurysm
	Iliac aneurysm
	Femoral aneurysm
	Popliteal arch aneurysm
Vein stripping	
Peripheral angioplasty	

when short occlusions or stenoses are dilated and distal run-off is good.

Balloon sizing and selection are crucial elements in successful peripheral artery angioplasty. Selection of a balloon that is too small may result in under-dilatation and early restenosis. A balloon that is too large may result in dissection of the vessel. Most physicians base their balloon selection on measurements from angiographic studies (allowing for magnification). Balloon length should be sufficient to extend 1–2 cm beyond the lesion (Figure 23-9).

The following represent considerations for peripheral artery angioplasty:

1. The diseased area of the artery should be approached cautiously. A variety of guidewires, catheters, and balloons may be necessary for proper repair.
2. Passage of a guidewire through a lesion is the most critical part of the procedure.
3. Once the dilatation has been performed, further passage of guidewires should be prohibited because of the known trauma at the dilatation site and the risk of thrombosis.
4. Detailed angiographic mapping should be performed before angioplasty to define the lesion properly.
5. Antegrade puncture of the common femoral artery is the best approach for most peripheral stenoses.
6. Aggressive steps to prevent and reverse spasm, such as the intra-arterial injection of nitroglycerine, should be employed during the procedure.
7. Close cooperation with vascular surgeons for alternative methods of therapy is essential.

The procedure for peripheral artery angioplasty is usually performed in the special studies room of the radiology department by a specially trained radiologist. The most common approach is through the ipsilateral femoral artery, but the **contralateral** approach is occasionally used.

Assuming that angiographic studies have already been done, the following are the procedural steps for peripheral artery angioplasty:

1. The femoral artery is punctured with an arterial needle/cannula assembly, and the needle/obturator is removed.
2. A guidewire is introduced through the cannula into the femoral artery.
3. A balloon-tipped angioplasty catheter is threaded over the guidewire and positioned across the peripheral vascular lesion.
4. The balloon is inflated.
5. The balloon is replaced with a selective diagnostic catheter and postangioplasty films are made to document the repair.

Intraluminal stents may be placed within the vessel after balloon angioplasty to maintain **patency** of the repair. The Palmaz stent may be delivered to the site of the arterial obstruction with a balloon angioplasty catheter. Once positioned, the balloon is inflated and the stent is

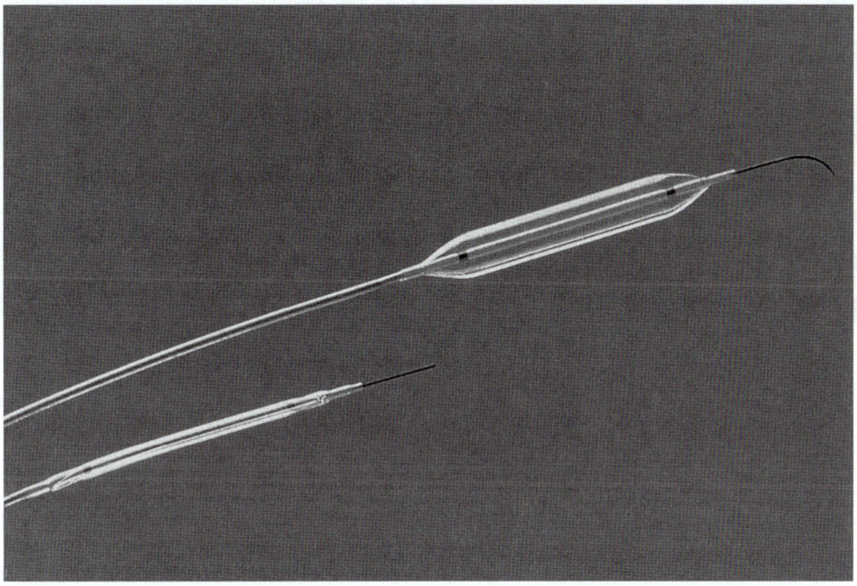

Figure 23-9 **Angioplasty balloon catheter** ***(Courtesy of Boston Scientific/Vascular)***

expanded against the arterial wall and left in place. Stents may be made of stainless steel mesh, titanium, polypropylene, or other inert materials.

BYPASS GRAFTING AND ENDARTERECTOMY

Surgery remains the treatment of choice in most patients with disabling claudication, pain during rest, or gangrene. Bypassing the occlusion with a synthetic or biologic graft and endarterectomy are the two basic reconstructive procedures utilized today. Endarterectomy, which is the excision of the thickened, atheromatous tunica intima of an artery, has certain advantages over bypass grafting. The patient's own vessels are preserved, little or no foreign material is introduced, and the procedure is more sound hemodynamically. However, extensive endarterectomy below the hypogastric level carries a high complication and failure rate. Endarterectomy is most often performed on the carotid artery.

Arterial bypass grafting is the popular alternative to endarterectomy. Biologic or synthetic grafts are required to bypass vascular obstruction or to reconstruct vessels. Grafts may be straight or Y-shaped. One end of the graft is sewn to a proximal, healthy portion of either the affected vessel or another vessel altogether. The other end of the graft is sewn to the distal portion of the affected vessel, bypassing the obstruction and serving as a substitute conduit for blood flow.

Autogenous saphenous vein remains the material of choice for distal bypasses of the lower extremity. It is pliable, easy to tailor, and amenable to fine suture technique. It remains supple when placed across the knee joint, and resists infection better than any other graft material. The saphenous vein may be used in reverse, nonreversed, or ***in situ*** fashion. The *in situ* technique (with the saphenous vein left in place in the lower extremity and only the proximal and distal ends dissected free for anastomosis) holds a number of advantages over the reversed saphenous vein method of bypass grafting. The structural integrity and function of the endothelium may be better preserved in the *in situ* technique with an attendant improvement in early and late graft patency. It also enables vessels too small for reversed grafting to be accommodated. Another advantage is that by having the larger proximal end of the vein attached to the larger proximal end of the artery and the smaller distal end of the vein attached to the smaller distal end of the artery, graft hemodynamics are enhanced and anastomoses are better matched (Figure 23-10). These advantages have led to better limb preservation, particularly for patients undergoing femoropopliteal reconstruction.

Synthetic grafts are made of various materials, including knitted polyester (Dacron), knitted velour (Dacron), woven polyester (Dacron), and polytetrafluorethylene (Gore-Tex, Impra) (Figure 23-11).

Knit polyester (Dacron) grafts are porous for rapid tissue ingrowth. However, this porosity also allows blood to seep through the material, requiring preclotting by the surgical team. Dacron functions reasonably well above the knee. Results of below-knee popliteal bypass have been less than satisfactory due to kinking of the graft across the knee joint. In addition, the anastomosis of a thick, stiff prosthetic

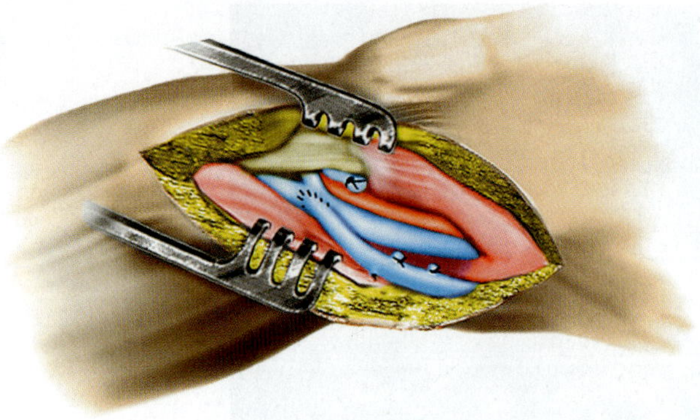

Figure 23-10 ***In situ* saphenous vein anastomosis**

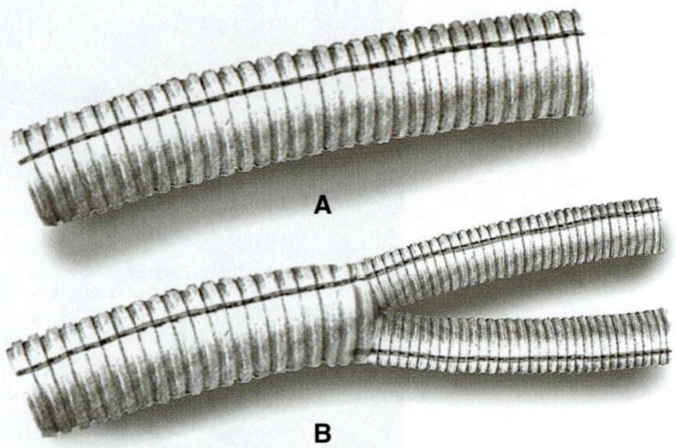

Figure 23-11 **Vascular grafts: (A) Tubular, (B) bifurcated**

to a small distal vessel is very difficult. Therefore, Dacron is no longer used for below-knee anastomosis.

Knitted velour polyester (Dacron) grafts are uniformly porous for good tissue ingrowth. One type of knitted velour graft, the exoskeleton (EXS) prosthesis, has a spiral polypropylene support within the graft, and was specially designed for use across the knee joint. Another type has the antibiotic amikacin impregnated into the prosthetic wall, making the graft impervious to leaks and obviating the need for preclotting.

Woven polyester construction of the Dacron graft is leak proof and does not need to be preclotted. Because of their inflexibility, however, these grafts are relegated to larger arterial bypass grafting.

Expanded polytetrafluorethylene (PTFE) can be taken across the knee joint without risk of kinking. Although effective at the popliteal level, PTFE may be less satisfactory for more distal bypasses. The microporous wall of PTFE serves as a lattice framework for tissue ingrowth, creating an ultra-thin layer for contact with blood and obviating the need for preclotting. The PTFE graft may have rigid rings built into the prosthetic wall for support.

A composite of synthetic and autogenous vein may substitute for an insufficient length of saphenous vein. These grafts retain the advantage of a distal vein-artery anastomosis, which is particularly important at the infrapopliteal level. Dacron-vein composites have been used in the past, but are liable to stenosis and false aneurysm at the intermediate anastomosis. PTFE-vein grafts appear to be less prone to this problem, and results have been superior to PTFE alone for infrapopliteal bypass.

FEATURES OF PERIPHERAL VASCULAR PROCEDURES

The structure of blood vessels and the solutions to pathological conditions are relatively similar throughout the body. Many of the features of peripheral vascular surgery are, therefore, common to all procedures in this field. These include preoperative routines, intraoperative monitoring, instrumentation, sutures, and drugs used in the sterile field.

PERIPHERAL VASCULAR PREOPERATIVE ROUTINES

Preoperative routines for the peripheral vascular procedures include a number of personnel and items. For the patient undergoing any peripheral vascular procedure, special consideration should be given to the patient's compromised circulation and general state of poor vascularization. Patients with peripheral vascular disease are often diabetic or are cigarette smokers. The anesthesia provider should review respiratory function tests before induction. The patient's chart should be checked for history and physical, consent, laboratory results, and diagnostic test results. Preoperative diagnostic arteriograms are done to assess the extent of the arterial lesion, and should be in the OR before the surgeon arrives.

INTRAOPERATIVE MONITORING

Intraoperative monitoring includes ECG, BP, and oxygen saturation. Transesophageal echocardiography may be necessary for certain abdominal aorta procedures, and electroencephalogram may be used during carotid endarterectomy. A cannula may be inserted into the radial artery for direct arterial pressure readings, and a Swan-Ganz catheter may be utilized for central venous or pulmonary wedge pressures. Urinary output is monitored with the use of a Foley catheter.

INSTRUMENTATION

Many ORs have vascular sets related to the size of the artery being worked on. For example, small arteries would require a minor set for soft tissue and exposure instruments, and an AV fistula set for the delicate vascular forceps, clamps, and scissors (ideal for smaller arteries). Arteries of medium size, such as the femoral or carotid arteries, may require a minor set and a carotid set. Large arteries, such as the aorta, would require a major laparotomy set and a general vascular set with larger and longer vascular instruments. Other facilities may have only small and large vascular sets.

Commonly used instrumentation for peripheral vascular procedures includes:

- Hemoclip applicators (Weck or Ethicon) of varying size and length are necessary for most vascular procedures.
- Weitlaner is the self-retaining retractor of choice for most superficial peripheral vascular procedures.
- For procedures on the aorta, a large Balfour retractor (or self-retaining abdominal retractor of the surgeon's choice) will be necessary in addition to the large retractors on the major laparotomy set.
- A Diethrich coronary set (vascular dilators, bulldogs, CV forceps [Figure 23-12 A and B], Potts coronary scissors, and vascular clamps) is useful for most vascular procedures.
- Castroviejo needle holders and DeBakey forceps are preferred by many surgeons for anastomoses.
- Rubber shods, also known as Prolene clamps (mosquito clamps with ¼-in. sections of a small-French red rubber catheter on the tips), are essential when double-armed polypropylene sutures are used.
- DeBakey angled vascular clamps are preferred for medium-sized artery occlusion (Figure 23-13A and B).
- Beaver knife handles and blades and tenotomy scissors are also frequently utilized for smaller arteries.

SUTURES

Typical suture gauges for peripheral vascular anastomoses are:

- *Aorta:* 3–0 or 4–0
- *Iliac:* 4–0 or 5–0
- *Femoral:* 5–0 or 6–0
- *Popliteal:* 5–0 or 6–0
- *Posterior tibial:* 6–0 or 7–0
- *Common carotid:* 6–0
- *Internal carotid:* 6–0 or 7–0
- *Brachial:* 6–0 or 7–0
- *Subclavian:* 6–0
- *Radial or ulnar:* 6–0 or 7–0

Suture for peripheral vascular procedures includes polypropylene, Dacron, polyester, and PTFE materials. Double-armed sutures on swaged needles are used for anastomoses. Silk ties and silk and polypropylene suture ligatures are frequently used.

DRUGS

Drugs handled by the STSR during peripheral vascular procedures include:

- Sodium heparin in sodium chloride for intra-arterial irrigation (1000 units in 500 mL saline is typical)
- Lidocaine with or without epinephrine for local procedures or postoperative anesthetic

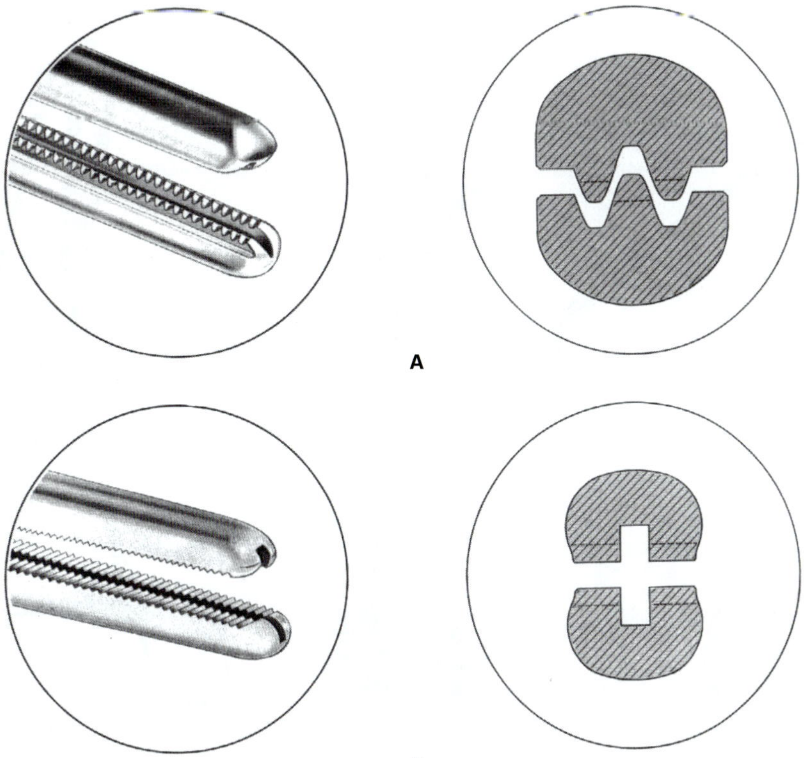

A

B

Figure 23-12 Atraumatic serrations for cardiovascular instruments: (A) DeBakey type serration, (B) Cooley type serration ***(Photos courtesy of Miltex, Inc.)***

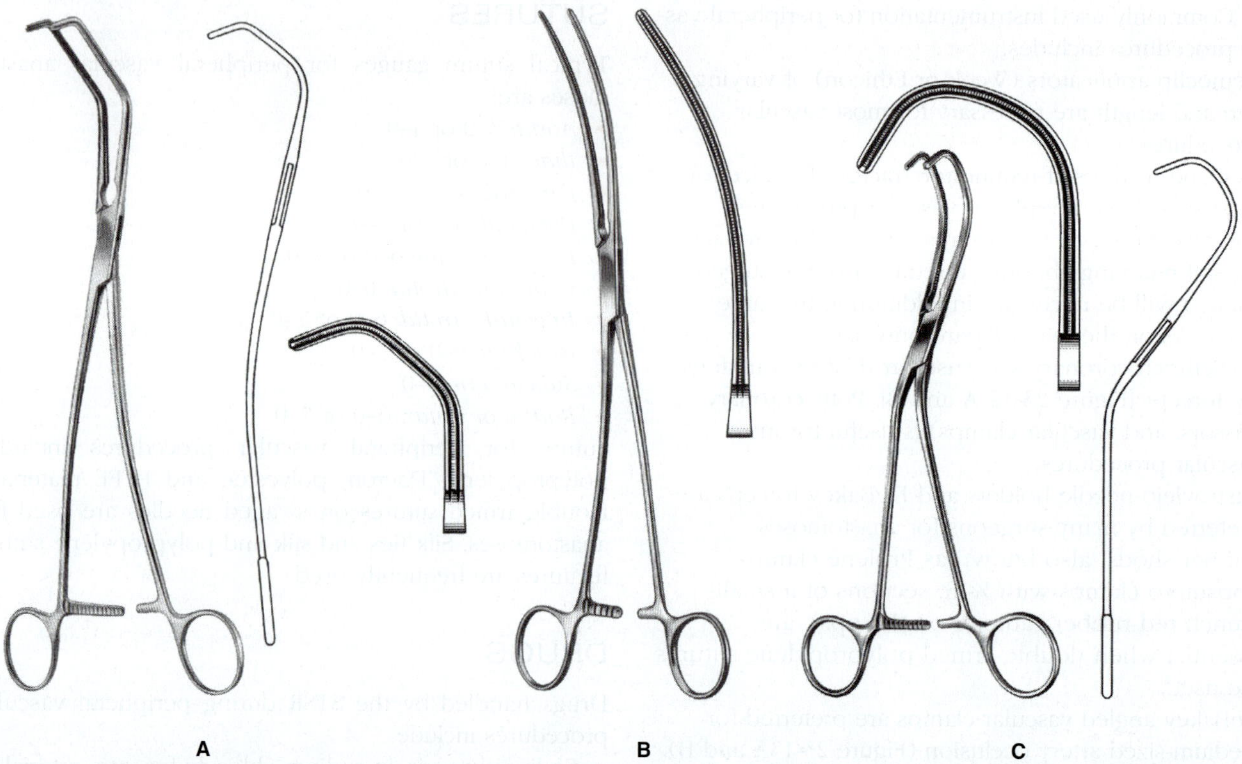

Figure 23-13A **Selected cardiovascular instruments: (A) DeBakey tangential occlusion clamp, (B) DeBakey vascular clamp for aortic aneurysm, (C) Lambert-Kay vascular clamp for aortic anastomosis** ***(Photos courtesy of Miltex, Inc.)***

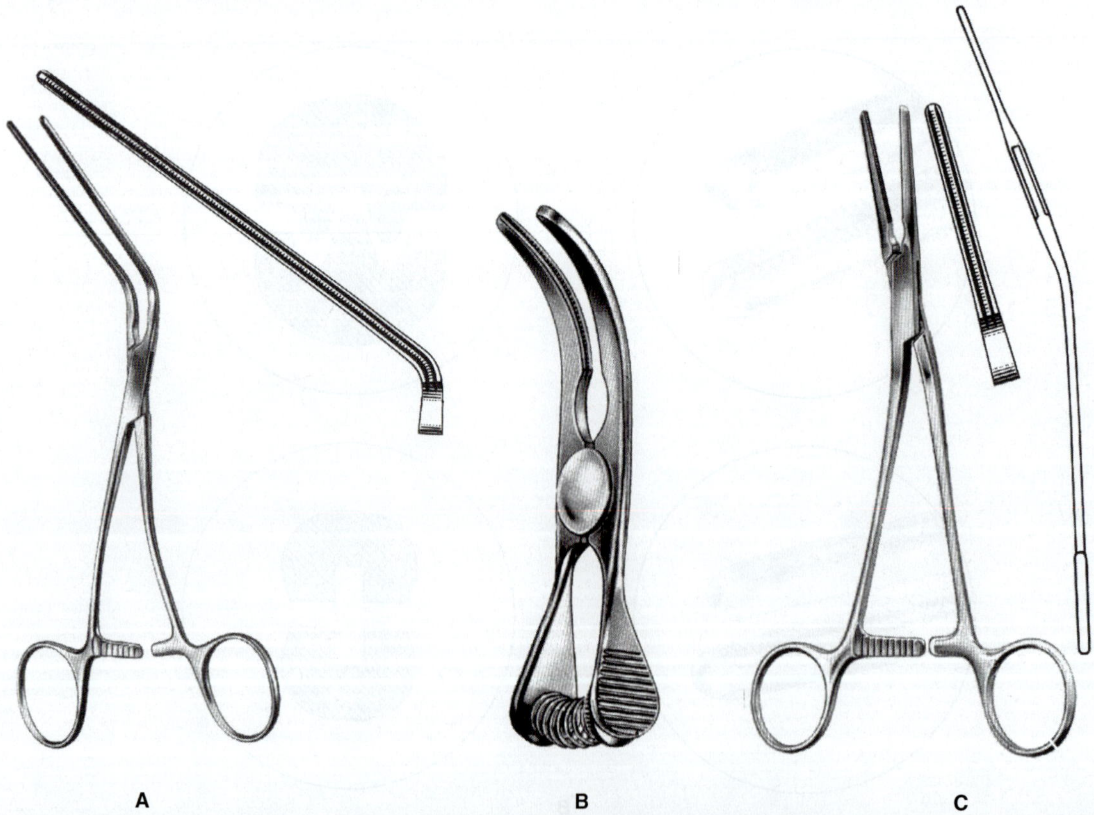

Figure 23-13B **Selected peripheral vascular instruments: (A) DeBakey peripheral vascular clamp, (B) Glover Bulldog peripheral vascular clamp, (C) DeBakey patent ductus and peripheral vascular clamp** ***(Photos courtesy of Miltex, Inc.)***

- **Papaverine** for the suppression of arterial vasospasm
- Antibiotic of surgeon's choice in sodium chloride for irrigation
- Hemostatic agents (Gelfoam soaked with topical thrombin, Surgicel, Avitene)
- Contrast solution for intraoperative arteriogram (Hypaque, Conray, Renografin, Cystografin, etc.)

AORTOFEMORAL BYPASS

Arterial obstructions due to atherosclerosis occur most frequently in the aortoiliac segment of the arterial system. Results of arterial bypass in this region are good because of its high flow rate and large-diameter vessels. The procedural steps are delineated in Procedure 23-1.

(Text continues on page 947)

PROCEDURE 23-1 Aortofemoral Bypass

Equipment

- Cell Saver
- Hypo/hyperthermia unit
- Electrosurgical unit
- Headlight and fiberoptic light source
- Doppler unit
- Suction system

Instruments

- Major vascular set
- Major laparotomy set
- Diethrich coronary artery set
- Balfour self-retaining retractor and blades
- Extra-wide Deaver retractors
- Harrington retractors
- Weitlaner self-retaining retractors
- Hemoclip applicators of various lengths and sizes
- Tunneler

Supplies

- Pack: laparotomy
- Basin set
- Gloves
- Blades (#20, #10, #11)
- Drapes: towels, adhesive drape, laparotomy drape
- Suture:
  - 4–0, 5–0, 6–0 Prolene
  - 2–0, 3–0, 4–0 silk ties, 18–32 in.
  - 2–0, 3–0 silk stick ties
- Drains: surgeon's preference; typically, Jackson-Pratt
- Dressings: Adaptic, 4 × 4s, ABD
- Drugs: heparin, antibiotic irrigation, contrast solution
- Miscellaneous:
  - Doppler probe
  - Fogarty embolectomy catheter (assorted sizes) with tuberculin or 3-cc syringe
  - Vessel loops and/or umbilical tape
  - Laparotomy sponges
  - Ray-Tec sponges
  - Surgicel, Avitene, Gelfoam
  - PTFE or Dacron polyester bifurcated grafts and patch material
  - Cell Saver suction tubing and regular suction tubing
  - Electrosurgical pencil
  - Electrosurgical extension
  - Hemoclips of various sizes
  - Butterfly needle
  - Extension tubing
  - Variety of syringes and hypodermic needles
  - Fogarty clamp inserts
  - 20-cc syringe and heparin needle or Angiocath cannula for intra-arterial irrigation
  - Kitner dissectors

Operative Preparation

Anesthesia
- General

Position
- Supine
- Patients with compromised circulation should not be positioned in such a way that superficial vessels or nerves are compressed
- Pressure points should be identified and padded as necessary

(continues)

PROCEDURE 23-1 Aortofemoral Bypass *(continued)*

Prep

- The patient is prepped from the mid-chest to the mid-thigh

Draping

- The groin is covered with a folded towel. The abdomen and inguinal areas are square-draped with towels and covered with plastic adhesive drape and fenestrated laparotomy drape. The laparotomy sheet is cut for exposure of the area over the femoral arteries

Practical Considerations

- STAC should ensure that blood for the patient is available
- Blood loss should be carefully monitored during the procedure. The STSR should keep accurate measurement of the amount of irrigation used
- The surgeon's hands should be moistened with saline from an Asepto before tying Prolene sutures

Operative Procedure	Technical Considerations
1. With the patient in the supine position, incisions are made in each groin lateral to the vascular axis with dissection of the profunda femoris down to the first perforating branch or beyond.	**1.** Dissection is accomplished using medium Metzenbaum scissors and tissue forceps. The STSR should have Weitlaner retractors ready for placement.
2. The inguinal ligament is partially excised at the upper limit of the incision for unlimited passage of the Dacron graft from the abdomen. The deep circumflex iliac vein is divided to make way for eventual tunneling.	**2.** Dissection will continue with the electrocautery and sharp and blunt techniques. Suction may be used intermittently.
3. The abdomen is opened from the xiphoid to the pubis, and the transverse colon and omentum are reflected superiorly. The small bowel is displaced over the right-hand wound margin and covered with warm moist packs.	**3.** A #20 blade on a #4 handle is typically used for this large incision. The STSR should have bowel bag or warm moist packs completely wrung and ready for coverage of small bowel.
4. The posterior peritoneum is incised and extended toward the aortic bifurcation.	**4.** The STSR should be prepared for sudden hemorrhage.
5. The portion of the aorta just below the renal arteries is isolated and cleared, and the left renal vein is mobilized.	**5.** 18-in. silk ties of 3–0 or 4–0 gauge are good for ligating small superficial vessels. For ligation of larger, deeper vessels, 2–0 or 3–0 silk ties of 30-in. length on carriers are necessary. Typical carriers are Schnidt tonsil clamps or Sarot clamps for deeper ligation.
6. A retroperitoneal tunnel is developed with a tunneling device or long clamp lateral to the vascular axis and behind the ureter.	**6.** A device for tunneling may be a Sarot clamp, uterine dressing forceps, or a specialty CV tunneler with a bullet tip that the graft end can be tied onto with heavy silk ties and pulled through the tunnel. If a clamp is used to create the tunnel, it can also be used to grasp the graft end and pull it through.
7. Blood is drawn from the vena cava, and a knitted Dacron graft is selected and preclotted.	**7.** Have various graft sizes available (but unopened) for inspection by the surgeon. (*Note:* PTFE grafts do not require preclotting.)

PROCEDURE

23-1 Aortofemoral Bypass *(continued)*

8. The patient is heparinized systemically, and a large vascular clamp is applied to the aorta just below the left renal vein. A 2–3 cm section of aorta is excised and the distal aortic stump is oversewn.

9. The proximal stump of the aorta is prepared for anastomosis, and the Dacron graft is sewn to the aorta in an end-to-end fashion with a continuous 4–0 Prolene suture.

8. Make sure the vascular clamps chosen are the proper size for the vessel being repaired or bypassed. The aorta is typically occluded with a large Fogarty or DeBakey aortic clamp.

9. If the aorta is friable, Teflon-coated **pledgets** may be used with the suture to reinforce the anastomosis, preventing the suture from tearing the tissue. The pledget is loaded by carefully folding the pledget in half with one hand, and placing the needle (loaded on a needle holder) through the top half of the fold (Figure 23-14).

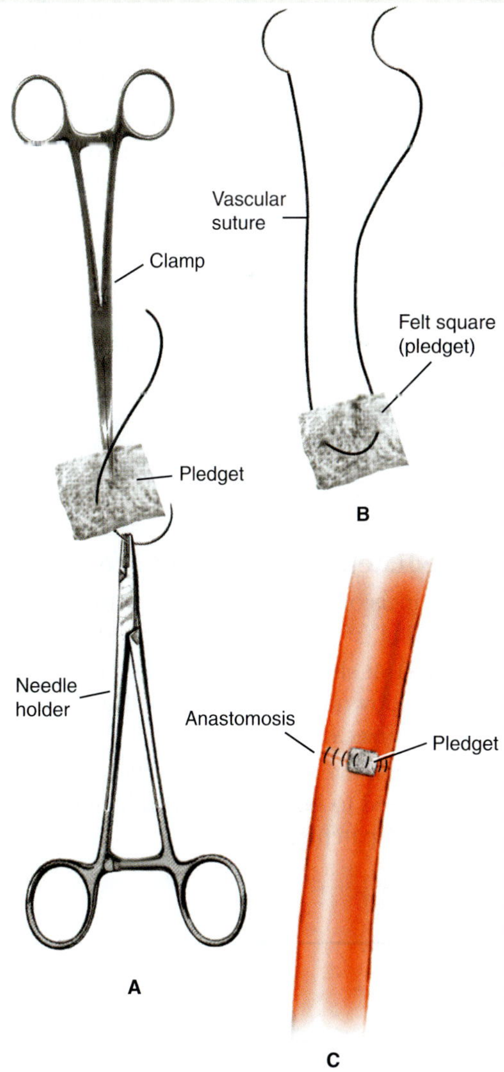

Figure 23-14 **Pledget preparation and use: (A) Loading the pledget, (B) pledget ready for use, (C) pledgeted suture incorporated in the anastomosis**

(continues)

PROCEDURE 23-1 Aortofemoral Bypass *(continued)*

10. A vascular clamp is applied to the common femoral artery. (*Note:* If the anastomosis site is further distal, clamps are applied to the superficial and deep femoral vessels.)

10. Angled vascular or offset-Potts clamps are frequently used for femoral artery occlusion. The superficial and deep femoral vessels are frequently occluded with bulldog vascular clamps.

11. An incision is made into the common femoral artery, and the graft is cut to the correct length and its end beveled.

11. Arteriotomy is begun with a #11 blade on a #7 handle. It is completed with Potts or coronary scissors. The Dacron graft is cut with straight Mayo scissors. A PTFE should be cut with a fresh knife blade.

12. The graft limb is anastomosed to the femoral artery utilizing a continuous, double-armed 5–0 or 6–0 Prolene suture. Just before the completion of anastomosis, the proximal and distal clamps are released to flush the graft, and the femoral suture line is flushed with heparinized saline.

12. The STSR should be familiar with the art of "running" polypropylene suture. A small basin may be useful to contain blood when graft is flushed to remove clotted blood and air. Heparin solution is prepared in advance of need.

13. The suture line is completed for the right side, and the same process is repeated for the left. The posterior peritoneum and pre-aortic fascia are closed over the graft, and the abdomen and groins are closed in layers.

13. Be prepared for an intraoperative arteriogram. Supplies needed are arterial needle (or butterfly needle), 20-cc syringe, X-ray cassette or C-arm drape, injectable saline, and contrast solution. Make sure that bubbles are completely removed from the syringe and tubing. Glass syringes are better than plastic for intra-arterial injection because they do not retain bubbles as badly as plastic. Three incisions are used. Be sure appropriate number of counts are carried out.

Postoperative Considerations

Immediate Postoperative Care

- The incisions will be dressed with a three-layer dressing (e.g., Adaptic, 4 × 4s, ABDs, and tape).
- The STSR should remain sterile, and should not break down the back table or Mayo tray until the patient has safely left the OR.
- Postoperative bleeding from the anastomosis site may need to be repaired with a single-armed Prolene patch suture.

Prognosis

- If arterial flow is reinstated before tissue damage has become too severe, then the prognosis for recovery is good.
- Anticoagulants are necessary to prevent clot formation postoperatively.

Complications

- Wound infection
- Failure of graft
- Amputation of a lower limb

PEARL OF WISDOM

The STSR should have a variety of atraumatic vascular clamps available for aortofemoral bypass. Anatomical variables require different shapes, angles, and curves for the vascular clamp. What may be sufficient for one vessel may not work for another.

ABDOMINAL AORTIC ANEURYSMECTOMY

Aneurysms are weakened areas in an arterial wall. They represent significant danger to the patient. They may rupture with significant hemorrhage or contribute to the formation of emboli. Aortic aneurysms are a significant threat to life due to the size of the vessel. Aneurysms are typically resected electively (Procedure 23-2).

(Text continues on page 950)

PROCEDURE 23-2 Abdominal Aortic Aneurysmectomy

Equipment

- Cell Saver
- Hypo/hyperthermia unit
- Electrosurgical unit
- Headlight and fiberoptic light source
- Doppler unit
- Suction system

Instruments

- Major vascular set
- Major laparotomy set
- Diethrich coronary artery set
- Balfour self-retaining retractor and blades
- Extra-wide Deaver retractors
- Harrington retractors
- Hemoclip applicators of various lengths and sizes

Supplies

- Pack: laparotomy
- Basin set
- Gloves
- Blades (#20, #10, #11)
- Drapes: towels, adhesive drape, laparotomy drape
- Suture:
  - 4–0, 5–0, 6–0 Prolene
  - 2–0, 3–0, 4–0 silk ties, 18–32 in.
  - 2–0, 3–0 silk stick-ties
- Drains: surgeon's preference
- Dressings: Adaptic, 4 × 4s, ABD
- Drugs: heparin, antibiotic irrigation, contrast solution
- Miscellaneous:
  - Doppler probe
  - Fogarty embolectomy catheter (assorted sizes) with tuberculin or 3-cc syringe
  - Vessel loops and/or umbilical tape
  - Laparotomy sponges
  - Ray-Tec sponges
  - Surgicel, Avitene, Gelfoam
  - PTFE or Dacron polyester tube grafts and patch material
  - Cell Saver suction tubing and regular suction tubing
  - Electrosurgical pencil
  - Electrosurgical extension
  - Hemoclips of various sizes
  - Butterfly needle
  - Extension tubing
  - Variety of syringes and hypodermic needles
  - Fogarty clamp inserts
  - 20-cc syringe and heparin needle or Angiocath cannula for intra-arterial irrigation
  - Kitner dissectors

(continues)

PROCEDURE

23-2 Abdominal Aortic Aneurysmectomy *(continued)*

Operative Preparation

Anesthesia
- General

Position
- Supine

Prep
- Axillary line to the mid-thigh

Draping
- Modified laparotomy

Practical Considerations

- The Dacron or PTFE graft will generally be bifurcated for anastomosis into the iliac arteries.
- If the aneurysm has ruptured, control of hemorrhage is the first consideration.

Operative Procedure	Technical Considerations
1. An incision is made from the xiphoid to the pubis, and the aorta is exposed as described previously.	**1.** The STSR should prepare a large self-retaining Balfour retractor for the abdominal wall, and large Deaver and Harrington retractors for the bowel.
2. The inferior mesenteric artery is isolated at the left border of the aneurysm with a vessel loop. The peritoneal incision is extended to the area over the common iliac arteries.	**2.** Vessel loops should be moistened and loaded onto hemostats before passing. Vessel loops may be red, white, or yellow for easy identification of different structures.
3. The external and internal iliac arteries are cleared for eventual vascular clamp placement. However, if the common iliac artery is aneurysmal, only the external iliac artery is mobilized. Often only one vascular clamp is applied to the distal portion of the common iliac artery bilaterally.	**3.** Atraumatic offset-Potts vascular clamps are frequently used to occlude the iliac artery.
4. The aorta is mobilized proximal to the aneurysm up to the level of the renal arteries, and cleared for eventual placement of a vascular clamp.	**4.** A large right angle may be useful to mobilize the aorta.
5. A bifurcated knitted Dacron graft is selected after sizing, and blood is drawn from the vena cava for preclotting. (If a PTFE or woven polyester is used as graft material, preclotting is not necessary.)	**5.** A 20-cc plastic syringe with a 20–23 gauge hypodermic needle is used to draw venous blood for preclotting. The STSR should have the graft in a metal bowl for saturation with blood.
6. The patient is given intravenous heparin, and vascular clamps are applied to the external and internal iliac arteries bilaterally (or to the common iliac arteries).	**6.** Note the time that the heparin is administered and the time of placement of proximal and distal vascular clamps.
7. An aortic vascular clamp is carefully applied to the aorta above the aneurysm.	**7.** The STSR should ensure that all anastomosis sutures are loaded and ready.
8. The aneurysm is opened longitudinally along the anterolateral wall and stopped just short of the aortic bifurcation. Thrombus material is removed from the interior of the aorta, and lumbar vessels are oversewn from within the aneurysm sac (Figure 23-15).	**8.** The aneurysm is opened with #11 blade on No.7 knife handle, and completed with Mayo scissors. Thrombus material should be saved for specimen.

PROCEDURE 23-2 Abdominal Aortic Aneurysmectomy *(continued)*

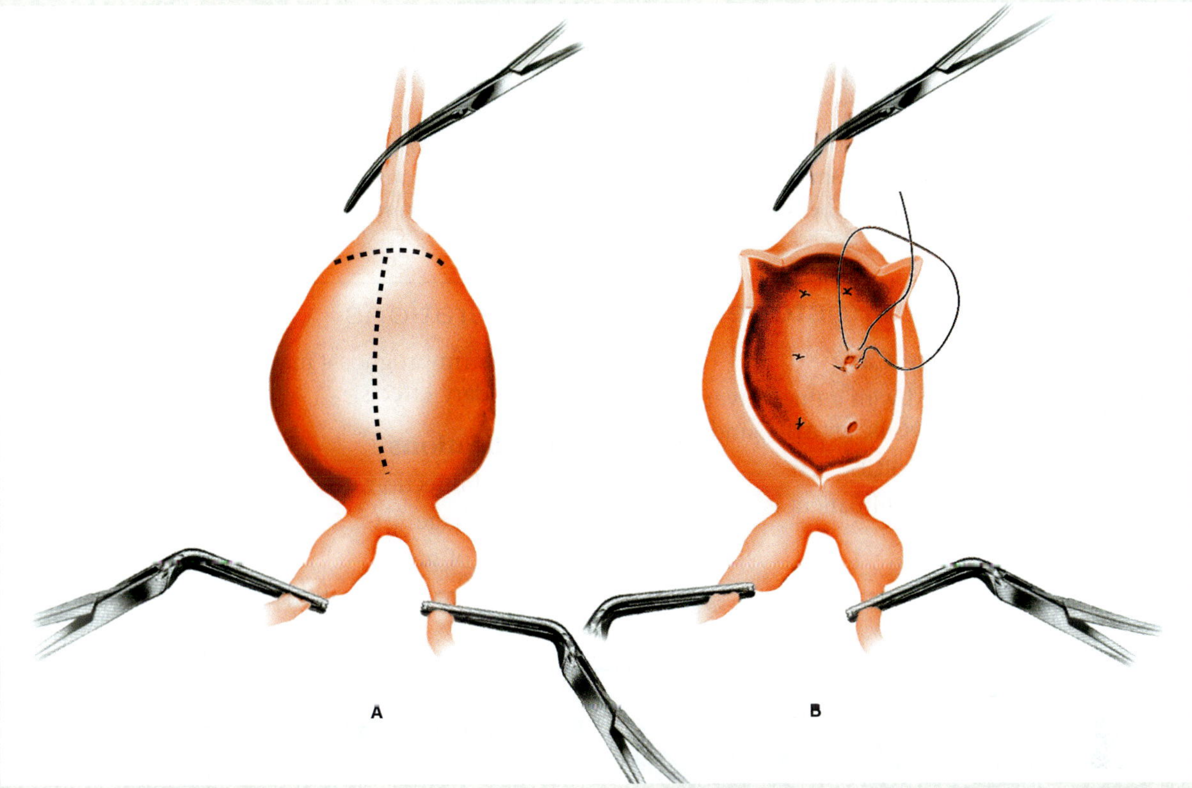

Figure 23-15 Aortic aneurysm: (A) Planned incision sites, (B) lumbar vessels oversewn

9. A T-shaped extension is cut into the proximal border of the aneurysm, and the anterior aneurysm wall is opened for copious irrigation with heparinized saline.
10. The proximal anastomosis is begun with a continuous, double-armed 4–0 Prolene suture and taper-cut needle.
11. A Fogarty clamp is placed across the graft immediately distal to the anastomosis, the aortic vascular clamp is released, and the two ends of the Prolene suture are tied together, completing the anastomosis.
12. The right limb of the graft is aspirated, brought down to the common iliac bifurcation, and cut to the correct length.
13. An arteriotomy is performed on the right common iliac vessel, and the graft limb is anastomosed in an end-to-side fashion with a double-armed 5–0 or 6–0 Prolene.

9. The "jet" action of the 20-cc syringe/heparin needle combination with heparinized saline forces small pieces of thrombus from the aortic wall.
10. 4–0 Prolene should be loaded onto a long, vascular needle holder with a narrow diamond jaw.
11. Any leaks in the proximal anastomosis are patched with interrupted, pledgeted Prolene sutures. Most patch sutures are single-armed, so the surgeon may ask the STSR to cut a double-armed Prolene suture in half.
12. Prepare to cut the graft to the appropriate size. An additional vascular clamp may be placed on the distal graft.
13. Don't try to remove knots from Prolene sutures. If a knot is found while loading the suture, simply discard the knotted Prolene and load another.

(continues)

PROCEDURE

23-2 Abdominal Aortic Aneurysmectomy *(continued)*

14. Before completion of the iliac anastomosis, the distal and proximal clamps are opened for flushing. The suture ends are tied, and circulation is opened.
15. The same process is repeated for the left side. The anterior wall of the aneurysm sac is sutured over the proximal aortic graft. The abdominal wound is closed in layers.

14. Wet the hands of the surgeon with saline before tying polypropylene sutures. Note time blood flow is restored to limb. Patch sutures may be needed.
15. Prepare closure suture. Note number of laps removed from abdominal cavity. Routine closure including counts is carried out.

Postoperative Considerations

Immediate Postoperative Care

- Wound is typically dressed with a three-layer dressing (e.g., Adaptic, 4 × 4s, an ABD, and tape).
- Transportation to PACU or SICU.
- Setup is to remain sterile until patient is transported from OR.

Prognosis

- Surgical prognosis is good.
- Long-term prognosis may vary depending on secondary effects.

Complications

- Wound infection
- Hemorrhage
- Failure of graft
- Secondary complications

PEARL OF WISDOM

For ruptured abdominal aneurysms, prepare those items that will allow access to the abdomen and exposure of the ruptured vessel first. Have a knife, cautery, Cell Saver suction, laparotomy sponges, and retractors ready to go. A Foley catheter with a 30-cc balloon may be utilized for hemorrhage control. A large aortic cross-clamp, such as a Fogarty aortic clamp, will be needed. Make sure that various size grafts are available for inspection.

FEMOROPOPLITEAL BYPASS

Although obstruction in the distal portion of the femoral artery can be adequately bypassed with synthetic graft material, the material of choice remains the autogenous saphenous vein, particularly for more distal obstructions. For *in situ* bypass, the valves of the vein must stripped for unimpeded flow of arterial blood. The procedural steps are delineated in Procedure 23-3. (*Note:* The procedure for femorotibial bypass is essentially the same as the one described here, except that the tibial artery is used as the distal anastomosis site rather than the popliteal artery.)

(Text continues on page 954)

PROCEDURE

23-3 Femoropopliteal Bypass (Unilateral)

Equipment

- Electrosurgical unit
- Suction system
- Doppler unit
- Headlight and fiberoptic light source

PROCEDURE

23-3 Femoropopliteal Bypass (Unilateral) *(continued)*

Instruments

- Minor set
- Vascular set (with instrumentation for medium and small vessels)
- Diethrich coronary artery set
- Valvulotome

Supplies

- Graft material will not be necessary for *in situ* bypass, but should be available
- Pack: laparotomy or extremity
- Basin set
- Gloves
- Blades (#10, #11, #15)
- Drapes: towels, ¾ sheet, 6-in. stockinet, laparotomy sheet
- Suture:
  - 5–0, 6–0 Prolene
  - 3–0, 4–0 silk ties, 18 in.
  - Closure suture of surgeon's choice
- Drains: optional
- Dressings: Adaptic, 4 × 4s
- Drugs: heparin, antibiotic irrigation, contrast solution
- Miscellaneous:
  - Doppler probe
  - Fogarty embolectomy catheter (assorted sizes) with tuberculin or 3-cc syringe
  - Vessel loops and/or umbilical tape
  - Laparotomy sponges
  - Ray-Tec sponges
  - Surgicel, Avitene, Gelfoam
  - Electrosurgical pencil
  - Hemoclips (small, medium)
  - Butterfly needle
  - Extension tubing
  - Variety of syringes and hypodermic needles
  - 20-cc syringe and heparin needle or Angiocath cannula for intra-arterial irrigation
  - Kitner dissectors
  - Disposable plastic bulldogs

Operative Preparation

Anesthesia

- General

Position

- Supine, with padding underneath the knees
- The affected leg should be externally rotated and abducted for access to the popliteal artery and saphenous vein

Prep

- Midabdomen to toes, with the leg prepped circumferentially
- A Foley catheter may be required

Draping

- A flat sheet is placed under the affected leg, and a folded towel is secured to the pubic area
- A 6-in. stockinet or towel wrap is placed onto the foot
- The femoral area is square-draped with towels
- Split sheets may be placed around the leg (with tails up and down), or the leg may be passed through the fenestration of a laparotomy sheet that is placed over the femoral area

Practical Considerations

- STAC should ensure that blood for the patient is available.
- Blood loss should be carefully monitored during the procedure.
- STSR should keep track of the amount of irrigation used.
- The surgeon's hands should be moistened with saline from an Asepto before tying Prolene sutures.

(continues)

PROCEDURE 23-3 Femoropopliteal Bypass (Unilateral) *(continued)*

Operative Procedure	Technical Considerations
1. The first incision is made over the distal portion of the popliteal artery, extending from the posterior border of the medial femoral condyle to just below the tibial tuberosity.	**1.** The STSR should keep contact with the exposed leg to a minimum. Weitlaner retractor will likely be used.
2. The saphenous vein is identified and inspected for size and quality, and is dissected free with its branches ligated and divided with 4–0 or 5–0 silk ties.	**2.** The STSR should have synthetic graft material available in case the saphenous vein is inadequate for grafting.
3. The distal popliteal artery is exposed by retracting the tendons of sartorius, gracilis, and semitendinosus superiorly. The gastrocnemius is retracted posteriorly.	**3.** Retractors for this phase may be U.S. Army, Richardson (small double-ended), Cushing, or vein.
4. The dissection continues distally toward the soleal arcade and the anterior tibial vein is identified, ligated, and divided.	**4.** The anterior tibial vein is ligated with 4–0 silk ties, 18 in. in length, and/or small or medium hemoclips.
5. A longitudinal incision is made into the groin over the saphenofemoral junction and the proximal portion of the saphenous vein is located, inspected, and dissected free.	**5.** Dissection is made with medium Metzenbaum scissors and medium DeBakey forceps. Handheld and/or self-retaining retractors will be necessary.
6. The tributaries of the saphenous vein are ligated with 4–0 or 5–0 silk ties and small clips.	**6.** Small, short hemoclip applicators are used with clips from the small (blue) carrier.
7. The common femoral vein is cleared in the area of its junction with the saphenous vein, and a small Satinsky partial-occlusion clamp is applied.	**7.** The partial-occlusion clamp allows blood flow to continue through the vessel because the clamp is applied to only the top portion of the vessel.
8. The saphenous vein and a small cuff of the common femoral vein is cut free from the saphenofemoral junction. The junction is closed with 6–0 Prolene suture.	**8.** 6–0 Prolene is frequently loaded onto a Castroviejo needle holder.
9. The patient is administered systemic heparin. The common femoral artery is exposed and clamped with a DeBakey angled vascular clamp.	**9.** The femoral artery will be isolated with vessel loops placed proximally and distally.
10. An arteriotomy is performed on the anterolateral portion of the common femoral artery, and the saphenous vein is anastomosed in an end-to-side fashion with a continuous 6–0 Prolene suture.	**10.** Arteriotomy is performed with #11 blade on No. 7 knife handle, and Potts coronary scissors.
11. The clamp is removed, and blood is allowed to flow up to the first valve.	**11.** Clamp will be replaced several times as procedure progresses.
12. The distal end of the saphenous vein is transected at the anastomosis site, and a Cartier valvulotome is introduced and passed through the full length of the vein.	**12.** The valvulotome will remove any valves that may prevent the flow of arterial blood to target tissues.
13. The arterialized saphenous vein is ligated at its distal end, and its medial side is marked to prevent torsion.	**13.** Marking of the vein is done with a purple marking pen so that the vein is anastomosed without a twist.

PROCEDURE 23-3 Femoropopliteal Bypass (Unilateral) *(continued)*

14. The knee is flexed and the popliteal artery is occluded with small vascular clamps.

14. Popliteal artery occlusion is usually accomplished with small bulldog vascular clamps or vessel loops tightened around the artery.

15. An incision is made into the popliteal artery and the spatulated saphenous vein is anastomosed with a continuous 6–0 or 7–0 Prolene suture. Before completion of the suture line, clamps are released to flush and the lumen is irrigated with heparinized saline (Figure 23-16).

15. Rubber shods (Prolene clamps) should be available for all vascular anastomoses. Heparin solution is prepared in advance.

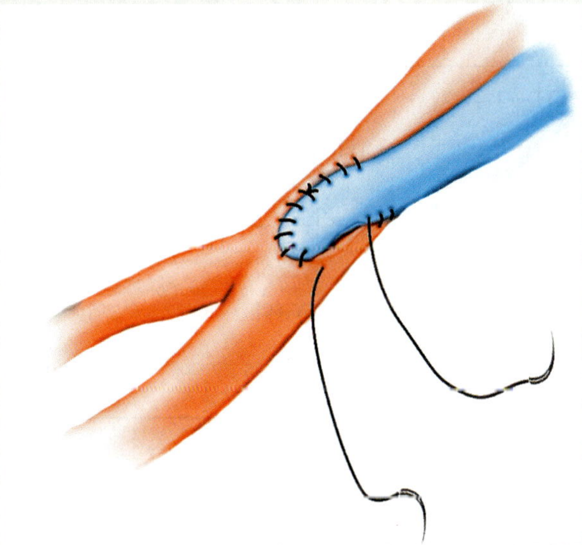

Figure 23-16 Popliteal artery—saphenous vein anastomosis

16. The suture ends are tied, and the anastomosis completed. The wounds are closed in layers.

16. Have the Doppler probe and unit available for postanastomosis vessel evaluation.

Postoperative Considerations

Immediate Postoperative Care

- The distal pulses will be evaluated by finger palpation and Doppler probe.
- STSR should maintain the sterile field until it is determined that the wound will not be reopened.

Prognosis

- Good, if blood flow has been restored to the extremity before damage to the tissue.
- Patients often suffer from diabetes and may have complications related to that disease.

Complications

- Wound infection
- Hemorrhage
- Failure of graft
- Amputation secondary to tissue damage

PEARL OF WISDOM

The STSR should be adept at handling small polypropylene sutures and small delicate needles. A white paper towel laid between the Mayo and the operative site, or on the Mayo tray itself, helps to visualize the blue suture. Needles should be returned from the surgeon directly to the STSR, because they are small and easily lost.

FEMOROFEMORAL BYPASS

A subcutaneous graft placed between the two femoral arteries is useful for any patient with unilateral iliac arterial occlusive disease or occlusion of an aortoiliac or aortofemoral prosthesis (Procedure 23-4). One iliac artery must be free of atherosclerotic plaque for this type of bypass to be successful.

PROCEDURE 23-4 Femorofemoral Bypass

Equipment

- Electrosurgical unit
- Suction system
- Doppler unit
- Headlight and fiberoptic light source

Instruments

- Minor set
- Vascular set (with instrumentation for medium and small vessels)
- Diethrich coronary artery set
- Tunneler

Supplies

- Graft material will not be necessary for *in situ* bypass, but should be available
- Pack: laparotomy
- Basin set
- Gloves
- Blades (#20, #10, #11)
- Drapes: towels, adhesive drape, laparotomy drape
- Suture:
  - 4–0, 5–0, 6–0 Prolene
  - 2–0, 3–0, 4–0 silk ties, 18–30 in.
  - 2–0, 3–0 silk stick-ties
- Drains: surgeon's preference
- Dressings: Adaptic, 4 × 4s, ABD
- Drugs: heparin, antibiotic irrigation
- Miscellaneous:
  - Doppler probe
  - Vessel loops and/or umbilical tape
  - Laparotomy sponges
  - Ray-Tec sponges
  - Surgicel, Avitene, Gelfoam
  - PTFE or Dacron polyester tube grafts and patch material
  - Electrosurgical pencil
  - Hemoclips of various sizes
  - Variety of syringes and hypodermic needles
  - Fogarty clamp inserts
  - 20-cc syringe and heparin needle or Angiocath cannula for intra-arterial irrigation
  - Kitner dissectors

Operative Preparation

Anesthesia

- General

Position

- Supine, with padding under each knee

Prep

- From mid-chest to mid-thigh
- A Foley catheter may be required

Draping

- Transverse laparotomy sheet
- Folded towel over groin—towel may be secured with towel clips or skin staples

PROCEDURE

23-4 Femorofemoral Bypass *(continued)*

Practical Considerations

- Blood loss should be carefully monitored during the procedure. The STSR should keep track of the amount of irrigation used
- The surgeon's hands should be moistened with saline from an Asepto before tying Prolene sutures

Operative Procedure

1. The procedure begins with incisions in each groin over the common femoral artery.
2. The common femoral, superficial, and deep femoral arteries are dissected free and isolated with vessel loops.
3. A subcutaneous, suprapubic tunnel is established between the two femoral arteries with a tunneling device and finger dissection.
4. A PTFE or Dacron graft is passed through the tunnel and cut to length. The patient is systemically heparinized.
5. Vascular clamps are placed on the common, superficial, and deep femoral arteries, and an incision is made into the common femoral artery.
6. The right side of the graft is anastomosed to the right common-deep femoral segment in an end-to-side fashion with a continuous 6–0 Prolene suture, and the same is done for the left side (Figure 23-17).

Technical Considerations

1. Incisions are made with a #10 blade on a No. 3 knife handle.
2. Moisten vessel loops and umbilical tapes and load them on a hemostat.
3. The tunnel is typically made with a Sarot clamp.
4. The STSR should watch closely to ensure that the graft is not twisted when placed through the tunnel.
5. DeBakey angled vascular clamps are used for the common femoral arteries, and bulldog vascular clamps are used for the smaller arteries.
6. The STSR should be prepared to follow the Prolene if necessary.

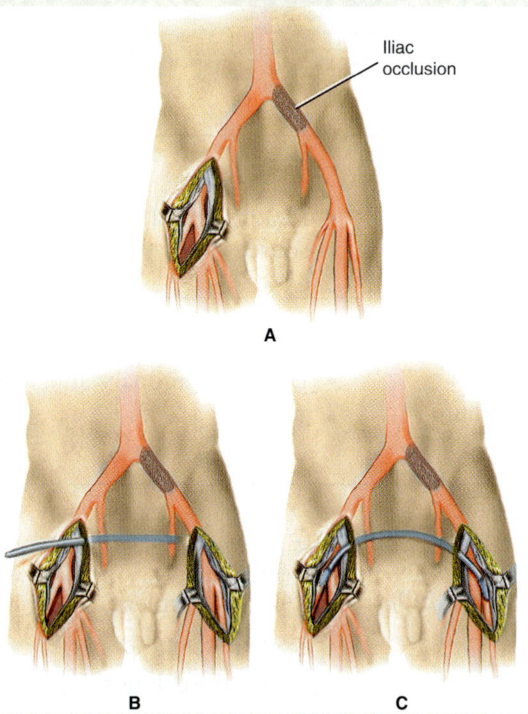

Figure 23-17 Femorofemoral bypass: (A) Occlusion site and primary incision, (B) secondary incision and creation of the tunnel, (C) graft positioned and blood flow restored to the left lower extremity

(continues)

PROCEDURE 23-4 Femorofemoral Bypass *(continued)*

7. The vascular clamps are removed, and the incisions closed.

7. The STSR should be ready for intraoperative arteriogram after the final anastomosis is completed.

Postoperative Considerations

Immediate Postoperative Care

- The two incisions are typically dressed with an inner contact layer and 4 × 4s.

Prognosis

- Good, if blood flow has been established in time.

Complications

- Wound infection
- Hemorrhage
- Failure of graft
- Amputation secondary to tissue damage

PEARL OF WISDOM

Be sure that the suture does not catch on any instrumentation that must remain on the field. It may be helpful to cover the rings of the Weitlaner with a towel.

AXILLOFEMORAL BYPASS

If abdominal surgery is contraindicated for aortoiliac reconstruction, subcutaneous passage of a tube graft prosthesis from the axillary artery to femoral artery is an option for consideration (Procedure 23-5).

PROCEDURE 23-5 Axillofemoral Bypass

Equipment

- Electrosurgical unit
- Suction system
- Doppler unit
- Headlight and fiberoptic light source

Instruments

- Minor set
- Vascular set (with instrumentation for medium and small vessels)
- Diethrich coronary artery set
- Tunneler

Supplies

- Pack: basic
- Basin set
- Gloves
- Blades (#10, #11, #15)
- Drapes: towels, adhesive drape, ¾ sheets, stockinet (4 in., 6 in.), split sheets
- Suture:
  - 5–0, 6–0 Prolene
  - 3–0, 4–0 silk ties, 18 in.
  - 3–0 silk stick-ties

PROCEDURE 23-5 Axillofemoral Bypass *(continued)*

Closure suture of surgeon's preference

- Drains: surgeon's preference
- Dressings: Adaptic, 4 × 4s
- Drugs: heparin, antibiotic irrigation
- Miscellaneous:

  Doppler probe

  Vessel loops and/or umbilical tape

  Laparotomy sponges

  Ray-Tec sponges

  Surgicel, Avitene, Gelfoam

  PTFE or Dacron polyester grafts and patch material

  Electrosurgical pencil

  Hemoclips of various sizes

  Variety of syringes and hypodermic needles

  Fogarty clamp inserts

  20-cc syringe and heparin needle or Angiocath cannula for intra-arterial irrigation

  Kitner dissectors

Operative Preparation

Anesthesia

- General

Position

- Supine
- Arm on the affected side may be extended on an armboard, and the shoulder elevated with a roll

Prep

- From the right shoulder and upper extremity to the mid-thigh of the affected side

Draping

- ¾ sheet is placed under the affected lower extremity and over the unaffected lower extremity
- A 6-in. stockinet is rolled up to the thigh
- Another ¾ sheet is placed under the upper extremity on the affected side
- A 4-in. stockinet is rolled up to the shoulder
- The area between the two incision sites is square-draped with towels, and a folded towel is secured to the groin. Split sheets are placed with tails up and down, exposing the area along and between the femoral incision site and the axillary incision site

Practical Considerations

- The STSR should be sure that various sizes and types of grafts are available for inspection by the surgeon
- Arteriogram studies should be in the room before the procedure begins

Operative Procedure

1. An incision is made in the groin for exposure of the common femoral artery to find a suitable anastomosis site.
2. An incision is made over the axillary artery, and the proximal segment of the axillary artery is dissected free and isolated with vessel loops.
3. A tunnel is developed between the axillary incision and the relay incision within the deep fascia of the chest wall, and extended to the groin subcutaneously.

Technical Considerations

1. The STSR should be ready with medium Metzenbaum scissors, medium DeBakey forceps, and a Weitlaner retractor.
2. The STSR should have a medium right angle ready to pass for placement of vessel loops.
3. Small incisions between the two primary incisions are referred to as "relay" incisions.

(continues)

PROCEDURE 23-5 Axillofemoral Bypass *(continued)*

4. An umbilical tape or heavy silk suture may be placed through the full length of the tunnel as a guide.

4. 0 silk is typically used to pull the graft from the axillary incision to the femoral incision.

5. The patient is heparinized, the axillary artery is clamped and incised, and a PTFE graft is anastomosed to the artery in an end-to-side fashion with a 5–0 or 6–0 Prolene suture (Figure 23-18).

5. DeBakey angled vascular clamps are typically used to occlude the axillary artery. A variety of bulldog vascular clamps should be available.

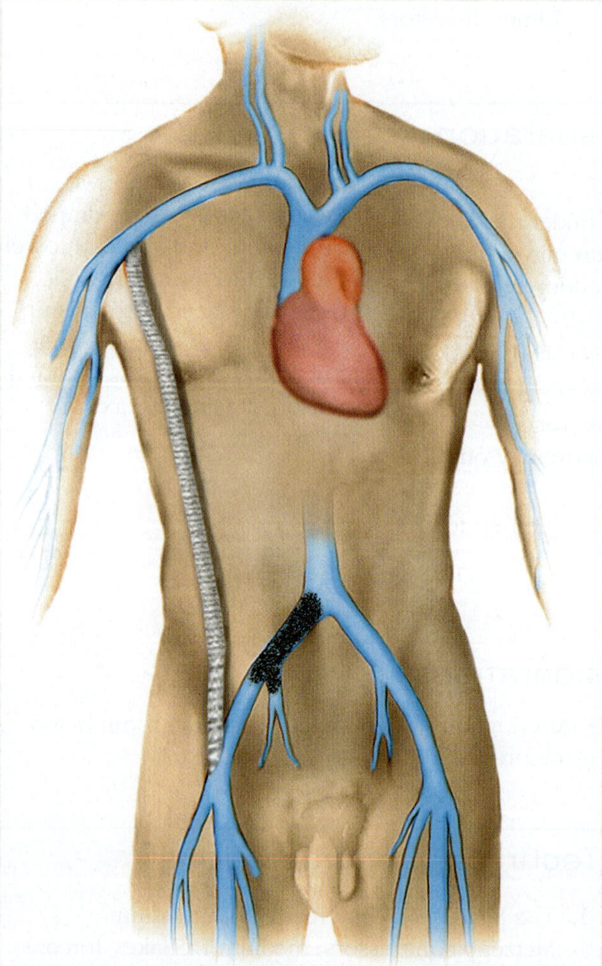

Figure 23-18 Axillofemoral bypass

6. The distal end of the graft is occluded with a heavy tie. The graft is filled with arterial blood and drawn through the tunnel to the femoral exposure.

6. The graft may be tailored to size. Be sure graft is not twisted or kinked.

7. The femoral anastomosis is carried out and the wounds closed.

7. Repeat anastomotic steps. Both wounds are closed and counts performed.

PROCEDURE

23-5 Axillofemoral Bypass *(continued)*

Postoperative Considerations

Immediate Postoperative Care

- The primary incisions are typically dressed with an inner contact layer and 4 × 4s.
- The relay incisions are dressed with small gauze pieces.

Prognosis

- Good, if blood flow has been reestablished in sufficient time.

Complications

- Wound infection
- Hemorrhage
- Failure of graft
- Amputation secondary to tissue damage

PEARL OF WISDOM

For procedures that involve tunneling for graft placement between two separate anastomosis sites, a particular pattern is typically followed. The anastomosis sites are exposed through two primary incisions. A tunneler of some sort that can create a space in the connective tissues between the primary incisions is utilized. Some specialty cardiovascular tunnelers are designed to accept one end of the synthetic graft after the tunnel has been made, so that it can be pulled through the tunnel to the destination site. If long clamps, such as the Sarot clamp, are utilized to create the tunnel, small relay incisions between the two primary incisions are necessary so that silk sutures can be tied together to create a relay for graft movement through the tunnel. Once positioned and checked for twisting, the graft can be sutured to the arteries.

CAROTID ENDARTERECTOMY

The primary indication for carotid endarterectomy is transient cerebral ischemia (Procedure 23-6). Small pieces of plaque break away from the common carotid or internal carotid artery and are flushed upstream to lodge in small cerebral vessels, temporarily blocking blood flow to that particular area of the brain. These forerunners to permanent stroke are referred to as transient ischemic attacks (TIAs). Patients suffering from TIAs often demonstrate a contralateral weakness that worsens over a series of episodes. They may exhibit confusion and/or speech difficulty that resolves or gets better a day or so following an episode. Both patients and their families are usually frightened by these episodes.

(Text continues on page 963)

PROCEDURE

23-6 Carotid Endarterectomy

Equipment

- Electrosurgical unit
- Suction system
- Electroencephalogram may be required, especially if no shunt is used

(continues)

PROCEDURE 23-6 **Carotid Endarterectomy** *(continued)*

Instruments

- Carotid set
- Minor set
- Javid shunt clamps
- Hemoclip applicators (short, medium, and small)

Supplies

- Pack: laparotomy or basic
- Basin set
- Gloves
- Blades (#10, #11)
- Drapes: towels, laparotomy drape, or pedi or thyroid sheet
- Suture:
  - 6–0, 7–0 Prolene
  - 3–0, 4–0 silk ties, 18 in.
  - Closure suture of surgeon's choice
- Drains: surgeon's preference; typically a ½-in. Penrose with safety pin
- Dressings: Adaptic, 4 × 4s
- Drugs: heparin for saline irrigation, antibiotic irrigation, Xylocaine 1% for carotid body injection
- Miscellaneous:
  - Vessel loops and/or umbilical tape
  - Laparotomy sponges
  - Ray-Tec sponges
  - Surgicel, Avitene, Gelfoam
  - Electrosurgical pencil
  - Hemoclips (small and medium)
  - Variety of syringes and hypodermic needles
  - 20-cc syringe and heparin needle or Angiocath cannula for intra-arterial irrigation
  - Javid shunts (available)

Operative Preparation

Anesthesia

- General

Position

- Supine position with the head turned approximately 45 degrees to the unaffected side
- Head should rest on a donut headrest or rolled 6-in. stockinet, and a shoulder roll may be necessary for neck extension
- Arms should be tucked at the patient's side. Protect the ulnar nerves
- If a saphenous vein patch graft is to be procured, the affected leg should be bent at the knee and externally rotated

Prep

- From the lower ear of the affected side, across the midline of the neck, to just below the clavicle
- If saphenous vein graft is to be procured, lower limb of choice must also be prepped

Draping

- Square-draping with towels and thyroid sheet or pediatric sheet
- A ¾ sheet or medium sheet may be placed over the feet
- If a saphenous vein graft is to be procured, a ¾ sheet should be placed under the affected leg and over the unaffected leg, and a 6-in. stockinet should be rolled over the foot up to the area of incision. A folded towel should be secured over the groin, and the laparotomy, pedi, or thyroid sheet should be folded under at the top of the pubis

Practical Considerations

- No synthetic graft material will be necessary
- A Javid or Argyle shunt is frequently used for shunting cerebral blood flow
- If a graft is necessary, a small portion of the saphenous vein is obtained and trimmed to size

PROCEDURE

23-6 Carotid Endarterectomy *(continued)*

Operative Procedure

1. An incision is made in the anterior line of the sternocleidomastoid, over the carotid bifurcation.
2. The common, internal, and external carotid arteries are dissected free and isolated with vessel loops.
3. Heparin is administered systemically, and clamps are applied first to the internal carotid, then to the external carotid, and finally to the common carotid artery (Figure 23-19).

Technical Considerations

1. Incision is made with a #10 blade on a No. 3 knife handle. Two folded sponges should be placed on opposite sides of the operative site. A magnetic mat placed over the chest is useful for procedures of the neck.
2. Dissection is accomplished with small or medium Metzenbaum scissors and small or medium DeBakey forceps.
3. Angled vascular and bulldog vascular clamps are used for occlusion. The internal and external carotid arteries may be occluded with vessel loops. Note time of heparin administration and vessel occlusion.

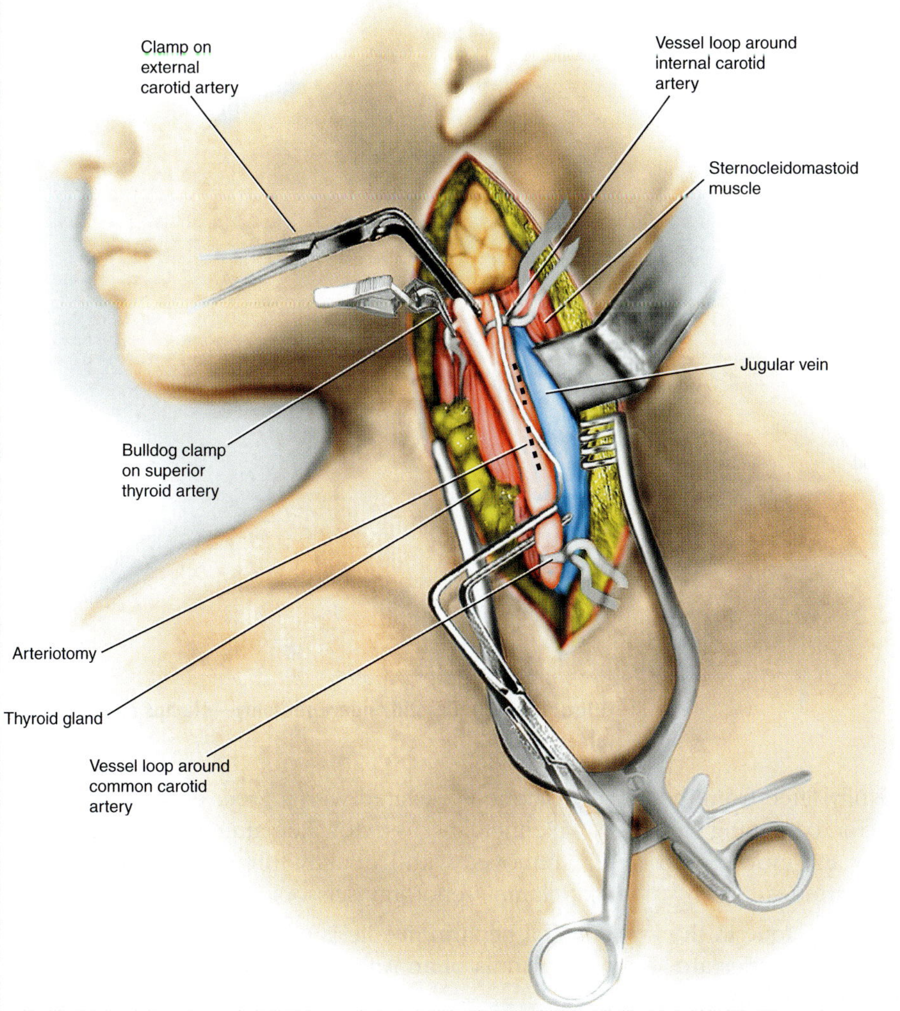

Figure 23-19 Restrictive devices applied to the common, external, and internal carotid arteries—line of arteriotomy is shown

(continues)

PROCEDURE

23-6 Carotid Endarterectomy *(continued)*

4. An arteriotomy is made along the lateral portion of the distal common carotid artery and, with the use of Potts coronary scissors, is extended into the internal carotid artery.

4. Arteriotomy is begun with a #11 knife blade on a No. 7 knife handle.

5. A Javid or Argyle shunt is placed into the common carotid and internal carotid artery. The Javid shunt is held in place with Javid shunt clamps. The Argyle shunt is held in place with clamped vessel loops or tapes (Figure 23-20).

5. If the surgeon prefers to proceed without shunting, the STSR should be prepared for a faster paced procedure. The surgeon will not dally with flow shutoff to one side of the brain.

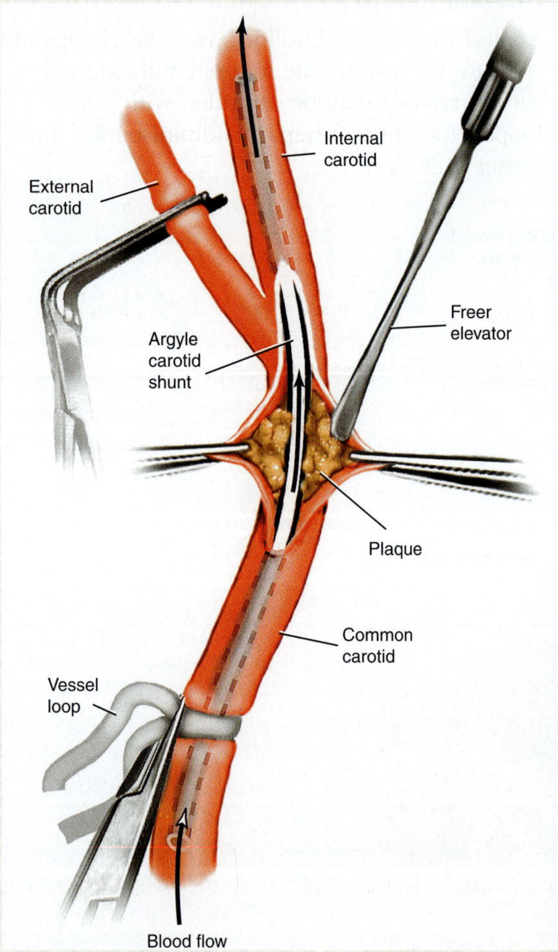

Figure 23-20 Carotid endarterectomy—clamps and shunt in place

6. The atheromatous core is carefully lifted from the arterial wall with a blunt dissector, beginning in the distal common carotid artery and moving into the external and internal carotid arteries.

6. Plaque is elevated with a Freer elevator or Penfield #4 dissector. Remaining pieces are removed with DeBakey forceps and mosquito clamp. Tenotomy scissors may also be used.

7. An end point is established for the plaque in the distal internal carotid artery, and the arteries are irrigated with heparinized saline to wash away any stray media or fibrin strands.

7. If a heparin needle is not available, the plastic cannula of an Angiocath needle works nicely.

PROCEDURE

23-6 Carotid Endarterectomy *(continued)*

8. The arteriotomy is closed directly with 6–0 and 7–0 Prolene sutures. (*Note:* An autogenous vein patch may be utilized for closure of the arteriotomy.)

9. The vascular clamps are removed from the common, external, and internal carotid arteries (in that order), a drain is placed and secured, and the wound is closed.

8. Note time blood flow is restored. Vein patch may be procured at this time, but it is likely that it has been secured prior to neck incision if its use is anticipated.

9. ½-in. Penrose drains are frequently used for procedures of the neck. The STSR should ensure that the Penrose drain is secured with a safety pin. Penrose drains require bulky 4 × 4 dressings for fluid absorption.

Postoperative Considerations

Immediate Postoperative Care

- The patient's neurological signs should be closely monitored for postoperative changes.

Prognosis

- If neurological signs are intact, the prognosis is good.

Complications

- Stroke
- Wound infection
- Hemorrhage

PEARL OF WISDOM

There is a typical procedural sequence to all endarterectomies after vessel exposure is achieved. The sequence represents a pattern that appears often in peripheral vascular surgery. It is as follows:

1. The vessel is dissected free from surrounding tissues.
2. A right-angle clamp is placed underneath the vessel and opened.
3. Vessel loops or umbilical tapes loaded onto hemostats are fed into the right-angle clamp proximally and distally.
4. The vessel loops are clamped with hemostats.
5. Vascular clamps are applied to the vessel proximally and distally.
6. Arteriotomy is begun with a #11 blade on a #7 handle, and continued with Potts scissors.

All patients who have been diagnosed with a lesion of the common/internal carotid artery should undergo transfemoral arteriography to outline the specific location of the lesion and to view intracerebral vasculature for possible occlusions. CT scan will rule out cerebral infarction.

Intraoperative cerebral protection is accomplished with balanced anesthesia for maximum blood pressure stability and reduced cerebral oxygen demands. Many surgeons prefer to divert cerebral blood flow with a Javid or Argyle shunt during the procedure; others feel that the shunt is unnecessary and cumbersome, especially if the surgeon works quickly and cerebral functions are closely monitored. Electroencephalogram may be utilized to monitor the patient for signs of cerebral hypoxia.

CASE STUDY

Thelma is a 65-year-old diabetic scheduled for a femoropopliteal bypass. The OR team knows her from past visits to the OR. Her overall health appears to them to be worsening.

1. What is the relationship between diabetes and the condition leading to this procedure?
2. What is Thelma's prognosis?
3. What are the complications related to the procedure and for which of these is Thelma at high risk?

QUESTIONS FOR FURTHER STUDY

1. What is meant by collateral flow?
2. What is the difference between ischemia and infarction?
3. Why aren't the neurological deficits associated with transient ischemia attacks permanent?
4. Describe the method for loading a pledget with a double-armed needle for use during an aortofemoral bypass.
5. Why is preclotting a PTFE or woven polyester graft not necessary?
6. What two surgical instruments are used to create the arteriotomy in the common carotid artery during an endarterectomy?

BIBLIOGRAPHY

Cameron, J. L. (1989). *Current surgical therapy* (3rd ed.). Burlington, Ontario: B. C. Decker.

Carter, D. C., & Dudley, H. (Eds.). (1985). *Rob & Smith's operative surgery* (4th ed.). St. Louis, MO: Mosby.

Cormier, J. M., & Ward, A. S. (1986). *Operative techniques in arterial surgery* (1st ed.). Chicago: Precept Press.

Edwards, W. H. (Ed.). (1976). *Vascular surgery* (1st ed.). Baltimore: University Park Press.

Grabowski, S. R., & Tortora, G. J. (1996). *Principles of anatomy and physiology* (8th ed.). New York: Harper-Collins.

Harvey, A. M., Johns, R. J., McKusick, V. A., Owens, A. H., & Ross, R. S. (Eds.). (1988). *The principles and practices of medicine* (22nd ed.). East Norwalk, CT: Appleton & Lange.

Hole, J. W. (1990). *Human anatomy and physiology* (4th ed.). Dubuque, IA: Wm. C. Brown.

McGuiness, A. M., et al. (2002). *Core curriculum for surgical technology* (5th ed.). Centennial, CO: Association of Surgical Technologists.

Sabiston, D. C., Jr. (1991). *Textbook of surgery. The biological basis of modern surgical practice* (15th ed.). Philadelphia: W. B. Saunders.

Sanders, T., & Scanlon, V. C. (1995). *Essentials of anatomy and physiology* (2nd ed.). Philadelphia: F. A. Davis.

Snelgrove, D. L. (1996). The carotid body tumor. *The Surgical Technologist 28,* 8–11.

Zelinskas, E. J. (1993). Abdominal aortic aneurysmectomy with graft bypass. *The Surgical Technologist 25,* 8–23.

Zelinskas, E. J. (1995). Carotid endarterectomy. *The Surgical Technologist 27,* 8–14.

CHAPTER 24

Neurosurgery

Paul Price
Ben D. Price

CASE STUDY

Katy is a 10-year-old girl who was admitted to the emergency room after falling from a school yard slide and sustaining an injury to her head. Katy initially lost consciousness, but awoke soon after complaining of nausea and a severe left-sided headache. She developed right-sided hemiparesis within minutes of the injury. On arrival at the emergency room, she was conscious and responding to verbal commands.

A neurosurgeon called to the emergency room examined Katy. During the examination, Katy's condition began to deteriorate rapidly. As she lost consciousness, her blood pressure rose rapidly and her pulse rate fell. Her left pupil became fixed and dilated. The neurosurgeon informed the OR that an emergency procedure should be scheduled and appropriate personnel summoned.

1. What is the suspected diagnosis?
2. Why did the neurosurgeon schedule an emergency procedure?
3. What procedure did the neurosurgeon schedule?

OBJECTIVES

After studying this chapter, the reader should be able to:

A 1. Discuss the relevant anatomy and physiology of the neurological system.

P 2. Describe the pathology that prompts surgical intervention of the neurological system and the related terminology.

3. Discuss any special preoperative neurological diagnostic procedures/tests.
4. Discuss any preoperative preparation procedures related to neurosurgery.

O 5. Identify the names and uses of neurosurgical instruments, supplies, and drugs.

6. Identify the names and uses of special equipment related to neurosurgery.
7. Discuss the intraoperative preparation of the patient undergoing the neurosurgical procedure.

8. Define and give an overview of the neurosurgical procedure.
9. Discuss the purpose and expected outcomes of the neurosurgical procedure.
10. Discuss the immediate postoperative care and possible complications of the neurosurgical procedure.
11. S Discuss any specific variations related to the preoperative, intraoperative, and postoperative care of the neurosurgical patient.
12. Discuss recent advances in neurosurgery.

SELECT KEY TERMS

1. abscess	7. CNS	14. ICP	20. radiculopathy
2. acute	8. decompress	15. integration	21. somatic nervous system
3. autonomic nervous system	9. dysraphism	16. meninges	22. sympathetic nervous system
4. cerebellum	10. epidural	17. osteophyte	23. TIA
5. cerebrum	11. extruded	18. parasympathetic nervous system	24. transphenoidal
6. circle of Willis	12. glioma	19. PNS	
	13. hematoma		

SURGICAL ANATOMY

Surgery on the nervous system involves the brain, spinal cord, peripheral nerves, and the protective structures that surround them.

DIVISIONS OF THE NERVOUS SYSTEM

The nervous system of the human body is divided into two systems: the central nervous system (**CNS**), comprised of the brain and spinal cord; and the peripheral nervous system (**PNS**), comprised of the nerves that link the various parts of the body to the CNS (Figure 24-1). The PNS includes the cranial nerves that originate from the brain, and the spinal nerves that originate from the spinal cord. The primary functions of the nervous system are:

1. *Sensory:* The nervous system detects alterations of internal and external stimuli.
2. *Integrative:* Sensory information is analyzed and appropriate behaviors are selected in response.
3. *Motor:* The appropriate behaviors are implemented.

The PNS can be divided into the **somatic nervous system** (SNS) and the **autonomic nervous system** (ANS). The SNS connects the CNS to skin and skeletal muscles via the cranial and spinal nerves, initiating voluntary responses; and the ANS connects the CNS to visceral organs via the cranial and spinal nerves, initiating involuntary responses. The ANS can be subdivided into the **sympathetic** and **parasympathetic nervous systems**. A sympathetic response prepares the body to deal with emergencies through the expenditure of energy (the "fight or flight" response), whereas a parasympathetic response restores homeostatic balance and conserves energy.

The surgical team is typically concerned with the following neurosurgical divisions: the cranium and its coverings, the brain and its protective coverings, the spinal cord and its protective coverings, the spinal column, and the peripheral nerves.

CRANIUM

The cranium encloses and protects the brain and is covered with skin, subcutaneous tissue, galea aponeurotica, and periosteum. Muscles of the cranium that are typically encountered during neurosurgery include the epicranius, consisting of two parts: the frontalis muscle, which covers the frontal bone, and the occipitalis muscle, which covers

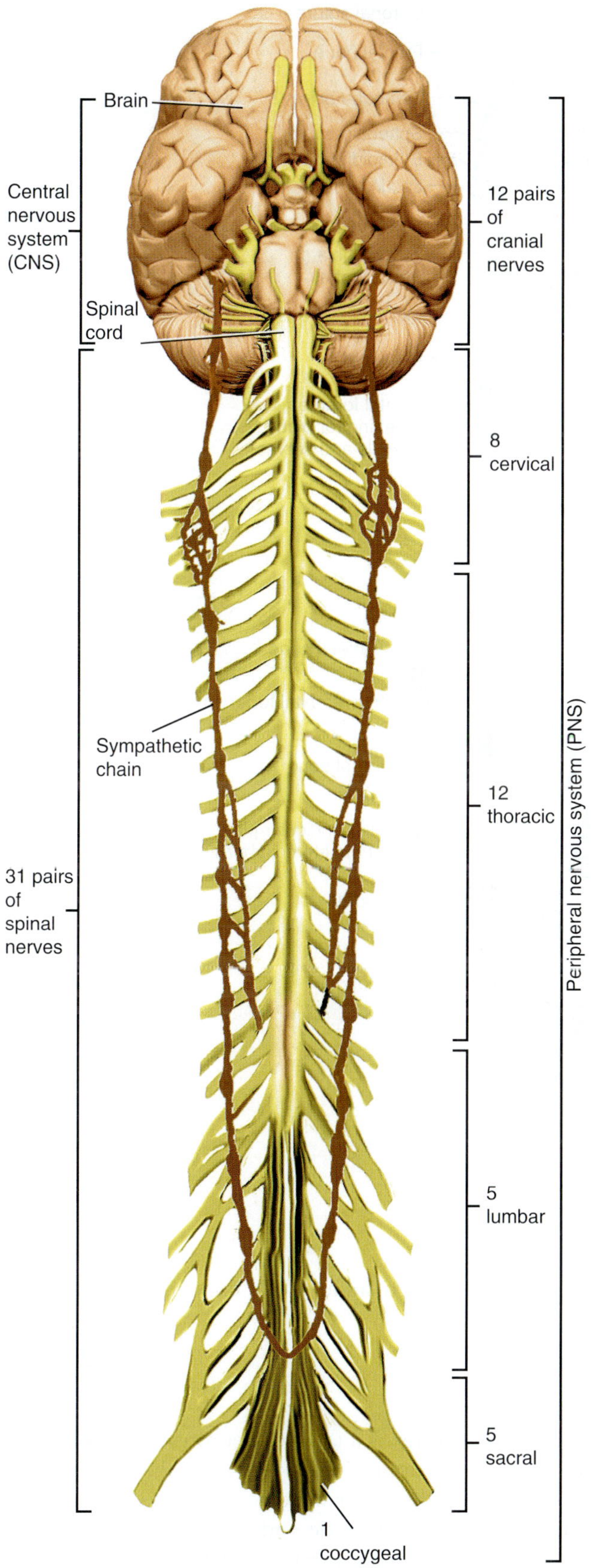

Figure 24-1 Divisions of the nervous system

the occipital bone; and the temporalis muscle, which lies over the temporal bone.

The cranium consists of eight bones:

- One frontal bone, forming the forehead, nasal cavity, and orbital roofs.
- Two parietal bones on each side of the skull; just posterior to the frontal bone, forming a large portion of the sides and roof of the cranium.
- One occipital bone, forming the back and a large portion of the floor of the cranium.
- Two temporal bones, forming a small portion of the sides and floor of the cranium.
- One sphenoid bone, forming portions of the base of the cranium, sides of the skull, and base and sides for the orbits.
- One ethmoid bone that forms portions of the roof and walls of the nasal cavity, the floor of the cranium, and walls of the orbits (Figure 24-2).

BRAIN

The human brain weighs slightly less than 3 pounds and is composed of approximately 100 billion neurons that communicate with each other through electrochemical pulses. These complex interactions are ultimately responsible for all human physical and mental functions. Neurons are the same as other body cells except that they are specialized to gather and evaluate information from the internal and external environment, and then coordinate a response to that information.

When sectioned, the brain reveals area of white and gray contrasts. The gray coloration, also known as gray matter, is a collection of large numbers of cell bodies. Examples of gray matter include the cerebral cortex on the surface of the brain and the basal ganglia deep within the brain. The white coloration, also known as white matter, is a collection of bundles of axons, covered in the protective sheath of myelin, leading away from the cell bodies through the brain. White matter consists of association fibers that transmit impulses between specific locations in the same hemisphere, commissural fibers that transmit impulses between specific locations between hemispheres, and projection fibers that transmit information back and forth between the **cerebrum** and deeper brain structures and the spinal cord.

Meninges

Three layers of protective tissue called the cranial **meninges** cover the brain and spinal cord. The outermost layer, referred to as dura mater, is composed of tough fibrous connective tissue. The dura mater extends between the cerebral hemispheres within the longitudinal fissure and is referred to as the falx cerebri. Dura mater also extends between the cerebellar hemispheres and is referred to as the falx cerebelli. The dural extension

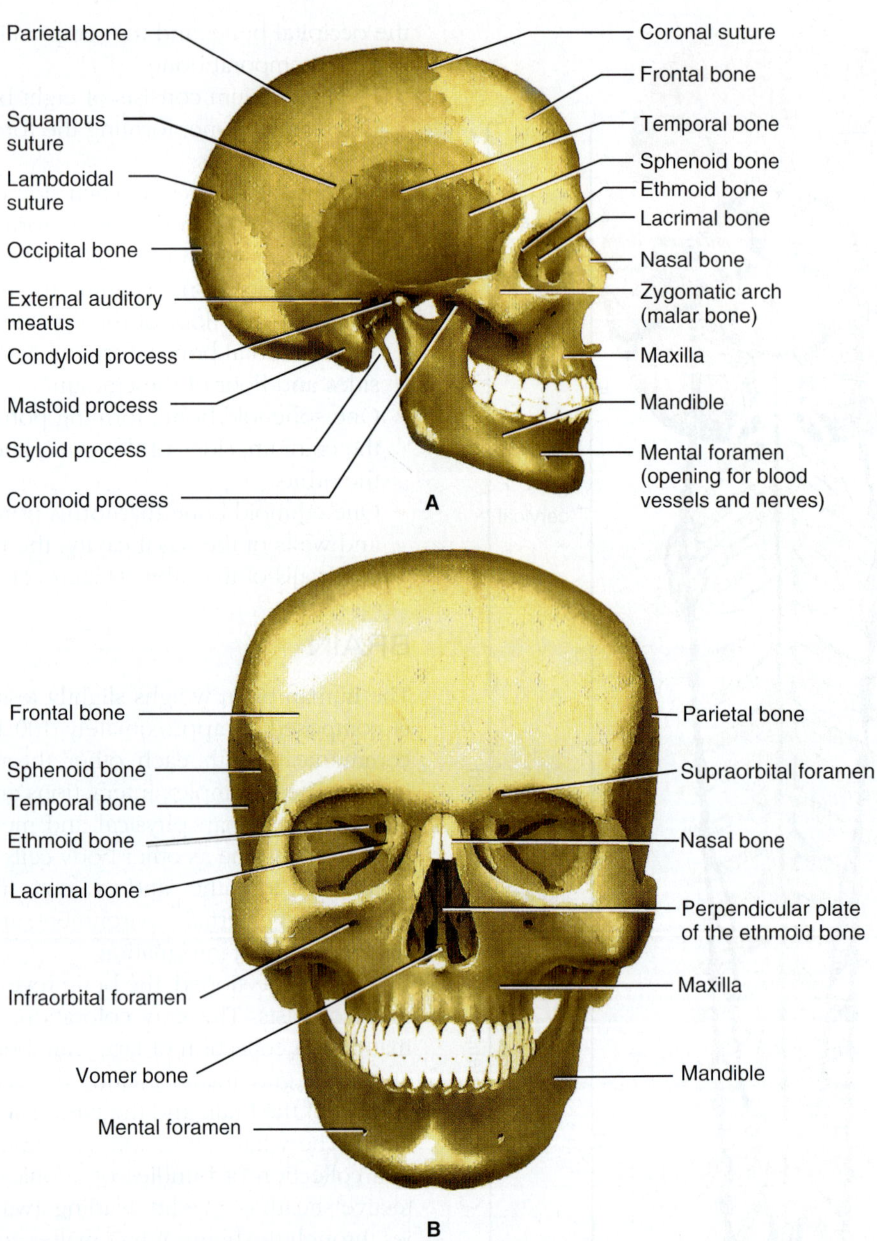

Figure 24-2 Cranial bones: (A) Lateral view, (B) anterior view

between the cerebrum and the **cerebellum** is called the tentorium cerebelli. In certain areas, the dura mater separates and creates channels for venous blood from cranial veins. These channels are called dural sinuses. The dura mater of the spinal cord does not attach directly to the bones of the vertebrae, but creates a space between bone and dura called the **epidural** space.

The middle meningeal layer is a thin, web-like membrane lacking blood vessels called the arachnoid mater. The innermost layer is the pia mater; it contains blood vessels and nerves for the nourishment of the neural tissue underneath. The space created between the arachnoid mater and the pia mater is referred to as the subarachnoid space, an area that contains cerebral spinal fluid (Figure 24-3).

Cortex

The cerebral cortex is a layer of neurons on the surface of the brain that is approximately 2–4 mm thick. These neurons are specialized for specific functions, and are distributed across layers in the cortex. Approximately 25% of the cortical neurons are located in definite regions and are in charge of processing specific stimuli and motor responses. The great majority of cortical neurons, however, have association properties; that is, they integrate infor-

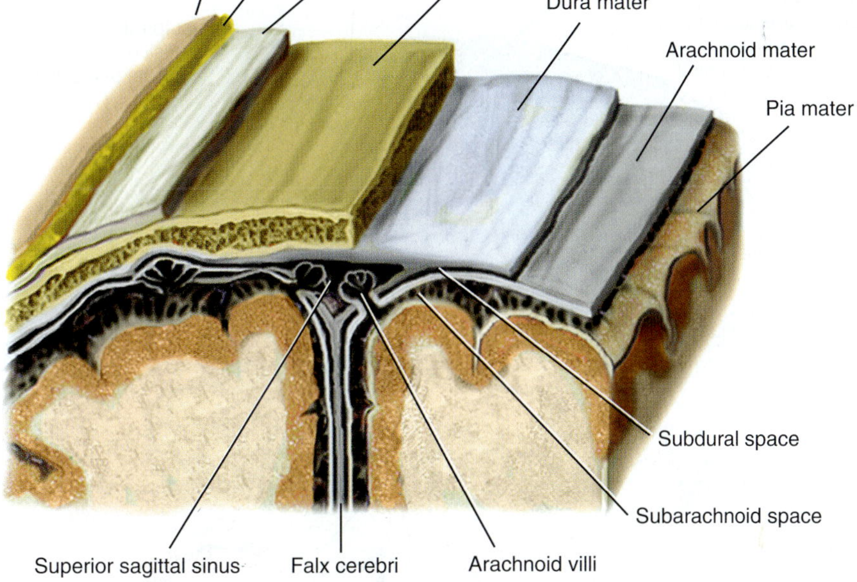

Figure 24-3 Meninges and related structures

mation from various portions of the brain into cohesive patterns. For example, the association areas of the parietal lobe process somatosensory data from the skin, muscles, tendons, and joints with data related to body posture and movements. These stimuli are integrated with stimuli from hearing and visual brain centers, allowing a conscious thought to be formulated about precise body location. The cerebral cortex represents the most recent evolutionary addition to the central nervous system, and ultimately separates humans from lower mammals.

Cerebrum

The cerebrum represents the largest portion of the human brain. Its surface is covered with convolutions (gyri) that are separated by shallow depressions (sulci) and deep grooves (fissures). The cerebrum is divided into two separate halves, or hemispheres, by a prominent central groove called the longitudinal fissure. The transverse fissure separates the cerebrum from the cerebellum.

Each hemisphere has important functional distinctions; for instance, the left hemisphere generally handles speech functions, while the right hemisphere deals with nonverbal, intuitive behaviors. Although both hemispheres share common functions of sensory **integration** and contralateral motor control, one hemisphere almost always "dominates" the other. For 90% of the population, the left hemisphere is the dominant hemisphere because it controls verbal, computational, and analytical skills.

The two hemispheres are connected by a thick bundle of commissural nerve fibers referred to as the corpus callosum and anterior and posterior commissures. These structures allow for communication between the two brain halves.

The cerebrum is divided by sulci and fissures into specific lobes, each with complex functions and named for the cranial bone that covers it. The anterior portion of the cerebrum is called the frontal lobe. Its posterior boundary is the central sulcus, also known as the fissure of Rolando, and its lateral boundary is the lateral sulcus, or fissure of Sylvius. Just posterior to the frontal lobe is the parietal lobe, separated from the frontal lobe by the fissure of Rolando. The occipital lobe forms the posterior region of the cerebrum and has no clear demarcation from the parietal lobe. The temporal lobe lies just inferior to the frontal lobe and is separated from it and the parietal lobe by the fissure of Sylvius (Figure 24-4).

The association areas of the frontal lobes are responsible for the elaboration of thinking, planning, problem solving, and judgment of consequences of behavior. The motor areas of the frontal lobes, located in the precentral gyrus just anterior to the central sulcus, control voluntary muscle movements. The parietal lobes contain sensory areas, located in the postcentral gyrus just posterior to the central sulcus, that are responsible for the sensation of touch, proprioception, temperature, and pain. The association areas of the parietal lobes help to interpret sensory information, make sense of speech, and formulate words with emotional content. The sensory areas of the temporal lobes are primarily responsible for hearing, and the association areas are used to understand speech, read printed words, and recall visual memory and

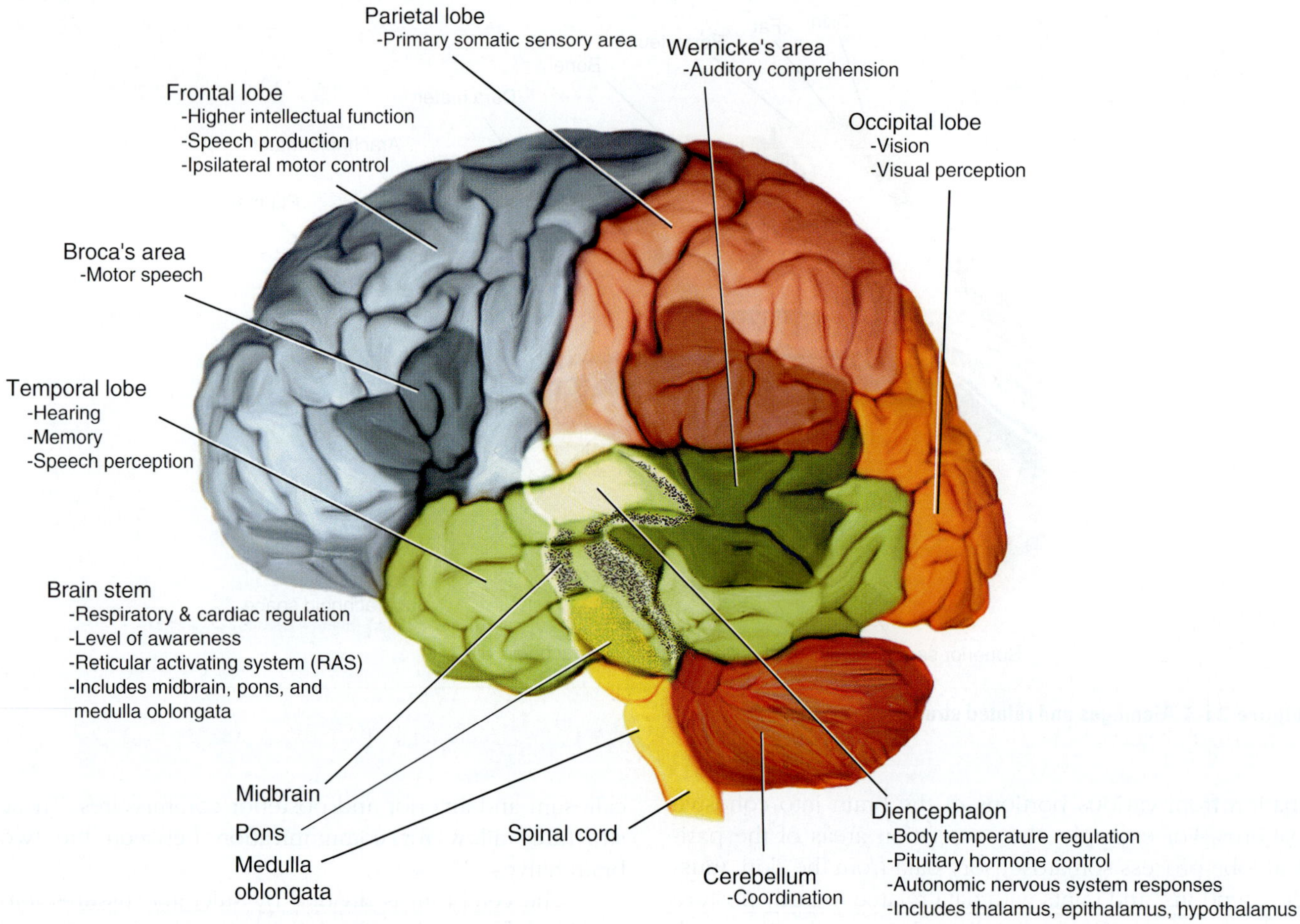

Figure 24-4 Functions of the cerebrum, brain stem, and cerebellum

music. The sensory areas of the occipital lobes are responsible for vision, and the association areas integrate visual patterns with other sensory stimuli.

Ventricles and Cerebral Spinal Fluid

Within the brain are a series of interconnected canals and cavities called ventricles. The first two ventricles are referred to as the lateral ventricles (right and left). The two large ventricles which are located in each cerebral hemisphere connect to the smaller third ventricle, located between the halves of the thalamus, by way of the interventricular foramen (foramen of Monro). The third ventricle connects to the even smaller fourth ventricle, located in the brain stem anterior to the cerebellum, by way of the cerebral aqueduct (aqueduct of Sylvius). The fourth ventricle is continuous with the central canal of the spinal cord (Figure 24-5).

The ventricles are filled with a clear, colorless fluid containing small amounts of protein, glucose, lactic acid, urea, and potassium, as well as a relatively large amount of sodium chloride. The fluid, known as cerebral spinal

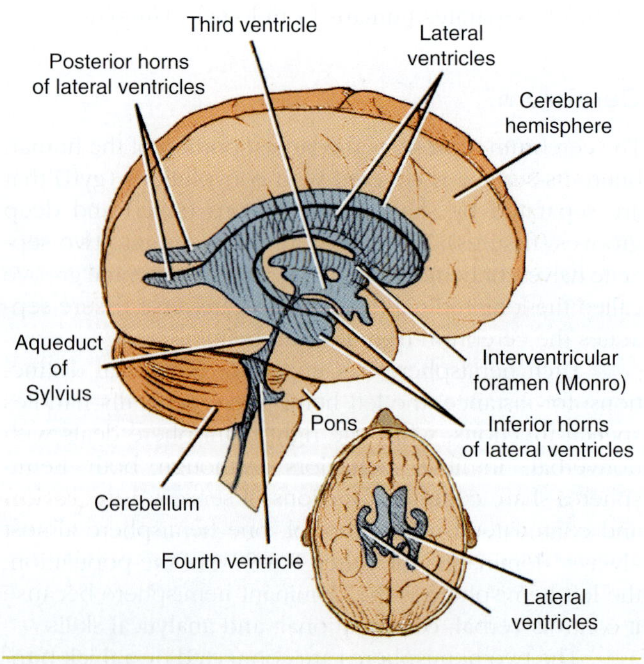

Figure 24-5 Ventricular system

fluid (CSF), helps to support and cushion the brain and spinal cord, and stabilizes the ionic concentration of the central nervous system. It also acts to filter the waste products of metabolism and other substances that diffuse into the brain from blood.

Approximately 800 mL of CSF is produced each day by specialized capillaries that project from the medial walls of the lateral ventricles and the roofs of the third and fourth ventricles. These specialized capillaries are called choroid plexuses, and they create CSF by filtration of blood plasma. The lateral ventricles, however, produce the largest amount of CSF. From the lateral ventricles, CSF flows through the interventricular canal into the third ventricle. From the third ventricle, CSF flows through the aqueduct of Sylvius into the fourth ventricle, where a small portion enters the subarachnoid space through the fourth ventricular wall. CSF flows from the fourth ventricle into the central canal of the spinal cord and around the cord's surface, eventually surrounding the brain and spinal cord. The CSF is reabsorbed by finger-like projections of the arachnoid that project into the dural sinuses called arachnoid villi. This reabsorption occurs at approximately the same rate that CSF is formed, allowing for a constant CSF pressure.

A blockage may occur in the narrow connections between the ventricles, and drainage of CSF into the subarachnoid space may be impeded. The obstruction could be caused by a tumor, scarring due to inflammation, injury, subarachnoid hemorrhage, or a congenital abnormality. As CSF is manufactured, it accumulates within the ventricles and causes the cavities to expand and compress nervous tissue. This condition is known as hydrocephalus. If hydrocephalus occurs in an infant whose fontanels have not yet closed, the cranium can grow to an extreme size.

Basal Ganglia

The basal ganglia are a collection of nuclei (gray matter) imbedded deep within the white matter of the cerebral hemispheres (Figure 24-6). They act with the cerebellum to modify movement from moment to moment. The cerebellum and basal ganglia receive information that is sent out from the motor cortex, which is located in the precentral gyrus of the frontal lobes. The information is modified and sent back to the motor cortex via the thalamus. The output of the cerebellum is excitatory, while the output of the basal ganglia is inhibitory. The balance between these three systems allows for smooth, coordinated movement.

The largest structure of the basal ganglia of the brain is the corpus striatum, which consists of the caudate nucleus and the lenticular nucleus. The lenticular nucleus is subdivided into the putamen and globus pallidus. Other structures of the basal ganglia include the substantia nigra and subthalamic nuclei.

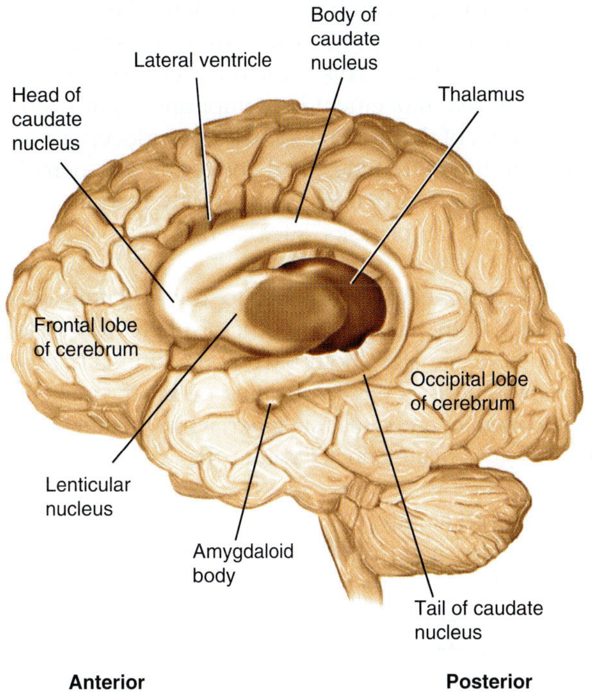

Figure 24-6 Basal ganglia

Lesions within the basal ganglia produce disorders of movement. Typically, disorders fall into one of two categories: unwanted movements and difficulty with intended movements. Parkinson's disease is a result of the gradual loss of dopamine producing nuclei within the substantia nigra. The three symptoms typically associated with Parkinson's are tremor at rest, rigidity (a result of the simultaneous contraction of extensors and flexors), and bradykinesia (the inability to initiate a movement).

Limbic System

The limbic system refers to a ring of gray matter nuclei on the inner border of the cerebrum that forms a border around the brain stem. The limbic system commands certain behaviors that are necessary for the survival of all mammals, such as the ability to distinguish between favorable or unfavorable outside stimuli, or the need to protect and care for offspring. The limbic system is also responsible for a portion of memory formation, emotional expression, and some aspects of personal identity. The structures of the limbic system include the parahippocampal and cingulate gyri within the cerebral hemispheres, the hippocampus on the floor of the lateral ventricle, the dentate gyrus, the amygdala, the septal nuclei, mammillary bodies, anterior nucleus of the thalamus, and olfactory bulbs.

Cerebellum

The cerebellum is the second largest structure of the brain and is located posterior to the medulla oblongata and inferior to the cerebrum's occipital lobe. It is separated from the cerebrum by the transverse fissure and the tentorium cerebelli. This structure acts to coordinate skeletal muscle movement by comparing input from the motor cortex of the frontal lobe with proprioceptive feedback from the extremities, and correcting any perceived problems. The cerebellum is also partly responsible for learning new motor tasks, such as throwing or catching a ball.

The cerebellum is similar to the structure of the cerebrum. Both consist of two hemispheres of approximately the same size. Both have convolutions (although the convolutions of the cerebellum are much smaller), an outer cortex of gray matter, inner white matter, and islands of gray matter nuclei within the white matter. Unlike the cerebrum, however, the cerebellum controls functions ipsilaterally.

The two hemispheres of the cerebellum are separated by a layer of dura mater called the falx cerebelli, and joined by a structure called the vermis. The cerebellum communicates with other structures of the central nervous system via the inferior, middle, and superior cerebellar peduncles. Input to the cerebellum is received via the spinocerebellar pathways, the inferior olive, and the pons, which transmits impulses from the cerebrum. The three deep nuclei of the cerebellum are the fastigial, interposed, and dentate nuclei. The dentate and interposed nuclei are concerned with voluntary movement; the fastigial nucleus is concerned with balance.

Diencephalon

The diencephalon is located between the midbrain and the cerebrum. It is composed of gray matter nuclei and surrounds the third ventricle. The primary structures of the diencephalon include the thalamus, hypothalamus, posterior pituitary gland, and pineal gland.

The thalamus acts as a relay station to the cerebral cortex for all sensory data from the cerebellum, brain stem, spinal cord, and other parts of the cerebrum. The thalamus decides which sensory data will make its way to the cortex for further action and interpretation, and then channels the data to the appropriate location. This structure of the diencephalon also produces a general awareness of the sensations of pain, touch, and temperature.

The hypothalamus is a collection of nuclei located just inferior to the thalamus. It regulates homeostasis of the body through coordination of activities of the autonomic nervous system. It releases neurosecretory substances that stimulate the anterior pituitary gland to release hormones; therefore, the hypothalamus serves as a link between the endocrine system and the nervous system. It also regulates emotional and behavioral patterns through connections with the limbic system. Other important functions of the hypothalamus include:

1. Glandular secretion control for the gastrointestinal tract
2. Wakefulness and arousal regulation
3. Control of water balance
4. Control of electrolyte balance
5. Hunger and thirst regulation
6. Regulation of body temperature
7. Regulation of heart rate and arterial blood pressure

Mesencephalon

The midbrain, or mesencephalon, is a section of the brain stem located between the diencephalon and the pons. It contains tracts of white matter and gray matter nuclei. The white matter tracts that connect the cerebral cortex with the pons, medulla, and spinal cord are called the cerebral peduncles. Other important structures of the midbrain include:

1. The superior cerebellar peduncles that connect the mesencephalon with the cerebellum
2. The corpora quadrigemina that serve as reflex centers for eye, head, and neck movement in response to visual stimuli, as well as movement of the head and trunk in response to auditory stimuli
3. The substantia nigra that control subconscious muscle movement (Dopamine-producing neurons within this structure may degenerate, resulting in Parkinson's syndrome.)
4. Red nuclei that coordinate muscular movements in conjunction with the basal ganglia and cerebellum

Brain Stem

The brain stem connects the diencephalon to the spinal cord and consists of the following (Figure 24-7):

1. The medulla oblongata, which forms the inferior portion of the brain stem, begins at the foramen magnum and ends at the inferior border of the pons. It contains all ascending and descending tracts (white matter) that connect the brain with the spinal cord. Five of the 12 cranial nerve nuclei are located in the medulla. The medulla also contains the nuclei responsible for breathing rhythm, heart rate, and blood pressure.
2. The pons, which lies superior to the medulla and anterior to the cerebellum, connects the brain with the spinal cord and other brain parts. The pons also contains the nuclei for 4 of the 12 cranial nerves, as well as nuclei that work with the medulla for the regulation of breathing.
3. The midbrain, located just below the thalamus, contains a center for visual reflexes, such as movement of the head and eyes.

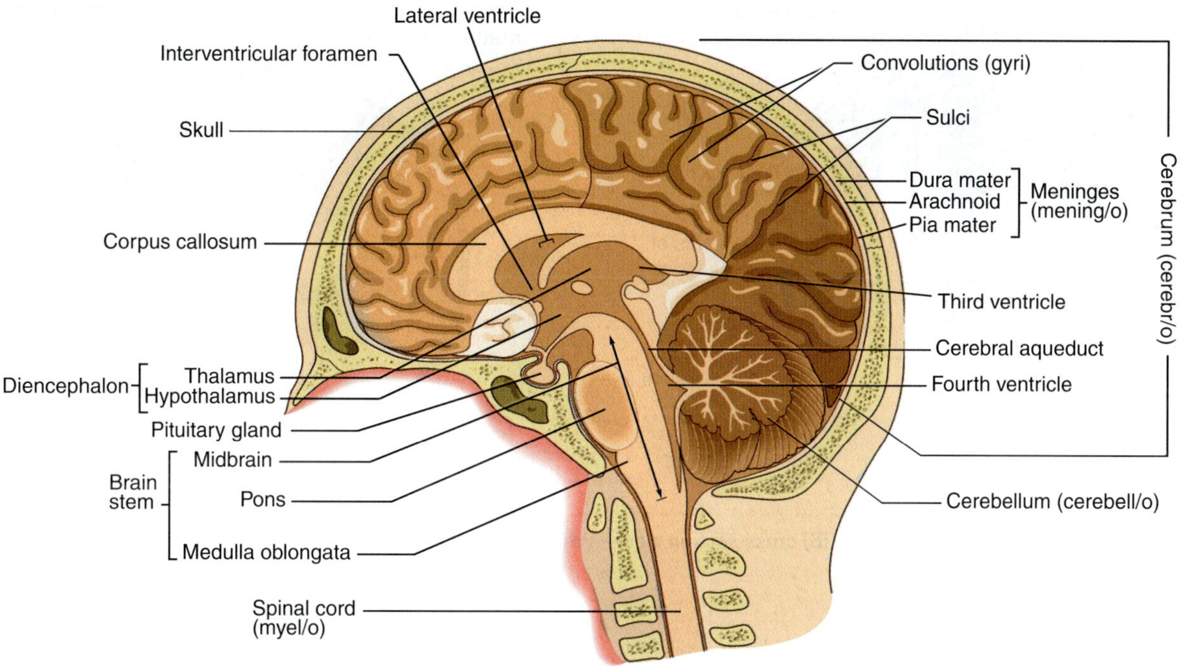

Figure 24-7 Cross-section of the brain

VERTEBRAL COLUMN

The vertebral column of a normal adult is comprised of 33 vertebrae and is part of the axial skeleton. These 33 individual bones are separated into five regions. They are, from superior to inferior: cervical, thoracic, lumbar, sacral, and coccygeal. They are commonly referred to by abbreviations. The first abbreviation stands for the region and the second lists the individual bone number in that particular region. Thus, the first cervical vertebrae is referred to as C1.

There are seven bones in the cervical region. The uppermost, or first, cervical vertebra (C1) is the atlas, which supports the skull. The second cervical vertebra (C2) is the axis, which is fused with the body of the atlas; it is responsible for allowing rotation, flexion, and extension of the head. The remaining five vertebrae (C3–C7), which are similar to each other in their structure, function in a supportive role of the skeleton.

There are 12 bones in the thoracic region (T1–T12). They are larger and stronger than the cervical vertebrae and are the main support for the thorax, as each of the 12 ribs forming the thoracic cage articulate with each of the thoracic vertebrae.

There are five lumbar vertebrae (L1–L5). The lumbar vertebrae have two main responsibilities. They provide support for a major portion of the weight of the body and allow for much of the flexibility of the trunk. Thus, the lumbar vertebrae are very large and have heavy bodies.

The sacrum is formed by five individual bones that fuse to form one bone in adulthood. The sacrum is considered part of the pelvic girdle.

The coccyx consists of four fused vertebrae. The coccyx serves as an important attachment for several hip and pelvic muscles.

The structure of individual vertebrae may vary, but there are many similarities typically shared by all vertebrae. Each vertebra has a body or centrum anteriorly. Posteriorly, a neural arch encircles the opening for the spinal cord called the vertebral foramen. As the neural arch extends from the body on each side of the vertebra, it is referred to as the pedicle. The lateral extensions of the pedicles are called the transverse processes, which support the facets. The facets provide the articulating surfaces between the vertebrae. The bony surface extending posteriorly from the facet is the lamina. Laminae that extend from each side of the vertebra connect to form the spinous process of each vertebra. The atlas is the exception to the rule, lacking both a centrum and a spinous process. In place of the centrum, the atlas has a mass of bone extending laterally to accept the condyles of the occipital bone of the cranium, and the structure in place of the spinous process is the posterior tubercle.

The spinal nerves pass through openings between adjacent vertebrae. These openings are referred to as the intervertebral foramina.

Intervertebral disks keep the individual vertebrae separated from one another. The disk itself is comprised of fibrous connective tissue. Its tough outer layer is termed the annulus fibrosis, and the soft core is called the nucleus pulposus. The intervertebral disks bear most of the stress, in the form of pressure from gravity (body weight and lifting objects), that is transmitted to the vertebral column.

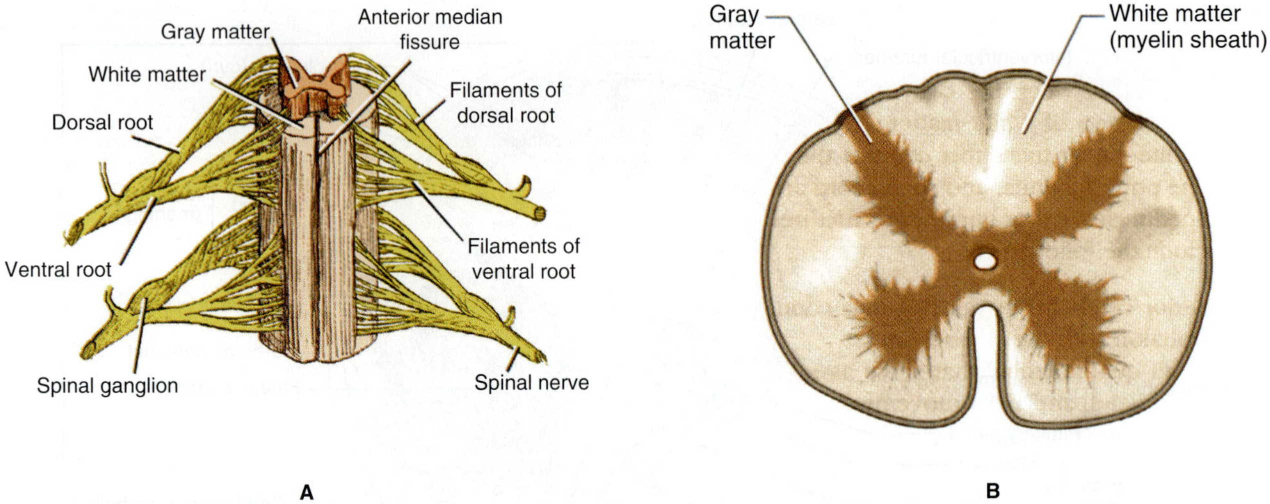

Figure 24-8 Spinal cord: (A) Anterior view, (B) cross-section view—white and gray matter

SPINAL CORD

The spinal cord is a column of nervous tissue that begins at the level of the foramen magnum and terminates at the level of the first and second lumbar disk. It runs within the vertebral canal of the vertebral column as a continuation of the medulla oblongata of the brain stem. The spinal cord is protected by the same three meningeal coverings as the brain (dura, arachnoid, and pia mater). Its function is to conduct impulses and serve as a spinal reflex center.

When cross-sectioned, the cord reveals central areas of gray matter (shaped somewhat like a butterfly) surrounded by white matter. The anterior extensions (the wings of the butterfly) of gray matter are called the ventral horns, and the posterior extensions are called the dorsal horns. A bridge of gray matter called the gray commissure connects the left and right ventral and dorsal wings (Figure 24-8).

The white matter of the cord consists of longitudinal nerve tracts that are axons from cell bodies located throughout the central nervous system. The ascending nerve tracts carry information from the body to the brain, and the descending tracts carry information from the brain to the body.

At the level of the first lumbar vertebra, a collection of spinal roots descends from the inferior spinal cord, resembling the hairs of a horse's tail. These nerves are known collectively as the cauda equina (Figure 24-9).

BLOOD SUPPLY

The internal carotid artery, branching from the common carotid artery, provides the brain with most of its blood. It divides into the anterior cerebral artery, which supplies blood to the cerebrum's medial surface, and the middle cerebral artery, which supplies blood to the lateral surface of the cerebrum.

Posteriorly, the two vertebral arteries unite to form the single basilar artery that divides to form the posterior cerebral arteries. The posterior cerebral arteries serve the occipital and temporal regions of the cerebrum.

The posterior cerebral arteries are connected to the internal carotid arteries by the posterior communicating arteries, forming the posterior portion of the **circle of Willis** (Figure 24-10). This circle is a ring of arteries that give rise to the various branches supplying blood to the brain. The anterior communicating artery connects the anterior cerebral arteries, forming the anterior portion of the circle.

The spinal cord receives its blood supply from the median anterior spinal artery that arises from the vertebral arteries, and paired posterior spinal arteries from the posterior inferior cerebellar arteries. Below the cervical level, the cord receives additional blood from the radicular arteries that branch from the intercostal and lumbar arteries. The cord is drained by the anterior and posterior spinal veins.

CRANIAL NERVES

With the exception of the first and second, the cranial nerves originate in the brain stem (Figure 24-11).

The cranial nerves can be divided into sensory (originating in the lateral brain stem), motor (originating in the medial brain stem), or mixed nerves. The cranial nerves and their functions are found in Table 24-1.

SPINAL NERVES

The spinal cord is made up of continuous nerve tracts and cell columns that can be divided into segments, each of

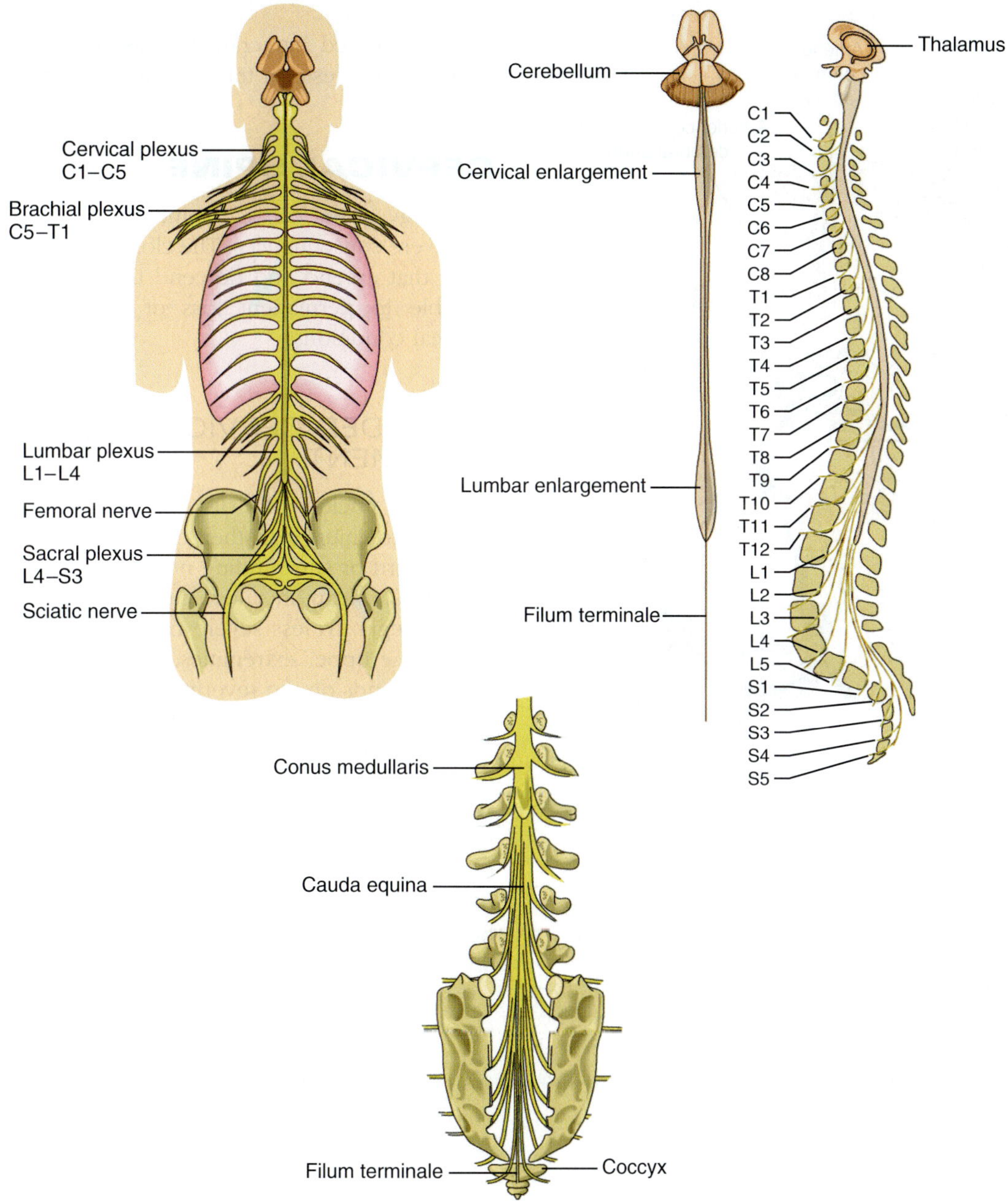

Figure 24-9 Spinal cord and spinal nerves

which gives rise to a pair of spinal nerves. There are 31 of these spinal nerve roots: 8 cervical, 12 thoracic, 5 lumbar, 5 sacral, and 1 coccygeal. At each segment, a root arises from the dorsal and ventral portions of the spinal cord and combines into one spinal nerve that exits outward from the vertebral canal through the intervertebral foramen. The ventral root deals with motor stimuli from the brain to the body, and arises from the axons of the motor neurons within the ventral horn (gray matter) of the spinal cord. The dorsal root arises from the gray matter dorsal horn. It handles sensory information from the body and is easily identified by an enlarged portion of the root called the dorsal root ganglion.

With the exception of the thoracic nerves, branches of the spinal nerves unite to form networks that combine fibers from neighboring nerves. These networks are called plexuses. The primary plexuses are the cervical, brachial, lumbar, and sacral plexuses.

The cervical plexus is formed on either side by the first four cervical nerves (C1–C4) with contributions from C5. These supply the skin and muscles of the head, neck, and top of the shoulders. Branches of the cervical plexus also combine with fibers from the 11th and 12th cranial nerves. The brachial plexus is formed by the spinal nerves C5–C8 and T1, and innervates the shoulder and upper limb. The lumbar plexus is formed by the spinal nerves

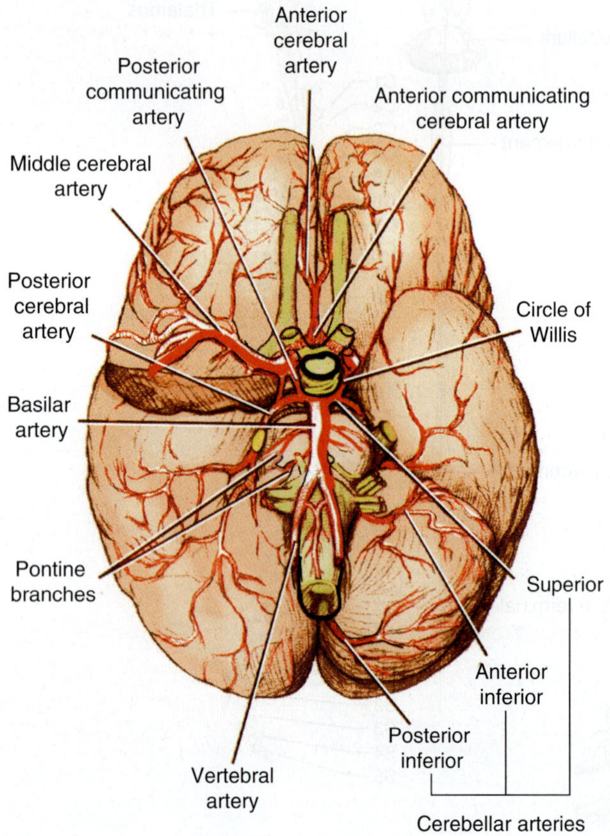

Figure 24-10 Circle of Willis

L1–L4. It innervates the anterolateral abdominal wall, external genitals, and portions of the lower extremities. The sacral plexus is formed by the spinal nerves L4–L5 and S1–S4 and innervates the buttocks, perineum, and lower extremities.

NEUROSURGICAL PATHOLOGY

Diagnosis in neurosurgical cases is arrived at after a thorough history and physical examination. Symptoms assist the physician in determining the type of disease, as well as the resultant neural deficit, if any. Specific symptoms assist in localization of the area of lesions, and are related to specific pathology such as **abscess**, tumor (neoplasm), or **hematoma**.

Symptoms that sometimes alert the physician to the necessity for neurosurgical intervention include seizures, elevated intracranial pressure, and coma. Other symptoms, such as headache, nausea, dizziness, and aphasia may also be present. The type of seizure, the preseizure aura, and the postictal state help the surgeon localize the lesion. Seizures are common in patients with tumors and cortical injuries. Tumors, abscesses, hematomas, or any other lesion that occupies space within the cranium can cause increased intracranial pressure. Coma may result from cerebral lesions, trauma, tumor, or stroke.

CERVICAL SPINE

Pathology of the cervical spine always has the potential for severe consequences. The closely packed neural pathways that ascend and descend the spinal cord are susceptible to permanent loss of function from several cervical conditions.

EXTRUDED CERVICAL DISK FRAGMENT

When the nucleus of a disk extrudes through the annulus due to injury or other cause, it may compress the spinal cord or surrounding nerves and nerve roots. This compression can, in severe cases, result in paraplegia or quadriplegia. In less severe cases, it may cause sensory loss in the upper extremities. The severity of the symptoms depends on the severity of the compression caused by the disk fragment. In some cases, the disk does not extrude, but simply degenerates. This causes narrowing of the joint space, causing the cartilage at the end plates of the adjacent vertebrae to wear more quickly. Sometimes an **osteophyte**, or bony spur, may develop due to this increased mobility. When osteophytes form within the spinal canal, the cord may be compressed by the bony structure. This formation of osteophytes is called spondylosis.

With cervical disk extrusion, symptoms may be chronic or **acute** (due to some injury). The patient may experience neck stiffness, soreness, and limited mobility, along with radicular symptoms. Some tenderness may occur over the brachial plexus. The normal curvature of the neck tends to be straightened somewhat in these patients.

When osteophytes have formed in the foramen, cervical discomfort may occur in episodes over a period of months or years before radicular symptoms become evident.

In some instances, radiographs will show narrowing in the disk space, indicating **extruded** disk, or disk degeneration (Figure 24-12). Radiographs will also show osteophytes that have formed.

Myelography and computed axial tomography are also used diagnostically to identify ventral extradural defects and to help differentiate osteophytes from extruded disk. MRI is used in identification of disk herniation and helps show the amount of spinal cord compression, if any. Electromyography (EMG) is useful in confirmation of the above diagnoses.

Many in the surgical community feel very strongly about treating cervical disk disease conservatively and using surgical intervention in only those cases that do not or will not respond to medical treatment.

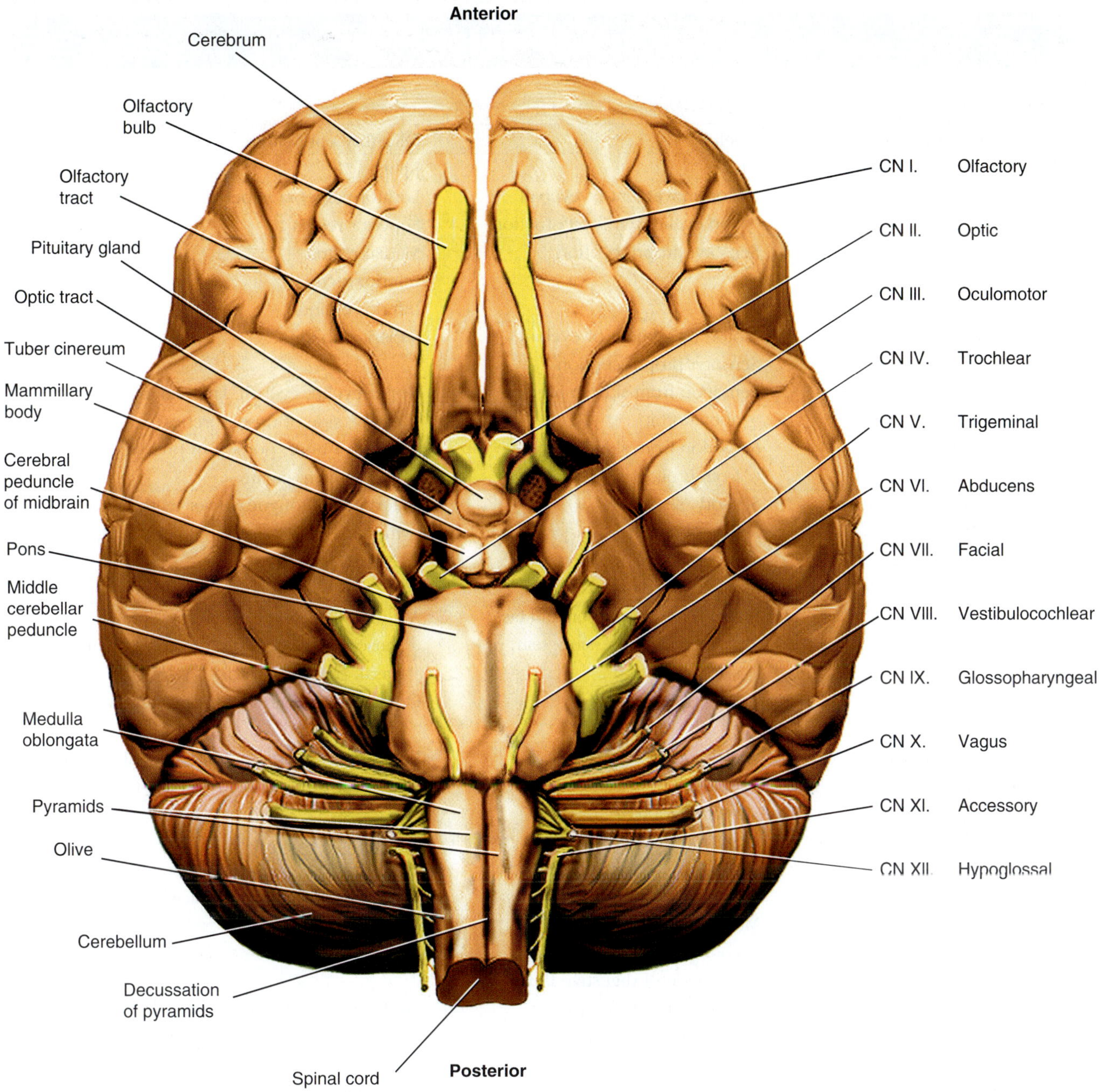

Figure 24-11 Cranial nerves and related structures

There are two primary surgical treatments for cervical disk disease:

1. Decompression of the nerve roots and/or spinal cord with a posterior cervical laminectomy and discectomy.
2. Anterior cervical discectomy and fusion. The anterior approach offers the advantage of a direct approach to the disk space without the removal of the lamina. After the disk is removed, the disk space is filled with cancellous and cortical bone (fusion), usually from the iliac crest.

THORACIC SPINE

Extruded thoracic disk is very similar in symptoms and treatment to cervical disk problems. The canal in the thoracic spine is small in relation to the size of the cord, increasing the likelihood of cord compression. When thoracic disk rupture occurs, paraplegia may result. Often, osteophyte formation secondary to disk degeneration causes spinal canal narrowing. In these cases, the extruded disk and/or osteophytes are removed surgically. When necessary, fusion is performed with bone or any of the several available plating and screwing systems. Fusion

Table 24-1 Cranial Nerves and their Function

NERVE (TYPE)	FUNCTION	TARGET
I. Olfactory (sensory)	Smell	Olfactory epithelium
II. Optic (sensory)	Vision	Retina
III. Oculomotor (mixed)	Motor: movement of eyeball and eyelid, pupil constriction Sensory: proprioception	Levator palpebra superioris Superior rectus Medial rectus Inferior rectus Inferior oblique
IV. Trochlear (mixed)	Motor: movement of eyeball Sensory: proprioception	Superior oblique
V1. Trigeminal ophthalmic (sensory)	Sensation from skin in region above orbit	Upper eyelid, eyeball, lacrimal glands, nasal cavity, side of nose, forehead
V2. Trigeminal maxillary (sensory)	Sensation from skin in region from orbit to mouth	Mucosa of nose, portion of pharynx, upper lip, upper teeth, palate
V3. Trigeminal mandibular (mixed)	Sensory: sensation Motor: chewing	Anterior ⅔ of tongue, lower teeth, mandibular muscles, cheek
VI. Abducens (mixed)	Sensory: proprioception Motor: movement of eyeball	Lateral rectus muscle
VII. Facial (mixed)	Sensory: proprioception and taste Motor: facial expression, tear, saliva secretion	Anterior ⅔ of tongue, facial, scalp, and neck muscles; lacrimal, sublingual, submandibular, nasal, palatine glands
VIII. Vestibulocochlear (sensory)	Hearing and balance	Organ of Corti, semicircular canals, saccule, utricle
IX. Glossopharyngeal (mixed)	Sensory: blood pressure regulation, taste, proprioception Motor: saliva secretion	Posterior ⅓ of tongue, pharynx, palate, carotid sinus, carotid body
X. Vagus (mixed)	Sensory: sensation from visceral organs, proprioception Motor: smooth muscle contraction and relaxation, secretion of digestive fluids	Pharynx, larynx, auricle, external auditory meatus, muscles of thoracic and abdominal organs
XI. Accessory (mixed)	Sensory: proprioception Motor: swallowing, head movements	Voluntary muscles of pharynx, larynx, palate; sternocleidomastoid, trapezius muscles
XII. Hypoglossal (mixed)	Sensory: proprioception Motor: tongue movement during speech, swallowing	Tongue muscles

is necessary when disk space narrowing results in joint instability or intractable pain.

LUMBAR SPINE

When disk material extrudes through the annulus due to degeneration or trauma in the lumbar region, nerve roots may be compressed. In cases where the entire cauda equina is compressed, the patient may experience complete loss of sensation and motor function that may also include the loss of bladder and bowel control. As with cervical and thoracic disk disease, loss of mobility may occur and osteophytes may form secondary to disk extrusion or degeneration (Figure 24-13).

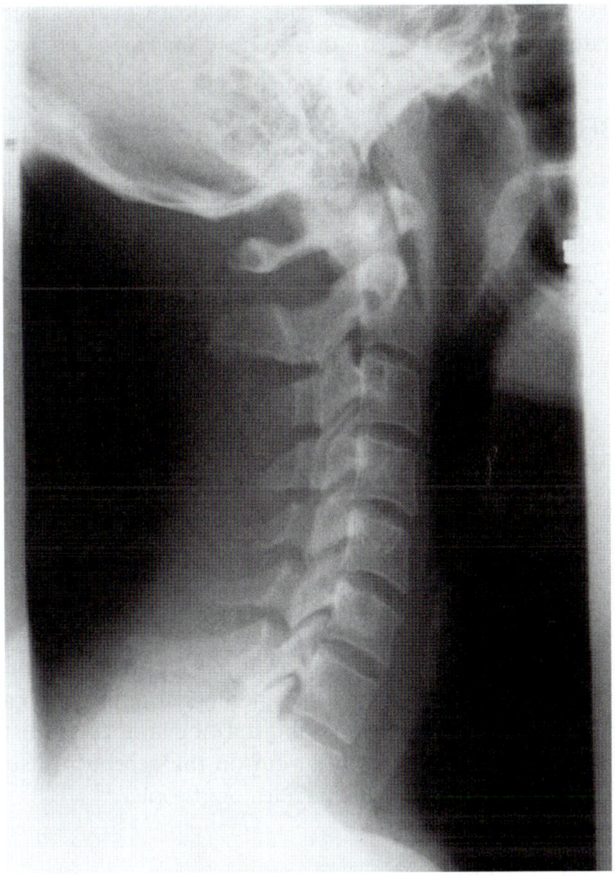

Figure 24-12 Lateral cervical X-ray

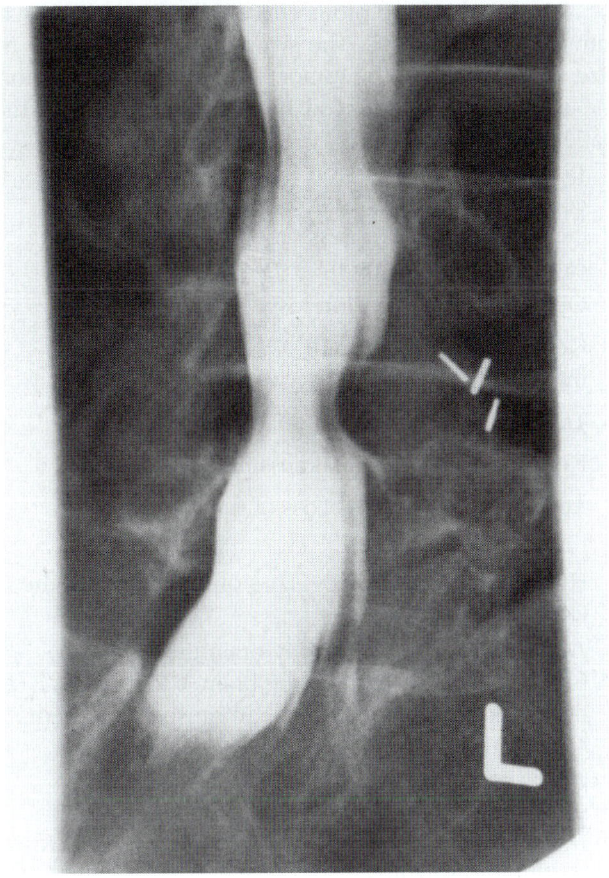

Figure 24-13 Lumbar myelogram depicting a herniated disk

A great majority of the problems in this region occur in the L4–L5 and L5–S1 intervertebral spaces. Problems associated with lumbar disk disease are as follows:

- *Lumbar spondylosis:* advanced lumbar disk disease
- *Lumbar stenosis:* advanced constriction of the spinal canal caused by spondylosis
- *Lumbar spondylolisthesis:* forward displacement of the upper vertebral body on the lower vertebral body

The patient usually experiences chronic pain, although pain may be acute in the instance of herniation due to injury. Back pain and leg pain may radiate into the buttock or posterior thigh (lumbar **radiculopathy**). Patients may complain that the pain is made worse by coughing, sneezing, or Valsalva's maneuver. Lying down usually relieves pain, while the sitting position typically exacerbates the condition. There is usually tenderness over the sciatic notch and back muscles may be in spasm. Raising the leg worsens back pain or radiculopathy. Patients may experience weakness in the quadriceps, great toe, or hand, depending on the level of the herniation.

For diagnosis, plain radiographic films of the spine are used to identify bony changes in the lumbar spine. CT or MRI scanning is useful in identifying lumbar disk herniations.

Surgical treatment is not indicated unless patients have progressive weakness in the extremities, sensory loss, or loss of sphincter control. Surgery may be indicated for patients with acute or chronic neurological deficit, or for patients whose deficit will increase over time. Surgery is also utilized to treat chronic disabling pain. As with thoracic and cervical disk degeneration, surgical treatment involves removal of the degenerated disk and fusion of the joint when necessary. This is usually achieved with a posterior approach and laminectomy.

NEOPLASMS

The nervous system is liable to damage from primary and secondary neoplasms. The primary neoplasms arise from neural tissues or the meninges. Secondary neoplasms are metastatic lesions from other parts of the body.

INTRACRANIAL TUMORS

Although the cause of brain tumors is still largely unknown, some patients with a familial history of tumors are known to be more prone to several types of intracranial tumors.

A variety of symptoms are evident in patients with intracranial neoplasms. The symptoms will vary with the size and location of the tumor. The following are among the symptoms experienced by most intracranial tumor patients:

- *Compression:* Tumors on the surface of the brain compress the brain itself, as well as surrounding cranial nerves. Compression of these nerves will cause specific symptoms:

  Optic nerve (II)—Vision loss

  Ocular muscle nerves (III, IV, VI)—Loss of eye movement

  Trigeminal nerve (V)—Numbness in the face

  Facial nerve (VII)—Weakness in the face

  Accessory nerve (XI)—Loss of function in the trapezius muscle

  Hypoglossal nerve (XII)—Loss of movement of the tongue
- *Destruction:* Tumors destroy brain tissue, and function in those parts of the brain is lost. This destruction of neural tissue may cause impairment, such as the loss of speech or comprehension (aphasia). Other symptoms may include loss of sensation, coordination, or mental abilities.
- *Irritation:* Tumors may irritate the cerebral cortex, resulting in seizures.
- *Increased intracranial pressure:* As tumors increase in mass, intracranial pressure increases. Symptoms include nausea, vomiting, and headaches. If pressure reaches a high enough level, the patient may become unconscious.

Tumors are diagnosed with CT (Figure 24-14) and MRI. High-resolution MRI allows the detection of very small tumors. Radiography is still used because it shows bone erosion and tumor calcification. Cerebral angiography is used to show the vascularity of tumors and aids in determining the type of tumor.

Benign tumors can usually be excised totally through craniotomy. These tumors include craniopharyngiomas, epidermoids, dermoids, hemangiomas, meningiomas, acoustic neuromas, and pituitary microadenomas. Malignant tumors, such as the astrocytomas or **gliomas**, usually cannot be totally excised, but as much tumor as possible is removed. Glioblastoma multiforme tumors are excised when there is only one tumor, but not when there are multiple tumors or the patient has a short life expectancy. A brief overview of the types of tumors is shown in Table 24-2.

HEAD INJURY

Head injuries that require surgical intervention include scalp injury, skull fracture, epidural hematoma, subdural hematoma, and brain injury. In persons up to 44 years of age, trauma is the leading cause of death in the United States. Of these, 50% are due to head injuries.

BRAIN INJURY

Brain injuries result from the effects of shearing and the rotational effects of a blow to the head, or from rapid acceleration or deceleration. If cerebral contusion has caused intracerebral hematoma, the area of the contusion may be evacuated via craniotomy.

Depressed skull fractures may require the elevation of depressed bone with wound debridement and closure.

HEMATOMA

A blow to the head or postoperative bleeding may result in the accumulation of blood in the subdural or epidural space. This collection of blood results in an increasing intracranial pressure and a distortion and shifting of the brain within the cranial cavity, and can be fatal if left untreated. Epidural hematomas are typically the result of a tear in a branch of the middle meningeal artery and can cause rapid deterioration. Subdural hematomas are usually the result of a tear in a vein on the cerebrum's surface, and can be acute, subacute, or chronic.

Epidural Hematoma

Epidural hematoma may result from a fractured skull. The pressure of blood from this arterial bleeding strips the dura away from the skull, causing more bleeding as the tiny veins from the dura to the skull are torn. As this bleeding occurs, a hematoma forms, putting pressure on the cerebral cortex. Epidural hematomas may form after a blow to the head, with subsequent loss of consciousness. When the patient regains consciousness, there may be a

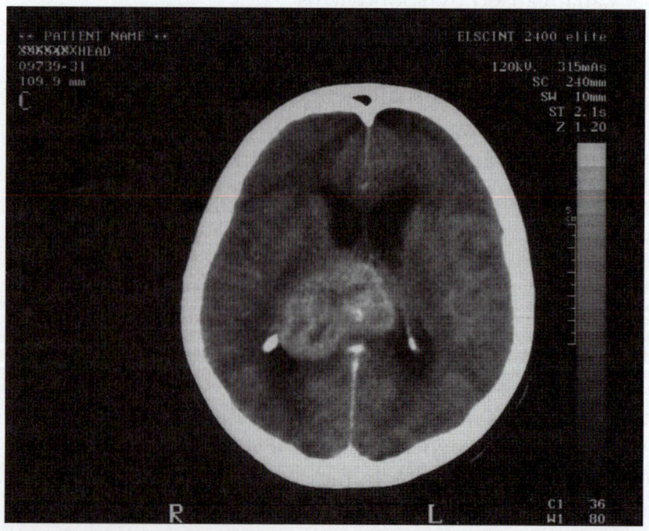

Figure 24-14 **CT scan depicting a brain tumor**

Table 24-2 Intracranial Neoplasms

DISORDER	INCIDENCE	SYMPTOMS	TESTS	TREATMENT	MORTALITY
All intracranial neoplasms		Headache, nausea and vomiting, personality changes, increased intracranial pressure	CT scan MRI		
Glioma	40% of primary brain tumors—majority are malignant		Above		
Astrocytoma, grades I and II	30% of gliomas; most common ages 30–40	Symptoms present for long period of time	Above	Excision and radiation	
Astrocytoma, grades III and IV	55% of gliomas; most common ages 50–60	Above symptoms present for up to 6 months	Above	Excision and radiation; chemotherapy	Glioblastoma survival usually less than 12 months
Oligodendroma	5% of gliomas; most common ages 30–50	Spontaneous hemorrhage in 40%; calcification present in 50%; occurs along with astrocytomas in 50%	Above	Excision and radiation; chemotherapy	
Ependymoma	7% of gliomas; most common in children and young adults			Excision and radiation	
Medulloblastoma	Most common in children			Excision; chemotherapy	
Meningioma			Marked enhancement on CT scan or MRI; angiography shows characteristic "blush"	Excision	Benign; these tumors recur if not completely excised
Acoustic neuroma	Increased incidence with familial history of neurofibromatosis	Loss of hearing, headache, vertigo, facial pain	MRI, CT, audiometry	Surgery	
Craniopharyngioma	Most common in the young	Headache, behavioral changes	MRI	Treated conservatively with surgery	Usually benign; location determines postoperative complications
Hemangioblastoma	Involves the cerebellum; occurs primarily in the young		MRI	Surgical excision; postoperative radiation when complete removal is not possible	

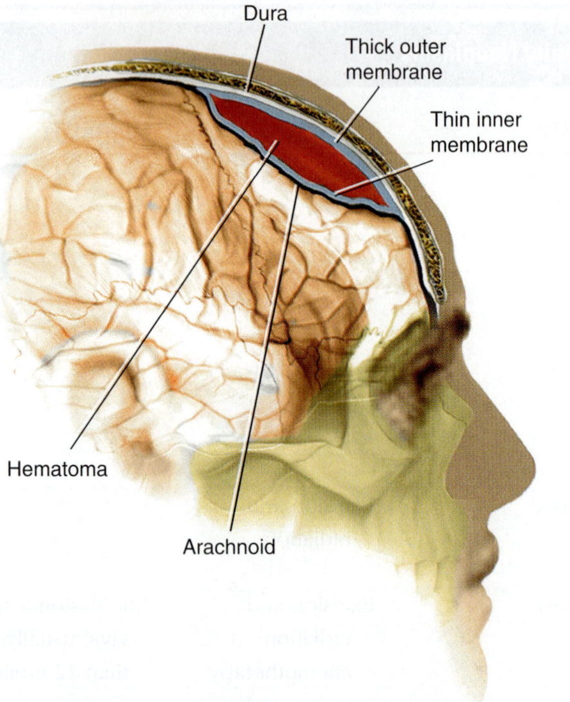

Figure 24-15 Subdural hematoma

symptomless period as the hematoma enlarges to a size sufficient to compress the cerebrum, resulting in a gradual loss of consciousness that can progress to coma and death without surgical intervention. The mortality rate for these lesions is high because patients may be seen by a physician during the symptomless period and released. Craniotomy is performed to relieve the resultant pressure of the hematoma, as well as to debride the area and control bleeding.

Subdural Hematoma

Acute subdural hematoma occurs in relation to severe head injuries (Figure 24-15). When veins bridging the cerebral cortex to the venous sinuses are torn or the cortex is lacerated, hemorrhage occurs. The resultant hematoma may be large, and is usually discovered by CT scanning. These patients typically enter the hospital in an unconscious state.

Subacute subdural hematoma does not become apparent for several days to several weeks after the causative injury. The patient shows progressive symptoms of lethargy, confusion, or other neural deficits. For subacute and acute subdural hematomas, craniotomy is performed to remove the hematoma, relieve pressure, debride the area, and provide hemostasis. In acute subdural hematoma, a significant neurological deficit may remain due to cerebral contusion and/or laceration.

Chronic subdural hematoma typically occurs after a minor head injury that results in a small initial hematoma that goes unnoticed. This type of hematoma is particularly common in infants and the elderly. Over time, the hematoma is encased in a fibrous membrane. As the lesion enlarges, it puts pressure on the cerebral cortex, resulting in neural deficits such as aphasia or ataxia. Headaches, confusion, and drowsiness may mark this period of hematoma enlargement. Occasionally, these patients are mistakenly diagnosed as suffering from Alzheimer's disease. Treatment for epidural or subdural hematoma involves craniectomy or bur holes for drainage.

SPINAL CORD INJURY

Injury may occur to the spinal cord from fracture or dislocation of the vertebra, herniation of the intervertebral disk into the spinal canal, or laceration from penetrating injuries such as gunshot wounds. The objectives of treatment for these injuries are to protect the undamaged structures, restore function, correct spinal alignment, and provide spinal stability. Reduction and immobilization of fractures is a top priority. Patients with complete cord injuries rarely recover function below the point of the lesion. Patients with incomplete cord injuries, however, show more improvement and can sometimes walk again if treatment is begun at an early stage.

In some cases, traction and bed rest alone can reduce fractures. Many cervical fractures are successfully reduced by the use of closed reduction and traction. However, when there is an inability to reduce the fracture and/or dislocation by the closed methods, or when there is compression of the spinal cord caused by an intraspinal mass even after closed reduction, surgery is indicated. Any penetrating injury, such as a gunshot or stab wound, also indicates a need for surgery, especially if there is a cerebrospinal fluid leak.

CEREBROVASCULAR DISEASE

Cerebrovascular disease is the third leading cause of death in the United States and is marked by cerebral ischemia or hemorrhage.

INTRACRANIAL ANEURYSM

Aneurysms are weak spots in the walls of arteries. Over the course of years, these weak spots balloon out from the arterial wall. When the walls have thinned sufficiently, they can rupture, causing severe bleeding in and around the brain.

Cerebral aneurysms are typically found at points of bifurcation in the arteries of the circle of Willis. More than 85% of aneurysms occur in the carotid circulation, 30% of these arising from the internal carotid near the origin of the posterior communicating artery. Others arise from the anterior communicating artery, and some are positioned at the first major branch point of the middle cerebral artery. They often occur in multiples, and vary in size from a small pea to a plum.

Patients with cerebral aneurysm are generally asymptomatic until rupture unless the defect is large enough to press on surrounding structures, such as the optic chiasma or optic nerves. If the aneurysm ruptures, the patient will typically present with signs of meningeal irritation, focal signs of cerebral damage, and uniformly bloody spinal fluid. Angiography will reveal the exact size and location of the aneurysm.

Patients with intracranial aneurysm usually present with a sudden and very severe headache, neck stiffness, and photophobia. Some patients experience back pain and nausea or vomiting. Patients with aneurysms large enough to put pressure on the brain or nerves may experience seizure, double vision, and hemiparesis. The primary danger to the patient with intracranial aneurysm is hemorrhage. Prevention is often impossible, because most aneurysms are not discovered until after their rupture.

ARTERIOVENOUS MALFORMATIONS

Arteriovenous malformations (AVMs) are congenital collections of abnormal vessels of the brain that increase in size with time, eventually stealing blood from adjacent areas of the brain. Most AVMs occur in the parietal or occipital lobes of the cerebral hemispheres, and half reach the cortical surface. AVM can also occur in the spinal cord. Most AVMs eventually rupture, so nonsurgical or surgical intervention becomes necessary. Many arteriovenous malformations have associated aneurysms, increasing the danger of hemorrhage.

Patients with AVM experience a sudden headache, usually associated with hemorrhage within the brain. They may also exhibit a loss of consciousness or neurologic deficit. Some patients experience seizures. High-resolution MRI confirms the existence of an AVM, but selective cerebral angiography is usually necessary to identify details of the lesion.

BRAIN HEMORRHAGE

Brain hemorrhages are typically the result of uncontrolled hypertension and atherosclerosis. Increased pressure against the arterial wall and atherosclerotic plaque can result in arterial dissection and hemorrhage. These spontaneous hemorrhages usually occur in the thalamus, cerebellum, putamen, or pons. Ruptured cerebral aneurysms and AVMs may also cause brain hemorrhage.

In cases of thalamic hemorrhage, the patient experiences sensory loss on one side of the body, followed by single-sided motor control loss. These patients also exhibit downward eye deviation and small, sluggish pupils.

Cerebellar hemorrhages present with sudden severe headache and dizziness, accompanied by vomiting and ataxia. This type of hemorrhage exerts pressure on the brain stem and may cause coma and death.

The patient with brain stem hemorrhage, the most devastating of the brain hemorrhages, presents with the classic "posturing," pinpoint pupils, and coma. A brain stem hemorrhage larger than 1 cm can be fatal.

Brain hematomas may be treated surgically by decompression through craniotomy. Those nearer the surface are the easiest to remove, and those that are larger than 3 cm in size usually indicate surgical treatment. It is important to remove cerebellar hematomas surgically to prevent brain stem compression.

ISCHEMIC DISEASE (STROKE)

Ischemia and subsequent infarction (stroke) may occur in any part of the brain. Ischemia is caused either by atherosclerotic stenosis in the large vessels or by emboli in the smaller vessels. Once ischemia has reached a point where infarction has occurred, there is no current medical or surgical treatment.

Patients with a history of transient ischemic attacks (**TIAs**) are at high risk of stroke, as are patients with hypertension. Patients who have had a stroke may exhibit hemiparesis or hemianesthesia, as well as dysphagia, weakness, and ataxia. Some patients may be unconscious or exhibit signs of decreased consciousness. These patients undergo CT or MRI to determine the degree of any infarction and to rule out brain tumors. CT or MRI also helps rule out subdural hematoma. After the CT or MRI, angiography is performed to determine viability of the circulatory system. Stroke patients also undergo such cardiac tests as an electrocardiogram to check for arrhythmias and atrial fibrillation. These disorders can cause thrombi to be ejected from the left atrium and into the cerebral vessels, obstructing blood flow to areas of the brain.

Because there is no medical or surgical treatment that is effective after a stroke has occurred, any surgical treatment is performed to prevent further strokes (prophylaxis). When angiography shows a stenosis of 70% or greater in the common or proximal internal carotid artery, carotid endarterectomy is performed. This procedure removes atherosclerotic plaque and increases circulation through the affected artery.

CONGENITAL ABNORMALITIES

Like all systems, the neurological system is liable to both acquired and congenital abnormalities. Congenital abnormalities may affect every tissue type in the nervous system. Some commonly seen conditions are reviewed here.

CRANIOSYNOSTOSIS

Craniosynostosis is a premature closure of the cranial sutures of an infant. These sutures should remain open up to the age of 2 to allow for brain expansion. If the sutures fuse too early, the brain may be damaged because of insufficient space for growth.

Craniosynostosis is believed to be the result of a secondary transmission of tensions from the skull base through the skull vault's dural and fascial attachments. The sagittal suture is the most commonly affected suture, creating a long and narrow skull. Bilateral coronal suture craniosynostosis creates a short, high head. Unilateral coronal suture involvement flattens the frontal bone and orbit.

Clinical diagnosis is made from the misshapen appearance of the head and is confirmed with radiographic studies.

The surgeon treats sagittal and lambdoidal deformities by creating an artificial suture by strip craniectomy. A Kerrison rongeur is typically used for the cut. Silastic strips are sutured along the edges of the craniectomy strip through small holes drilled with an air drill to prevent closure of bone. Coronal suture repair involves cuts in the skull base anteriorly with orbital ridge advancement.

HYDROCEPHALUS

The obstruction of the flow of CSF through the ventricular system and into the subarachnoid space (noncommunicating hydrocephalus), an increase in the amount of CSF normally produced (communicating hydrocephalus), or the improper absorption of CSF by the arachnoid villi causes CSF pressure to rise within the cranial cavity. Obstructive hydrocephalus in the infant may result from a congenital tumor or hemorrhage at the foramen of Monro, aqueduct of Sylvius, or the canal of exit from the fourth ventricle. Childhood hydrocephalus may be a result of meningitis, tumors, hemorrhage, or aqueductal stenosis. Hydrocephalus in adults may be caused by obstructive tumors, meningitis, or hemorrhage.

Infants with hydrocephalus have an enlarged head circumference and present with enlarged and distended scalp veins. Increased intracranial pressure may cause optic atrophy, and these patients sometimes appear to have "setting sun" eyes, where the only visible part of the eye is the tops of the irises. Symptoms are related to the pressure of the expanding ventricles against the cerebral cortex. While infants may have few neurological symptoms associated with this defect, older children and adults may experience headaches, nausea, and lethargy. Some patients experience decreased mental ability, behavioral changes, and endocrine disorders.

Hydrocephalus is diagnosed by the above symptoms and confirmed with CT scanning. When CT is unable to identify hydrocephalus, ventriculography may be employed.

SPINAL AND CRANIAL DYSRAPHISM

Dysraphism is an abnormal fusion of normally united parts. Included in this classification is a condition called spina bifida. Spina bifida is a failure of the bony structures around the neural tube to close properly during embryonic development. A less severe form of dysraphism is myelomeningocele, a condition that results in a partial closure of the neural tissue with epithelium. In certain cases, neural tissue actually lies outside the skin surface. Hydrocephalus is often associated with these conditions, although a separate syndrome causes it. Cranial dysraphism usually involves a failure of the meninges to close. This condition is referred to as a meningocele. It is interesting to note that in the Western Hemisphere, 90% of all meningoceles are in the occipital region and 10% are in the frontal-basilar region, while in the Eastern Hemisphere, the distribution is exactly the opposite. Most meningoceles do not have associated hydrocephalus, and most are covered with skin.

Physical and neurological examination usually reveals dysraphic states, whether spinal or cranial. Radiographic studies of the affected area help to diagnose spina bifida or cranial defects. MRI and myelography are sometimes employed.

Surgical treatment involves closure of open lesions and the preservation of neural tissue. Surgical treatment is usually started within 36 hours for infants with open lesions for the prevention of infection. Hydrocephalus is treated with shunting. In cranial dysraphism, it is usually necessary to resect exposed cerebral substance. Because of this, there is a high mortality or permanent mental disability rate.

INFECTION

Several types of infections lead to symptoms requiring surgical intervention. Osteomyelitis, epidural abscess, and subdural empyema call for surgical debridement and drainage in addition to antibiotic treatment. Brain abscess requires surgical drainage to relieve pressure if the abscess is not treated in its early stages. In cases of meningitis-induced hydrocephalus, increased pressure is sometimes relieved by the surgical insertion of a shunt. Postoperative infections sometimes must be surgically debrided.

ABSCESS

Brain abscess arises from any of several causative factors, among them secondary infection from a primary infection such as bacterial endocarditis, direct contamination of the brain from a penetrating wound, and bone fragments or debris from traumatic injury.

Patients with brain abscess will present with symptoms related to increased intracranial pressure, such as headache, neurological deficit, and changes in the level of consciousness. These patients may have little evidence of infection and may not run a fever. Some patients present with seizures.

CT and MRI scanning are both useful in detecting abscess, and subsequent lumbar puncture with culture of the CSF helps determine the specific organism causing the infection.

Brain abscess is treated with intravenous antibiotics and bur holes or craniotomy for the drainage of pus. Drainage surgically also reduces the mass of the abscess, thus reducing the pressure on the brain and the resultant symptoms. When abscess is discovered early, treatment with antibiotics alone may suffice. Surgical debridement is also the treatment for intracranial epidural abscess, although this condition is rare.

SUBDURAL EMPYEMA

Subdural empyema is an infection of the subdural space, usually forming as a complication of trauma, meningitis, sinusitis, or contamination of the subdural space intraoperatively.

Patients with subdural empyema present with rapid neurological deterioration that results from cerebral edema caused by the accumulation of pus around the brain.

Skull and sinus radiographs and CT or MRI are used to diagnose subdural empyema. In some rare cases, spinal subdural empyema occurs.

Surgical treatment of subdural empyema consists of procedures to drain the sinus or mastoid, when involved. With spinal empyema, laminectomy is performed, and the infection is debrided and drained along with subsequent antibiotic therapy.

POSTOPERATIVE INFECTION

Postoperative infection is usually treated surgically when a foreign body is involved or when the dura mater is not sealed from the environment. When a foreign body (such as a ventriculoperitoneal or ventriculoatrial shunt) becomes infected, it should be removed immediately or it will continue to harbor infection. To prevent meningitis, drainage of infected wounds involving the CNS cannot be performed unless the dura mater is sealed. Scalp infection may be debrided surgically to treat infection.

SPINAL TUMORS

The cause of spinal tumors remains largely unknown. As with intracranial tumors, the majority are benign. Most can be excised surgically. Spinal tumors are classified according to location (Table 24-3):

1. Intramedullary—within the spinal cord
2. Intradural—within the dura but outside the spinal cord
3. Extradural—outside the spinal cord

Spinal tumors are diagnosed through radiography of the level of the spine from which symptoms originate. Radiography reveals any bony destruction of the spine and any widening of the spinal canal. Following radiography, weighted MRI is used to identify tumors. CT scanning may be used if bony masses are involved.

Surgical treatment for spinal cord tumor involves bilateral, multilevel laminectomy for biopsy and tumor excision (Figure 24-16). Certain tumors are rarely completely removable and are therefore treated with radiation. These include intramedullary astrocytomas, extradural tumors that invade the bony spine, and certain metastatic tumors. Intramedullary ependymomas, intradural meningiomas, and neurilemomas can often be completely excised. Tumor excision also relieves myelopathy, or spinal cord compression. Removal of the tumor decompresses the cord and associated nerve roots.

PERIPHERAL NERVE DISORDERS

The PNS also suffers from various conditions. Like many surgical areas, surgeons from different specialties may be

Table 24-3 Spinal Cord Tumors

TUMOR CLASSIFICATION	TUMOR TYPES	SYMPTOMS
Intramedullary	Astrocytoma, ependymoma	Progressive weakness, sensory loss
Intradural	Meningioma, neurinoma	Progressive weakness, sensory loss due to cord compression, symptoms of nerve root compression (radiculopathy)
Extradural		Progressive weakness, sensory loss due to cord compression (myelopathy), numbness or weakness and pain (radiculopathy), bony tumors create spine pain

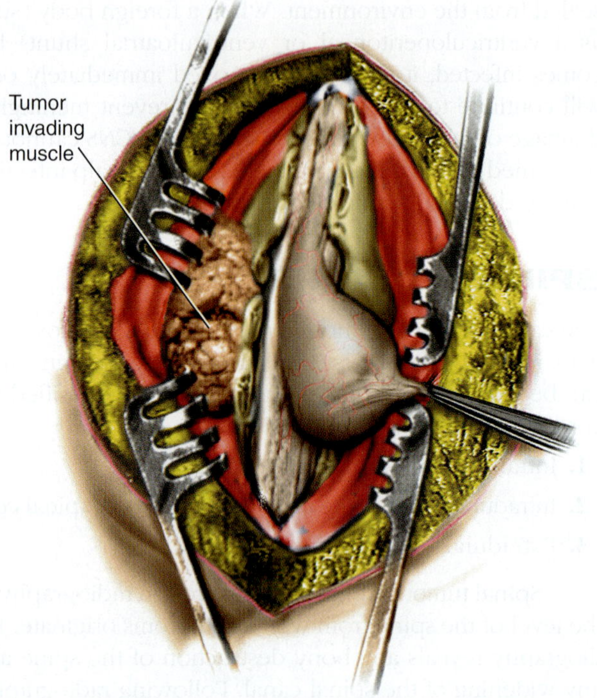

Figure 24-16 Spinal cord tumor

involved in peripheral nerve surgery. However, the neurosurgeon remains active in this area.

CARPAL TUNNEL SYNDROME

Carpal tunnel syndrome is compression of the median nerve at the level of the wrist. This condition may be due to swelling, a thickening of the transverse carpal ligament, or a deformity that may be congenital or acquired due to trauma.

The patient is aware of pain and numbness in the hand. Carpal tunnel syndrome is often the result of repetitive hand movement and is frequently associated with the patient's occupation.

The condition is diagnosed by patient history, physical examination, and electrical studies designed to measure nerve function. Arthroscopic or open carpal tunnel release is the surgical treatment of choice.

ULNAR NERVE COMPRESSION

The ulnar nerve can become entrapped or compressed at the level of the elbow by the ligament of Osborne. The patient typically presents with pain in the ring and small finger of the affected hand. Pain is sometimes accompanied by muscle weakness that is caused by inflammation from overuse or external trauma.

As with carpal tunnel syndrome, electrical nerve conduction studies as well as presentation with the above symptoms are evidence of this disorder. Ulnar nerve decompression or ulnar nerve transposition are the surgical interventions of choice for this disorder.

NEUROSURGICAL PROCEDURES

For the patient undergoing neurological surgery, special consideration must be given pertaining to neurological deficit such as aphasia or hemianopia. The patient is often fearful of intraoperative or postoperative death or loss of function. For some intracranial procedures that are performed under local anesthesia only, the patient receives no preoperative sedation because he or she needs to be alert throughout the operation. This can be an anxious experience for the patient, and the surgical team must make preparations to allay unnecessary anxiety.

The chart should be reviewed by surgical personnel for patient history and physical, consent, diagnostic findings, and laboratory results. Diagnostic tests for review include routine chest X-ray and electrocardiogram, electroencephalogram, cerebral arteriogram, and CT scan or MRI. The patient is generally typed and cross-matched for possible blood replacement, and OR personnel should check with the blood bank to be sure that blood has been ordered and is available.

The surgical team should ensure that all necessary equipment for positioning and for the procedure is in the room and working properly. The surgeon's preference card should be checked for any supplies or equipment that may not have been pulled. It is always a good idea to speak with the surgeon before setup begins for insight into any possible procedural variations.

Anesthesia for neurosurgical procedures should be performed by physicians who are specially trained in neurological anesthesia. The patient will require a high degree of monitoring intraoperatively and postoperatively.

SPECIAL INSTRUMENTATION, SUPPLIES, DRUGS, AND EQUIPMENT

Special equipment for neurosurgical procedures includes:

1. The standard operating microscope for increased illumination and variable magnification of the operative field. Microscopes can be mounted on floor stands or suspended from the ceiling. Sophisticated support stands allow for ease of movement of the scope, and some can be moved using mouth-controlled devices. Some companies are now offering microscopes that track the focal point of the scope and are programmed to convey that information on the patient's CT or MRI scan. Robotic surgical microscopes can be programmed to remember positions in space for automatic positioning.

2. Video camera, monitor, and recorder.
3. YAG or CO_2 laser. The CO_2 laser is able to deliver variable amounts of precise energy for removal of small amounts of tissue in tight places. The energy is delivered through a tube using a series of mirrors, and can be attached to the operating microscope. The neodymium:YAG (Nd:YAG) laser delivers diffuse energy for better coagulation of bleeding vessels around the target tissue. The laser's beam is delivered down a fiberoptic strand to a handheld device or an endoscope.
4. Positioning equipment, such as the Mayfield "horseshoe" headrest, or Gardner-Wells or Mayfield pin fixation device (Figure 24-17). The Wilson frame or Andrews table may be employed for posterior approaches to the thoracic or lumbar spine.
5. Operative ultrasound machine. This instrument emits sound waves that penetrate the brain and bounce back to the machine to generate an image. It is typically used to locate lesions that lie deep beneath the surface of the cerebrum and to evaluate the completeness of tumor resection.
6. Frame-based or frameless stereotaxis systems. These systems can precisely deliver an instrument to a target at any point within a defined space. The target space is defined by CT or MRI scanning with reference points attached to the head. Various monitoring devices and amplifiers are used in conjunction with these systems.
7. Cavitron ultrasonic aspirator (CUSA). This device emits a variable ultrasonic energy field that emulsifies abnormal tissue while preserving normal neural tissue. Saline ejected from the tip of the handheld unit liquefies the tissue, which is then aspirated back to the unit. This instrument is used when a moderate to large amount of tissue is to be removed.
8. Heating/cooling unit and temperature monitoring devices.
9. Bipolar and monopolar electrosurgical units.
10. Neuroendoscope, light source, recorder, and monitor.
11. Nitrogen source for power equipment (piped in or portable tank).
12. Mayfield overhead table.
13. Headlight and fiberoptic light source.
14. C-arm and monitor.
15. Fluid warming units and Cell Saver autotransfusion machine.

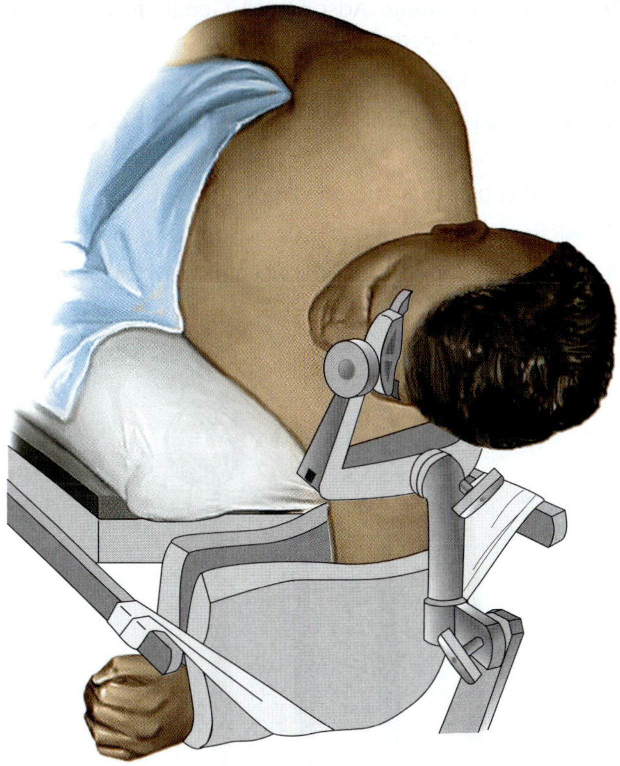

Figure 24-17 Pin fixation device

Instrument sets for spinal procedures include a basic neurological set or laminectomy set for posterior approaches, and an anterior cervical discectomy set that includes the instruments necessary for the exposure and removal of the anterior cervical disk and the excision and placement of a bone graft.

A minor set may be necessary if the laminectomy set is only supplied with bone and neurosurgical instruments. A basic orthopedic set is necessary for bone procurement for fusion after laminectomy. A specialty set of plates and screws may also be used.

Instrument sets for craniotomy include a minor set with basic clamps, scissors, forceps, towel clips, knife handles, needle holders, and retractors and a basic craniotomy set or neurological set. A basic neurological set is equipped with the following basic instruments:

1. Hudson brace with bits and attachments (Figure 24-18)
2. Gigli saw, handles, and guide for bone flaps (Figure 24-19)
3. Various bone rongeurs (Kerrison, Leksell, Stille-Leur, Adson)
4. Various pituitary rongeurs (straight, up-biting, down-biting)
5. Penfield dissectors (Figure 24-20)
6. Self-retaining retractors (Gelpi—shallow and deep), Weitlaner, Adson-Beckman, Adson cerebellar)
7. Manual retractors (Cushing, Meyerding, Army-Navy, Taylor)
8. Malleable brain spoons (Silastic, metal)

9. Bayonet, Cushing, Adson, and Gerald forceps, with and without teeth
10. Nerve hooks
11. Periosteal elevators (Adson, Langenbeck, Freer, Cushing)
12. Dural separators and elevators
13. Suction tips (e.g., Frazier or Adson) of various sizes
14. Scalp clip applicators or scalp gun (may be separate) (Figure 24-21)

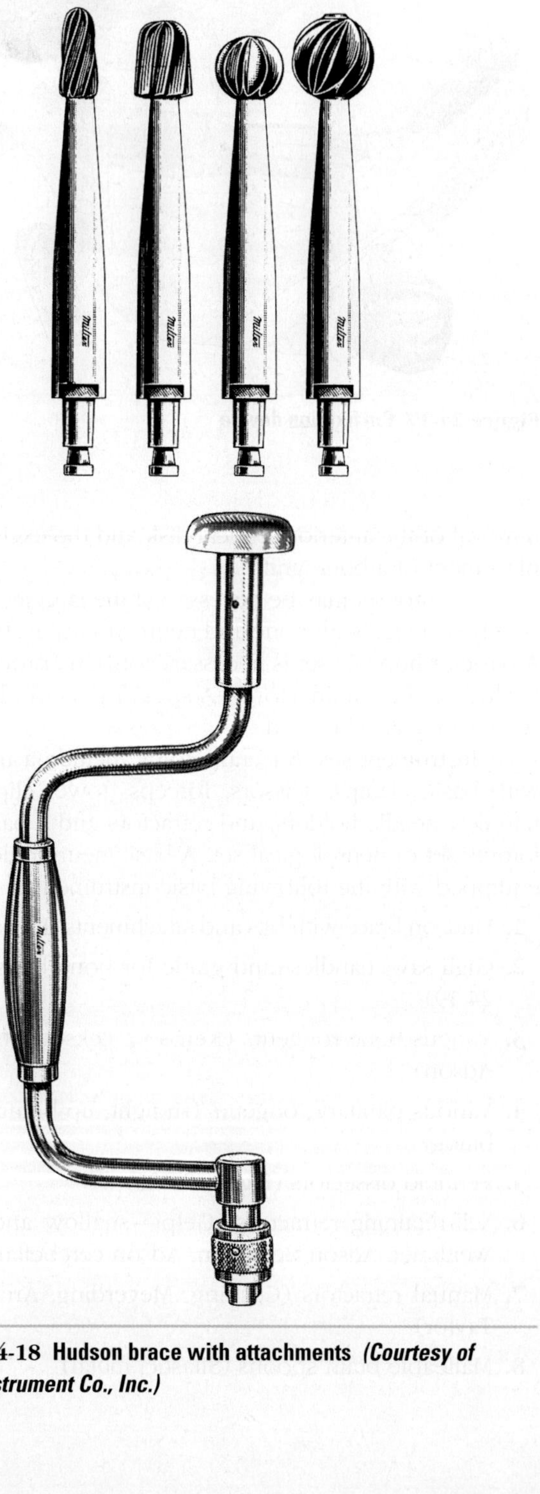

Figure 24-18 Hudson brace with attachments *(Courtesy of Miltex Instrument Co., Inc.)*

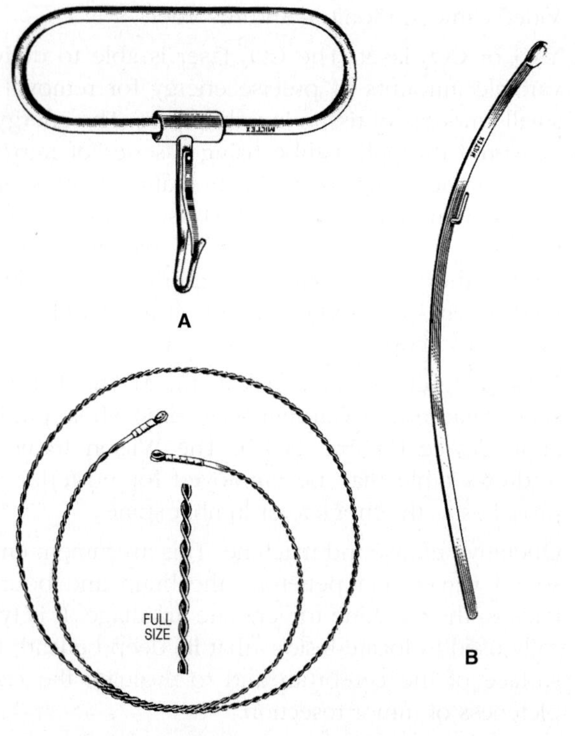

Figure 24-19 Gigli saw: (A) Handle, (B) guide, (C) blade ***(Courtesy of Miltex Instrument Co., Inc.)***

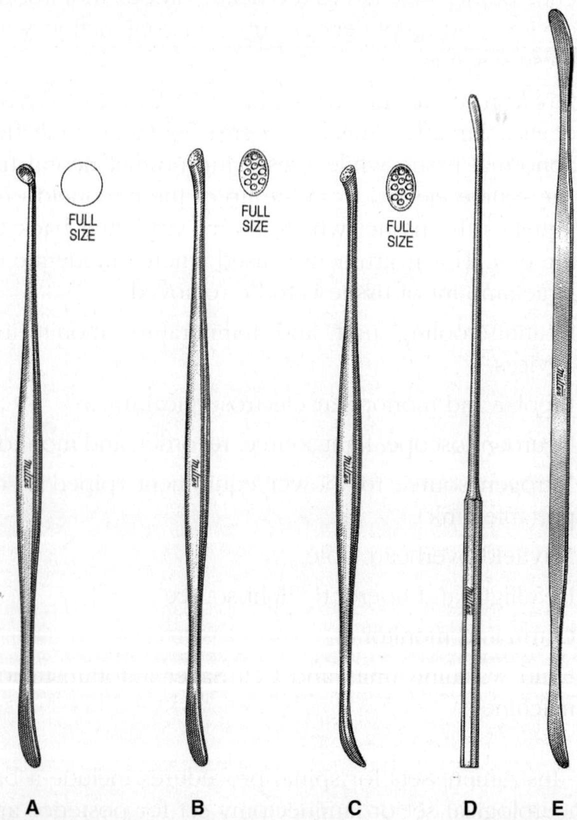

Figure 24-20 Penfield dissectors: (A) Style #1, (B) style #2, (C) style #3, (D) style #4, (E) style #5 ***(Courtesy of Miltex Instrument Co., Inc.)***

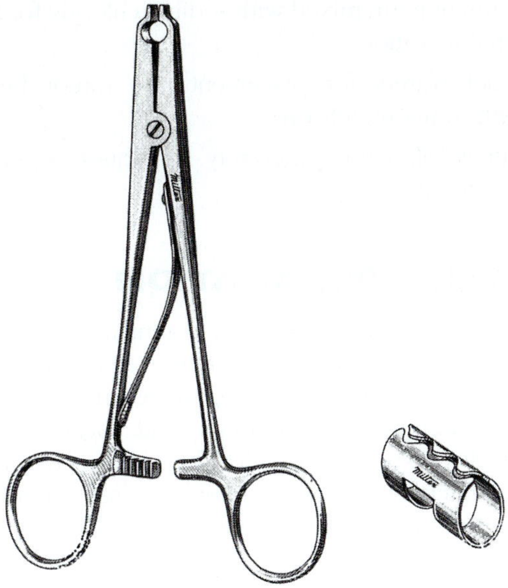

A B

Figure 24-21 **Raney scalp clip system: (A) Applicator, (B) clip *(Courtesy of Miltex Instrument Co., Inc.)***

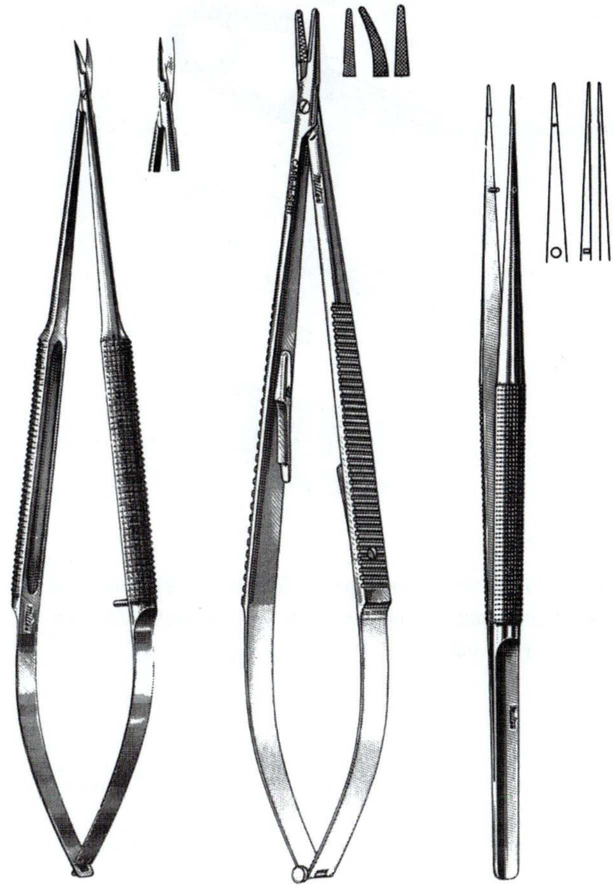

A B C

Figure 24-22 **Microsurgical instruments: (A) Microsurgery scissors, (B) Jacobson microvascular needle holder, (C) Rhoton micro forceps *(Courtesy of Miltex Instrument Co., Inc.)***

15. Leyla-Yasargil or Greenberg self-retaining retractor (may be separate)
16. Dandy clamps
17. Hemoclip applicators (short)
18. Bone curettes, gouges, and osteotomes (may be separate)
19. Bipolar forceps
20. Dura hooks
21. Pituitary spoons

Power instrumentation includes Midas Rex or Anspach pneumatic drill with attachments, burs, and bits; air-, battery-, or electric-powered cranial perforator and craniotome with dura guard; and wire-pass air drill with burs and bits.

Microsurgical instruments include arachnoid knife, micro forceps (bayonet-type), curettes, scissors, needle holders, dissectors, and bipolar forceps (Figure 24-22).

Fusion of the posterior spine typically requires the following specialty instrumentation for the removal of cancellous and cortical bone from the iliac crest:

1. Bone curettes of variable sizes, curved and straight
2. Osteotomes of various sizes, curved and straight
3. Gouges of various sizes, curved and straight
4. Large mallet
5. Oscillating saw (optional)
6. Gelpi self-retaining retractors
7. Army-Navy and/or Hibbs retractors
8. Periosteal elevator (Cobb, Key, Langenbeck)

Aneurysm repair requires the use of microsurgical instruments with aneurysm clips and applicators, such as those designed by Yasargil (Figure 24-23).

Transphenoidal procedures require a minor set for fascial resection, a basic neuro set, a nasal set, Cushing's speculum, enucleators, pituitary spoons, and dissectors.

Standard supplies for any neurological procedure include #10, #15, and #11 knife blades, disposable basin set, suction tubing, Ray-Tec sponges, laparotomy sponges, Asepto bulb syringes, syringes and needles (for preoperative injection of lidocaine with epinephrine), marking pen, and needle counter.

Draping supplies include towels, plastic adhesive drape, craniotomy drape for cranial procedures, laparotomy drape for most posterior spinal procedures, thyroid sheet for anterior cervical discectomy, and extremity sheet, ¾ sheet, and stockinette for peripheral nerve procedures.

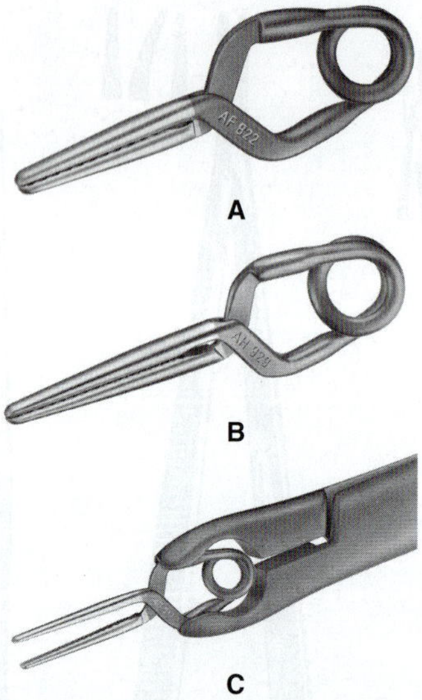

Figure 24-23 **Aneurysm clips: (A) Temporary, (B) permanent, (C) applicator loaded with aneurysm clip** ***(Courtesy of Miltex Instrument Co., Inc.)***

Specialty supplies for neurosurgical procedures include:

- Hemostatic agents (Gelfoam, Avitene, Surgicel, bone wax)
- Disposable bipolar cord (for attachment to nondisposable bipolar forceps)
- Monopolar electrosurgical pencil
- Radiopaque cottonoid strips of various sizes
- Raney scalp clips (for scalp clip gun or manual applicators)
- Hemostatic clips (MRI compatible)
- Rubber bands for Dandy clamps
- Shunt catheters, tubing, and connectors
- Cotton balls
- Drain (Hemovac)
- Nerve stimulator
- Telfa
- Microscope drape
- C-arm drape
- Ultrasound wand drape

Suture materials for neurological procedures include silk or braided nylon for the dura; polyester, polyglactin 910, or braided nylon for wound closure; and monofilament nylon or stainless steel clips for skin.

Intraoperatively used drugs and solutions include:

1. Antibiotic solution of surgeon's choice mixed with warm saline for irrigation
2. Topical papaverine for the prevention of vasospasm during intracranial arterial surgery
3. Thrombin for use with Gelfoam for hemostasis
4. Methyl methacrylate for cranioplasty procedures
5. Sodium heparin mixed with sodium chloride for intra-arterial irrigation
6. Gliadel wafers for placement into tumor bed of glioblastoma multiforme
7. Contrast solution (e.g., Conray, Hypaque) for cerebral arteriogram

PATIENT PREPARATION

Neurological pathology has such potentially devastating consequences that a full perioperative team approach is usually required. This includes registered nurses, physical therapists, occupational therapists, and social workers. The complexity of neurosurgical procedures requires a team approach in the OR. Equipment, instrumentation, and patient preparation are often very involved.

CRANIAL PROCEDURES

After transportation from the holding area, the patient is assisted in moving from the transport stretcher to the OR table. If unconscious, quadriplegic, paraplegic, or impaired in any way, the patient will have to be lifted by operative personnel. If the procedure is to be performed in the prone position, the patient is anesthetized and intubated on the transport stretcher, then repositioned on the OR table.

Monitoring equipment is prepared by anesthesia personnel and may include a Swan-Ganz catheter for central venous pressure recordings, arterial catheter for arterial blood gases, and ECG, EEG, pulse oximeter, thermometer, and blood pressure equipment. Fluid intake and output should be carefully monitored during cranial procedures. The Foley catheter with attached urinometer should be inserted just after induction and intubation and before positioning begins.

Positioning of the patient undergoing a cranial procedure can be complex because of the headrests, fixation devices, and stereotactic equipment used in neurosurgical positioning. Pillows, pads, sheets, blankets, wide tape, and chest rolls are all necessary for proper positioning. The surgical approach and type of procedure determine the position.

The supine position is the most common approach, allowing exposure of the frontal, parietal, and temporal lobes. This position may require a simple "donut" headrest for superficial tumor or clot removal, or a three-pin skull fixation system, such as a Gardner-Wells or Mayfield pin fixation device, for procedures that require complete immobilization of the head. Before the skull pins are placed into the skull, they are sterilized and then slipped into the skull clamp. The patient's head is prepped with iodophor, and the device is inserted into the skull, attached to the OR table, and locked into position.

The lateral or semilateral position may be utilized for exposure of the unilateral temporal lobe, occipital lobe, brain stem, or cerebellum. Stabilization of the body in the lateral position generally requires equipment, such as a bean bag or chest rolls, tape, and pillows. The head may be placed onto a headrest or into a fixation device, depending on the type of procedure.

The sitting position allows bilateral access to the occipital lobe, brain stem, or cerebellum. It requires the use of a three-pin skull fixation device attached to a frame that attaches to the side rails of the head end of the operating table.

The prone position may be utilized for bilateral access to the occipital lobe, cerebellum, or brain stem. Typically, chest rolls support the chest and pillows are placed under the legs and feet. A padded Mayfield horseshoe headrest that replaces the smaller, adjustable head of the operating table supports the patient's head. A pin fixation device may also be utilized. The patient is typically anesthetized and intubated on the stretcher and then rolled over onto an OR table that has been equipped with the Mayfield headrest.

For intracranial procedures that require a general anesthetic, hair is typically shaved in the OR after the induction of anesthesia to prevent undue discomfort and anxiety for the patient. Some surgeons prefer that hair be shaved in the holding area. Typically, only enough hair is removed to safely facilitate the incision, and any hair that is removed is saved in a plastic bag as the property of the patient. Hair should be shaved as close to incision time as possible to decrease the chance for infection, and great care must be taken to prevent small nicks in the scalp.

A small covered prep table equipped with electric or battery-powered hair clippers, straight or safety razor, 4 × 4s, and a bowl of water with a scrub brush is often used for shaving the head.

After the patient has been positioned and shaved, the circulator preps the patient with an iodophor scrub solution and blots with a sterile towel. Some surgeons prefer to paint the head with iodophor paint solution and alcohol from a sterile Mayo tray equipped with small bowls, 4 × 4 sponges, sponge sticks, marking pen, and a 10-cc syringe loaded with 1% lidocaine with epinephrine. After the prep, the physician marks the incision site with the marking pen and then injects with 1% lidocaine and epinephrine for hemostasis.

The patient is square-draped with towels and the towels are secured with small towel clips, skin clips, or 3–0 silk sutures. A craniotomy drape with a plastic adhesive sheet built into the round fenestration is placed so that the attached plastic bag hangs below the patient's head at the surgeon's feet. This bag collects the blood and irrigation fluid that runs down from the operative site and funnels it through suction tubing into a suction canister.

If the Mayfield table is to be used, it is placed over the patient with its edge just below the patient's chin before draping begins. The craniotomy sheet is placed over the table, and instrumentation is then brought up by the STSR and placed onto the draped Mayfield table. Suction tubing and bipolar and unipolar electrosurgical lines are passed off and hooked up, as are power equipment cords or hoses.

SPINAL PROCEDURES

For spinal procedures performed in the prone position, the patient is anesthetized on the transport stretcher and rolled onto either the Wilson or Andrews frame or chest rolls. The knee-to-chest position is occasionally used for surgery of the lumbar spine. For bilateral posterior cervical procedures, the Mayfield horseshoe headrest may replace the OR table's head section, with the patient positioned prone using chest rolls. Cervical procedures are still occasionally performed in the sitting position, with the head secured by pin fixation and arms extended onto padded armboards. Unilateral spinal procedures can be performed in the lateral position, with the affected side up.

Anterior cervical discectomy and fusion is performed in the supine position with the head turned away from the affected side and the hip slightly elevated for bone procurement. Anterior approaches to the lumbar spine are performed in the supine position, and the patient may be turned to the prone position to complete the procedure. The anterior thoracic spine may be approached via thoracotomy in the lateral position.

Monitoring equipment is prepared by anesthesia personnel and includes ECG, pulse oximeter, thermometer, and blood pressure equipment. Certain spinal procedures may require electrophysiological monitoring. Antiembolic stockings may be applied preoperatively.

After positioning, hair is typically shaved from the operative area. Posterior cervical procedures may require the removal of some head hair, so clippers should be available. The operative area is then prepped with iodophor scrub to the proper perimeters, and blotted with a sterile towel. The circulator or the surgeon then applies iodophor paint, and draping begins with four folded towels placed by the surgeon. An adhesive drape often follows, and then the laparotomy or thyroid sheet is positioned.

Suction tubing and bipolar, monopolar, and power cords are passed off by the STSR and hooked up by the circulator. The two Mayo stands (one for bone and one for soft tissue instruments) are positioned, and the incision is made.

CRANIOTOMY

Craniotomy involves incising the cranium for access to the brain, usually for the removal of blood clots or lesions, or for repair of aneurysm or arteriovenous malformation (Procedure 24-1).

(Text continues on page 997)

PROCEDURE

24-1 Craniotomy

Equipment

- Monopolar and bipolar electrosurgical units
- Fiberoptic headlight and light source (optional)
- Positioning devices (pin fixation device, Mayfield headrest, pillows, chest rolls)
- Operating microscope and/or loupes (optional)
- CUSA (optional)
- CO_2 or Nd:YAG laser (optional)
- Ultrasound machine and attachments (optional)
- Two suction systems
- Nitrogen source
- Mayfield overhead table
- Autotransfusion machine (optional)
- Temperature monitoring device

Instruments

- Craniotomy set, or basic neurological set
- Microsurgical instruments (optional)
- Anspach or Midas Rex power instruments with attachments, or cranial perforator and craniotome
- Air drill with bits and burs

Supplies

- Pack: basic
- Basin set
- Gloves
- Blades (#10, #11, #15)
- Drapes: towels, craniotomy drape
- Suture: 4–0 silk, 4–0 Nurolon
- Closure suture of surgeon's preference
- Drains: Hemovac
- Dressings: inner contact gauze (e.g., petroleum gauze), 4 × 4s, Kerlix
- Drugs:
  - Hemostatic agents (Gelfoam with topical thrombin, Surgicel, Avitene)
  - Antibiotic irrigation
  - Xylocaine 1% with epinephrine
- Miscellaneous:
  - Laparotomy sponges
  - Ray-Tec sponges
  - Control syringe
  - Hypodermic needles
  - Electrosurgical pencil
  - Bipolar cord for attachment to bipolar bayonet forceps
  - Suction tubing (2)
  - Radiopaque cottonoid strips of various sizes
  - Raney scalp clips (for scalp gun or manual applicators)
  - Hemostatic clips (MRI compatible)
  - Rubber bands for Dandy clamps
  - Cotton balls
  - Telfa for specimen
  - Microscope drape
  - Ultrasound wand drape
  - Asepto syringes

Operative Preparation

Anesthesia

- General

Position

- Depends on approach

Prep

- The area around the incision site should be shaved with an electric razor and straight or safety razor. Hair should be saved for the patient in a plastic bag
- Eyes and ears should be protected from prep solutions
- After the initial prep with iodophor scrub by the circulator, the surgeon may paint from a sterile Mayo with alcohol and/or iodophor paint

Draping

- Square-drape with towels that may be sutured in place with silk on a cutting needle
- Placement of the craniotomy drape with built-in adhesive drape over the fenestration

PROCEDURE 24-1 Craniotomy *(continued)*

Practical Considerations

- Make sure CT or MRI scans, arteriograms, or plain film studies are in the room before the procedure begins
- Always test drills and saws before the procedure
- Surgicel should be cut into strips and postage stamp-size squares. Microsurgical and vascular procedures may require smaller cuts
- Gelfoam is typically cut into postage stamp-size squares and 1–3 in. strips, placed into a container, and saturated with topical thrombin mixed and poured by the circulator. Microsurgical and vascular procedures may require smaller size pieces
- Frazier suction tips are easily clogged with debris. A 10-cc syringe filled with saline and attached to the proximal port completely flushes debris out of the tube
- Know how to drape microscopes, ultrasound devices, and C-arms. Wounds should be protected from non-sterile overhead X-ray units with sterile towels
- For emergency cranial procedures, think about what you will be doing first and prepare the items necessary to do those things. Decide what you will need to quickly get into the head and control hemorrhage
- Small dural needles and cottonoids are easily lost. Keep close track of these
- Make sure that the Mayfield horseshoe headrest and pin fixation devices are locked into place and the handle is secured to prevent slippage

Operative Procedure	Technical Considerations
1. Digital pressure is applied to each side of the marked incision line for hemostasis, a U-shaped incision is performed, and Raney scalp clips are applied over the upper skin edges.	1. Unless a Raney clip applicator gun is used, the STSR should quickly load the Raney scalp clips onto the applicators as they are received from the surgeon. Bleeding from the scalp can be profuse, and the surgeon will not want to wait while a clip is loaded.
2. Dandy hemostatic clamps may be placed onto the lower skin edges and secured with rubber bands around the handles.	2. If used, Dandy clamps should be passed to the surgeon with tips pointing downward.
3. The galea and periosteum are incised by electrosurgery, and the cranium is exposed.	3. Electosurgical smoke should be suctioned with a suction tip held close to the electrosurgical pencil.
4. After hemostasis has been achieved, the scalp flap is dissected away from the cranium, folded backward over a laparotomy sponge, and secured to the drape for retraction.	4. The STSR should be ready to pass a small towel clip, rubber band and/or Ray-Tec sponge, and hemostat for attachment of the scalp flap to the drape.
5. Muscle and periosteum are stripped away from the cranium with a periosteal elevator and retracted.	5. A U.S. Army or Cushing retractor will be needed at this step, and self-retaining Gelpi retractors will be placed at both ends of the incision.
6. Two or more bur holes are made into the cranium with an air-powered bur, such as the Midas Rex, or an electric, battery, or air-powered cranial perforator. Occasionally, bur holes are drilled manually with a Hudson brace and D'Errico bit (Figure 24-24).	6. As the surgeon drills the bur holes, the surgical assistant should irrigate the bit with normal saline to counteract the heat generated by friction, and to remove bone dust that accumulates in the hole.

(continues)

PROCEDURE 24-1 Craniotomy *(continued)*

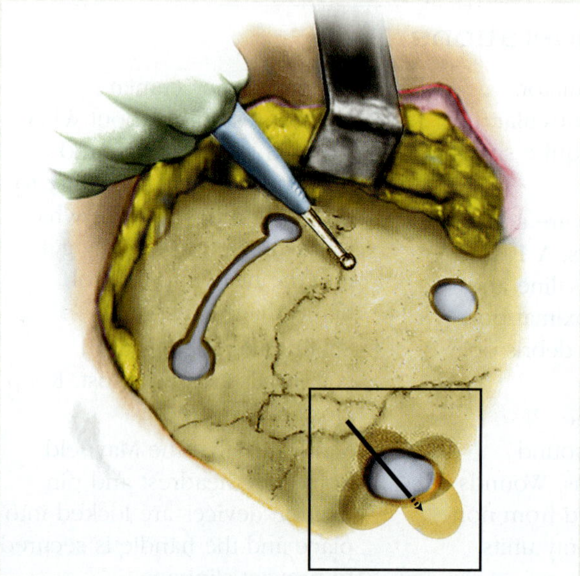

Figure 24-24 Bur holes

7. After the holes are drilled, they may be enlarged with a double-action rongeur or Kerrison rongeur. Any bleeding from the edges of the bur holes is controlled by bone wax and neurosurgical sponge.	**7.** Bone wax balls may be pressed against the tip of a #4 Penfield dissector by the STSR, and passed to the surgeon for placement against bur hole edges. Otherwise, the bone wax is smeared against bur hole edges by hand and a cottonoid pressed against the bone wax with bayonet forceps ensures hemostasis.
8. A small, straight bone curette is used to carve away the inner table and expose the dura.	**8.** As the curette is being used, the STSR should be preparing and testing the craniotome. If the Midas Rex or Anspach is used, the bur is removed and the craniotome blade is inserted with dural guard.
9. The dura around the bur hole is separated from the cranium by a #3 Penfield dissector to prevent tearing of the dura mater when the flap is turned.	**9.** Suction may be necessary. Pass dural separator or Penfield.
10. The cranium between the bur holes is cut with an electric-, battery-, or air-powered craniotome saw with dural guard attachment. Occasionally, the cranium is manually cut with a Gigli saw.	**10.** As with the cranial perforator, the craniotome bit should be irrigated to displace heat generated by friction and remove accumulated bone dust.
11. After each bur hole has been connected, the bone flap is carefully lifted away from the dura with a periosteal elevator (Figure 24-25).	**11.** If the mechanical craniotome fails, the Gigli saw may be used as a backup.
12. If muscle has been left attached, the bone flap is covered with a moistened laparotomy pad and retracted in a manner similar to the scalp flap; otherwise, it is removed.	**12.** The bone flap should be placed in a basin on the back table to soak in Betadine solution or normal saline and antibiotic.

PROCEDURE

24-1 Craniotomy *(continued)*

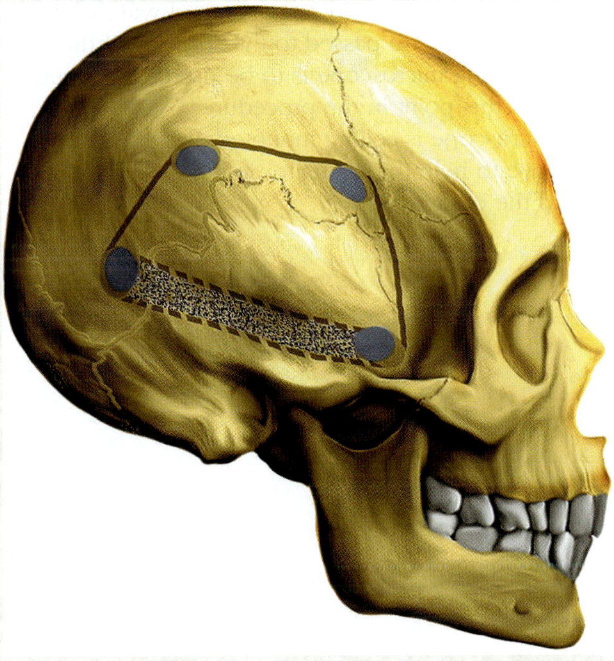

Figure 24-25 Temporal craniotomy

13. Bleeding around the bone edges is controlled with bone wax; bleeding from the dura is controlled with the bipolar forceps and thrombin-soaked Gelfoam.	**13.** After the bone flap is turned and the dura is exposed, the STSR should be ready with an Asepto filled with warm saline dura so that the dural bleeders may be identified.
14. Holes may be drilled along the edges of the cranial defect for epidural tacking to prevent postoperative epidural dead space.	**14.** Holes will be drilled with an air drill (e.g., Stryker Micro-Aire) or Midas Rex. The dura will be tacked with 4–0 braided nylon sutures.
15. Dural traction may be necessary to pull the dura away from the brain surface before incising.	**15.** Dural traction is achieved with 4–0 braided nylon traction sutures. Some surgeons prefer to use a dural hook instead.
16. A small incision is made into the dura.	**16.** The dura is incised with a #11 or #15 blade on a #7 knife handle, and the incision is extended with Metzenbaum or dura scissors and Cushing or Gerald forceps.
17. Cottonoid patties are placed under the dura with bayonet forceps as the dura is incised to protect delicate brain tissue underneath, and 4–0 dural traction sutures are placed along the dural edges and tagged with mosquito hemostats for retraction.	**17.** Dural sutures are placed in an interrupted fashion. The STSR should load one suture as the other is passed, and maintain close track of small dural needles as they are returned on the needle holders.

(continues)

PROCEDURE 24-1 Craniotomy *(continued)*

18. Brain spoons are placed and held manually or attached to the Leyla-Yasargil self-retaining retractor (Figure 24-26).

18. Brain spoons should be moistened with saline before they are passed to the surgeon. If the operating microscope is to be used, it is brought in at this point in the procedure. Unless the microscope is ceiling mounted, the STSR may have to help the circulator guide the microscope to the operative site.

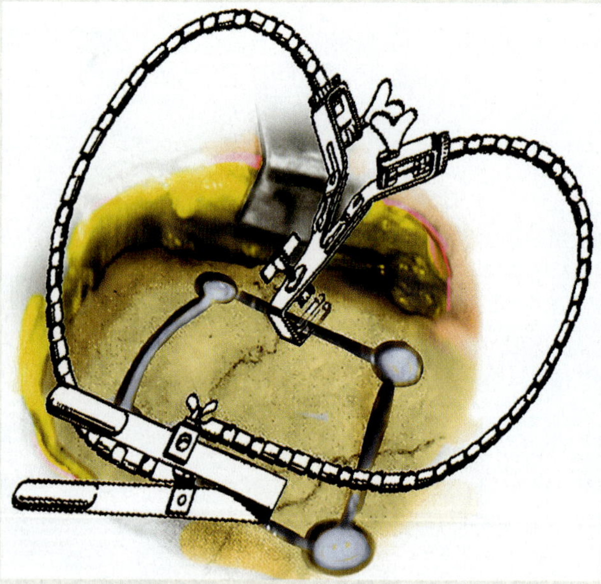

Figure 24-26 Self-retaining brain retractor

19. The pathological condition is treated, and hemostasis is achieved with warm saline irrigation, Surgicel, thrombin-impregnated Gelfoam, and the bipolar cautery.

19. Surgicel that is cut into various sizes may be placed onto a folded towel and presented to the surgeon. The surgeon selects the preferred size with bayonet forceps.

20. The brain is irrigated with copious amounts of warm saline and antibiotic, and the dura is closed in an airtight fashion with a running 4–0 braided nylon or silk suture.

20. At this point, copious amounts of saline will be used. Two Asepto syringes are necessary so that the surgeon does not have to wait as an Asepto is filled. The STSR should keep close track of the amount of saline that is used.

21. The Midas Rex or small air drill is used to place holes at strategic locations along the edges of the cranial defect and the bone flap, and the flap is secured to the cranium with titanium plates and screws. Some surgeons may prefer to wire the bone flap to the cranium with stainless steel wire.

21. A stainless steel brain spoon or periosteal elevator placed between the cranium and the dura prevents the drill from penetrating brain tissue.

22. A Hemovac drain is placed in the epicranium and brought up through the scalp through a small stab wound. The wound is closed in layers.

22. The Hemovac is secured with an 0 or 2–0 silk suture with cutting needle. The reservoir should be attached immediately to prevent clot formation within the drain.

PROCEDURE

24-1 Craniotomy *(continued)*

Postoperative Considerations

Immediate Postoperative Care

- Care must be taken not to drop the head when removing it from the pin fixation device.
- Operative personnel should take precautions when moving the patient to the transport stretcher or ICU bed. The patient will have monitoring lines, urinary catheter and drainage bag, wound drains, or other important lines that can be easily pulled.

Prognosis

- Prognosis depends on the pathological situation and the condition that the patient was in preoperatively.

Complications

- Complications that may occur postoperatively include wound infection, meningitis, neurological deficits related to the pathological condition, or intraoperative damage to vital structures, subdural or epidural hematoma, or intracerebral hemorrhage. Postoperative bleeding and intracranial pressure is monitored closely by ICU or recovery room personnel through Hemovac drainage and attention to neurological signs. If bleeding is deemed excessive, the patient is returned to the OR and the wound is reopened for hemorrhage control.

PEARL OF WISDOM

Make sure saline irrigation is always body temperature. Always test the temperature of the saline before handing it to the surgeon. Keep close track of the amount of irrigation used.

CRANIOTOMY FOR REMOVAL OF MENINGIOMA

Meningiomas are the most common of the slow-growing intracranial neoplasms, and, although they can arise from any part of the meninges, they typically favor certain locations. Because of their focal nature, these lesions are surgically treatable with a low probability of recurrence. Most meningiomas are extracerebral, in that they do not invade the brain but slowly displace brain tissue. Meningiomas are relatively vascular neoplasms, and the location of some of them can be very challenging for the surgical team.

The objective of the procedure is to remove the entire meningioma including its dural attachment and any bone that may be involved, with preservation of neurological function. The patient is started on steroidal medication 48 hours before the procedure to control cerebral edema. A central venous line is placed and urinary catheterization is achieved after induction. Ten to 20 mg of furosemide and 100 g of mannitol is administered intravenously at the beginning of the procedure. Positioning depends upon the location of the tumor.

The procedure follows the steps and requirements for a standard craniotomy. There are two significant technical considerations to be added to the routine craniotomy:

- A CUSA is normally used to **decompress** the tumor; it must be set up and checked prior to the scalp incision.
- Since many meningiomas have meningeal origination at the base of the skull, an operative microscope will be required on most cases.

CRANIOTOMY FOR ANEURYSM REPAIR

The goal of surgical treatment for cerebral aneurysm is to isolate the aneurysm from the parent vessel by placing a specially designed clip across the neck of the aneurysm (Procedure 24-2). If the aneurysm cannot be clipped in such a manner, the sac of the defect may be reinforced with synthetic materials such as methyl methacrylate or mesh gauze, or one of the feeding vessels may be ligated. Nonsurgical techniques include the placement of multiple coils of platinum wire into the aneurysm to cause thrombosis. Occasionally, the common carotid artery may be occluded to shut down the blood supply to one hemisphere.

PROCEDURE 24-2 Craniotomy for Aneurysm Repair

Equipment

- Monopolar and bipolar electrosurgical units
- Fiberoptic headlight and light source (optional)
- Positioning devices (pin fixation device)
- Operating microscope
- Suction system
- Nitrogen source
- Mayfield overhead table
- Autotransfusion machine (optional)
- Temperature monitoring device

Instruments

- Craniotomy set, or basic neurological set
- Anspach or Midas Rex power instruments with attachments, or cranial perforator and craniotome
- Air drill with bits and burs (not necessary if Anspach or Midas Rex are used)
- Microsurgical instruments
- Aneurysm clip applicators
- A self-retaining brain spoon retractor (e.g., Leyla-Yasargil)
- Carotid set for carotid artery exposure should be available for hemorrhage control

Supplies

- Pack: basic
- Basin set
- Gloves
- Blades (#10, #11, #15)
- Drapes: towels, craniotomy drape
- Suture:
  - 4–0 silk, 4–0 Nurolon
  - Closure suture of surgeon's preference
- Drains: Hemovac
- Dressings: inner contact gauze (e.g., petroleum gauze), 4 × 4s, Kerlix
- Drugs:
  - Hemostatic agents (Gelfoam with topical thrombin, Surgicel, Avitene)
  - Antibiotic irrigation
  - Papaverine
  - Xylocaine 1% with epinephrine for hemostasis
- Miscellaneous:
  - Laparotomy sponges
  - Ray-Tec sponges
  - Control syringe
  - Hypodermic needles
  - Electrosurgical pencil
  - Bipolar cord for attachment to bipolar bayonet forceps
  - Suction tubing (2)
  - Radiopaque cottonoid strips of various sizes
  - Raney scalp clips (for scalp gun or manual applicators)
  - Hemostatic clips (MRI compatible)
  - Aneurysm clips (temporary and permanent)
  - Rubber bands for Dandy clamps
  - Cotton balls
  - Telfa for specimen
  - Microscope drape
  - Asepto syringes

Operative Preparation

Anesthesia

- General

Position

- Supine with the head turned away from the affected side for a unilateral frontotemporal approach. A bifrontal approach is necessary for some aneurysms. A three-point pin fixation device will be secured to the head for complete stabilization

Prep

- The area around the incision site should be shaved with an electric razor and straight or safety razor.

Hair should be saved for the patient in a plastic bag

- Eyes and ears should be protected from prep solutions
- After the initial prep with iodophor scrub by the circulator, the surgeon may paint from a sterile Mayo with alcohol and/or iodophor paint

Draping

- Square-drape with towels that may be sutured in place with silk on a cutting needle
- Placement of the craniotomy drape with built-in adhesive drape over the fenestration

Practical Considerations

- Make sure CT or MRI scans, arteriograms, or plain film studies are in the room before the procedure begins
- Make sure saline irrigation is always body temperature. Always test the temperature of the saline before handing it to the surgeon
- Keep close track of the amount of irrigation used

Operative Procedure

1. The scalp and bone flaps are turned, and the dura is opened and retracted with dural sutures.
2. The Sylvian fissure is split by bipolar cautery dissection of meningeal layers for separation of the frontal and temporal lobes.
3. Brain spoons are placed and secured to the Leyla-Yasargil or Greenberg self-retaining retractor. The optic nerves and optic chiasma are visualized.
4. The operating microscope is brought in and positioned, and the feeding vessels and the neck of the aneurysm are exposed with microsurgical dissection of surrounding structures.
5. A temporary aneurysm clip may be utilized to test eventual placement of a permanent clip or to occlude the parent vessel if rupture occurs and the neck of the aneurysm cannot be visualized for clip placement (Figure 24-27).

Technical Considerations

1. Follow steps listed in Procedure 24-1 for entry into the cranium.
2. As the fissure of Sylvius is split with bipolar, the STSR should be preparing the brain spoons and self-retaining retractor for lobe retraction.
3. Microsurgical instruments should be brought up to the Mayo at this point. The STSR should make sure that the microscope is properly draped.
4. Aneurysm clip applicators should be ready for loading and temporary clips should be available for use. Aneurysm clips will be selected at this time.
5. Papaverine may be necessary to prevent vasospasm. The STSR should ensure that it is available.

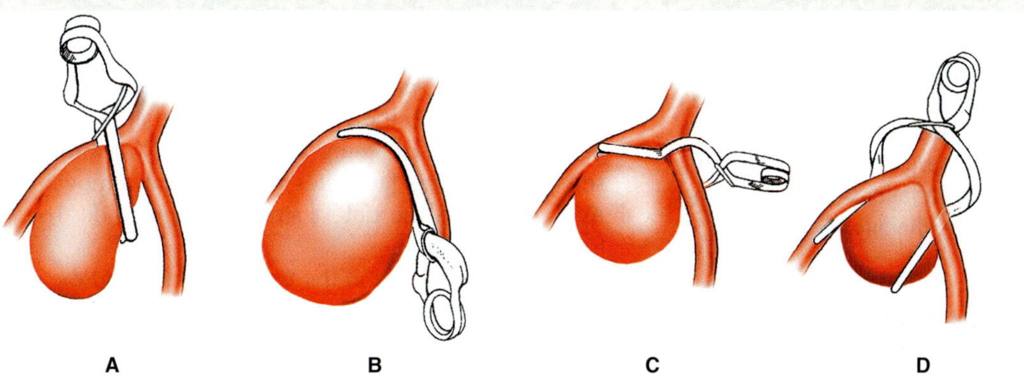

Figure 24-27 Cerebral aneurysm with clip—showing different configurations and types of clips

(continues)

PROCEDURE 24-2 Craniotomy for Aneurysm Repair *(continued)*

6. After the patient's blood pressure has been lowered by the anesthesiologist, an angled, curved, or straight aneurysm clip is applied across the neck of the defect.

6. The STSR should remember that once an aneurysm clip has been opened, it cannot be closed and used again.

7. The blood pressure is slowly raised, and the clip is checked for proper postioning and leakage. If necessary, an intraoperative angiogram can be performed with a C-arm.

7. The STSR should be prepared for hemorrhage control at this point.

8. The dura is closed, a drain is placed, and the bone flap and scalp flaps are secured in the usual manner.

8. Follow closure steps listed in Procedure 24-1.

Postoperative Considerations

Immediate Postoperative Care

- Care must be taken not to drop the head when removing it from the pin fixation device.
- Operative personnel should take precautions when moving the patient to the transport stretcher or ICU bed. The patient will have monitoring lines, urinary catheter and drainage bag, wound drains, or other important lines that can be easily pulled.
- Postoperative bleeding and intracranial pressure are monitored closely by ICU or recovery room personnel through Hemovac drainage and attention to neurological signs.

Prognosis

- Prognosis is good to excellent.

Complications

- Wound infection
- Meningitis
- Neurological deficits related to the pathological condition
- Intraoperative damage to vital structures
- Subdural or epidural hematoma
- Intracerebral hemorrhage

PEARL OF WISDOM

Cerebral aneurysm procedures illustrate a common problem for the STSR. The opening and closing of the craniotomy procedure is mostly concerned with bone, while the middle section is concerned with soft neural tissue. In this case, the concern is microscopic. The STSR must organize for wide variations in instrumentation, equipment, and passing technique.

CRANIOTOMY FOR REMOVAL OF ARTERIOVENOUS MALFORMATION

When feasible, AVMs are surgically excised to minimize the risk of bleeding. In young patients, resection of the AVM is advisable when the malformation is accessible. The surgery involves microsurgical resection of the malformation.

Nonsurgical techniques for the treatment of AVM include stereotactic focused irradiation and endovascular embolization. Focused irradiation is useful for small, low-flow, deeply seated lesions that cannot be safely excised surgically. Endovascular embolization involves passing tiny catheters into the cerebral vessels that feed the AVM and injecting a sclerosing agent that occludes those vessels. This process facilitates the eventual removal of the AVM, or makes the defect small enough to destroy with focused irradiation.

A flap is turned in the usual manner, and the dura is opened to expose the malformation. (The STSR should be prepared for bleeding from vessels that may be torn as the flap is lifted and the dura opened. Gelfoam squares, Surgicel, and bipolar are typically used for this.) The feeding vessels are identified and dissected to a distance below the AVM, where they are occluded with aneurysm clips or hemoclips. As vessels are dissected, oozing is imminent. Bleeding is controlled as it is encountered. Large feeding arteries are clipped. The remaining vessels are coagulated with argon laser or bipolar cautery, or occluded with clips. The draining veins are identified and clipped, and the site is checked for hemostasis.

CRANIECTOMY

For certain neurosurgical procedures, creation of a bone flap is not necessary. Instead, one or more bur holes are made with a Hudson brace, cranial perforator, or Midas Rex or Anspach bur, and enlarged with bone-biting instruments such as the Kerrison rongeur, Adson rongeur, or double-action Leksell rongeur. Craniectomy is typically used for posterior fossa procedures, epidural or subdural hematoma removal, ventriculostomy, intracranial pressure (**ICP**) monitor placement, or stereotactic cranial procedures. The bone that is removed is not replaced, and, if the defect is large, cranioplasty may be performed later (Figure 24-28).

CRANIECTOMY OR CRANIOTOMY FOR REMOVAL OF ACOUSTIC NEUROMA

Although tumors of the eighth cranial nerve are typically slow-growing neoplasms, their proximity to the cranial nerves and brain stem make them dangerous intracranial lesions. As these tumors grow, they press against the brain stem and adjacent cranial nerves, interrupting the normal function of those structures. At least 95% of vestibular schwannomas are unilateral, and most appear as encapsulated, rounded, single masses.

The ideal treatment for these tumors is total excision in a single stage with minimal morbidity and mortality and with preservation of neurological function, although subtotal resection may be indicated. When the facial nerve can be spared, the goal of the procedure should be preservation of hearing. The approach depends primarily upon tumor location and status of preoperative auditory function. The three approaches are as follows:

- The middle fossa approach is useful for small tumors arising from the superior vestibular nerve and situated in the internal auditory canal. This approach provides good extradural exposure and enables potential hearing preservation, but is less suitable for large tumors with intracranial involvement.
- The translabyrinthine approach is useful for ventral tumor exposure and allows easy identification and preservation of the facial nerve; however, this approach sacrifices hearing.
- The suboccipital or retrosigmoid approach allows for a wide exposure so the surgeon can identify vital structures, such as the brain stem, cranial nerves, and cerebral vasculature. It is suitable for small and large tumors, and for the smaller tumors allows for preservation of hearing.

During the procedure, facial nerve function is monitored with a continuous recording of electromyographic activity (Procedure 24-3).

(Text continues on page 1005)

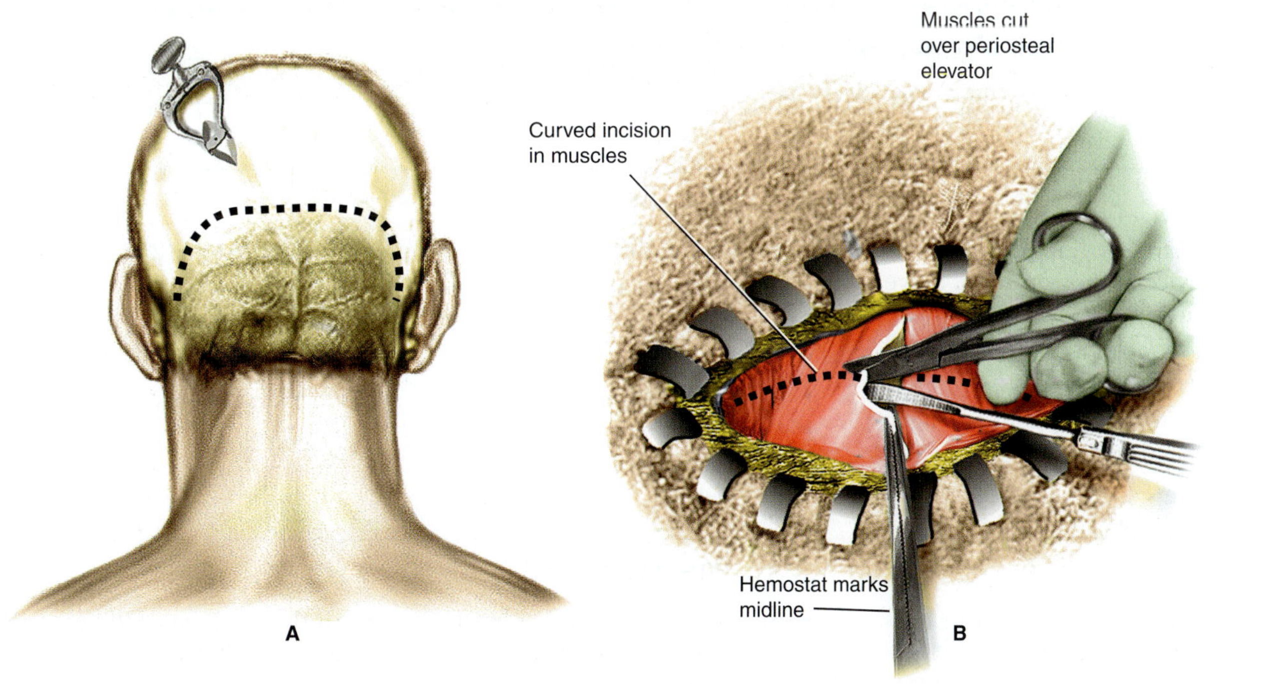

Figure 24-28 Posterior fossa craniectomy: (A) A transverse horseshoe incision is made over the occipital bone. (B) Scalp clips are placed and the muscle is cut.

(continues)

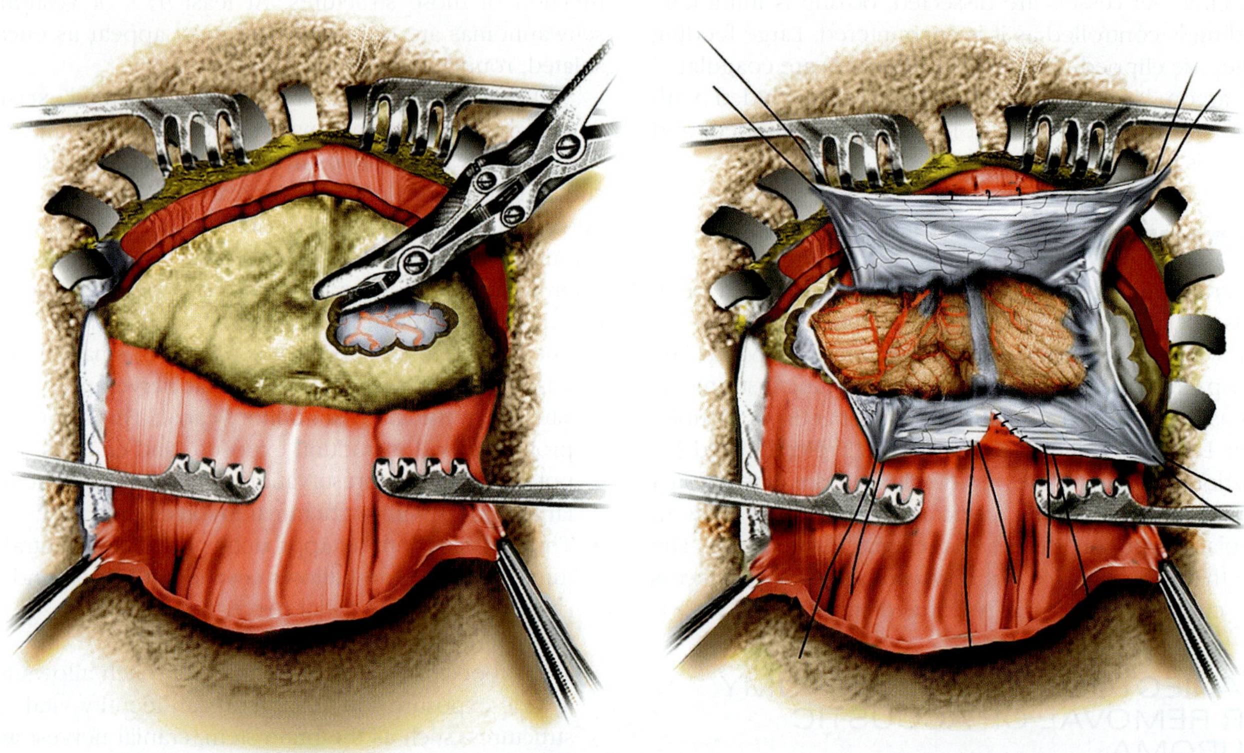

Figure 24-28 ***(continued)*** **(C) Retractors are positioned and bone is removed with a rongeur. (D) The dura is opened and retracted, exposing the cerebellar hemispheres**

PROCEDURE

24-3 Craniectomy or Craniotomy for Removal of Acoustic Neuroma

Equipment

- Electromyographic monitoring device to monitor facial nerve function
- Monopolar and bipolar electrosurgical units
- Fiberoptic headlight and light source (optional)
- Positioning devices
- Operating microscope and/or loupes
- CUSA
- CO_2 or Nd:YAG laser (optional)
- Ultrasound machine and attachments (optional)
- Suction system (2)
- Nitrogen source
- Mayfield overhead table
- Temperature monitoring device

Instruments

- Craniotomy set, or basic neurological set
- Microsurgical instruments (optional)
- Anspach or Midas Rex power instruments with attachments, or cranial perforator and craniotome
- Air drill with bits and burs (not necessary if Anspach or Midas Rex are used)

PROCEDURE 24-3 Craniectomy or Craniotomy for Removal of Acoustic Neuroma *(continued)*

Supplies

- Pack: basic
- Basin set
- Gloves
- Blades (#10, #11, #15)
- Drapes: towels, craniotomy drape
- Suture:
  - 4–0 silk, 4–0 Nurolon
  - Closure suture of surgeon's preference
- Drains: Hemovac
- Dressings: inner contact gauze (e.g., petroleum gauze), 4 × 4s, Kerlix
- Drugs:
  - Hemostatic agents (Gelfoam with topical thrombin, Surgicel, Avitene)
  - Antibiotic irrigation
  - Xylocaine 1% with epinephrine
- Miscellaneous:
  - Nerve stimulator for 7th cranial nerve identification
  - Laparotomy sponges
  - Ray-Tec sponges
  - Control syringe
  - Hypodermic needles
  - Electrosurgical pencil
  - Bipolar cord for attachment to bipolar bayonet forceps
  - Suction tubing (2)
  - Radiopaque cottonoid strips of various sizes
  - Raney scalp clips (for scalp gun or manual applicators)
  - Hemostatic clips (MRI compatible)
  - Rubber bands for Dandy clamps
  - Cotton balls
  - Telfa for specimen
  - Microscope drape
  - Ultrasound wand drape
  - Asepto syringes

Operative Preparation

Anesthesia

- General

Position

- The patient is typically placed in the semi-Fowler's position, with the head turned away from the affected side and the ipsilateral shoulder elevated. Three-point pin fixation devices are often used

Prep

- The area around the incision site should be shaved with an electric razor and straight or safety razor. Hair should be saved for the patient in a plastic bag
- Eyes and ears should be protected from prep solutions
- After the initial prep with iodophor scrub by the circulator, the surgeon may paint from a sterile Mayo with alcohol and/or iodophor paint

Draping

- Square-drape with towels that may be sutured in place with silk on a cutting needle
- Placement of the craniotomy drape with built-in adhesive drape over the fenestration

Practical Considerations

- Steroids are started 48 hours before the procedure to reduce cerebral edema, and intravenous antibiotics are given at the beginning of the procedure. After urinary catheterization, 10–20 mg of furosemide is given intravenously, and after dural exposure, mannitol is infused
- Make sure CT or MRI scans, arteriograms, or plain film studies are in the room before the procedure begins
- Make sure saline irrigation is always body temperature. Always test the temperature of the saline before handing it to the surgeon. Keep close track of the amount of irrigation used

(continues)

PROCEDURE 24-3 Craniectomy or Craniotomy for Removal of Acoustic Neuroma *(continued)*

Operative Procedure	Technical Considerations
1. A vertical incision centered 2 cm medial to the mastoid process is made; suboccipital muscles and fascia are incised with electrocautery, and stripped away from bone with the periosteal elevator.	**1.** Follow steps listed in Procedure 24-1 for entry into the cranium.
2. A bone flap over the lateral two-thirds of the cerebellar hemisphere is turned (or bur holes are made) and the dura is exposed. Additional bone is removed with double-action rongeur and Kerrison rongeur to expose the transverse sinus.	**2.** For craniectomy, the STSR should have available large Kerrison and Adson, Leksell, or Stille-Leur rongeurs for removal of thick bone.
3. The dura is opened and retracted with sutures. The cerebellum is elevated and the arachnoid opened to allow continuous drainage of CSF.	**3.** Brain spoons and self-retaining retractor should be prepared at this point in the procedure. The STSR should ensure that the microscope is properly draped.
4. Following the placement of self-retaining brain spoon retractors, the microscope is brought in and positioned. The removal of bone with an air-powered bur exposes the internal auditory canal.	**4.** The air drill should be loaded with the selected bur, hooked to the source, and tested before use.
5. The relationship of the tumor to the cochlear and vestibular nerves is assessed. The tumor is carefully rotated and the seventh cranial nerve is identified.	**5.** Nerve stimulator may be required at this point. If the CUSA is to be used, the STSR should have the sterile handpiece attached and ready to go.
6. After the location of each of these nerves is identified, internal decompression of the tumor is accomplished with ultrasonic aspirator, bipolar coagulation, and sharp dissection.	**6.** The OR may be darkened to enhance the surgeon's view of the operative field. Procedure may be long and tedious. Remain alert.
7. After the tumor has been removed, hemostasis is checked and the dura is closed in the usual fashion. Pericranial tissue may be used as a graft.	**7.** Care for specimen as directed by the surgeon. Body temperature irrigation will be needed. Prepare for closure.
8. The bone flap is replaced and secured, and muscle and fascia are closed in the usual manner. The skin is closed with nylon suture or stainless steel staples.	**8.** Follow closure steps listed in Procedure 24-1.

Postoperative Considerations

Immediate Postoperative Care

- As usual, the surgical technologist and the back table should remain sterile until the patient has safely left the OR.
- Care must be taken not to drop the head when removing it from the pin fixation device (if used).
- Operative personnel should take precautions when moving the patient to the transport stretcher or ICU bed. The patient will have monitoring lines, urinary catheter and drainage bag, wound drains, or other important lines that can be easily pulled.

Prognosis

- Prognosis is good to excellent.

Complications

- Hearing loss and facial hemiparesis resulting from damage to the seventh and eighth cranial nerves are the most common complications

PROCEDURE 24-3

Craniectomy or Craniotomy for Removal of Acoustic Neuroma *(continued)*

- Neurological deficits related to other cranial nerve dysfunction is also a possibility
- Wound infection
- Meningitis
- Neurological deficits related to the pathological condition, or intraoperative damage to vital structures
- Subdural or epidural hematoma
- Intracerebral hemorrhage

PEARL OF WISDOM

The cerebellopontine angle is an area rich with cranial nerves. Surgery there is dangerous because of the number of nerves and vessels and the pontine respiratory center. Movement in and around the field should be very quiet and controlled on these procedures.

VENTRICULOPERITONEAL AND VENTRICULOATRIAL SHUNT

The treatment for hydrocephalus involves the placement of a proximal, multi-holed draining catheter into the lateral ventricle that connects to a distal draining tube that is inserted into the right atrium of the heart or the peritoneal cavity (Figure 24-29). Between the ventricular catheter and the distal draining tube is a reservoir and valve system that directs the flow of CSF away from the ventricles toward the peritoneal cavity or right atrium. The reservoir is placed just above and behind the ear and is used to test patency of the system or flush an obstruction. The shunt system consists of the multi-holed ventricular catheter, a right-angled connector, the reservoir, a straight connector, and the peritoneal or atrial catheter (Procedure 24-4).

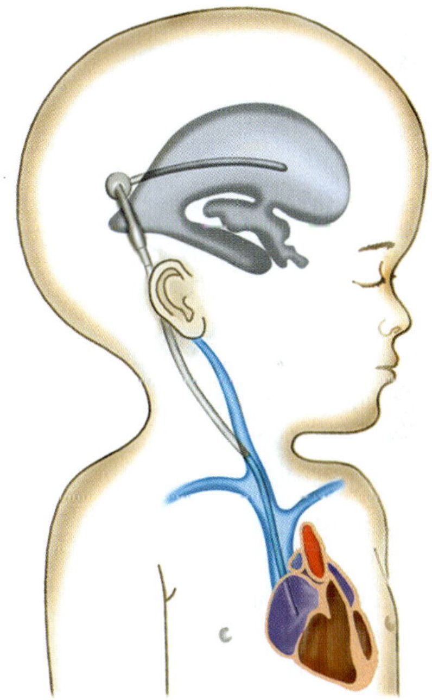

Figure 24-29 **Ventriculoatrial shunt**

PROCEDURE 24-4

Ventriculoperitoneal and Ventriculoatrial Shunt

Equipment

- Scales are often used for pediatric shunting procedures to weigh the soiled sponges to closely measure blood loss, as are heating pads to prevent hypothermia
- Monopolar and bipolar electrosurgical units

(continues)

PROCEDURE

24-4 Ventriculoperitoneal and Ventriculoatrial Shunt *(continued)*

- Fiberoptic headlight and light source (optional)
- Positioning devices (pin fixation device, Mayfield headrest, pillows, chest rolls)
- Two suction systems
- Nitrogen source
- Mayfield overhead table
- Temperature monitoring device

Instruments

- Midas Rex or Anspach systems are typically used to create a small bur hole. The craniotome is not needed
- A tunneling device of some sort is necessary to create tunnels from the bur hole to the peritoneum or upper thorax
- Craniotomy set, or basic neurological set
- Minor procedures set (soft tissue instruments are needed to place the catheter into the peritoneum or vascular instruments for placement into the jugular vein)

Supplies

- Pack: basic
- Basin set
- Gloves
- Blades (#10, #11, #15)
- Drapes: towels, craniotomy drape or split sheets
- Suture:
  - 4–0 silk, 4–0 Nurolon #1 silk ties for pulling the catheter through the tunnels
  - Prolene pursestring suture
  - Closure suture of surgeon's preference
- Dressings: inner contact gauze (e.g., petroleum gauze), 4 × 4s, Kerlix
- Drugs:
  - Hemostatic agents (Gelfoam with topical thrombin, Surgicel, Avitene)
  - Antibiotic irrigation
  - Xylocaine 1% with epinephrine
- Miscellaneous:
  - The shunt system of surgeon's choice
  - Laparotomy sponges
  - Ray-Tec sponges
  - Control syringe
  - Hypodermic needles
  - Electrosurgical pencil
  - Bipolar cord for attachment to bipolar bayonet forceps
  - Suction tubing (2)
  - Radiopaque cottonoid strips of various sizes
  - Raney scalp clips (for scalp gun or manual applicators)
  - Cotton balls
  - Manometer (available)
  - Asepto syringes

Operative Preparation

Anesthesia

- General

Position

- Supine with the head turned slightly. The patient's head typically rests on a "doughnut" or unrolled stockinette

Prep

- The area for the cranial incision site should be shaved. The prep should extend from the cranial incision site to the abdomen or upper chest
- Eyes and ears should be protected from prep solutions
- After the initial prep with iodophor scrub by the circulator, the surgeon may paint from a sterile Mayo with alcohol and/or iodophor paint

Draping

- Towels for square-draping from the head to the chest or abdomen are typically secured with a plastic adhesive drape. A nonfenestrated drape may be placed over the patient and holes cut in strategic locations for incision. Split sheets may be placed with tails up and down, or a fenestrated drape may be extended with scissors

PROCEDURE

24-4 Ventriculoperitoneal and Ventriculoatrial Shunt *(continued)*

Practical Considerations

- Pediatric patients can quickly become hypothermic
- Blood loss should be closely monitored (sponges should be weighed)
- Make sure CT or MRI scans, arteriograms, or plain film studies are in the OR before the procedure begins

Operative Procedure	Technical Considerations
1. A small linear incision is made, and a bur hole is drilled in the occipital or parietal bone with Hudson brace and D'Errico bit, cranial perforator, or Midas Rex or Anspach bur.	**1.** The STSR should ensure that all sponges are weighed for blood loss measurement during pediatric procedures. The shunt may be soaked in a saline and antibiotic mixture before use.
2. The dura is nicked and coagulated, and a ventricular catheter with stylet is placed into the posterior lateral ventricle. The stylet is removed, and a small bit of CSF is taken as specimen.	**2.** The STSR should be loading the stylet into the ventricular catheter as the dura is nicked. A rubber shod may be necessary to clamp the end of the catheter closed after it is placed to prevent CSF loss. ICP may be measured with the use of a manometer.
3. The proximal portion of the ventricular catheter is connected to the reservoir. A tunneling device is used to make a tunnel from the bur hole to the abdomen, and the distal end of the shunt system is threaded under the skin and soft tissues to an incision in the abdomen.	**3.** Tunneling devices may be hollow CV tunnelers, Sarot clamps, or uterine dressing forceps. Long, heavy silk sutures will be used to draw the shunt system under the skin to the abdomen.
4. The peritoneum is exposed and opened, and the abdominal catheter is placed into the peritoneal cavity and secured with a pursestring suture. The wounds are irrigated with antibiotic solution and closed after patency of the system is verified.	**4.** Small double-ended Richardson retractors are necessary for peritoneal exposure. A 3–0 or 4–0 PDS on a tapered needle is frequently used as a pursestring suture.
5. For ventriculoatrial shunts, an incision is made in the neck and the internal or external jugular vein is exposed.	**5.** Vascular instruments will be needed.
6. A tunnel is made from the bur hole to the neck incision, and the distal end of the shunt is threaded through the tunnel into the opened jugular vein, and into the right atrium.	**6.** An X-ray may be necessary to verify proper catheter placement.
7. The wounds are irrigated and the incisions are closed.	**7.** Several wounds may require closure and a variety of suture material will be needed.

Postoperative Considerations

Immediate Postoperative Care

- The incisions for these procedures are small, and are typically dressed with 4 × 4 pieces.
- The patency of the shunt must be determined before the patient leaves the OR.

Prognosis

- Good, if hydrocephalus has not been prolonged and severe.

Complications

- Shunts have a tendency to become infected.
- Small children will eventually outgrow the shunt, requiring revision.

PEARL OF WISDOM

There are many different kinds of shunts. They vary in their pumping technique and the pressure required to open the valve. The STSR should know the technical details of all the shunts used in his or her facility.

TRANSPHENOIDAL HYPOPHYSECTOMY

Tumors of the pituitary gland are usually benign, and are often responsible for the overproduction of specific pituitary hormones. For example, an excessive production of glucocorticoids by the adrenal glands (because of an increase in the production of adrenocorticotropic hormone by the pituitary gland) can cause fat to accumulate in the face, back, and chest. This is a condition referred to as Cushing's syndrome. Other symptoms include hyperglycemia, weakened muscles, weakened bones, and hypertension. Some pituitary tumors can cause acromegaly, an enlargement of the hands, feet, and face, by causing the pituitary gland to release excess amounts of growth hormone.

There are two basic approaches in the surgical treatment of pituitary tumors. Craniotomy is indicated if the tumor is large and pressing against the optic nerves and is similar to the technique previously described. Transphenoidal resection is indicated for smaller tumors (Figure 24-30).

The transphenoidal approach to pituitary tumor removal offers several advantages. The cranium is not opened, so recovery time is much shorter. Pain may be considerably less for the patient, as well. Complications associated with manipulating the brain and vital structures are avoided. The sella turcica is easily approached through the sphenoid sinus, and complete tumor removal is possible for most tumors (Procedure 24-5).

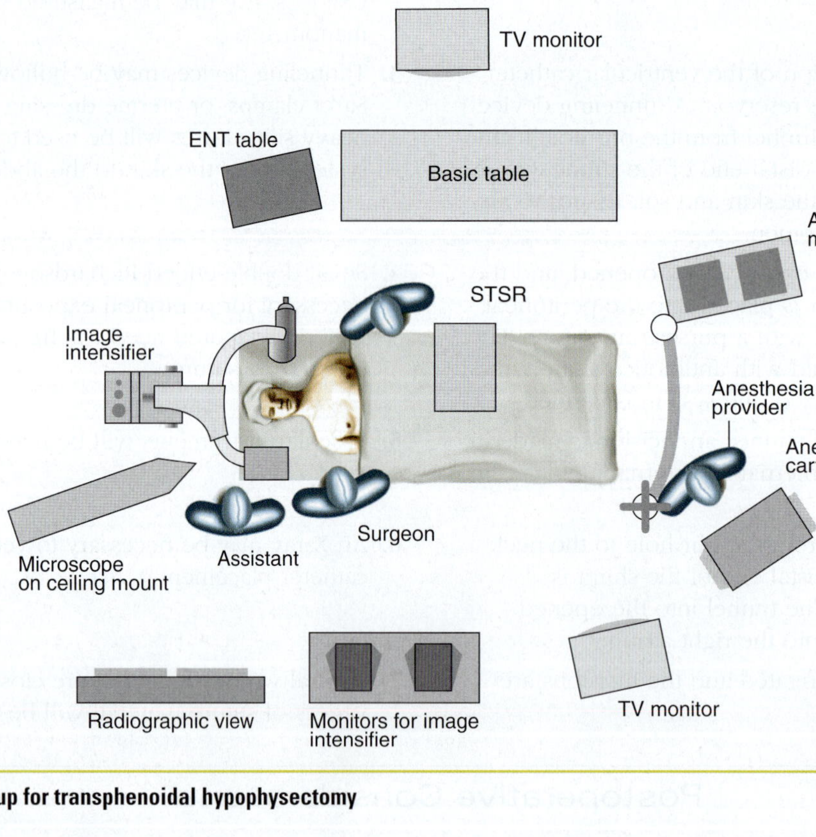

Figure 24-30 OR set up for transphenoidal hypophysectomy

PROCEDURE 24-5 Transphenoidal Hypophysectomy

Equipment

- Fiberoptic headlight and light source
- Suction system
- Monopolar and bipolar electrosurgical units
- Operating microscope
- C-arm and image intensifier with monitor

Instruments

- Craniotomy set
- Transphenoidal set
- Nasal set (optional)
- Minor set for graft procurement

Supplies

- Pack: basic, craniotomy
- Basin set
- Gloves
- Blades (#10, #11, #15)
- Drapes: towels, split sheet, medium sheet
- Suture:
  - 3–0 chromic
  - 3–0 Vicryl and staples for leg incision closure
- Drains: none
- Dressings:
  - inner contact layer and 4 × 4s for leg incision
  - Nasal packing
- Drugs
- Surgicel (4 × 8 in.)
  - Gelfoam with topical thrombin
  - Antibiotic irrigation
  - Xylocaine 1% with epinephrine
  - Cocaine solution
- Miscellaneous:
  - Suction tubing
  - Electrosurgical pencil
  - Bipolar cord (for attachment to bayonet bipolar forceps)
  - Ray-Tec sponges
  - Laparotomy sponges
  - Bone wax
  - Nasal packing
  - Asepto syringes
  - C-arm drape
  - Microscope drape
  - Bulb syringes

Operative Preparation

Anesthesia

- General

Position

- Semi-Fowler's

Prep

- The face and thigh are prepped with an antiseptic solution. The mouth and nose are usually not prepped, however

Draping

- The thigh is square-draped with towels and adhesive drape for removal of fascia and fat that will eventually pack the sellar cavity
- The face is draped exposed (split sheet to the mouth with tails up, and flat sheet across the brow). A hole is cut in the drape covering the thigh

Practical Considerations

- The nasal mucosa is typically injected with lidocaine and epinephrine for hemostasis. Cocaine may be applied to the nasal mucosa
- An image intensifier that has been covered with a sterile drape is positioned in the lateral tilt with the beam aimed directly into the sella turcica

(continues)

PROCEDURE 24-5 Transphenoidal Hypophysectomy *(continued)*

Operative Procedure	Technical Considerations
1. The surgeon injects the nasal mucosa and gingiva with lidocaine and epinephrine for hemostasis.	1. The STSR should have a 10-cc control syringe with lidocaine 1% with epinephrine ready for injection. An assistant may take the fascial graft from the thigh while the pituitary is being exposed. The graft should be kept on the back table in saline so that it does not dry out.
2. The surgeon may approach the sella turcica with an incision in the upper gum margin just under the upper lip, or through the nasal cavity.	2. The STSR should know which approach the surgeon will make in order to have the proper instruments available.
3. After elevation of soft tissues by periosteal elevator, the nasal septum is exposed and mucosa is separated from septal cartilage.	3. The STSR should ensure that the C-arm is properly draped for visualization of the sella turcica.
4. A special bivalved speculum designed for this procedure is inserted. After cartilage is resected and the floor of the sphenoid sinus is removed, the floor of the sella turcica is viewed.	4. The STSR should ensure that the microscope is properly draped at this point. All nasal instruments are kept isolated on a separate Mayo stand.
5. The microscope is brought in, and the sella turcica is punched with Kerrison rongeur and osteotome.	5. The STSR may be asked to gently tap on a small osteotome at the base of the sella turcica. This may be considered a task outside the scope of practice for the STSR.
6. The dura is incised and the tumor is removed with pituitary curette, dissector, enucleator, and suction.	6. Bayoneted hypophysectomy instruments will be used at this point. The STSR will be working around the C-arm, microscope, and other equipment during hypophysectomy. Be sure not to bump into the equipment and disturb the surgeon's view.
7. The sellar cavity is packed with fat and fascia from the thigh, and the gingival incision is closed with 3–0 chromic gut (Figure 24-31).	7. Refer to Chapter 17 for information on nasal surgery.

Postoperative Considerations

Immediate Postoperative Care

- Nasal packing with petroleum gauze will be the only dressing for the head. Petroleum gauze and 4 × 4s are typically used to dress the thigh incision.

Prognosis

- Excellent

Complications

- Wound infection
- CSF leakage
- Meningitis

PROCEDURE 24-5 Transphenoidal Hypophysectomy *(continued)*

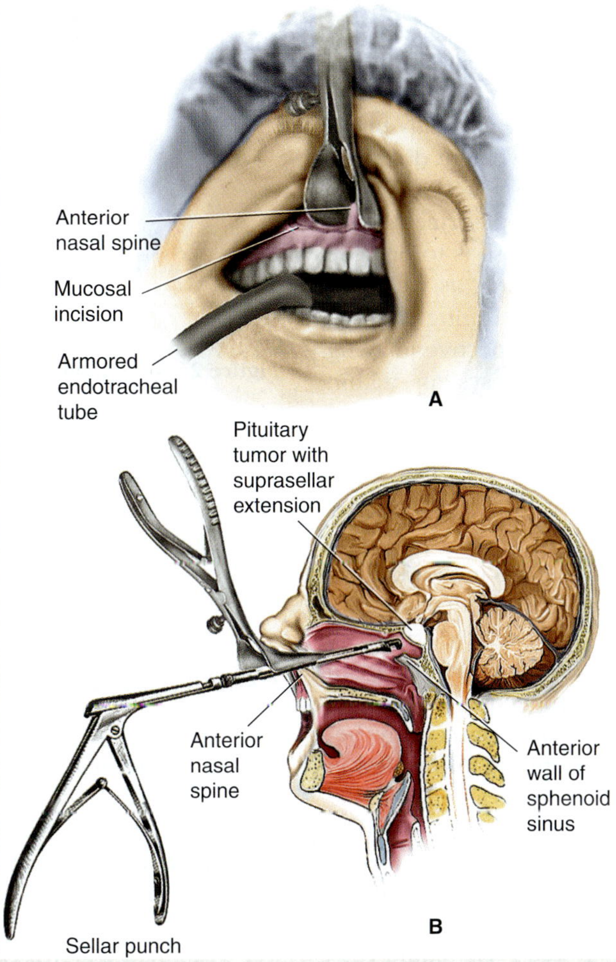

Figure 24-31 **Transphenoidal approach to hypophysectomy: (A) A bivalved speculum is inserted. (B) The floor of the sphenoid is removed with a sellar punch**

> **PEARL OF WISDOM**
>
> Prepare separate Mayo stands for the nasal/oral phase and the surgical phase. Be sure that nasal speculums are not placed on the wrong Mayo stand, thereby contaminating the sterile field.

STEREOTACTIC PROCEDURES

Craniotomy has historically involved large scalp and bone flaps for access to the brain. Neurosurgeons were forced to perform these procedures this way because they needed to be certain that a subcortical lesion could be localized and completely removed within the limits of the cranial opening. Localization methods for classical resection were imprecise, and the precise localization of subcortical targets contributes to the success of the cranial procedure. With the advent of computed axial tomography and magnetic resonance imaging, localizing intracranial lesions with pinpoint precision became a reality.

Stereotactic cranial surgery, used in conjunction with computed tomography, allows a probe to be guided to a specific location within the brain with minimal damage to normal neural tissue. Intracranial masses (tumor, hematoma, abscess) and vascular malformations (arteriovenous malformations) can be successfully treated using stereotactic techniques. Biopsy of intracranial tumors for treatment planning has been the primary focus of this technique, but stereotactic techniques are currently being utilized for the surgical treatment of movement disorders such as Parkinson's disease.

Stereotactic surgery requires the placement of a rigid head-mounted frame, whose purpose is to provide a marker system during computer imaging, as well as a rigid platform for mounting instruments during surgery. The marker set is visualized with the respective imaging modalities and provides a coordinate system within which targets appearing in the images may be localized (Figure 24-32).

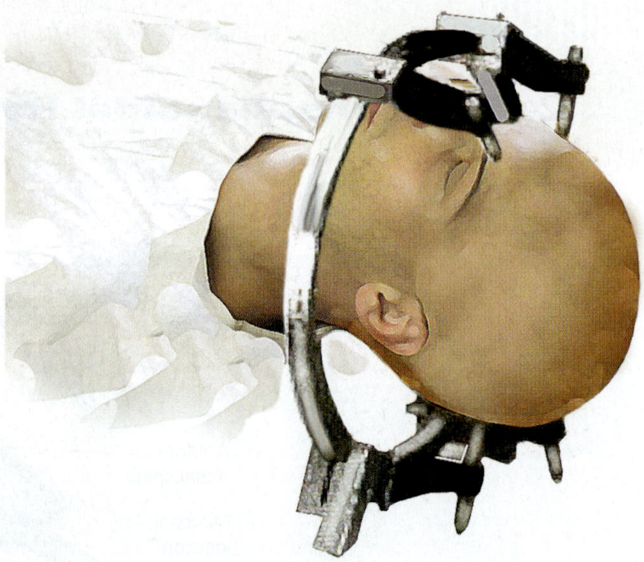

Figure 24-32 Stereotactic frame

CRANIOPLASTY

Cranioplasty is performed to repair defects in the skull resulting from a previous cranial procedure, trauma, or congenital anomaly. Various materials are available for repair, but the best is the patient's own bone flap that has been preserved from a previous cranial procedure. Typically, these bone flaps are not replaced after craniotomy because of cerebral edema, and are sterilized and stored in a bone bank within the facility. Bone grafts taken from the patient are equally reliable, but are typically removed in strips and must be molded to fit the defect. Methyl methacrylate is a reliable synthetic material that can be easily molded to fit the cranial defect, and can be used in conjunction with wire mesh, if necessary. Titanium plates are occasionally used, but are preformed and cannot be easily molded. Titanium screws or stainless steel wire are used to secure the implant to the cranium.

SPINAL PROCEDURES

Spinal procedures fall within the surgical scope of both the neurosurgeon and orthopedic surgeon. Neurosurgeons are almost always involved in cervical procedures, but both intervene in lumbar procedures. Often members from each specialty may form an operative team.

LAMINECTOMY

Laminectomy or hemilaminotomy is the surgical approach for herniated disk, spinal compression, or spinal cord tumor, and involves the removal of a vertebral lamina for exposure of the spinal cord and/or its nerve roots. The procedure is also used to provide exposure for insertion of pain control infusion pumps, cordotomy, and rhizotomy.

Laminectomy for discectomy is a common surgical procedure for the decompression of a nerve root that has been impinged by an extruded fragment of disk material in the cervical, thoracic, or lumbar region of the spine. Due to its weight-bearing configuration, the lower lumbar region is affected the most often. Surgical treatment is often necessary to remove the extruded fragment and decompress the nerve root (Procedure 24-6).

(Text continues on page 1016)

PROCEDURE 24-6 Laminectomy

Equipment

- Suction system
- Monopolar and bipolar electrosurgical units
- Wilson frame, Andrews table, or Mayfield horseshoe headrest
- Fiberoptic headlight and light source
- Nitrogen source
- Operating microscope (optional)

Instruments

- Laminectomy set
- Minor procedures set for soft tissue instruments
- Midas Rex, Stryker, or Anspach power instruments with burs and attachments

For fusion:

- Basic orthopedic set
- Power instruments (oscillating saw)
- Curettes
- Osteotomes
- Gouges

Supplies

- Pack: laparotomy
- Basin set
- Gloves
- Blades (#10, #11)
- Drapes: towels, adhesive drape, laparotomy drape
- Suture: closure sutures of surgeon's preference
- For intradural tumor removal, 4–0 silk or Nurolon is required
- Drains: Hemovac
- Dressings: inner contact layer, 4 × 4s, ABD
- Drugs:
  - Hemostatic agents (Gelfoam with topical thrombin, Avitene, Surgicel)
  - Antibiotic irrigation
  - Depo-Medrol
- Miscellaneous:
  - Electrosurgical pencil
  - Bipolar cord (for attachment to bayonet bipolar forceps)
  - Ray-Tec sponges
  - Laparotomy sponges
  - Kerlix (optional, for Taylor retractor)
  - Asepto syringes
  - Cottonoids of various sizes
  - Bone wax
  - Microscope drape (optional)

Operative Preparation

Anesthesia

- General

Position

- The patient is usually placed in the prone position for bilateral laminectomy, but the lateral position may be utilized for unilateral laminectomy. For fusion, the hip is slightly elevated for graft procurement

Prep

- Depends on the level of the spine to be operated on

Draping

- The area is square-draped with towels, and the laparotomy drape is placed and positioned

(continues)

PROCEDURE

24-6 Laminectomy *(continued)*

Practical Considerations

- Make sure that CT or MRI scans, myelograms, or plain film studies are in the OR before the procedure begins
- When positioning on the Wilson frame, make sure that bony prominences are well padded, and breasts or testicles are not impinged. The arms should be above the head on armboards
- The Wilson frame should be lowered completely before positioning
- For prone positioning with the Mayfield headrest (utilized for bilateral cervical laminectomy), the STSR should ensure that the horseshoe headrest is well padded, and that the Mayfield attachment for the OR table is locked and secured

Operative Procedure	Technical Considerations
1. The interspace of the affected levels of the spine is approached posteriorly via a midline or paramedian incision.	**1.** A #10 blade on a #3 knife handle is typically used for the incision. Electrosurgical pencil and Mayo scissors are used to expose the spine.
2. The paraspinous muscles are separated from the spinous processes and laminae in the area with periosteal elevator or osteotome. As the muscles are separated, sponges are packed around the margins to assist with hemostasis and to aid in blunt dissection.	**2.** Osteotome and periosteal elevator are used to strip the paraspinous muscles. The STSR should have 4 × 4 Ray-Tec sponges opened and folded lengthwise for packing around margins.
3. After the muscles have been reflected, a retractor is placed to provide exposure.	**3.** Martin-Meyerding, Taylor, Adson-Beckman, or angled Gelpi are examples of the types of retractors used for exposure.
4. The spinous process is removed and rongeurs are used to remove the margin of the lamina above the interspace, the ligamentum flavum, and the medial margin of the adjacent facet. Care is taken not to damage the epidural veins when incising the ligamentum flavum (Figure 24-33).	**4.** When necessary, hemostasis of bone may be achieved using minimal amounts of bone wax. Moistened cottonoids may be used to protect the dura if the electrosurgical pencil is used.

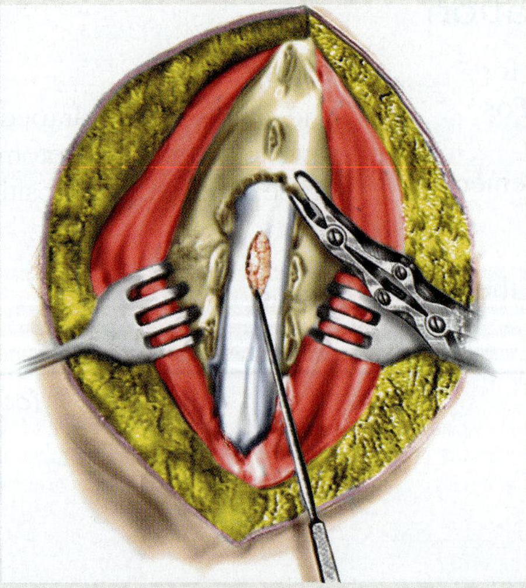

Figure 24-33 Completed bilateral multilevel laminectomy

PROCEDURE 24-6 **Laminectomy** *(continued)*

5. After the necessary amount of the lamina has been removed with a Kerrison rongeur, the dura and nerve root are carefully retracted medially with a nerve root retractor.	**5.** The STSR should remove bone from the rongeur with a Ray-Tec sponge, rolling it after each swipe. The Scoville or Love nerve root retractors are frequently used to retract the nerve root. The retractor should not be moved after placement to prevent damage to the nerve root.
6. Pituitary rongeurs are then used to remove extruded fragments of disk material.	**6.** The STSR will need to remove the disk material from the rolled Ray-Tec sponge and place it into a sterile specimen jar. Disk material, once removed, is retained by the STSR to be sent for pathological analysis. Extruded disk material is easily identifiable from bone and muscle material in that it tends to stick to instruments and has an appearance much like crabmeat.
7. Once the extruded disk material has been removed, the inner portion of the disk may be removed using rongeurs. Curettes are used in the intervertebral disk space to remove all remaining fragments of disk material. Care must be taken not to injure the aorta or vena cava that lie anterior to the vertebral column.	**7.** A major laparotomy and cardiovascular set should be readily available in case the aorta is nicked.
8. If the spine has been destabilized following laminectomy or laminotomy, fusion of the vertebrae may be performed. Fusion is achieved by placing struts of bone in and along the intervertebral spaces after curettage.	**8.** If a fusion is necessary, the STSR should have curettes, gouges, and osteotomes available for bone graft procurement. A basic ortho set and Gelpi and U.S. Army retractors are needed. The bone graft should be placed in a small metal basin; it may need to be trimmed with rongeur or bone cutter before use.
9. Curettage of the vertebral bodies assists in the formation of bony material after bone graft material is placed into the vertebral interspace. This bone is either taken from the iliac crest of the patient, or homogenous banked bone is used.	**9.** For certain pathological conditions or fractures, stability may not be achieved by simple bone grafting. In these cases, stability is achieved by using any of several implanted device systems. These systems involve rods, hooks, and screws attached to the nondamaged vertebra above and below.
10. Prior to wound closure, the wound is irrigated free of debris. All cottonoids and sponges are removed.	**10.** Hemovac drains are typically placed in the wound before closure. The reservoir should be attached immediately to prevent clot formation within the drain.
11. The paraspinous muscles are approximated with heavy-gauged polyglactin suture. The wound is closed in layers, and the skin is closed with monofilament nylon or stainless steel staples.	**11.** Heavy, interrupted sutures are usually best for closure. The count begins when the first closure suture is passed.

(continues)

PROCEDURE

24-6 Laminectomy *(continued)*

Postoperative Considerations

Immediate Postoperative Care

- The wound is dressed with an inner contact layer and 4 × 4s.
- The operative team should be careful when turning the patient back to the supine position. Injury to the patient or staff may occur.

Prognosis

- Depends on the factors. Simple extruded unilateral disks without foot drop are frequently treated successfully. Bilateral decompressive laminectomy for compression of the spinal cord or cauda equina may not be as successful.
- Generally, if decompression of the nerve root or spine is accomplished early enough, the results are favorable, especially if the spine is not destabilized. The more extensive the laminectomy, the less favorable the results.

Complications

- Wound infection
- Destabilization of the spine
- Nerve root damage
- Hemorrhage

PEARL OF WISDOM

For a laminectomy you will receive specimens that are bone and ligament. With the discectomy, you will receive disk material. Disk material looks and feels somewhat like crabmeat. Always check the specimen materials as you take them from the rongeur. Report any suspicious looking specimen (e.g., lumen) to the surgeon immediately.

LAMINECTOMY FOR REMOVAL OF SPINAL CORD TUMOR

The microscope is usually necessary for tumor removal. An ultrasonic aspiration device should be available, and microsurgical instruments will be necessary. Dural traction sutures (e.g., 4–0 braided nylon) will be needed for intradural tumor removal.

When laminectomy is performed for the excision of a spinal cord tumor, the patient is usually placed in the prone position on the Mayfield horseshoe headrest (for cervical laminectomy) or the Wilson frame (for lumbar laminectomy). Chest rolls may be employed if the prone position is preferred.

Typically, multilevel bilateral laminectomy is necessary for proper exposure. The STSR should have an ultrasonic aspirator, microsurgical instruments, and microscope ready for the surgeon.

Bilateral multilevel laminectomy is performed in the manner described for laminectomy above. Multilevel laminectomy requires the removal of a large amount of bone. Adson, Leksell, and Stille-Leur rongeurs will be the primary instruments for bone removal.

For removal of an intradural mass, the dura is incised with a #15 knife blade and dural scissors after exposure. A grooved director placed under the dura protects the spinal cord during dural incision. When necessary, 4–0 braided nylon or silk traction sutures on control-release dura needles are placed to assist in exposure of the cord.

The tumor mass is then dissected using small pituitary rongeurs, bipolar bayonet electrosurgical forceps, blunt dissection with cottonoids, or an ultrasonic aspirator. Bipolar bayonet coagulation is always used around the nerves and spinal cord for precision. After all tumor material is removed intradurally, the wound is irrigated, hemostasis is achieved, and the dura is closed in an airtight fashion with 4–0 braided nylon.

DISCECTOMY (ANTERIOR APPROACH AND ANTERIOR/POSTERIOR APPROACH)

Certain spondylitic lesions, some fractures, and procedures for correction of spinal stenosis may require an anterior approach to the spine. Extreme cases require an anterior approach followed by a posterior approach. The anterior approach is especially useful for treatment of spinal stenosis at the cervical and thoracic levels.

A thoracotomy approach is popular for discectomies in the thoracic region because of the small diameter of the thoracic spinal canal. An alternative approach is the removal of the medial segment of a rib and transverse process to expose the intervertebral disk. For these procedures, the rib is often used as autograft bone material and is packed into the disk space after the disk and cartilage plates have been removed and the vertebral bodies have been curetted. Special long rongeurs, curettes, and instruments are used for this approach due to the depth of the operative field.

An anterior/posterior thoracic approach may be utilized for the placement of rods and pedicle screws. The patient is first placed in a lateral thoracic position for the anterior approach, and a thoracic surgeon exposes the vertebral bodies through a thoracotomy. Screws and rods or fusion material is placed and secured, and the wound is closed in layers in the usual manner. The patient is then turned onto the Wilson frame to a prone position, prepped, and redraped. The posterior thoracic spine is exposed in the usual manner.

SURGICAL PROCEDURE FOR MENINGOCELE REPAIR

Meningocele, a type of spinal dysraphism, involves a herniation of the subarachnoid space into the surrounding tissues. Simple meningocele does not involve nervous tissue and accounts for 5% of spinal dysraphism. Left alone, these types of meningoceles will generally epithelialize on their own with no need for surgical intervention.

Myelomeningocele is a much more serious disorder because it involves the subarachnoid space and nervous tissue, as well. The spinal cord and roots are exposed through a skin defect, and some degree of permanent paralysis is common. This disorder has a 90% mortality rate associated with infection and hydrocephalus. Surgical intervention includes shunting for hydrocephalus and closure of the spinal lesion. Because of the high number of handicaps usually associated with this disorder (including paralysis, urinary incontinence, and mental retardation), a general opinion prevails that surgery should only be performed on babies with restricted sphincter control and limb movement. Surgery is generally performed in the first 24 hours of life to prevent infection of the exposed neural tube.

ANTERIOR CERVICAL DISCECTOMY AND FUSION

Removal of a disk that is compressing a cervical nerve root or cervical cord may be accomplished through an anterior approach. This approach is less traumatic for the patient because it does not involve laminectomy, although bone must be removed from the iliac crest for placement within the intervertebral space (Procedure 24-7).

PROCEDURE 24-7 Anterior Cervical Discectomy (Cloward Technique)

Equipment

- Suction system
- Monopolar and bipolar electrosurgical units
- Nitrogen source (optional for Stryker, Midas Rex, or Anspach power instruments)

Instruments

- The Cloward technique is frequently utilized for this procedure, and involves the use of Cloward instruments, which include:
  - Special hand retractors and self-retaining retractors with various detachable blades
  - Vertebral spreaders for proper exposure of the intervertebral space and graft placement
  - Cervical drill with guards
  - Bone dowel cutter for circular bone graft procurement
  - Bone graft holder and impactor
  - Bone curettes and rongeurs of various sizes
- A minor set is also necessary for additional soft tissue exposure instruments
- Angled and straight bone curettes are sometimes necessary to completely remove disk material and prepare the intervertebral disk space for graft placement

(continues)

PROCEDURE 24-7

Anterior Cervical Discectomy (Cloward Technique) *(continued)*

Supplies

- Pack: laparotomy or basic
- Basin set
- Gloves
- Blades (#10, #11, #15)
- Drapes: towels, adhesive drape, laparotomy drape, thyroid or pedi sheet
- Suture: closure sutures of surgeon's preference
- Drains: Hemovac for iliac crest
- Dressings: inner contact layer, 4 × 4s, ABD
- Drugs:

  Hemostatic agents (Gelfoam with topical thrombin, Avitene, Surgicel)

  Antibiotic irrigation
- Miscellaneous:

  A spinal needle will be utilized for proper disk level identification with X-ray

  Electrosurgical pencil

  Bipolar cord (for attachment to bayonet bipolar forceps)

  Ray-Tec sponges

  Laparotomy sponges

  Asepto syringes

  Cottonoids of various sizes

  Bone wax

Operative Preparation

Anesthesia

- General

Position

- The patient is positioned supine with a shoulder roll and the head turned slightly away from the affected side. The hip is slightly elevated for graft procurement

Prep

- The neck and iliac crest are prepped

Draping

- The neck should be square-draped with towels and then covered with a laparotomy, thyroid, or pediatric sheet
- The iliac crest should be square-draped with towels, then covered with a plastic adhesive drape and laparotomy sheet

Practical Considerations

- The STSR should be prepared for lateral X-ray for disc level identification
- If the surgeon chooses to obtain a bone graft without Cloward instruments, the STSR should obtain osteotomes, curettes, and gouges in addition to a basic ortho set

Operative Procedure	Technical Considerations
1. An incision is made over the cervical disk space at the medial border of the sternocleidomastoid muscle, and hemostasis is obtained with electrocautery.	1. A #10 blade on a #3 knife handle is used for the incision. Finger dissection and sharp dissection with small Metzenbaum scissors allows exposure.
2. The esophagus, carotid artery, and trachea are retracted medially. The periosteum of the anterior cervical vertebral bodies is stripped with periosteal elevator, and a spinal needle is inserted into the vertebral space.	2. Vital structures are retracted with Army-Navy or Cloward hand retractors. Adson or freer periosteal are used for periosteal stripping.

PROCEDURE 24-7

Anterior Cervical Discectomy (Cloward Technique) *(continued)*

3. A lateral C-spine X-ray is taken to identify the proper level.	**3.** The lateral cassette holder for cervical X-ray should be covered with a sterile medium sheet before placement against the OR table. The STSR should seek cover behind a lead shield to prevent exposure.
4. An incision is made over the iliac crest, and a bone graft is procured with a Hudson brace and dowel cutter.	**4.** Some surgeons may prefer to obtain the bone graft with osteotome and mallet, trimming to the necessary size with rongeur and/or bur.
5. Blades are chosen for the Cloward self-retaining retractor, and the retractor is placed.	**5.** The blades for the Cloward self-retaining retractor may be lined up within a kidney basin for choice by the surgeon.
6. An incision is made into the disk space, and disk material is removed with pituitary rongeur and sent for specimen.	**6.** The disk space is incised with a #15 blade loaded onto a #7 knife handle. Disk material should be removed from the pituitary rongeur with a Ray-Tec sponge, and preserved as specimen.
7. The vertebral spreader is placed into the disk space and opened to the desired width. Additional disk material is removed with small curettes, angled and straight.	**7.** A caliper may be used to ensure that the vertebrae are distracted to the proper distance.
8. Depth of the intervertebral space is measured, and the cervical drill guard is inserted into the space. A hole is drilled into the guide with the Cloward drill on Hudson brace, and the drill and guide are removed.	**8.** Prepare Cloward instrumentation according to the surgeon's specifications.
9. The bone dowel is trimmed for size with air drill and rongeur and placed into the disk space. The vertebral spreader is removed, and the bone graft is inspected for proper positioning.	**9.** An impactor and mallet are typically necessary to properly place the bone graft within the disk space.
10. Retractors are removed, and the wound is irrigated and closed in layers.	**10.** A lateral cervical X-ray may be obtained before closure to ensure proper bone graft placement.

Postoperative Considerations

Immediate Postoperative Care

- The incisions are dressed with inner contact layers, 4 × 4s, and an ABD for the iliac crest.
- The STSR should remain sterile, and should not break down the back table or Mayo tray until the patient has left the OR.

Prognosis

- Good

Complications

- Wound infection
- Nerve root damage

PEARL OF WISDOM

In the classic Cloward procedure, the graft taken is one millimeter greater in diameter than the drill bit that matches it. This allows the normal muscle tension of the neck to hold the graft in place. Always check to see that the drill bit will fit just inside the graft taker.

PERIPHERAL NERVE PROCEDURES

The PNS suffers from various conditions. Trauma and various compression syndromes often lead to surgery. Like many surgical areas, surgeons from different specialties may be involved in peripheral nerve surgery. However, the neurosurgeon remains active in this area.

CARPAL TUNNEL RELEASE

Carpal tunnel syndrome can be treated conservatively by having the patient decrease intensive repetitive hand activities (even to the extent of considering a permanent change of job), by employing wrist splints, or with the injection of steroids.

Carpal tunnel release is the name of the surgical procedure to correct carpal tunnel syndrome (Procedure 24-8). The procedure may be preformed by a number of specialists including the neurosurgeon, plastic surgeon, hand surgeon, and the orthopedic surgeon. It is usually an open procedure, but can also be accomplished endoscopically.

PROCEDURE 24-8 Carpal Tunnel Release

Equipment

- Arm table
- Sitting stools
- Monopolar and bipolar electrosurgical units
- Pneumatic tourniquet system

Instruments

- Hand set

Supplies

- Pack: extremity
- Basin set
- Gloves
- Blades (#15)
- Drapes: ¾ sheet, 4-in. stockinette, extremity sheet
- Suture: Closure suture of surgeon's choice
- Drains: none
- Drugs: Xylocaine 1%; Depo-Medrol
- Miscellaneous:
  - Esmarch bandage
  - Ray-Tec sponges
  - Bipolar cord with straight disposable forceps

Operative Preparation

Anesthesia

- Local, regional, or general

Position

- The patient is placed on the operating table in the supine position with the affected arm extended on an arm table

Prep

- The arm is prepped circumferentially with iodophor

Draping

- A ¾ sheet is placed on top of the hand table, and the arm is covered with a 4-in. stockinette up to the shoulder
- An extremity sheet is placed over the arm and spread to cover the patient
- A medium sheet may be used to cover the legs

PROCEDURE

24-8 Carpal Tunnel Release *(continued)*

Practical Considerations

- The use of a tourniquet is optional depending on surgeon's preference
- The surgeon and the assistant will sit

Operative Procedure

1. A small incision is made on the palmar surface of the hand.
2. Hemostasis is achieved and the transverse carpal ligament is either stretched or cut to release the pressure being exerted on the median nerve.
3. The wound is irrigated and a simple closure is done.

Technical Considerations

1. A #15 blade on a #3 handle is used for the incision.
2. Small Metzenbaum scissors and Adson forceps with teeth are used to incise the carpal ligament. Some surgeons prefer to incise the ligament with a #15 blade on a #3 handle.
3. The initial dressing is usually bulky and contains a splint to temporarily restrict movement of the wrist.

Postoperative Considerations

Immediate Postoperative Care

- The hand is dressed with a bulky dressing: inner contact layer, followed by 4 × 4s, super fluffs, and a Kerlix or Kling. An Ace bandage binds the bulky dressings.

Prognosis

- The overall results of carpal tunnel release are good and the patient can expect to return to normal activities in a few weeks.

Complications

- Median nerve damage
- Wound infection

PEARL OF WISDOM

The STSR will often be sitting opposite the surgeon with the affected arm between them. Be sure all instruments and supplies are positioned where you can reach them before sitting. Once seated, do not stand up until the procedure is complete.

ULNAR NERVE DECOMPRESSION AND TRANSPOSITION

To relieve discomfort from ulnar nerve pain, the patient may be asked to modify his or her activities, keep pressure off the nerve, and take anti-inflammatory drugs. If this fails to produce good results, surgery may be indicated.

Ulnar nerve pain can be relieved with surgical intervention from two different surgical procedures. The first, called ulnar nerve decompression, is accomplished by cutting the ligament of Osborne where the nerve passes through the medial aspect of the elbow. The second, called ulnar nerve transposition, is an actual relocation of the ulnar nerve to a slightly more anterior location in the elbow. Both of these procedures may be performed with the patient in the supine position under local, regional, or general anesthesia. Once the affected arm has been prepped circumferentially and draped, it is either suspended or laid across the patient's body for the procedure. Usually this is a soft tissue procedure, but the STSR should be prepared to assist with bone reshaping if necessary. The overlying tissues are closed with absorbable suture and the dressing is applied. The patient can expect a very restrictive dressing (including splint or cast material) to prevent flexing or extending the affected joint until the inflammation subsides and wound healing is complete. Most patients enjoy complete pain relief following ulnar nerve decompression/transposition.

ADVANCES IN NEUROSURGERY

Neurosurgery has seen important advances in intraoperative patient care in the last two decades. For example, laser technology and the operating microscope have greatly improved patient outcomes, and advances in computer technology have led to the use of less invasive techniques that allow more accurate procedures and shorten hospital stays.

Recent neurosurgical applications include intraoperative MRI, three-dimensional reconstruction for brain tumor resection, radiosurgery, minimally invasive techniques, stereotaxis, intraoperative ultrasound, brain mapping, endoscopic neurosurgery, and deep brain stimulation.

In the near future, molecular medical advances will allow the diagnosis of most neurological problems without the need for open biopsy. Malignant tumors that are now incurable will be managed through genetic engineering and targeting strategies. Stem cells will be routinely implanted by neurosurgeons to repair damaged portions of the central nervous system.

INTRAOPERATIVE MRI

Intraoperative MRI scanning allows direct evaluation of patients and their tumors during the surgical procedures. This is helpful to establish the margins of a tumor to ensure that all possible portions are removed. The intraoperative MRI is different from the type used for clinical diagnosis. It has a magnetic field between two "donuts" that allows the patient's head to be freely accessed by the surgeon during the procedure, an important design that allows for image guidance and tumor resection.

THREE-DIMENSIONAL RECONSTRUCTION

The capacity to work from three-dimensional images for brain tumor resection is a major advance in neurosurgery. New systems allow three-dimensional creation of a holographic model of the brain that can be superimposed on the patient's head during surgery (with the use of laser scanning technology). The superimposed image can be used as a guide for surgical resection, which is particularly useful for tumors around critical areas of the brain (such as the motor strip) that cannot sustain damage. This superimposition of data from CT scans, MRI images, and angiograms allows for presurgical planning of a safe route to the tumor.

RADIOSURGERY

Until recently, neurosurgeons and radiologists used a special radiation device called a gamma knife to focus small beams of radiation into brain tumors. The gamma knife minimized damage to surrounding healthy brain while the tumor was more selectively targeted for destruction. But the gamma knife device is limited to use in brain tumors.

The newly developed "X-knife" is superior to the gamma knife because it can be used to treat tumors outside of the skull, can deliver different thresholds of radiation exposure, and can deliver smaller, repeated doses.

X-knife radiosurgery is a powerful tool for the treatment of intracranial metastatic tumors, recurrent gliomas, and meningiomas. The X-knife utilizes non-coplanar arcs to target a lesion that has been localized by CT scanning and three-dimensional reconstruction. The patient has a stereotactic base ring applied and a CT scan is done that demonstrates the abnormality. The tumor is then targeted with precise, focused beams of radiation.

MINIMALLY INVASIVE TECHNIQUES

Neurosurgery is rapidly evolving toward a minimally invasive approach for access to neurological lesions that increases accuracy and reduces morbidity. Minimally invasive neurosurgery refers to a more precise craniotomy for access to brain lesions and also to a more precise trajectory to the lesion that will not injure critical adjacent brain structures. Radiosurgery with a gamma knife or X-knife is the least invasive neurosurgical technique and combines radiation techniques with computer-assisted stereotaxis.

STEREOTAXIS

Stereotaxis refers to a system of navigating to any point within the brain, with the aid of imaging techniques that concurrently display external reference landmarks and neural structures (including the brain lesions). As discussed previously in this chapter, the system requires the use of an external head frame attached to the patient's skull just before a CT scan or MRI image is made. The frame provides reference points for the calculation of trajectories and depths to a target point within the image brain. This type of approach replaces large-exposure craniotomies that increase morbidity and neurological deficit caused by access to a deep lesion. Disruption of normal cortex is minimized with this approach, and navigation is more precise.

The latest generation of stereotactic systems can be used with CT, MRI, and cerebral angiographic localization. The frame is specially designed to allow easy access to the head for stereotactic craniotomies.

INTRAOPERATIVE ULTRASOUND

Intraoperative ultrasound has aided the development of minimally invasive surgery and is used either alone (during a traditional craniotomy) or during a stereotactic procedure. When used alone, the ultrasound wand can be used over unopened dura to pinpoint the exact location of a lesion, sparing healthy brain tissue in the process. It can also be used to guide a biopsy needle to an exact location within a brain lesion.

Ultrasound provides the neurosurgeon with real-time information about a brain lesion. Image information previously available to the neurosurgeon at the time of the procedure for stereotactic navigation may be hours or even days old. In the meantime, the lesion's location may have changed slightly after injection with mannitol (to shrink the brain) or after drainage of CSF during the procedure, making previous stereotactic measurements inaccurate. Ultrasound in conjunction with stereotaxis during the procedure confirms lesion location and shape.

BRAIN MAPPING

Critical areas of the brain (those dealing with speech, movement, or visual functions) must be preserved during craniotomy, but they are often adjacent to a brain lesion. In the past, neurosurgeons were forced to rely on anatomical landmarks to determine these critical brain areas, but those landmarks were often unreliable. Brain mapping is a more accurate method for determining the location of these critical areas.

Intraoperative brain mapping can be carried out under local anesthesia. The brain's cortex is stimulated electrically for mapping critical motor and sensory areas. Once identified, the critical areas are marked and avoided. Mapping can be used with stereotaxis and ultrasound to provide a highly accurate map for the neurosurgeon, and it provides critical information for the preservation of neurological functions.

ENDOSCOPIC NEUROSURGERY

Rigid and flexible fiberoptic endoscopes introduced through a bur hole are used in pediatric neurosurgery for the placement of shunts, fenestration of cysts, and creation of third ventriculostomies. Endoscopes give neurosurgeons access to areas that have been difficult to approach in recent years; for example, third ventricular tumors are now routinely approached endoscopically. The endoscopic removal of pituitary tumors has been particularly successful. Laser and various other instruments (including biopsy instruments) can be attached to the endoscope to aid in the procedure.

DEEP BRAIN STIMULATION

Abnormalities in cells of the basal ganglia of the brain create movement disorders (known as tremors) that are classified as essential or Parkinsonian. Parkinson's tremor differs from essential tremor in two ways: Parkinson's tremor occurs at a lower shaking frequency when the body or limbs are at rest, and ceases during purposeful movement. Essential tremor has a higher shaking frequency and is most obvious during intentional movement.

Deep brain stimulation is a treatment for tremor that consists of a multielectrode lead implanted into the ventrolateral nucleus of the thalamus. An extension wire from the electrode lead is threaded from the scalp area under the skin to the chest where it is connected to the pulse generator. The pulse generator produces a high-frequency, pulsed electric current that is sent along the electrode to the thalamus, effectively blocking the essential tremor. (Parkinsonian tremors do not respond as well, but patients are often able to decrease their medication after treatment.)

CASE STUDY

Jamal is a 33-year-old truck driver. He went to his family physician because his right leg and buttock were hurting. The family physician examined him and referred him to a neurosurgeon. Jamal was examined again. He did not know of an incident that started the pain. Moving his legs with the knees bent did not bother him but lifting the leg with the knee straight caused sharp pain. Jamal had an MRI and was diagnosed with an L4–L5 herniated disk. He was scheduled for a lumbar discectomy.

1. Are a laminectomy and a discectomy the same thing? Discuss your answer.
2. What instruments will be used on a discectomy? Will a microscope be used?
3. What are the complications associated with lumbar surgery?

QUESTIONS FOR FURTHER STUDY

1. What is the difference between a subdural and an epidural hematoma?
2. Which is the most dangerous type of intracranial hematoma and why?
3. What is the difference between a craniotomy and a craniectomy?
4. Which approach is used for exploration of the posterior fossa and why?
5. Why is a multilevel, bilateral laminectomy usually necessary for removal of an intradural spinal tumor?

BIBLIOGRAPHY

Adams, R. D., & Victor, M. (Eds.). (1993). *Principles of neurology* (5th ed.). New York: McGraw-Hill.

Allen, M. B., & Miller, R. H. (Eds.). (1995). *Essentials of neurosurgery: A guide to clinical practice*. New York: McGraw-Hill.

Anthony, C. P., & Thibodeau, G. A. (1979). *Textbook of anatomy and physiology* (10th ed.). St. Louis, MO: Mosby.

Black, P. M. (2002). *Advances in neurosurgery*. Available from *http://virtualtrials.com/black.cfm*

Bonaroti, E. A., Kondziolka, D., & Lunsford, L. D. (No date). Pallidotomy for Parkinson's disease [Online]. Available from *http://www.neuronet.pitt.edu/group/sctr-image/ssfind[baseline character]sp.html*

Caruthers, B. L. (1993). The frontal lobes: Key to moral thinking. *The Surgical Technologist, 25,* 8–13.

Caruthers, B. L. (1997). The eyes have it: A guide to a critical portion of the neurological trauma examination. *The Surgical Technologist, 29,* 24–31.

Chan, K. (No date). Gross anatomy of spinal cord and spinal nerves: A web based tutorial [Online]. Available from *http://www.uq.edu.au/anatomy/gmc/spinal/*

Continuum Health Partners. (No date). Operating room [Online]. Available from *http://www.bethisraelny.org/inn/webtour/microscopes.html*

Cosgrove, G. R., & Eskander, E. (1998). Thalamotomy and pallidotomy [Online]. Available from *http://neurosurgery.mgh.harvard.edu/pallidt.htm*

Davis, J. H., & Sheldon, G. F., et al. (1987). *Surgery: A problem solving approach* (2nd ed.). St. Louis, MO: Mosby.

Goldman, M. A. (1988). *Pocket guide to the operating room*. Philadelphia: F. A. Davis.

Grabowski, S. R., & Tortora, G. J. (1996). *Principles of anatomy and physiology* (8th ed.). New York: HarperCollins.

Hole, J. W. (1987). *Human anatomy and physiology* (4th ed.). Dubuque, IA: Wm. C. Brown.

Iacono, R. P. (2002). *Deep brain stimulation*. Available from *http://www.pallidotomy.com/deep_brain_stimulation.html*

Jackler, R. K., & Pitts, L. H. (1998). Treatment of acoustic neuromas. *The New England Journal of Medicine, 339,* 1471–1473.

Jennett, B., & Lindsay, K. W. (1994). *An introduction to neurosurgery* (5th ed.). Oxford: Butterworth-Heinemann.

Junge, T. (1996). Microvascular decompression for control of essential hypertension. *The Surgical Technologist, 28,* 10–15.

Lindsay, K. W., Bone, I., & Callander, R. (1997). *Neurology and neurosurgery illustrated*. Edinburgh: Churchill Livingstone.

McGuiness, A. M., et al. (2002). *Core curriculum for surgical technology* (5th ed.). Centennial, CO: Association of Surgical Technologists.

Ogilvy, C. S. (No date). Combined modality treatment in the management of brain arteriovenous malformations [Online]. Available from *http://neurosurgery.mgh.harvard.edu/v-s-93-4.htm*

Ojemann, R. G. (1992). Management of cranial and spinal meningiomas. *Clinical Neurosurgery, 40,* 321–383.

Ondra, S. L., Troup, H., George, E. D., & Schwabb, K. (1990). The natural history of asymptomatic arteriovenous malformations of the brain: A 24 year follow-up assessment. *J. Neurosurg., 73,* 387–391.

Pribram, K. H. (1969). The primate frontal cortex. *Neuropsychologia, 7,* 259–66.

Sabatini, R. M. E. (No date). The history of the electroencephalogram [Online]. Available from *http://www.epub.org.br/cm/n03/tecnologia/eeg.htm*

Shepard, G. M. (1988). *Neurobiology* (2nd ed.). New York: Oxford University Press.

Solomon, E. P., Schmidt, R. R., & Adragna, P. J. (1990). *Human anatomy & physiology* (2nd ed.). Ft. Worth, TX: Saunders.

University of Southern California. (1998). A new way of looking at stroke [Online]. Available from *http://www.usc.edu/hsc/neurosurgery/stroke/stroke.html*

Vincent, J. F. (1996). Stereotactic-ct biopsy. *The Surgical Technologist, 28,* 8–11.

Washington University in St. Louis. (No date). Neuroanatomy: coronal and horizontal sections [Online]. Available from *http://thalamus.wustl.edu/course/corhor.html*

Washington University in St. Louis. (1998). Basal ganglia and cerebellum [Online]. Available from *http://thalamus. wustl.edu/course/cerebell.html*

Wills, R. E. (1997). Transphenoidal approach to pituitary tumors. *The Surgical Technologist, 30,* 27–35.

Appendix A

Anatomy Plates

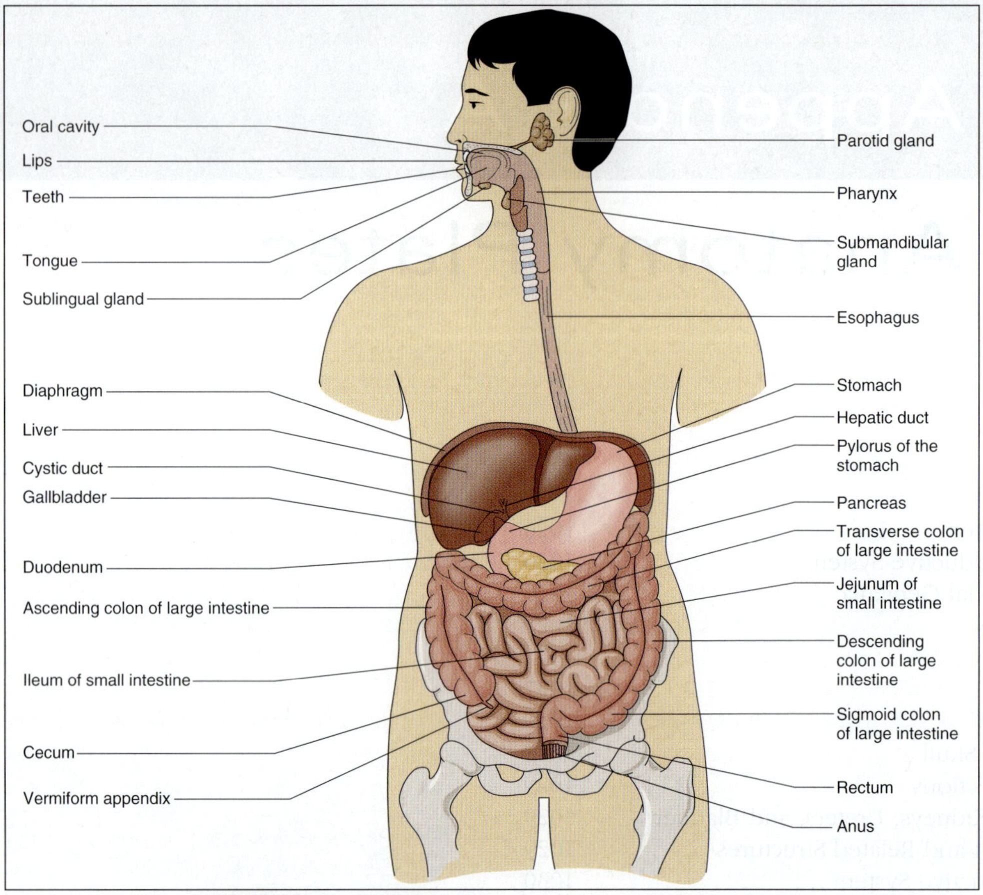

Plate 1 Digestive System

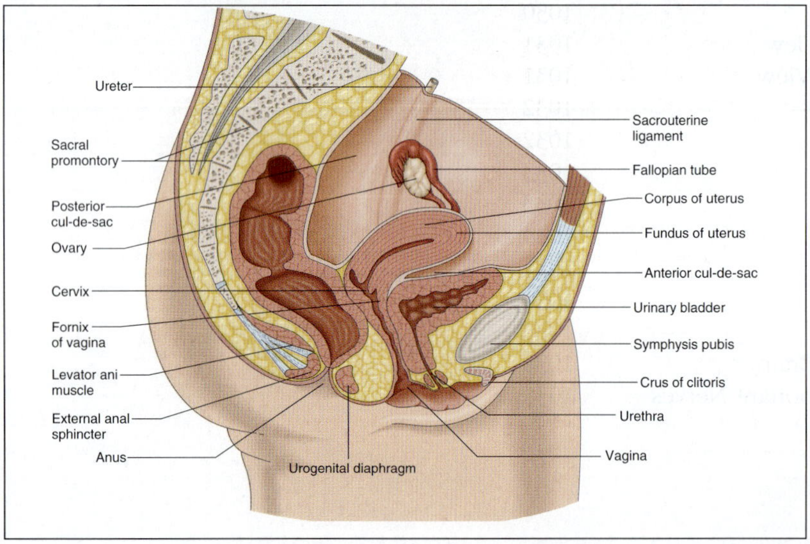

Plate 2A Female Reproductive System

Plate 2B Female External Genitalia

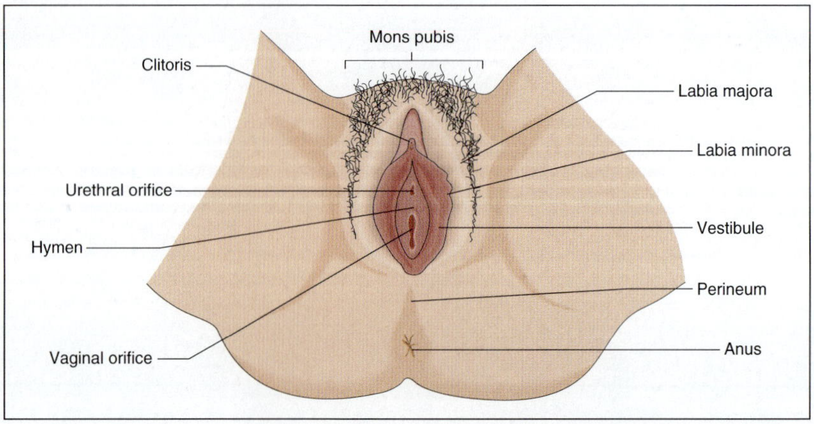

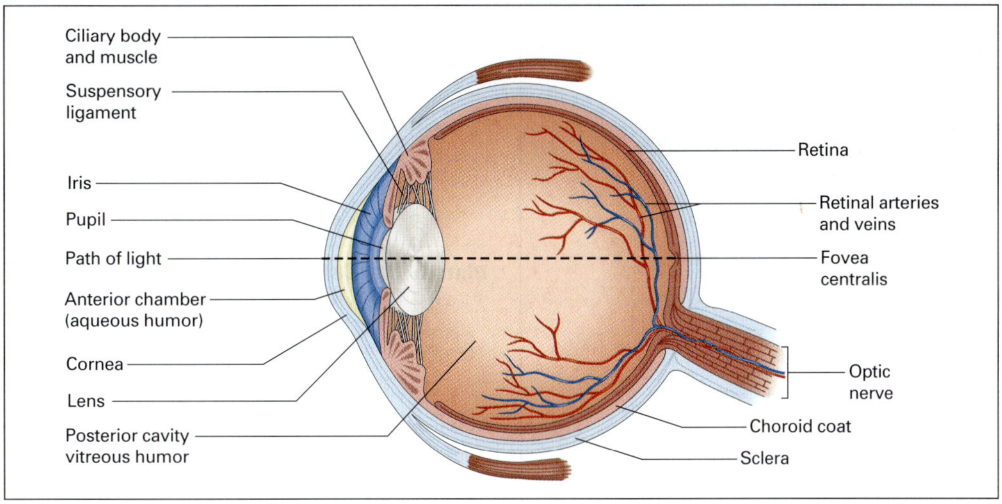

Plate 3 Eye Structure

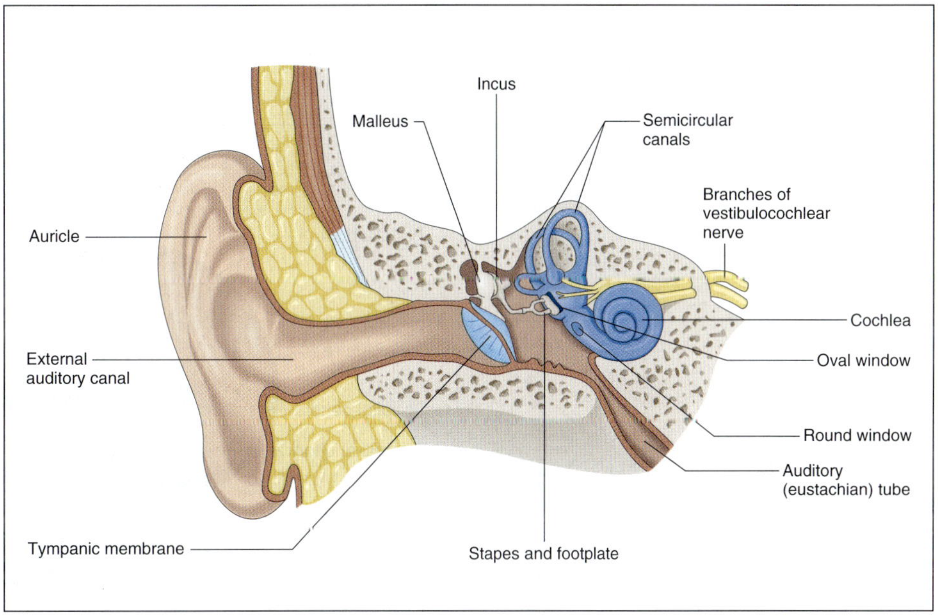

Plate 4 Ear Structure

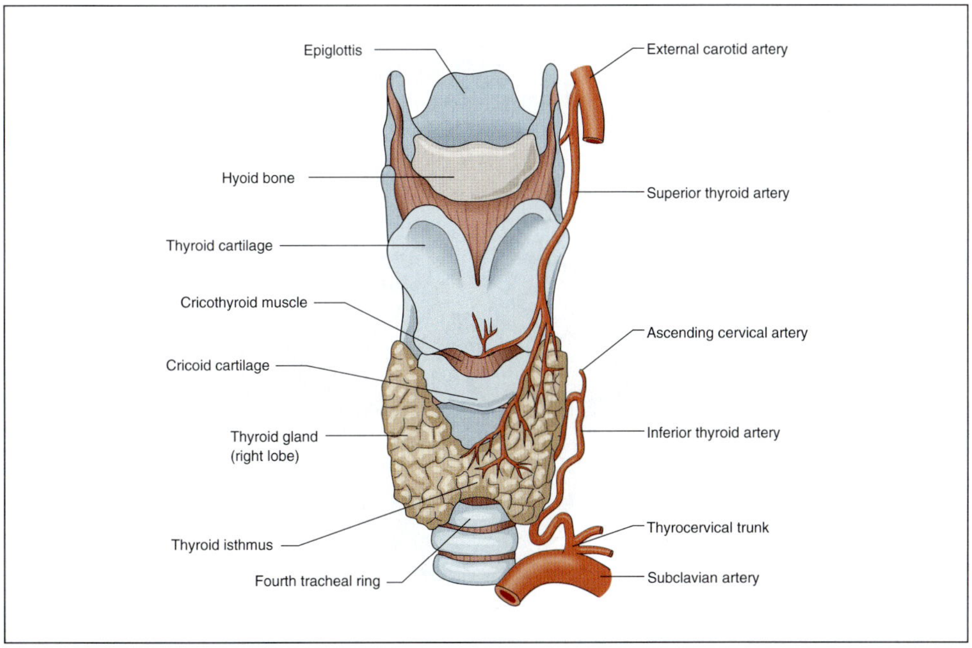

Plate 5 Thyroid

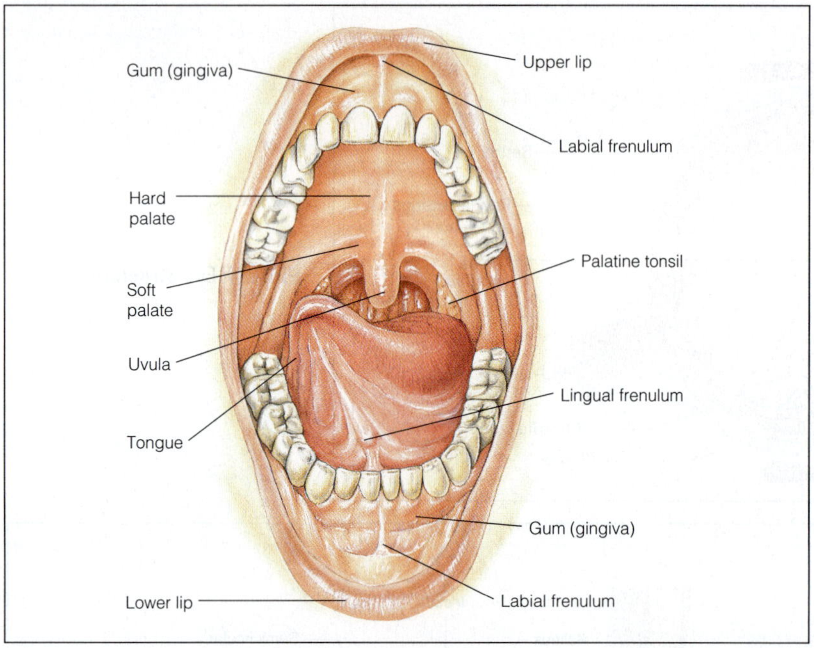

Plate 6 Oral Cavity

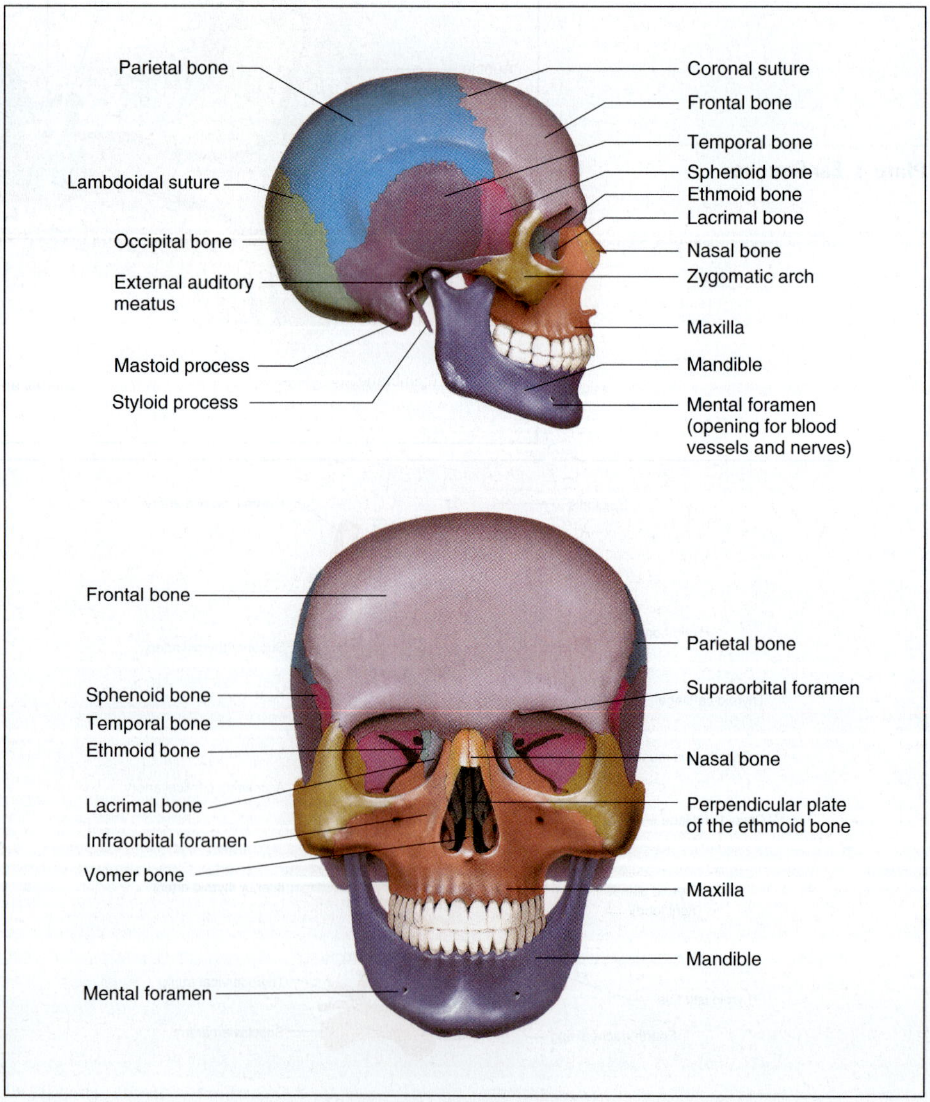

Plate 7 Bones of the Skull

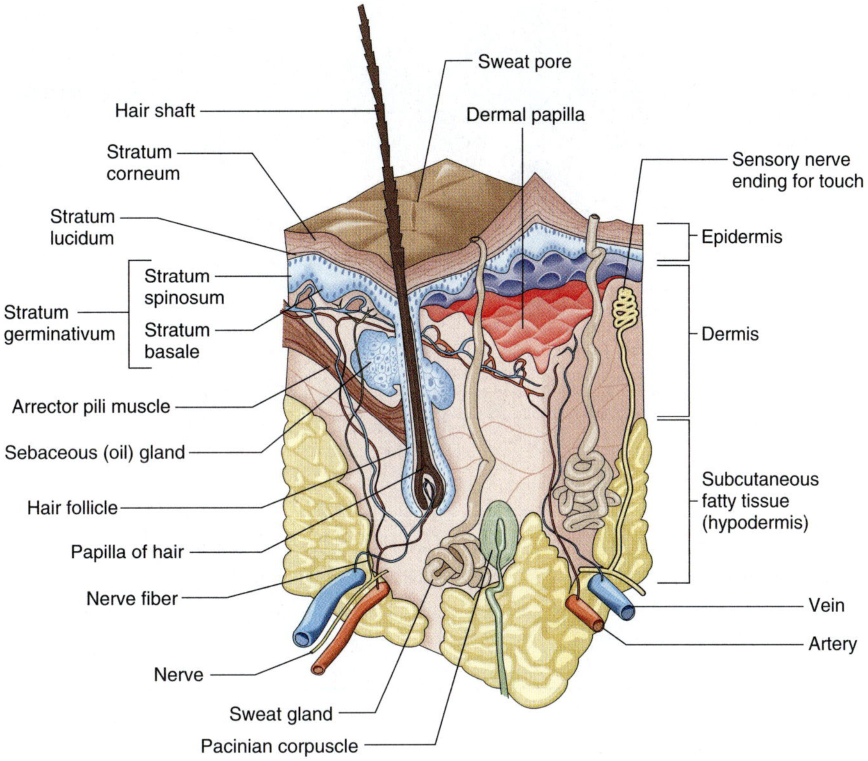

Plate 8 Skin Cross Section

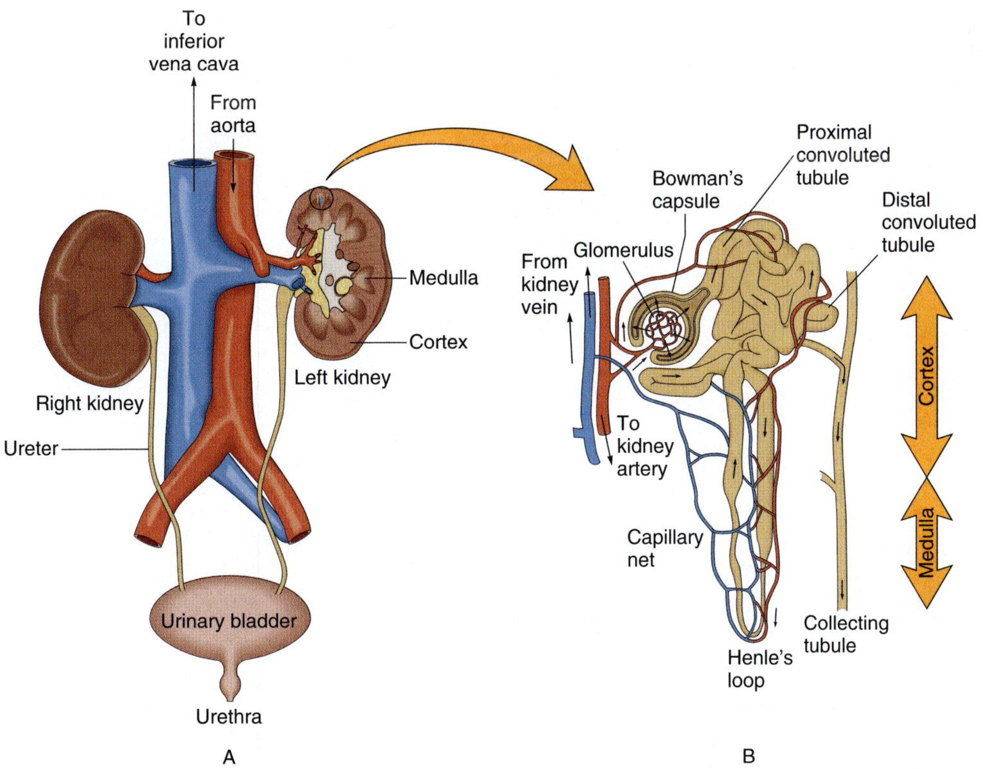

Plate 9A View of the Kidneys, Ureters, and Bladder

Plate 9B Nephron Unit and Related Structures (Arrows indicate the flow of blood through the nephron.)

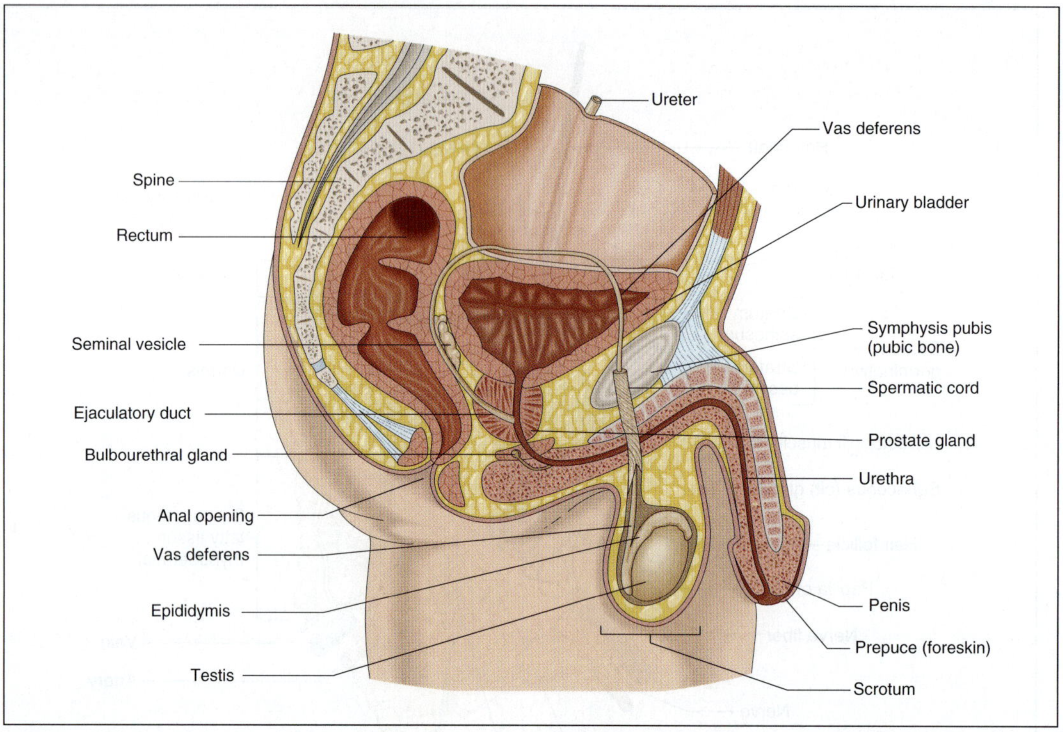

Plate 10 Male Reproductive System

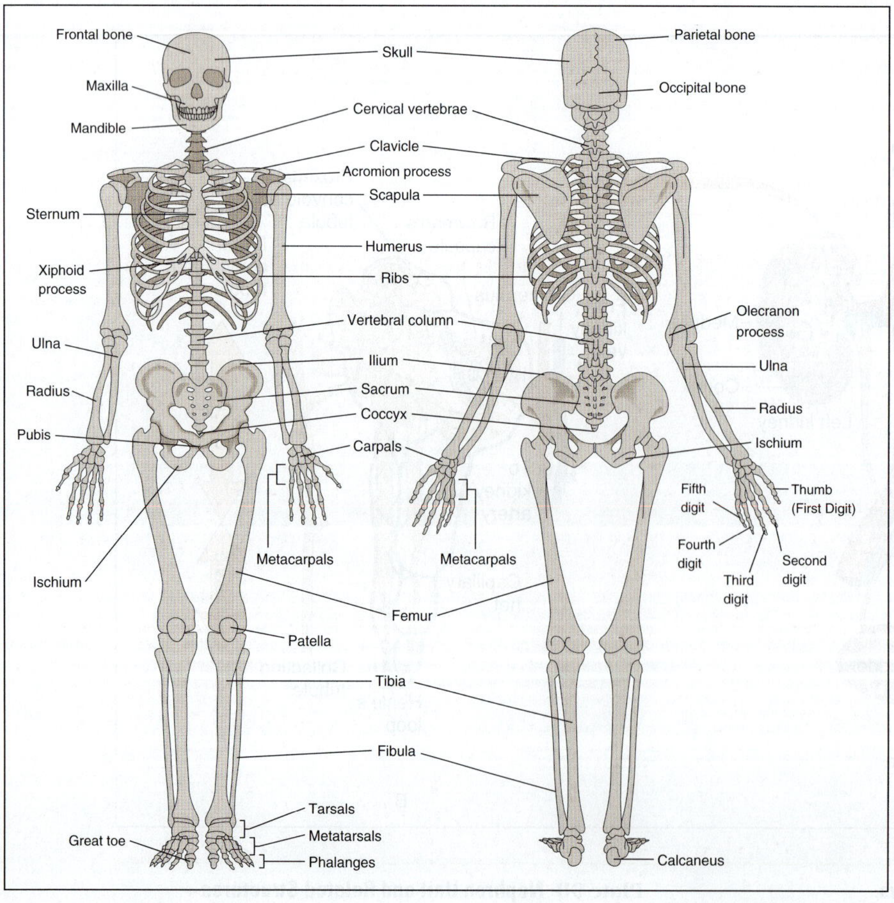

Plate 11 Skeletal System

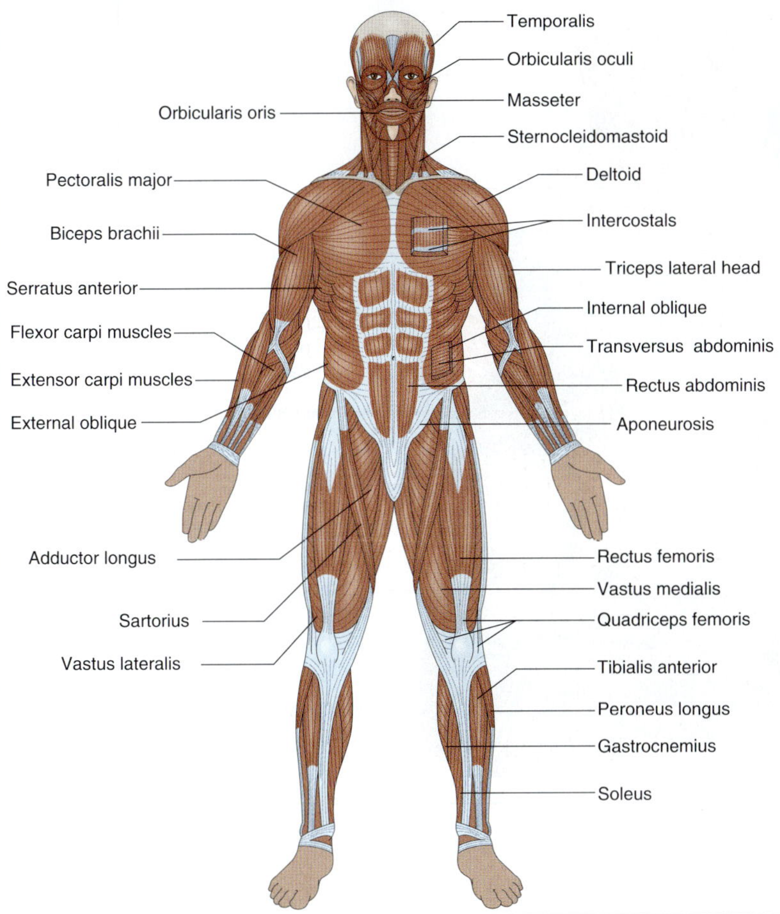

Plate 12A Skeletal Muscles—Anterior View

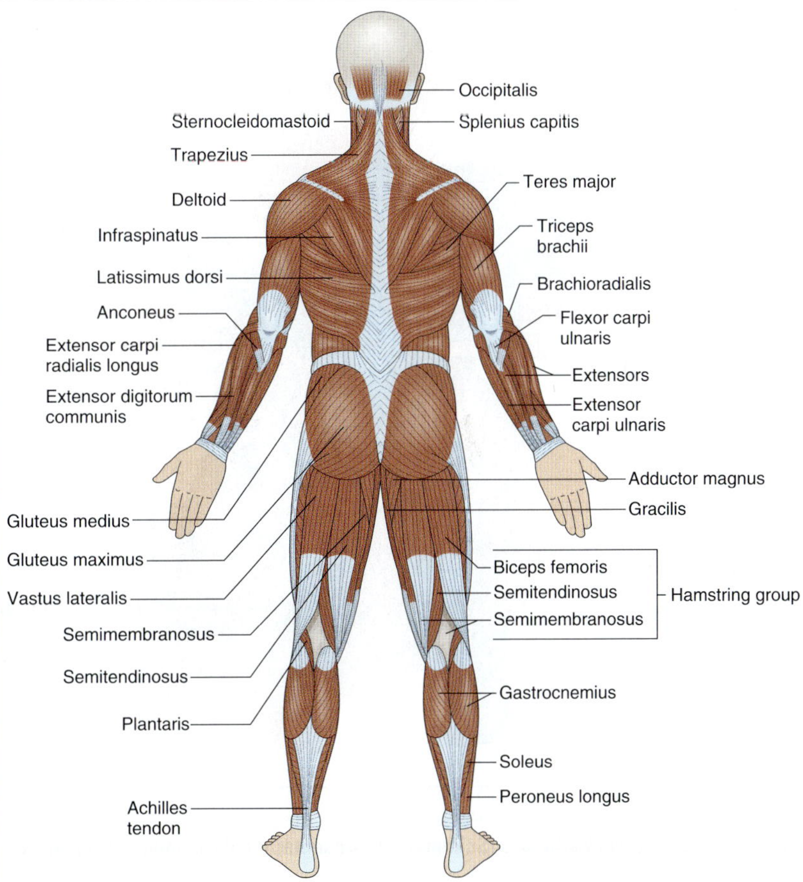

Plate 12B Skeletal Muscles—Posterior View

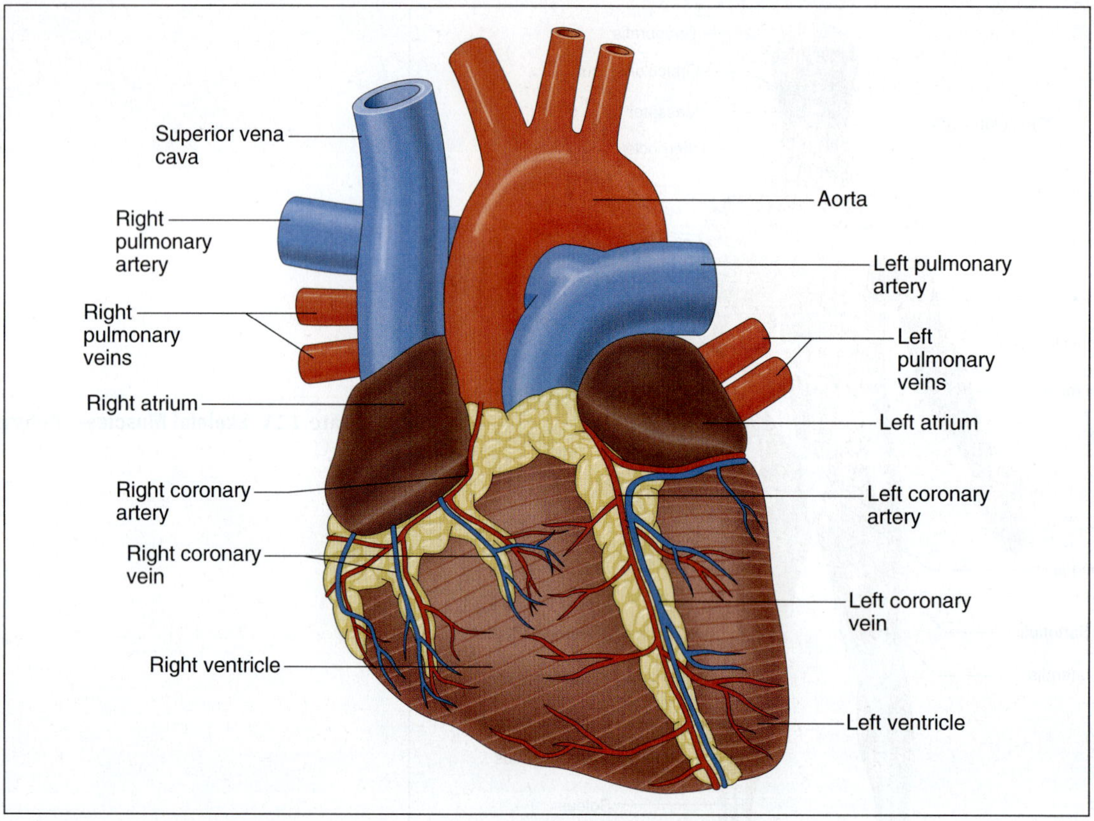

Plate 13A Heart—Anterior View

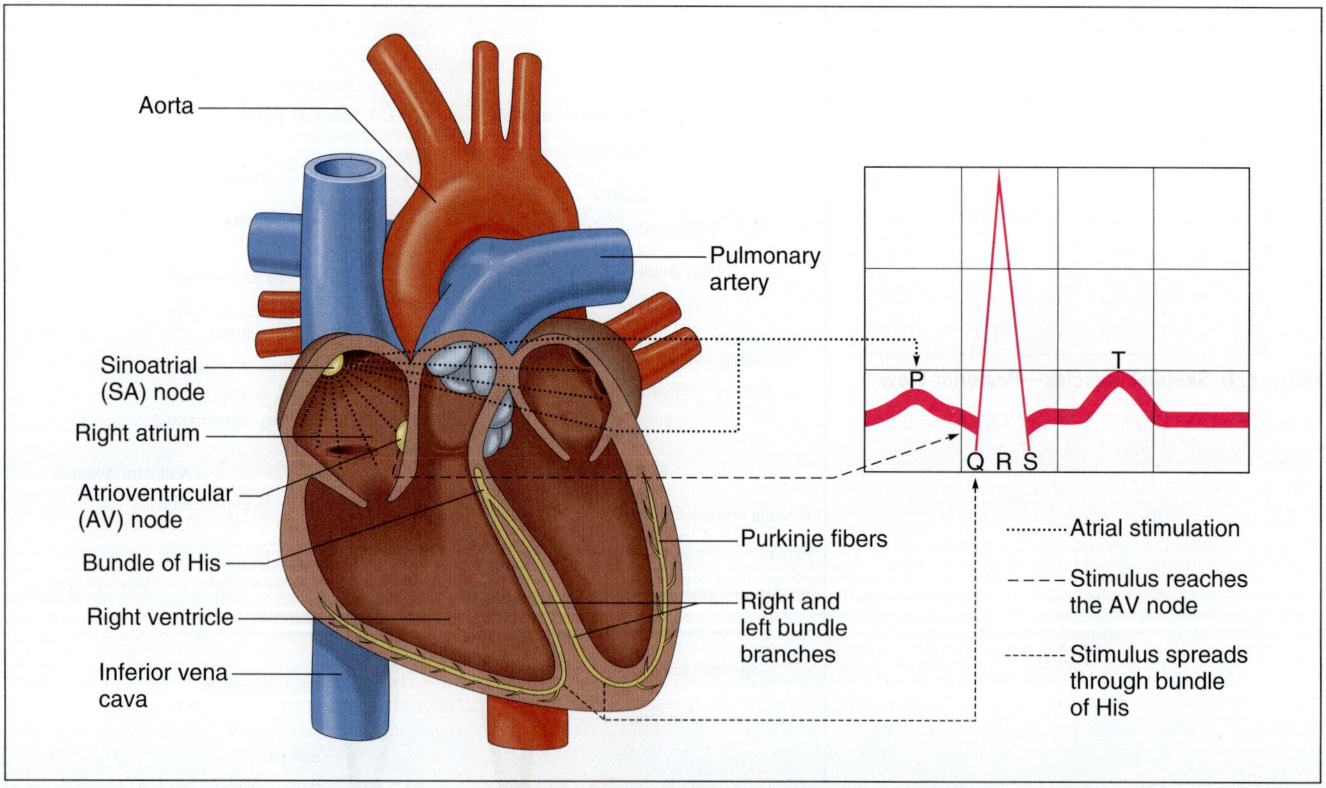

Plate 13B Conductive Pathways (Schematic representation of the impulses is shown on the right.)

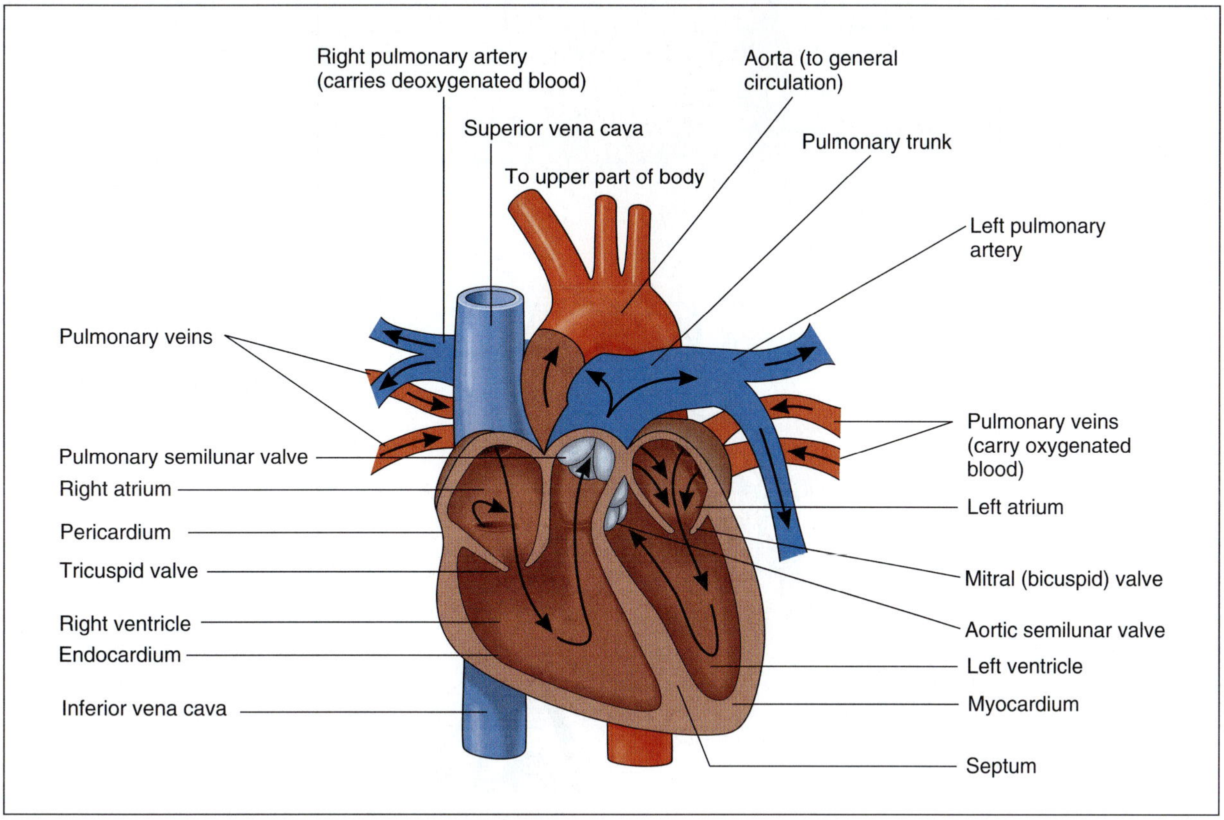

Plate 13C Pulmonary Circulation

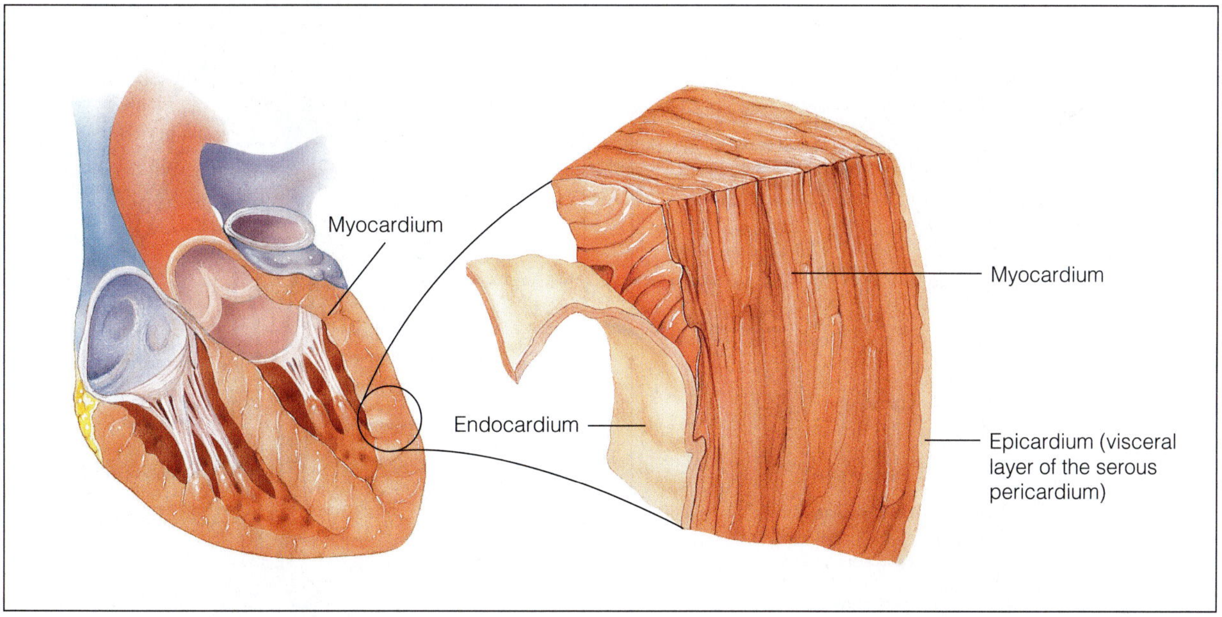

Plate 13D Wall of the Heart

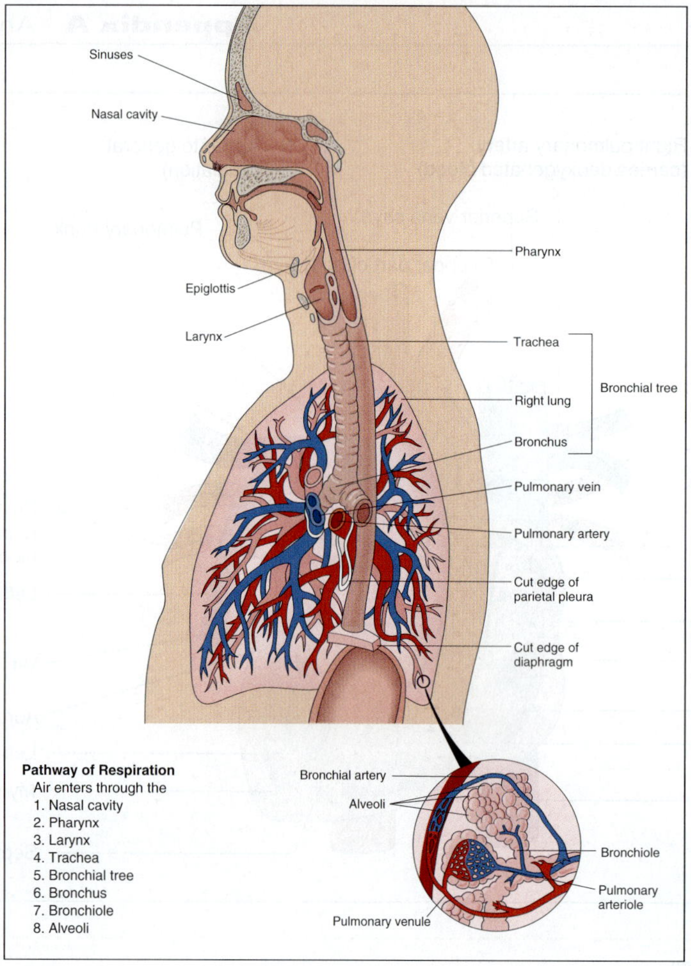

Plate 14 Respiratory System

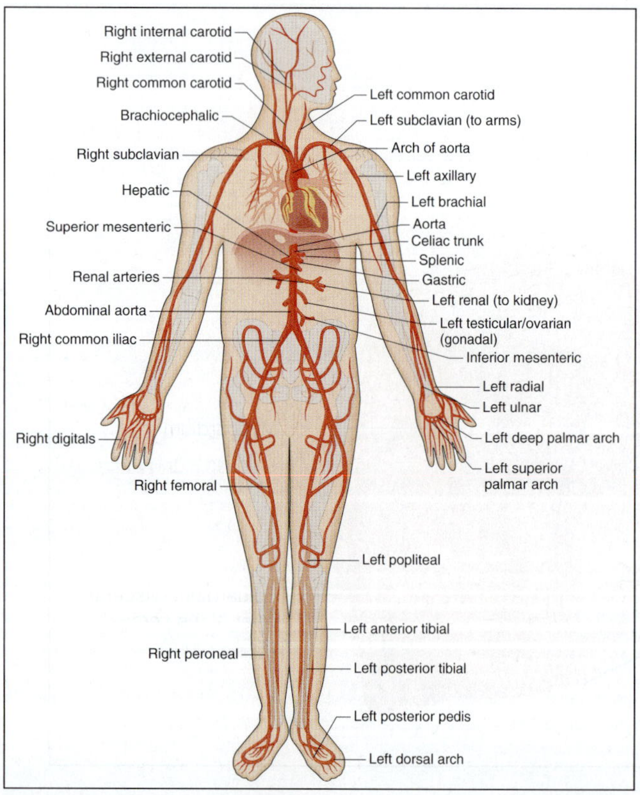

Plate 15A Arterial Circulation

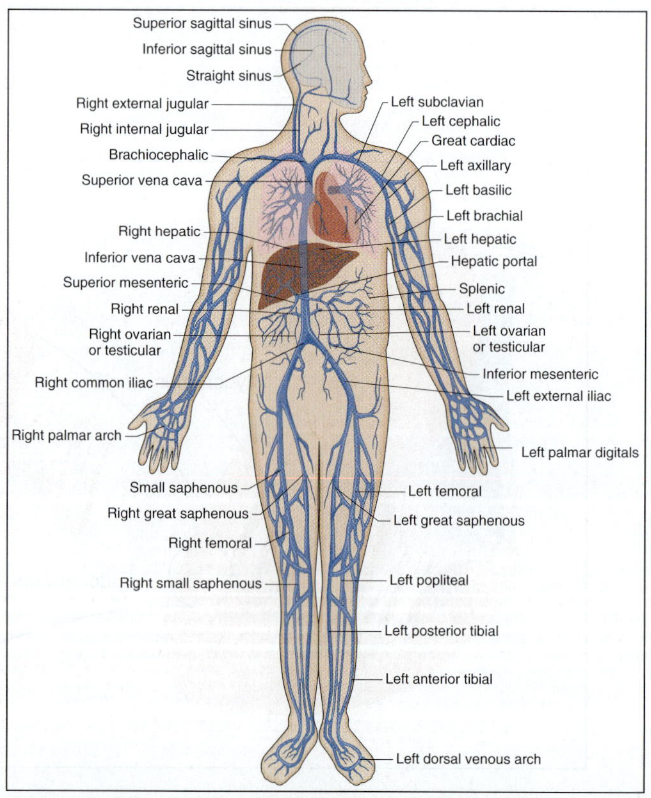

Plate 15B Venous Circulation

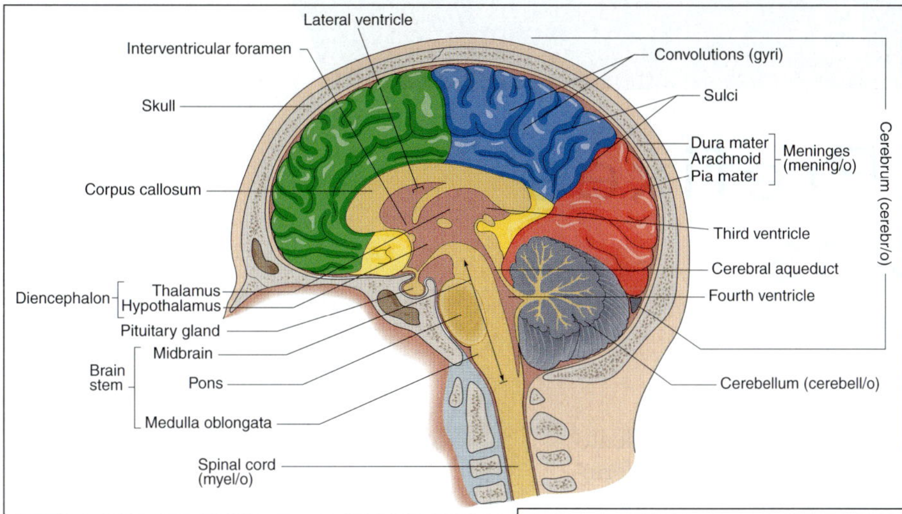

Plate 16A Cross Section of the Brain

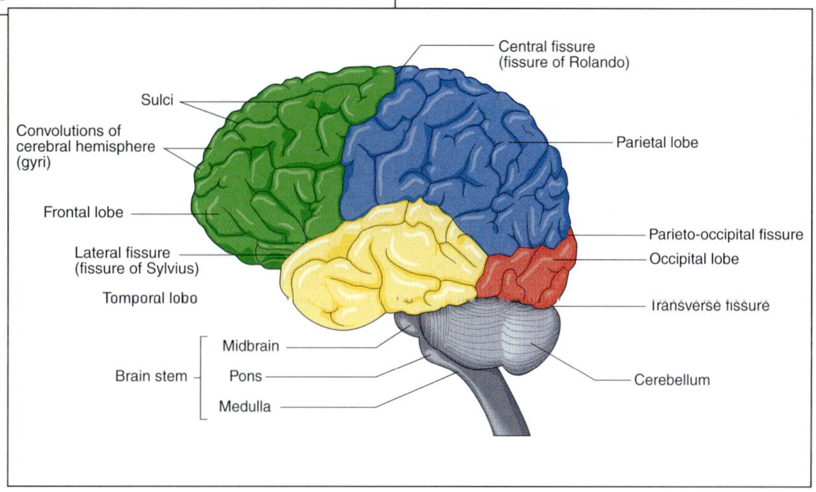

Plate 16B Lateral View of the Human Brain

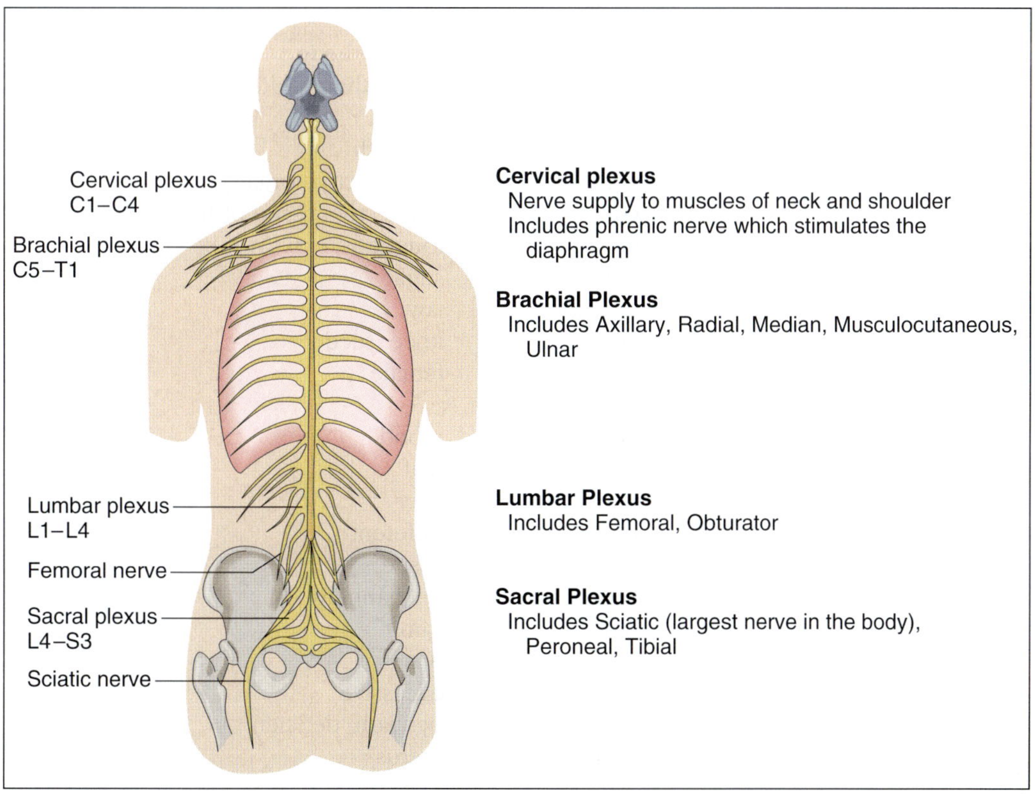

Plate 17 Spinal Nerve Plexus and Important Nerves

Appendix B

Common Prefixes and Suffixes

PREFIXES

a-, an-	absent or deficient
ab-	away
ad-	toward
adeno-	gland
af-	toward
angio-	vessel
ante-	before
antero-	ahead, in front
anti-	against
arthro-	joint
aur-	ear
auto-	self
bi-	two
brachi-	arm
brachy-	short
brady-	slow
bucc-	cheek
carcin-	cancer
cardi-	heart
cephalo-	head
cerebro-	brain
cervi-	neck
cheilo-	lips
chole-	bile, gall
chondr-	cartilage
circum-	around
colpo-	vagina
contra-	opposed
cost-	ribs
counter-	against
cranio-	skull
cryo-	cold
crypt-	hidden
cut-	skin
cysto-	bladder, sac
cyto-	cell
dactyl-	digits
de-	remove
dento-	tooth
derm-	skin
di-	twice
dia-	across, through
diplo-	double
dis-	apart
dorsi-	back
dys-	difficult, painful
ecto-	external
ef-	toward
endo-	within
entero-	intestine
epi-	upon
erythro-	red
eu-	good, well
ex-	away from, outside
extra-	beyond, in addition to
fasci-	fibrous tissue
fibro-	fibers, thread-like
gastro-	stomach
genito-	reproductive organs
glio-	connective tissue of the CNS
gloss-	tongue
glyco-	sugar
gnatho-	jaw
gon-	knee, seed
gyn-	female
hem-	blood
hemi-	half
hepato-	liver
hetero-	different
histo-	tissue
homeo-	unchanging
homo-	same
hydro-	water
hyper-	excessive
hypo-	beneath, deficient
hyster-	uterus

idio-	self
im-	into
in-	lacking
infra-	below
inter-	between
intra-	within
ipsi-	same
iso-	equal, same
juxta-	next to
kerat-	cornea, keratin
lacri-	tear
lacto-	milk
later-	side
leuko-	white
litho-	calculi
macro-	large
mal-	abnormal
malacia-	softening
mast-	breast
mega-	unusually large
meningo-	membranes covering the CNS
meno-	menstrual function
meso-	middle
meta-	beyond, change
micro-	small
mono-	one
muco-	mucous
multi-	many
myco-	fungi
myelo-	marrow, spinal canal (cord)
myo-	muscle
necro-	death
neo-	new
nephro-	kidney
neuro-	nerve
nocti-	night
noso-	disease
ocul-	eye
oligo-	few, deficient
onycho-	nails
oo-, ovi-, ovo-	ovum
oophoro-	ovary
ophthalm-	eye
ortho-	normal, straight
oseo-	bone
oto-	ear
ox-	pertaining to oxygen
pan-	all
para-	near
path-	disease
ped-	child, foot
per-	excessive, through
peri-	around
phag-	ingest
phleb-	vein
photo-	light
pleuro-	membranous lining of thoracic cavity
pneumo-	air, lung
pod-	foot
poly-	many
post-	following
pre-	before
presby-	old
pro-	in front of
procto-	rectum
pseudo-	false
psych-	mind
pulmo-	lung
pyelo-	pelvis of kidney
pyo-	pus
radio-	emission of radiation
re-	again
ren-	kidney
retro-	backward, behind
rhino-	nose
salpingo-	tube
sclero-	hard
scolio-	twisted
semi-	partial
sep-	poison
somato-	body
sono-	sound
sta-	stand still
sten-	narrow
sub-	under
super-	excessive
supra-	above
sym-	together
syn-	together
tachy-	rapid
thermo-	heat
tox-	poison
trach-	windpipe
trans-	through
tri-	three
ultra-	excessive
uni-	one
vas-	duct, vessel
viscero-	internal organs
xero-	dry

SUFFIXES

-algia	pain
-ase	enzyme
-cele	enlarged cavity, swelling
-centesis	removal of fluid via a surgical puncture
-cide	cut, kill, destroy
-clast	break
-dynia	pain
-ectasis	enlargement or stretching
-ectomy	surgical removal
-emia	relating to blood or a blood condition
-esthesia	sensation
-ferent	to carry
-gen	produces, originates
-glia	connective tissue of the CNS
-gram	written or recorded
-graph	writing or recording instrument
-graphy	the process of recording
-ia	state of
-ism	state of
-itis	inflammation
-lysis	breaking down, destruction, separation
-malacia	abnormal softening
-megaly	large
-meter	measure
-oid	like
-ology	study of
-oma	mass or tumor
-osis	abnormal condition, disease state
-ostomy	surgically creating a mouth or opening
-otomy	incision
-oxia	pertaining to oxygen
-penia	lack of
-pexy	fixation
-plasty	surgical repair
-pnea	related to breathing
-ptosis	drooping or prolapsed
-rrhagia	excessive flow
-rrhaphy	surgical repair of a defect
-rrhea	flow or discharge
-rrhexis	rupture
-sclerosis	abnormal hardening
-scopy	visual examination
-stenosis	abnormal narrowing
-taxia	order
-tripsy	to crush
-trophic	nutrition
-tropic	influencing change
-uria	related to urination or urine

Appendix C

Measurements

WEIGHTS, MEASURES, AND EQUIVALENTS

APOTHECARIES' SYSTEM	
Weight	
1 dram (ʒ) =	60 grains (gr)
1 ounce (℥) =	480 grains
=	8 drams
1 pound (lb) =	16 ounces
Volume	
1 fluid dram =	60 minims (m)
1 fluid ounce =	8 drams
1 pint (pt) =	16 ounces
1 quart (qt) =	2 pints

METRIC SYSTEM	
Weight	
1 gram (gm) =	1,000 milligrams (mg)
1 kilogram (kg) =	1,000 grams
Volume	
1 liter =	1,000 cubic centimeters (cc)

APPROXIMATE EQUIVALENTS

HOUSEHOLD, METRIC, AND APOTHECARIES'		
1 teaspoon (tsp)	= 4 cc	= 1 fluid dram
1 tablespoon (tbsp)	= 15 cc	= ½ ounce
1 teacup	= 120 cc	= 4 fluid ounces
1 tumbler	= 240 cc	= 8 fluid ounces

WEIGHTS

Metric	Apothecaries'	Metric	Apothecaries'
0.4 mg =	1/150 grain	30 mg =	½ grain
0.6 mg =	1/100 grain	60 mg =	1 grain
1.0 mg =	1/60 grain	1 gm =	15 grains
10.0 mg =	⅙ grain	15 gm =	4 drams
15.0 mg =	¼ grain	30 gm =	1 ounce

POUNDS TO KILOGRAMS CONVERSION

1 lb = 0.4536 kg	*1 kg = 2.2 lb*
lb	kg
5	2.3
10	4.5
20	9.1
30	13.6
40	18.1
50	22.7
60	27.2
70	31.7
80	36.3
90	40.8
100	45.5
110	49.9
120	54.4
130	58.9
140	63.5
150	68.0
160	72.6
170	77.1
180	81.6
190	86.2
200	90.7
210	95.3
220	99.5
230	104.3

LINEAR MEASURES

1 millimeter (mm) =	0.04	inch (in.)
1 centimeter (cm) =	0.4	inch
1 decimeter (dm) =	4.0	inches
1 meter (m) =	39.37	inches
1 inch =	2.54	centimeters
1 foot =	30.48	centimeters

CELSIUS (CENTIGRADE) FAHRENHEIT EQUIVALENTS

Celsius	*Fahrenheit*	*Celsius*	*Fahrenheit*
36.0	96.8	39.0	102.2
36.5	97.7	39.5	103.1
37.0	98.6	40.0	104.0
37.5	99.5	40.5	104.9
38.0	100.4	41.0	105.8
38.5	101.3	41.5	106.7

- To convert kilograms to pounds:
  Multiply weight in kilograms by 2.2
- To convert pounds to kilograms:
  Divide weight in pounds by 2.2
- To convert centimeters to inches:
  Divide length in centimeters by 2.54
- To convert inches to centimeters:
  Multiply length in inches by 2.54
- To convert degrees Fahrenheit to degrees Centigrade:
  Subtract 32, then multiply by 5/9
- To convert degrees Centigrade to degrees Fahrenheit:
  Multiply by 9/5 then add 32

Glossary

abandonment To leave a patient alone who is still in need of patient care or observation

Abbreviated Burn Severity Index (ABSI) A scale used to assess the severity of a burned patient's condition based on the age and sex of the patient, presence of inhalation injury, depth of burn according to degree, and the percentage of the total body surface that has been burned

abdominoplasty Surgical procedure that is performed for the purposes of thinning the upper abdominal fat, tightening the abdominal muscles, and removing fat and excess skin from the mid to lower abdomen

abduction Move away from the midline or turn outward

ablation Use of intense heat to vaporize or erode tissue

abortion Termination prior to completion

abscess Area of broken-down tissue containing pus and liquefied tissue

absorbable suture Suture that is capable of being broken down by the body's fluids and tissues

absorption To take in or soak up

AC joint *See* acromioclavicular joint

accessory structures The hair, nails, sudoriferous glands, and sebaceous glands

accountability Obligation to disclose details for evaluation; commonly used to mean "to be held responsible for"

accreditation Process whereby businesses, educational institutions and programs, and health care organizations are determined to meet standards and performance criteria as established by an accrediting agency

Accreditation Review Committee on Education in Surgical Technology (ARC-ST) A committee on accreditation that is under the large umbrella of the Commission on Accreditation of Allied Health Education Programs (CAAHEP), which oversees the accreditation processes of surgical technology education programs

acne vulgaris An inflammatory disease of the skin that causes the formation of pustules (or more commonly called pimples). It is caused by the blockage of the sebaceous glands and bacteria that infect the blocked passageway

acromioclavicular joint (AC joint) A part of the pectoral girdle located at the top of the shoulder that is an articulation between the lateral end of the clavicle and the flattened, small process located on the border of the acromion

acronym A word formed by the initial letters of the principal components of a compound term

ACTH *See* adrenocorticotropic hormone

active electrode Transfers concentrated electrical current into another medium, e.g., electrical current transformed into thermal energy

acute Severe, short-term condition

acyanotic defect A congenital heart defect that does not produce blue color of the skin, usually due to cyanosis. Complications include right ventricular failure and an abnormal increase on the load of the pulmonary circulation

Addison's disease The adrenal glands fail to produce the hormones necessary to maintain fluid balance and blood pressure or they inhibit the response to stress; also called *adrenal insufficiency*

adduction Move toward the midline or turn inward

adenocarcinoma Renal cell carcinoma, the most common type of kidney cancer, which causes a malignant change to cells lining the renal tubule, producing hematuria, flank pain, and presence of a palpable mass

adhesion Abnormal attachment of two surfaces or structures that are normally separate

adhesive Type of surgical drape that is typically made of a thin, clear plastic material that has an adhesive backing and is applied to the skin; the drape may be impregnated with an antimicrobial iodine agent

adjustable suture surgery An alternative surgical procedure for the correction of strabismus that allows more accurate alignment and placement of the field of vision

adnexa Appendages or accessory structures of an organ

Adrenocorticotropic hormone (ACTH) A hormone secreted by the anterior pituitary gland that stimulates the growth of the adrenal gland cortex and the secretion of corticosteroids. An increase in secretion is in response to a low level of circulating cortisol and to stress, fever, surgery, and hypoglycemia

adrenalectomy Surgical removal of an adrenal gland

advance directive Written instructions expressing the patient's wishes concerning the types and amount of medical treatment to be rendered in the event the patient can no longer make those types of decisions

adventitia The outermost layer of an artery composed of elastic connective tissue

adverse effect Undesirable response to pharmacologic therapy or other treatment

aeger primo "The Patient First"

aerobe Microorganism that requires oxygen to sustain life

aerodigestive tract Medical term for the throat

aerosol Substance suspended in a gas

aesthetic Visually pleasing

afferent Carrying toward a given point

affidavit Voluntary statement of facts sworn to be true before an authority

agonist Refers to an agent that stimulates or prolongs the response of a drug or a physiologic action

airborne Transported or spread by air; the surgical technologist is primarily concerned with airborne bacteria

-algia Suffix meaning painful

alveolar process The part of the mandible or maxilla that forms the dental arch which contains the sockets for the teeth

alveoli The terminal end of the bronchioles that are grape-like clusters within the lung where the exchange of carbon dioxide and oxygen takes place

ambulatory surgical facility Facility where patients are treated and released the same day; also known as out-patient surgery center or same day surgery

American National Standards Institute (ANSI) Organization of industry experts who promote and facilitate voluntary consensus standards in technical fields

American Society for Testing and Materials (ASTM) An organization of industry experts who develop and provide voluntary consensus standards for medical equipment by testing the equipment

amnesia Lack of recall

amphiarthrosis A joint that is slightly movable

ampule Small hermetically sealed glass container usually containing medication intended for parenteral use

anaerobe Microorganism that sustains life in the absence of oxygen

analgesia Reduction in sensibility to pain without the loss of consciousness

analgesic Refers to an agent or method used to reduce the sensibility to pain without the loss of consciousness

anaphylaxis An immediate hypersensitivity reaction to a foreign protein or other specific substance

anastomosis Pathological, surgical, or traumatic formation of an opening between two normally separate organs or spaces

anatomic position A position in which the body is upright, facing forward, arms slightly outward from body with palms facing forward, and feet forward

ancillary A supplement or secondary feature that is not necessary, but enhances the performance or looks of an item

anesthesia Absence of sensation

anesthesia cart Portable unit containing supplies needed for administration of the anesthetics

anesthesia machine Device that contains equipment needed to administer the anesthetic, monitor the patient's vital signs, and provide supportive measures during a surgical procedure

anesthesia provider A physician or certified registered nurse anesthetist (CRNA) who is a nonsterile surgical team member who administers the anesthetic, monitors the patient's vital signs, and provides supportive measures during a surgical procedure

anesthesia screen Attachment to the operating table that is used to create a barrier between the sterile and nonsterile area following placement of the drapes on the patient and to aid in keeping the drapes off the patient's face

anesthetic Agent that produces anesthesia

aneurysm A sac formed by localized dilatation of the walls of an artery due to structural weakening

angina Intermittent or continuous cardiac pain caused by anoxia of the myocardium

angioplasty The surgical reconstruction of blood vessels damaged by disease or trauma

angle closure glaucoma An abnormal condition of elevated pressure within an eye caused by the obstruction of the outflow of aqueous humor; angle closure refers to an eye with a narrow angle between the iris and cornea. The pupil is abnormally dilated, causing the iris to block the exit of the aqueous humor from the anterior chamber

anoxia Absence of oxygen

antagonist Refers to an agent used to block the action of another drug or physiological action without producing any effect of its own

anterior Toward the front

anterior chamber The cavity of the eye located anterior to the iris and containing the aqueous humor

antibiotic Refers to an agent used to destroy or suppress the activity of microorganisms

antibody Protein produced in the blood in response to a specific foreign antigen

anticipate To foresee or prepare for a situation before it occurs, such as the surgical technologist anticipating the surgeon's needs

anticoagulant Refers to an agent used to delay or counteract blood clotting

antigen Foreign substance that stimulates antibody production, initiating the immune response

antimicrobial Refers to an agent capable of killing some microorganisms and suppressing the growth of other types of microbes

antimuscarinic/anticholinergic Refers to an agent used to block parasympathetic effects such as salivation and bradycardia

antiseptic Refers to an agent used to interfere with the growth and development of microorganisms

aortic semilunar valve The heart valve between the left ventricle and aorta; as pressure increases in the left ventricle, the valve opens and oxygenated blood enters the aorta for distribution to the rest of the body

aperture An opening

apical pulse The pulse taken at the apex of the heart

apnea Cessation of breathing

apocrine sweat glands One of two types of sweat glands that are larger than merocrine sweat glands. Location is limited to external genitalia and axillae; ducts open through the hair follicles and are especially active at puberty. They are stimulated by pain, emotional stress, and sexual arousal

apposition To fit together or place side by side; to make contiguous

approximated Returned to proximity; to bring together sides or edges

aqueous Solution prepared with water

aqueous humor A clear liquid located in the anterior and posterior chambers of the eye

ARC-ST *See* Accreditation Review Committee on Education in Surgical Technology

armboards An attachment to the operating table for placement of the patient's arms

arrhythmia Absence of cardiac rhythm

arterial blood gases (ABGs) A method of monitoring blood oxygenation levels

arteriovenous (AV) fistula A surgical procedure that involves creating an access site for hemodialysis in which a direct connection is created between the radial artery and cephalic vein

arthrodesis Surgical fixation of a joint to relieve pain and provide support

arthroplasty The surgical replacement or reconstruction of a diseased or worn joint in order to restore mobility

arthroscopy Surgical procedure in which a special type of endoscope is used to view a joint internally for diagnostic purposes

arthrotomy Incision into a joint

articulate To form a joint

ascites Abnormal collection of fluid in the abdominal cavity

asepsis Absence of microorganisms

aspiration Drawing in or out by suction

Association for the Advancement of Medical Instrumentation (AAMI) Organization that establishes standards that reach across the spectrum of the health care field, including sterilization, electrical safety, use of medical devices, and levels of device safety

Association of Surgical Technologists (AST) The nonprofit national professional membership organization for surgical technologists and surgical assistants

asystole Absence of cardiac contractions

atheroma An abnormal buildup of fat and lipids that deposit in an arterial wall forming a mass

atherosclerosis A disorder of the arteries characterized by the buildup of yellow-colored plaque in the inner layers of the arterial wall. The plaque gradually becomes thick and calcified, and the lumen of the vessel narrows, resulting in a reduced blood flow to the organ supplied by the artery

atraumatic Causes little or no trauma

atria (pl.); atrium (sing.) Upper chambers of the heart that receive blood from the superior vena cava and inferior vena cava veins and the coronary sinus

atrial fibrillation A cardiac arrhythmia characterized by uneven electrical activity in the atria, causing the atria to quiver instead of rhythmically pumping blood into the ventricles

atrial flutter Atrial tachycardia with heart rate of 230 to 380 beats per minute. The two types, typical and atypical, are differentiated by their heart rates and electrocardiographic patterns

atrial septal defect An abnormal opening in the wall between the two atria that results in a shunting of oxygenated blood from the left atrium into the right atrium, resulting in pulmonary hypertension, enlargement of the pulmonary artery, and enlargement of the right side of the heart

atrioventricular node Located in the septum of the heart and between the two atria; receives the electrical conduction impulse from the sinoatrial node and provides the conduction pathway between the atrial and ventricular syncytium

atrioventricular orifice An opening through which the atrium on each side of the heart communicates with its corresponding ventricle

augmentation Process of increasing; refers to size, quantity, degree, or severity

augmentation mammoplasty Plastic reconstruction that increases the size of the breasts

auscultation Use of the unaided ear or a stethoscope to listen to sounds within the body

autoclave Device to accomplish steam or gas sterilization

autoimmune diseases A disease that attacks the body's own tissues such as rheumatoid arthritis

autologous From oneself

autonomic nervous system (ANS) Involuntary motor portions of the nervous system responsible for smooth muscle contraction

back table Large movable table that is covered with a sterile drape for placement of sterile instruments, supplies, and equipment for surgical procedures

bacteriostasis Situation in which bacterial growth is inhibited (static), but the microorganisms are not killed

balanced salt solution (BSS) An irrigant used for the eye during eye procedures

barrier Item used to prevent or reduce environmental transmission or migration of microorganisms

behavior Actions or conduct of a living organism; influenced by beliefs, emotions, ethics, feelings, morals, and values; may indicate mental state

benign Not malignant or recurrent

benign prostatic hypertrophy (BPH) Abnormal enlargement of the prostate gland that usually occurs in men over the age of 50; it is not a malignant or inflammatory condition

bifurcation Division into two branches; "Y" shaped

bilateral Pertaining to both sides

bile A secretion of the liver that emulsifies fats preparing them for further digestion and absorption in the small intestine

bioburden Amount of gross organic debris or the number of microorganisms on an object at any given time

bioethics Study of the ethical implications of biological research and application, especially in medicine

biohazard Biologic material, which may be infective, that threatens humans or the environment

biological indicator A method for testing the sterilization capability of a sterilizer; contains microorganisms that are killed when exposed to a sterilization process; only method of guaranteeing the sterility of an item(s)

biopsy Removal of tissue or fluid from the body for pathological examination to determine a diagnosis

biotechnology The newest source of drugs from the laboratory that are genetically engineered; also referred to as recombinant DNA technology

biotransformation Metabolism of a substance that generally occurs in the liver

bipolar electrosurgery For this type of electrosurgery, both the active electrode and return electrode functions are performed at the site of surgery. The two tines of the forceps perform the active and return electrode functions. Only the tissue grasped is included in the electrical circuit. Because the return function is performed by one tine of the forceps, no patient return electrode is needed

bladder A muscular sac that serves for the collection of urine

blepharochalasis Lack of tone or relaxation of the skin of the eyelid causing the lid to appear thin and wrinkled; most often affects young people

blepharoplasty Surgical repair or plastic surgery of the eyelid performed to remove excess skin or fat deposits from the lower or upper eyelids

blood pressure (BP) Force of circulating blood against the blood vessel wall

blood, urea, nitrogen (BUN) Three items in which the concentration of each in urine is measured; part of a urinalysis

blunt dissection Technique of separating tissues with the finger(s) or nonsharp surgical instrument

bolster Device used to support, maintain, or prevent pressure; often used in reference to suture bolsters

bolus Soft, rounded mass such as chewed food or a concentrated amount of a drug usually administered intravenously

bone wax Beeswax that has been processed and sterilized for use on bone to control bleeding

bony pelvis The four bones of the pelvis that make up the lower part of the trunk of the body that serves to support the upper body and protect the pelvic organs

Bowie-Dick test Specifically designed for use with a prevacuum steam sterilizer to test for air entrapment

Bowman's capsule A double-layered cup-shaped end of a renal tubule that is the site of filtration along with the glomerulus in the kidney

brachial artery The primary artery of the upper arm that is continuous from the axillary artery; it has three branches and terminates at the bifurcation into the radial and ulnar arteries

bradycardia Slow heart rate; less than 60 beats per minute

breakpoints Points in the operating table that indicate where a section can be moved up or down

breech Intrauterine position of a fetus in which the buttocks or feet first present

bronchial tree Refers to the trachea, bronchi, and bronchioles

bronchioles The division of the bronchus resulting in smaller branches that terminate at the alveoli

bronchoscopy Endoscopic procedure that involves the insertion of a rigid or flexible bronchoscope through the trachea into the bronchus for the evaluation of hemoptysis, infection, carcinoma of the lung, damage to the lungs due to smoke inhalation, or laser treatment of endobronchial tumors or for removal foreign objects lodged in the airway

bronchospasm Sudden involuntary muscle contraction of the bronchus

BSS *See* balanced salt solution

buccal Pertaining to the cheek or mouth

bundle of His Located in the upper portion of the septum of the heart between the ventricles and divides into left and right bundle branches that course along the septum toward the apex of the heart. It is the only electrical connection between the atria and ventricles. The bundle receives the electrical impulse from the AV node and the impulse is then transmitted to the Purkinje fibers via the bundle. Also called the *atrioventricular bundle*

CABG *See* coronary artery bypass graft

calculi (pl.); calculus (sing.) Abnormal hard mass composed of minerals and salts; commonly referred to as a stone

calvarial Pertaining to the superior portion of the cranium where the fontanels of the infant are situated

cancellous bone A type of bone tissue found at the ends of bone and lining the medullary marrow cavity; composed of columns of trabeculae with large spaces in between; also referred to as spongy bone due to its appearance

cancer Malignant neoplasm

cannulation The placement of cannulas into the right atrium or vena cava for draining venous blood to the pump oxygenator; and into the ascending aorta for return of arterial blood from the pump oxygenator

capillary The smallest blood vessel composed of a single layer of endothelial cells where oxygen and carbon dioxide exchange occurs

capillary action Action by which liquid travels along an established path; often used in reference to suture in which infectious fluid travels along the length of the suture strand placed in a wound; also referred to as wicking

capnography Used in the anesthetic setting to provide a breath-by-breath analysis of expired carbon dioxide (end-tidal CO_2)

cardiac conduction system The system that coordinates and transmits the electrical impulses throughout the myocardium of the heart

cardiac cycle One cycle includes everything that occurs within the heart during a single heartbeat

cardiac dysrhythmias Refers to any type of abnormal heart rhythm

cardiac output The amount of blood ejected from the left ventricle into the aorta, or from the right ventricle into the pulmonary artery. Cardiac output equals the stroke volume times the number of heartbeats per minute

cardiac tamponade The accumulation of blood in the pericardial sac that produces pressure on the heart. Signs and symptoms include distended neck veins, hypotension, tachypnea, weak peripheral pulses, decreased heart sounds, and decreased left atrial pressure

cardiomyopathy Any disease of the heart that affects its normal function and anatomical structure

cardiopulmonary resuscitation (CPR) The act of manually providing chest compressions and ventilations to patients in cardiac arrest in an effort to provide oxygenated blood to the brain and vital organs, and reverse the processes that lead to death

cardioversion The use of the defibrillator pads to restore the normal sinus rhythm of the heart

carina The inferior tracheal cartilage that projects from the tracheal cartilage and bifurcates into the two primary bronchi

C-arm Type of portable fluoroscope that is named for its configuration

carpal bones The eight short bones of the wrist; proximally the bones articulate with the distal radius and the distal radioulnar joint to form the wrist

carpal tunnel A canal in the wrist through which the flexor tendons and the median nerve pass

carrier One who harbors an infective agent, but does not show symptoms of disease and is capable of transmitting the disease to others

cartesian coordinate geometry Refers to the 16th-century philosopher Renes Descartes who invented coordinate geometry; also called *rectangular coordinate geometry*

cartilage A nonvascular fibrous connective tissue that is located in the joints, larynx, trachea, thorax, nose, and ear

cataract A pathological condition in which the crystalline lens has become opaque due to age or trauma

catheter A hollow, cylindrical tube that allows for the removal of fluids or air from the body, injection of fluids, removal of obstruction from ducts, or intravascular monitoring; may be plain tipped or may contain a retention balloon

catheterization The use or act of placing a catheter

caudad Toward the tail; inferior

caudal Toward the distal end of a structure or the body

cavitation Mechanical process used by ultrasonic cleaners during which air pockets implode to dislodge debris and soil from the crevices and serrations of surgical instruments and equipment

cell Functional unit of a living organism consisting of a nucleus, cytoplasm, and plasma membrane

central nervous system (CNS) The system composed of the brain and spinal cord, responsible for processing information to and from the peripheral nervous system. It is the main component that coordinates and controls the activities of the body

central processing unit (CPU) Silicon chip located within the computer case that is responsible for coordinating the operations of the computer, manages the computer systems, and facilitates the exchange of data with the computer memory

central sterile department The department responsible for the primary decontamination of instruments, supplies, and equipment; assembly and sterilization of instrument sets; and storage and distribution of supplies and equipment

central venous pressure The venous blood pressure within the right atrium, indicating the efficiency of the blood leaving the heart; therefore, indicating the patient's fluid status

cephalad Toward the head; superior

cephalopelvic disproportion (CPD) An obstetric complication in which the pelvis/birth canal is too small for a vaginal delivery, or the baby's head is too large to pass through the birth canal

cerebellum The portion of the brain located in the posterior cranial fossa posterior to the brainstem and consisting of two lobes; functions in coordinating voluntary muscular activity

cerebrospinal fluid (CSF) The fluid that flows through the ventricles of the brain, subarachnoid space, and spinal canal; serves to protect these structures

cerebrum The largest section of the brain, divided by a fissure into the right and left cerebral hemispheres; at the bottom of the fissure the hemispheres are connected by the corpus callosum, and the surface of the hemispheres is convoluted and lobed; functions include motor functions, sensory functions, and functions associated with the many mental activities of the individual

cerumen Earwax

ceruminous gland Third type of sweat gland found only in the external auditory canal that produces cerumen

cesarean section (C-section) A surgical procedure in which the abdomen and uterus are incised to deliver a baby

chalazion A small, red, and inflamed lump that can be located on the inner or outer surface of the eyelid; caused by an inflammatory reaction to material trapped inside the meibomian gland in the eyelid

cheilo- Combining form that means lip

cheiloplasty Surgical procedure performed to repair a cleft lip

cheiloschisis Cleft lip

chelation A method of cleaning instruments in which the chosen cleaning solution uses the process of binding ions, such as iron and magnesium, in the solution to prevent their deposit on the surface of surgical instruments

chemical indicator Internal or external monitor that changes color when exposed to the sterilization process; only indicates that the sterilization process has occurred, it does not guarantee the sterility of the item

chemotherapy Treatment with multiple drugs, often referring to cancer treatment

cholangiography A preoperative and intraoperative diagnostic tool in which a catheter is inserted into the common bile duct and contrast medium is injected to outline potential calculi under fluoroscopy

chole- Combining form that means bile

cholesteatoma A mass composed of cholesterol and epithelial cells that is either congenital or occurs as a complication of chronic otitis media; located in the middle ear

chordae tendineae Fibrous cords that originate from papillary muscles that project outward from the walls of the muscle and are attached to the cusps on the ventricular side; the chordae tendineae prevent the cusps of the atrioventricular valve from folding back into the atrium, causing incomplete closure of the valve and allowing blood back into the atrium

choroid A thin, dark-brown highly vascular membrane that makes up the posterior five-sixths of the eye

chromic A suture material manufactured from the submucosa of sheep intestine or serosa of beef intestine treated with chromium salts to delay the rate of absorption

chromic gut *See* chromic

chronic Condition that persists for an extended period of time

chronic pulmonary disorder (CPD) Persistent diseases of the lung, such as asthma or bronchopulmonary dysplasia, that interfere with normal breathing

chronic wound Wound that persists for an extended period to time

chyle A white liquid that consists of products of digestion, chiefly emulsified fats, that passes through the small intestine and into the lymphatic system

chyme The thick, semifluid contents of the stomach formed during digestion

cicatrix Scar

ciliary body Similar in structure to the choroids, but contains larger vessels; it is the thickened portion of the vascular tunic of the eye that joins the iris with the anterior portion of the choroids

ciliary muscle Smooth muscle fibers attached to the choroid of the eye that bring the ciliary process inward, causing the lens to become more convex and adjusting the eye to view objects that are close-up

circle of Willis A complex vascular network located at the base of the brain and formed by the following interconnected arteries: internal carotid, anterior cerebral, posterior cerebral, basilar, anterior communicating, and posterior communicating

circuit The path which electricity travels between an energy source and its usage device(s)

circulator Nonsterile surgical team member who moves about the periphery of the sterile field

circumcision Surgical removal of the foreskin

circumferentially Circular, or movement completely around an item, such as the circumferential prep of an extremity

claudication Severe pains in the muscle of the lower leg caused by poor circulation of blood to the muscle; usually caused by atherosclerosis

clean-catch sample A urine sample in which a midstream sample is obtained for urinalysis

cleft Cleave, crack, or fissure

clinical ladder program An established method of allowing a surgical technologist to ascend to positions of increased responsibility within an organization by demonstrating necessary skills and competencies

closed gloving Method of self-donning sterile surgical gloves when wearing a sterile surgical gown

CNS *See* central nervous system

coagulant Agent, physical or chemical, that acts to promote or accelerate blood clotting

coagulation Refers to blood clotting

coarctation of the aorta Localized narrowing of the aorta. In adults the narrowing is usually distal to the left subclavian artery or just distal to the ligamentum arteriosum. In infants the obstruction is proximal to the ductus arteriosus

code of ethics Guidelines, usually formed in a series of statements, that provide ethical standards of conduct for a profession

cognition Mental process involving awareness, perception, reasoning, and judgment; critical thinking

cold potassium cardioplegia solution A solution administered into the coronary arteries via the aortic root that inhibits myocardial contraction and is infused at frequent intervals during the surgical procedure

Colles' fracture Angled fracture of the distal radius

colonization The growth and collection of microbes into a group that lives in a particular area, such as the colonization of *S. aureus* in the nares of humans

colporrhaphy Surgical procedure to relieve stress incontinence in the female by elevating the base of the bladder through elimination of redundant and weakened vaginal tissue

comitant A form of strabismus in which the amount of misalignment stays the same, no matter which direction the eyes are pointed

comminuted fracture A type of bone fracture consisting of three or more fragments

community-acquired infection Infection acquired outside of a hospital in the general population

competency (1) Skill; (2) Ability; (3) Statements that establish the level of skill or quality needed to be able to perform the job duties of a profession

competent Qualified and capable to perform; competency may be measured by a test or level of skill

compound fracture A fracture in which a bone fragment punctures the skin and exposes the bone; also referred to as an *open fracture*

compress To apply pressure

conduit Channel or pipe for conveying fluids

condyle Rounded projection/process at the epiphysis of a bone that articulates with another bone, and serves as the point of attachment for ligaments

congenital Present at birth

congenital nephroblastoma (Wilms' tumor) A malignant tumor that primarily affects children; it is a mixed cell tumor that originates in the kidney and eventually replaces most of the involved kidney, causing hemorrhage and eventual necrosis

conjunctiva The mucous membrane that covers the eye

conscious sedation A type of anesthesia in which the patient's level of consciousness is pharmacologically depressed while the patient retains the ability to breath independently and respond to verbal or physical stimulation

consent Term that refers to permission being given for an action

contaminated Soiled with gross debris or by the presence of microbes

contracture Abnormal shortening of a muscle or tendon resulting in a deformity that is resistant to stretching

contraindication A reason why a specific procedure or drug may be undesirable or improper in a particular situation

contralateral The opposite side

contrast media Solutions injected into arteries, veins, or ducts during a radiographic exam that are radiopaque and therefore stand out in contrast to the surrounding tissues

controlled substance Drugs with a high potential to cause psychological and/or physical dependence or abuse

cor pulmonale An alteration in the structure and function of the right ventricle caused by a primary disorder of the respiratory system

core curriculum The recommended appropriate curriculum template for an educational program that provides the expected base of knowledge for entry level into the chosen profession

cornea Transparent part of the external tunic of the eye that forms the anterior one sixth of the globe

corona Crown-like projection or circular structure

coronal flap An incisional technique that begins with the development of a skin flap; the incision extends from one temporal region to another, and horizontally across the frontal bone

coronary artery bypass graft (CABG) Open heart surgery to replace one or more blocked coronary arteries to restore the oxygenated blood supply to the heart muscle

coronary sinus A small vein that empties into the right atrium, draining blood from the wall of the heart

corpus luteum A small mass of yellow-colored tissue that develops on the ovary and that grows within the ruptured ovarian follicle after ovulation; responsible for secreting progesterone to maintain the high level of vascular supply to the uterine endometrium for the purposes of implantation and pregnancy

corpus spongiosum One of two lengths of spongy tissue that forms the penis

cortex Outermost part of a structure

cortical bone Type of bone tissue that is hard and dense, and that surrounds the marrow cavity; also referred to as *compact bone*

cortical nephrons The nephrons located in the cortex of the kidney that do not extend into the medulla

cottonoid Another name for neurosurgical sponge used to protect delicate neural tissue and to assist with hemostasis

count Term used to describe the act of counting items used intraoperatively that could potentially be left in a surgical wound

CPD *See* chronic pulmonary disorder

CPR *See* cardiopulmonary resuscitation

craniosynostosis Premature closure of the cranial sutures of an infant

craniotomy Incision into the cranium

credentialing Process by which an agency or organization establishes a minimum knowledge base for a given health care profession and awards a credential to individuals that meet the minimum knowledge level

cross-contamination Contamination of a person or object by another

cryo- Prefix or combining form meaning cold

cryptorchidism The failure of one or both testicles to descend into the final anatomical position in the scrotum after the first year of life

crystalline lens A transparent, biconvex body, held in place by suspensory ligaments, that directs light into the eye; situated behind the pupil and in front of the vitreous body

CSF *See* cerebrospinal fluid

culture (1) Cultivation of microorganisms in a nutrient medium for the purpose of identifying a type of microbe; (2) Beliefs, customs, and values particular to a group or society

curettage Removal of tissue with a blunt or sharp curette by scraping the surface; performed to remove abnormal tissue, to obtain tissue for examination and diagnostic purposes, or to remove tissue from infected areas

current Flow of air, fluid, or electricity

Cushing's syndrome A rare condition that results from a pituitary tumor that causes an overproduction of cortisol by the cortex of the adrenal gland

cutaneous membrane Medical term for the skin

cyanosis Bluish discoloration of the mucous membranes and skin due to hypoxemia

cycloplegics A group of paralytic agents used to dilate the pupil by paralyzing the sphincter muscle of the iris and the accommodation mechanism

cylindrical Object with a tubular shape

cystectomy Surgical removal of the bladder

cysto- Prefix or combining form meaning bladder

cystoscopy The insertion of an endoscope through the urethra and into the bladder for the purpose of viewing for treatment and diagnosis

cytotoxin Substance poisonous to a cell

dacryo- Prefix meaning the lacrimal apparatus of the eye

dacryocystitis Inflammation of the lacrimal sac most often due to an obstruction of the nasolacrimal duct

dacryocystorhinostomy Surgical procedure that establishes a new pathway between the lacrimal sac and nose to assist in the drainage of tears and secretions into the middle meatus of the nose

dead space A space remaining in the tissues as a result of failure of proper closure of a surgical wound

debridement Removal of devitalized tissue and contaminants

decompress To remove pressure

decontamination Elimination of contamination (such as gross organic debris or blood and body fluids) from a person or object

decontamination room Room that typically contains sinks for gross decontamination, an ultrasonic washer, and a washer-sterilizer to decontaminate instruments and equipment

defamation Injury to an individual's reputation or character caused by false statements to a third party; libel and/or slander

defendant Individual whom legal action is brought against

defibrillator Electronic device used to deliver an electric shock to the heart to treat atrial or ventricular fibrillation

deflect Deviate from or move away from a given course

degrees of freedom The number of ways in which a robotic manipulator moves

dehiscence Partial or total separation of a layer or layers of tissue after closure of the wound

delivery forceps Surgical instrument used to grasp the head of a baby to aid in a vaginal delivery

dentition The development of teeth, including their arrangement, type, and number

deontological approach An ethical approach that concerns itself with the ideas of obligation and duty, including the duty to the patient as an individual and the outcome of the care provided

deposition Method of pretrial discovery in which questions are answered under oath

depressed fracture A type of fracture in which bone is driven into bone

De Quervain's stenosing tenosynovitis Painful condition caused by inflammation of the tendons in the first dorsal compartment of the wrist

derma-carrier A flat piece of plastic on which a harvested skin graft is placed and consequently inserted through a mesh graft device; the purpose of the carrier is to keep the graft flat and to allow it to smoothly pass through the mesh device; one side of the carrier is smooth, and the other has ridges that determine the size of openings to be placed in the harvested skin

dermachalasis Relaxation and hypertrophy of the eyelid skin linked to sun exposure and age

dermatome Powered or manually operated surgical instrument used to cut thin slices of skin for grafting purposes

dermis The deeper layer of the skin located beneath the epidermis that contains the blood vessels, nerves, hair follicles, sebaceous glands, and sudoriferous glands; also referred to as the *stratum corium*

desiccation Dehydration of a substance

detritus Loose fragments formed by disintegration

DeVega annuloplasty Surgical procedure performed to resolve a tricuspid valve that has become leaky, resulting in tricuspid regurgitation. The repair involves the placement of a pursestring suture around the circumference of the annulus to reduce the backflow of blood from the right ventricle into the right atrium

devitalized Deprived of life; necrotic

diabetes mellitus A disorder of the endocrine system that affects the production of insulin in the pancreas; either Type I (in which the pancreas produces little or no insulin) or Type II (in which the pancreas produces different amounts of insulin)

diabetic nephropathy A disease that causes sclerosis to the glomerular apparatus of the kidney, accompanied by an excess of hyaline; the disease is caused by uncontrolled diabetes mellitus that eventually leads to the damage of many body systems; also called *Kimmelstiel-Wilson disease* and *diabetic glomerulosclerosis*

dialysate The solution in a dialysis machine that is responsible for collecting the excess fluid and waste products for discarding

diameter Thickness or width

diaphoresis Profuse perspiration

diaphragm A dome-shaped muscular structure that extends transversely across the upper half of the body, dividing the thoracic cavity from the abdominal cavity; it plays an important role during respiration by moving up and down to aid in forcing air in and out of the lungs

diarthrosis Freely movable joint

diastole Pertains to the resting phase of the cardiac cycle

diathermy The use of high frequency electromagnetic currents to cauterize blood vessels and destroy neoplasms

disease Deviation or interruption of normal structure or function of any body part, organ, or system

disinfectant Substance, physical or chemical, used to kill vegetative forms of microorganisms or vectors; usually cannot destroy spores; generally applied to fomites

disinfection Destruction of microorganisms or vectors by direct exposure to a chemical or physical agent

disinfection, high-level Agent capable of killing all microorganisms including some spores

disinfection, intermediate-level Agent capable of killing most microorganisms but not spores

disinfection, low-level Agent capable of killing some microorganisms

dispersive (inactive) electrode A device that safely conveys any leaking electrons to a neutral location or scatters them over an area to prevent electrical shock or burn; also called a *grounding pad*

displaced fracture Fracture in which bone fragments are out of alignment

dissect To separate, as in the separation of tissue layers

dissecting aneurysm A dilation of an artery, characterized by a longitudinal dissection between the adventitia and tunica media layers of the artery wall

dissection, blunt To separate tissue without the use of a sharp instrument, i.e., fingers or sponge placed on a sponge stick

dissection, sharp Separate tissue with the use of a sharp instrument, i.e., knife blade or scissors

distal Farther from the point of reference or origin of a structure

distal convoluted tubule A portion of the renal tubule located between Henle's loop and the collecting duct

divide Separate

DO *See* Doctor of Osteopathy

docho- Combining form meaning intestine

Doctor of Osteopathy (DO) A physician who treats patients in a holistic manner and emphasizes the use of manipulative techniques for correcting abnormalities thought to cause disease and inhibit recovery

donning To put on or dress in

donor site Site from which a skin or bone graft is taken

Doppler Ultrasonic device used to identify and assess vascular status of peripheral arteries and veins by magnifying the sound of the blood moving through the vessel

dormant Resting or inactive stage

dorsal Toward the back

dorsal carpal ligament The ligament that covers the six dorsal compartments of the hand that is a thick fibrous band of tissue attached to the lower end of the radius and to the styloid process of the ulna

double-lumen endotracheal tube An endotracheal tube that utilizes two tubes, one for the tracheal lumen and another for the bronchial lumen, so that the affected lung can be collapsed during the surgical procedure without interfering with the unaffected lung's ventilation

drain Hollow, cylindrical device that is used to evacuate air and/or fluids from a surgical wound; may be passive or active

droplet Small mass of liquid

drug Agent used as a medicine for the diagnosis, treatment, cure, mitigation, or prophylaxis of a disease or condition

drug interaction Occurs when two or more agents are prescribed and administered concurrently, causing a modification of the action of one or both substances

DUB *See* dysfunctional uterine bleeding

ductus arteriosus A fetal blood vessel that joins the aorta and pulmonary artery

ductus deferens The duct that continues from the epididymis, traveling from the scrotum and joining the seminal vesicle to form the ejaculatory duct; serves to transport sperm and semen; also called the *vas deferens*

ductus venosus The vascular channel in the fetus that travels through the liver and joins the umbilical vein. It is responsible for transporting oxygenated blood to the placenta as part of the fetal circulation. Just after birth, as pulmonary circulation is established, it closes

Dupuytren's disease A contraction of the palmar fascia that causes restricted movement and impaired function of the hand

dye Agent used to stain tissue

dynamic equilibrium The ability of the individual to adjust to displacements of the center of gravity of the body

dysfunctional uterine bleeding (DUB) Abnormal uterine bleeding that is not due to a tumor, pregnancy, or infection, and occurs when menstruation is not taking place

dyspnea Difficult or labored breathing

dysraphism Incomplete closure or faulty fusion

dysrhythmia Abnormal cardiac rhythm

dystocia Difficult labor due to various reasons, such as cephalopelvic distortion, fetus size, or condition or position of fetus

ECG *See* electrocardiograph

-ectomy Suffix meaning removal of

edema Abnormal fluid accumulation in the intercellular/interstitial space

EEG *See* electroencephalography

efferent Carrying away from a given point

ejaculatory ducts Thin-walled ducts that are formed by the unification of the vas deferens and seminal vesicles; the ducts are contained within the prostate gland and open into the prostatic urethra

elective surgery Pertaining to a surgical intervention that does not require immediate intervention; the patient "elects" to have the surgery at a specific time

electrical charge Electrical charge is too many or too few electrons or an atom creating a positive or negative charge and an electrical current is the movement of the electrical charge

electrical current A flow of electrical charge along a conductor consisting of electrons flowing along a path with an opening for escape

electrocardiogram (ECG) A record of the electrical activity of the heart

electrocardiograph (ECG or EKG) A device used for recording the electrical activity of the heart to detect transmissions of the electrical cardiac impulse through the tissues of the myocardium

electroencephalogram (EEG) A record of the electrical activity of the brain

electroencephalography (EEG) Display and recording of the electrical activity of the brain by measurement of changes in electric potentials

electrons The negatively charged particles circling the nucleus of an atom

electrosurgical unit (ESU) Mechanical device which produces an electric current that is converted into thermal energy (heat) for the purpose of cutting or coagulating tissue

elixir Sweetened alcohol solution

elliptical Curved or crescent shaped

embolus A piece of tissue, thrombus, air, or gas that circulates in the circulatory system until it becomes lodged in a vessel

embryo Developing fetus *in utero;* generally refers to a pregnancy from the second through the eighth week of development

emergent Surgical pathology that is life threatening

empyema An abnormal condition of blood or pus from a chest injury that is not properly drained from the pleural cavity; the fluids coagulate and form a fibrin layer over the visceral and parietal pleura that interferes with the proper expansion of the lung

emulsification A method of cleaning instruments in which the chosen cleaning solution acts by dispersing two liquids that are not capable of being mixed to remove organic and inorganic soil

emulsion Combination of two liquids that cannot mix; the droplets of one liquid are suspended throughout the other liquid

en bloc Removal as a whole

endocardial leads One of two types of electrodes available for permanent pacemaker implantation that are placed through the subclavian vein into the right ventricle or atrium

endocardial tubes Two separate tubes that originate from mesodermal cells that develop during the third week of gestation. One end of each tube represents the eventual arterial component of the heart, and the other end represents the venous component. The two tubes will eventually fuse to form one tube called the *primitive heart tube*

endocardium The inner lining of the heart wall that lines all of the heart's chambers and valves; composed of endothelial tissue

endocrine glands Several types of ductless glands that are responsible for producing and secreting hormones into the circulatory and lymph systems

endogenous Originating within or caused by factors from within

endoscope A general term used to describe the various types of flexible or rigid scopes used to view the internal structures of the body

endotracheal Within the trachea

end-stage renal disease (ESRD) A term that refers to the final stages of many types of kidney diseases; renal failure is defined as kidneys functioning at less than 10% of their normal capacity

enterocolitis Inflammation of the small intestine and colon

enucleation En bloc removal of a structure; usually refers to the removal of the eye

epicardium The outer tissue layer of the heart that provides protection

epidemiology The study of disease and its control

epidermis The outer layer of the skin that consists entirely of epithelial cells, has five layers, and contains no blood vessels or nerves

epididymis A pair of long ducts that carries sperm and semen from the seminiferous tubules of the testes to the vas deferens

epidural Above or outside the dura mater

epiglottis The small cartilaginous structure that acts like a lid and closes the passageway to the larynx to prevent food from entering the larynx and trachea during the act of swallowing

epiphysis The proximal portion of a long bone

episiotomy The surgical incision of perineum to enlarge the vaginal opening and prevent tearing of the perineum and muscles during delivery

epispadias The congenital abnormality in which the anterior wall of the urethra is absent and the urethral meatus is located on the dorsum of the penis

epistaxis Nosebleed

ergonomics The study of how to fit a job or duty to a person's anatomical, physiological, and psychological characteristics to enhance efficiency and safety

erythrocyte Red blood cell

Esmarch bandage Elastic wrap applied to an extremity to act as a tourniquet or to exsanguinate prior to application of a tourniquet

ESRD *See* end-stage renal disease

ESU *See* electrosurgical unit

ESWL *See* extracorporeal shockwave lithotripsy

ethics Branch of philosophy dealing with good conduct and moral values

ethylene oxide (EtO) Liquid chemical converted to a gas for sterilization purposes

event-related sterility Sterility determined by how a sterile package is handled rather than time elapsed; the package is considered sterile until opened, or until the integrity of the packaging material is compromised

evisceration Interruption of a closed wound or traumatic injury that exposes the viscera

excision Surgical removal

exenteration Refers to total removal of; usually used in reference to the surgical procedure of total pelvic exenteration, which involves the removal of the vagina, uterus and cervix, fallopian tubes, ovaries, bladder, and rectum for surgical treatment of cancer

exogenous Originating outside or caused by factors from outside

exposure To lay open or subject to

exsanguinate Extensive loss or removal of blood

extracapsular cataract extraction A method for surgically removing a cataract through an incision in the side of the cornea and replacing the diseased lens with an intraocular implant

extracorporeal shock wave lithotripsy (ESWL) A noninvasive method that uses shock waves generated by an electrical discharge through water to pulverize calculi of the kidney

extravasation Escape of blood, lymph fluid, or serum from a vessel into the tissue or body cavity

extrinsic muscles The six muscles of the eye that come from the bones of the orbit and function to move the eye in various directions

extruded Forced out of position

fasciculation Involuntary twitching or contraction of muscle fibers that may be strong enough to be visible; often follows administration of a depolarizing neuromuscular blocking agent

fenestration Opening

fetus Developing young *in utero;* generally refers to a pregnancy from approximately the eighth week of development until birth

fiberoptics Conveyance of light or an image through fine, flexible, transparent tubes using internal reflection

fibrillation Series of twitches or rapid ineffective muscle contractions

fimbria Finger-like structures that form on the edge such as the fimbria of the fallopian tubes

first-degree burn A classification of a burn that affects just the epidermis; characterized by erythema with no blisters

first intention Type of healing that occurs with primary union that is typical of an incision opened under ideal conditions; healing occurs from side to side in which dead space has been eliminated and the wound edges are accurately approximated

fiscal Pertaining to the finances of an individual or organization

fistula Abnormal communication between two normally separate internal structures, or an abnormal communication between an internal structure and the body surface

fixation To prevent or stabilize

flash sterilization A process of quickly sterilizing unwrapped items (such as a surgical instrument that has been dropped on the floor and is needed right away) using prevacuum or gravity steam sterilizers

flexion Bending of a joint

focal point Convergence of interest or energy

Fogarty catheter A type of catheter that is small in diameter and is balloon-tipped; used to facilitate the removal of an embolus

fomite Inanimate object on which microorganisms may be harbored and conveyed

font A style of lettering, such as Times New Roman or Arial

footboard Attachment to the operating table that may be inserted horizontally (to add length to the table) or vertically (to prevent foot drop or slippage from the table)

foramen ovale An opening between the two atrial chambers of the fetus that remains until birth and closes on birth, leaving a depression in the interatrial septum called the *fossa ovalis*. The foramen ovale is a passageway for blood from the right atrium into the left atrium, diverting blood from the fetal lungs

foreign body Any type of substance or object located or lodged in the tissue or organ that does not belong under normal circumstances

formalin A liquid preservative for tissue specimens

formalism A general ethical approach to right or wrong in which an act is not judged by its consequences, but rather is itself in accord with what is right or wrong

fossa ovalis A slight depression in the interatrial septum formed when the foramen ovale closes at birth

fourth-degree burn A classification for burns that damage blood vessels, nerves, muscles, tendons, and bone

Fowler's position Modification of the supine position; the patient is sitting

fracture Breaking of a part, commonly refers to bone

fray To break apart or start to fragment

free electrons The outermost electrons in the atom's orbit that can most easily be attracted away from the nucleus

free flap reconstruction A type of reconstruction mammoplasty; involves the complete removal of the tissue to be transferred from its original location for transplantation on the chest

free-tie Length of suture for ligation that is not threaded onto or attached to a needle

French-eyed needle A type of needle in which the suture must be threaded by pulling the strand into a V-shaped area just above the eye

friable Easily torn or crumbled

frontal Directional term that indicates a plane perpendicular to the midline that divides the body into anterior and ventral segments

frozen section A pathological method of diagnosis that involves freezing a tissue sample, slicing it into thin sections, staining it, and then viewing it under a microscope

full-thickness skin graft (FTSG) A graft composed of the epidermis and all of the dermis (may also include some of the subcutaneous tissue)

ganglion cyst A benign lesion filled with synovial fluid that can arise from any tendon sheath or joint in the hand or wrist; may be a result of trauma or tissue degeneration

gangrene Tissue death often accompanied by bacterial infection

Gelfoam Type of absorbable gelatin hemostatic agent that is made from purified pork skin gelatin; available in either pad or powder form, it is placed over an area of bleeding to control hemorrhage

general anesthesia Anesthesia during a surgical procedure in which the patient is unconscious and the muscles completely relaxed; assisted breathing is necessary

generator Devices that convert mechanical energy to electric energy

generic Nonproprietary name for a drug that is often a shortened version of the chemical name and may include a reference to the intended use

Gerota's fascia A fibrous capsule that encircles the kidney to aid in keeping the kidney in the correct anatomical position and to cushion it from injury

gestation Length of time that begins when conception occurs and continues up to birth (pregnancy)

Gibson incision A surgical incision that begins medial to the anterosuperior iliac spine and curves downward and medially, to slightly above the symphysis pubis; specifically designed for access to the lower portion of the ureter

glans penis The tip of the penis and the opening to the urethra; located at the tip of the glans penis. The widest part of the glans penis (called the corona glandis) is located around the base of the proximal portion

glenoid fossa The socket in which the head of the humerus articulates to form the shoulder joint; a ball-and-socket joint

glioma Group of malignant tumors composed of glial cells

globe The eyeball in its entirety

glomerulus A portion of the renal corpuscles that consists of a network of capillaries

glottis The small opening between the true vocal cords

glutaraldehyde Liquid disinfectant and sterilizing agent

gnath- Combining form meaning jaw

goblet cells A specialized epithelial cell that secretes mucus and forms the epithelial layer of the stomach, GI, and respiratory tracts

golden hour Concept of medical treatment for a trauma victim that provides treatment within the first hour following injury to improve patient outcomes

-gram Suffix meaning written record

Gram stain Laboratory method of identifying bacteria; bacteria that stain purple are referred to as *gram-positive,* and bacteria that do not retain the stain and appear red in color are referred to as *gram-negative*

granulation tissue Tissue that is grainy in appearance and fills a wound that is left to heal by second intention

granuloma Neoplasm that appears to consist of many small particles (grains)

-graph Suffix meaning producing a drawing or writing

gravida Refers to the pregnant female; the first pregnancy is referred to as gravida I; additional pregnancies are numbered sequentially

greenstick fracture Fracture that occurs in only one cortex of the bone; an incomplete fracture that commonly occurs in children

grounding Method to prevent the passage of an electrical current through a person or object by directing the current to the ground

grounding pad A pad that is placed on a patient to complete the pathway for the electrical current back to the electrosurgical unit; also called the *dispersive electrode*

ground wire A separate wire that safely conveys any leaking electrons to a neutral location to prevent electrical shock

gurney Stretcher for transporting a patient

gynecomastia Abnormal excess development of male breast tissue, often seen at the time of puberty

halon fire extinguisher A special type of fire extinguisher that uses the chemical halon; used for laser fires due to its low toxicity

hamper Four-wheeled stand that can be lined with a biohazardous bag for the collection of linen or trash

handwash The mechanical and chemical washing of the hands to aid in removing transient microorganisms, dirt, and debris

hard palate Anterior portion of the palate that consists of the palatine processes of each maxilla and the palatine bones

HCG *See* human chorionic gonadotropin

headboard Attachment to the operating table for placement of the patient's head; may be angled or flexed

headlamp Device worn by the surgeon to precisely illuminate the surgical site

health maintenance organization (HMO) Health care organization that serves as both the insurer and provider of medical services; typically, a group of physicians provides services to a population of clients who voluntarily enroll in the program

hematoma Localized collection of extravasated blood that is often clotted

hemodialysis The removal of excess fluids and waste products from the body with the use of the dialysis machine

hemodynamics Study of the movement of blood and the forces responsible for circulation

hemolysis The destruction of erythrocytes

hemorrhage Discharge of blood; often used in reference to excessive bleeding

hemostasis The arrest of the escape of blood through natural or artifical means

hemostat A device or agent used as a coagulant

HEPA filter *See* high efficiency particulate air (HEPA) filter

herniation Abnormal protrusion of an organ or other body structure through an opening in a covering membrane or muscle

heterograft *See* xenograft

heterologous From a dissimilar species

high efficiency particulate air (HEPA) filter Filter that is capable of removing bacteria as small as 0.5-5 μm; utilized in the operating room to aid in preventing the patient from acquiring a postoperative wound infection

hilum The medial border of the kidney that is convex and receives the renal blood vessels

hirsutism Abnormal hairiness, especially in women

HIV *See* human immunodeficiency virus

HMO *See* health maintenance organization

homeostasis The reactions in the body that act and counteract to maintain the body in a normal physiological state

homograft A graft obtained from the same species, such as from another person or cadaver

homologous From the same species

hopper Device that looks somewhat like the standard toilet, except larger; used for the disposal of certain fluids, especially body fluids

host (1) Organism that harbors and/or nourishes another organism; (2) Recipient of a transplant

human chorionic gonadotropin (HCG) A component of the urine of pregnant females;

stimulates the corpus luteum to secrete estrogen and progesterone

human development The various stages of human growth, both psychological and physical

human immunodeficiency virus (HIV) The virus that causes acquired immune deficiency syndrome (AIDS)

hyaline cartilage An elastic connective tissue that covers the ends of bones, supports the trachea and larynx, and connects the ribs to the sternum. It is covered by the perichondrium and calcifies as the individual ages

hydraulic pressure The pressure of liquid at any given depth

hydrops Abnormal accumulation of clear watery fluid in the tissue or a body cavity such as the middle ear; formerly called *dropsy*

hypercapnia Excessive carbon dioxide

hyperosmotic drugs Drugs that increase the concentration of osmotically active components

hypertension Chronic high blood pressure

hyperthermia Abnormally high body temperature

hypertrophy Enlargement or overgrowth of a structure due to an increase in the size of its cells

hypnosis Altered state of consciousness that may be achieved by suggestion of another, an individual's own concentration, or with the use of a substance

hypnotic Agent that alters the state of consciousness

hypospadias A congenital abnormality characterized by the urethral opening located on the underside of the penis or on the perineum of the male, or in the vagina of the female

hypotension Abnormally low blood pressure

hypothermia Abnormally low body temperature typically defined as a core body temperature that is below 35°C

hypovolemia Abnormally decreased volume of circulating blood in the body

hypovolemic shock A state of shock produced when hypovolemia exists, either internally or externally; the body compensates by attempting to divert blood to the vital organs

hypoxemia Below normal level of oxygen in the arterial blood

hypoxia Below normal level of oxygen in the tissues

IABP *See* intra-aortic balloon pump

iatrogenic Adverse patient condition or injury resulting from the action of a health care provider

ICP *See* intracranial pressure

idiosyncratic Peculiar reaction to an action, idea, or substance, i.e., drug or food

ileal conduit Surgical procedure performed when the entire bladder is removed and the ureters are implanted onto the ileum

illness Sickness

immersion Placing an item in a container so it is completely covered by a liquid, such as immersing a surgical instrument in glutaraldehyde

immunocompetence Degree of function of an immune system that is designed to keep a patient from infection by pathogens

immunosuppressed patient Patient whose immune system has decreased due to disease, or intentionally decreased with immunosuppressive drugs for organ transplant patients to prevent organ rejection

impacted fracture The broken end of a bone that is forced into the bone on the other side of a fracture

in situ At the site of origin, or in its normal place

inanimate Nonliving

incident report Mechanism for reporting an incident, usually by completing a document describing what happened, related to any adverse patient occurrence

incision Cut made with a sharp instrument

incomitant A form of strabismus in which the amount of misalignment changes as the eyes move to view objects in different directions; the two types of incomitant strabismus are restrictive and paralytic

incontinence Inability to control excretory functions

indication A reason to perform a specific procedure or prescribe a certain drug

indicator Tape, paper, vial, or other item used to confirm that a specific reaction has taken place (such as the chemical indicators for steam sterilization)

induction The second phase of general anesthesia in which the patient is given induction drugs and intubated

induction charging One of two processes by which static charge buildup can occur when an item or person is near an electrostatic field

indwelling A substance or item that remains in place either permanently or for a period of time

inert Substance or agent that causes little or no tissue reaction

inertia A property of matter that causes it to resist a change in motion

infarction An area of dead tissue caused by an inadequate supply of oxygenated blood

infection Invasion by pathogenic organism

inferior Below a point of reference or the origin of a structure

inferior pedicle breast reduction A method of reduction mammoplasty in which the primary incision line resembles a keyhole, and the finished wound resembles the shape of an anchor

infiltrate Accumulation or diffusion of a foreign substance into tissue

inflammation The body's protective response to injury or tissue destruction

inflammatory response The response of the body to infection or injury that includes signs of inflammation: pain, heat, redness, and swelling; serves to destroy, dilute, or wall off the injured tissue

informed consent A situation in which a patient gives voluntary permission to another party (surgeon and anesthesia provider) to perform the procedures that have been explained; includes the risks, benefits, possible complications, and alternative treatment options

infrared waves Waves in the electromagnetic spectrum that are longer than visible light, but shorter than microwaves

innominate An unnamed structure; for example, the innominate artery that branches from the arch of the aorta and divides into the right common carotid and right subclavian artery

instrument room A separate room for storage of nonsterile equipment and instrumentation; instrument sets may be assembled after decontamination in this type of room

insufflation To force powder, gas, or vapor into a body cavity

insulator Material that inhibits the flow of free electrons; typically prevents electron leakage and directs the flow to a destination

integration Processing information and bringing together several components or functions to facilitate harmony

integrity Complete, no breaks or tears

integumentary Pertaining to or composed of skin

intercellular Between cells

intermediate-level disinfection Level of disinfection in which most microorganisms are killed except spores

interphalangeal joint (IPJ) A synovial hinge-type of joint formed between the phalanges

interrupted suture A type of suture placement in which each suture strand is separately placed, tied, and cut

interstitial Between structures of an organ or tissue

intima Inner layer of the arterial vessel wall

intra-aortic balloon pump (IABP) Mechanical device designed for circulatory support after cardiac procedures. Insertion of the device may increase cardiac output to a level that would permit separation from the pump oxygenator and allow time for the heart to recover

intra-arterial measurement A method of ECG monitoring in which the intra-arterial catheter is inserted directly into the artery

intra-articular Within a joint

intracapsular cataract extraction A method for surgically removing a cataract by injecting alpha chymotripsin into the posterior chamber to digest the suspensory ligament so that the diseased lens can be removed in its entirety

intracellular Within a cell

intracoronary thrombolysis Surgical procedure that involves injecting streptokinase to break down thrombi within a vessel

intracranial pressure (ICP) Pressure produced within the cranium; when elevated, represents a space-occupying lesion or brain edema

intramuscular Within the muscle

intraocular lens (IOL) Lens implant that replaces the excised crystalline lens during a cataract procedure

intraoperative Occurs during the surgical intervention

intrathecal Within the subdural space

intravenous (IV) Within a vein

intravenous urogram (IVU) Diagnostic study that involves the injection of a contrast medium into a vein; the radiopaque material is filtered through the kidney and excreted, providing an outline of the entire urologic system; formerly called *intravenous pyelogram* (IVP).

IOL *See* intraocular lens

ionizing radiation Process by which energy either directly or indirectly induces ionization of radiation-absorbing material or tissues; X-rays

IPJ *See* interphalangeal joint

ipsilateral On the same side

iridectomy Surgical removal of the iris

iridotomy Incision of the iris for the creation of a new aperture in the iris when the pupil is closed

iris The middle colored part of the eye that is thin, circular shaped, and contractile; it is suspended in the aqueous humor posterior to the cornea and anterior to the crystalline lens, and perforated in the center by the pupil

irrigation Washing with a stream of fluid

ischemia Lack of oxygenated blood supply to an area or organ of the body

isotope scanning Involves the intravenous injection of a radioactive isotope into the patient prior to an imaging study; also referred to as *nuclear medicine study* or *radionuclide imaging*

IV *See* intravenous (IV)

IV stand Portable pole with hooks on which intravenous fluid containers are hung

IVU *See* intravenous urogram

jackknife position Another name for the Kraske patient position

JCAHO *See* Joint Commission on Accreditation of Healthcare Organizations

job description Description of the tasks, functions, and responsibilities of a position within an organization

Joint Commission on Accreditation of Healthcare Organizations (JCAHO) An independent, nonprofit national organization that develops standards and performance criteria for health care organizations

Julian date Calendar days are sequentially numbered through the year; often used when maintaining sterilization records, i.e., February 1 would be the 32nd day of the Julian calendar

juxtamedullary nephrons Nephrons that extend deep into the medulla of the kidney

Kaposi's sarcoma A cancer that produces external and internal lesions that are painful; internally, the lesions can cause complications, such as difficulty in swallowing (if present in the esophagus) or bowel obstruction (when present in the intestine)

keloid Abnormal scar that results from increased collagen deposits; scar appears firm, raised, red, and thick

keratin A hard protein that is the chief component of the epidermis, nails, hair, and enamel of teeth

kerato- Combining form or prefix indicating a relation to horny substances or to the cornea

kick bucket Small portable stand on wheels that can be maneuvered into place with the foot for the purpose of placing used surgical sponges

kidney Bilateral bean-shaped organs that are responsible for eliminating wastes and forming urine

kidney lift Metal cross bar portion of the operating table that may be raised to elevate the kidney area when the patient is in the kidney position

kidney position Modification of the lateral position in which the operating table is flexed to better expose the flank area of the patient

kidney rests Attachments to the operating table that slide onto the kidney lift to aid in stabilizing the patient in the kidney position; the larger rest is placed anteriorly, and the smaller rest is placed posteriorly

kidneys, ureters, bladder (KUB) An anterior/posterior X-ray view of the urinary system that provides basic information about the size, shape, and position of the organs and certain types of calculi that may be visible

kinematics An attempt to understand the mechanism of injury and the action and effect of a particular type of force on the human body

knee-chest position A position in which the patient is resting on the knees on the operating table, and the knees are pulled upward toward the chest to elevate the lower back and buttock region

Kraske position A position in which the patient is placed in the prone position, and the operating table is flexed in the middle (lowering the head and feet and elevating the hip and buttock region); also known as the jackknife position

KUB *See* kidneys, ureters, bladder

labia (pl.); labium (sing.) Lips; a fleshy border

laceration Cut or tear

lacrimal A facial bone that, along with the zygomatic bone and palate, helps to form the orbit of the eye

lacrimal system Consists of the lacrimal gland and excretory ducts that convey fluid to the surface of the eye that is carried away by the ducts into the cavity of the nose

laminar air flow The unidirectional positive-pressure flow of air that captures microbes to be filtered

lap sponge A type of surgical sponge that is the largest and most absorbent of the sponges

laryngo- Combining form meaning larynx

laryngospasm Sudden involuntary contraction of the larynx capable of causing partial or total occlusion of the larynx

laser *L*ight *a*mplification by *s*timulated *e*mission of *r*adiation; a machine that emits a focused and amplified beam of light that can be used for a variety of surgical procedures

lateral Toward the side, away from the middle or midline

lateral position A position in which the patient is positioned on his or her side

latex Substance made from natural rubber harvested from trees found in warm tropical climates; used to produce many types of medical patient care products, including gloves

latissimus dorsi musculocutaneous flap A flap technique used for reconstruction mammoplasty in which the latissimus dorsi muscle is used to reconstruct the breast

lavage To wash out, particularly a hollow body cavity or organ, i.e., gastric lavage

LCC-ST *See* Liaison Council on Certification for the Surgical Technologist

LEEP *See* loop electrosurgical excision

leukocyte White blood cell

liability (1) An obligation to do or not do something; (2) An obligation potentially or actually incurred as a result of a negligent act

liable Legally responsible; obligated

Liaison Council on Certification for the Surgical Technologist (LCC-ST) National credentialing organization that offers national certification examinations for the surgical technologist and surgical assistant

libel A statement, verbal or written, that damages an individual's reputation or character

licensure Legal right granted by a government agency in compliance with a statute that authorizes and oversees the activities of the profession

ligament A band of fibrous tissue composed of collagen that connects bone to bone

ligamentum venosum The ligament of the liver that originated from the ductus venosus

ligate The placement of a suture tie around a vessel or other anatomical structure for the purpose of constriction, i.e., to control hemorrhage from a blood vessel

linen hamper Four-wheeled stand that can be lined with a biohazardous-marked bag for the collection of nondisposable linen during a surgical procedure

liposuction Surgical procedure in which fat deposits are vacuumed from specific areas of the body to contour those areas that have not responded to changes in diet and exercise

Lister Joseph Lister, an English surgeon in the 19th century and the "father of antiseptic surgery"; applied Pasteur's principles to surgical practice. His contributions led to the establishment of the principles of asepsis in the operating room

load The weight supported or force imposed

loop electrosurgical excision (LEEP) Surgical procedure that uses the electrosurgical unit coupled to a loop electrode on the cautery pencil; used to excise a cone of tissue to remove the area of neoplasia

loop of Henle A portion of the renal tubule that is U shaped and consists of descending and ascending portions; performs a significant role in urine concentration

lumen The opening in a tube or vessel

lung One of a pair of organs located bilaterally in the thoracic cavity that is composed of spongy, elastic tissue; the main organ of respiration

lysis Dissolution, loosening, or destruction of

magnification Process of enlarging the size of an object with the use of a device such as a micro scope

major calyces Two or three ducts that drain the superior, middle, and inferior portions of the kidney into a common renal pelvis

malar bone Cheek bone

malignant Extremely destructive or harmful; often used to refer to a condition that is invasive and metastatic

malignant hyperthermia A fulminant hypermetabolic crisis triggered by an anesthesia agent or combination of agents; characterized by a sudden increase in end-tidal carbon dioxide, an increase in body temperature, muscle rigidity, tachycardia, and uncontrolled hemorrhaging of the capillaries

malocclusion Abnormal alignment of the teeth of the upper jaw with those of the lower jaw

malpractice Professional misconduct that results in harm to another; negligence of a health care professional

mammoplasty Plastic reconstruction of the breast

marrow Semisolid tissue found in the spaces of cancellous bone; there are two types: red bone marrow and yellow bone marrow

marsupialization Incision of a closed cavity with the suturing of the opened edges to the wall of the wound to form an open wound that will heal by second intention

mask A cover worn over the mouth and nose by surgical personnel to prevent blood and body fluids from splashing into those areas; also protects the patient from the surgical personnel's secretions

Maslow's hierarchy of needs A model developed by Maslow that expresses human development and progression using developmental stages that prioritize needs

mass The property of a body that causes it to have weight in a gravitational field

Material Safety Data Sheets (MSDS) Technical information sheets provided by the manufacturer that give all the pertinent information about chemicals or other types of agents purchased by an institution; must be kept readily available in the department(s) in which the substance is being used

maxillofacial Pertaining to the face and maxilla

Mayo stand Small portable stand with a tray on top that is covered with a sterile drape and on which the instruments, equipment, and supplies that are most frequently used for the surgical procedure are placed; it is most often positioned over the legs of the patient

medial Toward the middle of a patient or object

median nerve A nerve that branches into two sections to innervate the skin of the lateral two-thirds of the hand, flexor muscles of the forearm, and several intrinsic muscles of the hand

mediastinoscopy An endoscopic procedure that involves the insertion of a mediastinoscope through the pretracheal fascia and into the superior mediastinum; performed for the evaluation of nodal involvement or mediastinal masses in patients with carcinoma of the lung

mediastinum The area in the thoracic cavity in the middle of the thorax between the lungs

medulla Innermost part of a structure

membranous urethra The duct that leads from the bladder to an external opening; serves to transfer urine and empty the bladder during micturation

memory Ability of an item, such as a surgical drape or a suture, to retain its configuration after removal from a package

meninges Three tissue membranes (called *dura mater, arachnoid, pia mater*) that enclose the brain and spinal cord

meniscus A type of tissue made of cartilage that is fibrous; located in joints, spinal column, and bony pelvis, it serves to cushion and protect bone

mentoplasty Plastic surgery of the chin

merocrine sweat glands One of two types of sweat glands that are distributed over most of the body; open directly onto the skin surface through the pores, and stimulated to produce sweat by heat or emotional stress

mesh graft device A manually operated device used to expand the size of a skin graft

metacarpals The bones of the palm of the hand; there are five bones in each hand, and they are long and cylindrical in shape

metacarpophalangeal joint (MPJ) A synovial hinge-type joint consisting of a metacarpal that articulates with a phalange; commonly referred to as a knuckle

metaiodobenzylguanidine (MIBG) Nuclear medicine study that is specifically designed to detect and locate pheochromocytoma

metastasis Ability of a disease to spread from its original site to another location

methyl methacrylate (MMA) A chemical compound composed of a mixture of liquid and powder used for cementing prostheses during total joint arthroplasties; also referred to as bone cement

MIBG *See* metaiodobenzylguanidine

microorganism Organism that can only be seen with the use of a microscope

minimally invasive direct coronary artery bypass procedures (MID-CAB) Minimally invasive surgery performed to treat certain types of coronary artery lesions. The heart is not stopped, and only a 4-inch incision is required for access to the coronary vessels

minor calyces The initial portions of the system of extrarenal ducts; the minor calyces empty into the major calyces

miotics A class of drugs that constricts the pupil by stimulating the sphincter muscle of the iris

mitigate Reduce the effects

mitral valve The heart valve located between the left atrium and left ventricle that prevents blood in the left ventricle from backing up into the left atrium

MMA *See* methyl methacrylate

modem A communications hardware device that enables the sending and receiving of data over a telephone line or cable; typically used to send e-mail or to access the Internet

monitor A visual interface for computers

monofilament suture Suture that is manufactured from one strand of natural or synthetic material

monopolar cautery Monopolar electrocautery in which the electrical circuit completes a path from the generator, to the patient, and then back again to the generator

moral principles Guides for ethical decision making that include the concern that we have for the well-being of others, respect for individual autonomy, basic justice, prevention of harm to others, and refusal to take unfair advantage

morbidity Pertaining to disease

mortality Pertaining to death

mouse A hand device used to move a cursor on a computer monitor and select a file or function

mouth prop A self-retaining retractor used to keep the mouth open during oral or dental procedures

MPJ *See* metacarpophalangeal joint

multifilament suture Suture that is made of several strands of natural or synthetic material that is braided or twisted together

mustache dressing A type of wound dressing that involves the placement of a small folded sponge just above the upper lip that is held in place with surgical tape

mydriatics A class of paralytic drugs that dilates the pupil by paralyzing the sphincter of the muscle of the iris

myocardium The muscle of the heart that is composed of specially constructed cardiac muscle cells that contract and force blood from the heart's chambers

myoma A benign fibroid tumor of the uterus

myringo- Combining form referring to the tympanic membrane

narcotic Controlled agent that aids in relieving the perception of pain, dulls the senses, and/or induces sleep

National Fire Protection Agency (NFPA) Organization whose mission is to reduce the frequency of fires through the establishment of fire prevention standards, research, and public fire safety education

National Institute for Occupational Safety and Health (NIOSH) Organization whose responsibilities are similar to OSHA but are more research oriented in establishing permissible exposure limits for chemical vapors and gases

Nd:YAG Neodymium:yttrium aluminum garnet; a laser that has a wavelength of 1064 nm, with a beam that is located in the near-infrared region of the light spectrum

necrosis Tissue death

negligence Omission or commission of an act that a reasonable or prudent person would not do under the same conditions

neonate Pediatric patient (defined as from birth to the 28th day of life)

neoplasm New growth

nephrectomy Surgical removal of the kidney

nephrons The functional unit of the kidney

neurorrhaphy Surgical repair of a nerve

neutral zone An area designated within the sterile field in which sharps may be safely placed by one person and retrieved by another

neutrons Subatomic particles equal in mass to protons but without an electrical charge

nonabsorbable suture Suture that is not broken down by the fluids of the body and remains permanently in the body

nonsterile Item that has not been subjected to a sterilization process or is contaminated

nosocomial infection Hospital-acquired infection
NPO Nothing by mouth; Latin acronym for *nil per os*
oblique Angle; slanted
oblique fracture Fracture that occurs at an angle or slant across the bone
obstruction Hindrance or blockage of a passage
occiput anterior The most common relationship between the presenting fetal part and the maternal body pelvis
occlusion An obstruction
Occupational Safety and Health Administration (OSHA) Federal organization that is dedicated to protecting the health of workers by establishing standards that address issues related to safety in the workplace
ocutome A cutting system for posterior vitrectomy
olfaction Sense of smell
-oma Suffix meaning tumor
oncogene Gene responsible for the transformation of a normal cell into a malignancy
open gloving Method of self-donning sterile gloves when not wearing a sterile gown; method used by the STSR when assisting a team member who is wearing a sterile gown to apply sterile gloves
open mitral commissurotomy Surgical procedure used to treat mitral stenosis; requires a median sternotomy and CPB
open pneumothorax An emergency condition that results from a large penetrating wound to the chest that exposes the pleural space to atmospheric pressure. As the diaphragm contracts, air is sucked into the wound
opportunistic microbe Microorganism that normally does not cause disease unless given the opportunity (such as when entering an open wound to cause an infection)
optional Surgical intervention that does not have to be performed in order to preserve life or limb
OR attire The items worn by the surgical personnel to protect the patient and surgical personnel from microorganisms; consists of the scrub suit, hair cover, mask, protective eyewear, and shoe covers
orbicular Refers to something round
orchiectomy Surgical removal of a testicle
orchiopexy Surgical fixation of a testicle
oropharynx Pertaining to the oral cavity and pharynx
OSHA *See* Occupational Safety and Health Administration
osteogenesis Development of bone tissue
osteomalacia Abnormal condition characterized by softening of the bone due to a loss of calcification of the bone matrix; occurs as a result of an inadequate amount of phosphorus and calcium in the blood for the mineralization of bone, caused by a deficiency of vitamin D
osteophyte An abnormal bony growth
osteotomy Incision into a bone
-ostomy Suffix meaning to create a new opening
oto- Combining form meaning ear
-otomy Suffix meaning to make an incision into
oxygenated Saturated with oxygen
pacing modes One of two types of pace modes for a permanent pacemaker pulse generator: (1) fixed (asynchronous) rate that fires at a preset rate; (2) demand (standby) mode that senses the patient's heartbeats and is stimulated to fire when the rate drops below a preset standard
packing Sterile fine-mesh gauze that is loosely placed in a chronic wound or one that has been left open to heal by second intention
PACU *See* postanesthesia care unit
palate Roof of the mouth that functions to separate the nose from the mouth
palatoplasty Surgical procedure performed to repair a cleft palate
palatoschisis Cleft palate
palliative Intended to ease pain or reduce severity, but is not a cure
palpation To examine by touch
pan- Combining form meaning all
panniculectomy Removal of the apron of abdominal fat in the obese patient
panniculus Sheet or layer of tissue
papaverine A drug that is a smooth muscle relaxant used in the treatment of cardiovascular spasms
para Refers to the number of live births; first birth is referred to as para I, and additional live births are sequentially numbered
parasympathetic Division of the autonomic nervous system that responds by restoring homeostatic balance and conserving energy
parasympathetic nervous system (PNS) A division of the autonomic nervous system that slows the heart rate, relaxes sphincters of the body, and increases peristalsis in the GI tract
parenteral Injection other than enteral
parietal (1) Refers to the outer portion of a cavity or organ; (2) Pertaining to the parietal bone of the cranium; (3) Pertaining to the parietal lobe of the cerebrum
parietal pleura A thin serous membrane composed of a single layer of flattened mesothelial cells on top of a thin layer of connective tissue; the parietal pleura lines the chest wall, covers the diaphragm, and reflects over the structures contained in the mediastinum
parity The classification used to indicate the number of live and stillborn births that a female has delivered at more than 20 weeks of gestation
pars radiata The tubules located in the innermost portion of the cortex of the kidney
parturition Act of giving birth
Pasteur French chemist in the 19th century who is known as the "father of microbiology, virology, and

immunology" due to his many discoveries made in those science fields

patency The condition of being wide open

patent Open; unobstructed

patent ductus arteriosus (PDA) Failure of PDA to close at the time of birth. During fetal life, the ductus arteriosus connects the pulmonary artery to the aorta to shunt oxygenated blood directly into the systemic circulation, bypassing the lungs

pathogen Microorganism that is capable of causing disease

pathological fracture Fracture that occurs without trauma as a result of a disease of the bone; also referred to as spontaneous fracture

pathology The study of the characteristics, causes, and effects of disease on the human body

pathology department The department responsible for testing and processing specimens, tissues, and body fluids to obtain a diagnosis

patient The person receiving medical treatment

Patient's Bill of Rights Developed by the American Hospital Association, the rights that established the patient as a consumer of goods who has the right to make decisions concerning his or her care, including the right to refuse treatment

PDA *See* patent ductus arteriosus

pectus carinatum A congenital deformity of the chest wall that results in a prominent sternum, caused by an upward curve of the lower costal cartilages. Occasionally the manubrium and upper ribs are pushed outward with a posteriorly angulated body that suddenly projects anteriorly

pectus excavatum Congenital deformity of the chest that results in a funnel-shaped, asymmetrical depression due to a posterior displacement of the sternal body; symptoms include bronchospasm, exercise intolerance, dysrhythmias, chest pain, and dyspnea

pedicle The extension of the vertebrae that connects the spinous process to the lamina; or the attachment of an organ (such as the kidney pedicle)

pedicle flap reconstruction A type of reconstruction mammoplasty in which the tissue is relocated via a tunnel under the skin layer, allowing it to remain attached to its blood supply

penetrating keratoplasty A surgical procedure in which the full thickness of a cornea is replaced to restore vision

penetrating trauma A foreign object that passes through tissue, such as a bullet or knife

penis The external reproductive organ of the male that serves a dual function: transport of sperm and semen during the act of sexual intercourse and transport of urine during micturition

percutaneous transluminal coronary angioplasty (PTCA) Surgical procedure involving the placement of a catheter with a balloon tip into a blocked coronary artery; the balloon is inflated to compress the atheroma against the wall of the coronary artery with minimal risk of arterial dissection

perfusion To force blood or fluid through a vascular bed or lumen

perfusionist The individual responsible for running and maintaining the cardiopulmonary bypass machine during open heart procedures

pericardiectomy Surgical procedure in which decortication is performed to remove fibrous scarring of the heart as a result of constrictive pericarditis

pericardium A thin serous sac that surrounds the heart; it consists of the serous pericardium and fibrous pericardium

perineal prostatectomy The removal of the prostate gland through a perineal approach

perineum The area between the posterior portion of the vagina or scrotum and the opening to the anus

periodic table A table consisting of the elements, listed by their specific properties and atomic weight

perioperative The term used to refer to the preoperative, intraoperative, and postoperative periods of surgery

peristalsis Rhythmic contractions of smooth muscle layers that force food through the GI tract, urine through the ureters, and bile through the common bile duct

peritoneal dialysis The placement of a catheter into the peritoneal cavity to facilitate dialysis

peritoneum A thin serous membrane that lines the abdominal cavity

permanent specimens Tissue that is sent to pathology in a preservative solution, such as formalin

permeability The condition of being permeable; capable of allowing the passage of fluids or substances

personal protective equipment (PPE) Attire worn to protect against exposure to physical and biological hazards

Pfannenstiel Surgical transverse incision made in the lower abdomen, usually employed when performing a cesarean section

pH Indicates the relative acidity or alkalinity of a solution

phacoemulsification A variation of the irrigation/aspiration technique that uses ultrasonic energy to fragment the lens, while simultaneously irrigating and aspirating the lens fragments

phagocytosis The process used by leukocytes to engulf bacteria, foreign particles, or dead cells

phakic lenses A type of intraocular lens that is implanted without removing the eye's natural lens

phalanges The bones of the fingers; each hand has 14 phalanges

pharmacodynamics The interaction of drug molecules with the target cells resulting in biochemical and physiological actions

pharmacokinetics The study of the movement of drugs through the body, involving absorption, distribution, biotransformation, and excretion

pharmacology The study of drugs and their actions

pharyngotympanic tube An open tube that links the middle ear to the nasopharynx; it releases pressure pushing against the tympanic membrane and allows the membrane to vibrate

pheochromocytoma A tumor affecting the medulla of the adrenal gland, causing an overproduction of adrenaline

phimosis A condition in which the foreskin cannot be retracted over the glans penis, caused by a thin band of skin at the opening of the foreskin; the condition can cause pain, particularly on erection

photon Smallest particle of light

phrenic Pertaining to the diaphragm

PKD *See* polycystic kidney disease

plaintiff Individual who files a lawsuit or complaint

plasma (1) Liquid portion of body fluid; (2) An ionized gas made primarily of free electrons and having a neutral charge

platelet Thrombocyte, necessary component of the blood clotting process

platelet aggregation Clumping together of thrombocytes; part of the blood clotting process

pledget Small squares of Teflon sutured over a hole in a vessel; they exert external pressure over any small needle holes to prevent bleeding and to promote clotting; often used in peripheral vascular surgery

plethysmography An instrument for determining and registering variations in the volume of an extremity and in the amount of blood present in the extremity or passing through it; useful in patients with diffuse, small-vessel arterial disease

pleura A thin serous membrane that encloses the lung, composed of a single layer of mesothelial cells on top of a thin layer of connective tissue; it is divided into the visceral and parietal pleural layers

pliable Flexible; easily manipulated

plume Smoke produced by laser or electrocautery that has been shown to contain biological material

pneumatic Pertaining to air

pneumonectomy Surgical removal of an entire lung

pneumothorax Abnormal accumulation of air in the pleural cavity

PNS *See* parasympathetic nervous system

podocytes A special type of epithelial cell located in the inner visceral layer of Bowman's capsule that sends out multiple branches that adhere to the capillaries of the glomerulus; the branches create a filter through which many substances must pass before entering Bowman's capsule

polycystic kidney disease (PKD) Disease that occurs when the kidney parenchyma is replaced by multiple fluid-filled benign cysts. There are three types of the disease; two are inherited forms and the other develops in patients with long-term kidney disorders

poly- prefix meaning many or much

polydactyly A duplication of the digits that usually only involves the phalangeal bones

polyp Growth that protrudes from a mucous membrane; often precancerous growths

polysomnography Diagnostic test during which physiological variables are measured and recorded during sleep; often administered to individuals who suffer from some type of sleep disorder

polytetrafluoroethylene (PTFE) A synthetic coating used on certain types of nylon suture material to reduce the drag through tissue

portal venous system Venous system that carries blood to a second capillary bed prior to returning the blood to general circulation

positive-pressure air By means of ventilation, air pressure in the OR that is kept at a higher level than that of the surrounding corridor, preventing the rushing of air from the corridor into the OR when the door is opened

postanesthesia care unit (PACU) Area where immediate postoperative care of the patient takes place before transfer to the hospital room or ICU

posterior Toward the back

posterior chamber The area behind the iris, but in front of and behind the lens

postoperative Period of time after surgery when the patient is recovering

PPE *See* personal protective equipment

preceptor Instructor or tutor who demonstrates the general rules of conduct and procedures and guides the students while they are practicing or performing

preference card Information sheet, either handwritten or computer generated, listing the surgeon's required instruments, equipment, and supplies for each procedure the surgeon performs

premature ventricular contraction (PVC) Contraction of the ventricle that occurs before it is expected in a normal series of cardiac cycles

preoperative Period of time before the surgical procedure begins

preoperative check-in unit Also referred to as same-day check-in unit; patients enter this area on arrival to the hospital and are provided a private room and locker for clothes change in preparation for surgery

preoperative holding area A designated quiet room or area in or near the surgery department where patients wait before entering the OR; certain actions can be completed in this area, such as the skin shave prep and insertion of IV lines

prep Preparation, such as the skin prep of the patient

prep stand Small movable table where the patient skin prep tray is opened; the circulator works from this stand to perform the surgical skin prep

prepuce A fold of skin that forms a cover that can be pulled back, such as the foreskin of the penis and the fold around the clitoris

pressure The force per unit of area; applied evenly over a surface

primary suture line Main suture that approximates the wound edges for first intention healing to occur

principles of asepsis Concepts and standards that establish the basis for the practice of aseptic technique, with the goal of keeping the microbial count within the sterile field to an irreducible minimum and protecting the patient from postoperative infection

prioritize To complete in order of importance

professional An individual who has special education and experience in a given field and who meets certain competency-based and ethical criteria

prolapse To fall or slip out of normal anatomical position

prone A position in which the patient lies face downward

prophylaxis Prevention of a disease or condition

proprietary Organization or company that is owned and operated by an individual or corporation with the intent of making a profit that is returned to the investors; the profit is taxable

prostate A seminal tract accessory gland of conical shape that lies under the bladder; the prostatic tubules lead to prostatic ducts that empty into prostatic sinuses on both sides of the urethral crest

prostate-specific antigen (PSA) A protein produced and secreted by the prostate; elevated levels in the bloodstream may indicate cancer or another disease of the prostate

prostatectomy Surgical removal of the prostate

prostatic urethra The portion of the urethra that travels through the prostate gland

prosthesis Artificial device used to replace a body structure, aid bodily function, or give a cosmetic appearance; may be permanent or removable

protons An elemental particle with a positive charge equal to the negative charge of the electron

proud flesh Abnormal scar that results from the buildup of excess granulation tissue

proximal Nearer to the origin of a structure

proximal convoluted tubule A portion of the renal tubules that is near the renal corpuscle; it increases surface area and aids in reabsorption and secretion

PSA *See* prostate-specific antigen

psychological need A mental requirement or necessity for fulfillment as a person

PTCA *See* percutaneous transluminal coronary angioplasty

pterygium An abnormal, thick, small piece of tissue that extends from the medial border of the cornea to the inner canthus of the eye

PTFE *See* polytetrafluoroethylene

ptosis Abnormal drooping of one or both eyelids, due to congenital or acquired weakness of the levator muscle or a paralyzed third cranial nerve

puboprostatic ligament An extension of the endopelvic fascia that originates from the neck of the bladder and the base of the prostate; it attaches to parietal fascia on the rear of the pubis and superior fascia of the pelvic diaphragm; the ligament anatomically supports the inferior portion of the bladder

pulse Rhythmic expansion of an artery due to the force of the contracted heart

pulse generator The portion of a permanent pacemaker that controls energy output, heart rate, and pacing modes; it is powered by a lithium source

pulse oximeter A device that measures the percentage of blood oxygenation level; a small clip is placed on the finger, toe, or earlobe, and a light passes through the tissues to determine the optical density of the blood

pump oxygenator The machine used in cardiac surgery to remove unoxygenated blood from the venous system, oxygenate and filter it, and return it to the arterial system. By assuming the roles of the heart and lungs, the machine allows the heart to be stopped so that cardiac procedures can be performed

Purkinje fibers Large-diameter conduction fibers in the heart that receive the electrical impulse from the bundle of His and spread the action potential to the apex of the left ventricle and upward to the remainder of the ventricular myocardium, resulting in ventricular contraction

pursestring suture Suturing technique in which a strand of suture is circumferentially passed through tissue around a hollow structure, and then pulled taut like a drawstring

pus Fluid consisting of bacteria, dead bacterial cells and leukocytes, and tissue debris that forms in infected tissue

PVC *See* premature ventricular contraction

pyrexia A fever or febrile condition

quarks The subatomic particles that make up nucleons (protons and neutrons)

radial artery A branch of the brachial artery that travels along the radius and supplies the lateral aspect of the forearm

radial hypoplasia A congenital condition caused by the failure of the radius and adjacent soft tissue to develop, causing the hand to be medially deranged; typically associated with deformities of the thumb; also referred to as radial dysplasia

radial nerve A nerve that travels along the radius and innervates the skin of the forearm, hand, and extensor muscles of the forearm

radiation therapy Treatment of malignant neoplasms utilizing ionizing radiation or radionuclides

radical nephrectomy The surgical removal of the kidney, adrenal gland, perirenal fat, upper ureter, and Gerota's fascia en bloc; regional lymph nodes may also be removed

radiculopathy Pain, numbness, as tingling in an extremity due to compression of a spinal nerve root

radiopaque Opaque to any form of radiation; appears as a white area on exposed X-ray film

ramus Smaller branch of a structure that extends from a larger branch that divides into two parts, such as the rami of the pubis

recession Surgical procedure to correct strabismus in which the vertically acting muscles of the eye are resected and reattached at a point posterior to their original attachment

recipient site Site in which the skin or bone graft will be placed

red blood cell Erythrocyte responsible for transporting heme that binds oxygen for transport to the tissues of the body

reduction Correction or placement of a body structure back into normal anatomical position

reduction mammoplasty Plastic surgery performed to reduce the size of the breasts either by liposuction or removal of breast tissue

refraction The bending of a light ray as it passes through a substance

regional anesthesia Technique of anesthesia in which the nerves are blocked from transmitting impulses in a regional area of the body; involves a larger area, as compared to local anesthesia

registration Formal process by which qualified individuals are listed in a registry

regurgitation Backward flow of fluid, the opposite of a normal direction

renal corpuscle One of several small round bodies located in the cortex of the kidney that communicates with a renal tubule that is part of the filtering system; also called *malpighian corpuscle*

renal pelvis Funnel-shaped structure that passes inferiorly and medially beyond the hilum; as it nears the inferior border of the kidney, the extrarenal pelvis narrows and continues as the ureter

renal tubule A portion of the nephron that travels from the glomerulus to the collecting tubules; it consists of a loop and two convoluted sections; the tubule resorbs substances back into the blood and secretes, collects, and transfers urine

replantation The replacement of an organ or other structure to the site from which it was previously lost or removed; also known as reimplantation

resect Partial excision of a section of tissue

resection Surgical procedure to correct strabismus in which a section of the vertically acting muscles is removed and the muscle reattached

resident organisms Microorganisms that live on and within the body and that are beneficial for health; typically refers to bacteria that live below the skin surface in hair follicles and glandular openings; also referred to as *normal* or *resident flora*

resistance (1) Opposing or counteracting force; (2) A force that delays or impedes action

respiration Exchange of oxygen and carbon dioxide between the atmosphere and the body cells; the act of breathing

respondeat superior Legal principle that states the employer is responsible for the actions of his or her employees

restricted area The areas of an operating department (including the sterile storage areas of the surgery department) that require proper OR attire, including the wearing of a mask

retention suture Secondary suture line that supports and reinforces the primary suture line and obliterates any dead space

retina The delicate nervous membrane that makes up the inner tunic of the eye and on which images are received

retinal detachment A pathological emergency that occurs secondary to a retinal tear; the liquid from the vitreous cavity passes through the tear and travels under the retina, separating it from the choroid of the eye

retract To draw back; expose

retrobulbar Behind the eyeball or pons

retrograde urogram The injection of contrast medium into the ureters with the use of a cystoscope; required due to an obstruction that is preventing the antegrade process from occurring

retroperitoneal Referring to the space between the peritoneum and the posterior abdominal wall

retropubic prostatectomy The surgical removal of the prostate through a retropubic approach; a prostatic capsulotomy is performed between two stay sutures

reverse Trendelenburg's position A position in which the patient is placed in the supine position and the operating table is tilted foot downward-head upward to approximately 45° (or the desired angle)

Revised Trauma Score (RTS) A scoring system used to assess the severity of a traumatic wound and to determine the condition of a patient

Rh (Rhesus) factor Genetically determined blood group antigen that is present on the surface of erythrocytes of some individuals; if the antigen is present the individual is Rh+ (positive) and if absent Rh- (negative)

rheostat Devise for controlling the amount of electrical current entering a circuit

rheumatic fever An inflammatory disease that can develop due to an infection by group A beta-hemolytic streptococcus in the upper respiratory tract. It can cause calcium deposition and fibrous tissue formation on the leaflets of the mitral valve, resulting in an immobile valve and a narrowing of the atrioventricular orifice between the left atrium and left ventricle

rheumatoid arthritis An autoimmune disease of unknown etiology that attacks the synovial tissues, causing inflammation and damage to cartilage and bone

rhino- Combining form that means nose

rhinoplasty Surgical reshaping of the nose

rhytidectomy Facelift

ring stand A stand that is designed with one or two circular bands at the top to hold sterile basins

risk management The efforts of a health care provider organization to collect and utilize data to decrease the chance of harm to patients or staff, or damage to property

Roentgenography Radiography; X-rays

role interactions The recognition by an individual that interactions with others revolve around our understanding of rules that pertain to certain social or professional roles

rotation advancement A method of cheiloplasty in which incisions are made on both sides of a cleft lip, and the tissue from the cheek is rotated into position to eliminate the defect

Rule of Nine A method used to estimate the body surface area that has been burned in a burn patient; uses increments of 9%

running suture Series of stitches placed with one long continuous strand

Safe Medical Device Act Established in 1990, this act requires medical device users to report to the manufacturer and/or FDA incidents that reasonably suggest that there is a probability that a medical device has caused or contributed to the death, serious injury, or illness of a patient

sagittal Directional term that indicates a plane parallel to the midline that divides the body into right and left segments

scalpel Another name for the surgical knife handle on which knife blades are attached

scar The mark left after a wound that was closed with suture or staples (or by second intention healing) heals; the scar of wounds that healed by primary intention consist of collagen tissue

-schisis Root word pertaining to split or cleft

Schlemm's canal A tiny canal at the angle of the anterior chamber of the eye that is responsible for draining the aqueous humor and funneling it into the bloodstream

sclera The firm fibrous membrane that maintains the globe shape of the eye; the visible white portion of the eye

scleral buckle A surgical procedure used to treat retinal detachment in which a small piece of silicone sponge or solid silicone is placed to close the retinal break

-sclerosis Suffix relating to hardening of a structure or tissue due to a pathological occurrence

scope of practice Professional duty limits based on state and federal law and on an individual's education and experience

scrotum The pouch that contains the testes and a portion of the spermatic cord. It is divided into two lateral cavities and has two layers, the skin and dartos tunic

scrub (sterile) attire Sterile garment and gloves donned during a surgical procedure

sebaceous glands Glands that produce the oily substance called sebum that reaches the skin through ducts that enter the hair follicle

sebum Oily substance produced by the sebaceous glands that reaches the skin through ducts that enter the hair follicle; aids with fluid regulation and acts to keep the skin and hair soft and pliable

second-degree burn A burn that affects the epidermis and dermis in varying degrees; characterized by blisters, the burns generally heal on their own with no scarring, but deeper burns take longer to heal and leave a hypertrophic scar

second intention Healing that occurs when a wound fails to heal by primary union, or the wound is left open and allowed to heal from the inside to the outside by filling with granulation tissue

secondary suture line Sutures placed to support and ease the tension on the primary suture line, thus reinforcing the wound closure and obliterating any dead spaces

sedation State of being calm, usually effected by means of a sedative drug

sedative Agent that produces a soothing or quieting effect but does not cause the person to sleep

seeding (1) Implantation of cancer cells at a new site that have broken away from the main tumor; (2) Implantation of radionuclide particles near cancerous tissue in the body to destroy cancer cells

segmentectomy Surgical removal of an individual bronchovascular segment of a lung due to bronchiectasis, cysts, blebs, or benign lesions

semi-Fowler's position A position in which the operating table is manipulated to resemble a chair and the patient is placed in a semisitting position; also referred to as the "beach chair" position

seminal vesicles Structures that lie on the fundus of the bladder and that narrow at the prostatic end to unite with the vas deferens

seminiferous tubules Convoluted tubes that lie between the septa of the testis and unite to form the straight seminiferous tubules

semirestricted area Area beyond the "red line" on the floor in which proper OR attire must be worn, including hair cover; the mask is not required

sepsis Presence of pathogenic microorganisms in the blood or tissues

septic shock A state of shock produced by septicemia, when the body is overwhelmed by the pathogenic microorganisms and cannot adequately fight the infection

septicemia Systemic infection by pathogenic microorganisms that are distributed to other areas of the body by the circulatory system

septum A wall or partition dividing a body space or cavity; usually refers to the muscular wall within the heart that separates the chambers of the heart into right and left portions. The septum between the atria is called the *interatrial septum;* the septum between the ventricles is called the *interventricular septum*

serrations Grooves located on the jaws of surgical instruments that are either longitudinal, cross-hatched, or horizontal

shelf life Amount of time that a stored item remains safe to use

shock Failure of the circulatory system to adequately perfuse the vital organs, due to a variety of causes such as severe hemorrhaging

shoulder joint The ball-and-socket joint composed of the head of the humerus that rests in the glenoid fossa

shunt A prosthetic tube surgically implanted in the body to redirect body fluid to another part of the body or to provide access to vessel(s)

side effect Undesirable consequences that accompany the therapeutic responses to a drug

sign Indication of a disease or condition perceived by the examiner

simple fracture A type of fracture in which the bone fragments are aligned within the fracture site

Sims' position A position in which the patient is placed on his or her left side (with the left leg kept straight and the left hip moved back toward the edge of the operating table), the right leg is flexed, the left arm placed behind the patient along the back, and the right arm flexed in front of the patient

sinoatrial node (SA node) The pacemaker of the heart and the conduction system's key component; located in the right atrial wall just inferior to the opening of the superior vena cava. The SA node fires an electrical impulse that spreads into the myocardium and stimulates cardiac muscle fibers to contract in a rhythmic manner

sinus A dilated channel for venous blood

sinus tachycardia Rapid heart rate characterized by an atrial and ventricular rate of 100 beats per minute or more; often associated with the ingestion of nicotine, alcohol, or caffeine. It is a normal response to fear, excitement, or physical exertion. Also associated with hyperthyroidism, hypovolemia, or hypotension

slander A verbal statement that is false and malicious that is damaging to another person's reputation

SMR *See* submucous resection

social need A need to fit into society and to be accepted by one's peers

soft palate The posterior portion of the palate that is composed of fat, muscle, and mucous membrane; terminates with the uvula at the fauces

solution Solute (i.e., drug) dissolved in a liquid (solvent)

somatic nervous system (SNS) Voluntary motor portions of the nervous system responsible for skeletal muscle movement

specimen Tissue, fluid, or foreign body removed from a patient

spermatic cord An anatomical structure that extends from the deep inguinal ring in the abdomen into the scrotum. Each cord contains arteries, veins, nerves, lymphatics, and the vas deferens

sphygmomanometer Device used to measure blood pressure, either manually or automatically; consists of an inflatable cuff that is placed around the upper arm

spinal anesthesia A type of regional anesthesia in which the anesthetic agent is injected intrathecally through the dura mater into the subarachnoid space, usually in the lumbar region of the spine; used to anesthetize the lower portion of the body

spiral fracture A type of fracture in which the fracture line curves around the bone, due to a twisting action that produced the fracture

spiritual need A need for a connection with a higher order

splenectomy Removal of the spleen

splenomegaly Abnormal enlargement of the spleen

splint A rigid device that is placed on one side of an extremity to immobilize and support while healing takes place; available in many forms (plastic, wood, metal, plaster)

split-thickness skin graft (STSG) A graft that involves the epidermis and approximately half the dermis; used when a large surface area needs to be covered

spongy urethra The third division of the male urethra that is about 15 cm long; it enters the bulb of the penis just after the perineal membrane has been crossed and terminates at the external urethral meatus

spore Resistant form of certain types of bacterial species that is formed when harsh environmental conditions are present; a method of self-preservation until normal conditions return that are conducive to survival

SSI *See* surgical site infection

stainless steel A type of metal that is a combination of carbon, chromium, iron and other metals; most often used in the manufacture of surgical instruments

Stamey procedure Endoscopic procedure in which the bladder neck is suspended for the treatment of stress incontinence affecting a female; accomplished by suspending the facial attachments of the bladder to the rectus fascia with sutures that are placed with the use of a Stamey needle and supported with Dacron bolsters

standard Established authoritative model, rule, or criteria for measurement and comparison

Standard Precautions Guidelines established by the Occupational Safety and Health Administration and the Centers for Disease Control and Prevention to reduce the risk of disease transmission from blood and body fluids

-stasis Suffix meaning stoppage or reduction of the flow of bodily fluids

stenosis Narrowing or constriction

stent (1) Device inserted to support luminous structures while still allowing passage of fluid; (2) External device applied to secure a skin graft or dressing in place

sterilant Agent, physical or chemical, capable of killing all microorganisms including spores

sterile Free of all living microorganisms including spores

sterile field Area of sterility maintained by the surgical team during a procedure

sterile team member Member of the surgical team who has performed a surgical scrub, donned the sterile gown and gloves, and works within the sterile field

sterile technique Methods used to prevent contamination of the sterile field and prevent the patient from acquiring a postoperative wound infection

sterilization (1) Procedure to render an individual incapable of reproduction; (2) Process by which all microorganisms, including spores, are destroyed

sterilizer Machine used in the destruction of all microorganisms, including spores

sternum The long flattened bone located in the middle of the thorax that provides support for the clavicles; the first seven pairs of ribs attach to it; divided into three sections: manubrium, body, xiphoid process

stick tie Length of suture for ligation that is threaded on or swaged to a needle; also referred to as *suture ligature*

stirrups Patient positioning devices attached to the sides of the operating table to secure the patient's legs in the lithotomy position

stockinet A stretchable tube that is open at one end; composed of either cloth or impermeable plastic material packaged in a roll and unrolled over an extremity for draping purposes

stoma An incised opening that is kept open for drainage or other purposes

strabismus A pathological condition that is a misalignment or deviation of the eyes that normally work simultaneously to track visual objects

strata Layers

stratum basale The innermost reproductive layer of the epidermis that contains the pigment melanin

stratum corneum The outermost layer of the epidermis that consists of several layers of cells in various stages of disintegration

stratum granulosum Third layer of the epidermis where the process of keratinization begins

stratum lucidum Fourth layer of the epidermis located underneath the stratum corneum; only present in thick skin areas such as the palms of the hands and soles of the feet

stratum spinosum Second layer of the epidermis located underneath the stratum granulosum; this layer receives the daughter cells produced by mitosis in the stratum basale

streptokinase A fibrinolytic enzyme that is produced by strains of streptococci and is commercially produced for use in breaking down thrombi within arteries

stricture Narrowing

strike-through contamination Penetration of a sterile item or field causing contamination, usually referring to moisture penetrating through a sterile drape or cover

STSG *See* split-thickness skin graft

STSR *See* surgical technologist in the scrub role

subcutaneous layer Located beneath the dermis, serves to anchor the skin to the underlying structures; consists of adipose and loose connective tissue, providing insulation and protection to the internal organs; also called the *hypodermis*

submucous resection (SMR) A surgical procedure to restore normal breathing; involves incising the mucous membrane lining of the nasal cavity, lifting the underlying perichondrium, removing underlying mucous membrane structures, and placing the mucous membrane back into position; also called a *septoplasty*

subpoena Court order to appear and testify or produce required documents

substerile room A workroom located next to one or more ORs that usually contains a sink, steam sterilizer, blanket, and solution warmer; used for a variety of reasons, it is separated from the OR by a door

subungual Under the fingernail

suction The act of sucking up air or fluids through a device, such as a tonsil suction tip

suction apparatus Mechanical device that utilizes a vacuum to remove fluids from the surgical site or patient's airway

suction canisters Small containers placed in the suction apparatus that collect the blood and body fluids that are suctioned from the patient during a surgical procedure

suction outlet A wall or ceiling connection for a suction device

sudoriferous glands Sweat glands

summons A legal order to appear in a particular place such as a court room

superior Toward the head or toward the upper portion of an anatomical structure

supine position A position in which the patient lies on his or her back, face upward, with arms usually placed on arm boards with the palms facing up

suprapubic cystostomy An alternate method of catheterizing the bladder for drainage when a catheter cannot be placed through the urethra; it involves the surgical placement of the cystostomy tube into the bladder just above the symphysis pubis, performed in men experiencing acute urinary retention due to an obstruction of the urethra caused by an enlarged prostate

suprapubic prostatectomy The surgical removal of the prostate gland that uses a suprapubic incision and a cystotomy to gain access to the gland

suprapubic vesicourethral suspension Surgical procedure performed vaginally for the placement of sutures to elevate the bladder for the treatment of stress incontinence in females; also called *Marshall-Marchetti-Kranz procedure*

suprarenal glands Endocrine glands that rest on the superior portion of the kidneys; consist of a cortex and medulla; the cortex secretes steroid-type hormones essential to the control of fluid and electrolyte balance, and the medulla secretes epinephrine and norepinephrine

surgeon Sterile surgical team member who performs the surgical procedure; credentials can include MD (medical doctor), DO (doctor of osteopathy), DPM (doctor of podiatric medicine), and DDS (doctor of dental science)

surgeon's preference card A list of the equipment, supplies, and surgical instrument set(s) that a surgeon prefers for each surgical procedure performed; used as a guide in collecting the items to be used for the surgical procedure; most surgery departments now have the cards stored on a computer, eliminating the need for hand-written cards

surgical assistant Sterile surgical team member who assists the surgeon by providing visualization of the surgical site through retraction of tissue, suctioning and sponging, and hemostasis; also sutures body planes

surgical conscience The basis for the practice of strict adherence to sterile technique by all surgical team members; involves a level of honesty and moral integrity that must be upheld

surgical scrub A hand and arm wash that is performed prior to donning the sterile gown and gloves; used for the purpose of removing as many microorganisms as possible and for arresting the growth of others; accomplished with the use of chemicals and mechanical action

surgical site infection (SSI) An infection of the surgical wound that was acquired during the course of the surgical procedure

surgical technologist in the scrub role (STSR) Functions as a member of the sterile surgical team and performs many nonsterile duties in preparation for surgical procedures

surgically clean As free of microorganisms as possible, but not sterile

suspension Solid particles suspended in a liquid

suture (1) Thread-like material used to approximate and secure the edges of a surgical or traumatic wound; (2) Refers to immovable fibrous joint found between the bones of the skull

suture ligature Refers to a stick tie

swaged Strand of suture material with an eyeless needle attached by the manufacturer; the needle is continuous with the suture strand

Swan-Ganz catheter A catheter inserted into the pulmonary artery that indirectly measures left atrial and left ventricular pressures by assessing right atrial, right ventricular, and pulmonary artery wedge pressures. Also used to monitor central venous pressure

switch A device used to open or close a circuit, thereby controlling the flow of electricity

sympathetic nervous system Division of the autonomic nervous system that is responsible for the "fight or flight" mechanism

symphysis A joint in which the two bony surfaces are joined by fibrocartilage (meniscus)

symptom Indication of a disease or condition perceived by the patient

syndactyly Webbed digits; congenital abnormality that occurs when the digits of the hands or feet fail to separate

synovial membrane Thin layer of tissue that lines the articular capsule of freely movable joints; secretes the thick fluid called *synovium* that lubricates the joint to aid in movement

synovium A synovial membrane

synthesis The formation of a new entity out of previously existing ones

syrup Sweetened aqueous solution

systemic Pertaining to a whole rather than just one part

systole Represents the contraction phase of the cardiac cycle

T&A *See* tonsillectomy and adenoidectomy

table break Hinged areas between segments of the operating table

tachycardia Fast heart rate that is greater than 100 beats per minute

tagging Marking an anatomical structure or area with suture or other material for easy identification at a later point in the surgical procedure

tamponade Pathological compression of an anatomical part

teeth Small projections from the tip(s) of the jaw of certain surgical instruments; used to aid in grasping tissue or vessels

temporomandibular joint (TMJ) The joint formed by the mandible that articulates with the glenoid fossa in each temporal bone

tendon sheath A protective covering that contains the tendons of the fingers and thumbs and is lined with synovium

tendonitis Inflammation of a tendon

tenorrhaphy Surgical repair of a tendon

tensile strength Amount of pull or tension that a suture strand will withstand before breaking; expressed in pounds

tension pneumothorax Condition in which air escapes from a bronchus into the pleural cavity, but cannot regain entry back into the bronchus. Increasing air pressure within the pleural cavity causes collapse of the lung, decreased venous return due to mediastinal shift, and eventual cardiovascular collapse

testicular torsion A serious condition in which the spermatic cord twists on itself, causing pain and obstructing the blood flow to the testicle; resolved by surgically rotating the cord and by performing an orchiopexy

tetralogy of Fallot Common cyanotic congenital heart defect in children characterized by four defects: (1) ventricular septal defect, (2) infundibular or pulmonary valve stenosis, (3) aorta that overrides the ventricular septal defect, (4) right ventricular hypertrophy. Results in cyanosis and if not immediately treated by surgery can result in other life-threatening complications

theft Taking the property of another; larceny

third-degree burn A life-threatening burn that penetrates the full thickness of the skin; appears charred or white colored

third intention Healing that occurs when two granulated surfaces are approximated; also referred to as *delayed primary closure*

thoracic outlet syndrome Term used to refer to a variety of symptoms associated with compression of the brachial plexus nerve complex and subclavian vessels at the superior aperture of the thorax; may be caused by a drooping shoulder girdle, adventitious fibrous band, cervical rib, continual hyperabduction of the arm, or most commonly, an abnormal first rib

thoracocentesis The placement of a needle into a posterior portion of the pleural space for the analysis of pleural effusion. Performed as an aid in diagnosing inflammatory or neoplastic diseases of the pleura or lung. Fluid can be removed from within the thoracic cavity for therapeutic purposes

thoracoscopy Endoscopic examination of the thoracic cavity using a rigid thoracoscope that is inserted into the cavity for examination of the pleura, mediastinum, thoracic wall, sympathetic chain, diaphragm, and pericardium. Biopsies of the lung, mediastinal nodes, or pleura may be taken through the scope

thrombocyte Platelet

thrombolytic Agent capable of dissolving a thrombus

thrombus Stationary blood clot within a blood vessel

TIA *See* transient ischemic attack

tie-on-a-pass(er) Suture strand (tie) that has one end secured in the jaws of an instrument to facilitate the placement of the tie around a deep vessel for ligating

tincture Solution prepared with alcohol

TMJ *See* temporomandibular joint

tonsillectomy and adenoidectomy (T&A) Surgical removal of the tonsils and adenoids

topical As pertaining to anesthesia, an agent that is applied to the surface of the skin or anatomical structure (such as the eye) to produce a loss of feeling or sensation in the area of application; blocks the nerve conduction of superficial nerves

torsion A condition of being twisted

tort A civil wrong; may be intentional or unintentional

tort law Describes any civil wrong independent of a contract; allows for a remedy in the form of an action for damages

torticollis An abnormal contracted state of a muscle(s)

tourniquet Device placed around an extremity and tightened to temporarily slow or stop the flow of arterial blood

trabeculoplasty Plastic surgery procedure used to treat glaucoma; involves the use of a laser to open the trabecular network to allow the aqueous fluid to drain from the eye

trachea Cylindrical tube located in the neck that is primarily composed of cartilage; it extends from the larynx to where it divides into the two primary bronchi and transports air to the lungs; also called the *windpipe*

tranquilizer Agent that acts to reduce tension and anxiety

transect To cut across

transient ischemic attack (TIA) Intermittent episodes of cerebrovascular insufficiency associated with partial blockage of an artery by plaque or an embolism

transient organisms Organisms that reside on the surface of the skin and are easily removed by handwashing

transphenoidal Across or through the sphenoid bone

transurethral resection of the prostate (TURP) The partial or full removal of the prostate gland with a resectoscope that is placed through the urethra

transverse Directional term that indicates a plane horizontal to the midline, dividing the body into superior and inferior segments

transverse carpal ligament A broad, flat ligament that is attached to the tubercle of the scaphoid and crest of the trapezium; located on the anterior side of the hand that covers the passageway that is surrounded on three sides by carpal bones and nine flexor tendons; the median nerve passes through this tunnel

transverse fracture Fracture line of bone that is perpendicular to the long axis of the bone

transverse rectus abdominis musculocutaneous (TRAM) flap A flap technique in which the transverse rectus abdominis muscle is used to reconstruct the breast; the muscle is transferred through a tunnel made under the skin layer and rotated into position to form the new breast

Trendelenburg position The patient is placed in the supine position and the operating table is tilted head downward to the desired angle

trephine A cylindrical saw for cutting a circular piece of bone

triage System for classifying patients according to the severity of their condition or injury; most often used during mass casualty situations to determine who will first receive medical and/or surgical treatment

triangular flap method A method of cheiloplasty that uses the Z-plasty technique in which, on closure of the mucous membrane layer and the muscle tissue, the skin flaps are overlapped and interlocked to close the lip defect

triboelectrification One of two processes by which static electricity can build; occurs by friction between two surfaces

tricuspid atresia Absence of the tricuspid valve and orifice, resulting in no opening between the right atrium and right ventricle

trigger finger A type of stenosing tenosynovitis caused by painful inflammation of the synovial sheath, enlargement of the tendon, and narrowing of the annular band; patient experiences pain on snapping of the fingers

truncus arteriosus Abnormal condition characterized by having a single artery from both ventricles. The pulmonary arteries usually arise from one of several positions on a truncal vessel

tube A hollow, cylindrical device that can be used for gastrointestinal decompression, administration of anesthetic gases, or evacuation of air and fluids from body cavities

tumescent liposuction Involves injecting a mixture of local anesthetic (for pain control), epinephrine (for vasoconstriction), Wydase, and saline; the mixture also liquefies the fat, making it easier to suction out

tumor Abnormal swelling, growth, or enlargement of tissue; neoplasm

tunic An investing membrance

tunica albuginea A thick connective tissue that covers the testes and turns into the testicular substance at the posterior border, forming a mesh-like mediastinum testis

tunica vaginalis testis An invaginated serous sac that covers most of the testis, epididymis, and lower end of the spermatic cord

TURP *See* transurethral resection of the prostate

UA *See* urinalysis

ulcer A crater-like lesion that is usually circular in shape and penetrates the skin; may be very deep, resulting from infections or malignant disease processes

ulnar artery A branch of the brachial artery that supplies the medial side of the forearm and descends along the ulna

ulnar nerve A nerve that innervates the skin of the medial one-third of the hand and some flexor muscles of the hand and wrist

ultrasonic washer A machine used to remove minute organic particles and soil from the areas of instrumentation hardest to reach by manual or other mechanical methods of cleaning; the washer utilizes the process of cavitation for cleaning instruments

ultrasonography The use of high-frequency waves that are directed into the body and are reflected from the tissues to record an image for diagnostic purposes

ultraviolet radiation The damaging component of sunlight

unilateral Pertaining to or affecting one side only

Universal Precautions Set of standards defined by the CDC in 1996 that combines Universal Precautions and body substance isolation rules as an aid in reducing the risk of transmission of pathogens from blood and body fluids

unrestricted area Located near entrance of the operating department, this area contains the dressing rooms, offices and main desk of the operating department; street clothes are allowed to be worn in this area

UPPP *See* uvulopalatopharyngoplasty

ureter A thick-walled muscular tube with a small lumen that conducts urine from the kidney to the bladder

ureteral Pertaining to the ureters that exit the kidney and transport urine from the kidney to the bladder

urethra The tube that transports urine from the bladder to the exterior of the body during micturation

urethral Pertaining to the urethra, which travels from the bladder to the exterior of the body

urethral meatus Opening of the urethra; on males it is located at the tip of the glans penis and on females it is located just superior to the vaginal opening

urgent Surgical pathology requiring treatment within a relatively short period of time

urinalysis (UA) Laboratory examination of a urine specimen for diagnostic purposes

urinary tract infection (UTI) Inflammation or infection of one or more organs or structures of the urinary system

urine output Amount of urine collected and measured from a patient over a given amount of time; indicator of kidney function

UTI *See* urinary tract infection

utilitarianism A belief that the end result is a necessary condition for evaluating an action; and that the action must produce the greatest good for the greatest number

uvulopalatopharyngoplasty (UPPP) Surgical procedure to treat intractable snoring and obstructive sleep apnea; involves removal of the redundant tissue of the fauces, tonsils, and a portion of the soft palate, including the uvula

valgus Bent or twisted away from the midline

valve A membranous fold in a passage that prevents backflow of material passing through it

varus Bent or twisted toward the midline

vasectomy Partial removal of the vas deferens; used to render a male sterile

vasovasostomy Microsurgical procedure to reattach a previously resected vas deferens during a vasectomy; used to provide the male with the ability to pass sperm during sexual intercourse

vector Carrier of an infective agent, usually an insect or rodent

venous compression device A device used for patients who are prone to the development of thrombophlebitis; a patient is fitted with intermittent venous compression boots that inflate and deflate every few seconds to promote the movement of venous blood in the leg(s)

ventral Toward the front or abdominal surface

ventricles The lower chambers of the heart that receive blood from the atria

ventricular fibrillation Abnormal condition of the heart characterized by rapid, uncoordinated ventricular contractions; the walls of the fibrillating ventricles are completely ineffective at pumping blood; unless corrected, results in death

ventricular septal defect (VSD) An abnormal opening in the wall between the right and left ventricle of the heart. The opening allows a certain amount of oxygenated blood from the left ventricle to be shunted through the defect to the right ventricle

ventricular tachycardia Abnormal condition that happens when three or more premature ventricular contractions occur in succession, usually at a rate of 140 to 250 beats per minute. The two types of tachycardia are sustained or nonsustained

Vesalius Father of modern anatomy who openly challenged and corrected the scientific anatomical writings of Galen by dissecting cadavers to illustrate anatomy

vesical trigone An important anatomical landmark of the bladder formed by the two ureteral openings at the posterolateral angles, and the urethral opening at the inferior angle

vessel loop Thin strips made of silicone that can be placed around a vessel, nerve, or duct for the purposes of retracting or isolating; the loops are colored for easy identification of the retracted structures

vestibule An opening that serves as the entrance to a passageway, such as the vestibule of the vagina

viable Able to live, grow, develop, and reproduce

viewing box A device in the operating room that is lighted and positioned at eye level for the viewing of X-rays, CT scans, MRIs, etc.; also referred to as an X-ray view box

viscera Any organ of a body cavity; usually refers to the abdominal organs

viscoelastic agents A class of agents that are thick, jelly-like substances injected into the eye during certain types of ophthalmic procedures

vital signs Measurements of bodily functions essential to life, including temperature, pulse, respiration (TPR), and blood pressure

volatile agents A group of liquids that easily evaporate, and when inhaled produce general anesthesia through interaction with the CNS

volume The amount of space occupied by an object

VSD *See* ventricular septal defect

waste anesthetic gases Vapors that escape from the anesthesia machine and tubing into the atmosphere

weight A measurement of gravitational force based on an object's mass and the earth's gravity

white blood cell Leukocyte

Wilson frame operating table A special type of operating table used for procedures in which the patient may need to be repositioned from the supine to the prone position

wound Injury to the body's structure(s); may be intentional, traumatic, or chronic

wraparound-style gown Sterile surgical gown that "wraps" around the individual to enclose the body from the neck to middle of the lower leg, and is kept in place by ties and Velcro strips

xenograft Graft obtained from dissimilar species

X-rays High energy electromagnetic radiation produced by the collision of a beam of electrons with a metal target in an X-ray tube

zygote Cell that results when an ovum is fertilized

Index

('b' indicates boxed material; 'i' indicates an illustration; 't' indicates a table)

A

B

C

D

E

M

Q

R

T